Veterinary Nursing of Exotic Pets and Wildlife

Veterinary Nursing of Exotic Pets and Wildlife

THIRD EDITION

Simon J. Girling
BVMS (Hons) PhD DZooMed, DipECZM (ZHM), CBiol FRSB, FRCVS, Royal College of Veterinary Surgeons Recognised Specialist in Zoo and Wildlife Medicine, EBVS® Recognised European Veterinary Specialist in Zoo Health Management

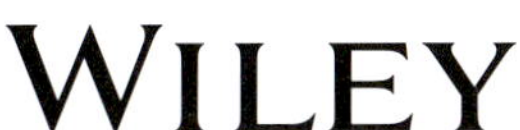

This edition first published 2025

Edition History
Blackwell Publishing Ltd, (1e, 2003; 2e, 2013)

Registered Offices
John Wiley & Sons, Inc., 111 River Street, Hoboken, NJ 07030, USA
John Wiley & Sons Ltd, New Era House, 8 Oldlands Way, Bognor Regis, West Sussex, PO22 9NQ, UK

For details of our global editorial offices, customer services, and more information about Wiley products visit us at www.wiley.com.

Wiley also publishes its books in a variety of electronic formats and by print-on-demand. Some content that appears in standard print versions of this book may not be available in other formats.

Printed in Singapore
M120670_171224

Library of Congress Cataloging-in-Publication Data Applied for:
Paperback: 9781119868620

Cover Design: Wiley
Cover Image: Courtesy of Simon J. Girling

Set in 9/12pt MinionPro by Straive, Pondicherry, India

Contents

Foreword

Veterinary Nursing of Exotic Pets has been a core textbook for veterinary nurses for over 20 years. The book is an invaluable resource for Registered Veterinary Nurses (RVN), Certified Veterinary Technicians and student vets and nurses both in the UK and internationally. This 3rd edition provides a timely update sharing current best practice across all key species; small mammals, birds, reptiles and amphibians with the addition of a new and much needed wildlife chapter. The addition of this new chapter supports nurses with their knowledge and understanding of wildlife and crucially includes wildlife emergency and critical care medicine as well as the wildlife rehabilitation and release considerations, that need to be made when nursing wildlife. The book provides veterinary nurses all that they will need to support them in the nursing care of these different species. The new appendices are an excellent addition to the book, the first, providing example care plans which can be used as templates to support delivery of care to exotic pets and wildlife. The second appendix is also very important as it provides readers with a list of relevant legislation and guidelines for exotic pets and wildlife to ensure that veterinary nurses, when caring for these different species are working within the scope of their practice within clear legislative frameworks.

Dr Andrea Jeffery Ed.D, MSc,
FHEA, DipAVN (Surg), Cert.Ed, RVN

Abbreviations

ACE	angiotensin-converting enzyme
ACP	acepromazine
ACTH	adrenocorticotropic hormone
AI	avian influenza
ALSV	avian leukosis and sarcoma virus
ALT	alanine aminotransferase
APH	African pygmy hedgehog
APHA	Animal and Plant Health Agency
APV	avian polyomavirus
AST	aspartate aminotransferase
AVT	arginine vasotocin
BMR	basal metabolic rate
CDV	canine distemper virus
CK	creatine kinase
CNS	central nervous system
COX	cyclooxygenase
CPDA	citrate/phosphate/dextrose/adenine
CPK	creatine phosphokinase
CPR	cardiopulmonary resuscitation
CRF	chronic renal failure
CT	computed tomography
DEFRA	Department of the Environment, Farming and Rural Affairs
ECF	extracellular fluid
EDTA	ethylenediaminetetraacetic acid
EFA	essential fatty acid
EPEC	enteropathogenic *Escherichia coli*
ERE	epizootic rabbit enteropathy
ET	endotracheal
$ETCO_2$	end-tidal carbon dioxide
FMR	field maintenance requirement
FSH	follicle-stimulating hormone
GALT	gut-associated lymphatic tissue
GFR	glomerular filtration rate
GGT	gamma-glutamyltransferase
GLDH	glutamate dehydrogenase
GnRH	gonadotropin-releasing hormone
HPAI	high pathogenic avian influenza
IBD	inclusion body disease
IPPV	intermittent positive pressure ventilation
LCMV	lymphocytic choriomeningitis virus
LDH	lactate dehydrogenase
LDL	low-density lipoprotein
LPAI	low pathogenic avian influenza
MAC	minimum alveolar concentration
MBD	metabolic bone disease
MCV	mean cell volume
MER	maintenance energy requirement
MHV	mouse hepatitis virus
MRI	magnetic resonance imaging
MuHV	murid herpesvirus
NALT	nasal-associated lymphatic tissue
NSAID	non-steroidal anti-inflammatory drug
NSHP	nutritional secondary hyperparathyroidism
PBA	post-brumation anorexia
PBFD	psittacine beak and feather disease
PBT	preferred body temperature
PCR	polymerase chain reaction
PCV	packed cell volume
PDD	proventricular dilatation disease
PHV	pigeon herpesvirus
PMV	paramyxovirus
POTZ	preferred optimum temperature zone
RER	resting energy requirement
RHD	rabbit haemorrhagic disease
RHDV	rabbit haemorrhagic disease virus
SARS-CoV-2	severe acute respiratory syndrome coronavirus 2
SCUD	septicaemic cutaneous ulcerative disease
SMEC	specific minimum energy cost
SMR	standard metabolic rate
SVL	snout-to-vent length
TPeC	*Treponema paraluisleporidarum* ecovar Cuniculus
VHS	vertebral heart score
YPDS	young pigeon disease syndrome

Part I Small Mammals

Chapter 1 Basic Small Mammal Anatomy and Physiology

Classification of small mammals

The commonly seen species of small mammals in veterinary practice are classified in Table 1.1.

RABBIT

Biological average values for the domestic rabbit

Table 1.2 gives the biological parameters for domestic rabbits.

Musculoskeletal system

The skeletal system of rabbits is light. As a percentage of body weight, the rabbit's skeleton is 7–8%, whereas the domestic cat's skeleton is 12–13%. This makes rabbits prone to fractures, especially of the spine and the hindlimbs.

Skull

Unlike many rodents the mandible is narrower than the maxilla, and the temporomandibular joint has a wide surface area, allowing lateral movement of the mandible in relation to the maxilla. The hemimandibles are fused rostrally with a fibrocartilaginous ligament which is also unusual for many rodents.

Axial skeleton

The spinal formula is generally C7, T12, L7, S4, Ca16 (where C represents cervical vertebrae; T, thoracic vertebrae; L, lumbar vertebrae; S, sacral vertebrae; Ca, coccygeal vertebrae). However, many rabbits have 13 thoracic and 6 lumbar while some have 13 thoracic and 7 lumbar vertebrae so there is considerable breed and individual variation. The cervical vertebrae are box-like and small and give mobility. The thoracic vertebrae possess attachments to the 12 (usually) paired ribs, which are flattened in comparison to cat's ribs. The first seven pairs of ribs articulate directly with the sternum. The last five pairs do not, with the most caudal three pairs being unconnected to the rest and so are free floating. The pelvis is narrow and positioned vertically. The iliac wings meet the ischium and pubis at the acetabulum, where an accessory bone unique to rabbits, called the os acetabuli, lies. The pubis forms the floor of the pelvis and borders the obturator foramen which is oval in rabbits.

Appendicular skeleton

The scapula is slender and there is a hooked supra-hamate process projecting caudally from the hamate process. The scapula articulates with the humerus which in turn articulates with the radius and ulna. In rabbits, the ulna fuses to the radius in older animals and the two bones are deeply bowed. The radius and ulna articulate with the carpal bones, which in turn articulate with the metacarpals and the five digits.

The femur is flatter than a cat's ventrodorsally, and the tibia and fibula are fused in the rabbit. The tibia articulates distally with the tarsal bones where there is a prominent calcaneus bone. The tarsals articulate with the metatarsals which articulate with the four hindlimb digits.

The hindlimbs are well muscled and powerful.

Respiratory anatomy

Upper respiratory tract

Rabbits, like horses, are nasal breathers, with the nasopharynx permanently locked around the epiglottis. For this reason, upper respiratory disease or evidence of mouth breathing is particularly problematic. The nasolacrimal ducts open onto the rostral floor of the nasal passage. The epiglottis is not visible easily from the oral cavity, making direct intubation difficult. It is narrow and elongated and leads into the larynx which has limited vocal fold development. The larynx leads into the trachea which has incomplete C-shaped cartilage rings for support.

Lower respiratory tract

The trachea bifurcates into two primary bronchi. There are two lungs, which are relatively small in proportion to the overall rabbit's body size. This means that even minor lung disease may cause serious problems. Each lung has three lobes (although the right lung caudal lobe is subdivided into medial and lateral segments), with the cranial ones being the smallest (see Figure 1.1). Rabbits do not have respiratory bronchioles leading to alveoli rather they have so-called vestibules that contain the alveoli (Cruise and Brewer, 1994).

Respiratory physiology

The main impetus for inspiration derives from the muscular contraction and flattening of the diaphragm. The lung parenchyma possesses a cellular population that is well supplied with anaphylactic mediating chemicals. These are strong enough to cause fluid extravasation and blood pooling, as well as spasms within the walls of the main pulmonary arterial supply, leading to rapid right-sided heart failure when their release is triggered.

Digestive system

Oral cavity

The dental formula is:

$$I2/1 C0/0 Pm3/2 M3/3.$$

Veterinary Nursing of Exotic Pets and Wildlife, Third Edition. Simon J. Girling.

Table 1.1 Classification of commonly seen small mammals.

Order	Lagomorpha	Rodentia							Eulipotyphla	Didelphimorphia	Diprotodontia	Carnivora
Sub-order		Myomorpha		Hystricomorpha			Sciuromorpha					Caniformia
Family	Leporidae	Muridae	Cricetidae	Caviidae	Chinchillidae	Octodontidae	Sciuridae		Erinaceidae	Didelphidae	Petauridae	Mustelidae
Species	Domestic rabbit (*Oryctolagus cuniculus*)	Rat (*Rattus norvegicus*) Mouse (*Mus musculus*)	Gerbil (*Meriones unguiculatus*) Syrian hamster (*Mesocricetus auratus*) Russian hamster (*Phodopus sungorus*) Chinese hamster (*Cricetulus griseus*)	Guinea pig (*Cavia porcellus*)	Chinchilla (*Chinchilla lanigera*)	Degu (*Octodon degus*)	Siberian chipmunk (*Eutamias sibiricus*) Eastern chipmunk (*Tamias striatus*)	Black-tailed prairie dog (*Cynomys ludovicianus*)	African pygmy hedgehog (*Atelerix albiventris*)	Virginia opossum (*Didelphis virginiana*)	Sugar glider (*Petaurus breviceps*)	Domestic ferret (*Mustela putorius furo*)

Table 1.2 Biological parameters for the domestic rabbit.

Biological parameter	Domestic rabbit
Weight (kg)	1.5 (Netherland dwarf) to 10 (New Zealand whites and Belgian hares)
Rectal body temperature (°C)	38.5–40
Respiratory rate at rest (breaths per minute)	30–60
Heart rate at rest (beats per minute)	130 (New Zealand whites) to 325 (Netherland dwarf)
Gestation length (days)	29–35 (average 31)
Litter size	Typically 5–8
Birth weight (g)	30–100
Weaning age (weeks)	4–6
Age at sexual maturity (months)	
Male	5–8
Female	4–7
Lifespan (years)	6–13

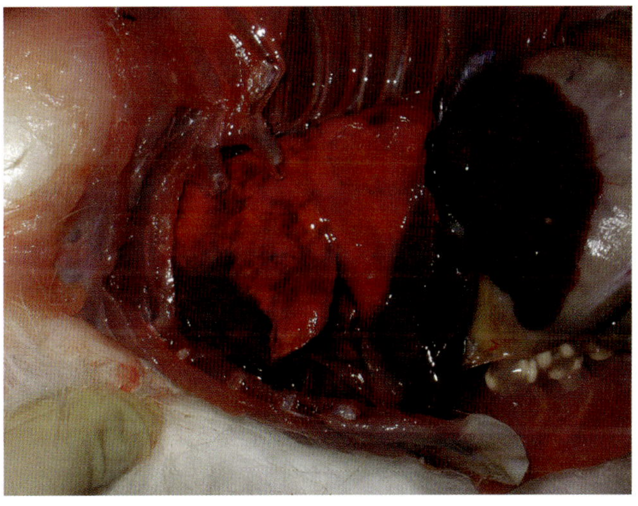

Figure 1.1 Lateral post-mortem view of a rabbit with the chest wall removed. The structures from left to right (cranial to caudal) are the dark-red heart, bright-red lungs (three lobes), darker brown diaphragm and liver, and pale cream stomach (Fraser and Girling, 2009).

The premolars and molars look physically similar and are often referred to simply as 'cheek teeth'. It should be noted that some breeds of rabbit, particularly the lop breeds, may have fewer cheek teeth in the maxilla (five instead of six on each side).

All rabbit teeth are elodont, growing continuously throughout life and the root apices are open (aradicular) with germinal tissue located at the apices producing the new tooth enamel and dentine. The premolar/molar enamel is folded providing an uneven occlusal surface with the ipsilateral jaw which allows interlocking (so-called interlocking lophs). Wear is kept even by the lateral movement of the mandible across the maxilla, allowing independent left and right arcades to engage in mastication. The incisors help differentiate Lagomorpha from Rodentia as rabbits, pikas and hares have two smaller incisors, or 'peg teeth', behind the maxillary incisors, whereas rodents have only two upper incisors. The larger (rostral) incisors only have enamel on the labial surface, whereas the smaller (caudal) maxillary peg teeth have enamel on the labial and lingual sides. This creates a wedge-shaped bite-plane where the lower incisors close immediately behind the upper large incisors and fit into a groove made by the peg teeth. The permanent rostral incisors are present at birth, although the peg teeth are replaced by permanent peg teeth at around the second week of life. The deciduous premolars present

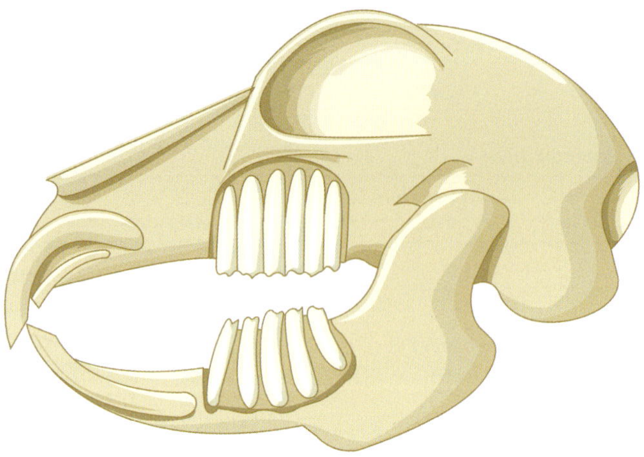

Figure 1.2 Lateral diagram of a normal rabbit skull showing the presence of the diastema, the smaller maxillary incisors (peg teeth) caudal to the main maxillary incisors and the relationship of the incisor and cheek teeth roots to the eye socket and jawbones.

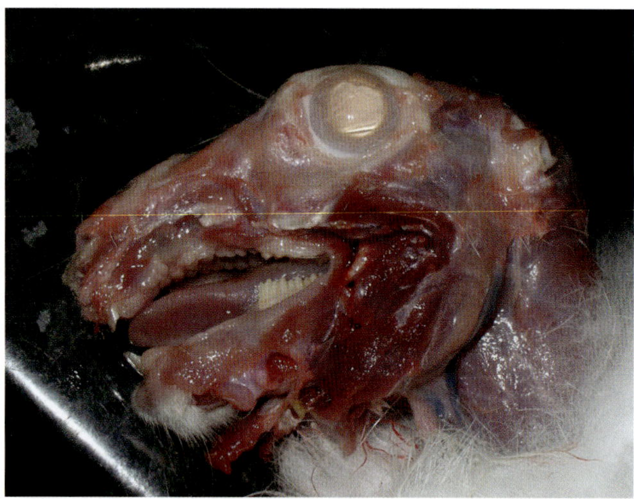

Figure 1.3 Lateral post-mortem view of a rabbit skull with the skin removed showing the presence of the diastema, and the occlusal surface of the cheek teeth demonstrating interlocking lophs.

at birth are replaced and joined by permanent molars by the fourth week of life. There are no canines; instead, there is a gap, or diastema, between the incisors and premolars (see Figures 1.2 and 1.3).

Stomach

The stomach is a large, simple structure, with a strong cardiac sphincter (see Figure 1.1). This makes vomiting in the rabbit virtually impossible. There is a main body, or fundus, and a pyloric section with a well-formed pyloric sphincter. The lining of the wall of the fundus contains acid-secreting and separate pepsinogen-secreting cells. The pH of the stomach contents is surprisingly lower than that of a cat's or dog's at 1.5–1.8. In addition, a healthy rabbit's stomach never truly empties of food.

Small intestine

The total length of the small intestine in the average rabbit may be some 2–3 m. It is difficult to determine the divisions between duodenum, jejunum and ileum as they all have a similar diameter. The duodenum is however split into descending, transverse and ascending segments. It receives the bile duct and pancreatic duct at separate sites.

Caecum and large intestinal anatomy

At the junction of the ileum and caecum lies the sacculus rotundus. This is a swelling of the gut infiltrated with lymphoid tissue and a common site for foreign body impactions. The caecum is large, sacculated and spiral-shaped, finishing in a blind-ended, thickened, finger-like projection known as the vermiform appendix, which also contains lymphoid tissue. The bulk of the caecum is thin-walled and possesses a semi-fluid digestive content where bicarbonate ions are secreted to buffer volatile fatty acid (VFA) production by the bacteria it contains.

The start of the large intestine is the ampulla coli which sits near to the sacculus rotundus and caecum. It is a smooth-walled portion of the gut with some lymphoid infiltration of its walls, unlike the rest of the large intestine. It is also distinguished by bands of fibrous tissue (known as taeniae) that create sacculations (each one also known as haustra). The surface area of the lining of the haustra is further increased by small projections (known as warzen or warts). At the end of the proximal colon, the taeniae and haustra cease, and the gut is then known as the fusus coli. Its walls are thickened and smooth because of the presence of large numbers of nerve ganglia which act as pacemakers for contraction waves in the large bowel. The distal descending colon has no haustra and continues through the pelvis to empty via the rectum and anus. The whole of the caecum and large intestine occupy around half of the abdominal cavity, predominantly on the right-hand side. There are a couple of para-anal glands just inside the anus, one on either side, that empty their secretions onto the faecal pellets.

Large intestinal physiology

Two types of faecal pellets are produced by the rabbit. One is a true faecal pellet, comprising waste material in a dry light-brown spherical form. The other is a much darker, mucus-covered pellet known as a caecotroph. The caecotroph is eaten directly from the anus, as soon as it is produced, which in the wild is during the middle of the day when the rabbit is underground. In captivity, they are often produced overnight, but may be produced at any time. The caecotroph contains plant material from which all of the nutrients have yet to be extracted and the mucus covering it protects the contents from the acidic pH of the stomach, allowing some further fermentation to occur while the caecotroph is still in the stomach before it eventually breaks down and the bacterial proteins are released. Caecotrophs are therefore a significant source of microbial protein (24.4–37.8%), accounting for 15–25% of the total amino acid requirement and 9–15% of the digestible energy needs (Griffiths and Davies, 1963; Lebas, 1989).

The large bowel can produce two types of pellets due to waves of contraction in the large intestine and caecum. The proximal colon can separate out food because the haustra or sacculations of the colon hold on to the smaller particles. The larger particles (often 0.5 mm or more) are pushed towards the lumen of the colon. The haustra then push the small particles (generally 0.3 mm or less) towards the caecum by contracting, and the segmental contractions of the colon itself propel the larger particles towards the rectum producing a waste pellet. When caecotrophs are produced, the haustra dramatically reduce their contractions, and instead the segmental activity drives material from the caecum through the distal colon where it is covered in mucus and then eaten directly from the anus. The caecum is thus the powerhouse filled with microbes that turn the ingesta into VFAs that can either nourish the caecal epithelium (butyrates) or be absorbed and converted to glucose by the liver (acetates). A high-fibre diet is important for maintaining the balance of VFAs, which should comprise predominantly acetates followed by butyrates and then propionates. Decreased levels of fibre increase butyrates and propionates at the expense of acetates, resulting in a reduction in normal gut peristalsis and leading to hypomotility disorders and ileus or gut stasis, as well as the growth of increased amounts of harmful bacteria such as *Clostridium* spp.

Liver

The rabbit liver has four main lobes, a right and left (each of which is divided into anterior and posterior lobules), a quadrate lobe caudal to the gall bladder, and a caudate lobe near the right kidney which is prone to torsions. The gall bladder has an opening separate from the pancreatic duct into the proximal descending duodenum, where there is a mild dilatation immediately distal to the pylorus of the stomach. The main bile pigment is biliverdin, rather than bilirubin as seen in cats and dogs.

Pancreas

The pancreas is split into a left lobe along the greater curvature of the stomach and a more diffuse organ, suspended in the loop of the duodenum. There is one single accessory pancreatic duct, separate from the bile duct, emptying into the intestine at the junction of the transverse and ascending duodenum. The main pancreatic duct regresses during *in utero* development.

Urinary anatomy

Kidney

The kidneys are bean-shaped and unipapillate (one papilla and one calyx entering the ureter) similar to rodents. The right kidney is more cranial than the left and close to the quadrate lobe of the liver. The kidneys are often separated from the ventral lumbar spine by large fat deposits. The number of glomeruli actually increases after birth and some become ectopic forming small cysts, some of which can be seen with the naked eye, in the adult rabbit (Moffat and Fourman, 1964).

A single ureter arises from each kidney and traverses the abdominal cavity to empty into the urinary bladder.

Bladder

The bladder lining is composed of transitional cell epithelium. The urethra in the male rabbit exits through the pelvis and out through the penis. In females, the urethra opens onto the floor of the vagina.

Renal physiology

Rabbit's urine is predominantly alkaline with a pH varying between 6.5 and 8, but it will become acidic if the rabbit has been anorectic for 24 hours or more. Volumes of urine production average around 50–75 mL/kg body weight in a normally hydrated rabbit (Gillett, 1994). The urine contains varying amounts of calcium often in the form of calcium carbonate. This is because rabbits have limited ability to alter how much calcium is absorbed from the gut as they can absorb calcium, assuming dietary levels are sufficient, in the absence of vitamin D. However, supplementary vitamin D will increase the level of calcium absorbed. Any excess calcium must be excreted by the kidneys into the urine. When this occurs it can be seen as a tan-coloured silt in the urine. Porphyrin pigments may also be seen in rabbit's urine. These are plant pigments and make the urine appear anywhere from a dark yellow to a deep wine-red in colour. This may mimic haematuria; therefore, to diagnose blood in the urine, it is necessary to examine it microscopically to visually determine if erythrocytes are present.

Cardiovascular system

Heart

The rabbit heart is small in relation to body size. The right atrioventricular valve usually has only two cusps instead of three. The pulmonary artery also has a large amount of smooth muscle in its wall which can contract vigorously during anaphylactic shock, causing immediate right-sided cardiac overload and failure.

The coronary arterial anatomy of the rabbit heart has significant variability. The main coronary artery is the left but typically half of all rabbit hearts show bifurcation and half trifurcation of the left main coronary artery. Some publications suggest that this is an oversimplification of the anatomy of the rabbit heart, which is commonly used to investigate human cardiac disease, for example suggesting that the right coronary artery may be the major supplier of blood to the myocardium in many rabbits (Morrissey *et al*., 2017).

Rabbits are often used to study atherosclerosis in humans as they rapidly develop hyperlipidaemia, mainly due to low-density lipoproteins (similar to humans) after being fed high-fat diets. However, they do not naturally form atherosclerotic plaques as humans do, but will develop lipid mural deposits, which will often mineralise in the walls of major vessels such as the aorta in the presence of high calcium-containing diets or advanced kidney disease.

Blood vessels for sampling

Vascular access sites in rabbits include the following.

Lateral ear vein

This runs along the lateral margin of either ear. It may be accessed using a 25 or 27 gauge needle or catheter and used for slow intravenous injections and small volume blood sampling.

Cephalic vein

This runs in a similar position to that seen in cats and dogs. It may be split into two in some individuals, but may be used for intravenous fluids and sampling although it is often a small vessel (see Figure 1.4).

Saphenous vein

This runs across the lateral aspect of the hock, as in cats and dogs, and may also be used for venepuncture.

Jugular vein

The external jugular veins are prominent in the rabbit and form the major part of the drainage of blood from the head and orbit of the eye

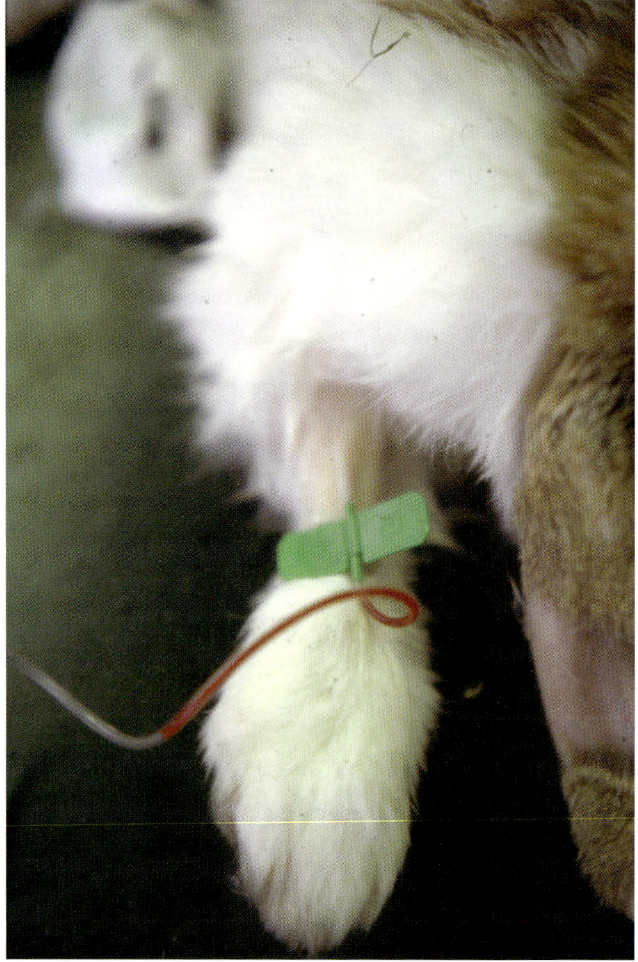

Figure 1.4 Cephalic vein access in a rabbit using a pre-heparinised butterfly catheter.

and have few anastomoses with the internal jugular veins. If a haematoma or thrombus forms in the external jugular vein(s) and blocks the lumen, severe orbital swelling and head oedema may occur, with possible damaging effects.

Lymphatic system

Spleen

The spleen is a flattened structure, oblong in nature and attached to the greater curvature of the stomach and is thus found predominantly on the left side. It is relatively small in comparison to body size, possibly because almost half of lymphatic tissue is found in the intestines as gut-associated lymphatic tissue (GALT).

Thymus

The thymus is a large structure in the cranial thoracic compartment even in the adult rabbit. It provides the body with the T-cell lymphocytes.

Lymph nodes

The root of the mesentery supporting the digestive tract is well supplied with lymph nodes, as is the hilar area of the lungs where the two main bronchi diverge to supply each lung. In addition, there are superficial lymph nodes in the popliteal, prescapular and submandibular areas. Large amounts of GALT exist in the small intestine, sacculus rotundus and vermiform appendix.

Reproductive anatomy

Male

The paired testes can move from an inguinal position within the thin-skinned scrotal sacs to an intra-abdominal position through the open inguinal canal. The scrotal sacs are sparsely haired and lie on either side of the anogenital area.

The accessory sex glands in the buck attached to the urethra in the caudal abdomen include the dorsal and smaller ventral prostate, the bilobed vesicular gland, the bilobed coagulating (sometimes referred to as seminal) gland and a bilobed bulbourethral gland. The prepuce has numerous small preputial glands in the dermis, and there are a couple of inguinal glands situated on either side of the penis which secrete a brown-coloured sebum clearly seen adjacent to the anus.

Female

The ovaries are supported by the ovarian ligament and lie caudal to each respective kidney. The ovarian artery often splits into two parts after leaving the aorta, and it, along with the rest of the reproductive tract, is frequently encased in large amounts of fat.

The uterus is duplex – there is no common uterine body. Instead, there are two separate uteri with separate cervices emptying into the vagina (see Figure 1.5). The vagina is large and thin-walled, with the urethra opening onto its floor cranial to the pelvis. The vulva therefore is a common opening for the reproductive and urinary systems unlike many rodents. It lies just cranial to the anus and is flanked on either side by the inguinal glands, as with the buck.

The doe has on average four pairs of mammary glands extending from the inguinal region to the axillary areas.

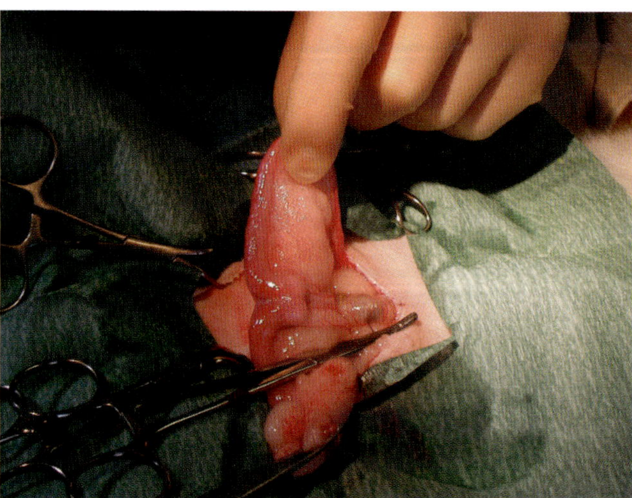

Figure 1.5 Intraoperative view of the uterus and ovaries of a domestic rabbit. Note the significant amount of fat deposition and the two cervices and two separate uterine horns.

Reproductive physiology

Male

The buck rabbit has similar reproductive hormones to those in cats and dogs, but they are on a seasonal time clock triggered by the lengthening daylight of spring. This is mediated through the pineal gland in the brain which has neural links from the eyes and controls the hormone melatonin. It in turn controls the pituitary release of follicle-stimulating and luteinising hormones which then act upon the testes.

Female

Does are induced ovulators. Waves of follicles swell and regress during the course of the season, starting to increase in activity in early spring. If not mated, these follicles will often dominate the cycle for 12–16 days at a time. There is no real anoestrus phase in does; instead, a slight waning in activity for 1–2 days occurs before a return to heat. During peak sexual activity, the vulva is often deeply congested and almost purple in colour and considerably enlarged.

Once mated, the male's semen may form a copulatory plug, which is a gelatinous accumulation of sperm that drops out of the doe's vagina 4–6 hours after mating. Gestation lasts from 29 to 35 days, with the fetus forming a haemochorial placenta (where the outer chorion layer of the fetal placental membrane burrows into the lining of the uterus so that it directly attaches to the blood in the intrauterine vessels) at about day 13. This is a common time for abortions to occur. A pregnant doe will remove fur from her ventrum to line the nest in the latter few days prior to parturition.

Parturition is often referred to as 'kindling'. Dystocia is uncommon. The doe only nurses the kittens once a day for 20 minutes or so, often in the early morning. It is therefore not uncommon for owners to think that the doe is neglecting her young as she will often spend the rest of the time eating and away from the litter.

Pseudopregnancy often occurs after an unsuccessful mating or mounting activity by another buck or doe. A corpus luteum forms and this lasts for 15–17 days during which time the doe may produce milk and build a nest. At this time, the doe is susceptible to mastitis.

Neonatology

The young kits or kittens are altricial in nature, that is, they are totally dependent on the mother for nutrition and survival for the first few weeks of life. They are born blind, deaf and furless. Fur growth appears around day 5–6, the eyes open at day 8–10 and the ears at 11–12. When nursing from the mother kits only suckle once a day consuming 35% of their body weight rapidly over a few minutes (Hudson and Distel, 1983). Weaning occurs around 4–6 weeks of age, with the young taking solid food from 2 to 3 weeks.

Sexing

The young may be sexed from 4 to 5 weeks of age. Gentle pressure is placed on either side of the reproductive or anal area to protrude the vulva or penis. The vulva of the young doe is rounded and has a central slit in midline and projects cranially. The penis of the young buck is more conical and pointed, with no central slit and tends to project caudally when protruded. Once the buck is older, the testes descend into the scrotum.

Skin

Lop breeds, particularly does, have extra skin folds called 'dewlaps' around the ventral neck region. In addition, extra folds of skin may also be found around the anogenital area, leading to increased risk of urine and faecal soiling. The skin is thin and can tear easily.

Rabbits do not have keratinised footpads. Instead they have thick fur covering the areas of the toes and metatarsals which are pressed flat to the ground.

In addition to the para-anal scent glands mentioned above there are a series of discrete submandibular chin glands. These are used to mark territory and also, in the case of does, to mark their young to distinguish them from others. Rabbits also have inguinal scent glands dorsal to the urogenital opening on each side of the anus.

The rabbit has no skin sweat glands except a few along the margins of the lips. This means that they are very prone to heat stress at temperatures greater than 28°C.

The presence of many vibrissae or sensitive hairs around the lips and chin are important since rabbits cannot see anything immediately below their mouths, and so rely on touch to manipulate food towards the mouth.

Eyes

Rabbits have prominent eyes, which allow a near 360° field of vision. There is a prominent third eyelid, which moves from the medial canthus of the eye and possesses a large amount of reactive lymphoid tissue within its structure and a Harderian tear gland at its base. This is often enlarged in the buck during the breeding season and possesses two lobes in both the sexes. The optic disc is above the horizontal midline of the eye unlike the domestic cat or dog and the retina has no tapetum lucidum.

There is a significant orbital venous plexus that makes enucleation of the globe complicated. A retrobulbar plexus also exists which can become engorged with increased mediastinal pressure (such as a thymic tumour) resulting in bilateral exophthalmos (Wagner *et al.*, 2005). Tears drain from the eye via the nasolacrimal duct which starts at a single ventromedially located punctum, rather than the paired openings seen in cats and dogs. There is a small lacuna or swelling of the duct shortly after its start, located medial to the canthus of each eye. The duct then moves ventral to the root of the main maxillary incisor on each side before opening onto the floor of the rostral nasal passage. This path around the root of the maxillary incisor means occlusion of the duct can occur with dental disease or with incisor root elongation, resulting in epiphora and dacryocystitis.

Haematology

The most notable feature is the esosinophilic staining of the rabbit neutrophil, making it easily mistaken for an eosinophil and meaning it is often referred to as the pseudoeosinophil. Many rabbits have more lymphocytes than pseudoeosinophils, resembling other mammals such as cattle, rather than cats and dogs, in which the neutrophil is the commonest white blood cell. Romanowsky-stained blood smears from rabbits, as with other small mammals, often show significant polychromasia and anisocytosis as the lifespan of the erythrocyte is short, 57 days, indicating a relatively high turnover of red cells.

RAT AND MOUSE

Biological average values for the rat and mouse

The normal biological values for the rat and mouse are given in Table 1.3.

Musculoskeletal system

Skull

The skull of both species is elongated. The eyes are laterally situated, and there is a long snout and a shallow cranium. The maxilla is narrower than the mandible. The temporomandibular joint is elongated craniocaudally, allowing the mandible to move rostrally and caudally in relation to the maxilla. This allows the incisors to be engaged for gnawing, while the molars are disengaged. Alternatively, the molars may be engaged for mastication prior to swallowing, while the incisors are disengaged. The two procedures cannot occur at the same time. The rostral symphysis, joining each half of the mandible, is also articulated allowing movement of each hemimandible independently of the other.

Axial skeleton

The pelvis of the female mouse is joined at the pubis and ischial areas midline by fibrous tissue. This allows separation of the pelvis during parturition in the mouse. There are no fibrous areas to the pelvis of the female rat and consequently no pelvic separation occurs.

The vertebral formula of the domestic rat is:

$$C7, T13, L6, S3-4, Ca27-36$$

The vertebral formula of the domestic mouse is:

$$C7, T13, L6, S4, Ca26-34$$

Table 1.3 Biological parameters for the rat and mouse.

Biological parameter	Average range rat	Average range mouse
Weight (g)	400–1000	25–50
Rectal body temperature (°C)	37.6–38.6	37–38
Respiration rate at rest (breaths per minute)	60–140	100–280
Heart rate at rest (beats per minute)	250–450	500–600
Gestation length (days)	20–22	19–21
Litter size	6–16	8–12
Birth weight (g)	6–8	0.5–1.5
Weaning age (days)	21 (average)	21 (average)
Age sexual maturity (weeks)		
Male	8	6
Female	10	4–7
Oestrus interval (days)	4–5	4–5
Lifespan (years)	3–4	2–3

Appendicular skeleton

The scapula articulates at its coracoid process with the clavicles as well as the humerus. There are four metacarpal bones in the rat, with four digits. Occasionally the vestigial remnant of digit 1 is present. Mice have five metacarpal bones and five digits in the forelimbs.

The hindlimbs have a strong laterally bowed fibula in both species. The tibia articulates with five metatarsal bones at the hock joint. Consequently there are five digits in the hindlimbs of both of these species. Rats and mice are plantigrade in their stance, meaning they walk with the whole of the metatarsal bone area flat to the ground.

Male rats may still have open growth plates in many of their long bones well into the second year of their lives, whereas mice close their growth plates in the first 3–4 months of life.

Respiratory system

The nares of both species are prominent and surrounded by an area of hairless skin containing some sweat glands.

There is a vomeronasal organ in the floor of the nasal passages, accessed via two small stoma in the roof of the mouth just caudal to the maxillary incisors. This organ is responsible for detecting pheromones secreted by other individuals. At the junction of the nasopharynx lie significant amounts of lymphoid tissue referred to as nasal-associated lymphatic tissue (NALT).

The right lung of the rat is divided into three distinct lobes, the right lung of the mouse into four lobes and the left lung in both species is undivided. The chest cavity itself is smaller in proportion to the abdominal cavity than is the case in cats and dogs, meaning that rats and mice have little respiratory reserve.

Digestive system

Oral cavity

The lips of mice, and particularly rats, are deeply divided exposing the upper incisors, with large areas of loose folds of skin forming the cheeks.

Both species have pigmented yellow/orange enamel coating the labial aspect of the incisors. The maxillary incisors are one-third to one-quarter of the length of the mandibular incisors. There is a chisel shape to their occlusal surfaces due to the absence of enamel on the lingual aspect of the incisors making them wear quicker on this side. The mandibular incisors are also mobile and loosely rooted in the lower jaw. Their dental formula is

$$I1/1 C0/0 Pm0/0 M3/3.$$

There is no evidence of any deciduous or 'milk' teeth being present in either species. The molars have a limited period of growth with long narrow roots (varying between three and five per tooth depending on the species and molar) being brachydont in nature. Unlike rabbits there is no overlap between maxillary and mandibular molar occlusal surface, each molar occluding fully with the corresponding molar in the ipsilateral jaw.

Both species have a diastema. In the case of rats, this gap is particularly noticeable and large enough to allow them to draw their cheeks into the gap to effectively close off the back of the mouth. This enables them to gnaw, without consuming the material they are nibbling.

The tongue is relatively mobile and its surface is covered with small, backward-pointing papillae.

Stomach

The stomach of the mouse and rat is elongated and narrow. In the rat, in particular, the stomach is divided into two regions: cranial is the proventricular region, covered by a thin whitened lining of aglandular mucosa; caudal is the pyloric region, covered by a redder, thicker, glandular mucosa. The oesophagus enters the stomach halfway along the length of its lesser curvature and has an abdominal section. This, combined with a strong cardiac sphincter, makes vomiting extremely difficult. Both species have separate hydrochloric acid-secreting (parietal) and pepsinogen-secreting (chief) cells with additional mucin-secreting cells.

Small intestine

The small intestine comprises the largest portion of the gastrointestinal tract. In the rat the bile duct enters the first part of the duodenum direct from the liver, which has no gall bladder. The mouse does have a gall bladder which empties into the first part of the duodenum. The ileum is most easily distinguished by the presence of lymphoid deposits (Peyer's patches).

Large intestine

The ileum enters the large intestine at the junction of the caecum and the large intestine on the left side of the abdomen. The caecum is a medium-sized organ in the mouse and rat, reflecting their omnivorous nature, and forms a blind-ended pouch which is flexed back on itself and is approximately one-third the total length of the large intestine.

Liver

The liver is divided in both species into four lobes. There is a gall bladder present in the mouse but not in the rat. The liver sits cranial to the stomach. Biliverdin is the prominent bile pigment in rats and mice.

Pancreas

The pancreas lies along the proximal aspect of the duodenal loop. In both species, it empties through a series of ducts into the bile duct. Its function appears to be the same as in cats and dogs, producing both insulin and glucagon for glucose homeostasis and the digestive enzymes amylase, lipase and trypsinogen.

Urinary system

Kidney

The kidneys are bean-shaped. The right kidney sits in a depression in the right lobe of the liver, and the left kidney is slightly more caudal. Each empties through its ureter which enters the bladder at the trigone area. Mice often excrete urine drop by drop as it is generally highly concentrated and small in volume (1.5–2 mL per day). Mouse urine also contains an inherently high level of the so-called mouse urinary protein (MUP), whose function is believed to be pheromone transport. Male mice excrete greater levels of MUP than female mice.

Bladder

The bladder, which is lined with transitional epithelium, empties through the urethra. In the female mouse and rat, the urethra empties through a separate urinary papilla rather than onto the floor of the vagina as it does with higher mammals. The female mouse and rat therefore have three orifices caudoventrally: the anus most caudally, the reproductive tract entrance next cranially and the urinary papilla the most cranial of the three.

Cardiovascular system

Heart

The heart of the mouse and rat has four chambers, as in other mammals. As with rabbits, the chest compartment is relatively small in comparison to the abdomen, and the heart therefore appears relatively large in relation to the rest of the chest. The heart occupies the fourth to sixth rib spaces.

Blood vessels for sampling

Useful vessels from which to sample blood are the lateral tail veins. These are best accessed after first warming the tail, or lightly sedating the mouse or rat to allow dilation of the vessels. A 25–27 gauge needle or butterfly catheter is required. Some mild pressure at the tail base allows further dilation.

In the rat, the femoral vein may also be used for sampling. This is found on the medial aspect of the thigh, close to its junction with the inguinal area, just caudal to the femur. This vessel is best used only under anaesthetic due to the difficulty of accessing it in a conscious rat.

For small capillary samples, a microcapillary tube may be gently pushed into the medial canthus of the eye socket in the anaesthetised rat or mouse. This collects blood from the orbital sinus.

Lymphatic system

Spleen

The spleen of male mice is often twice the size of that in females. In both species, it is a strap-like organ sitting along the greater curvature of the stomach.

Thymus

The thymus is an obvious organ in the cranial chest, and may be split into several smaller islands of tissue. It is frequently still present in the adult rat or mouse.

Lymph nodes

The lymph nodes follow similar patterns to those seen in the rabbit. The mesenteric lymph nodes can become very prominent in certain bacterial infections.

Reproductive anatomy

Male

The male rat and mouse reproductive systems are nearly identical in design.

The testes are large and can move between the abdomen and the scrotal sacs, although somewhat inhibited by a large fat body attached to the tail of each testicle extending through the open inguinal canal. Each testis descends into the scrotum around the fifth week of age in the rat and the third to fourth week in the mouse.

The vasa deferentia are joined by the opening of the small ampullary glands which open into a swelling of the vas deferens known as the ampulla just before they join the urethra. Other accessory sex glands, including the vesicular glands, the coagulating glands (which are joined together) and the two parts of the prostate (the ventral and dorsal lobes), open into the urethra itself. As the urethra exits the pelvic canal, a paired bulbourethral gland also empties into its lumen.

These accessory sex glands produce nutrients and supporting fluids for the spermatozoa. In addition, the coagulating glands are responsible for allowing a plug of sperm to form in the female's vagina immediately after mating. The penis has an os penis in both species. There is a preputial gland in the small prepuce that is used for territorial marking. Male mice and rats have no nipples.

Female

The rat uterus has two separate uterine horns which come together at a single cervix, but with separate cervical canals for each horn. From the outside these appear to merge to form a common uterine body, and so it is sometimes referred to as bicornuate in nature. The vagina itself has no lumen in the immature rat. Instead, at puberty, the solid mass of tissue forms its own lumen, breaking through to the surface at the time of the first ovulation.

The mouse uterus is almost exactly the same except that the two separate uterine horns do fuse just before the cervix, making it truly bicornuate and there is just the one cervical opening into the vagina. The vagina is also non-patent in the immature state.

Mammary tissue is extensive in both female rats and mice. In mice there are normally five pairs of mammary glands, three in the axillary region, with mammary tissue extending dorsally nearly to midline. The other two pairs of glands are in the inguinal region, with mammary tissue extending around the anus and tail base. In rats there are more commonly six pairs of mammary glands. Three are located in the axillary region, again with some tissue moving onto the lateral chest wall. The other three glands are inguinally located.

Reproductive physiology

The female rat and mouse are non-seasonally polyoestrus. The commonest time for heat to occur is during the night. The first cycling activity occurs around 8 weeks of age in the female rat, with the cycle lasting 4–5 days in total. Ovulation is spontaneous and occurs towards the end of the 12-hour-long heat. There is a reduction in reproductive activity in the female rat over 18 months of age.

During mating, the semen deposited in the female rat's vagina forms a copulatory plug which sits in the cranial vagina, blocking the cervix. This dries and falls out within a few hours of mating, but seems to play an important role in the success of mating. It is often eaten rapidly after being passed.

Gestation length is around 21 days. The placentation of the rat and mouse is discoidal and haemochorial – the area of attachment is disc-like with the chorion of the placenta in contact with the bloodstream of the dam's uterus. There may be a bloody mucous discharge from the vagina around 14 days, which is normal. This stops within 2–3 days. Mammary development occurs at around days 12–14 and at that stage the fetuses may be palpated.

Parturition is rarely complicated. There is no separation of the pelvis in the female rat, although the female mouse's pelvis does separate at the ischial and pubic sutures. Parturition occurs in the afternoon and is followed by a postpartum oestrus.

Pseudopregnancy is seen in both rats and mice. During this time the female may build a nest; there may be some mammary development and no signs of a heat for up to 2 weeks.

There are a couple of important physiological reproductive phenomena in mice and rats. One of these is the Whitten effect. This is when a group of anoestrus females will all come into heat spontaneously some 72 hours after being exposed to the pheromones of a male. This has beneficial effects when it comes to successful rapid breeding. The other is the Bruce effect. This is when a female in the early stages of gestation will reabsorb the embryos and come back into heat when presented with a new male. By preferentially allowing successful mating with a new male, this is thought to have a beneficial effect on genetic diversity. The Lee–Boot effect occurs when mature female mice, kept in large groups in the absence of males, exhibit suppressed oestrus cycles, leading to prolonged dioestrus and the spontaneous development of pseudopregnancy.

Neonatology

Rat and mouse pups are altricial. They are born blind, deaf and hairless. The ear canals open around days 4–5 and the eyes at around 2 weeks of age. The first few hairs are also seen in the first week of life. The pups are born without teeth, the incisors becoming visible at 1–2 weeks of age with the molars developing later.

The female rat and mouse are prone to cannibalism if disturbed with their young in the first few weeks after parturition. It is therefore important to leave the female rat and mouse alone during this period, only disturbing them to replenish food and clear the worst of any cage soiling.

Sexing

Sexing may be done from 4 to 6 weeks of age. In males the urinary papilla is slightly larger than the female and further away from the anus. It may be possible in the sexually mature female to see the small reproductive tract entrance as a transverse slit between the anus and urinary papilla. Also, in male mice and rats, no nipples are visible. In mature males, if the rat or mouse is gently suspended in a vertical position with the head uppermost, the testes will often descend into the scrotal sacs and are then obvious.

Skin

Rats and mice possess no generalised sweat glands and so are prone to heat stress at temperatures above 26–28°C. There are some sweat glands present on the soles of the feet as well as the nares.

There is a layer of brown fat between the shoulder blades dorsally; its function is not clearly known, but it decreases with age and may play a role in thermoregulation.

The tails of rats and mice are relatively hairless. As rats age, there is an increasing number of coarse skin scales present on the tail surface making blood sampling difficult. Rats should not be grasped by the tip of the tail as the skin may slough in this region. Sensory innervation of the hairless skin of the forepaws in mice is up to three times greater than the innervation to the hairless skin of the hindlimbs.

White fur will often yellow in rats as they age, and most rats will show evidence of a yellow hue to the skin on the back with time.

The vibrissae around the lips and nose are important for detecting vibrations and determining where food is due to their inability, as with rabbits, to see food immediately below their mouths. The vibrissae are innervated by the trigeminal nerve.

Eyes

Rats and mice have a prominent set of small eyes located laterally. Both species have a third eyelid located at rest in the medial canthus of the eye. The albino breeds lack pigment in their irises or retinas, and so their eyes appear pink red. These albino breeds should therefore be exposed to dimmed lighting during the day otherwise retinal damage can occur. Both species have the ability to see in the ultraviolet light spectrum. There are three main tear glands: the Meibomian (producing an oil film to stabilise tears); the lacrimal (two forms producing aqueous tears); and around the base of the third eyelid, the Harderian gland (producing aqueous tears and porphyrin pigments).

Haematology

The haematological parameters are similar to those seen in cats or dogs, except that the lymphocyte, as opposed to the neutrophil, is the most common white blood cell. Basophils are rarely seen in mice in the circulation. Erythrocyte turnover is high, with the average lifespan of the mouse erythrocyte being 30–40 days; therefore, as with rabbits, when a blood smear is stained using Romanowsky stains, a high degree of polychromasia and anisocytosis is considered normal. Howell–Jolly bodies (leftover fragments of nuclear DNA) are also commonly seen in erythrocytes.

GERBIL AND HAMSTER

Biological average values for the gerbil and hamster

Table 1.4 gives the average normal biological values for gerbils and hamsters.

Musculoskeletal system

Skull

The skull of the gerbil is not dissimilar to that of the rat or mouse; in the hamster, the skull is shortened, particularly in the Russian and Chinese hamster subspecies. The mandibular symphysis of adult hamsters often does not fuse allowing some independent hemimandible movement when chewing.

Axial skeleton

The axial skeleton is much the same as for the rat and mouse, except the hamster has far fewer coccygeal vertebrae.

The vertebral formula of the Syrian hamster is

$$C7, T13, L6, S4, Ca6-14$$

The vertebral formula of the gerbil is

$$C7, T12/13, L6/7, S4, Ca14-26$$

Appendicular skeleton

Gerbils have a longer femur and tibial length, giving them longer hindlimbs equipped for jumping. Their normal stance is bipedal, standing erect on their hindlimbs. Hamsters are a much shorter-legged creature, stockier in build, and walk predominantly on all fours.

The forelimbs have four digits, and the hindlimbs have five in both species.

Respiratory system

As with rats and mice, the chest cavity is small in relation to the abdomen, but the situation is not so pronounced as that seen in rats. Hamsters have a single left lobe and four to five right lobes to the

Table 1.4 Biological parameters for the gerbil and hamster.

Biological parameter	Russian hamster	Syrian hamster	Gerbil
Weight (g)	30–60	90–150 (male larger)	70–120 (male larger)
Rectal body temperature (°C)	36–38	36.2–37.5	37.5–39
Respiration rate at rest (breaths per minute)	60–80	40–70	80–150
Heart rate at rest (beats per minute)	300–460	250–400	250–400
Gestation (days)	Average 16 (Chinese hamster 21)	15–18	24–26 (up to 42 days with delayed implantation)
Litter size	4–8	4–12	2–6
Birth weight (g)	1–1.5	2–3	2.5–3.5
Weaning age (days)	20–24	21–28	21–30
Age at sexual maturity (weeks)			
Male	5–6	6–8	8–9
Female	6–8 (Chinese hamster 14)	8–12	9–10
Oestrus interval (days)	3–4	4	4–6
Lifespan (months)	18–24	24–36	36–60

lungs. Gerbils have three lobes to the left lung and four to the right (Williams, 1974).

Digestive system

Oral cavity

The incisors in both species are continuously erupting (open rooted), and both species have orange pigmentation of the enamel surfaces. The dental formula is

I1/1C0/0Pm0/0M3/3.

Hamsters are born with the incisors fully erupted and use them to grasp the nipples of the female enabling them to suck effectively.

The molars do grow continually for a limited part of the early life of the rodent, with multiple, short, narrow tooth roots (so-called brachydont). In addition, there appears to be no evidence of deciduous teeth (monophyodont). All species possess a diastema. The mandible is generally wider than the maxilla and the occlusal surfaces of the molars are flat. Hamsters have small cusps to the occlusal molar surfaces but gerbils do not.

The cheek pouches of the hamster are its most distinguishing feature. These are not present at birth, but rather develop during the second week of life from a solid cord of cells which disintegrate, creating the cavities. The entrances to the cheek pouches open into the diastema. Each cheek pouch extends caudal to the respective ear. They are lined with stratified squamous epithelium and have a reduced local immune system and lymphatic function, although they have a high incidence of mast cells. This can be a problem if the cheek pouch becomes infected.

Stomach

The stomach of the hamster has two separate areas. The oesophagus enters the proximal portion. This portion is non-glandular and has a bacterial population that allows limited microbial breakdown of food. It is sharply divided by a deep groove from the distal area of the stomach, which is glandular, with a redder lining composed of the acid- and pepsinogen-secreting cells that start the process of enzymatic digestion.

The gerbil has two areas to the stomach but they are less clearly demarcated, and the proximal portion does not support a significant microbial population.

Small intestine

The hamster's small intestine is extremely long, being three to four times its own body length. The gerbil has a similar layout to the mouse.

Large intestine

In the hamster the caecum is a sacculated and enlarged organ sitting in the ventral left portion of the abdomen at the ileocaecal junction. Its connection with the ileum is complicated by a series of four valves in the hamster. The hamster caecum has fine divisions within it, which may function to increase its surface area and aid fibre fermentation. It also has a semi-lunar valve separating the caecum into basal and apical portions. The gerbil has a similar layout to the mouse.

Liver

The liver in both species is divided into four main lobes (although two of the lobes are further partly divided into two). In both hamsters and gerbils, a gall bladder is present. A bile duct empties into the duodenum accompanied by the pancreatic ducts.

Pancreas

The pancreas is found adjacent to the descending duodenum. It has a similar structure and function to that seen in the rat and mouse. The hamster pancreas has three lobes (gastric, splenic and duodenal). The common bile duct merges with the three pancreatic ducts before emptying into the duodenum similar to many other rodents.

Urinary system

Kidney

The kidneys are similar to the rat and mouse kidney. The gerbil is very good at concentrating its urine, being a desert-dwelling species, and to do this it has a large number of nephrons (over 96% of the total) with long loops of Henle containing the countercurrent multiplier system for water reabsorption (Ichii *et al.*, 2006). In the hamster, the renal papilla is particularly long and protrudes from each kidney into its ureter.

Bladder

The bladder of gerbils and hamsters is essentially the same as that seen in rats and mice.

Cardiovascular system

Heart

The heart is similar in form to the rat and mouse heart.

Blood vessels for sampling

The hamster has very few accessible external vessels for blood sampling. This is principally due to its much reduced tail length, which provides the main vascular access in the rat and mouse. The skin covering the gerbil's tail can slough easily, making tail vein blood sampling potentially hazardous. However, the lateral tail veins have been used in research settings as with mice and rats. Other vessels used include the jugular veins and the femoral veins, both of which require the hamster or gerbil to be sedated or anaesthetised. Capillary samples may be taken from the orbital sinus as described in the rat and mouse.

Lymphatic system

Spleen

The structure and position of the spleen is much the same for both species as that seen in the rat.

Thymus

The thymus is again a prominent organ in the cranial chest and often persists in the adult. It provides the T-cell lymphocytes.

Lymph nodes

The presence of lymphatic tissue is the same as that seen in the mouse and rat.

Reproductive anatomy

Male

The male hamster has a smaller fat body attached to the testicle than has the rat. The testes are freely moveable between the abdominal cavity and the scrotal sacs. A small os penis is present in the penile structure. Accessory sex glands, from proximal to caudal, include paired ampullae, seminal vesicles, coagulating glands, a trilobed prostate, and paired bulbourethral glands.

The male gerbil is similar to the male rat and mouse. The main difference is the slightly smaller size of the testes in relation to the overall body size and the presence of a pigmented scrotum.

Female

The hamster uterus is bicornuate. It has two separate canals combining to a single cervix that then opens into a common vagina. The vagina is, as with the rat, not patent at birth. It opens after day 10 of life, rather than at puberty as in the rat.

The gerbil reproductive tract is similar to that of the mouse. The main difference is that while there is only one cervical opening into the vagina, the division between the left and right uterine lumens persists to within a few millimetres of this single cervical orifice.

The female hamster has four pairs (in the Djungarian hamster up to seven pairs) of mammary glands stretching in a continuous band from the axillary region to the inguinal and perianal region.

The female gerbil has four pairs of mammary glands. Two pairs are found in the axillary region and two pairs in the inguinal region.

Reproductive physiology

The female hamster is seasonally polyoestrus with cycling and fertility dropping off during the winter period. The reproductive cycle is short, lasting 4 days. The female hamster develops a creamy white vaginal discharge around the first day following oestrus. This may be mistaken for a pathological discharge as it has an odour. Ovulation is spontaneous and generally occurs overnight. Phantom pregnancy does occur in the hamster, postponing oestrus for 7–13 days. Gestation itself lasts for 15–18 days in the Syrian hamster, an average of 21 days in the Chinese hamster and an average of 16 days in the Russian hamster. Successful mating is followed by the presence of a copulatory plug of coagulated semen 24 hours later. Pregnancy can be confirmed by failure to produce the copious white discharge 5 days after mating, and an increase in weight at around day 10. There is no evidence of pelvic separation at parturition. There is reduced fertility in the female hamster after 1 year of life. Male Syrian hamsters need exposure to more than 12.5 hours daylight per day for breeding to occur.

Gerbils form a monogamous pair, that is they pair for life. The female gerbil is seasonally polyoestrus and a spontaneous ovulator. The oestrus cycle lasts for 4–6 days. Oestrus lasts for 24 hours and may occur within 14–20 hours of parturition. Gestation lasts an average of 26 days but may take up to 42 days if mating has occurred at the postpartum heat as when the female is still feeding the young, the fertilised ova will not implant, so prolonging the interval from mating to parturition.

Neonatology

The young hamster is altricial. The pale pink colour of the skin is replaced by some darker pigmentation after the first 2–3 days, with the eyes opening at 2 weeks of age. Weaning occurs around 3–4 weeks of age, with the female hamster becoming sexually mature at 6–8 weeks (up to 14 weeks for the Chinese hamster) and the male at 8–9 weeks.

The young gerbil is also altricial. The skin is a pale pink at birth but darkens by the end of the first week with the appearance of the first few hairs. The teeth erupt in the first few days of life. The eyes open at 2 weeks of age and the ears around days 4–5. Weaning occurs at 3–4 weeks of age. The female gerbil becomes sexually mature at 9–10 weeks of age when the vaginal opening becomes patent. The male gerbil becomes sexually mature at 8–9 weeks of age, with the testes descending into the scrotal sac at 5 weeks.

It is inadvisable to disturb the female hamster with her young as cannibalism can occur. However, a common protective action of the female is to place the young into her cheek pouches to move them, and this may look as if she is 'eating' the young. Gerbils are less prone to abandoning or abusing their young if disturbed.

The placenta of gerbils and hamsters is haemochorial in form, similar to other rodents.

Sexing

This may be performed from 4 weeks of age. In the immature gerbil and hamster, the differences are determined by anogenital distances as with the rat and mouse. In the sexually mature hamster, the male has a pointed outline to its rear, owing to the descended testes, whereas the female has a more rounded appearance. In both, it is relatively easy to determine the sex once mature if the individual is supported in a vertical position with the head uppermost. In this position, the testes will descend into the scrotal sacs where they are clearly visible.

Skin

Hamster and gerbil skin has no sweat glands. Gerbils, however, can tolerate wider temperature ranges, up to 29–30°C, although if the humidity increases above 50% they will rapidly suffer from heat exhaustion.

In hamsters, there is a pair of oval, raised scent glands situated on each flank cranial to the thigh region. In the mature adult, particularly the male, they may become darkly pigmented. The secretions of these glands may matt the sparsely covered fur, increasing their prominence. Male and female hamsters also have a glandular sac in the region of the umbilicus.

In gerbils, there is a large ventral sebaceous scent gland in the region of the umbilical scar that secretes a yellow sebaceous fluid and which is more prominent in males. This area is devoid of fur and is predisposed to the development of adenocarcinoma in adults. The tail of gerbils is fully furred, but has a series of fracture planes in the middle and caudal sections allowing a degloving injury if a gerbil is grasped by the tail. The soft tissue structure never regrows, and the denuded vertebrae will die off leaving a stump. Gerbils should therefore never be restrained by the end of the tail. Gerbils also produce a number of secretions from the Harderian gland (see next section) including lipids and pigments, some of which drain through the tear ducts to the nose, are mixed with saliva and are then transferred to the fur of the coat. If the gerbil does not have dry (<50% humidity), dusty conditions (e.g. a sand bath or fine shavings) to bathe in and help remove these secretions, the coat may become dull and matted.

Eyes

In hamsters, as with mice, a significant orbital venous sinus exists and has been used as a means of blood sample collection, using a fine lithium heparin-coated capillary tube under anaesthesia. Female Syrian hamsters secrete between 100 and 1000 times more porphyrins from the Harderian gland than males (Buzzell, 1996).

Haematology

The lifespan of the gerbil erythrocyte is short, even by rodent standards, lasting only 10 days. This is why so many gerbil red cells show degenerative basophilic speckling when stained with Romanowsky stains. Gerbil blood is often lipaemic, and this has been blamed on their high-fat (sunflower seed) diet; they are often used as a cholesterol model for humans. They are resistant to atherosclerosis but not hepatic lipidosis. In addition, the blood parameters vary depending on the sex: the male gerbil has a higher packed cell volume, and white blood cell and lymphocyte count than the female. Hamster haematology is similar to that seen in mice.

GUINEA PIG, CHINCHILLA AND DEGU

Biological average values for the guinea pig, chinchilla and degu

The average normal values for guinea pigs, chinchillas and degus are given in Table 1.5.

Table 1.5 Biological parameters for the guinea pig, chinchilla and degu.

Biological parameter	Guinea pig	Chinchilla	Degu
Weight (g)	600–1200	400–550	200–300
Rectal body temperature (°C)	37.2–39.5	37.8–39.2	36–37.9
Respiration rate at rest (breaths per minute)	60–140	50–60	60–100
Heart rate at rest (beats per minute)	100–180	120–160	240–300
Gestation length (days)	59–72 (average 63)	111 (average)	90–95
Litter size	1–6 (average 3)	1–5 (average 2)	4–10 (average 6)
Birth weight (g)	45–115	30–50	10–16
Weaning age (weeks)	2–4	6–8	4–5
Age at sexual maturity (months)			
Male	2–3	6–7	3–4
Female	1.5–2	8–9	3–4
Oestrus interval (days)	16	30–50	16–26
Lifespan (years)	3–8	6–10	5–9

Musculoskeletal system

Guinea pig

Skull

The skull is rodent shaped, with an elongated nose, low forehead and widely spaced eyes. There are moderately large tympanic bullae which house the middle ear and are clearly visible on radiographs. All hystricomorphs have a flared angular process to the mandible to which the large masseter muscles attach, with a large infraorbital foramen through which the medial masseter muscle passes. The mandible is wider than the maxilla.

Axial skeleton

The vertebral structure is the same as that seen in the rat and mouse, except the number of coccygeal vertebrae (four to six) is much reduced and they are less mobile. There are 13–14 pairs of ribs depending on the number of thoracic vertebrae; the last two are more cartilaginous than mineralised and the last three to four are not attached to the rest (floating). Guinea pigs also possess vestigial clavicles. The vertebral formula for the guinea pig is

$$C7, T13/14, L6, S2/3, Ca4-6$$

The pelvis of the female is joined at the pubis and ischium by a fibrocartilaginous suture line, allowing separation of the pelvis prior to and during parturition. If the female guinea pig has not had a litter by the time she has reached 1 year of age, this suture line mineralises and prevents future separation. Female guinea pigs not mated before 1 year should therefore not be mated for the rest of their life as dystocia problems are common.

Appendicular skeleton

The forelimbs and hindlimbs are relatively long in comparison to the rat and mouse, but the same bone formulas exist. The main difference is that the guinea pig has four digits on each forelimb and only three digits on each hindlimb. Like other hystricomorph rodents, the guinea pig has an unfused tibia and fibula.

Chinchilla

Skull

The bones of the skull are more domed than the guinea pig, although still distinctly rodent-like (see Figure 1.6). The chinchilla has very large tympanic bullae, larger than the guinea pig, which are clearly visible as coiled, snail-shell-like features on radiographs. The mandible is wider than the maxilla.

Axial skeleton

The vertebral structure is similar to that in the rat and mouse. Chinchillas are fine-boned and prone to fractures. The vertebral formula is C7, T13, L6, S2, Ca20–25 with 13 pairs of ribs.

Appendicular skeleton

The hindlimbs in particular have very long femurs and tibias. The chinchilla has the usual four digits on each forelimb, but, unlike the guinea pig, has five digits on each hindlimb as well, although digits 1 and 5 are rudimentary. Chinchillas have an obvious and long tail often held erect.

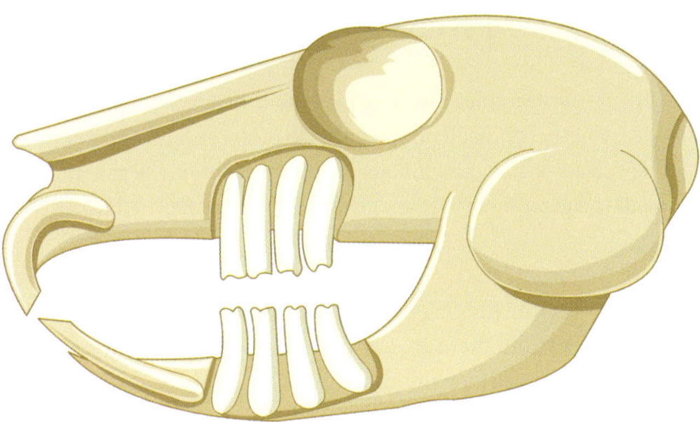

Figure 1.6 Lateral diagram of the skull of a normal chinchilla showing the relation of tooth roots to the orbit and jawbones. Note how close the roots of the third and fourth cheek teeth are to the inner aspect of the eye; hence, root elongation often causes watering of the eyes.

Degu

Skull

The bones of the skull are similar to those of the chinchilla and so more domed than the guinea pig. The tympanic bullae are more developed than guinea pigs but less developed than chinchillas. Other features (pronounced masseter muscles, flared masseter muscle attachments on the mandible) are also present. The mandible is wider than the maxilla.

Axial skeleton

The vertebral structure is similar to that seen in the chinchilla. Metabolic bone disease is relatively common, and there are reports of vertebral fractures and paresis/paralysis.

Appendicular skeleton

This is similar to the chinchilla, with elongated slender hindlimbs. The fibula and tibia are fused proximally.

Respiratory system

The lung structure of the guinea pig is similar to that seen in the rat and mouse. The left lung is divided into three lobes, and the right into four. Chinchillas follow a similar pattern. Degus have the same numbers of lobes, but in the left lung instead of a cranial/middle, caudal and accessory lobe they have a cranial, middle and caudal lobe.

Digestive system

Oral cavity

The dental formula for chinchillas, guinea pigs and degus is

I1/1C0/0Pm1/1M3/3.

In all three species, all of the teeth – incisors, premolars and molars (cheek teeth) – are elodont ('open rooted') and therefore continuously growing. This can lead to malocclusion, particularly in chinchillas and degus, if an inappropriate diet low in calcium, vitamin D_3 and fibre is fed. Degus have cheek teeth that in cross-section resemble the figure '8' (hence their scientific name *Octodon degus*). The incisors of the chinchilla are orange/yellow pigmented on their enamel surfaces, but those of the guinea pig are often white. In both cases, a diastema is present. The occlusal surface of the cheek teeth in guinea pigs is oblique as the mandible is wider than the maxilla, with the occlusal plane sloping from dorsolateral to ventromedial. In chinchillas and degus the occlusal surface of the cheek teeth is horizontal. In all species the occlusal surface of the cheek teeth has a folded, rough appearance due to alternating bands of cementum and dentin. Most texts describe rodents including guinea pigs as being monophyodont – they only develop one permanent set of teeth during their lifetime (having no deciduous teeth) (Hargaden and Singer, 2012; Lennox *et al.*, 2021). They are also often born with only the permanent incisor teeth fully erupted, the permanent cheek teeth erupting over the ensuing 1–6 weeks of life postpartum.

Hystricomorphs also have a palatal ostium creating an entrance through the soft palate, allowing communication of the oropharynx with the pharynx. It exists because the soft palate is actually connected with the base of the muscular tongue, the epiglottis achieving access to the nasopharynx through a hole (the palatal ostium) in the soft palate.

Stomach

The whole stomach of the guinea pig is covered with a glandular epithelium containing acid- and pepsinogen-secreting cells and is usually full of food material. It has a strong cardiac sphincter, making vomiting a rare and grave occurrence. The stomach of the chinchilla and degu is much the same. Stomach emptying time is around 2 hours in the guinea pig.

Small intestine

The small intestine of both species is relatively long and pink in colour, measuring anywhere up to 50–60 cm in the chinchilla and degu and more than 120 cm in the adult guinea pig.

Large intestine

The large intestine starts at the ileocaecal junction on the left side of the abdomen where the ileum enters the caecum. The caecum is a large sacculated organ, measuring 20 cm in length, and in the guinea pig it contains 60–70% of all the gut contents. It is attached to the dorsal abdomen and has a series of three smooth muscle bands running along its length known as taeniae coli. These produce the sacculations of the caecum known as haustra. In the chinchilla, the caecum is smaller, containing only 20–25% of gut contents, but it is more folded. The degu caecum has both taenia and haustra. The caecum itself forms a blind-ending sac at one end and empties into the colon near to the ileocaecal junction.

The colon is on average twice as long as the small intestine and is dark brown. In the chinchilla, the proximal section of the colon possesses taeniae and haustra, whereas in the guinea pig the whole of the colon is smooth surfaced. The degu proximal colon has taenia but no haustra. The latter half of the colon can be distinguished by the presence of faecal pellets in its lumen. The large intestine of the guinea pig has a complicated series of coils, which form a spiral of bowel on the right cranial ventral aspect of the abdomen. The chinchilla's colon is much more simply arranged, and not as long.

Hystricomorphs such as the guinea pig, chinchilla and degu all exhibit coprophagy.

Liver

The liver of the guinea pig has six lobes. There is also an obvious gall bladder, unlike the rat. The gall bladder empties through one bile duct into the small intestine. Just before it empties into the small intestine there is a small ampulla or swelling of the duct that has a sphincter proximally to prevent bile regurgitating up the bile duct towards the liver. The guinea pig liver does not possess the enzyme L-gluconolactone oxidase and therefore preformed vitamin C is required in the diet.

The chinchilla's liver has four lobes with a gall bladder present between the right and median lobes.

Pancreas

The pancreas has two limbs in the guinea pig and lies alongside the stomach and proximal duodenum. It empties via one duct into the mid-descending duodenum and performs the same functions as in other mammals.

Urinary system

Kidney

As with the hamster, the guinea pig has a relatively long renal papilla. Both kidneys in the guinea pig are surrounded by large amounts of fat, making them difficult to see at laparotomy; the chinchilla's kidneys have fewer fat deposits. The chinchilla and the degu originate from arid environments in the wild and appear to be able to produce highly concentrated urine. One study concluded that during the dry Chilean summers, wild degu urine osmolarity could be as high as 3137 ± 472 mosmol/kg, whereas urine produced during the wetter winter months was around 1123 ± 472 mosmol/kg (Bozinovic *et al.*, 2003). Chinchilla urine commonly has a specific gravity in the region of 1.045 or greater (Hrapkiewicz and Medina, 2007).

Lower urinary tract

The urine of the guinea pig is often yellow and cloudy in nature. Like all herbivore urine, it is alkaline under normal conditions and may contain calcium carbonate or calcium oxalate crystals. In the female guinea pig, the urethra empties just caudal to the vagina, but without a urinary papilla, giving the false impression of a common urogenital opening.

In the female chinchilla, cloudy alkaline urine is common. The urethra of the bladder, however, opens through a separate orifice from the vagina. The urinary papilla is a large structure in the female chinchilla and may easily be confused with the male penis.

Cardiovascular system

Heart

In all three species, the thoracic cavity appears relatively small in comparison with the abdominal cavity; therefore, the heart appears relatively large in comparison with the lung field. Chinchillas have only a left coronary artery.

Blood vessels for sampling

The jugular veins are the vessels commonly used for blood sampling in all three species. Small doses of intravenous medications may be administered through the ear veins, which are clearly visible on the non-furred ears, or via the cephalic or saphenous veins, which occupy the same positions as in other species. Cephalic veins may be accessed for blood sampling and intravenous injections but are small, requiring 25 gauge or smaller-sized needles and catheters.

Lymphatic system

Spleen

The spleen of the guinea pig is a wide structure attached to the greater curvature of the stomach on the left side of the cranial abdomen.

The spleen of the chinchilla is a smaller strap-like organ attached again to the greater curvature of the stomach on the left side.

Thymus

In guinea pigs, the thymus is prominent in the cranial thorax in the immature stage, but there are often only remnants left in the adult. A similar situation exists in the chinchilla and degu.

Lymph nodes

The guinea pig is prone to *Streptococcus zooepidemicus* infections of the cervical lymph nodes, which run in a chain along the ventral aspect of the neck. Chinchillas, guinea pigs and degus have prominent mesenteric lymphoid deposits.

Reproductive anatomy

Male

Guinea pig

The male guinea pig is often referred to as a boar. Its testes are prominent and occupy the scrotal sacs on either side of the anus. Each testis has a large fat body projecting through the open inguinal canal into the abdomen. The vas deferens opens, with the accessory sex glands (vesicular glands, coagulating glands and ventral and dorsal prostate lobes), into the proximal urethra. The vesicular glands are the most prominent, curving cranially into the abdomen for 10 cm or more. The paired bulbourethral glands lie dorsal to the urethra just before it passes into the penis, which is Z-shaped, moving cranioventrally from the caudal brim of the pelvis and then caudoventrally so to point caudally at rest. The penis is a large structure by rodent standards and possesses a glans structure distally. There is an os penis which sits dorsal to the urethra when the penis is erect and pointing cranially. Ventral to the distal urethra is the intromittent sac that contains two invaginated spurs, which, when the penis is erect, project from the end of the glans as two slender spurs 4–5 mm in length. Their function is not fully known but they may aid in locking into similar grooves in the female reproductive system. The whole penis is contained in a prepuce, which possesses sebaceous glands, and is partly formed from a fold of perineal skin.

Chinchilla

There is no true scrotum. The tail of the epididymis sits lateral to the anus, while the testis occupies an inguinal position. A fat body projects from each testis into the abdominal cavity. The vas deferens opens into the urethra caudal to the bladder neck along with the accessory sex glands. These include the ventral and dorsal paired lobes of the prostate as well as the paired, frond-like vesicular glands. The urethra then passes caudally through the pelvis, becoming ensheathed in the ischiocavernosus muscles that control the movement of the penis and pelvic floor. The bulbourethral glands lie dorsal to the urethra in this area. The urethra then passes out of the pelvis and into the penis, which is tubular and blunt-ended and points caudally when relaxed. The penis forms a Z-like flexure, similar to the guinea pig, and contains a small approximately 1-cm long os penis in its most caudal portion. The glans has small backward-pointing spines on its surface.

Male chinchillas are often prone to fur rings. This is when a band of fine fur becomes wound around the penis inside the prepuce. This may constrict and so may cause ischaemic damage to the penis.

Degu

The male degu has no scrotum as the testes are intra-abdominal to inguinal in position with a wide inguinal canal. Sexual maturity can be inferred by the presence of two cornified spikes in the inside of an invagination of the skin of the glans penis. The penis has an os penis dorsal to the distal urethra. The accessory sex glands are similar to those of the chinchilla, and include a prostate, paired seminal vesicles, and bulbourethral glands.

Female

Guinea pig

The female guinea pig is often referred to as a sow. Its uterus is bicornuate. It has two uterine horns, a short uterine body and a single cervix. The ovaries are closely associated with the respective kidneys. The periuterine tissues and cornuate ligaments are sites for the same fat deposition that is seen in the female rabbit. The vagina opens just cranial to the urethral opening. A small clitoris sits just ventral to the urethral opening, and the two are enclosed in skin folds to create a Y-shaped slit. The entrance to the vagina is sealed by epithelial tissues at all times other than at oestrus and immediately prior to parturition. A perineal sac sits between the vagina and the anus and contains a large number of sebaceous glands that produce an oily fluid.

The female guinea pig has two mammary glands in the inguinal region (the male has two vestigial glands as well).

Chinchilla

The female chinchilla has a uterus like the rabbit. There are two uterine horns but no common uterine body. Instead two separate cervices open into the vagina. The entrance to the vagina is sealed at all times except during oestrus and just prior to parturition, although a faint transverse line can be seen in this area at other times. The urethra opens through a separate, cranially located, urinary papilla.

The female chinchilla has three pairs of mammary glands, two thoracic and one inguinal.

Degu

The uterus is bicornuate, similar to the guinea pig. The entrance to the vagina is sealed with a membrane except for a few days during oestrus and immediately prior to parturition. The urethra opens through a separate, more cranial, urinary papilla.

The female degu has four pairs of mammary glands.

Reproductive physiology

Guinea pig

The female guinea pig is non-seasonally polyoestrus. The cycle lasts for around 16 days, oestrus lasting for 6–12 hours, and ovulation is spontaneous. Immediately after mating (1–2 hours), a copulatory plug may be found in the cage. It is possible that this is necessary to prevent leakage of sperm back out of the reproductive tract, but it could also prevent another male from successfully mating the female. Gestation lasts on average 63 days, although it may take up to 67 days for small litters and 59 days for large ones. The average litter contains three young. Pregnancy may be detected by gentle palpation from 3 weeks. The entrance to the vagina is closed at all times other than immediately before parturition, and for 2–3 days around oestrus. There is a postpartum heat within 10 hours of parturition at which the female may be successfully re-mated.

In the last 2 days of gestation, hormones such as relaxin and progesterone allow the pelvic ligaments to separate the pubis and ischium by up to 2 cm, allowing the passage of the relatively large young. This occurs only if the female is less than 1 year of age or has had her first litter before 1 year. Nulliparous females more than 1 year of age have a fused pelvis, and dystocias are therefore common. Many female guinea pigs will breed through to 2 years of age.

The guinea pig placenta is haemochorial – the membranes of the placenta (chorion) are in contact with the blood of the mother. This allows for large amounts of immune system exchange between mother and fetus during gestation.

Chinchilla

The chinchilla is seasonally polyoestrus. The reproductive season stretches from November to May (in the northern hemisphere) and from May to November (in the southern hemisphere), and the cycle lasts on average 40 days with oestrus being 2–3 days in duration. The entrance to the vagina opens at oestrus, which lasts for 12–24 hours, and stays patent for 3–4 days. At this stage, the perineum may darken in colour, and clear mucus may be seen from the vaginal opening. It also opens 2–3 days prior to parturition and remains open for the commonly seen postpartum oestrus. Interestingly, male chinchillas in captivity can produce viable spermatozoa throughout the year.

Chinchillas are spontaneous ovulators. A copulatory plug is frequently found the day after a successful mating. Gestation lasts on average 111 days, with typically two kits being born. Pregnancy may be diagnosed by palpation from day 60. Female chinchillas may continue to breed up to 10 years of age.

The chinchilla placenta is haemochorial.

Degu

The degu is a spontaneous ovulator and in the wild seasonally polyoestrus (during the rainy season) but in captivity will often breed all year round. The oestrus cycle varies from 16 to 26 days (averaging 21) and, like the chinchilla, the vaginal opening is covered by a membrane at all times except at oestrus for 1–3 days and just prior to parturition. Gestation is typically 90–95 days with four to six young being born in primiparous females and 6–10 young thereafter. Female degus become noticeably less fecund after 4 years of age.

The degu placenta is haemochorial.

Neonatology

Guinea pigs, chinchillas and degus are precocial – they are born fully furred, with eyes and ears open, and often start to eat small amounts of solid food from day 1. Weaning generally occurs at 6 weeks in guinea pigs, 6–8 weeks in chinchillas and 4–5 weeks in degus. Sexual maturity occurs at 2–3 months in the guinea pig, 3–4 months in degus and 6–8 months in the chinchilla.

Sexing

Guinea pig

Sexing of male and female guinea pigs is relatively simple and may be performed from the first few weeks of life. The female anogenital area is oval in nature. The anus is closest to the tail base, and cranial to this is a Y-shaped slit housing the small clitoris and the entrance to the urinary and genital tracts. In the male, the distance between the anus and urogenital system is larger, and gentle pressure on either side of the prepuce will allow protrusion of an obvious penis.

Chinchilla

The female chinchilla has a large urinary papilla making identification difficult. The identification is made on the distance between the anus and the urinary papilla. The female's urinary papilla is close to the anus, and if examined closely it may be possible to observe the transverse slit which marks the sealed (when not in heat) entrance to the reproductive tract lying between the anus and urinary papilla. The male's prepuce, which resembles the female's urinary papilla, is much larger and more cranial, and the penis may be protruded in compliant individuals. See Figures 1.7 and 1.8 for comparison of female and male chinchillas.

In chinchillas, females are larger than males – the reverse of many other rodents. Female chinchillas also have three pairs of mammary glands, two thoracic pairs and one inguinal pair.

Degu

The female degu has a large urinary papilla that makes identification difficult as it can be mistaken for a phallus in very young animals, similar to the chinchilla. Caudal to this, the genital opening is covered with a membrane except during oestrus and immediately prior to parturition. Protrusion of the phallus in compliant males is possible and allows sex identification. The sexually mature male degu has two cornified spikes in the inverted sac of the glans penis that can easily be everted. These become apparent from 2.5 months of age, with all showing evidence at 3.5 months of age. The testes are inguinally located but can be easily retracted intra-abdominally.

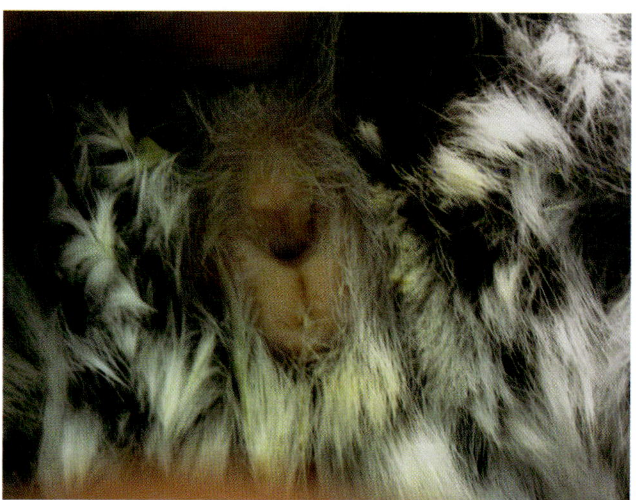

Figure 1.7 External genitalia of a female chinchilla. Note the prominent urinary papilla at the top. Immediately below is the entrance to the reproductive tract and then the anus.

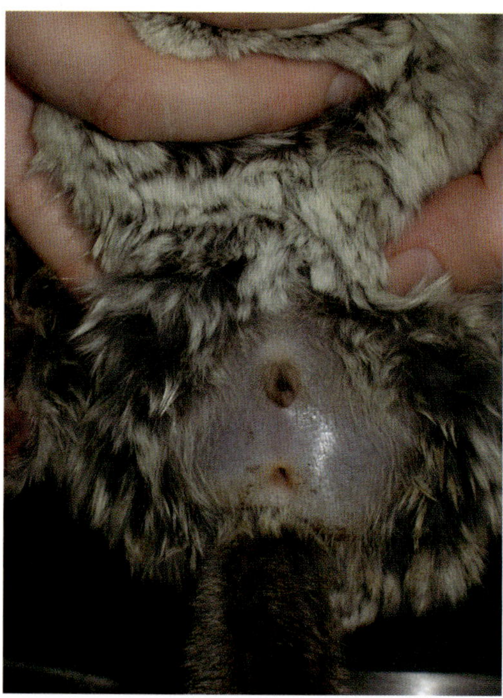

Figure 1.8 External genitalia of a male chinchilla. Note the prepuce towards the top and the greater distance from this to the anus with no evidence of an entrance between.

Skin

The fur patterns of guinea pigs differ significantly between breeds, with the Peruvian having the longest fur, Abyssinians having short fur in whorls and rosettes, Silky breeds having medium length soft fur and the English and American breeds having short smooth fur. The guinea pig has a prominent sebaceous gland on its back, cranial to the tail base which is more developed in the male. This secretes a yellow waxy material which frequently matts the fur in this area. There are additional glands emptying into the anal sacs in the folds of skin which enclose the anus and genitalia. These can produce a creamy white, strong-smelling discharge in the boar. Guinea pig fur is often relatively coarse in nature.

The fur colourations of chinchillas vary considerably. The 'wild-type' chinchilla fur colour was yellow-grey but captive breeding has selected predominantly for a blue-grey colour (Donnelly and Brown, 2004). Other colourations are now commonly seen in the pet trade including white, beige, ebony (all associated with dominant genes), sapphire and violet (associated with recessive genes). The coat of the chinchilla is renowned for its soft silky nature with a high density of hairs emerging from each pore (on average 50–60 soft wool hairs and a single longer guard hair). It responds badly to moisture, requiring dust baths for cleaning. In addition, the chinchilla may experience a feature known as 'fur slip'. This is when a section of fur drops out due to fright or stress, and the fur in this alopecic area may take several weeks to regrow. Breeding for a recessive trait of velvet, shorter fur is also common in the pet trade (Donnelly and Brown, 2004).

Significant vibrissae are present around the rostral upper lips in chinchillas, with less prominent vibrissae seen in guinea pigs, thought to be associated with the more nocturnal nature of the chinchilla.

In both chinchillas and guinea pigs, the ears are prominently furless, with the chinchilla in particular having the largest pinnae.

The guinea pig has a prominent subcutaneous fat pad over the scruff region of the neck, which makes large injections at this site painful.

The chinchilla has very small claws on each digit. In comparison, the guinea pig has prominent claws on every digit. Both have defined leathery pads at the ends of each digit and an area of thickened skin on the hindlimbs up to the hock joint with a tarsal pad to accommodate their more plantigrade stance.

Eyes

The eyes of the guinea pig are small in comparison to the size of its head. There is a prominent third eyelid tear gland which may prolapse. The chinchilla on the other hand has large prominent eyes, and a vertical slit-like pupil which allows the chinchilla to virtually close off all light reaching the retina. This reflects the more nocturnal nature of the chinchilla.

Haematology

The morphology of the red and white cells is similar to that seen in other rodents. There are predominantly more lymphocytes than neutrophils in the white cell count. In the guinea pig, an intracellular inclusion known as the Kurloff body may be seen in circulating monocytes, which are thus known as Kurloff cells. These are rare in juvenile and male guinea pigs, but common in adult females particularly during gestation, and they may play a role in the physiological immunity relationship between mother and fetus. Their origin is not clear but they are thought to come from the thymus or spleen.

CHIPMUNKS AND PRAIRIE DOGS

Biological average values for the chipmunk and prairie dog

The normal values for the basic biological parameters for the chipmunk and black-tailed prairie dog are given in Table 1.6.

Table 1.6 Biological parameters for the chipmunk and black-tailed prairie dog.

Biological parameter	Chipmunk	Black-tailed prairie dog
Weight (g)	55–150	500–2000 (males much larger than females)
Rectal body temperature (°C)	37.8–39.6 (when not hibernating)	38–39 (when not in torpor)
Respiration rate at rest (breaths per minute)	60–90	65–120
Heart rate at rest (beats per minute)	150–280 (drops to 3–6 during hibernation/torpor)	150–250
Gestation (days)	28–35	30–35 (average 34)
Litter size	2–10 (average 4)	2–10 (average 5)
Birth weight (g)	3–5	10–30
Weaning age (weeks)	5–7	5–7
Age at sexual maturity (months)		
Male	8–9	18–24
Female	9–12	18–24
Oestrus interval (days)	Average 14 (breeding season March–September in northern hemisphere)	Monoestrus (breeding season February–April in northern hemisphere)
Lifespan (years)	8–12 (may be shorter in captivity)	8–10

Musculoskeletal system

The musculoskeletal system has many similarities to the rat as outlined above.

Skull

The skull is typically rodent-like in its long and flattened form.

Axial skeleton

The spinal vertebral layout is similar to the rat.

The vertebral formula of the chipmunk is

$$C7, T12-13, L6-7, S3, Ca26-31$$

The vertebral formula of the black-tailed prairie dog is

$$C7, T12, L7, S4, Ca12-18$$

Appendicular skeleton

In the chipmunk each forelimb has four and each hindlimb five digits. The chipmunk's gait is a jumping sinuous movement, which makes them excellent climbers, with forelimbs and hindlimbs a similar length. The chipmunk body form is more elongated than that of rats or mice, and their long prehensile tail is used for balance and support. The chipmunk bone structure is lightweight and more bird-like than the heavier structure of the rat.

The prairie dog is a terrestrial rodent and has a body form that is heavier than the chipmunk family. It is however still identifiably squirrel-like in appearance. They have five digits on both fore and hind feet.

Respiratory system

In chipmunks the left lung is variably divided into two or three lobes and the right lung into four.

In the prairie dog the lungs are divided into four lobes on the right side with the left side being undivided. Their thoracic cavity is larger in relation to the abdomen than is the case in many other rodents.

Digestive system

Oral cavity

The incisors are open rooted or continuously growing, and malocclusions are not uncommon.

The dental formula for Siberian chipmunks and prairie dogs is

$$I1/1C0/0Pm1-2/1M3/3.$$

They both have a diastema. The mouth is narrow, and the tongue fleshy and fixed firmly at the base, although the rostral tip is mobile. In both species there are small cheek pouches, communicating with the diastema of the oral cavity and extending back to the ear base. These are frequently sites for abscess formation if sharp seeds, such as unhusked oats, are fed.

Stomach

The stomach is of a simple glandular design. There is a strong cardiac sphincter which normally prevents regurgitation.

Small intestine

The small intestine is relatively long in both species. The duodenum receives a duct from the gall bladder just after the pyloric sphincter and one further on from the pancreas. In prairie dogs, other smaller openings of the pancreas may enter the duodenum in the descending limb.

Large intestine

In chipmunks the initial part of the large intestine at the ileocaecal junction has a small blind-ending caecum with some sacculations, or haustra.

In prairie dogs, the large intestine starts at the ampulla coli where a swelling and valve system exists. From this area the caecum extends across the ventral abdomen and is a significant organ reflecting the species' herbivorous (largely grass-based) natural diet. The ascending large intestine has taenial bands and haustra.

Liver

The liver has four main lobes in both species and possesses a gall bladder and common bile duct which joins the descending duodenum.

Pancreas

The pancreas is found along the descending duodenum and the edge of the stomach. In chipmunks it empties through one duct which empties into the proximal descending duodenum. In prairie dogs there also appear to be numerous smaller ducts in addition to the main one and these open directly into the duodenum.

Urinary system

Kidney

The kidneys are a typical bean shape in both species. Fat deposits are often found in this area during the late summer and early autumn. Each kidney has the usual ureter passing caudally to the urinary bladder.

Bladder

Both species' urine is usually alkaline in nature and may contain calcium crystals (calcium carbonate, calcium oxalate). However, chipmunks may also produce acidic urine due to their more omnivorous nature (they eat insects, eggs, etc.).

Cardiovascular system

Heart

The heart is similar to that seen in the rat and mouse.

Blood vessels for sampling

The jugular veins make the best vessels for blood sampling in both species. The ventral or lateral tail veins may be used in chipmunks but care should be exercised and the chipmunk should be sedated as the tail skin can deglove and slough relatively easily. Similarly, the cranial vena cava may be used in both species but this procedure should only be carried out under general anaesthesia. The saphenous and cephalic veins, although small, may be used in the larger prairie dog using a 23 or 25 gauge needle or catheter.

Lymphatic system

Spleen

The spleen is a small strap-like organ on the greater curvature of the stomach to the left side of the cranial abdomen in both species.

Thymus

The thymus is a prominent organ in the juvenile, and persists in the cranial thorax of the adult. It is described as bilobed in prairie dogs.

Reproductive anatomy

Male

In chipmunks the testes sit in a caudally placed scrotum, but only during the reproductive season. During the quiescent period, the testes are retracted into the abdomen. The scrotum and testes thus enlarge during the breeding season from January to September.

In prairie dogs, there is no true scrotum, the testes sitting more inguinally. The testes enlarge during the breeding season (February–April in the northern hemisphere).

Seminal vesicles, bulbourethral (Cowper's) glands and a prostate are reported as accessory sex glands in both species.

Female

Both species have a bicornuate uterus with a single cervix.

The female chipmunk has four pairs of mammary glands, two inguinal and two thoracic. The female prairie dog has four to six pairs of mammary glands.

Reproductive physiology

The chipmunk is seasonally polyoestrus, cycling between March and September. Chipmunks are spontaneous ovulators, with an oestrus cycle length of around 14 days. There is no evidence of a postpartum oestrus, and gestation length averages 31–32 days. Mammary development becomes prominent 24–48 hours prior to parturition. Reproductive success drops dramatically after 6–7 years of age in the female chipmunk.

The prairie dog is seasonally monoestrus, breeding once in the period February–April (in the northern hemisphere). Females will generally only breed in captivity in a colony situation as their social structure and behaviour is complex. The gestation length is around 30–35 days with an average of five young being born.

Neonatology

Chipmunk young are altricial and so are born blind, deaf and hairless. Fur starts to appear around 7–10 days of age, and the eyes open at 4 weeks. The age at weaning is 5–7 weeks. Sexual maturity is reached at 8 months in the male and 10 months in the female.

Prairie dog young are similarly altricial. Eyes open around 33–37 days of age. Weaning in the wild is typically around 7 weeks. Sexual maturity varies from 18 months to 2 years of age, but most prairie dogs are still growing up until 15 months of age or so.

Sexing

The male chipmunk has a clearly visible penis which points caudally. During the breeding season, the scrotum is noticeably enlarged. The female has a urogenital papilla, but the distance from anus to papilla is less than the distance from anus to prepuce in the male.

The male prairie dog also has testes that enlarge with the breeding season and are more inguinally located (there is no true scrotum). The female has a small urinary papilla which is closer to the anus than the prepuce is in the male, similar to other rodents.

Skin

Chipmunks have soft fur covering the whole of their bodies. Sebaceous glands exist around the anus in both sexes. They have five digits on their forepaws and four on the hind, which possess small pads and claws. The ears are small and furred.

Prairie dogs fur is short and soft. They have trigonal anal sacs that empty just inside the anal sphincter via three small papillae which may be everted for scent marking and in times of stress.

AFRICAN PYGMY HEDGEHOG

Biological average values for African pygmy hedgehogs

African pygmy hedgehogs are found from the southern Sahara through Central and East Africa. Their biological parameters can be found in Table 1.7.

Table 1.7 Biological parameters for African pygmy hedgehogs.

Biological parameter	African pygmy hedgehog
Weight (g)	250–700
Rectal body temperature (°C)	35.4–37
Respiration rate at rest (breaths per minute)	25–50
Heart rate at rest (beats per minute)	180–280
Gestation (days)	34–37 (average 35)
Litter size	1–9 (average 6)
Birth weight (g)	10–18
Weaning age (weeks)	4–6
Age at sexual maturity (months)	
Male	2–6
Female	2–6 (can be sexually mature at 2 months but not recommended to breed before 6 months)
Oestrus interval (days)	13–17
Lifespan (years)	4–6

Musculoskeletal system

The muscles that allow the hedgehog to roll into a ball while erecting its spines are perhaps some of its most unusual musculoskeletal adaptations. Panniculus muscles help erect the spines, while an orbicularis muscle that runs around the edge of the area containing spines helps the hedgehog to roll into a ball. Additional muscles over the skull (frontodorsalis) and dorsal rump (caudodorsalis) help to pull the spine-covered skin over the skull and rump, respectively.

Skull

The skull is narrow and elongated. There are strong jaw muscles as African pygmy hedgehogs, although predominantly insectivorous, are more typically omnivorous in nature. There is a significant vomeronasal organ in the hard palate.

Axial skeleton

Hedgehogs of all species can roll themselves into a ball when threatened. This behaviour is facilitated by a spinal column that can undergo hyperflexion and by an orbicularis muscle running around the ventral edge of the skin that contains the spines and which when contracted acts like a drawstring and pulls the head and rear together and ensures the hedgehog forms a tight ball; simultaneous contraction of the panniculus muscle erects the skin spines. The animal can remain rolled into a tight ball for many hours without much difficulty or effort. African pygmy hedgehogs have no tail.

Appendicular skeleton

The radius and ulna are fused distally. There are five toes on the forelimbs. The tibia and fibula are fused distally. There are, unusually for hedgehogs, only four toes on the hindlimbs. The stance of the hedgehog is plantigrade.

Respiratory system

The left lung is undivided and the right lung is divided into a cranial, middle, caudal and accessory lobe.

Digestive system

Oral cavity

The permanent dental formula is

I3/2C1/1Pm3/2M3/3

Incisors are used to grasp insects and so are pointed in nature. Premolars and molars have a flattened occlusal surface for crushing food items. African pygmy hedgehogs do have deciduous teeth (diphyodont) that appear around 3 weeks of life with the adult dentition appearing around 7–9 weeks of age.

Stomach

The stomach is simple in form and has separate hydrochloric acid- and pepsinogen-secreting cells. African pygmy hedgehogs can vomit.

Small intestine

The small intestine is divided into the usual duodenum, jejunum and ileum, although the latter two segments are difficult to distinguish from each other. The duodenum is larger in diameter and has a descending and ascending portion with a limb of the pancreas between the two. Total gut transit times are relatively short, around 12–16 hours (Ivey and Carpenter, 2012).

Large intestine

There is no caecum and the large intestine has no taenia or haustra, being smooth in nature. There are anal glands although they are not well developed.

Pancreas

The main limb of the pancreas is the descending limb along the descending duodenum. The structure of the pancreas is similar to that of other mammals.

Liver

There are six lobes to the liver and a gall bladder is present.

Urinary system

The kidneys resemble rodent kidneys and are bean-shaped. The right kidney is cranial to the left and sits in close proximity to the liver. A ureter connects each kidney to the urinary bladder which empties through the urethra. A combined urogenital opening is present in the female. The male urethra empties through the phallus which is housed in the prepuce located on the ventral body wall caudal to the umbilicus.

Cardiovascular system

Heart

The heart is similar to that of rodents such as the domestic rat.

Blood vessels for sampling

Blood vessels that may be used for sampling include the jugular veins (only under anaesthesia but larger volumes may be collected than other vessels), cephalic, lateral saphenous and femoral (again under anaesthesia).

Reproductive anatomy

Male

The prepuce is located on the ventral abdominal wall caudal to the umbilicus. The testes are usually located intra-abdominally, although in hot weather they may descend into an inguinal para-anal location and may be palpated in sexually mature males. There is no true scrotum. The phallus has a significant glans with two laterally located horns.

Male hedgehogs have a number of accessory sexual glands including a bilobed prostate, paired seminal/vesicular vesicles and bulbourethral glands.

Female

The female has a bicornuate uterus with a single cervix. The uterine and ovarian suspensory ligaments are typical fat deposition sites. Female African pygmy hedgehogs have three pairs of mammary glands.

Reproductive physiology

Female pygmy hedgehogs can start to breed from 2 months of age but generally the recommendation is to not let them breed before they reach 6 months of age. Female pygmy hedgehogs are spontaneous ovulators, although there is some evidence that they may be induced based on ovulation occurring after injection with human chorionic gonadotropins (Bedford *et al.*, 2000). If allowed they can breed twice per year. They are sexually active, once sexually mature, the whole year round. Once mated a female will rarely allow further mating and a copulatory plug similar to rodents will be formed.

Neonatology

Young hedgehogs are often called piglets or hoglets. They have closed eyes and ears until around 2–3 weeks of age and so are completely altricial in nature. When born the spines are underneath the skin surface but then erupt within hours of birth. These initial spines (also called 'nest spines') are shed after around a month of age. Weaning typically takes 4–6 weeks.

Sexing

Male African pygmy hedgehogs have a prepuce located on the ventral body wall, whereas the common urogenital opening of the female is close to the anus. Therefore an assessment of the distance between anus and urinary opening can be used to determine the sex.

Skin

When hedgehogs are born they have so-called nest spines that lie underneath the skin and push through a few hours after being born (Banks *et al.*, 2010). Nest spines are moulted at around 1 month old and are then replaced with permanent spines that are subsequently replaced one at a time from 18 months of age onwards. The permanent spines are made from keratin (as is hair/fur) and are hollow and have a narrowing in their diameter at skin surface level which means a spine is more likely to break off when pulled, rather than the whole spine including the root being pulled out. Adult hedgehog spines are replaced every 18–24 months or so and are erected by contraction of the panniculus muscle.

In the areas of the skin containing spines (dorsal head and body) there are no sebaceous glands. There are plentiful sweat and sebaceous glands in the ventrum of the feet and the skin without spines. Underneath the skin covered by spines sits a fat layer and although the epidermis is thin, the dermis has significant amounts of collagen fibres.

Haematology

Hedgehogs have similar cell lines as other mammals. The predominant white blood cell is the neutrophil (Okorie-Kanu *et al.*, 2015).

PET MARSUPIALS

Biological average values for some pet marsupials

Table 1.8 gives the basic normal biological values for sugar gliders (*Petaurus breviceps*) and Virginia opossums (*Didelphis virginiana*), two of the more commonly kept marsupial pets.

Sugar gliders may enter a stage of torpor when faced with starvation in an attempt to lower energy demands. Virginia opossums may sham death when attacked (the derivation of 'playing possum').

Table 1.8 Biological parameters for the sugar glider and Virginia opossum.

Biological parameter	Sugar glider	Virginia opossum
Weight (g)		
Male	115–160	4000–5000
Female	95–135	2000–2500
Cloacal body temperature (°C)	34–35	32.2–35
Respiratory rate at rest (breaths per minute)	16–40	25–40
Heart rate at rest (beats per minute)	200–300	70–100
Gestation length (days)	16	12–13
Litter size	1–2	8–20 embryonic young (average 13)
Birth weight (g)	0.2	0.13
Weaning age (weeks)	15–17	12–16
Age at sexual maturity (months)		
Male	12–14	6–8
Female	8–12	6–8
Oestrus cycle length (days)	29	28
Oestrus length (days)	1–2	1–2
Lifespan (years)	12–14	3–5

Musculoskeletal system

The sugar glider has five digits on front and rear limbs, but the second and third digits of the rear limbs are part fused together into a grooming comb. The first digit of the hindlimb is opposable.

The Virginia opossum has five digits, including opposable thumbs on both front and rear limbs. The majority of marsupials have no claw on the first digit of the hindlimbs.

Most marsupials have extra pubic bones that project cranially from the floor of the pelvis and are thought to help to support the pouch in females and abdominal muscles in both sexes. They are, however, absent in sugar gliders.

Both the sugar glider and the Virginia opossum have prehensile tails.

Respiratory system

The respiratory tract is similar to that of eutherian mammals. Respiratory rates for the sugar glider are around 16–40 breaths per minute and for the Virginia opossum around 25–40 breaths per minute.

Digestive system

The sugar glider's dental formula is

$$I3/1C1/0Pm3/4M4/4.$$

The incisors are specialised to gouge the bark of acacia trees to release their sap.

The Virginia opossum's dental formula is

$$I5/4C1/1Pm3/3M4/4.$$

The sugar glider has an enlarged caecum which may help to digest its natural diet of acacia gum. Otherwise the digestive system of omnivorous marsupials is similar to that of many omnivorous rodents with the exception that marsupials have a cloaca, similar to that in a bird or reptile as a common opening for the urinary, reproductive and digestive systems. Most male marsupials have anal glands just inside the cloaca (females have pouch glands), but the Virginia opossum has cloacal glands in the female as well. In the Virginia opossum, the secretions of this gland are green.

Urinary system

The urinary tract is similar to that of eutherian mammals, except the ureters pass between the lateral and medial vaginal canals.

Cardiovascular system

Heart

As marsupials have a heart rate around half that of a comparatively sized eutherian mammal, their heart is around 30% heavier than a comparatively sized eutherian mammal's heart.

Blood vessels for sampling

In the sugar glider, the cephalic, lateral saphenous, femoral, and ventral or lateral tail veins may be used to collect blood samples. The cranial vena cava has also been used as has the medial tibial artery. All blood sampling is best performed under general anaesthesia.

In the Virginia opossum, the cephalic, jugular, saphenous, and ventral or lateral tail veins may be used to collect blood samples. In addition, the female has pouch veins. Blood sampling is best performed under general anaesthesia.

Endocrine system

Most marsupials are unable to thermoregulate when born. This ability develops around halfway through their time in the pouch and coincides with the development of the thyroid gland.

The adrenal glands of the female marsupial are around twice the size of the male's in milligrams per kilogram body weight. This difference increases during lactation due to development of the cortex of the adrenal gland (the 'X' zone), which is due to the production of a testosterone-like hormone.

Reproductive anatomy

Male

The reproductive system of the male is much more similar to that of eutherian mammals than is that of the female. The main differences in the male are external rather than internal and comprise a bifurcate (bifid) penis which is posterior to the scrotum inside the cloaca. When flaccid, the penis is held in an S-shaped curve withdrawn into the body and lies on the ventral cloacal floor. The scrotum is obvious and pendulous.

The testes have epididymides, and the vas deferens when it leaves the scrotum enters the body and joins the large disseminated prostatic gland and one or more pairs of bulbourethral glands (Cowper's glands). The duct of the bulbourethral gland enters the urethra on the ventral surface. Marsupial males lack seminal vesicles and coagulating glands.

Female

Female marsupials have a double reproductive system. Each side comprises, from cranial to caudal, an ovary, an oviduct and a uterine body. The caudal half of the reproductive tract is composed of paired lateral and one median vaginal canals. All marsupials give birth through the central (median) vaginal canal. In some species, for example the brushtail possum, there is a septum that blocks the median canal and that is breached during birth, and which subsequently re-forms; in others, for example the grey kangaroo, this median canal remains open permanently. Caudal to the three vaginal canals is the urogenital sinus that also contains the urethral opening on its ventral floor. This then empties into the cloaca.

The female sugar glider has a well-developed pouch during the breeding season and has an average of four nipples inside, although some may only have two.

The female Virginia opossum has a well-developed cranial opening pouch in which 13 nipples are arranged in an open circle with one in the centre, although there may be some variation in this layout between individuals.

Reproductive physiology

Female sugar gliders are polyoestrus with a cycle averaging around 29 days. Females may produce two litters a year. In captivity there appears to be no specific breeding season. Gestation is on average 16 days.

Female Virginia opossums are polyoestrus with a cycle of around 28 days and are in full oestrus for 1–2 days. Generally the breeding season starts in December to January in the northern hemisphere with a second peak of breeding in the early spring, with an average of 110 days separating the two litters. Gestation is on average 12–13 days.

Females tend to have a postpartum oestrus during which breeding and fertilisation can occur, although if there are joeys in the pouch then development and implantation of the fertilised egg is halted until the young have been weaned or die. This is known as fetal diapause (similar to delayed implantation in some mammals, although the placenta of marsupials never actually implants during fetal development).

Neonatology

Marsupial milk changes in consistency during the period of development of the young. However, maternal immunoglobulins are absorbed across the neonate's gut right up until weaning. This makes up for the lack of placental transfer of immunity.

In all neonates, a strong shoulder girdle of cartilage (metacoracoid) exists at birth to aid their struggle to the pouch. This regresses once the journey is made and becomes the coracoid process of the scapula. The teat once in the neonate's mouth swells up, and the neonate becomes firmly attached.

The sugar glider in the wild lives in nests containing up to seven males and females and their young as an extended family. The young weigh around 0.19 g at birth and usually two are born. They first detach from the nipple at around day 40 or life and first leave the pouch around day 70. They are reported to become weaned from day 111.

The Virginia opossum's young are very underdeveloped but have impressive claws which they use to climb from the mother's birth canal to the pouch. They are only 10 mm long when born and weigh on average 0.13 g. Generally around 13 young are born but as many as 56 have been reported! As there are only around 13 mammary glands, more than 13 rarely survive. The young release their grip on the mammary glands around 50 days of age and will leave the pouch for short periods from day 70 onwards. They are completely weaned and independent of the mother around 3–4 months of age with sexual maturity occurring around 6–8 months.

Sexing

The female sugar glider has a well-developed cranial opening pouch with usually four mammary glands. The male has an obvious pendulous scrotum cranial to the cloaca that contains the phallus. The phallus is bifid.

The female Virginia opossum has an obvious pouch with around 13 mammary glands within. The male has a pendulous scrotum cranial to the cloaca containing the bifid phallus.

Skin

One of the most striking features of the sugar glider is the patagium, which stretches from the fifth digit of the forelimb to the tarsus of the ipsilateral hindlimb. The sugar glider has multiple scent glands on the head (often creating a bald patch in males), the chest and in the paracloacal area. Smaller scent glands are found around the corners of the mouth, on the paws and the inside of the ears. The female has scent glands inside her pouch which is located ventrally over the cranial abdomen and cranially facing. The fur is soft with no guard hairs and the tail is well furred.

In the Virginia opossum, the fur consists of a soft underfur with white-tipped guard hairs that are unique to the family Didelphidae. The first tenth of the tail is covered with fur and the rest is naked skin. The male has a sternal scent gland that mats the fur overlying it in the sexually mature animal.

Haematology

Red and white cell morphologies are similar to those of eutherian mammals. The predominant white cell is the lymphocyte.

FERRET

Biological average values for the domestic ferret

Table 1.9 gives the basic normal biological values for the domestic ferret.

Musculoskeletal system

Skull

The skull is rodent-like, in that it is pointed and flattened dorsoventrally. The eyes are forward-facing, giving binocular vision for prey detection. The mandible is narrower than the maxilla and the articular surface of the maxilla into which the mandible fits has an extra process to it to prevent jaw/mandibular dislocation.

Axial skeleton

The vertebral formula for the ferret is similar to that of most mammals and comprises the usual seven cervical vertebrae, with the extended 15 thoracic (occasionally 14), five to seven lumbar, three sacral and, on average, 18 coccygeal vertebrae, thus

$$C7, T14-15, L5-7, S3, Ca18$$

Appendicular skeleton

The form is basically similar to that seen in the cat. The forelimbs and hindlimbs each have five digits.

Respiratory system

The trachea is supported by C-shaped cartilages. Ferret lungs are split into two lobes on the left side and four on the right. The entrance to the thoracic cavity is very small and is bounded by the first ribs.

Table 1.9 Biological parameters for the domestic ferret.

Biological parameter	Domestic ferret
Weight (kg)	
Male	1–2
Female	0.5–1
Rectal body temperature (°C)	37.8–40
Respiration rate at rest (breaths per minute)	40–80
Heart rate at rest (beats per minute)	180–250
Gestation length (days)	41–42
Litter size	2–14 (average 8)
Birth weight (g)	6–12
Weaning age (weeks)	6
Age at sexual maturity (months)	
Male	4–6
Female	4–8 (spring following birth)
Lifespan (years)	5–10

Digestive system

Oral cavity

The ferret has a set of deciduous teeth, which appear at 3–4 weeks of age. These are replaced by permanent teeth at 7–11 weeks of age. The dental formula for the adult is

$$I3/3C1/1Pm3/3M1/2.$$

The deciduous formula for the ferret is

$$I3-4/3C1/1Pm3/3.$$

The most prominent teeth are the canines, which are responsible for holding onto the prey. The molars and premolars are shearing teeth. The tongue is fleshy and mobile.

Stomach

The stomach is of simple form, lined with glandular epithelium containing both acid- and pepsinogen-secreting cells. It has a weak cardiac sphincter, allowing easy vomition, and a pronounced pyloric sphincter. The stomach can dilate markedly when full.

Small intestine

The descending duodenum begins at the pylorus of the stomach and passes across to the right side of the abdomen. It is entered into, after the first 5 cm or so, by the common bile and pancreatic duct.

The jejunum and ileum are almost impossible to tell apart being of similar diameter and structure grossly.

Large intestine

The large intestine is not easily differentiated from the small intestine since it is the same width and colour, although the mesenteric lymph node marks the junction between the two. There is no caecum in the ferret. The terminal portion of the rectum has two anal glands attached which, when emptied, can give off the very unpleasant odour associated with a frightened ferret. The removal of these glands is considered an unnecessary mutilation by the Royal College of Veterinary Surgeons in the UK and so should not be done unless there is a medical reason to do so.

Liver

The liver is relatively large in relation to body size and is divided into six lobes. The right lobe has the usual renal fossa to accommodate the right kidney. A gall bladder is present and empties via a common duct with the pancreas.

Pancreas

The pancreas is a prominent organ with two main lobes, one along the descending duodenum and the other along the pyloric axis. A single duct merges with the bile duct to provide a common entrance to the duodenum.

Urinary system

Kidney

The kidneys are the traditional kidney-bean shape. The right kidney sits more cranially, in a fossa in the right lobe of the liver. The left kidney is more caudal and freely suspended.

Bladder

The bladder is similar to that seen in cats or dogs. The urethra passes through the penis in the male ferret, which contains a J-shaped os penis. This makes urinary catheterisation of the male difficult.

Ferret urine is naturally acidic in nature due to its carnivorous diet.

Cardiovascular system

Heart

The heart occupies rib spaces 6–8. Its tip is connected to the sternum by a ligament which frequently contains fat, making the heart appear elevated off the sternal floor on radiographs.

Blood vessels including those for sampling

Blood vessels for sampling include the jugular, cephalic and lateral saphenous veins. These are found in similar places as for the cat, although sampling in the conscious animal is rarely possible. A technique of sampling the cranial vena cava has also been described. The ferret is anaesthetised and placed in dorsal recumbency. A 1.25-inch, 23 gauge needle is inserted through the thoracic inlet on the left side at a 45° angle on a line towards the right hind leg. As the needle is slowly advanced, negative pressure is applied to the plunger allowing blood to flow when the vessel is entered.

The ferret also has an unusual series of arteries not used for routine blood sampling that branch from the main aortic trunk. In cats and dogs, two separate carotid arteries arise from the aortic trunk. In the ferret, a single vessel (the brachiocephalic or innominate artery 1) leaves the aortic arch. This then divides into the left and right carotid arteries, as well as into the right subclavian artery at the thoracic inlet. This prevents restriction of blood flow to the head which could occur due to the narrow chest inlet.

Lymphatic system

Spleen

The spleen varies greatly in size between individuals and is attached to the greater curvature of the stomach on the left side. Its ventral tip may extend across the floor of the abdomen and back up to meet the right kidney.

Thymus

The thymus is a prominent organ in the cranial thorax of the young ferret. It dwindles to a few islands of tissue in the adult.

Lymph nodes

The lymph nodes of the ferret are comparable to those of the cat, but they are greater in their individual size in relation to the ferret's overall body size. The most notable lymph node is the mesenteric node, which can be used to differentiate between small and large intestine.

Reproductive anatomy

Male

The male ferret is known as a hob. The testes are situated in a perineally located scrotum and enlarge in the breeding season (March to September). There is no movement of the testes from scrotal sac to abdomen.

The prostate lies at the neck of the bladder and opens into the lumen of the urethra. The urethra passes caudally through the pelvis before bending ventrally and cranially to exit at the ventrally located prepuce. The os penis is J-shaped.

Female

The female ferret is known as a jill. The ovaries are found close to the caudal poles of the respective kidneys. The uterus is bicornuate and similar to that seen in the cat, with two long uterine horns and a short uterine body. There is a single cervix opening into the vagina. The urethra opens into the floor of the vagina, so there is a common urogenital opening at the vulva, cranial to the anus.

Reproductive physiology

The female ferret is seasonally polyoestrus and an induced ovulator. Ovulation occurs 1–2 days after mating. The breeding season runs from March to September. Oestrus is demonstrated by the obviously swollen vulva, which returns to normal 2–3 weeks after a successful mating.

Gestation lasts on average 42 days. The placenta is zonary, similar to that seen in cats and dogs.

The most important point about the female ferret's reproductive cycle is that if she is not mated, or brought out of heat in some way, the persistent exposure to oestrogen can cause a fatal bone marrow suppression in one season. Female ferrets should therefore be mated by entire or vasectomised males, or treated with progesterone hormone therapy or gonadotropin-releasing hormone (GnRH) agonists to suppress oestrus.

The male ferret starts his breeding season in late January in the northern hemisphere. Testes increase in size during the breeding season and regress in size from September into winter.

Overall body weight of both sexes may decrease during the breeding season and increase during the non-breeding season.

Neonatology

The young ferret is known as a kit. They are born altricial, blind, furless and deaf. The average litter size is eight kits. The fur starts to appear around the second day after birth and is pronounced by 2 weeks. The eyes open around 3 weeks and the ears around 10 days. The kit is born with a prominent fat pad on the dorsum of the neck, providing some energy reserves during the early stages of life. The female ferret is sexually mature at 4–8 months of age and the male at 4–6 months, usually in the spring following birth.

Sexing

The male ferret has an obvious prepuce on the ventral abdomen similar to that seen in the domestic dog (see Figure 1.9). In addition, the male has a caudally located scrotum with obvious testes. The female has a vulval orifice just ventral to the anus.

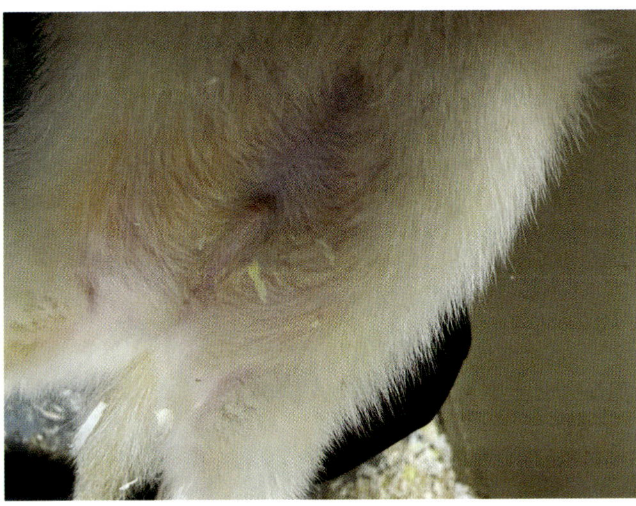

Figure 1.9 The male ferret (hob) has a prepuce located on the ventral abdomen.

Skin

The claws are not retractable. The odour of a ferret originates primarily from the normal sebaceous glands present within the skin, giving it the characteristic musky smell. These glands are particularly well concentrated around the mouth, chin and perineum. The odour of the male ferret is particularly strong due to the action of testosterone on these glands and the tendency to spray and empty the anal glands to mark territory. Neutering reduces this latter problem.

Haematology

One noticeable aspect of the ferret blood count is the consistently high packed cell volume, often in the 48–63% range in healthy adults. The white cell count on the other hand tends routinely to be lower than that seen in cats and dogs. The neutrophil is generally the predominant white cell seen.

References

Banks, R.E., Sharp, J.M., Doss, S.D. and Vanderford, D.A. (2010) Chapter 13 Hedgehogs. In: *Exotic Small Mammal Care and Husbandry*, pp. 143–155. Wiley-Blackwell, Ames.

Bedford, J.M., Mock, O.B., Nagdas, S.K. *et al.* (2000) Reproductive characteristics of the African pygmy hedgehog, *Atelerix albiventris*. *Journal of Reproduction and Fertility*, **120**, 143–150.

Bozinovic, F., Gallardo, P.A., Visser, G.H. and Cortes, A. (2003) Seasonal acclimatization in water flux rate, urine osmolality and kidney water channels in free-living degus: molecular mechanisms, physiological processes and ecological implications. *Journal of Experimental Biology*, **206**, 2959–2966.

Buzzell, G.R. (1996) Sexual dimorphism in the Harderian gland of the Syrian hamster is controlled and maintained by hormones, despite seasonal fluctuations in hormone levels: functional implications. *Microscopy Research and Technique*, **34**, 133–138.

Cruise, L.J. and Brewer, N.R. (1994) Anatomy. In: *The Biology of the Laboratory Rabbit* (eds P.J. Manning, D.H. Ringler & C.E. Newcomer), 2nd edn, pp. 47–61. Academic Press, San Diego.

Donnelly, T.M. and Brown, C.J. (2004) Guinea pig and chinchilla care and husbandry. *Veterinary Clinics of North America: Exotic Animal Practice*, **7**, 351–373.

Fraser, M.A. and Girling, S.J. (2009) *Rabbit Medicine and Surgery for Veterinary Nurses*. Wiley-Blackwell, Oxford.

Gillett, C.S. (1994) Appendix: Selected drug dosages and clinical reference data. In: *The Biology of the Laboratory Rabbit* (eds P.J. Manning, D.H. Ringler & C.E. Newcomer), 2nd edn, pp. 467–472. Academic Press, San Diego.

Griffiths, M. and Davies, D. (1963) The role of the soft pellets in the production of lactic acid in the rabbit stomach. *Journal of Nutrition*, **80**, 171–180.

Hargaden, M. and Singer, L. (2012) Part III Guinea pigs, Chapter 20 Anatomy, physiology and behavior. In: *The Laboratory Rabbit, Guinea Pig, Hamster and Other Rodents* (eds M.A. Suckow, K.A. Stevens & R.P. Wilson), pp. 575–602. Elsevier, London.

Hrapkiewicz, K. and Medina, L. (2007) Chinchillas. In: *Clinical Laboratory Animal Medicine*, pp. 180–197. Blackwell Publishing, Ames.

Hudson, R. and Distel, H. (1983) Nipple location by newborn rabbits: behavioural evidence for pheromonal guidance. *Behaviour*, **85**, 260–275.

Ichii, O., Yabuki, A., Ojima, T. *et al.* (2006) Species specific differences in the ratio of short to long loop nephrons in the kidneys of laboratory rodents. *Experimental Animals*, **55**, 473–476.

Ivey, E. and Carpenter, J.W. (2012) African hedgehogs. In: *Ferrets, Rabbits, and Rodents: Clinical Medicine and Surgery* (eds K.E. Quesenberry & J.W. Carpenter), 3rd edn, pp. 411–428. Saunders-Elsevier, St. Louis.

Lebas, F. (1989) Nutrient requirements of various categories of rabbits. *Proceedings of the First International Feed Production Conference, Piacenza*, p. 297. Facolta de Agraria, Piacenza.

Lennox, A., Capello, V. and Legendre, L.F. (2021) Small mammal dentistry. In: *Ferrets Rabbits and Rodents: Clinical Medicine and Surgery* (eds K.E. Quesenberry, C.J. Orcutt, C. Mans & J.W. Carpenter), 4th edn, pp. 514–535. Elsevier, St Louis, Missouri.

Moffat, D.B. and Fourman, J. (1964) Ectopic glomeruli in the human and animal kidney. *Anatomical Record*, **149**, 1–12.

Morrissey, P.J., Murphy, K.R., Daley, J.M. *et al.* (2017) A novel method of standardized myocardial infarction in aged rabbits. *American Journal of Physiology. Heart and Circulatory Physiology*, **312**(5), H959–H967. doi: 10.1152/ajpheart.00582.2016.

Okorie-Kanu, C.O., Onoja, R.I., Achegbulu, E.E. and Okorie-Kanu, O.J. (2015) Normal haematological and serum biochemistry values of African hedgehog. *Journal of Comparative Pathology*, **24**, 127–132. doi: 10.1007/s00580-013-1870-x.

Wagner, F., Beinecke, A., Fehr, M. *et al.* (2005) Recurrent bilateral exophthalmos associated with metastatic thymic carcinoma in a pet rabbit. *Journal of Small Animal Practice*, **46**(8), 393–397.

Williams, W.M. (1974) *The Anatomy of the Mongolian Gerbil (Meriones unguiculatus)*. Tumblebrook Farm, Inc, West Brookfield, MA.

Chapter 2 Small Mammal Housing, Husbandry and Rearing

DOMESTIC RABBIT

Breeds

There are many different breeds of rabbit, varying from the miniature breeds such as the Netherland dwarf, weighing 0.5–0.75 kg, to the New Zealand whites and the Belgian hares at 8–10 kg. Other commonly seen breeds include the lop-eared crosses, the angora breeds, the Rex and the traditional Dutch rabbits.

Cage requirements

Size and construction

The traditional hutch is a common feature of rabbit husbandry but can have many problems (see Figure 2.1). The provision of a wooden enclosure that is sufficiently large to provide sleeping quarters, a feeding area and a toilet area is common. In general, a rough guide to a minimum width of a rabbit hutch is three times the length of the rabbit to be housed when it is stretched out at rest. The depth should be one rabbit length, and the height equal to that of the rabbit standing on hind legs. Anything smaller and the rabbit must be provided with an outside run, or allowed out of the hutch for regular exercise periods every day. Indeed current recommendations suggest that all rabbits should have an exercise area, fully protected from predator attack, to ensure adequate environmental enrichment and exercise. The Rabbit Welfare Association and Fund recommends minimum cage dimensions of 3 × 2 × 1 m (width × depth × height). Cooping up a rabbit in an excessively small hutch is cruel; it will also lead to muscular and skeletal atrophy and increase the risk of spontaneous spine and limb fractures when the rabbit overexerts itself. However, many commercially available hutches are in fact too small for the adult rabbit.

Wooden hutches are the standard and are satisfactory in many cases. Their disadvantage is that they will tend to rot with the absorption of urine and rain unless properly protected. Care should be taken with wood preservatives to ensure an animal-friendly preservative is chosen. The roof may be further protected with the felt material used to roof garden sheds and should slope to the rear of the hutch to avoid rain dripping into the front, or pooling on the roof. The hutches should also be raised off the floor on legs to avoid the bottom rotting from the damp ground surface. A ramp should therefore be supplied if the rabbits are to be allowed in and out of the hutch of their own accord. Wooden hutches are also much more easily destroyed by gnawing.

In commercial fur- and meat-producing situations, rabbits are kept in wire mesh hutches suspended above a solid floor. The wire mesh 'hutch' has one major advantage in that it prevents soiling of the fur by urine and faeces. However, it can cause abrasions of the hocks in older overweight rabbits and is not advised for housing pet rabbits.

Substrates

Substrates used for cage floor covering include straw, hay, shavings and newspaper. Many rabbits will preferentially select hay and straw for bedding over shavings and paper. One of the advantages of the former is that they allow urine to drop through the fibre framework and away from the rabbit, so reducing the likelihood of urine scalding in older and arthritic rabbits.

Positioning

Care should be taken to avoid overheating of the hutch, as rabbits cannot sweat and temperatures above 26–28°C will rapidly cause hyperthermia and death. Hutches should therefore be positioned out of direct sunlight, particularly in the summer months. An ideal environmental temperature range would typically be 16–21°C. Rabbits will shiver when cold, although they can tolerate cold better than heat. Care should still be taken to ensure that the hutch is not overly draughty or exposed during the winter months. Bringing it into a shed or garage is often advisable in the worst weather (but see discussion on vitamin D issues in the section on outdoor runs).

Food and water bowls

Feeding bowls should be ceramic or metal. The former are preferable, as they are heavier and harder to knock over. Plastic feed bowls should be avoided as they are easily chewed.

Historically, water feeders with ball valve drip dispensers were commonly recommended as they allow less contamination of the water with food, urine and faeces than an open bowl. Care should be taken with these feeders, though, as some rabbits reared with water bowls will not drink from them. In addition, the ball valve often leaks and this will lead to excessively damp substrate and mould growth. Drip feeders will also suffer from bacterial build-up and need careful cleaning once or twice a week, or even daily if a large number of rabbits are housed. Finally, one study has found that rabbits drink up to 40% more from open water bowls than from sip feeders, suggesting that open water bowls may be preferable for preventing chronic dehydration (Tschudin *et al.*, 2011). The same study also indicated that diets with only dry feed led to an overall lower water intake, indicating that rabbits did not completely compensate for the lack of water when compared with diets containing some fresh vegetables. The

Veterinary Nursing of Exotic Pets and Wildlife, Third Edition. Simon J. Girling.

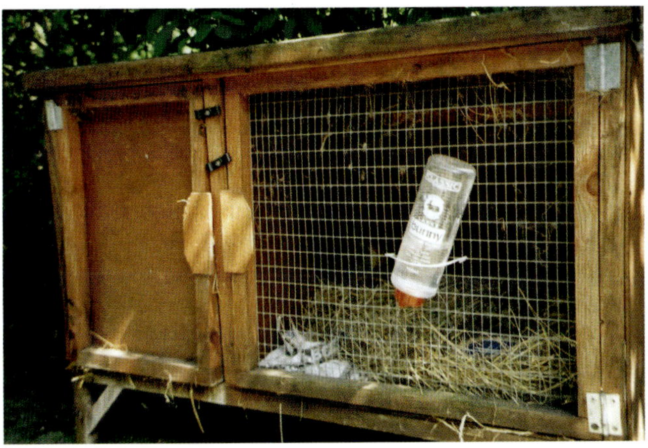

Figure 2.1 Traditional wooden rabbit hutch. Care should be taken to ensure that access is given to a run to ensure adequate exercise, enrichment and daylight exposure (the bigger the better).

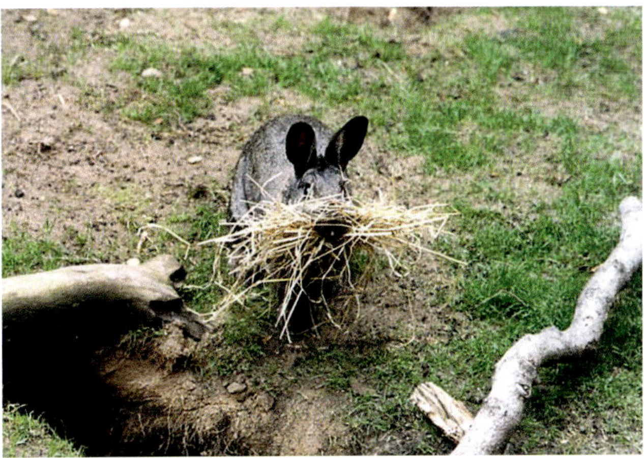

Figure 2.2 While an extensive open housing system outside is often positive for behavioural needs, rabbits will dig and may be able to escape as well as evade daily monitoring.

conclusion was to offer diets with a high fresh food component plus open water bowls to ensure good hydration. In order to minimise contamination, and if the housing allows, it may help to locate open water bowls in an elevated area accessible to the rabbit, rather than on the floor of the hutch.

Outdoor runs

It is advisable to provide outside runs attached to the hutch in the summer months. This allows the rabbit access to unfiltered sunshine, which is important for vitamin D_3 synthesis as well as for stimulating normal annual rhythms of behaviour. During the winter, sufficient protection from the weather should be afforded. However, denying the rabbit access to natural sunlight can result in a significant decline in vitamin D production if supplementation in the form of a dietary source of preformed vitamin D_3 is not provided and this can lead to metabolic bone and dental problems, particularly in young rabbits (Fairham and Harcourt-Brown, 1999).

Fresh grass is also the food item rabbits are supremely adapted to eat. In particular, the silicate and fibre content is vital, respectively, for wear of the teeth and stimulation of normal gut motility. Grass should not be cut first and then offered however, as this rapidly ferments and can produce colic.

Care should be taken when securing outside runs to make them both rabbit proof and predator proof. For this reason, it may be necessary to bury the wire sides to any run a foot or so beneath the ground surface as does in particular will burrow regularly (see Figure 2.2). To prevent foxes and cats gaining access to the run, a meshed roof should be provided. Finally, all outdoor rabbits should be vaccinated against myxomatosis, the viral condition spread by fleas and mosquitoes from wild rabbits, and rabbit viral haemorrhagic disease as well.

House rabbit

Many rabbits are now kept as house rabbits, with sleeping quarters and a litter tray. Rabbits can be toilet-trained relatively easily. The first steps in this are to keep the rabbit in a small area with a sleeping area, the litter tray and a feeding area. Once the litter tray has been associated with urination in particular, the rabbit may then be allowed more freedom to roam.

Dietary provision of preformed vitamin D_3 and adequate calcium needs to be considered for rabbits who do not receive exposure to unfiltered sunlight, otherwise metabolic bone and dental disease may develop, particularly in young growing animals.

Hazards in the home include electrical cabling, which should be hidden beneath carpets or protected inside heavy-duty cable trunking, which is available from hardware stores. Houseplants are another problem. Many of the exotic tropical houseplants are poisonous, for example African violet, *Dieffenbachia*, cheese plant and spider plant.

Social grouping

Rabbits are in general a social species, preferring to live in a group rather than singly. Problems arise though with keeping a number of entire males together, as bullying and sexual harassment will occur. Neutering is therefore advised where more than one male is to be kept and may be performed in bucks at 4–5 months of age. Mixed sex groups will work well if the does are spayed. This may be safely done at 5–6 months of age and is advisable even in solitary does due to the high risk of developing a malignant uterine cancer, known as a uterine adenocarcinoma, in middle age.

Some owners advocate the grouping of guinea pigs with rabbits. This is to be discouraged for two important reasons. One is that the rabbit has very powerful hind legs, and the guinea pig a long and fragile spine. Consequently, one well-placed kick from the rabbit can do a great deal of damage. The other reason is that rabbits are frequently asymptomatic carriers of the bacterium *Bordetella bronchiseptica* in their airways. This organism can cause a severe pneumonia in guinea pigs. Other domestic pets are not advised to be mixed with rabbits, as both cats and dogs are potential predators.

Behaviour

Rabbits are a prey species and therefore communicate in a very different manner from the more commonly understood cats and dogs. Indeed, it may seem that rabbits are very poor at communicating their feelings to their owners, when in fact they may be communicating, but in a much more subtle manner.

Affection is shown by mutual grooming of a companion, or owner, with licking of the hands in the latter case common. Other signs of relaxation include coming to the owner to be fed treats, following an owner around the house and, in many rabbits, making a buzzing noise from the larynx. This may be mistaken for a disease problem by inexperienced owners as it can be quite loud.

Aggression is shown by scratching, boxing with the front legs and biting. Aggression may be initiated because of a hormonal state, such as coming into season or bucks fighting for territory in the early spring, or it may be fear or pain driven. Aggression may also become a learnt behaviour if an act of aggression results in a desired effect, such as immediate backing off by the victim or replacement of a rabbit that has just been picked up by an owner.

Fear is shown initially by the regular thumping of the hind legs. This is a warning signal. As the object of fear approaches, the rabbit will either then freeze and remain motionless or suddenly bolt towards an exit.

Chewing of almost everything in the rabbit's environment is a perfectly normal behaviour and no amount of training will alter this fact. Owners of house rabbits should be warned of this and take appropriate action to prevent chewing of electric cables and other hazardous items of household furnishing.

Fostering

Rabbit kittens are difficult to hand-rear. Many females will not foster a strange doe's kittens, but does kept together and lactating at the same time will often allow another doe's young to suckle. This is the best scenario if another known lactating doe is available. If not, as is often the case, hand-rearing may be attempted.

A rearing formula has been derived (Okerman, 1998): 25 mL of whole cow's milk to 75 mL of condensed milk and 6 g of lyophilised skimmed milk powder. To this a vitamin supplement may be added. The kitten is fed only twice a day, from 2 to 10 mL depending on its age. This should continue until the kitten is 2 weeks old when more and more good-quality hay and pellets should be introduced, aiming to wean the kitten at 3 weeks. The anogenital area should be stimulated with a piece of damp cotton wool after every feed to stimulate urination and defecation for the first 2 weeks.

RAT AND MOUSE

Varieties

Rat

The common albino laboratory rat is widely domesticated. Other common varieties include the hooded rat and Rex groups. These are all variations on the *Rattus norvegicus* species, and the fancy rat numbers are ever increasing.

Mouse

As with rats, there are many different varieties of domesticated mouse. These vary from albinos through to the Rex, whole body colour types, etc.

Cage requirements

Construction and temperature

These are similar for both rats and mice. The traditional solid, plastic-bottomed and wire mesh upper cages are advisable. These allow good air circulation at the level of the rat or mouse's nose. The fish-tank style of housing is much less ventilated and allows the build-up of ammonia from urine-soaked bedding, particularly in rats who produce copious amounts of urine. Ammonia is a heavy gas and sits just above substrate level, that is at the rat's or mouse's nose level, and is thus inhaled often in high concentrations in this style of housing. Ammonia is highly irritant to the sensitive mucous membranes of the airways and will inflame and damage them, allowing secondary bacterial infection. This leads to the all-too-common problem of pneumonia seen in these species.

Environmental temperatures should range from 18 to 26°C. Because they lack skin sweat glands, temperatures above 28–29°C will rapidly induce hyperthermia and death in rats and mice. Rats can tolerate cooler temperatures better than mice, because of their lower surface area to body mass ratio and deposits of brown fat beneath the skin. However, temperatures consistently below 10°C will lead to poor health and hypothermia.

Substrate

Wood shavings are well tolerated by rats and mice, but be aware that many pine and coniferous woods contain resins which may cause skin and airway irritation. Alternatively, newspaper or paper towelling may be used. Straw and hay may be used, but again be aware that parasites may be introduced from wild rodents inadvertently with these bedding materials.

Cage furniture

As with hamsters, wheels are enjoyed by mice in particular. However, these should be solid in construction rather than open wired to avoid damage to limbs. Rats are less keen to use wheels, although they do enjoy climbing and hiding inside cardboard tubes and other enclosed items.

Food and water bowls

As with rabbits, sip feeders are ideal, as they lead to minimal wastage and contamination. Ceramic or stainless steel bowls are preferable to plastic.

Social grouping

Rat

Male rats may be kept with other males, particularly if reared together from an early age, without fighting. Females may also be paired with other females and seem to benefit from the company. Intersex groups also work well, although care should be taken to neuter the males (which may be performed at 3–4 months of age) if unwanted pregnancies are to be avoided. If breeding is intended, male rats may be 'paired' with one to six females. The pregnant female should be removed to a separate cage from the male rat 4–5 days prior to parturition to avoid disturbing the female at this sensitive time.

Mouse

Females may be kept in groups, particularly if reared together from a young age. Males should always be housed singly, as severe fights and even death may result from aggression between sexually mature males. If breeding is intended, male mice may be 'paired' with one to six females. It is then advised to remove the pregnant female from the male some 4–5 days prior to parturition.

Behaviour

Rat

Rats are generally docile and rarely do they bite. Female rats are prone to cannibalism of the young if disturbed in the first few days following parturition. Food and water should therefore be provided prior to whelping, to last for the following 7–10 days, and the female then left. The female rat builds a relatively poor nest in comparison to other members of the rodent family.

Mouse

Mice are generally relatively docile, although male mice may be more aggressive than females. The latter though will be aggressive in the defence of her young. In addition, although cannibalism towards her young is rare, a female mouse should be left undisturbed for a minimum of 2–3 days after birth. It is advisable to remove the female to a separate tank once she has mated to allow her to give birth and rear her young undisturbed.

Fostering

It is extremely difficult to rear young rats and mice successfully. Attempts may be made using a 1 : 1 dilution of evaporated milk to previously boiled water fed every 2 hours for the first 1–2 weeks. Weaning may be performed at 3 weeks. Stimulation of the anogenital area should be performed to encourage urination and defecation.

GERBIL AND HAMSTER

Varieties

Gerbil

There seems to be one main breed common in captivity, although a separate species known as the fat-tailed gerbil (*Pachyuromys duprasi*), has become more popular recently. There are however several different fur colour types, with albinos, black variants and greys as well as the normal tan colouration now available.

Hamster

There are four main species kept as pets: Syrian, European, Chinese and Russian. There is also a European hamster that is five to six times larger than the Syrian and although it was commonly kept as a laboratory animal is rarely kept as a pet. Within the pet species there are many colour variations, from albino to red to black, with differing fur types such as the fluffy 'teddy bear' version of the Syrian hamster in addition to the more common short-coated varieties.

Cage requirements

Cages and substrates

Gerbil

These enjoy tunnelling through deep litter substrates. It is important that the environment is kept dry, as humid conditions lead to poor fur quality and increased skin and respiratory infections. Shavings are an ideal substrate and should be at least 10–15 cm deep (see Figure 2.3). Placing ceramic or cardboard tubes through the substrate can help tunnel formation and provide environmental enrichment. However, peat and other soil substrates should be avoided because they are more likely to encourage damp. Environmental temperatures are usually kept around 20–25°C if possible.

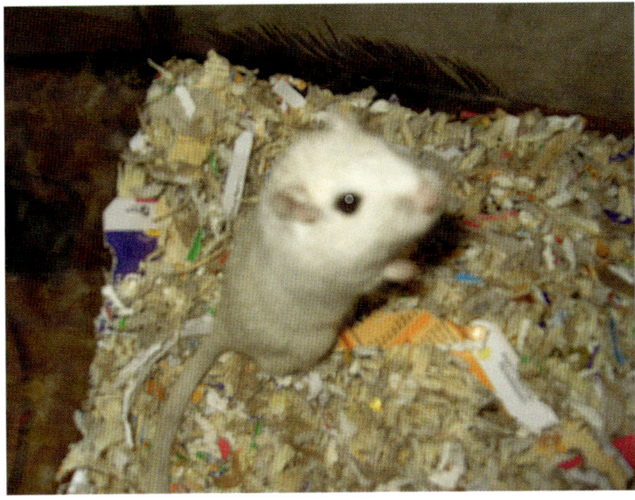

Figure 2.3 Deep substrate using shavings or paper is important for gerbils to allow burrowing.

Hamster

Cages for hamsters are best constructed of solid walls. The Rotastak®-style cage is ideal, with multiple tunnels for the hamster to manoeuvre from enclosed space to enclosed space. Wire cages are not so good, as hamsters have a habit of climbing up the sides, and then across the roofs of these cages. They will often lose their grip and suffer back injuries or compound fractures of the tibia as they land on the cage floor. It is advised to keep housing temperatures between 18 and 26°C. Temperatures less than 5–6°C will result in the hamster hibernating. In this state, respiration and heart rate slow considerably, making it difficult in many instances to detect if the hamster is still alive. Temperatures above 29–30°C will result in hyperthermia and death. Minimum cage requirements for dwarf hamsters have been suggested, ranging from 75 × 30 × 30 cm to 75 × 40 × 30 cm (Keeble, 2009). Chinese and Syrian hamsters must be kept alone (solitary) whereas the dwarf hamsters may be kept in small groups of same-sex litter-mates (Hedley *et al.*, 2023).

Cage furniture

Hamsters enjoy wheels very much, but these should be of a solid type, rather than the open wire format. This is to prevent the inadvertent damaging or even fracturing of a hind leg if it gets pushed between the wire slats. Tubes are ideal for entertaining gerbils as mentioned above.

Food and water bowls

Food bowls for both species are best made of a ceramic material, as these resist gnawing, are easily cleaned and difficult to tip over. Water is usually supplied in the traditional drip feeders, although care should be taken especially with gerbils that the valve is not leaky, as this leads to excessively wet substrate conditions and resultant dermatitis.

Social grouping

Gerbil

Gerbils are best housed singly, as a female pair or a neutered male and female pair. In the wild they will often bond, male to female, for life. Males housed together though will fight, inflicting severe wounds.

Female gerbils will rarely cannibalise their young, unlike hamsters, although care should still be taken not to disturb the female and young too much in the first week after birth.

Hamster

Males of the European, Chinese and Syrian species will fight. To a certain extent males of the Russian species will also fight, although this is lessened somewhat if they are reared from a young age together. Females may also be aggressive and so it is advised that hamsters in general be housed individually. For breeding purposes it is better to introduce a male hamster to a female's cage, rather than the other way around, to minimise fighting. A female hamster that has recently given birth should not be disturbed for a minimum of 10 days as the incidence of cannibalism of the young is high. To avoid this, enough food, water and bedding material (too little bedding is another reason for a female hamster killing the young) should be placed in the female's cage a few days prior to parturition and the female left undisturbed for the next 10–14 days.

Behaviour

Gerbil

Gerbils can be difficult to handle if not acclimatised to it from an early age. They will often bite if frightened or handled roughly. They are rarely vocal, but will communicate their alarm through regular drumming of the floor of the cage with one hind foot, in much the same way as a rabbit will do. Gerbils spend the day dozing and they are most active at night; that is, they are nocturnal.

Hamster

Hamsters are frequently accused of being aggressive. They will certainly bite readily if handled roughly, disturbed or frightened. Chinese and Russian hamsters are more aggressive than Syrian and European ones. Hamsters are also nocturnal and much of the aggression is due to being disturbed from their nest during the day. Therefore, they really do not make good pets for children. Females may be aggressive towards their young if disturbed.

Fostering

Gerbil

See the fostering section under rats and mice. Young gerbils are extremely difficult to rear artificially.

Hamster

See the fostering section under rats and mice. Young hamsters are extremely difficult to rear artificially. They do not foster well onto another female in any of the species, except perhaps the Russian hamster where a lactating female may accept another's young.

GUINEA PIG, CHINCHILLA AND DEGU

Breeds

Guinea pig

There are several different varieties of domesticated guinea pig: the Abyssinian, which possesses whorls of fur over the body and head; the Peruvian, which is particularly long-furred; the English or short-furred variety; and the Rex varieties, with short fuzzy fur. Colour variations are many and varied, from whole body colours of tan, white and black, through mixtures of two or three colours and albinos.

Chinchilla

There are just two subspecies of chinchilla recognised. *Chinchilla lanigera* is the standard domestic long-tailed chinchilla, which comes in a variety of colours from silver to white to champagne to black. Some authorities also recognise a subspecies known as *Chinchilla chinchilla*, which is a short-tailed larger version of the above.

Degu

There is one species of degu (*Octodon degus*). Their coat colouration is a red-brown.

Cage requirements

Guinea pig

A hutch system similar to that outlined for rabbits is advised, although the whole structure should be on one level. The same substrate and bedding materials are offered. In addition, it is often advised that lengths of tubing, such as drainpipe, should be offered as bolt holes for the guinea pigs to use when frightened. Access to grazing is useful, and guinea pigs cannot climb or dig so pen requirements are easier to provide than for rabbits. Care should be taken to ensure that any steps or ramps are not so steep that a guinea pig could fall, as their long and fragile backbone is easily damaged. Guinea pigs are expert chewers so, if allowed access to the home, precautions should be observed as with rabbits. Bowls and drinkers for food and water are as for rabbits.

Chinchilla

Space requirements for chinchillas are greater than for guinea pigs as they are extremely active. Recommendations include enclosures in excess of 2 m^3. They appreciate vertical space, unlike the ground-dwelling guinea pig. Cage construction should be of wire mesh, with a solid or mesh floor. This is because chinchillas are particularly good at chewing wood, and rapidly destroy wooden hutches. Chinchillas prefer an actual nest box rather than plentiful substrate. This should ideally be 20 cm^3 or more in size and can be lined with hay or straw, although the rest of the cage is often left bare. The floor is often a wire grid structure, to prevent any fluid accumulating, as this may lead to damage of the fur. The provision of lengths of drainpipe tubing is also advised, as for guinea pigs, to allow the shy chinchilla to hide from public gaze.

Water can be provided in the traditional drip feeders. Chinchilla fur mats very quickly when wet, so care should be taken to prevent the cage from becoming damp from any leakage. Because of this tendency to mat easily, chinchillas should not be allowed to bathe in water, but instead provided with daily access to a fine pumice sand and fuller's earth mixture as a dust bath. This can be provided in a metal box which may be clipped onto the inside of the cage or in a cat litter tray. The latter is less satisfactory as the chinchilla may chew the plastic. The sand bath should only be provided for short periods each day as otherwise the chinchilla tends to spend all day in the bath! Environmental temperatures should not exceed 20–22°C as heat stress may occur with that thick fur coat.

Degu

Tubing and nest boxes are recommended and many owners and institutions provide solid wheels for degus to exercise in as they are very active rodents. Dust baths, as with chinchillas, are also recommended to encourage scent marking and good fur maintenance. Most degus are housed in small groups or opposite sex pairs; for two to three individuals minimum space requirements should be around 45 × 30 cm floor space with vertical height of 20–25 cm.

Substrates such as pine or cedar shavings may result in irritation and so if shavings are used they should be from well-seasoned wood with low resin levels. Alternatively, shredded paper or corn may be used. Most prefer a 12-hour day and night cycle, with an environmental temperature of 17–20°C. Relative humidity ranges are typically 30–60%.

Social grouping

Guinea pig

Guinea pigs are a social species, and they live a much more contented life in the presence of other guinea pigs. Entire males can fight, although this is less likely if they are reared together from an early age. Even so, males will form a hierarchical system, and subordinate males may be bullied and bitten on a regular basis. Females live happily together, and the sexes may be mixed, although castration of the males (which may be done at 4–5 months of age) is advised to prevent unwanted pregnancies. In addition, females are unusual among the species so far discussed in that they will allow the nursing of other young than their own.

Chinchilla

Chinchillas will often form bonded pairs, although they will equally live happily in multi-sex and multi-chinchilla groups. If breeding is to be prevented, one or both of the sexes should be neutered. Males may be castrated at 5–6 months of age and females speyed at 6–7 months.

Degu

Degus are social creatures and enjoy physical contact with other degus and so should not be housed alone. Typically, housing two to three same-sex individuals is recommended, preferably from weaning to avoid aggression between sexually mature males in particular.

Behaviour

Guinea pig

Guinea pigs make good pets for the older child. They are docile and easily handled and rarely bite. Unlike many of the other species discussed here, they are very vocal. Their normal, contented vocal sounds include a series of chirrups and chattering noises which are low pitched. When alarmed, though, they will emit higher-pitched squeaks of warning. They will also run around the perimeter of their enclosure at high speed when stressed, and may flatten any younger guinea pigs in the process.

Chinchilla

Chinchillas are shy and retiring creatures. They are very affectionate and will make chirruping noises when contented. When frightened they will bite, bark and often exhibit fur-slip, where fur will drop out leaving alopecic areas that last for many weeks. When distressed, many chinchillas will urinate at the handler. This includes females who, having a large urinary papilla, can direct their urination as accurately as males.

Degu

Degus are relatively vocal and will produce a range of whistles, whines, snorts and squeaks during bonding, during periods of aggression (particularly between sexually mature males) and between mother and offspring. They will also communicate through tooth chattering and foot thumping similar to many other rodents. They will also communicate through pheromones particularly in their urine, again as with many other rodent species, although females tend to be more enthusiastic about scent marking than males which is different.

Fostering

Guinea pig

Use of a foster mother for any orphaned guinea pigs is advisable, even though they are precocious and may start to eat solids from day 3 after birth. Even so, it is still advisable to feed rearing milk formulas. Recipes for these include commercial feline weaner formulas, or using a 1 : 2 mixture of evaporated milk to previously boiled and then cooled water, thickened with a proprietary vegetable baby food powder (Richardson, 1992). This may be given through a kitten-rearing feeder every 2 hours for the first week, but the young should be encouraged to take solids as early as possible as a high incidence of cataracts is noticed in young guinea pigs fed for too long on cat, dog or cow's milk replacers. For the first 7–10 days the anogenital area of the young guinea pig should be stimulated with damp cotton wool to encourage urination and defecation.

Chinchilla

Even though young chinchillas are precocious at birth, they can be difficult to rear successfully. A rough guide to a rearing formula is to feed a 50 : 50 mix of a commercial cat- or dog-rearing formula added to evaporated milk. Alternatively, a 1 : 2 mix of evaporated milk with cooled, previously boiled water, thickened with a little fruit or vegetable baby food (Milupa or Farex) may be used. This should be fed through a kitten feeder every 2 hours for the first week, reducing to every 3–4 hours once the young chinchilla starts nibbling small volumes of solid. Chinchillas may be weaned early at 4 weeks if eating sufficient dry foods. Their weight should be measured daily to ensure regular gains. After each meal, the anogenital area should be stimulated with a piece of damp cotton wool to stimulate urination and defecation, although this is really only necessary for the first 7–10 days.

Degu

Natural degu milk, as with many species, is high in lipids (17.3 ± 5.5%) and protein (4.4 ± 0.4%) (Veloso and Kenagy, 2005). A number of commercially available products have been used, including Esbilac® diluted one part to five parts water as an artificial rearing milk. Feeding regimens are every 2 hours in pups less than 7 days of age, reducing to every 3–4 hours once the degu starts to take solids at around 2–3 weeks. Weaning can be carried out around 4–6 weeks of age. After each meal, the anogenital area should be stimulated with a piece of damp cotton wool to stimulate urination and defecation, although this is really only necessary for the first 7–10 days.

CHIPMUNK AND PRAIRIE DOG

Breeds

Chipmunk

The two main species seen in captivity are the Siberian chipmunk and, to a lesser extent, the North American chipmunk. The coat variations are limited, but the basic pattern is a light brown base coat with darker longitudinal body stripes. Albinos do exist.

Prairie dog

The main species in captivity is the black-tailed prairie dog (*Cynomys ludovicianus*). Coat colouration is a red-brown.

Cage requirements

Chipmunk

Cages and substrates

Chipmunks appreciate a combination of cage environments. The enclosure itself resembles more closely an aviary system designed for cage birds, with a wire mesh wall. The most successful examples combine a deep litter floor with bark chippings to allow foraging for food for environmental enrichment and roost boxes attached a few feet off the ground. These are constructed along similar lines to bird boxes. The cage may be further enhanced by stringing ropes from side to side to create aerial walkways.

Positioning

It is important not to house chipmunks near any source of electrical power in the 50–60 Hz range. This includes equipment such as television sets and many strip lights and computer terminals. The radiation given off by these electrical appliances causes high degrees of stress to the chipmunks, which will exhibit manic behaviour. This occurs even when the electrical equipment is turned off but still plugged in to the mains socket.

Prairie dog

Cages and substrates

Prairie dogs originate from North America and are a semi-fossorial species. They have been kept as pets in North America and Europe for many years, although at varying times their sale has been suspended, most notably in the USA because of a monkeypox virus outbreak (a zoonotic and legally notifiable disease). Ideally any housing should allow them to dig, as this is a natural behaviour and so should have depth of earth or other substrate. They are not good climbers but they do like some vertical height as a look-out point. Because of their burrowing behaviour their enclosure should ideally have an outside component and have a mesh floor sunk below ground level that provides a barrier preventing their escape (see Figure 2.4). Any mesh used to contain them should be no larger than 2.5 cm (1 inch) square. Prairie dogs will designate a latrine or use a litter tray if provided.

Typical environmental temperatures should range from 18 to 29°C, with an environmental humidity of 40–70%. In zoos they are commonly kept in groups, mimicking their natural social structure.

Positioning

As mentioned, an outside section to the enclosure is preferable to allow digging. Ensuring that the temperature range and humidity can be met may require shelter from the sun in an outdoor enclosure.

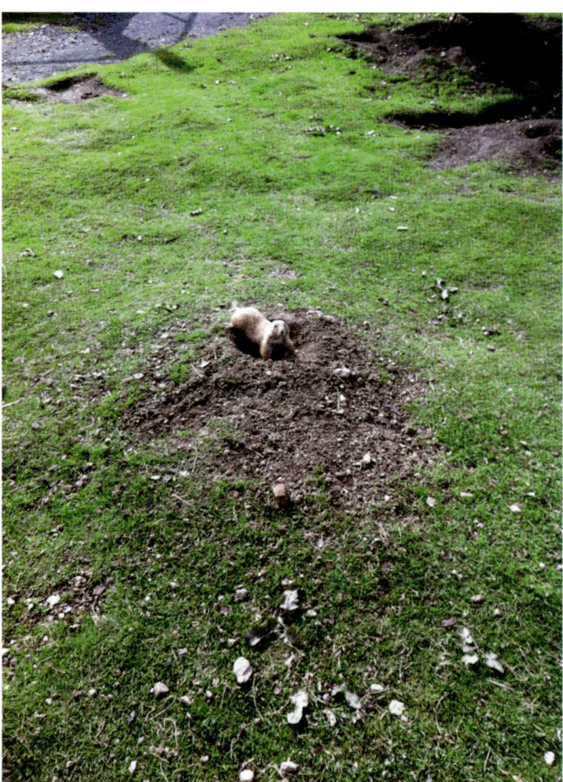

Figure 2.4 Prairie dogs are ground-dwelling species and form considerable complex burrow systems meaning that in order to prevent escape any outside enclosure should have a mesh floor sunk below ground level.

Social grouping

Chipmunk

Chipmunks prefer to be grouped together. Males are territorial and will fight during the breeding season, but females will tolerate each other well. In general, family groups are preferred, but the parents will chase away the young when weaned.

Prairie dog

The prairie dog is a social species and so ideally should be kept as such. However, they are commonly sold as individuals. Ideally, one male with two to four females makes a relatively stable group, although same-sex female groups work well. Same-sex male groups may fight, even when neutered, unless kept together from a juvenile age.

Behaviour

Chipmunk

Chipmunks are extremely nervous and highly strung creatures. They will bite if handled, and are difficult to tame, even when hand-reared. They will chatter excitedly to each other when stressed and often emit high-pitched squeaks. Some will also drum their hind legs as a warning signal. Tail flicking occurs almost continually, but becomes even more excited when stressed.

Prairie dog

Common behaviour for a prairie dog is to jump and then emit a yip when an owner enters the room. This natural behaviour is usually exhibited when a predator has disappeared and so is often viewed as an 'all-clear' signal. Prairie dogs are a social species and can become aggressive and show abnormal defensive behaviours such as self-mutilation when kept alone.

Fostering

Young abandoned chipmunks and prairie dogs are difficult to rear. A rearing formula has been proposed using a mixture of one part evaporated milk to two parts water, adding vegetable baby foods to this as the chipmunk ages. Minerals and vitamins may then be added, and the whole fed through a kitten-rearing feeder every 4 hours for the first 2 weeks of life, reducing to every 8 hours from 3 weeks until they are weaned at 5–6 weeks. The young chipmunk or prairie dog should be stimulated to urinate and defecate with a piece of damp cotton wool rubbed over the anogenital area immediately after feeding.

AFRICAN PYGMY HEDGEHOG

Cage requirements

Cage sizes per hedgehog would typically be around 60 × 90 cm floor space as a minimum. They do not regularly climb and so do not need vertical height. However, they can climb and so if the walls of an enclosure are made of mesh, an internal overhang should be created to prevent them climbing out. Alternatively, ensure the walls are smooth and their height is more than 1.5 times the length of the largest hedgehog housed. Substrate should be of non-irritant shavings (avoid resinous pine and cedar) or shredded paper to a depth of around 10 cm. Hide boxes are preferred as they are a solitary species and so if more than one individual is housed together there should be enough hide boxes to provide one for each hedgehog. Solid exercise wheels have been used to encourage activity and reduce obesity and seem to be enjoyed by pygmy hedgehogs. The species is nocturnal so dimmed lighting is preferred. As a semi-arid species, a lower relative humidity (<40%) is recommended with a temperature range of 24–30°C. African hedgehogs do not normally hibernate in the wild, but they can go into torpor in cool conditions (<18°C), which may result in immunosuppression if long in duration. Captive environmental temperatures are therefore recommended to be kept above 18°C.

Social grouping

African pygmy hedgehogs are a solitary species naturally and males when housed together will fight. If keeping multiple individuals together, a separate hide for each hedgehog must be provided.

Behaviour

African pygmy hedgehogs are solitary and nocturnal in the wild. They will dig burrows and hide under logs, rocks, tree roots and buildings and therefore hides must be supplied in captivity. When frightened they will hiss and, of course like other hedgehogs, roll into a ball making examination difficult. All hedgehogs can exhibit 'self-anointing' behaviours. This is where when presented with a new olfactory stimulus/smell the hedgehog will lick its spines and cover itself in its own saliva.

A variety of noises are typically made by African pygmy hedgehogs, including snuffling sounds when searching for food; high-pitched clicking sounds from mothers to offspring or sometimes males during courtship; tweeting/twittering noises made by neonates; whistling noises when the neonates have made contact with the mother; snorting, grunting and general guttural sounds when interrupted or disturbed or meeting a strange hedgehog; and screaming noises when in distress.

Fostering

Natural milk composition for African pygmy hedgehogs is a protein level of 16%, fat of 25.5% with a trace of carbohydrates (Ivey and Carpenter, 2012). Goat's milk and Esbilac have in practice been used to successfully rear hedgehog infants (Robinson, 2002; Dierenfield, 2009). Hand-reared infants are expected to gain weight at a minimum rate of 1.5 g/day until they are weaned at around 4 weeks (Robinson, 2002).

MARSUPIALS

Cage requirements

Sugar glider

Minimum cage dimensions for an adult pair would be 2 × 2 m floor space with a height of 1.8 m. Mesh size should be 1 cm^2. A nest box should be provided such as a wooden cylinder with a narrow opening. Branches should also be provided within the enclosure as sugar gliders are arboreal in nature. Additional heating is usually required to maintain environmental temperatures above 25°C with humidity of 60–80%. Substrate can be shredded paper or shavings.

Virginia opossum

Minimum cage dimensions should be 2 × 2 m unless they are regularly allowed out of their cages. Rabbit hutches and runs may be adapted for use but some facility for climbing should be provided. Substrate can be shredded paper, shavings or bark. Environmental temperature range of 12–25°C should be achieved with relative humidity levels above 60%.

Social grouping

Sugar glider

They are social animals and should not be kept singly as self-mutilation may occur. The most suitable group structure is to keep an adult male and an adult female together plus young. The young in a breeding pair of adults will usually comprise last year's joeys plus the current year's joeys in the pouch. When the former are sexually mature and need to be removed from the group, then the latter will have been weaned.

Virginia opossum

These are usually kept as pairs or individuals. Young should be removed 4–6 weeks after weaning. Neutered adults can be kept together in larger groups assuming sufficient space is allowed.

Behaviour

Sugar glider

These are very vocal when frightened and will make small barking noises as well as screeches. They will vigorously scent-mark and are very territorial, particularly the males.

Virginia opossum

These are very vocal and will hiss, click and growl as well as making a screeching sound when frightened. They can also feign death when threatened, called 'playing possum'

Fostering

Orphaned joeys must first be brought up to the correct body temperature (35–37°C) before being fed. Any milk replacer should be warmed to 35°C before being offered. Frequency depends on maturity, with non-furred joeys being fed every 2–3 hours and furred ones every 4–6 hours. Volumes fed should be between 10 and 20% of the joey's body weight over a 24-hour period. Teats on feeding bottles should have small needle holes and be long and thin in shape.

MacPherson (1997) derived a formula for sugar gliders using one scoop of Puppy Esbilac powder to three scoops of Pedialyte® (or equivalent small animal electrolyte replacer). A similar replacer can be used using one part Puppy Esbilac to three to five parts water.

FERRET

Cage requirements

Cages and substrates

Many ferrets are kept in outside hutches in a fashion similar to rabbits in the UK, particularly during the summer months (see Figure 2.5). It is also commonplace for ferrets to be kept as house pets. The problem with wooden hutches is that the often strong-smelling urine of the ferret will penetrate the wood. This is not so bad in ferrets that are kept outdoors, but for indoor ones this may be a considerable downside. Therefore the use of steel-bottomed and wire upper cages is preferred for indoor ferret keeping, as this type of cage can be easily disinfected. The size of the ferret cage should be a minimum of two ferret lengths in each direction. Ferrets like to make use of vertical space, so the provision of a shelf and raised sleeping quarters is useful. Care should be taken to ensure that the wire mesh is no larger than 2.5 cm^2 to avoid smaller ferrets escaping. Substrate in the cage may be newspaper, hay, shavings or straw. The nest box is best lined with towelling or a similar material. Ferrets enjoy hiding in plastic tubing and investigating every nook and cranny of a house. It is therefore essential not to allow a ferret access to rooms where there are holes in the walls for pipes, such as the kitchen, as they usually end up disappearing down them.

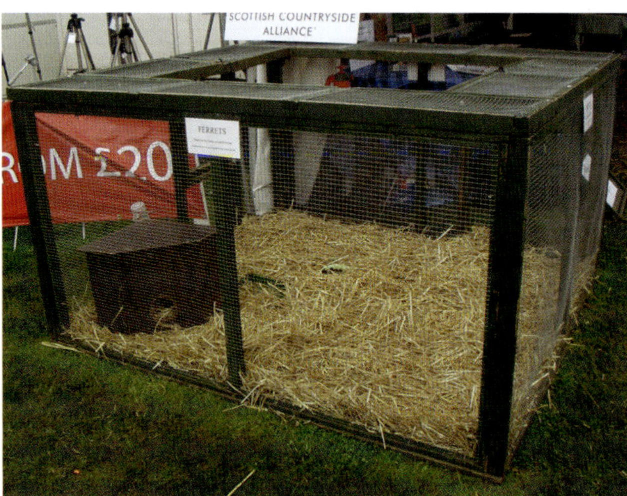

Figure 2.5 A typical temporary outside ferret run and housing for the summer months.

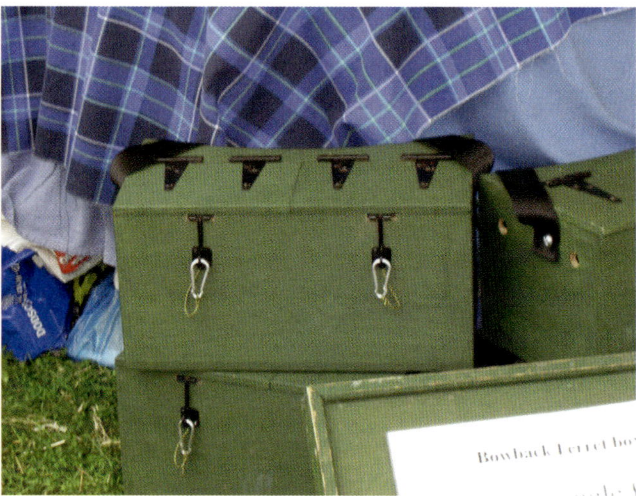

Figure 2.6 A typical working ferret hacking box to carry the ferret to and from the area of rabbiting.

Hacking boxes

These are used for transporting working ferrets to and from the area of rabbiting (see Figure 2.6). They tend to be capable of carrying two ferrets separately and are of a simple design in wood with ventilation holes and a shoulder strap for carrying. They are not designed for keeping a ferret in for any length of time.

Social grouping

Female ferrets get on well together, and ferrets in general like company, so it is often advisable to house them together. However, male ferrets (hobs) may fight and so care should be taken when housing multiples. Chemical neutering of male ferrets using deslorelin implants is advised on the grounds that it makes the animals more malleable and less likely to fight and also reduces odour. The female ferret (jill) is not susceptible to cannibalism of the young if disturbed, although care should be exercised when interfering with the young as the jill will defend them vigorously if she feels threatened.

Behaviour

Ferrets are extremely inquisitive creatures and will explore everything and anything. They are generally docile when reared in the company of humans, but they can give a ferocious bite when frightened, from which it may be difficult to disengage.

Management

Ferrets are currently kept in the UK mainly as working pets, for hunting, chiefly, of rabbits. Ferrets may be 'trained' to flush out rabbits from their warrens, although this is merely taking advantage of their natural hunting tendency.

Ferrets may be walked on a harness, and they can be litter trained with perseverance.

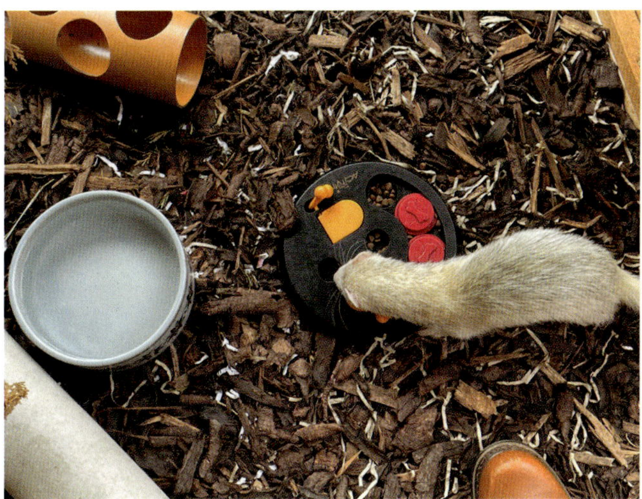

Figure 2.7 Environmental enrichment including puzzle feeders, deep substrate, toys and tunnels all encourage activity and reduce the incidence of obesity in pet ferrets.

Captive pet ferrets may be prone to obesity and boredom and so addition of puzzle feeders as well as toys, deep substrates and tunnels or tubes can all help mentally stimulate them and reduce weight gain (see Figure 2.7).

The odour of ferrets is reduced where hobs are castrated. However this has now been shown to be associated with adrenal gland neoplasia, and therefore the use of gonadotropin-releasing hormone agonists such as deslorelin has been advocated instead. The removal of the anal glands is prohibited in the UK as an unnecessary mutilation.

Fostering

Care should be taken to ensure correct nursing of the kit after failure of the jill to nurse, produce milk or when mastitis occurs. This is best done by fostering the kits onto another lactating jill, but this is often difficult. If the affected jill is still well enough the kits should be left with her to gain what little milk they may. Supplemental feeding may then be given using a proprietary feline milk replacer enriched with whipping cream to increase the fat content. A rough guide is two to three parts feline milk replacer to one part whipping cream. This needs to be fed every 2 hours or so via a nipple feeder, preferably warmed prior to feeding. Weaning may be brought forward to 3 weeks, and the kits trained to drink milk replacer from a saucer. Generally, kits cannot manage to survive on solid foods alone until they are over 5 weeks of age. As with neonatal cats and dogs, kits require stimulation of their anogenital areas with damp cotton wool after each feed to encourage urination and defecation.

References

Dierenfield, E.S. (2009) Feeding behavior and nutrition of the African pygmy hedgehog (*Atelerix albiventris*). *Veterinary Clinics of North America: Exotic Animal Practice*, **12**, 335–337.

Fairham, J. and Harcourt-Brown, F.M. (1999) Preliminary investigation of the vitamin D status of pet rabbits. *Veterinary Record*, **145**, 452–454.

Hedley, J.E., Pettitt, A. and Abeyesinghe, S.M. (2023) Preliminary investigation into the housing of dwarf hamsters. *Veterinary Record*, **193**(4), e3170. doi: 10.1002/vetr.3170.

Ivey, E. and Carpenter, J.W. (2012) African hedgehogs. In: *Ferrets, Rabbits, and Rodents: Clinical Medicine and Surgery* (eds K.E. Quesenberry & J.W. Carpenter), 3rd edn, pp. 411–428. Saunders-Elsevier, St. Louis.

Keeble, E. (2009) Rodents biology and husbandry. In: *Manual of Ferrets and Rodents* (eds E. Keeble & A. Meredith), pp. 1–17. BSAVA, Cheltenham, UK.

MacPherson, C. (1997) *Sugar Gliders, A Complete Pet Owner's Manual.* Barrons Educational Series, Inc, Hauppauge, NY.

Okerman, L. (1998) Breeding problems. In: *Diseases of Domestic Rabbits*, 2nd edn, pp. 113–120. Blackwell Science, Oxford.

Richardson, V.C.G. (1992) *Diseases of Domestic Guinea Pigs*. Blackwell, Oxford.

Robinson, I. (2002) Hedgehogs. In: *Hand-rearing Wild and Domestic Mammals* (ed. L.J. Gage), pp. 75–80. Iowa State Press, Ames, IA.

Tschudin, A., Clauss, M., Codron, D. *et al.* (2011) Water intake in domestic rabbits (*Oryctolagus cuniculus*) from open dishes and nipple drinkers under different water and feeding regimes. *Journal of Animal Physiology and Animal Nutrition (Berlin)*, **95**(4), 499–511. doi: 10.1111/j.1439-0396.2010.01077.x.

Veloso, C. and Kenagy, G.J. (2005) Temporal dynamics of milk composition of the precocial caviomorph *Octodon degus* (Rodentia: Octodontidae). *Revista Chilena de Historia Natural*, **78**, 247–252.

PART I: SMALL MAMMALS

Chapter 3 Small Mammal Handling and Chemical Restraint

It is known that anaesthesia mortality rates for small mammals are reported as higher than those for dogs and cats, for example the domestic rabbit is seven times more likely to die under general anaesthesia than a dog or cat (Brodbelt *et al.*, 2008). Reasons for this are many and include lack of familiarity with the species' anatomy and physiology, but underlying disease and the fact that many of the species described here are prey species and so cover their illnesses well also play a part. Before attempting to restrain a small mammal patient, we must first be sure that it is necessary. Points to be considered include the following.

- Is the patient severely debilitated and/or in respiratory distress? Examples include the pneumonic rabbit with obvious oculonasal discharge and dyspnoea, or the chronic lung disease so often seen in older rats. Excessive or rough handling of these patients is contraindicated.
- Is the species a tame one? Examples of the more unusual small mammals that may be kept include chipmunks, sugar gliders, prairie dogs, marmosets and raccoons. All of these are potentially hazardous to handlers and themselves as they will often bolt for freedom when frightened or turn and fight.
- Is the small mammal suffering from a metabolic bone disease? This is often seen in small primates, young rabbits and, to a lesser extent, guinea pigs. The diet may have been deficient in calcium and vitamin D_3 and exposure to natural sunlight may be absent. Therefore, long-bone mineralisation during growth will be poor leading to easily fractured bones.
- Does the small mammal patient require medication or physical examination, in which case restraint may be unavoidable?

Handling techniques

Because of the wide range of species grouped under the heading small mammal, this section is easier if considered under related taxonomic groups of small mammals. Always approach small mammals from the sides and keep hands low to avoid mimicking the swooping action of a bird of prey.

Domestic rabbit

The majority of domestic rabbits are docile. In the occasional aggressive rabbit, the main dangers are from the claws, which can inflict deep scratches, and the incisors, which can produce deep bites. Aggression is worse at the start of the breeding season in March and April, or when the rabbit is frightened. In addition, a struggling rabbit may lash out with its powerful hindlimbs and fracture or dislocate its spine. Severe stress can even induce cardiac arrest in some rabbits. Rapid and safe restraint is therefore essential.

If aggressive, the lagomorph may be grasped by the scruff with one hand while the other supports the hind legs. If the rabbit is not aggressive, then one hand may be placed under the thorax, with the thumb and first two fingers encircling the front limbs, while the other is placed under the hind legs to support the back (see Figure 3.1).

When transferred from one room to another the rabbit must be held close to the handler's chest. Non-fractious individuals may also be supported with their heads pushed into the crook of one arm, with that forearm supporting the length of the rabbit's body. The other hand is then used to place pressure on or grasp the scruff region (see Figure 3.2).

Once caught, the rabbit may be calmed further by wrapping it in a towel so that just the head and ears protrude. There are also specific rabbit papooses that encircle the rabbit, but leave the head and ears free. This allows ear blood sampling and oral examinations, but controls their powerful hindlimbs. It is important not to allow them to overheat in this position, as rabbits do not have significant sweat glands and do not actively pant. They can therefore overheat quickly with fatal results if their environmental temperature exceeds 23–25°C.

Rat and mouse

Mice will frequently bite an unfamiliar handler, especially in strange surroundings. First, grasp the tail near to the base and then position the mouse on a non-slip surface. While still grasping the tail, the scruff may now be grasped firmly between thumb and forefinger of the other hand.

Rats will rarely bite unless roughly handled. They are best picked up by encircling the pectoral girdle immediately behind the front limbs with the thumb and fingers of one hand, while bringing the other hand underneath the rear limbs to support the rat's weight (see Figure 3.3). The more fractious rat may be temporarily restrained by grasping the base of the tail before scruffing it with thumb and forefinger.

Under no circumstances should mice or rats be restrained by the tips of their tails as de-gloving injuries to the skin covering them will occur.

Gerbil and hamster

Hamsters can be difficult to handle. If the hamster is relatively tame, cupping the hands underneath the animal is sufficient to transfer it from one cage to another.

Some breeds of hamster are more aggressive than others, with the Russian hamster (also known as the Djungarian or hairy-footed hamster) being notorious for its short temper. In these cases, the hamster should be placed onto a firm flat surface, and gentle but firm pressure placed onto the scruff region with finger and thumb of one hand. As much of the scruff should then be grasped as possible, with the pull in a cranial direction, to ensure that the skin is not drawn tight around the eyes (hamsters have a tendency to proptose their eyes if

Veterinary Nursing of Exotic Pets and Wildlife, Third Edition. Simon J. Girling.

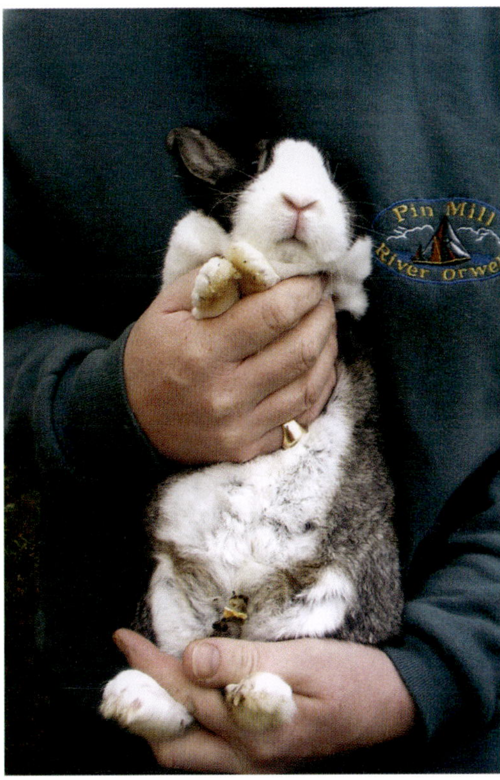

Figure 3.1 Method of restraining a tame rabbit for examination.

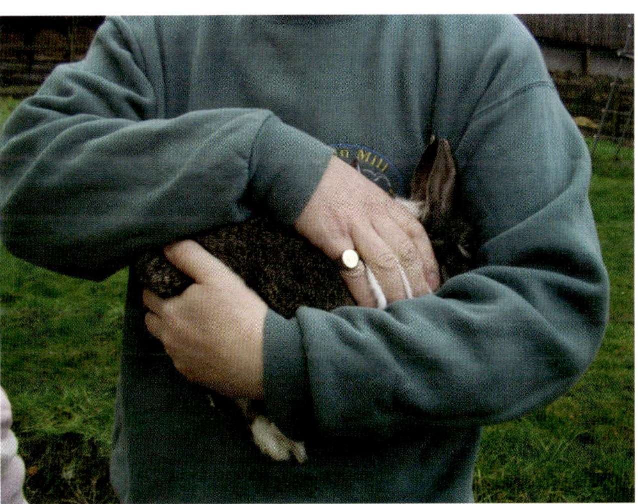

Figure 3.2 Method of transporting a rabbit from one place to another.

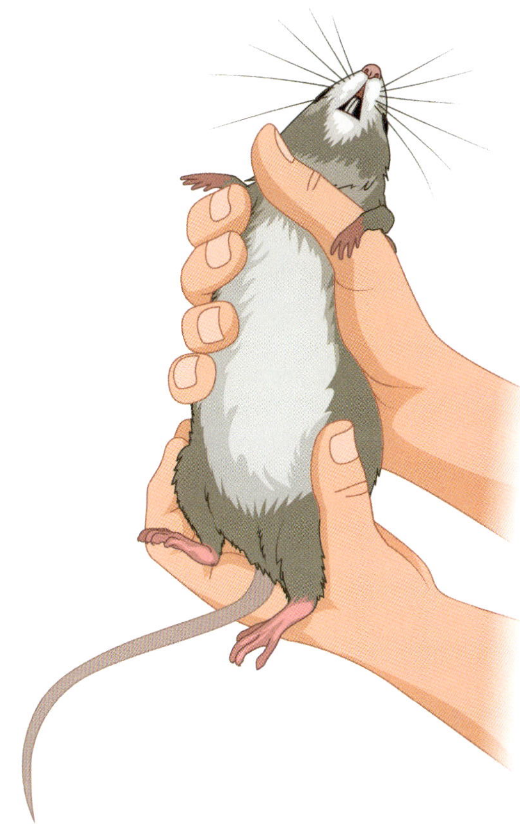

Figure 3.3 Method of restraining a hand tame rat. Note support of hindquarters with free hand.

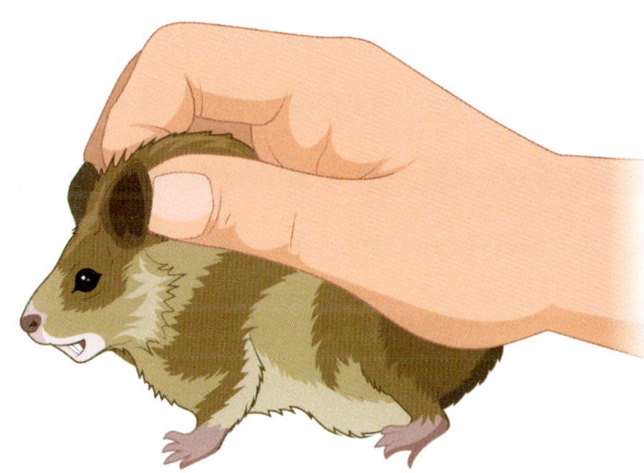

Figure 3.4 Method for restraining a hamster. Note the large amount of loose skin which must be grasped and the high position at which it is grasped immediately behind the ears to avoid eye proptosis.

roughly scruffed) (see Figure 3.4). If a very aggressive animal is encountered, the use of a small glass or Perspex container with a lid for examination and transport purposes is useful.

Gerbils are relatively docile, but can jump extremely well when frightened and may bite. For simple transport they may be moved from one place to another by cupping the hands underneath them. For more rigorous restraint, the gerbil may be grasped by the scruff between thumb and forefinger of one hand after placing it onto a flat level surface. It is vitally important not to grasp a gerbil by the tail. The skin will strip off, leaving denuded coccygeal vertebrae exposed, and the skin will never regrow. Jirds and jerboas are related species and handling techniques are the same.

Guinea pig, chinchilla and degu

Guinea pigs are rarely aggressive, but they are highly stressed when separated from their companions and normal surroundings. Dimming the lighting, and reducing noise and other stress can aid in control.

The guinea pig should be grasped behind the forelimbs from the dorsal aspect with one hand, while the other is placed beneath the hindlimbs to support its weight. This is particularly important as the guinea pig has a large abdomen but slender bones and spine. Without supporting the rear end, spinal damage is risked.

Chinchillas are equally timorous and rarely if ever bite. They too can be easily stressed and reducing noise and dimming room lighting can be useful. When restrained they must not be scruffed under any circumstances as this will result in the loss of fur at the site held. This fur-slip will leave a bare patch which will take many weeks to regrow. Chinchillas may actually lose some fur due to the stress of restraint, even if no physical gripping of the skin occurs. Some chinchillas, when particularly stressed, will rear up on their hind legs and urinate at the handler with surprising accuracy! It is therefore essential to pick up the chinchilla calmly and quickly with minimal restraint, placing one hand around the pectoral girdle from the dorsal aspect just behind the front legs, and the other hand cupping the hind legs and supporting the chinchilla's weight. Degus may be handled in a similar fashion, although they are less prone to fur-slip.

Chipmunk

Chipmunks are highly strung, and the avoidance of stress and fear aggression is essential to avoid fatalities. They are difficult to handle without being bitten, unless hand-reared, when they may be scruffed quickly, or cupped in both hands. To catch them in their aviary-style enclosures the easiest method is to use a fine-meshed aviary or butterfly net, preferably made of a dark material. The chipmunk may then be safely netted and quickly transferred to a towel for manual restraint, examination, or injection or induction of chemical restraint.

Prairie dog

Prairie dogs that are used to being handled may be held in a manner similar to a domestic rat. However, those that are frightened or not used to being handled can be challenging to safely manually restrain. A thick towel can be used to temporarily contain the prairie dog before administration of a sedative or general anaesthetic agent to allow a more detailed examination.

African pygmy hedgehog

African pygmy hedgehogs, like any hedgehog species, will rapidly curl into a ball when threatened. Due to the tendency to curl into a ball and because of the spines, it is recommended that handlers wear suitable gloves such as gauntlets or gardening gloves to protect their hands from the spines. Care should be taken however not to overzealously restrain them as it can be difficult to assess the strength of a grip when wearing such gloves and the African pygmy hedgehog is a small and potentially fragile species. Stroking the dorsum from cranial to caudal with a gloved hand may encourage the animal to uncurl as may gently holding it by the caudal body with its cranial body suspended just above the table top/floor to encourage it to place its forefeet down. However, a detailed examination of an African pygmy hedgehog is likely to require sedation or general anaesthesia.

Marsupials

Sugar gliders are very docile and may be restrained with minimal force. If they need to be held firmly for any reason, one hand can hold the base of the tail and the other the dorsal aspect of the neck. For Virginia opossums that are tame, one hand may be used to grasp around the pectoral girdle and the other to support the rear end in a similar fashion to that described for domestic rats. For more aggressive animals leather gardening gloves/gauntlets should be used. They may also be wrapped in towels in a fashion similar to rabbits.

Ferret

Ferrets can make excellent house pets and many are friendly and hand-tame. However, in the UK, ferrets are most frequently kept for rabbit hunting; hence, many ferrets are not regularly handled and so may be aggressive.

For excitable or aggressive animals, a firm grasp of the scruff, high up at the back of the neck is advised. The ferret may then be suspended while stabilising the lower body with the other hand around the pelvis. In tamer animals, they may be suspended with one hand behind the front legs, cupped between thumb and fingers from the dorsal aspect, with the other hand supporting the hindlimbs. This hold may be varied somewhat in more lively individuals by placing the thumb of one hand underneath the chin, so pushing the jaw upwards, and the rest of the fingers grasping the other side of the neck. The other hand is then brought under the hindlimbs as support.

Aspects of chemical restraint

Chemical restraint may be necessary for a number of reasons in small mammals:

- Sample collection, such as blood testing or urine collection
- For procedures such as radiography
- Oral examinations
- Nervous or aggressive individuals or species difficult to examine because of their behaviours (e.g. African pygmy hedgehogs curling into a ball).

Is the patient fit enough for chemical restraint?

It is important to assess whether the patient is fit enough for a chemical restraint before it is attempted. Factors that should be considered prior to the anaesthesia of small mammals are outlined below.

Low-grade respiratory infections

Many small mammals (e.g. rodents and rabbits) suffer from low-grade respiratory infection all of their lives. Most will cope with this, but when anaesthetised the respiratory rate slows and respiratory secretions, already thickened or increased due to chronic infection, become more tenacious. This can cause physical blockage of the airways and hypoxia.

Respiratory system anatomy

The majority of the species considered are nose breathers, with their epiglottis locked into their nasopharynx. Therefore, if the patient has a blocked nose, whether due to pus, blood, tumours or abscesses, then respiratory arrest is made much more likely under anaesthesia.

Hypothermia

Because of their small size and resultant high body surface area to volume ratios, small mammals are prone to hypothermia during anaesthesia. This is heightened due to the cooling effect of the inhaled gases and reduced muscular activity. It is dangerous, therefore, to anaesthetise a patient that is already hypothermic without first treating this condition.

Dehydration

Respiratory fluid losses during drying gaseous anaesthetic procedures are much greater than in cats, dogs or larger species, again due to their increased surface area to volume ratio. Therefore, putting a severely dehydrated small mammalian patient through an anaesthetic without prior fluid therapy is not advisable.

Pre-anaesthetic management

Weight measurement

It is vitally important to weigh the patient accurately. A mistake of just 10 g in a hamster, say, will lead to an under- or over-dosage of 10%. The use of scales that will read accurately down to 1 g in weight is therefore essential.

Blood testing

Blood testing prior to general anaesthesia should be considered in every clinically unwell or senior patient where a sufficiently large sample may be obtained and the patient is amenable to physical restraint for the procedure. Sites for venepuncture are detailed below.

Rabbit: A 25–27 gauge needle may be used in the lateral ear vein. Prior to sampling, apply a local anaesthetic cream to the site and warm the ear. Alternatively, the cephalic or the jugular veins may be used. The latter should be used with caution as it is the only source of blood drainage from the eyes, and so, if a thrombus forms in this vessel, ocular oedema and permanent damage or even loss of the eye may occur.

Rat and mouse: The lateral tail veins may be used. These run on either side of the coccygeal vertebrae and are best seen when the tail is warmed as for the lateral ear vein in lagomorphs. A 25–27 gauge needle is required.

Guinea pig, chinchilla and degu: The jugular veins are the most accessible. One handler holds both front limbs with one hand and brings the patient to the edge of the table, raising the head with the other hand. The other operator may then take a jugular sample with a 23–25 gauge needle. Lateral saphenous veins may be used in guinea pigs, but chinchillas and degus rarely have any other peripheral vessel large enough to sample.

Gerbil and hamster: These are difficult and not often attempted with only physical restraint due to their more fractious nature and poor accessibility of peripheral veins. With care (particularly in gerbils) the lateral tail veins may be used but watch as the tail should not be roughly handled or grasped as the skin easily sloughs. Frequently cardiac puncture under anaesthesia is often necessary to obtain a sufficient sample.

Chipmunk and prairie dog: Jugular blood samples may be taken, but in nearly every case anaesthesia is required first.

African pygmy hedgehog: This species is not easy to blood sample with physical restraint only due to its tendency to curl into a ball. Jugular veins are the preferred vessels to use once anaesthetised.

Marsupials: The lateral or ventral tail, cephalic or lateral saphenous veins may be used. Anaesthesia may be required first though due to the small size of some and potential aggression of others.

Ferret: The jugular vein is the easiest to access, but may be difficult in a fractious animal. One handler holds onto both front limbs with one hand, clamping the body with forearm and elbow, the other hand placed under the chin and raising the head. Towel restraint may also be used to papoose the ferret. Cephalic veins may also be accessed. Needles of 23–25 gauge suffice.

Fasting

Rabbit: These do not need to be fasted prior to anaesthesia, as they have a very tight cardiac sphincter preventing vomiting. Starving may actually be deleterious to the patient's health as it causes a cessation in gut contractility and subsequent ileus. It is important, though, to ensure that no food is present in the mouth at the time of induction, hence a period of 30–60 minutes starvation should be ensured.

Rat and mouse: Because of their high metabolic rate and likelihood of hypoglycaemia, rats and mice need only be starved a matter of 40–60 minutes (mice) to 45–90 minutes (rats) prior to anaesthetic induction.

Guinea pig, chinchilla and degu: These may be starved for 3–6 hours prior to surgery to ensure a relatively empty stomach and reduce pressure on the diaphragm. Again, prolonged starvation (>4 hours) will lead to hypoglycaemia and gut stasis and is not recommended.

Gerbil and hamster: As for Muridae, a period of 45–90 minutes is usually sufficient. Any longer than 2 hours and postoperative hypoglycaemia is a real problem.

Chipmunk: Periods of fasting of 2 hours have been reported as safe.

Prairie dog: As with other herbivorous rodents, prolonged fasting is not typically required as they rarely if ever vomit. A short period without food of 1–2 hours will ensure less pressure on the diaphragm.

African pygmy hedgehog: APHs do not vomit easily and have a relatively quick digestive tract transit time, meaning starvation of more than 2–4 hours is rarely required. However, it is not recommended that any live invertebrates are fed in the 12 hours prior to a planned anaesthetic.

Marsupial: Smaller marsupials may be starved for 1 hour with larger ones requiring 3–6 hours.

Ferret: These may be starved for 2–4 hours. Many older ferrets have insulinomas and will develop hypoglycaemia if starved for longer than 4 hours. Also, mustelids have a high metabolic rate and short gut transit times.

Pre-anaesthetic medications

Pre-anaesthetic drugs are used to help provide a smooth induction and recovery from anaesthesia, and in some cases to ensure a reduction in airway secretions, act as a respiratory stimulant or prevent serious bradycardia. Pre-anaesthetic fluid therapy and analgesia is dealt with later in this chapter but clearly should be considered on a case-by-case basis.

Alpha-2 drugs

Alpha-2 sedatives such as medetomidine and dexmedetomidine are commonly used as premedicants in larger domestic mammals. Xylazine historically has also been used, but due to its poor reversibility and greater deleterious side-effects it is not recommended for small mammals and as such will not be considered further in this chapter. The use of medetomidine and dexmedetomidine in small mammals as premedication drugs, as opposed to their use as part of a combination with ketamine for anaesthesia, has been reported, particularly in rabbits and ferrets. In these two species they are often combined with a partial opiate agonist such as butorphanol or buprenorphine. It should be noted that use of alpha-2 drugs should not occur where underlying cardiovascular disease or significant electrolyte disturbances (such as hyperkalaemia) are present as this is likely to lead to arrhythmias and potential cardiac arrest as well as exacerbating tissue hypoxia in less severely affected cases.

In rabbits doses of 0.1 mg/kg medetomidine on its own subcutaneously or intravenously may be used to provide very light sedation. Typically, dexmedetomidine dosages are half those quoted for medetomidine. Dexmedetomidine (0.02 mg/kg) can be combined with full opiates such as methadone (1 mg/kg) or fentanyl (0.03–0.3 mg/kg) intramuscularly to provide premedication and analgesia.

In rodents, medetomidine is not often used as a premedicant, rather it tends to be combined with a dissociative anaesthetic such as ketamine for full general anaesthesia.

In ferrets, medetomidine has been used as a premedicant on its own at 0.08–0.2 mg/kg (typically 0.1 mg/kg) (Cantwell, 2001). It may also be used at 0.08 mg/kg with butorphanol 0.1 mg/kg to produce a deep sedation (Marini and Fox, 1998).

Antimuscarinics

Atropine is used in some species such as African pygmy hedgehogs, guinea pigs and chinchillas where oral secretions are high and intubation is difficult. Doses of 0.05 mg/kg have been used subcutaneously 30 minutes before induction. It has been used in ferrets at 0.02–0.04 mg/kg and sugar gliders at 0.01–0.02 mg/kg where a concern over heart block has been reported with underlying cardiovascular disease as atropine also acts to prevent excessive bradycardia, which often occurs during the induction phase.

Atropine is not useful in lagomorphs, as around 60% of rabbits have a serum atropinesterase that breaks down atropine before it has a chance to work. Glycopyrrolate, another parasympatholytic, may be used instead in rabbits at doses of 0.01–0.1 mg/kg subcutaneously although most typically 0.01–0.02 mg/kg in my experience. It has also been used in African pygmy hedgehogs, sugar gliders and most rodents at 0.01–0.02 mg/kg.

Tranquillisers

Tranquillisers are used to reduce the stress of induction. Many species will breath-hold during gaseous induction, to the point where they may become cyanotic. In rabbits, the 'shock' organ is the lungs, and during intense stress the smooth muscle in the vessel walls of the pulmonary circulation can go into spasm, resulting in right-sided heart failure.

Acepromazine: Acepromazine (ACP) can be used at doses of 0.2 mg/kg in ferrets and marsupials, 0.5 mg/kg in rabbits, 0.5–1 mg/kg in rats, mice, hamsters, prairie dogs, chinchillas, degus and guinea pigs and 0.1–1 mg/kg in African pygmy hedgehogs. In general, it is a very safe premedicant even in debilitated animals. However, it is advised that it not be used in gerbils as ACP reduces the seizure threshold, and many gerbils suffer from hereditary epilepsy. I typically use a dose of 0.2 mg/kg ACP in combination with 0.05 mg/kg atropine as a premedication for example in chinchillas.

Diazepam: Diazepam is useful as a premedicant in some species. In rodents, doses of 0.5–3 mg/kg can be used, even in gerbils. In rabbits, the benefits are somewhat outweighed by the larger volumes required. In addition, as the drug is oil based, the intramuscular route may be painful and result in rhabdomyolysis.

Midazolam: Midazolam can be used in a similar fashion to diazepam and being aqueous tends to result in less tissue irritation post injection. Doses intramuscularly of 0.25–0.5 mg/kg in marsupials and ferrets, 0.3–0.4 mg/kg in African pygmy hedgehogs and 2–5 mg/kg in most rodent species have been used. In rabbits and hedgehogs midazolam may be used at 0.2–0.5 mg/kg combined with butorphanol at 0.3–0.5 mg/kg or with buprenorphine at 0.03–0.05 mg/kg intramuscularly as a premedication and sedative. It may also be combined with fentanyl and fluanisone in rodents and rabbits to induce general anaesthesia. Midazolam has been used intranasally to provide mild sedation in some species of small mammal, for example African pygmy hedgehogs at 1–2 mg/kg and sugar gliders at 0.1–0.5 mg/kg (Doss and de Miguel Garcia, 2022).

Neuroleptanalgesics

The fentanyl/fluanisone combination sold as Hypnorm® (VetaPharma Ltd., UK) has been used historically at varying doses as a premedicant, a sedative or as part of an injectable full anaesthesia and was widely discussed in the first two editions of this text. Unfortunately it has not been commercially available for a few years now and so is not discussed further in this edition.

Fluid therapy

Fluid therapy is a vitally important pre-anaesthetic consideration and will be mentioned below and elsewhere in the book.

Induction of anaesthesia

Injectable agents

Table 3.1 outlines some of the advantages and disadvantages of injectable anaesthetics in small mammals.

Table 3.1 Advantages and disadvantages of injectable anaesthetics.

Advantages	Disadvantages
Easily administered	Delay in reversal
Minimal stress	Hypoxia and hypotension common
Prevent breath-holding	Tissue necrosis
Inexpensive	Organ metabolism required

Propofol

It may be used in ferrets at 2–8 mg/kg after the use of a premedicant such as ACP. However, in rabbits and hystricomorphs, apnoea can be a problem, and because it must be given intravenously it is difficult to use in the smaller rodents. Doses intravenously of 2–6 mg/kg post premedication and 7.5–15 mg/kg without premedication have been used intravenously in rabbits.

Alfaxalone

Alfaxalone is currently (2023) licensed for use in rabbits in the UK (Alfaxan®, Jurox Pty Ltd.) and has been recommended at an initial dose of 2 mg/kg given intravenously via a previously placed intravenous lateral ear vein catheter to induce anaesthesia. This may need to be increased to 4 mg/kg in premedicated rabbits or 5 mg/kg in non-premedicated rabbits to induce stage III anaesthesia but the current recommendation is to start at 2 mg/kg and increase to effect. In all cases it must be given slowly as apnoea can result and the manufacturer recommends quarter dosages to be administered over roughly 15 seconds, so taking a full minute to deliver the total dose.

In ferrets it has been used at 9–12 mg/kg intravenously and intramuscularly, usually higher doses for the latter. In rodents dosages of 20 mg/kg intramuscularly have also been used. Apnoea is seen where rapid intravenous administration occurs.

Ketamine

Ketamine is a dissociative anaesthetic commonly used in small mammals.

Rabbit: Ketamine is used in healthy rabbits with no underlying disease issues at a dose of 15 mg/kg in conjunction with medetomidine at 0.25 mg/kg and butorphanol at 0.4 mg/kg to provide surgical anaesthesia of 30–40 minutes with recumbency for 90–240 minutes (Flecknell, 2006). Buprenorphine may substitute butorphanol in this regimen at 0.03 mg/kg if longer-lasting analgesia is required (giving 6–8 hours as opposed to 1–2 hours for butorphanol). The advantages of this intramuscular 'triple' drug combination are its simplicity and speed of administration, but the combination will cause blueing of the mucous membranes due to peripheral shutdown associated with the alpha-2 drug medetomidine, making detection of hypoxia difficult. Respiratory depression may become a problem and intubation and additional oxygen supply is advised. Ketamine at 15 mg/kg intramuscularly has been used with just medetomidine at 0.25 mg/kg. Alternatively an intravenous triple combination of 3–5 mg/kg ketamine plus 0.05–0.1 mg/kg medetomidine plus 0.05–0.1 mg/kg butorphanol has been used which provides a light plane of anaesthesia that requires volatile gaseous anaesthetic agents to deepen and maintain. Dexmedetomidine may be substituted for medetomidine in this last regimen at 0.025–0.05 mg/kg (i.e. half the medetomidine dosage in mg/kg). Medetomidine may be reversed using atipamezole at 1 mg/kg.

Rat, mouse, gerbil and hamster: Ketamine may be used at 75 mg/kg in combination with medetomidine at 0.5 mg/kg in gerbils (Keeble, 2001) and rats (Orr, 2001). Mice may require as much as 1 mg/kg medetomidine (Orr, 2001). The advantages of the alpha-2 agonists are that they produce good analgesia (which ketamine does not) and that they may be quickly reversed with atipamezole at 1 mg/kg. Their disadvantages include severe hypotensive effects, and that once administered they are more difficult to control than a gaseous anaesthetic. Alpha-2 agonists also increase diuresis, promote hyperglycaemia and may exacerbate renal dysfunction by altering renal perfusion.

Guinea pig, degu and chinchilla: Ketamine at 40 mg/kg may be used with medetomidine at 0.5 mg/kg for guinea pigs (Flecknell, 2001), or ketamine at 30 mg/kg with medetomidine at 0.3 mg/kg for chinchillas (Mason, 1997). These doses may be reversed with 1 mg/kg atipamezole. The response to both of these combinations may be improved after an ACP premedication of 0.25 mg/kg. Alternatively, for chinchillas, a ketamine (40 mg/kg) and ACP (0.5 mg/kg) combination can be used (Morgan *et al.*, 1981). Induction takes 5–10 minutes and typically lasts for 45–60 minutes, but recovery may take 2–5 hours for the non-reversible ACP combination, hence reducing the dose of this drug and using the reversible alpha-2 antagonists may be beneficial. I use a combination of 0.2 mg/kg ACP plus 0.05 mg/kg atropine as a premedication followed by 2–4 mg/kg ketamine and 0.02–0.04 mg/kg medetomidine as induction in chinchillas which is suitable for radiography, dental examinations/molar burring and minor invasive procedures with appropriate additional analgesia.

Sugar glider: Ketamine has been used at 2–3 mg/kg with medetomidine at 0.05–0.1 mg/kg intramuscularly for general anaesthesia (Ness and Johnson-Delaney, 2012).

African pygmy hedgehog: Ketamine may be used intramuscularly at 5 mg/kg with medetomidine at 0.1 mg/kg (or alternatively with dexmedetomidine at 0.05 mg/kg) to induce general anaesthesia. Intramuscular injections may be given in the lateral thigh if it can be accessed or in the orbicularis muscle around the ventral edge of the spine-covered skin. Better analgesia and greater muscle relaxation can be gained using 2 mg/kg ketamine with 0.2 mg/kg medetomidine and 0.1 mg/kg fentanyl subcutaneously (Banks *et al.*, 2010). The medetomidine can be reversed with 1 mg/kg atipamezole and the fentanyl with 0.16 mg/kg naloxone.

Ferret: Ketamine may be used alone for chemical restraint in the ferret at doses of 10–20 mg/kg but, as with cats and dogs, the muscle relaxation is poor and salivation can be a problem so it is not recommended. More often, ketamine is combined with other drugs such as the alpha-2 agonists medetomidine and dexmedetomidine. Dosages of 5–8 mg/kg ketamine plus 0.08–0.1 mg/kg medetomidine (or 0.04–0.05 mg/kg dexmedetomidine) have been suggested (Johnson-Delaney, 2009; Morrisey, 2013). Alternatively, a triple combination of 5 mg/kg ketamine plus 0.08 mg/kg medetomidine plus 0.1 mg/kg butorphanol has also been recommended (Evans and Springsteen, 1998).

Gaseous agents

Table 3.2 gives some advantages and disadvantages of gaseous anaesthetics in small mammals.

Table 3.2 Advantages and disadvantages of gaseous anaesthetics.

Advantages	Disadvantages
Faster alteration of depth of anaesthesia possible	Increased drying effect on respiratory membranes
Recovery times shorter	Hypothermic effect from drying
Less organ metabolism	Difficulty in some species which breath-hold
Delivered in 100% oxygen so better oxygenation than injectables on their own	May be considerably more expensive

Isoflurane

Usually a premedication is used as due to its mildly irritant effects on mucous membranes, breath-holding is common, particularly in rabbits. Its advantage over previous gases such as halothane is in its safety for the debilitated patient. Less than 0.3% of the gas is metabolised hepatically, the rest merely being exhaled for recovery to occur. Recovery is therefore rapid.

Induction levels vary at 2.5–4% and maintenance usually is 1.5–2.5% assuming adequate analgesia. Breath-holding can still be a problem, even with premedication, but the practice of supplying 100% oxygen to the patient for 2 minutes prior to anaesthetic administration helps minimise hypoxia. Isoflurane is then gradually introduced, first 0.5% for 2 minutes, then, assuming regular breathing, increased to 1% for 2 minutes and so on until anaesthetic levels are reached. This allows a smooth induction. Isoflurane is considered the anaesthetic of choice for induction and maintenance in species such as sugar gliders and hedgehogs (Ivey and Carpenter, 2012; Ness and Johnson-Delaney, 2012).

Minimum alveolar concentrations (MAC) for isoflurane are reported as 1.41% in the mouse, 1.38% in the rat and 2.05% in the domestic rabbit (Mazze *et al.*, 1985; Flecknell, 1996; Valverde *et al.*, 2003). As with other species, it should be noted that premedication will reduce the MAC, for example the use of butorphanol as a premedicant in the domestic rabbit reduced the MAC for isoflurane from 2.49 to 2.3%, although interestingly in the same study the use of meloxicam did not reduce the MAC (Turner *et al.*, 2006).

With both isoflurane and sevoflurane usage in the domestic ferret, splenic congestion resulting in a reduction in the packed cell volume and plasma proteins will occur (Marini *et al.*, 1997; Lawson *et al.*, 2006).

Sevoflurane

This gaseous anaesthetic is used commonly in small mammals and has an advantage over isoflurane in that, when it is used as an induction agent, breath-holding is much reduced particularly in rabbits. MAC in rabbits has been reported as 3.7% (Scheller *et al.*, 1988). At levels exceeding 4% on induction it can still induce breath-holding, so it is preferable to use it at 4% for induction and 2–3% for maintenance. In guinea pigs, profuse lacrimation as well as salivation occurs with both isoflurane and sevoflurane and therefore it is advisable to use atropine or glycopyrrolate as a premedicant. In ferrets, the differences in physiological responses such as heart rates, recovery times and indirect blood pressure assessments between isoflurane and sevoflurane were not considered significant (Lawson *et al.*, 2006).

Maintenance of anaesthesia

Intubation

As with all gaseous anaesthetics, the placement of an endotracheal tube for maintenance after induction is to be recommended whenever possible. This is relatively straightforward in ferrets, being much the same procedure as for cats.

In rabbits of 1.5–3 kg, the use of a number 1 Wisconsin flat-bladed paediatric laryngoscope and a 2–3 mm tube is advised. The rabbit is first induced either with an injectable anaesthetic or with an inhalational one. Two different procedures can then occur: the animal can be placed in dorsal recumbency, allowing the larynx to fall dorsally and into view, the tongue pulled out to one side and the laryngoscope and endotracheal tube inserted (see Figure 3.5); alternatively the animal may be kept in sternal recumbency but the soft palate needs to be pushed dorsally to allow the epiglottis to fall into the oropharynx. In both cases a guide wire may first be passed through the laryngeal opening and, once in, the endotracheal (ET) tube is threaded over the top and the wire withdrawn to facilitate intubation.

If the rabbit and so the ET tube is of sufficient size, a rigid endoscope may be inserted through the ET tube like a guide wire, and then the insertion into the trachea can be directly visualised (see Figure 3.6).

Alternatively the rabbit may be intubated blindly. This is performed in sternal recumbency, after initial induction. The head is lifted vertically off the table and the ET tube is inserted orally in the midline until slight resistance and a cough is elicited. It is then advanced slowly, and air passage through the tube checked to ensure correct placement.

Use of supraglottic devices has also become commonplace in rabbits and indeed, where suitable, other small mammals. Such devices (e.g. **v-gel**® Advanced Rabbit; Docsinnovent Ltd. www.docsinnovent.com) come in a range of sizes to match breed and age variations in rabbits. They function as a normal ET tube, except instead of the tube passing through the glottis and into the trachea, the end of the tube sits above the glottis with an inflatable cuff that

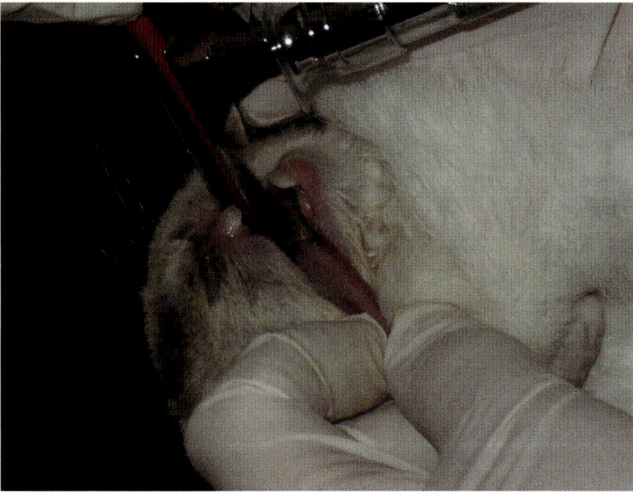

Figure 3.5 Insertion of a laryngoscope and ET tube in an already anaesthetised rabbit in dorsal recumbency. Note the careful lateral displacement of the tongue to avoid laceration on the incisors.

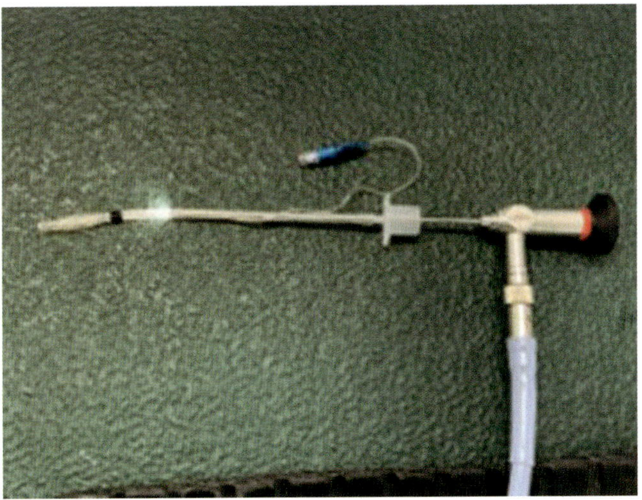

Figure 3.6 For sufficient sized ET tubes, an endoscope may be inserted through them like a guide wire to allow direct visualisation of its insertion into the trachea.

secures the airway. A distal segment to the device plugs the oesophagus to minimise the chance of air moving into the stomach and so reducing diaphragmatic movement which may impede respiration (see Figures 3.7 and 3.8). A capnograph should always be attached to the device to ensure the anaesthetist is aware of any airway occlusion as clearly movement of the patient in relation to the device can lead to occlusion of the airway as the device does not enter the trachea.

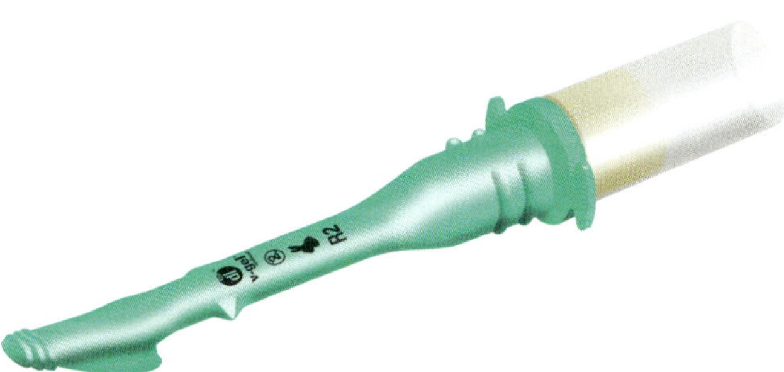

Figure 3.7 **v-gel** Advanced Rabbit airway device. *Source:* Courtesy of Docsinnovent Ltd. www.docsinnovent.com.

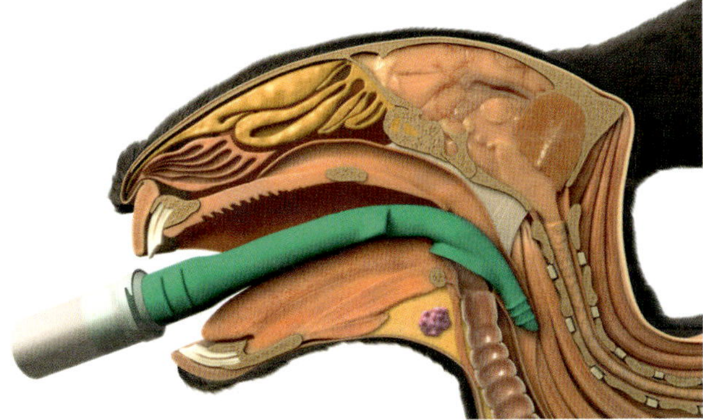

Figure 3.8 Diagram of the **v-gel** Advanced Rabbit airway device inserted correctly so that it sits above the glottis. *Source:* Courtesy of Docsinnovent Ltd. www.docsinnovent.com.

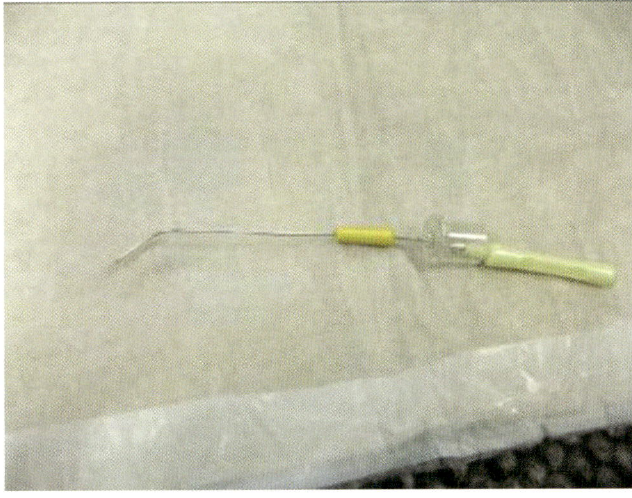

Figure 3.9 A guide wire is a flexible wire that is inserted through the ET tube to stiffen it and facilitate the tube's insertion through the glottis and into the trachea. Once the ET tube with wire is inserted into the trachea, the wire is then withdrawn leaving the ET tube in place which may then be connected to the anaesthetic circuit.

Intubation is a specialised procedure for rodents such as rats and mice where rigid guide tubes and wires and smaller scopes are used to guide the tube into the larynx. If intubation is not possible, then oxygen on its own or with an anaesthetic gas may be supplied via an intranasal catheter as rodents are obligate nose breathers.

Intubation of chinchillas, guinea-pigs and degus can be difficult not only because of their small size but also because of the palatal ostium. Effectively the soft palate is continuous with the base of the tongue and the epiglottis is locked into the nasopharynx through a hole in the soft palate known as the palatal ostium. In order to intubate such hystricomorphs, a guide wire can assist by pushing the soft palate rostral to the epiglottis dorsally to attempt to 'pop' the epiglottis into the oral cavity (see Figure 3.9).

Intubation of omnivorous marsupials is more straightforward as they have a large oral opening. However, the small overall body size of the sugar glider may still make it a challenge. Similarly the African pygmy hedgehog has a large gape and so visualisation of the glottis is relatively straightforward; however, their small size can still make it complicated and use of a thin guide wire can facilitate insertion of the tube.

Intubation of ferrets is similar to that for cats. They should be first induced or if injectable anaesthesia is used, deepened by face mask with a gaseous anaesthetic before intubation is attempted.

In rabbits and ferrets it is helpful to use xylocaine spray on the larynx to reduce laryngospasm and aid intubation (see Figure 3.10). Where the glottis cannot be visualised, spraying the end of the endotracheal tube can assist in removing post-anaesthetic irritation.

Intermittent positive pressure ventilation

Intermittent positive pressure ventilation (IPPV) may be necessary in some individuals that breath-hold during induction. The patient should receive ventilation at their resting respiratory rate. If intubation is not possible then three options are available:

1. Ensure a tight-fitting face mask and use an Ayres T-piece, Mapleson C or modified Bain circuit with 0.5-L bag attached to attempt ventilation.

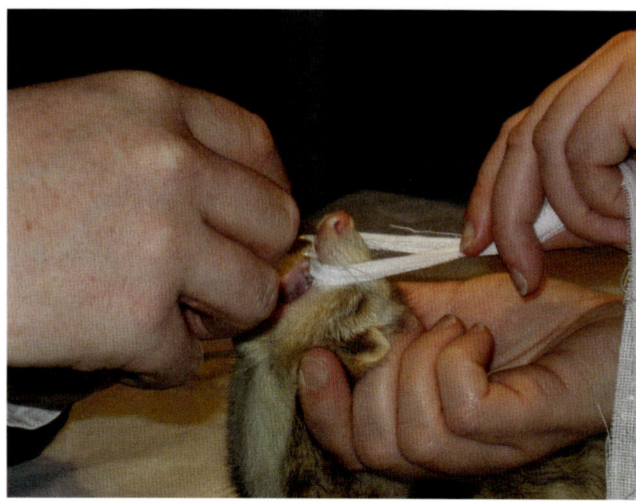

Figure 3.10 Spraying the larynx, which is easily visualised, is advised prior to inserting an ET tube in the ferret.

2. Place a nasopharygeal tube, via the medial meatus of the nose, into the pharyngeal area. Then supply 4 L or so of oxygen (to combat the resistance of the small diameter tubing of 1–2 mm) via this route. This cannot be done in mammals smaller than a young guinea pig.
3. Perform an emergency tracheostomy, in the case of a small rodent, with a 25–27 gauge needle attached to the oxygen outlet, placing the needle between the supporting C-shaped laryngeal cartilages ventrally.

Anaesthetic circuits

Most of the small mammals described here are less than 2 kg in weight. For this reason an Ayres T-piece (equivalent to a Mapleson E), modified (mini) Bain (equivalent to mini-Mapleson D) or Mapleson C circuit are the best ones to use as they provide the minimum of dead space. For larger rabbits, an Ayres T-piece is usually sufficient.

Tidal volumes for the domestic rabbit are typically 4–6 mL/kg body weight.

Supportive therapy during and after anaesthesia

Recumbency

For most surgical procedures, the positioning for restraint or recumbency will be dependent upon the area being operated on. This may necessitate the patient being placed in dorsal recumbency. Because small herbivores rely on their gut flora to aid digestion, most of them have developed an enlarged hindgut. When in dorsal recumbency there is a lot of weight on the diaphragm, and as the majority of small mammals considered here are diaphragm breathers, the hindrance to inspiration is significant. During lengthy surgical procedures, this may lead to apnoea and hypoxia. Therefore, place the patient with its cranial end elevated above the caudal when in dorsal recumbency by placing it on a tilted table or on a foam wedge. This allows gravity to draw the intestines, liver and stomach away from the diaphragm.

Maintenance of body temperature

Maintenance of core body temperature is vitally important in all patients to ensure successful recovery from anaesthesia, but is particularly important in small mammals. This is primarily due to their increased surface area to volume ratio, allowing more heat to escape per gram of animal. To help minimise this, the following actions may be taken:

- Perform minimal surgical scrubbing of the site, and minimal clipping of fur from the area. Do not use surgical spirit as this rapidly cools the skin.
- Ensure the environmental room temperature is around 20°C.
- Place the patient onto either a water-circulating heat pad or a hot air blanket, or use nitrile gloves/hot water bottles grouped around the patient (making sure that the containers are not in direct contact with the patient as skin burns may ensue).
- Administer warmed isotonic fluids subcutaneously, intravenously or intraperitoneally prior to and during surgery.

Anaesthetic gases in oxygen have a rapidly cooling effect on the oral and respiratory membranes, and so patients maintained on gaseous anaesthetics or supplemental oxygen will cool down quicker than those on injectable ones. This effect will worsen as the length of the anaesthesia increases.

It is worth noting, however, that hyperthermia may be as bad as hypothermia. Small mammals generally have few or no sweat glands, so heat cannot be lost via this route. In addition, very few actually pant to lose heat, so if over-warmed the core body temperature rises and irreversible hyperthermia will occur. A rectal thermometer is useful for monitoring body temperature and where large enough an oesophageal thermometer may also be used. Normal body temperature ranges are given in Table 3.3.

Table 3.3 Normal body temperatures for selected small mammals.

Species	Normal body temperature range (°C)
Rabbit	37–39.4
Guinea pig	37.2–39.5
Chinchilla	37.8–39.2
Degu	36–37.9
Rat	37.6–38.6
Mouse	37–38
Gerbil	37.5–39
Hamster (Syrian)	36.2–37.5
Chipmunk	37.8–39.6
Prairie dog	38–39
African pygmy hedgehog	35.4–37
Marsupial	34–35 (sugar glider) 32.2–35 (Virginia opossum)
Ferret	37.8–40

Fluid therapy

Preoperative, intraoperative and postoperative fluid therapy is important in small mammals, even for routine surgery. The small size and relatively large body surface area in relation to volume of these patients mean that they will dehydrate much faster, gram for gram, than a larger cat or dog. Studies have shown that the provision of maintenance levels of fluids to small mammals during and immediately after routine surgery improved anaesthetic safety levels by as much as 15% in some cases, with higher levels if the surgery was being performed on severely debilitated animals.

It is therefore recommended that all small mammal patients receive fluids during and after an anaesthetic be it routine or not. For further information see Chapter 6.

Monitoring anaesthesia

No one factor will allow you to assess anaesthetic depth. Indeed, in small mammals many of the useful techniques used in cats and dogs are irrelevant. Eye position, for example, should not be used to assess depth of anaesthesia in small mammals. Instead, a useful method is to assess the response to noxious stimuli such as pain.

The first reflex lost is usually the righting reflex – the animal is unable to return to ventral recumbency.

The next reflex to be lost, for example in rabbits and guinea pigs, is the swallow reflex. However, this may be difficult to assess. Palpebral reflexes (the response of blinking when the periocular area is lightly touched) are generally lost early on in the course of anaesthetic, but rabbits may retain this reflex until well into the deeper planes of surgical anaesthesia. The palpebral reflex is also affected by the anaesthetic agent used. Most inhalant gaseous anaesthetics cause loss of the reflex early on, but it is maintained with ketamine.

The pedal withdrawal reflex is useful in small mammals, with the leg being extended and the toe firmly pinched. Loss of this reflex suggests surgical planes of anaesthesia, but again rabbits will retain the pedal reflex in the forelimbs until much deeper (and often dangerously deep) planes of anaesthesia are reached. Other pain stimuli such as the ear pinch in the guinea pig and rabbit are useful. Loss of this indicates a surgical plane, as does the loss of the tail pinch reflex in rats and mice.

Monitoring of the pulse, heart and circulation may be done in a conventional manner, with stethoscope and femoral pulse evaluation, or, in the larger species, an oesophageal stethoscope may be used. Use of an electrocardiogram (ECG) may also be helpful in assessing heart rates (see below). Increases in respiratory and heart rates can indicate lightening of the plane of anaesthesia, but tachycardia may occur immediately prior to arrest, often following a period of brief bradycardia.

Pulse oximetry may be used in rabbits, but many oximeters will not read heart rates above 250 beats per minute, so care should be taken in the reliance on these, especially in smaller rodents with faster heart rates. The ear artery may be used with pulse oximeters, as may the ventral tail artery or a toe artery in larger rabbits. If the tongue is available then this may also be used. As with cats and dogs, the aim is to achieve 100% saturation, and levels below 93% would indicate significant hypoxaemia and the initiation of assisted ventilation.

Other forms of cardiac monitoring include the ECG. The recording devices can be adapted to minimise trauma by substituting fine needle probes for alligator forceps, or by blunting the alligator teeth or more commonly by using sticky contact pads. Oesophageal ECG probes are generally too large to be of use in most small mammals. ECGs are particularly useful for detecting heart block, which is common in a wide range of small mammals during anaesthesia, and where hyperkalaemia is present (e.g. with urinary obstruction). If detected early on in stage 1 heart block (elongation of the P–QRS interval) then reversal with a parasympatholytic may prevent progression to stage 2 (not every P wave is followed by a QRS) or stage 3 (disconnection between P and QRS complexes) which become increasingly difficult to reverse and eventually result in cardiac arrest.

Doppler probes that can detect blood flow in the smallest of vessels up to the heart itself are also useful. The Doppler probe converts blood flow into an audible signal, which is transmitted through a speaker device. This can then be assessed by the anaesthetist during surgery for changes in strength of output and heart rate. Doppler probes can also be used to measure non-invasive blood pressures in species large enough (such as the domestic rabbit and ferret). The principles are the same as those used in domestic cats, with a cuff (40% of the limb diameter) being placed distal to the elbow and the Doppler probe placed proximal to the ventral carpus. An average of five readings is usually taken and typical systolic blood pressure in normal rabbits and ferrets is 90–130 mmHg. Alternatively, direct blood pressure monitoring can be carried out by catheterising a peripheral artery such as the central ear artery in the rabbit (although this can be associated with occlusion of the vessel and loss of the ear tip and so is less commonly performed).

Respiratory monitors may be used if the patient is intubated and many pulse oximeters have outlets for these. Their use allows assessment of respiratory rates, which for rodents are typically 50–100 breaths per minute and for rabbits and ferrets around 40–50 breaths per minute. A reduction by 50% or more in this rate would give cause for concern.

Capnographs can also be used but obviously neither these, nor respiratory monitors, are useful for patients maintained on face masks or on injectable anaesthetics alone. In addition, because of the small lung capacity and the need to minimise dead space, only side-stream capnographs can be used and these may not always give accurate readings. However, changes in the trend can still be more useful than relying on absolute figures. Capnography is important where supraglottic devices are being used, in particular as they can give early warning of airway occlusion. The majority of species considered here have an end-tidal carbon dioxide level of 35–45 mmHg when normal cardiorespiratory function is present.

Blood sampling during anaesthesia using a point of care analyser can be helpful in ensuring any serious physiological changes are rapidly identified and corrected. Table 3.4 lists some normal blood parameters for anaesthetised small mammals.

Recovery and analgesia

Recovery

Recovery from anaesthesia is hastened and improved with the use of suitable reversal agents, if available. Examples include atipamezole after medetomidine/dexmedetomidine anaesthesia or sedation, and naloxone, butorphanol or buprenorphine after full opiate agonist (including fentanyl) anaesthesia or sedation. Gaseous

Table 3.4 Normal blood parameters for anaesthetised selected small mammals.

Parameter (arterial blood)	Rabbits (Ardiaca *et al.*, 2013)	Guinea pigs (Bar-Ilan and Marder, 1980*; Sanchez-Aparicio *et al.*, 2009†)	Rats (Brun-Pascaud *et al.*, 1982)
pH	7.358–7.502	*7.444 ± 0.032 †7.28–7.55	7.47 ± 0.02
PCO_2 (mmHg)	29.1–36.8	*35.7 ± 4.4 †28–44	34.5 ± 3
PO_2 (mmHg)	75–101	*91.9 ± 7.3 †18–70	90 ± 5.5
SpO_2 (%)	93–96	–	–
HCO_3^- (mmol/L)	17.5–27.6	*24.4 ± 2.8	25.5 ± 1.5
Total CO_2 (mmol/L)	18–29	–	–
Base excess (mmol/L)	−12	*+0.4 ± 2.1	–
Na (mmol/L)	136–142	†124–141	141–145
K (mmol/L)	3.5–5.1	†3–7.5	3.3–3.9
iCa (mmol/L)	1.67–1.85	†0.52–1.47	–
Haematocrit (%)	23–42	†27–49	–
Glucose (mg/dL)	106–205	†64–211	–
Lactate (mg/dL)	–	†0.3–6.6	–

anaesthesia, particularly with isoflurane, tends to result in more rapid recovery than injectable anaesthetics, but recovery from all forms of anaesthesia is improved by ensuring adequate maintenance of body temperature and fluid balance during and after anaesthesia.

Most small mammals will benefit from a quiet, darkened and warm recovery area. Subsequent fluid administration the same day is also beneficial, as many of these creatures will not be eating as normal for the first 12–24 hours.

Recovery temperatures of 24–26°C are recommended for most small mammals where a degree of cooling has occurred. This should be reduced to their normal thermal range (see Chapter 2) as soon as they are recovered to prevent hyperthermia developing.

Analgesia

Recognising pain in small mammals

This can be one of the most challenging aspects of small mammal medicine. The species that we are dealing with here are all prey species and as such there is a survival benefit in not showing signs of illness or pain. When in pain, many small mammals will become anorexic and due to their high metabolic rates will rapidly lose weight. Heart and respiratory rates will often increase – but remember that small mammals in strange surroundings with a fear response will also have elevated respiratory and heart rates. Additionally, as most rodents will have a heart rate in excess of 300 beats per minute, this can be a difficult parameter to measure with accuracy.

The following clinical signs may indicate pain in rodents (Miller and Richardson, 2011):

- Abnormal appearance, including lack of grooming, piloerection, hunched position and porphyrin staining in rats; facial changes in mice, for example orbital tightening, nose bulges and cheek bulges.
- Changes to normal behaviour: for example a decrease in normal exploratory behaviours – such as walking, sniffing – and an increase in sleeping; also, a decrease in food and water consumption.
- Guarding behaviour with alteration in body posture, preventing contact with the affected area.
- Self-mutilation with excessive grooming, licking, biting, scratching of the painful area.
- Vocalisation when the painful area is palpated. In guinea pigs, there may be a reduction in vocalisation with pain.
- Specific behaviour changes: for example belly pressing (particularly rats and mice with abdominal pain), abdominal contractions, twitching, back arching, raised tail (particularly mice) and increased aggression.

In addition to these, grimace scales have been derived for rabbits, rats and mice. These focus on the shape of the animal's face, particularly looking at eye opening, ear position, mouth outline and nose. The Grimace Scale for rabbits for example grades increasing levels of pain associated with wrinkling of the skin over the dorsal nasal area, narrowing of the ocular aperture, flattening of the ears to the head and caudal drawing of the corners of the mouth (Keating *et al.*, 2012). Scales based on similar physical features have been derived for mice (Langford *et al.*, 2010) and rats (Sotocina *et al.*, 2011). More recently, a different rabbit pain scale has been derived by Bristol University focusing on six parameters: demeanour, locomotion, posture, ear position, eyes and grooming. This is combined with four intensities of pain (0, 1, 2 and 3) giving a total score of 0–18 (Benato *et al.*, 2022).

A new pain scoring system has been devised in guinea pigs that uses a complex multidimensional scale composed of 14 descriptors grouped into four categories (appearance, function, physiology and

Table 3.5 Analgesics used in small mammals.

Drug	Rabbit	Myomorph rodent	Chinchilla and degu	Guinea pig	Chipmunk and prairie dog	Marsupial	African pygmy hedgehog	Ferret
Butorphanol (IM)	0.1–0.5 q2–4h	0.2–2 q4h mice, rats 1–5 q4h gerbils, hamsters, mice	0.5–2 q4–8h	0.5–1 q4–8h	1–5 q4h	0.2–0.5 q4h	0.3–0.5 q4h	0.3 q4h
Buprenorphine (IM)	0.01–0.05 q8–12h	0.02–0.05 q8–12h (NB: may be as high as 0.5 q8h in hamsters and rats)	0.01–0.05 q8–12h	0.01–0.05 q8–12h	0.01–0.05 q8–12h	0.01–0.03 q8–12h	0.01–0.05 q8–12h	0.01–0.03 q8–12h
Carprofen (PO, IM)	2–4 q24h	5 q24h	2–5 q24h	2–5 q24h	1–4 q24h	–	1 q12–24h	1–2 q24h
Fentanyl (IM, IV, transdermal)	0.03–0.3 q4–6h IM 7.5 μg/kg q20 min IV 30–100 μg/kg/hour by continuous rate infusion IV during anaesthesia 12–25 μg/hour transdermal	Rats: initial loading dose 5–10 μg/kg IV; 10–30 μg/kg/hour as continuous rate infusion IV during anaesthesia 1.25–5 μg/kg q1h IV postoperatively 3.5 q12h (mice slow-release formulation subcutaneously, some sedation)	–	Initial loading dose 5–10 μg/kg IV; 10–30 μg/kg/hour as continuous rate infusion IV during anaesthesia 1.25–5 μg/kg q1h IV postoperatively	–	–	–	Initial loading dose 5–10 μg/kg IV; 10–30 μg/kg/hour as continuous rate infusion IV during anaesthesia 1.25–5 μg/kg q1h IV postoperatively
Gabapentin (PO)	15–30 q8h	30 q8h (rats) 50 q24 (hamsters)	–	–	30 q8h (prairie dogs)	–	–	10 q8h
Meloxicam (IM, PO)	0.3–0.6 q12–24h	0.5–1 q24h 1–5 q24h (rats and mice)	0.3–0.6 q24h	0.3–0.6 q24h	0.3–0.6 q24h	0.2–0.4 q24h	0.2 mg/kg q24h	0.2 q24h
Methadone (IM)	0.2 q4–6h	0.5–3 q4–6h (rats)	0.2 q4–6h	0.2 q4–6h	0.2 q4–6h	0.2 q4–6h	0.1–0.2 q4–6h	0.2–0.5 q2–3h
Morphine (IM)	2–5 q3–4h	2–5 q3–4h	2–5 q3–4h	2–5 q3–4h	2–5 q3–4h	2–5 q3–4h	2–5 q3–4h	2–5 q3–4h (NB: even at 0.1–0.3 vomiting has been observed)
Tramadol (PO)	10–15 q12–24h	25 q8–12h (in mice, may not be sufficient analgesia)	5–10 q8–12h	5–10 q8–12h	5–10 q8–12h	5–10 q12h	5–10 q12h	10 q8–12h

Values are in mg/kg body weight unless stated otherwise.
q4h, every 4 hours; q8h, every 8 hours, and so on. PO, per os (orally); IM, intramuscularly; IV, intravenously.
Sources: data from Oates and Tarbert (2023), Ozawa *et al.* (2023), Petritz and de Matos (2023), Kapaldo and Esher (2022), Hawkins (2015), Brust and Pye (2013), Carpenter and Marion (2013), Mayer (2013), Fiorello and Divers (2013), Morrisey (2013), Banks *et al.* (2010), Johnson-Delaney (2010), Flecknell (1998, 2006) and Mason (1997).

behaviours). A score ranging from 0 to 3 is given to each item with a maximum total score of 26 (Benedetti et al. 2024).

Analgesia is vitally important to a quick and smooth recovery process. The time taken to return to normal activities such as grooming, eating and drinking has been shown to be considerably shortened following adequate analgesia. Dosages for analgesics frequently used in small mammals are given in Table 3.5. The administration of analgesia prior to the onset of pain makes for the most effective control. In the case of non-steroidal anti-inflammatory drugs (NSAIDs), cyclooxygenase (COX)-2 inhibitors are preferable, for example meloxicam or carprofen. Meloxicam has been used at 1.5 mg/kg once daily orally for 5 days with no significant changes in biochemistry or detectable deterioration in the health of the rabbit (Turner *et al.*, 2006). Indeed, there is evidence that the routinely published doses of meloxicam are not sufficient for post-surgical analgesia in rabbits. Meloxicam at 1 mg/kg per os post surgery followed by 0.5 mg/kg once daily on the following 2 days produced a significant reduction in some pain-associated behaviours associated with ovariohysterectomy (Leach *et al.*, 2009). As always, care should be exercised in the use of NSAIDs in renally compromised animals.

There are a number of issues when considering analgesia in small mammals, not least of which is the lack of reliable pharmacokinetic, safety and efficacy data for many drugs routinely used in domestic animals such as cats and dogs.

Full opioid agonists may slow intestinal motility and therefore their use in hindgut fermenters such as rabbits, chinchillas and guinea pigs should be accompanied by gut motility-enhancing medications. They can of course also produce respiratory suppression. Buprenorphine does have some of these effects but as a partial agonist they are significantly less than those of morphine, fentanyl or methadone. Tramadol has been used successfully at 10 mg/kg in the rabbit. However, pharmacokinetic data suggested that 11 mg/kg orally did not achieve the necessary levels in the bloodstream to provide analgesia in humans (Souza *et al.*, 2008).

Multimodal analgesia is also important as with other mammals, as the combination of NSAIDs and opioids is of greater benefit than the sum of their individual parts. The use of facilitating drugs such as low-dose ketamine (1 mg/kg) and alpha-2 drugs such as medetomidine (0.01 mg/kg) to facilitate other analgesics such as opiates is well known in domestic animals such as cats and dogs and is being used increasingly in the small mammals discussed here. Maropitant, a neurokinin-1 receptor antagonist, has also been used in dogs and cats to control visceral pain as well as to prevent vomiting, its main effect. It may also be useful in small mammals such as rabbits and guinea pigs where visceral pain exists, although it should be avoided where underlying cardiac disease is present due to its mechanism of action through binding to calcium and potassium channels. It may have some benefit in cases of ulcerative skin disease associated with pruritus in rodents such as mice (Le, 2017).

Local anaesthesia may be used in rabbits and rodents at a maximum of 2 mg/kg lidocaine. This is useful for head surgery where infraorbital nerve, mental nerve, mandibular nerve, maxillary nerve and palatine nerve blocks may be performed as with cats and dogs.

Choice of analgesic depends on the level of pain and other factors, such as concurrent disease processes. Flunixin, for example, is not a good analgesic to use in dehydrated animals or those with renal disease. Any NSAID should be used with caution where underlying renal disease or gastric ulceration is present or suspected as previously mentioned. Opioids depress respiration and so may be contraindicated in cases of severe respiratory disease. Buprenorphine frequently requires two to three times daily administration, while carprofen and meloxicam have been shown to be useful when given only once daily; however, with some rodents and even rabbits, more frequent administration may be required in more severe pain situations. Gabapentin has been shown to be particularly useful in a range of species where neuropathic and chronic pain is experienced. It is believed to work by decreasing central nervous system sensitivity to stimulation by binding to calcium channels in the dorsal horn of the spinal cord and may also bind to *N*-methyl-D-aspartate (NMDA) receptors. Tramadol is a weak opiate but also inhibits serotonin and noradrenaline (norepinephrine) reuptake.

References

Ardiaca, M., Bonvehi, C. and Montesinos, A. (2013) Point-of-care blood gas and electrolyte analysis in rabbits. *Veterinary Clinics of North America: Exotic Animal Practice*, **16**(1), 175–195.

Banks, R.E., Sharp, J.M., Doss, S.D. and Vanderford, D.A. (2010) Chapter 13 Hedgehogs. In: *Exotic Small Mammal Care and Husbandry*, pp. 143–155. Wiley-Blackwell, Durham.

Bar-Ilan, A. and Marder, J. (1980) Acid base status in unanesthetised, unrestrained guinea pigs. *Pflügers Archiv*, **384**, 93–97.

Benato, L., Murrell, J. and Rooney, N. (2022) Bristol Rabbit Pain Scale (BRPS): clinical utility, validity and reliability. *BMC Veterinary Research*, **18**(1), 341. doi: 10.1186/s12917-022-03434-x.

Benedetti, F., Pignon, C., Muffat-es-Jacques, P. *et al.* (2024) Development and validation of a pain scale in guinea pig (*Cavia porcellus*). *Journal of Exotic Pet Medicine*, **50**, 36–41. doi: 10.1053/j.jepm.2024.06.002.

Brodbelt, D.C., Blissitt, K.J., Hammond, R.A. *et al.* (2008) The risk of death: the confidential enquiry into perioperative small animal fatalities. *Veterinary Anaesthesia and Analgesia*, **35**(5), 365–373.

Brun-Pascaud, M., Gaudebout, C., Blayo, M.C. and Pocidalo, J.J. (1982) Arterial blood gases and acid–base status in awake rats. *Respiratory Physiology*, **48**(1), 45–57.

Brust, D.M. and Pye, G.W. (2013) Sugar gliders. In: *Exotic Animal Formulary* (ed. J.W. Carpenter), pp. 439–455. Elsevier Saunders, St. Louis, Missouri.

Cantwell, S.L. (2001) Ferret, rabbit and rodent anesthesia. *Veterinary Clinics of North America: Exotic Animal Practice*, **4**, 169–191.

Carpenter, J.W. and Marion, C.J. (2013) Hedgehogs. In: *Exotic Animal Formulary* (ed. J.W. Carpenter), pp. 456–476. Elsevier Saunders, St. Louis, Missouri.

Doss, G. and de Miguel Garcia, C. (2022) African pygmy hedgehog (*Atelerix albiventris*) and sugar glider (*Petaurus breviceps*) sedation and anesthesia. *Veterinary Clinics of North America: Exotic Animal Practice*, **25**, 257–272.

Evans, A.T. and Springsteen, K.K. (1998) Anesthesia of ferrets. *Seminars in Avian and Exotic Pet Medicine*, **7**, 48–52.

Fiorello, C.V. and Divers, S.J. (2013) Rabbits. In: *Exotic Animal Formulary* (ed. J.W. Carpenter), 4th edn, pp. 518–560. Elsevier, St Louis, Missouri.

Flecknell, P. (1996) *Laboratory Animal Anaesthesia*, 2nd edn. Academic Press, New York.

Flecknell, P.A. (1998) Analgesia in small mammals. *Seminars in Avian and Exotic Pet Medicine*, **7**(1), 41–47.

Flecknell, P. (2001) Guinea pigs. In: *Manual of Exotic Pets* (eds A. Meredith & S. Redrobe), 4th edn, pp. 52–64. BSAVA, Quedgeley, UK.

Flecknell, P.A. (2006) Anaesthesia and perioperative care. In: *Manual of Rabbit Medicine and Surgery* (ed. P. Flecknell), 2nd edn, pp. 154–165. BSAVA, Cheltenham, UK.

Hawkins, M.G. (2015) Advances in exotic mammal therapeutics. *Veterinary Clinics of North America: Exotic Animal Practice*, **18**, 323–337.

Ivey, E. and Carpenter, J.W. (2012) African hedgehogs. In: *Ferrets, Rabbits, and Rodents: Clinical Medicine and Surgery* (eds K.E. Quesenberry & J.W. Carpenter), 3rd edn, pp. 411–428. St. Louis, Saunders-Elsevier.

Johnson-Delaney, C. (2009) Ferrets: anaesthesia and analgesia. In: *Manual of Rodents and Ferrets* (eds E. Keeble & A. Meredith), 1st edn, pp. 245–253. BSAVA, Quedgeley, UK.

Johnson-Delaney, C. (2010) Marsupials. In: *Manual of Exotic Pets* (eds A. Meredith & C. Johnson-Delaney), 5th edn, pp. 103–126. BSAVA, Quedgeley, UK.

Kapaldo, N. and Esher, D. (2022) Ferret sedation and anesthesia. *Veterinary Clinics of North America: Exotic Animal Practice*, **25**, 273–296.

Keating, S.C.J., Thomas, A.A., Flecknell, P.A. and Leach, M.C. (2012) Evaluation of EMLA cream for preventing pain during tattooing of rabbits: changes in physiological, behavioural and facial expression responses. *PLoS One*, **7**(9), e44437. doi: 10.1371/journal.pone.0044437.

Keeble, E. (2001) Gerbils. In: *Manual of Exotic Pets* (eds A. Meredith & S. Redrobe), 4th edn, pp. 34–46. BSAVA, Cheltenham, UK.

Langford, D.J., Bailey, A.L., Chanda, M.L. *et al.* (2010) Coding of facial expressions of pain in the laboratory mouse. *Nature Methods*, **7**(6), 447–449. doi: 10.1038/nmeth.1455.

Lawson, A.K., Lichtenberger, M., Day, T. *et al.* (2006) Comparison of sevoflurane and isoflurane in domestic ferrets (*Mustela putorius furo*). *Veterinary Therapeutics*, **7**, 207–212.

Le, K. (2017) Maropitant. *Journal of Exotic Pet Medicine*, **26**(4), 305–309.

Leach, M.C., Allweiler, S., Richardson, C. *et al.* (2009) Behavioural effects of ovariohysterectomy and oral administration of meloxicam in laboratory housed rabbits. *Research in Veterinary Science*, **87**(2), 336–347.

Marini, R.P. and Fox, J.G. (1998) Anesthesia, surgery, and biomethodology. In: *Biology and Diseases of the Ferret* (ed. J.G. Fox), pp. 449–484. Williams and Wilkins, Philadelphia.

Marini, R.P., Callahan, R.J., Jackson, L.R. *et al.* (1997) Distribution of technetium 99m-labeled red blood cells during isoflurane anesthesia in ferrets. *American Journal of Veterinary Research*, **58**, 781–785.

Mason, D.E. (1997) Anaesthesia, analgesia and sedation for small mammals. In: *Ferrets, Rabbits and Rodents* (eds E.V. Hillyer & K.E. Quesenberry), pp. 378–391. W.B. Saunders, Philadelphia, PA.

Mayer, J. (2013) Rodents. In: *Exotic Animal Formulary* (ed. J.W. Carpenter), pp. 477–517. Elsevier Saunders, St. Louis, Missouri.

Mazze, R.I., Rice, S.A. and Baden, J.M. (1985) Halothane, isoflurane, and enflurane MAC in pregnant and nonpregnant female and male mice and rats. *Anaesthesiology*, **62**, 339–341.

Miller, A.L. and Richardson, C.A. (2011) Rodent analgesia. *Veterinary Clinics of North America: Exotic Animal Practice*, **14**, 81–92.

Morgan, R.J., Eddy, L.B., Solie, T.N. and Turbe, C.C. (1981) Ketamine–acepromazine as anaesthetic agent for chinchillas (*Chinchilla laniger*). *Laboratory Animals*, **15**, 281–283.

Morrisey, J.K. (2013) Chapter 10 Ferrets. In: *Exotic Animal Formulary* (ed. J.W. Carpenter), pp. 560–594. Elsevier Saunders, St. Louis, Missouri.

Ness, R.D. and Johnson-Delaney, C.A. (2012) Sugar gliders. In: *Ferrets, Rabbits and Rodents: Clinical Medicine and Surgery* (eds K.E. Quesenberry & J.W. Carpenter), 3rd edn, pp. 393–410. Saunders Elsevier, St Louis.

Oates, R. and Tarbert, D.K. (2023) Treatment of pain in rats, mice and prairie dogs. *Veterinary Clinics of North America: Exotic Animal Practice*, **26**, 151–174.

Orr, H. (2001) Rats and mice. In: *Manual of Exotic Pets* (eds A. Meredith & S. Redrobe), 4th edn, pp. 13–25. BSAVA, Cheltenham, UK.

Ozawa, S., Cenani, A., Guzman, D. and S.-M. (2023) Treatment of pain in rabbits. *Veterinary Clinics of North America: Exotic Animal Practice*, **26**, 201–227.

Petritz, O.A. and de Matos, R. (2023) Treatment of pain in ferrets. *Veterinary Clinics of North America: Exotic Animal Practice*, **26**, 245–255.

Sanchez-Aparicio, P., Mota-Rojas, D., Verduzco-Mendoza, A. *et al.* (2009) Reference values for blood gas analysis, electrolytes and critical biochemical variables for short-hair-English and Duncan-Hartley guinea pigs anaesthetized with xylazine-ketamine. *Journal of Animal and Veterinary Advances*, **8**(10), 1893–1899.

Scheller, M.S., Daidman, L.J. and Partridge, B.L. (1988) MAC of sevoflurane in humans and the New Zealand white rabbit. *Canadian Journal of Anesthesia*, **35**, 153–156.

Sotocina, S.G., Sorge, R.E., Zaloum, A. *et al.* (2011) The Rat Grimace Scale: a partially automated method for quantifying pain in the laboratory rat via facial expressions. *Molecular Pain*, **7**, 55. doi: 10.1186/1744-8069-7-55.

Souza, M.J., Greenacre, C.B. and Cox, S.K. (2008) Pharmacokinetics of orally administered tramadol in the domestic rabbit (*Oryctolagus cuniculus*). *American Journal of Veterinary Research*, **69**(8), 979–982.

Turner, P.V., Kerr, C.L. and Healy, A.J. (2006) Effect of meloxicam and butorphanol on minimum alveolar concentration of isoflurane in rabbits. *American Journal of Veterinary Research*, **67**, 770–774.

Valverde, A., Morey, T.E., Hernandez, J. and Davies, W. (2003) Validation of several types of noxious stimuli for use in determining the minimum alveolar concentration for inhalation anesthetics in dogs and rabbits. *American Journal of Veterinary Research*, **64**, 957–962.

Chapter 4 Small Mammal Nutrition

Classification

One way of classifying small mammals is according to their diet. There are three main categories of the commonly seen small mammals as defined by their diet.

Carnivores

The main carnivore seen in small mammal practice is the ferret, which, like the cat, is totally carnivorous. To cope with this diet, the ferret has developed sharp shearing teeth and powerful crushing jaws. In addition, because its diet consists of highly digestible fats and proteins, it has a very short gastrointestinal tract and a rapid digestive tract transit time of around 4 hours.

Herbivores

A variety of species, from lagomorphs such as the domestic rabbit to rodents such as the prairie dog, guinea pig, chinchilla and degu, are herbivores. Their cheek teeth are grinding in nature. Some species have continually growing/erupting premolars, molars and incisors, and their gastrointestinal tracts are long and often sacculated. This increases their volume and allows the bacterial fermentation that assists digestion of the relatively indigestible cellulose, which forms a large part of their diet in the wild.

Omnivores

Some rodents will eat a mixed diet. Rats and chipmunks will consume meat and eggs if offered, but both species are primarily herbivorous by preference, and true omnivores, such as humans, are uncommon among the small mammals seen routinely. The two species of marsupials we have looked at so far, the sugar glider and the Virginia opossum, are both omnivores as is the African pygmy hedgehog and although the latter is predominantly insectivorous it will readily eat vegetables.

Individual species have become highly evolved to cope with certain types of food. In addition to the above generalisations, we also know that in the wild, many of these creatures have a changing food supply throughout the year.

General nutritional requirements

Water

Maintaining good water quality is important. Many small mammals will dunk food in their water supply or, if the water feeders are poorly situated (in bowls rather than in sip-feeders), some animals may actually defecate in their water bowls. This can cause massive bacterial population explosions which may lead to gastroenteritis. Enriching the water with mineral and vitamin supplements will also allow rapid bacterial growth. It should be noted, however, that whilst nipple water feeders reduce the level of contamination and potentially spillage (the latter is important for arid-preferring rodents such as gerbils that do not like a damp environment), studies have shown that they reduce the overall levels of water consumption and so may increase the risk of urolithiasis and chronic dehydration in rabbits (Tschudin *et al.*, 2011). The recommendation by the authors of this study was that rabbits were given access to an open topped water bowl ad libitum to maximise water intake.

The amount of water an individual small mammal consumes will obviously depend on the diet being offered and the species considered. On dry biscuit or seed-based diets, water consumption will be much higher than for small mammals such as rabbits and guinea pigs, which consume large amounts of fruit and vegetables. A gerbil, for example, is a desert, seed-eating rodent and may only drink 5–10 mL of water in a 24-hour period whereas an average 2 kg rabbit may drink 200 mL or more. Sugar gliders have been reported to require 103 mL water per kilogram body weight on a daily basis either as free water or more usually as part of the wet food they consume (Hume, 1999).

Maintenance energy requirements

Every species has a level of daily energy consumption that is needed to satisfy basic maintenance requirements. It is the energy used purely to maintain current status under minimal activity and hence is frequently the lowest energy requirement during that mammal's life. As with other species a formula has been derived that relates maintenance energy requirements (MER) in kilocalories per day to basal metabolic rate (BMR, the energy requirement when at complete rest) as follows:

$$\text{MER} = \text{constant}(k) \times (\text{body weight})^{0.75}$$

The constant, *k*, varies with family groups and has been estimated at 100 for adult rabbits, increasing to 200 for growth and 300 for lactation (Carpenter *et al.*, 2010). Other small mammals are similar, having much higher metabolic rates than their larger dog and cat counterparts. A generalised formula has also been derived for rodents that varies from the above (Robbins, 1983):

$$\text{BMR} = 358.53 \times (\text{weight in kg})^{0.54}$$

Veterinary Nursing of Exotic Pets and Wildlife, Third Edition. Simon J. Girling.

This has been shown to work well for rodents such as degus (Edwards, 2009). A typical domestic rat would therefore require around 100 kcal/day (419 kJ/day).

The adult domestic ferret has an MER of between 200 and 300 kcal/day (837–1255 kJ/day) (Carpenter *et al.*, 2010).

Marsupials have much lower energy requirements and their *k* factor is around 40–60, which means that obesity is common as owners often feed them the equivalent amount of food that would be fed to a similar-sized eutherian mammal. Studies by Dierenfield *et al.* (2006) suggest that young male sugar gliders require energy levels of between 105 and 147 kJ/day.

Energy requirements give a guide to what a small mammal must consume per day in order to continue to maintain good health and body weight. Hence, if the foods offered are so low in energy content that the small mammal has to eat more of it than will fit into its digestive system in 24 hours, the animal will rapidly lose condition.

An example is that of meat-based foods such as rodent prey which have an energy content of 19–21 kJ/g dry matter (6.3–7.5 kJ/g real or wet weight), whereas high water-content vegetable foods such as lettuce have a lower energy density of 12.5 kJ/g dry matter (0.75 kJ/g real or wet weight). The latter is therefore unlikely to meet the needs of a high-energy-demanding ferret (irrespective of the fact it is a carnivore!) which has a requirement of 837–1255 kJ/kg per day (Carpenter *et al.*, 2010).

Conversely, many pet small mammals will continue to eat until their digestive tracts are full. If all they are offered are the energy-dense seed types (the all-sunflower seed diet) or in the case of African pygmy hedgehogs high-fat invertebrates such as mealworms, then they will rapidly achieve their MER and then exceed it, leading to obesity.

Protein and amino acids

The 10 essential amino acids required by birds and reptiles are also needed by the small mammals considered here, and the concept of biological value of a protein is just as applicable. In addition, it is known that an extra supplement of the amino acid glycine is required for diets low in the amino acids methionine or arginine.

For small mammals, levels of dietary protein on a dry matter basis have been shown to vary from maintenance to reproductive needs (Hillyer *et al.*, 1997; Dierenfield *et al.*, 2006; Dierenfield, 2009; Edwards, 2009), and from species to species:

- 35% for ferrets (likely maintenance as levels above this improved fertility in jills; Bell, 1999)
- 14–20% in most average rodents
- 18–20% in guinea pigs
- 13–18% in rabbits (lower end for maintenance, upper for growth and lactation)
- 16–20% for chinchillas and guinea pigs
- 13.5% in degus
- 30% for African pygmy hedgehogs
- as low as 7% but advised to be 19–25% for sugar gliders.

The majority of this protein in granivorous rodent diets seems to come from seeds. Some seeds are very high providers of certain amino acids. Sunflower seeds, white millet and rapeseed, for example, provide high levels of the sulphur-containing amino acids methionine and cysteine, useful when moulting. In rabbits and other grazing herbivores, the majority of the proteins are from plant sources such as clover, alfalfa hay and good-quality grass hays. Care should be taken with diets that focus on one or two specific food types as this will lead to problems with amino acid deficiencies (amongst other things), for example soya is deficient in methionine and corn is deficient in tryptophan and lysine.

Deficiencies in amino acids have been shown to cause certain diseases. An example of this is urolithiasis seen in ferrets that are fed on sources of plant protein, which is deficient in several essential amino acids. In addition, the lack of arginine in plant proteins will cause the young growing ferret to develop hyperammonaemia and neurological signs such as fitting (Bell, 1993). Lack of taurine, an important amino acid for carnivores such as ferrets, but not an essential amino acid for herbivores such as guinea pigs, chinchillas and rabbits, can lead to cardiac disease such as dilated cardiomyopathy.

Fats and essential fatty acids

Fats provide high concentrations of energy, but also supply the small mammal with essential fatty acids (EFAs). These are required for cellular integrity and as the building blocks of cellular constituents such as prostaglandins, which play a part in reproduction and inflammation.

Fats also provide a carrier mechanism for the absorption of fat-soluble vitamins such as vitamins A, D, E and K.

The primary EFA for small mammals is linoleic acid, as it is for larger mammals, with the absolute dietary requirement being 1% of the diet. For herbivores such as the degu, levels of 1.1% are typically quoted for non-reproductive females but rise to 5.5% for lactating females and their pups (Edwards, 2009). If the diet becomes deficient, a rapid decline in cellular integrity occurs. This is manifested clinically by the skin becoming flaky and dry and prone to recurrent infections. Fluid loss through the skin is also increased, even to the extent of causing polydipsia. It is, however, unlikely that any seed-eating small mammal will be deficient in linoleic acid as it is widely found in sunflower seeds and safflower seeds among others. It is also present in the animal protein fed to ferrets.

Ferrets also need access to arachidonic acid as they are strict carnivores and this preformed fatty acid is only found in animal fats and not plants. A deficiency in arachidonic acid results in a number of life-threatening issues as well as skin diseases, associated with intense pruritus. Ferrets have an overall fat requirement of 20–30% of dry matter fed. Rabbits require no additional dietary fat other than the 2–5% provided in their vegetable-based diet, similar to the other herbivorous rodents. Sugar gliders have been typically fed fats at 6–14% dry matter (Dierenfield *et al.*, 2006) and African pygmy hedgehogs around 10–20% (Dierenfield, 2009).

Another EFA which is thought to be important for rodents and which they cannot manufacture is alpha-linolenic acid which is necessary for some prostaglandin and eicosanoid synthesis.

The problem of overconsumption of fats in small mammals which are not exercising regularly is well known, and high-fat oil seeds are the prime culprits in this case. Obesity can also be a problem for overfed, underworked often house-pet ferrets and is very common in African pygmy hedgehogs. Saturated animal fats provide cholesterol, often in excessive amounts, to ferrets, and hepatic lipidosis can be the result. Because rodents and rabbits have a much lower requirement for fat, excess plant fats and overall calorific intake can also cause severe hepatic lipidosis and, in rabbits, atherosclerosis in major blood vessels.

Carbohydrates

Carbohydrates are primarily used for rapid energy production. This is particularly important for herbivorous small mammals that constantly demand rapid supplies of energy for their often hyperactive and high-metabolic-rate lives. Small mammals that are debilitated in some way will particularly benefit from the supply of high carbohydrate foods. Ferrets have no requirement for carbohydrates (similarly to cats) with blood glucose being provided by hepatic gluconeogenesis from amino acid sources.

Complex carbohydrates (fibre)

Dietary fibre does not seem to be important for ferrets. Indeed, their extremely short gastrointestinal tract and minimal bacterial microflora show an inability to cope with any fibre at all. Herbivorous small mammals, particularly the prairie dog, guinea pig, degu, chinchilla and the rabbit, rely more heavily on fibre. Fibre in these species is important for a number of reasons.

First, it provides a source of abrasive food, as most of the fibre-providing foods, such as grasses, contain silicates, which wear down the teeth. This is important as these species have open-rooted or continually growing teeth that need to be kept in check (see Figures 4.1–4.3).

Second, the fibre is essential for stimulating gut motility. These species are hindgut fermenters and rely on the microflora of the hindgut to digest food by breaking down the cellulose. Fibre is converted by the intestinal microflora into volatile fatty acids, which decrease the pH of the caecum and large bowel, so preventing bacterial overgrowth and minimising enteritis problems. Without sufficient fibre, the hindgut fermenting species develop a mucoid enteropathy, with intermittent constipation, diarrhoea and colic.

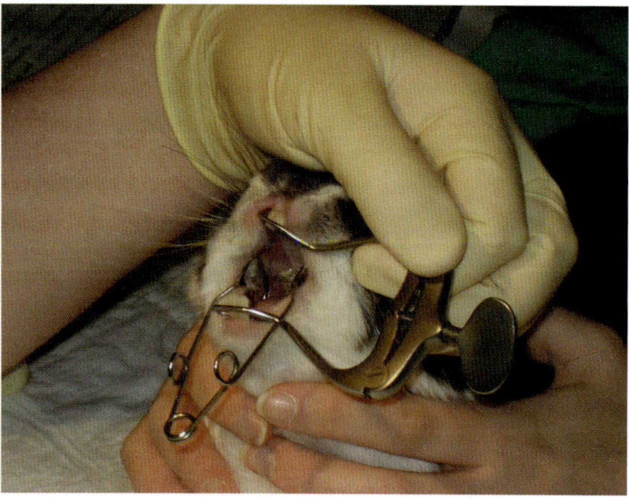

Figure 4.1 Cheek teeth in rabbits are elodont or 'open-rooted' and continually growing, designed to cope with the abrasive wearing nature of grass-based foods. The maxilla is wider than the mandible and so with poor-fibre diets, often exacerbated by poor calcium and vitamin D in the growing rabbit, elongation of the buccal aspect of the maxillary cheek teeth (as here) and lingual aspect of the mandibular cheek teeth can occur.

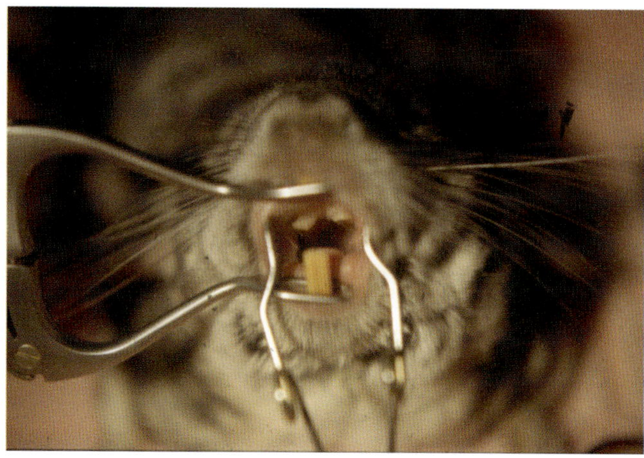

Figure 4.2 Intraoral view of a chinchilla showing bilateral maxillary cheek tooth elongation leading to buccal ulceration and anorexia.

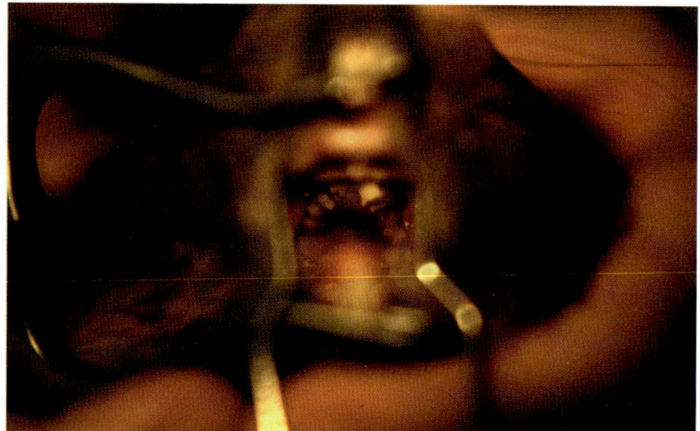

Figure 4.3 Intraoral view of a guinea pig showing maxillary cheek tooth elongation and uneven wear due to a poor-fibre diet.

Rabbits on low-fibre diets may also be inclined to overgroom themselves, consuming large volumes of fur as a 'fibre source' and so developing fur balls (trichobezoars) that may completely block the stomach. Rabbits have a minimal requirement for 12–16% crude fibre, which is similar to guinea pigs. However, many authors have suggested that crude fibre levels in rabbits should be nearer 18–25% to maintain good gut health and dental wear and minimise obesity (Lowe, 2020). Chinchilla dietary fibre levels have been quoted as varying from 15 to 35% and for degus around 20% (Hoefer, 1994; Langer, 2002). The high levels for chinchillas and degus are explained by their natural diet, which is chiefly composed of poor-quality, highly abrasive and fibrous grasses. The lack of such fibre in a diet may well account for the degu's and chinchilla's common susceptibility to molar malocclusion problems but so has an inverse calcium/phosphorus ratio of the diet (see below). It is recommended that these species are fed good-quality hay, dried grass or dried grass pellets as 30–50% of their diet as a minimum. The sole feeding of pelleted and dry mix foods currently available can lead to a fibre shortage which leads to lack of dental wear, gastrointestinal upsets and obesity.

Unlike rabbits and other species, it appears that guinea pigs do not eat until their calorific requirements are satisfied and then stop, but instead eat until their digestive system is full, irrespective of how diluted the energy of the diet is by increased fibre. Recommended minimum crude fibre levels for guinea pigs are 10%, with an average of 13% being routinely offered (Hillyer *et al*., 1997).

In African pygmy hedgehogs, there is no requirement for dietary plant fibre. However, they are prone to obesity in captivity and the use of plant-based fibre, which they cannot digest, as a 'bulking' agent to reduce the overall calorific intake can be helpful.

Vitamins

Fat-soluble vitamins

Vitamin A: In small herbivores the diet frequently contains only the vitamin A precursors, as carotenoid plant pigments, whereas in ferrets, vitamin A itself is obtained from animal proteins and does not need to be synthesised. In small herbivores, the most important form of these precursors, in terms of how much vitamin A can be produced from it, is beta-carotene. Because it is fat-soluble, vitamin A can be stored in the body, primarily in the liver.

Hypovitaminosis A is an uncommonly seen problem in herbivorous and omnivorous small mammals. This is because green vegetables are good providers of the beta-carotenes. A problem can arise with rodents that develop an addiction to seeds such as sunflower seeds and peanuts. Hypovitaminosis A in rabbits can cause infertility, fetal resorption, abortion, stillbirth and neurological defects such as hydrocephalus. In ferrets it can cause infertility, poor coat and fluid retention (anasarca) and has been associated with home-formulated diets of predominantly skeletal meat without supplementation or whole-prey feeding. The recommendation for minimum dietary levels of vitamin A in rabbits is 7000 IU/kg feed (Carpenter *et al*., 2010), although some authors recommend higher levels of 10 000–16 000 IU/kg (Lebas, 1980; Cheeke, 1987; Mateos *et al*., 2020). An upper limit of 16 000 IU/kg of food offered in rabbits has been recommended by the National Research Council to avoid toxicity issues such as hyperostosis and epidermal necrosis (National Research Council, 1987). In practice, Mateos *et al*. (2020) believe that levels of 6000 IU/kg feed for growing rabbits and 10 000 IU/kg feed for breeding rabbits is sufficient, in commercially kept rabbits. The low levels may be met by as little as 200 g of carrot per day for a 2 kg rabbit, but would require 70 kg of oats to provide the same levels! In rats levels of 0.7 mg/kg feed as retinol have been suggested as adequate (National Research Council, 1995).

Hypervitaminosis A rarely occurs naturally, but may be induced by overdosing with vitamin A injections at 1000 times or more the daily recommended doses. If this occurs, acute toxicity develops with mucous membrane and skin sloughing, liver damage and, frequently, death within 24–48 hours. It may also be seen in ferrets fed predominantly the livers of prey items. In these cases excess bony production may occur similar to the syndrome seen in cats as well as epidermal necrosis. National Research Council (1987) as stated recommends a maximum dietary level of 16 000 IU/kg feed offered.

Vitamin D: This vitamin is primarily concerned with calcium metabolism but also has important immune-system functions. Cholecalciferol is manufactured in the small mammal's skin, a process enhanced by ultraviolet light in many species. Small mammals kept indoors therefore produce much less of this compound, and this can lead to deficiency. Cholecalciferol must then be activated in the liver and kidneys before it can function in calcium metabolism. Once formed into its active metabolite it acts in concert with parathyroid hormone to increase reabsorption of calcium at the expense of phosphorus from the kidneys, to increase absorption of calcium from the intestines and to mobilise calcium from the bones, all of these functions increasing the blood calcium level.

Hypovitaminosis D_3 causes problems with calcium metabolism and leads to rickets. This is exacerbated by low-calcium-containing diets, a typical sufferer being a small mammal kept indoors, fed an all-seed diet in the case of a rodent or an all meat and no calcium supplement diet for a ferret. This leads to well-muscled heavy rodents or ferrets, with poorly mineralised bones, flaring of the epiphyseal plates at the ends of the long bones and concomitant bowing of the limbs, especially the tibiotarsal bones. Hypovitaminosis D_3 can also result in hypophosphataemia in rabbits (Harcourt-Brown, 2002). Recommended minimum levels are 3.5–9 IU/g feed for rodents and lagomorphs (Wallach and Hoff, 1982a,b) and 0.5–1.5 IU/g dry matter for sugar gliders.

Hypervitaminosis D_3 occurs due to oversupplementation with D_3 and calcium and leads to calcification of soft tissues, such as the medial arterial walls, and the kidneys, creating hypertension and causing organ failure. Recommended maximum levels are 2000 IU/kg dry matter of food for most small mammals (Wallach and Hoff, 1982a,b) but in rabbits, because of their efficient absorption of dietary calcium, maximum dietary levels of 1000–1300 IU/kg feed have been recommended (Mateos *et al*., 2020).

Vitamin E: This compound is found in several active forms in plants, the most active being alpha-tocopherol. It is used as an antioxidant and in immune system function.

Hypovitaminosis E in ferrets results in a yellow discolouration of body fat deposits, haemolytic anaemia and a progressive paresis of the limbs. In addition, a series of firm swellings underneath the skin in the inguinal area may be seen. In rabbits a similar disease is seen, with hindlimb paresis and white muscle degeneration. In hamsters, deficiencies have been reported as causing muscular weakness, ocular secretions and death, often due to cardiac muscle damage. Hypovitaminosis E may occur due to a reduction in fat metabolism or absorption as can occur in small intestinal, pancreatic or biliary diseases, or due to a lack of green plant material, the chief source of the compound, in the diet. Recommended levels for rabbits are 40 mg/kg dry matter of food offered (National Research Council, 1995) or 50 mg/kg of food fed (Carpenter *et al*., 2010).

In addition, feeding diets high in unsaturated fats (such as oily fish) may use up the body's reserves of vitamin E and so induce signs of hypovitaminosis E. This has occurred in ferrets and mink fed such a diet.

Hypervitaminosis E is extremely rare

Vitamin K: Because of its production by bacteria, it is very difficult to get a true deficiency of vitamin K, although absorption will again be reduced when fat digestion or absorption is reduced, for example in biliary or pancreatic disease. Levels of 2 mg/kg of food fed have been recommended for rabbits (Lowe, 2020).

Ferrets eating prey which has been killed by warfarin will show signs of deficiency. Rabbits and guinea pigs eating large amounts of sweet clovers can also experience a relative deficiency. The signs of disease that are seen are due to increased internal and external haemorrhage, but vitamin K also has some function in calcium/phosphorus metabolism in the bones and this may also be affected.

Water-soluble vitamins

Vitamin B_1 (thiamine): Hypovitaminosis B_1 is uncommon, but may be seen in ferrets fed raw saltwater fish or fish that has been frozen and defrosted, all of which contain thiaminases. When a relative deficiency occurs, neurological signs such as opisthotonus, weakness and head tremors are seen. Ferrets can suffer from a condition known as Chastek syndrome. The symptoms may include salivation, paralysis, incoordination, pupillary dilation and easily induced convulsions, which are characterised by strong ventral flexion of the neck. Evidence of dilated cardiomyopathies is seen at post-mortem. The recommended minimum level for most small mammals is around 6–7 mg/kg of diet dry matter (Wallach and Hoff, 1982a,b). Sugar gliders fed primarily on pollen/nectar replacers may develop thiamine deficiencies owing to the low levels of thiamine in these food sources. Clinically this can present with seizures. Ensuring adequate mineral vitamin preloading of insects in the sugar glider diet will prevent this.

Vitamin B_2 (riboflavin): Hypovitaminosis B_2 is very rare and produces growth retardation, roughened coat, alopecia, excess scurf and cataract formation.

Vitamin B_3 (niacin): Rodents fed a high proportion of one type of seed such as sweetcorn can become deficient in niacin. They exhibit blackening of the tongue (known as pellagra) and oral mucosa, retarded growth, poor coat quality and scaly dermatitis. Rats may also have anaemia and porphyrin-encrusted noses.

Vitamin B_6 (pyridoxine): This vitamin is essential for manufacturing coenzymes involved in amino acid as well as glycogen (the carbohydrate stored in the liver) and fatty acid metabolism. Deficiencies manifest as anaemia, dermatitis and neurological disease including paresis, seizures and paralysis. Typical minimum values are around 6 mg/kg food fed for rodents such as rats and mice (Kumar *et al.*, 2021).

Vitamin B_7 (biotin): Deficiency may occur in animals fed large amounts of unfertilised, raw eggs, the whites of which contain the anti-biotin vitamin avidin. This can be seen in ferrets and chipmunks when greater than 10% of the diet is composed of raw egg. Deficiency produces exfoliative dermatitis, toes may become gangrenous and slough off and ataxia may be observed. The recommended minimum requirement is 0.12–0.34 ppm food as dry matter for small mammals (Wallach and Hoff, 1982a,b).

Vitamin B_9 (folic acid/folate): Deficiency occurs mainly because of the folic acid inhibitors that are present in some foods such as cabbage and other brassicas, oranges, beans and peas. The use of trimethoprim sulfonamide drugs also reduces gut bacterial folic acid production. Deficiency causes a number of problems, such as failure in reproductive tract maturation, macrocytic anaemia due to failure of red blood cell maturation and immune system cellular dysfunction.

Choline: The need for choline is dependent on the levels of folic acid and vitamin B_{12}. Because of these interactions, a deficiency may be caused if folic acid and vitamin B_{12} are inadequate, as may occur in an animal fed a diet high in fats. Deficiency causes retarded growth, disrupted fat metabolism and fatty liver damage. Recommended minimum requirements for small mammals are 880–1540 mg/kg food as dry matter.

Vitamin C: There is no direct need for this vitamin in commonly kept small mammals other than the guinea pig, as vitamin C may be synthesised from glucose in the liver. In some marsupials it can be synthesised in the kidney. In the sugar glider it is not currently known whether it can synthesise vitamin C, but the Virginia opossum can do so in its liver. The guinea pig lacks the enzyme L-gulonolactone oxidase and therefore cannot convert glucose to ascorbic acid, so has a dietary requirement for vitamin C. However, during disease processes, particularly those conditions that affect liver function, it may be beneficial to the recovery process in all species to provide a dietary source of vitamin C.

Vitamin C is required for the formation of elastic fibres and connective tissues and is an excellent antioxidant, similar to vitamin E. Deficiency leads to scurvy, signs of which include poor wound healing, increased bleeding due to capillary-wall fragility, gingivitis and bone alterations. These include the swelling of long bones close to joints (the epiphyseal plates), which become very painful. In addition, crusting occurs at mucocutaneous junctions such as the eyes, mouth and nose, as well as loosening of the teeth due to periodontal ligament weakening.

Vitamin C also helps in the absorption of some minerals, such as iron, from the gut.

The daily recommended requirement for guinea pigs is 10 mg/kg body weight for maintenance, increasing to 30 mg/kg body weight during gestation, although recommended treatment of scurvy suggests levels of 50–100 mg/kg until resolution of clinical signs (Harkness and Wagner, 1995). This may be given by injection, or soluble human vitamin C tablets may be placed in the drinking water each day if the guinea pig is still drinking adequately. In addition, fresh fruit and vegetables, as well as a specific supplemented guinea pig diet, should always be fed. Many deficiencies occur due to guinea pigs being housed with rabbits and therefore fed only dry rabbit food which has no supplemental vitamin C.

Minerals

Macrominerals

Calcium: Calcium has a wide range of functions, the two most obvious being its role in the formation of the skeleton and mineralisation of bone matrix, and its use in muscular contraction. The active form of calcium in the body is the ionic double-charged molecule Ca^{2+}. Low levels of this form, even though the overall body reserves of calcium may be normal, lead to hyperexcitability, fitting and death.

Calcium levels in the body are controlled by vitamin D_3, parathyroid hormone and calcitonin.

The ratio of calcium to phosphorus is very important. As one increases the other decreases and vice versa. A ratio therefore of 2 : 1 calcium to phosphorus is desirable in juvenile and lactating small mammals and 1.5 : 1 for adults. Excessive dietary calcium (>1%) reduces the body's ability to utilise proteins, fats, phosphorus, manganese, zinc, iron and iodine. In rabbits, this is exacerbated by their unique method of calcium control, in that they have no ability to reduce calcium absorption from the gut, as do other species. Instead, all available calcium is absorbed from the diet, and any excess must then be excreted through the kidneys. When there is excess dietary calcium, therefore, this leads to excess calcium excretion into the urine, the formation of calcium carbonate crystals and urolithiasis. In addition, as rabbits are herbivorous, their urine pH is alkaline, and as calcium carbonate (limestone) is less soluble in alkaline environments it precipitates more readily in the urine, forming crystals. Levels of calcium above 4% dry matter for rabbits will lead to soft tissue mineralisation in sites such as the aorta and kidneys. Excessive levels of calcium may occur in adult herbivores fed alfalfa (lucerne) hay as this legume contains higher levels of calcium than grass hay.

Calcium deficiency and metabolic bone disease problems are common in omnivorous marsupials such as the sugar glider, which consumes sap and insects in large quantities, both of which are deficient in calcium. Hypocalcaemic tetany has also been reported in sugar gliders. Evidence and logical common sense suggests that in any growing animal an increased predisposition to dental disease and cheek tooth malocclusions occurs where dietary calcium to phosphorus ratios are less than 2 : 1 due to poor mineralisation of the jawbones and teeth and this has been reported in rabbits, chinchillas and degus (Harcourt-Brown, 1998; Muszczynski *et al.*, 2010; Jekl *et al.*, 2011).

Phosphorus: Like calcium, phosphorus is used in bone formation, but it also has a role in cell structure and energy storage. It is widespread in plant and animal tissues, but in the former it may be bound up in unavailable form as phytates. Levels of phosphorus are controlled in the body as for calcium, the two being in equal and opposite equilibrium with each other. Therefore, if dietary phosphorus levels exceed calcium levels appreciably (a maximum of twice the calcium levels on average) the parathyroid glands become stimulated to produce more parathyroid hormone in an effort to restore the balance. This causes nutritional secondary hyperparathyroidism which leads to progressive bone demineralisation and then renal damage due to the high circulating levels of parathyroid hormone. High dietary phosphorus also reduces the amount of calcium that can be absorbed from the gut, as it complexes with the calcium present there. This can be a big problem for ferrets that are fed pure meat diets with no calcium or bone supplement, and in rodents that are predominantly seed eaters, as cereals are high-phosphorus/low-calcium foods. Feeding green vegetables or supplementation with calcium powders may therefore be necessary. In the case of ferrets a standard ferret complete diet, or whole rodent prey, should be fed to avoid this.

Potassium: As with larger mammals, this is the major intracellular positive ion. Rarely is there a dietary deficiency. Severe stress can cause hypokalaemia due to increased kidney excretion of potassium due to elevated plasma proteins, as can persistent diarrhoea. Hypokalaemia can lead to cardiac dysrhythmias, muscle spasticity and neurological dysfunction. Other symptoms are stunted growth, ascites, abnormally short hair and reduced appetite. Potassium is present in high amounts in certain fruits, such as bananas. It is controlled in equilibrium with sodium by the adrenal hormone aldosterone which promotes sodium retention and potassium excretion.

Sodium: This is the main extracellular positive ion and regulates the body's acid–base balance and osmotic potential. In conjunction with potassium, it is responsible for nerve signals and impulses. Rarely does a true dietary deficiency occur, but hyponatraemia may occur due to chronic diarrhoea or renal disease. This disrupts the osmotic potential gradient in the kidneys and water is lost leading to further dehydration. Excessive levels of sodium in the diet (>10 times recommended) lead to poor coat, polyuria, hypertension, oedema and death.

Chlorine: This is the major extracellular negative ion and is responsible for maintaining acid–base balance in conjunction with sodium and potassium. Deficiencies are rare, but if they do occur, retarded growth and kidney disease are commonly seen.

Microminerals (trace elements)

Copper: Copper is used in haemoglobin synthesis, collagen synthesis and the maintenance of the nervous system. Copper toxicosis has been reported in ferrets as a possible hereditary storage disease. The symptoms are of liver disease, as seen in Bedlington Terriers (Brown, 1997). Deficiency has been reported in hamsters as a cause of poor coat quality and generalised alopecia. Minimum recommended levels are 13–20 ppm (Wallach and Hoff, 1982a,b).

Iodine: Iodine's sole function is in thyroid hormone synthesis, which affects metabolic rate. Deficiency causes goitre, and has knock-on effects on growth causing stunting, stillbirths and neurological problems. It is a relatively uncommon finding in small mammals but may occur in species such as rabbits that are fed large volumes of goitrogenic (iodine-inhibiting) plants such as cabbage, kale and Brussel sprouts.

Iron: This is essential, as with larger mammals, for the formation of the oxygen-carrying part of the haemoglobin molecule. Absorption from the gut is normally relatively poor, as the body is very good at recycling its own iron levels. Vitamin C enhances iron uptake from the gut. In sugar gliders Dierenfield *et al.* (2006) recommend iron levels of less than 50 μg/g of dry diet to avoid iron storage disease, which can damage the liver in this species.

Manganese: Deficiency has been reported as causing poor bone growth, with limb shortening as a consequence. Recommended daily requirements are 40–120.7 ppm with the higher dosages for guinea pigs (Wallach and Hoff, 1982a,b).

Selenium: The main role of selenium is as part of the antioxidant enzyme glutathione peroxidase, with which vitamin E is also involved. Its functions are therefore similar to those of vitamin E in that it helps keep peroxidases from attacking polyunsaturated fats in cell membranes. A general deficiency in both selenium and vitamin E will lead to liver necrosis, steatitis and muscular dystrophy. The selenium content of plants is dependent on where they were grown and the levels of selenium in the soil. Recommended minimum requirements are still not clearly defined for small mammals in general.

Zinc: This is a vital trace element for wound healing and tissue formation, forming part of a number of enzymes. Deficiencies can occur in young, rapidly growing guinea pigs and chinchillas fed on plant material high in phytates such as cabbage, wheat bran and beans. In addition, high dietary calcium decreases zinc uptake. Deficiency produces retarded growth and poor skin quality with increased scurf and hyperirritability. Zinc deficiency alopecia is particularly seen at about day 50 of gestation in chinchillas, with hair regrowth occurring 2–3 weeks after parturition (Smith *et al.*, 1977). Minimum recommended requirements are 20–122 ppm for small mammals (Wallach and Hoff, 1982a,b). Zinc toxicosis has been reported in ferrets, with anaemia, lethargy and hindlimb paresis, and was associated with feeding from zinc galvanised buckets (Donnelly, 1997).

Requirements for young and lactating small mammals

Rabbit

Neonatal rabbits nurse for only 3–5 minutes at a time once or twice in a 24-hour period and are totally dependent on their mother's milk up to day 21 postpartum (Okerman, 1994). At this time they should be weighed, as solid foods offered will be increasingly consumed, and weight losses may be seen if they do not eat enough of this. The doe may be offered increasingly more pelleted dry foods before weaning, as her energy demands increase to 3.5 times maintenance by peak lactation. Ad-lib dry food is therefore often advocated for the doe at this stage. It should be noted though that levels of food for the doe should not start to be dramatically increased until 5–7 days after parturition. Early overfeeding can cause excessive milk production, and mastitis will result if the kits do not have sufficient appetite to empty the mammary glands at each sitting. For hand-rearing formulas, see the section on fostering rabbits in Chapter 2.

Growing kits require higher levels of vitamin D_3 and calcium than their adult counterparts. To ensure that this is received, a balanced diet should be offered, combining pelleted food, good-quality grass hay and some greens. Dry foods should be carefully chosen. Many are balanced nutritionally, but only if the rabbit consumes all parts equally. Rabbits are concentrate selectors – they will preferentially pick out those foods containing the highest calories in their environment and eat them first. Therefore, if offered one of the 'muesli'-type diets, it will eat all of the fatty, carbohydrate foods first, and, if provided ad-lib, they will not get around to eating the high-fibre, calcium-containing grass pellets. Hence, it is advised either to use a homogenous pelleted diet where all of the pellets are exactly the same, or to feed enough in 24 hours so that the bowl is completely emptied before offering more. Access to unfiltered natural sunlight is also advised, even if for only 15–20 minutes daily, to ensure sufficient vitamin D_3 synthesis. Lactating does will also have higher calcium requirements, and so their consumption of pelleted diet and grass products (both high in calcium) will increase. Care should be taken, though, not to overdo pelleted diets at the expense of good-quality hay/grass, as excessive amounts of calcium and vitamin D_3 can occur, leading to renolithiasis and urolithiasis as well as soft tissue mineralisation.

Rodents

The guinea pig sow has a requirement for vitamin C which increases from 10 to 30 mg/kg per day when she is lactating. She also has the usual increases in calcium, energy and protein demands. The demands for increased calories are particularly important, as the long gestation of the guinea pig (average 63 days) and the frequent litter size of three to four piglets place huge stresses on the sow. If these increased requirements are not met, then a condition known as pregnancy toxaemia, or ketosis ensues. This is when a lack of available calories leads to increased fat mobilisation. If this is combined with a glucose deficit the fats are converted into chemicals known as ketones. These produce metabolic acidosis in addition to the hypoglycaemic state. Death can follow within 24 hours. Prevention is geared towards avoiding obesity and sudden dietary change, both of which set up the condition.

Young guinea pigs are frequently not hungry for the first 12–24 hours after birth because they have brown fat reserves. They should not be force-fed during this time. Young chinchillas and guinea pigs eat solid foods practically from day 1 after parturition. It is important therefore to ensure high-fibre foods are offered preferentially at this stage so as to avoid them developing into fussy eaters in later life.

Rodents such as rats and gerbils have been quoted as needing a dietary protein level of 20–26% during and prior to pregnancy and lactation, as opposed to their more usual 16–18%.

For rearing formulas see the section on fostering rats and mice in Chapter 2

Omnivorous marsupials

Energy requirements increase significantly in sugar gliders from around 46 kJ/day as basal requirements to 229 kJ/day for growth and activity. Lactation has much higher demands on the female marsupial than gestation, due to the altricial nature of the joeys when born. Many insectivorous marsupials can enter a state of torpor when food sources (mainly the insects which provide most of the protein, fats and calories) are scarce to conserve energy. Their body temperature will drop and they will appear to be unrousable. It is not uncommon for these periods to last up to 11 hours.

For hand rearing formulas see the section on fostering sugar gliders and Virginia opossums in Chapter 2.

African pygmy hedgehog

It is reported that a female African pygmy hedgehog that gains more than 50 g in weight 3 weeks after being introduced to a male is likely to be pregnant (Dierenfield, 2009). During lactation, females should be given ad-lib feed in order to maintain weight (Larson and Carpenter, 1999).

For hand rearing formulas see the section on fostering African pygmy hedgehogs in Chapter 2.

Ferret

Young ferrets have a higher calorific requirement than adults, as do lactating jills, needing 1.5–2 times maintenance adult calorie levels. The protein requirement is a minimum of 35% in young growing ferrets and lactating jills with a fat level of a minimum of 20–25% as dry matter (Kupersmith, 1998).

For hand rearing formulas see the section on fostering ferrets in Chapter 2.

Requirements for debilitated small mammals

In general, requirements for debilitated animals will vary from 1.5 to 3 times maintenance levels, with the lower levels being for mildly injured or infected animals and the upper levels for burns victims and cases of serious organ damage or septicaemia.

Fluid therapy as additional support is essential, particularly for the herbivorous mammals, which have very high maintenance requirements when compared with cats and dogs (on average 80–100 mL/kg per day). Also, herbivore gut contents are voluminous and need to be kept fluid. For further details see Chapters 6 and 8.

Rabbit

The debilitated rabbit may be supported with nasogastric or oral syringe feeding of vegetable-based baby foods (lactose-free varieties) or, for preference, with a gruel composed of ground dry rabbit pellets and water as this will supply a better fibre level for gut stimulation. Amounts suggested to feed at any one sitting vary from 3 to 15 mL four to six times daily.

A nasogastric tube (more correctly a naso-oesophageal tube as the tubing must not allow reflux of acid stomach contents into the oesophagus) is placed after first spraying the nose with lidocaine (lignocaine) spray. A 3–4 French tube is premeasured from the extended nose to the seventh rib or caudal end of the sternum and then inserted. Sterile water should be flushed through the tube before and after feeding to ensure it is correctly placed and does not become blocked. The tube may then be glued, taped or sutured to the dorsal aspect of the head and a bung inserted when not in use. It may be necessary to put an Elizabethan collar on the rabbit to prevent removal.

The use of cisapride at a dose of 0.5 mg/kg orally every 8–24 hours (Smith and Bergmann, 1997) is to be advocated in rabbits to stimulate large bowel activity and encourage the return of normal appetite.

Older rabbits often do better on lower protein (14%) and higher fibre (18–25%) diets as these reduce the risk of obesity and kidney and liver damage.

Rodents

Syringe feeding orally or using a straight avian crop tube to administer liquid food directly into the oesophagus are advised. The latter may be stressful, as the rodent must be scruffed prior to administration. Volumes suggested vary from 0.5 mL for a mouse up to 2.5 mL for a rat at any one sitting, the dose to be repeated six to eight times daily to ensure correct calorie administration. Diets such as dry rodent pellets ground in a coffee grinder and then added to water to form gruel, or vegetable-based lactose-free baby foods may be used. Guinea pigs and chinchillas benefit from the use of oral cisapride to stimulate gut motility, as well as the use of gruels made from higher-fibre chinchilla or rabbit pellets. Naso-oesophageal tubes can be attempted for the larger individuals of these two species.

Marsupials

For sugar gliders a typical diet would include the following (Johnson-Delaney, 2010): 15 mL of Leadbeater's mix (which is made of 150 mL warm water plus 150 mL honey plus one shelled, hard-boiled egg plus 15 g of baby rice-based cereal plus 5 g of powdered avian vitamin and mineral supplement); 15 g of an insectivore/carnivore diet; and then various additions as treats such as chopped fruit and live gut fed insects, which should not exceed 10% of the diet. The practice of gut-loading insects with vitamin/mineral supplements is useful and should be familiar to anyone keeping reptiles.

African pygmy hedgehog

Hedgehogs can be a challenge to syringe feed if they refuse to cooperate. Any assistance should avoid foods containing lactose as they are generally intolerant. They are highly susceptible to *Salmonella* spp. and so raw eggs and meat should be avoided as well. If a hedgehog is obese, a rapid reduction in calories should also be avoided as this can precipitate hepatic lipidosis. Commercially available diets designed for omnivores are currently available.

Ferret

Historically it was common for the debilitated ferret to be supported with nasogastric or oral syringe feeding of meat-based baby foods, or commercially prepared liquid meat-based formulas designed for cats and dogs such as Reanimyl® and Hill's a/d. Alternatively, carnivore support formulas have been specifically devised by companies such as Lafeber and Oxbow and these may be more appropriate. Amounts suggested for feeding at any one sitting based on maximum gastric volumes vary from 2 to 10 mL and so to ensure the correct nutritional energy supply may require administration from three to six times daily. It is vitally important that no debilitated ferret goes longer than 4 hours without nutritional support, as they will become rapidly hypoglycaemic, particularly if they are older animals as the incidence of insulinomas is common.

A 3 French nasogastric tube can easily be placed via the nostril after first spraying the area with lidocaine spray in a sedated or anaesthetised ferret. The tube should be premeasured to extend from the nose tip to the level of the seventh rib (i.e. it is really a naso-oesophageal tube, to avoid the acid contents of the stomach refluxing and causing an oesophagitis) and cut to this length. It may then be secured with tissue glue, or taped or sutured to the skin over the forehead. It is advised to fit an Elizabethan collar to prevent the ferret removing the tube. The tube should be flushed with sterile water before and after feeding to ensure the tubing is in the correct position and does not block.

Probiotics and prebiotics

The use of oral probiotics is recommended for small herbivores to encourage normal digestive function by providing enzymes and to encourage normal pH conditions. Probiotics are best added to the drinking water but may be added to the syringed food to ensure consumption.

Prebiotics are mixtures of nutrients that support the normal microflora of the gastrointestinal system and so encourage these commensal bacteria to outcompete potentially harmful bacteria such as *Clostridium* spp. and include oligosaccharides such as fructo-, alpha-galacto-, transgalacto-, mannan and xylo-oligosaccharides (Falçao-e-Cunha *et al.*, 2007). Prebiotics are often present in commercially available probiotic formulations.

References

Bell, J. (1993) Ferret nutrition and diseases associated with inadequate nutrition. In: *Proceedings of the North American Veterinary Conference*, pp. 719–720. Orlando, FL.

Bell, J.A. (1999) Ferret nutrition. *Veterinary Clinics of North America: Exotic Animal Practice*, **2**(1), 169–192.

Brown, S.A. (1997) Basic anatomy, physiology and husbandry. In: *Ferrets, Rabbits and Rodents: Clinical Medicine and Surgery* (eds E.V. Hillyer & K.E. Quesenberry), pp. 3–13. W.B. Saunders, Philadelphia, PA.

Carpenter, J.W., Wolf, K.N. and Kolmstetter, C.M. (2010) Feeding small exotic mammals. In: *Hill's Nutrition*, pp. 1215–1236. Mark Mervis Institute, Marceline, MO.

Cheeke, P.R. (1987) Vitamins. In: *Rabbit Feeding and Nutrition*, pp. p136–p153. Academic Press, London.

Dierenfield, E.S. (2009) Feeding behavior and nutrition of the African pygmy hedgehog (*Atelerix albiventris*). *Veterinary Clinics of North America Exotic Animal Practice*, **12**, 335–337.

Dierenfield, E.S., Thomas, D. and Ives, R. (2006) Comparison of commonly used diets on intake, digestion, growth and health in captive sugar gliders (*Petaurus breviceps*). *Journal of Exotic Pet Medicine*, **15**(3), 218–224.

Donnelly, T.M. (1997) Basic anatomy, physiology and husbandry. In: *Ferrets, Rabbits and Rodents: Clinical Medicine and Surgery* (eds E.V. Hillyer & K.E. Quesenberry), pp. 147–159. W.B. Saunders, Philadelphia, PA.

Edwards, M.S. (2009) Nutrition and behavior of degus (*Octodon degus*). *Veterinary Clinics of North America: Exotic Animal Practice*, **12**, 237–253.

Falçao-e-Cunha, L., Castro-Solla, L., Maertens, L. *et al.* (2007) Alternatives to antibiotic growth promoters in rabbit feeding: a review. *World Rabbit Science*, **15**, 127–140.

Harcourt-Brown, F.M. (2002) Diet and husbandry. In: *Textbook of Rabbit Medicine*, pp. 19–51. Butterworth-Heineman, Edinburgh.

Harcourt-Brown, F.M. (1998) Calcium deficiency, diet and dental disease in pet rabbits. *Veterinary Record*, **139**(23), 567–571.

Harkness, J.E. and Wagner, J.E. (1995) *The Biology and Medicine of Rabbits and Rodents*, 4th edn. Lea and Febiger, Philadelphia, PA.

Hillyer, E.V., Quesenberry, K.E. and Donnelly, T.M. (1997) Biology, husbandry and clinical techniques. In: *Ferrets, Rabbits and Rodents: Clinical Medicine and Surgery* (eds E.V. Hillyer & K.E. Quesenberry), pp. 243–259. W.B. Saunders, Philadelphia, PA.

Hoefer, H.L. (1994) Chinchillas. *Veterinary Clinics of North America: Small Animal Practice*, **24**, 103–111.

Hume, I. (1999) Metabolic rates and nutrient requirements. In: *Marsupial Nutrition*, pp. 1–34. Cambridge University Press, Cambridge.

Jekl, V., Gumpenberger, M., Jeklova, E. *et al.* (2011) Impact of pelleted diets with different mineral compositions on the crown size of mandibular cheek teeth and mandibular relative density in degus (*Octodon degus*). *Veterinary Record*, **168**(24), 641. doi: 10.1136/vr.d2012.

Johnson-Delaney, C. (2010) Marsupials. In: *Manual of Exotic Pets* (eds A. Meredith & C. Johnson-Delaney), 5th edn, pp. 103–126. BSAVA, Quedgeley, UK.

Kumar, S., Rajput, M.K. and Yadav, P.K. (2021) Laboratory animal nutrition. In: *Essentials of Laboratory Animal Science: Principles and Practices* (ed. P. Nagarajan), pp. 373–403. Springer Nature Singapore Pte Ltd.

Kupersmith, D.S. (1998) A practical overview of small mammal nutrition. *Seminars in Avian and Exotic Pet Medicine*, **7**(3), 141–147.

Langer, P. (2002) The digestive tract and life history of small mammals. *Mammal Review*, **32**(2), 107–131.

Larson, R.S. and Carpenter, J.W. (1999) Husbandry and medical management of African hedgehogs. *Veterinary Medicine*, **94**(10), 877–888.

Lebas, F. (1980) Les recherches sur l'alimentation du lapin: Evolution au cours des 20 dernieres annees et perspectives d'avenir. *Proceedings of the 2nd World Rabbit Congress*, **2**, 1–17.

Lowe, J.A. (2020) Pet rabbit feeding and nutrition. In: *The Nutrition of the Rabbit* (eds C. de Blas & J. Wiseman), 3rd edn, pp. 317–366. CABI Publishing, Oxfordshire, UK.

Mateos, G.G., Garcia-Rebollar, P. and de Blas, C. (2020) Minerals vitamins and additives. In: *Nutrition of the Rabbit* (eds C. de Blas & J. Wiseman), 3rd edn, pp. 126–158. CABI, Wallingford, Oxford.

Muszczynski, Z., Sulik, M., Ogonski, T. and Antoszek, J. (2010) Plasma concentration of calcium, magnesium and phosphorus in chinchilla with and without tooth overgrowth. *Folia Biologica (Krakow)*, **58**(1–2), 107–111. doi: 10.3409/fb58_1-2.107-111.

National Research Council (1987) *Vitamin Tolerance of Animals*. National Academy of Science, National Research Council, Washington, DC, USA.

National Research Council (1995) *Nutrient Requirements of Laboratory Animals.*, 4th edn, p. 192. National Academy Press, Washington, DC.

Okerman, L. (1994) Inherited conditions and congenital deformities. In: *Diseases of Domestic Rabbits*, 2nd edn, pp. 109–112. Blackwell, Oxford.

Robbins, C.E. (1983) *Wildlife Feeding and Nutrition*. Academic Press, San Diego (CA).

Smith, D.A. and Bergmann, P.M. (1997) Formulary. In: *Ferrets, Rabbits and Rodents: Clinical Medicine and Surgery* (eds E.V. Hillyer & K.E. Quesenberry), pp. 392–403. W.B. Saunders, Philadelphia, PA.

Smith, J.C., Brown, E.D. and Cassidy, W.A. (1977) *Zinc and Vitamin A: Interrelationships of Zinc Metabolism. Current Aspects in Health and Disease.* Alan R. Liss, Inc., New York.

Tschudin, A., Clauss, M., Codron, D. *et al.* (2011) Water intake in domestic rabbits (*Oryctolagus cuniculus*) from open dishes and nipple drinkers under different water and feeding regimes. *Journal of Animal Physiology and Animal Nutrition (Berlin)*, **95**(4), 499–511. doi: 10.1111/j.1439-0396.2010.01077.x.

Wallach, J.D. and Hoff, G.L. (1982a) Nutritional diseases of mammals. In: *Non-infectious Diseases of Wildlife* (eds G.L. Hoff & J.W. Davis), pp. 133–135. Iowa State University Press, Ames IA, 143-144.

Wallach, J.D. and Hoff, G.L. (1982b) Metabolic and nutritional diseases of reptiles. In: *Non-infectious Diseases of Wildlife* (eds G.L. Hoff & J.W. Davis), pp. 155–168. Iowa State University Press, Ames, IA.

Chapter 5 Common Diseases of Small Mammals

DISEASES OF THE DOMESTIC RABBIT

Skin disease

Skin problems in rabbits are commonly reported and, after respiratory and dental disease, make one of the commonest reasons for a pet rabbit being seen for veterinary treatment. In one study, skin disease comprised 31.02% of rabbit cases presented for veterinary treatment (Tokashiki *et al.*, 2019).

Ectoparasitic

Mites

Cheyletiella parasitivorax produces dense, white scurf along the dorsum, starting around the nape of the neck and spreading outwards and caudally. The fur drops out and new fur regrows rapidly. The condition may not appear pruritic, although in severe cases rabbits will self-traumatise. Microscopically it appears as a large mite, with mouthparts that have claws, and the ends of the legs possess combs rather than suckers (see Figure 5.1). Owners may be bitten by this mite often in the classical pattern of three bites grouped together.

Psoroptes cuniculi lives in the external ear canal of rabbit, where it irritates the lining making it weep serum. The serum dries in brown crusts which in severe cases may obliterate the lumen completely (see Figure 5.2). Infestation can lead to serious secondary bacterial ear infections which can lead to middle ear and then vestibular disease. The mites are large enough to be seen with the naked eye. Microscopically they have pointed mouthparts and conical suckers to the ends of the legs.

Leporacarus (Listrophorus) gibbus is generally a non-pathogenic fur mite of rabbits but can cause a moist dermatitis over the back, rump and inguinal region in animals debilitated with other diseases. It is an oval mite with short legs, and so may be distinguished from the above two mites on clinical signs and the absence of a 'waist' and having conical suckers and combs on the end of its legs.

Neotrombicula autumnalis is the harvest mite. It is not a true parasite, but the juvenile (six-legged) bright orange-red mite may irritate the skin of rabbits which have access to hay, grass or straw. It causes irritation of the skin surface chiefly over the palmar/plantar aspect of the feet, the face, and ears. Its typical orange-red colour is visible to the naked eye, and its six-legged form distinguishes it from other mites.

All of the above mites are surface-dwelling and may therefore be harvested for identification using a flea comb, or Sellotape® strip applied to the affected area and then stuck to a microscope slide for examination.

Burrowing mites are uncommon but may affect rabbits, the two main ones being *Sarcoptes scabiei* and *Notoedres* spp. They produce intensely pruritic skin lesions and are diagnosed after skin scrapings and microscopic examination.

Demodex cuniculi may be recovered from rabbits on a skin scraping but rarely cause disease. Other mites reported include *Ornithonyssus bacoti* a blood-sucking mite often associated with wild birds or rodents and these may cause pruritus, anaemia and scaling skin disease with fur loss.

Lice

Haemodipsus ventricosus is a louse of domestic rabbits, and belongs to the sucking (Anoplura) family. It is slender and often blood-filled and may cause significant anaemia in young kits.

Fleas

The rabbit flea is *Spilopsyllus cuniculi* and is the chief vector for the serious viral disease of rabbits, myxomatosis. It tends to concentrate around the ears of the rabbit where it stays plugged into a blood supply and may be distinguished from the cat and dog flea by the presence of obliquely arranged genal ctenidium (see Figure 5.3). These are the fronds which line the mouthparts of the flea, and which are horizontal in the cat and dog fleas.

Blowfly

Blowflies cause a condition called myiasis ('fly strike').

This horrible condition is common in outdoor rabbits that have perineal soiling due to urine scalding or diarrhoea. It is caused by flies including the blue (*Calliphora* spp.), black (*Phormia* spp.) and green (*Lucilia* spp.) bottle families. These lay their eggs on the skin of the rabbit. In warm conditions these eggs hatch into larvae within 2 hours. The larvae then mature and burrow into the rabbit.

In some parts of the world, *Cuterebra* spp. flies (so-called botflies) may also lay their eggs on rabbits. These develop into larvae which burrow into the skin, leaving a breathing hole through the skin surface to allow air to reach the developing larva. Multiple larvae can cause serious skin damage and discomfort and occasionally the larvae can migrate through other vital organs such as the central nervous system.

Other parasites

Coenurus serialis, which is the intermediate stage of the adult tapeworm of dogs *Taenia serialis*, may form large fluid-filled cysts in subcutaneous sites containing the scolices of the tapeworm.

Veterinary Nursing of Exotic Pets and Wildlife, Third Edition. Simon J. Girling.

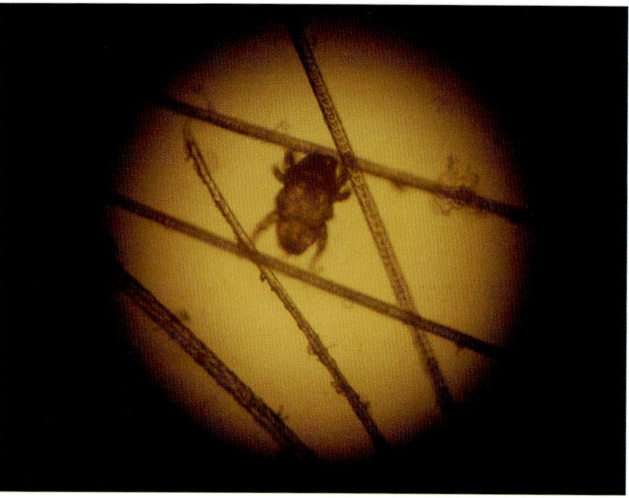

Figure 5.1 Microscope image of *Cheyletiella parasitivorax*.

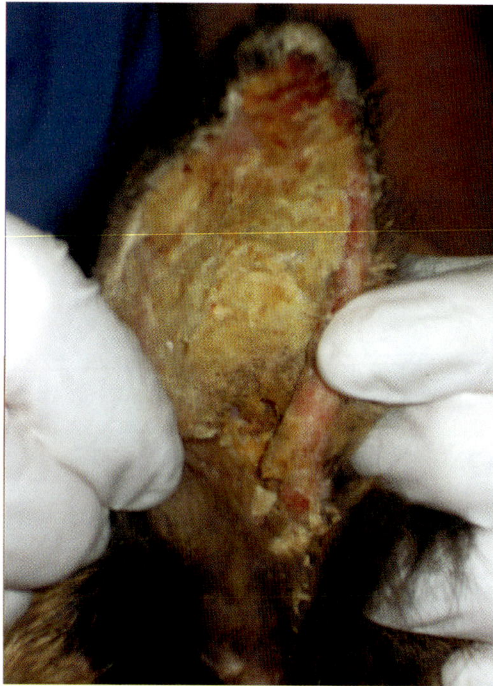

Figure 5.2 *Psoroptes cuniculi* infection in a rabbit. Note the extensive tan-coloured crusting and ulceration inside the pinna.

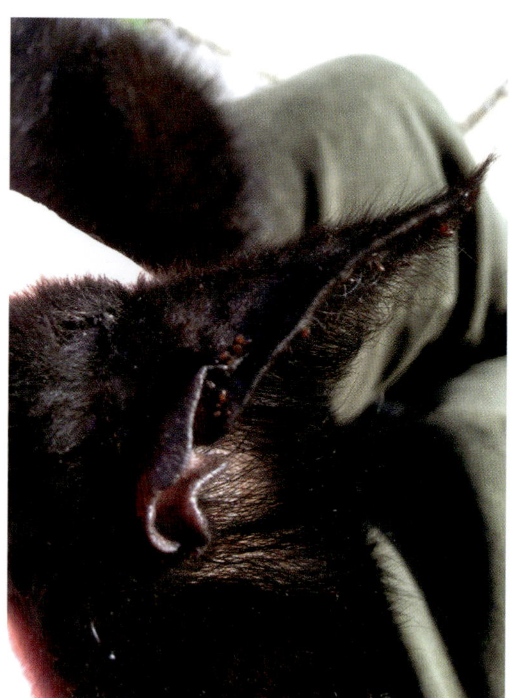

Figure 5.3 The rabbit flea *Spilopsyllus cuniculi* tends to stay along the ear margins of rabbits (and in this case a domestic cat) feeding off the blood in the ear veins.

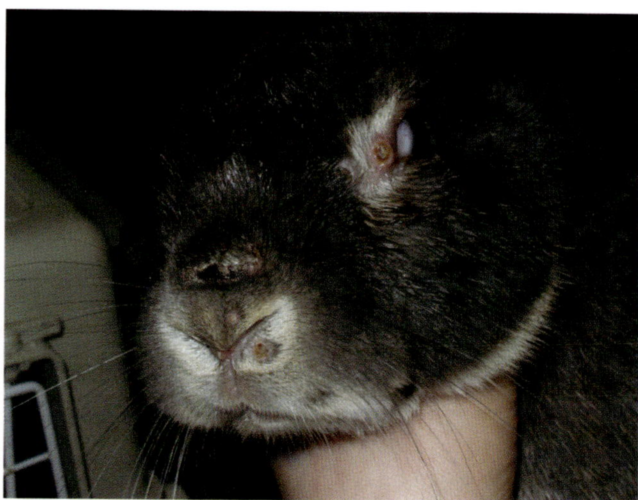

Figure 5.4 Myxoma lesions on the nose of a rabbit with partial immunity to myxomatosis.

Ticks such as *Ixodes ricinus*, *Dermacentor* spp. and *Haemaphysalis* spp. may attach to outdoor rabbits and may result in anaemia, abscess site reactions and the transmission of diseases such as myxomatosis.

Passalurus ambiguus, the oxyurid pinworm of rabbits, may cause rectal prolapse and perineal irritation in significant infections particularly in younger animals.

Viral

Myxomatosis

In rabbits with partial immunity, myxomatosis produces crusting nodules on the skin of the nose, lips, feet and base of the ears (see Figure 5.4). In these rabbits, death can still occur up to 40 days after the initial signs, but many will recover. The acute form of myxomatosis causes oedema of the periocular region, the base of the ears and the anal and genital openings. The virus attacks internal organs as well, and in the unvaccinated domestic rabbit is almost invariably fatal, running a course of 5–15 days (see Figure 5.5).

The myxomatosis virus is a member of the poxvirus family, and is transmitted by biting insects, chiefly fleas, but mosquitoes and lice may also provide a source of infection. In densely stocked situations, it is possible that the virus can be transferred by aerosol from one rabbit directly to another.

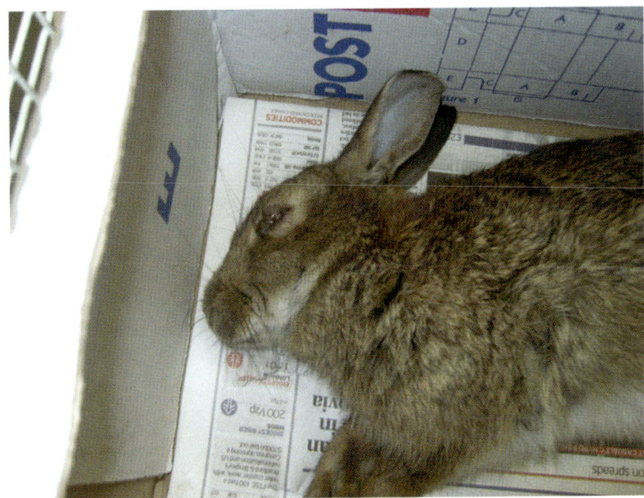

Figure 5.5 Myxomatosis in an unvaccinated rabbit. Note the swelling around the eyes, muzzle and base of the ears.

Other viruses

Rabbit (Shope) papillomavirus and rabbit (Shope) fibromaviruses may be seen in North America where they can cause papillomas and subcutaneous fibromas (sometimes with skin ulceration), respectively. There is also a rabbit oral papillomavirus that can cause oral papillomas and is discussed in the section on digestive disease.

Bacterial

Rabbit pus is thick and inspissated. Abscesses are common in the head where they are invariably associated with dental disease. Bacteria involved include *Pasteurella multocida* and *Staphylococcus aureus* although, after prolonged antibiotic treatment, many anaerobic bacteria will flourish.

'Blue fur disease' is caused by *Pseudomonas aeruginosa*, which produces a blue pigment, staining the fur, and is common in outdoor rabbits or those kept in damp conditions. It will infect damaged skin, such as occurs in the dewlap area of many lop breeds, where wet skin chafes.

Rabbit syphilis, due to *Treponema paraluisleporidarum* ecovar Cuniculus (TPeC), affects the anogenital area, nose, periocular areas and lips, producing brown crusting lesions. These may progress over the rest of the face and forepaws (see Figure 5.6). It may also result in abortions, metritis and neonatal mortality. This bacterium is thought to be passed from doe to young during parturition and may be sexually transmitted from buck to doe and vice versa. It has a prolonged incubation period of 10–16 weeks. It is not infectious for humans.

Rarely, infections with *Fusobacterium necrophorum* (so-called necrobacillosis) can occur, associated with skin wounds contaminated with faeces and therefore typically affecting the perineum, feet and head producing ulcers and necrotic tissues.

Fungal

The two most commonly seen dermatophytes are *Microsporum canis*, which will fluoresce under ultraviolet Wood's lamp, and *Trichophyton mentagrophytes*, which does not. Lesions associated with infection are dry and scaly, with often grey plaques appearing over the head initially, but then spreading to the feet and the rest of the body. Culturing brushings of the lesions on dermatophyte medium is advised for definitive diagnosis.

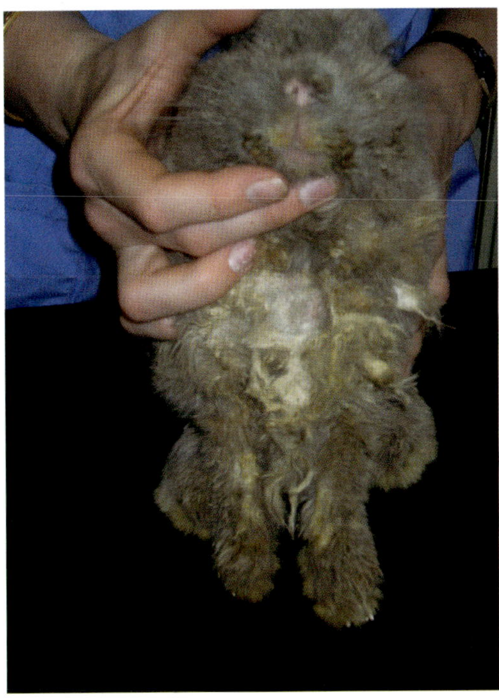

Figure 5.6 Tan-coloured crusting lesions around the nose, mouth and anogenital area are commonly seen with TPeC infection, lesions which may be transferred to the paws and rest of the body through grooming.

Neoplasia

Various skin neoplasms have been reported in rabbits with perhaps the most commonly seen being T-cell lymphoma (see Figure 5.7). Others include squamous cell carcinomas (often around the ear tips particularly in light-furred and albino rabbits), basal cell tumours, sebaceous carcinomas, adenomas and melanomas. Subcutaneous neoplasms such as leiomyomas, leiomyosarcomas, myxosarcomas, rhabdomyosarcomas, lipomas and liposarcomas have also been reported. Adenocarcinomas may be primary neoplasms of the skin or, in un-neutered females with uterine adenocarcinomas, the skin can be a metastasis site (see Figure 5.8).

Managemental

The fur of fine and long-haired breeds, such as the Angoras, mats easily, particularly when the animal is bedded on straw, hay or shavings. Owners are advised to keep them on paper or wire mesh, and to groom their rabbit once or twice daily.

Overgrown claws are common, particularly in hutch-kept rabbits with little access to the outside. Claws should be regularly assessed and, if necessary, trimmed on a 4–6-week basis. Overgrown claws can lead to lateral twisting of digit joints and deformity of the foot.

Perineal soiling may be due to faecal soiling from diarrhoea, or inability to consume the caecotrophs which are softer than the faecal pellet. Urine scalding is also common. Older rabbits may have spinal arthritis, which prevents them from positioning correctly to urinate, and lop breeds have excessive folds of skin around the urogenital area.

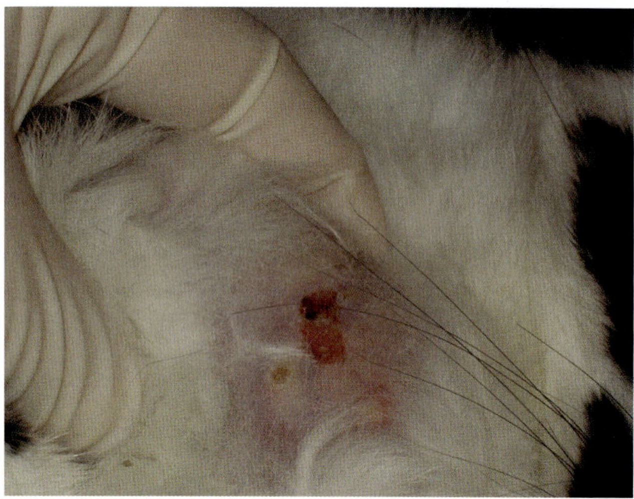

Figure 5.7 T-cell lymphoma is a common skin neoplasm causing raised plaques that may ulcerate.

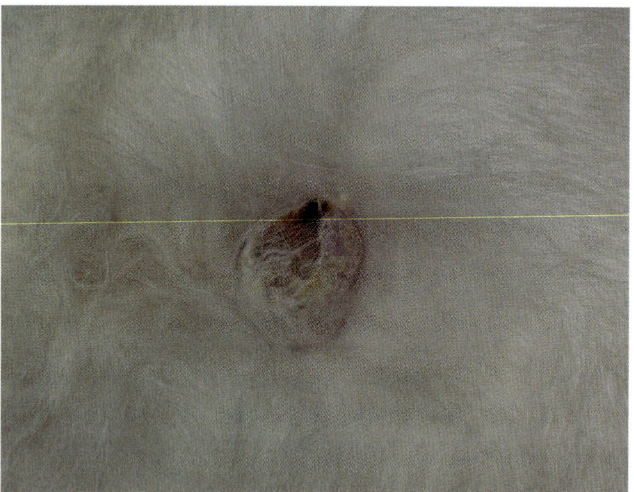

Figure 5.8 Adenocarcinomas are sometimes reported in rabbits and may be of primary skin origin or metastasis from another site such as the uterus.

For mild cases, provision of absorbent bedding underneath a deep layer of straw is advised. Attention to cage and rabbit hygiene on a daily basis is essential to prevent blowfly strike and secondary bacterial skin infections. To prevent blowfly strike, topical treatment such as cyromazine should also be considered in such cases.

Pododermatitis is relatively common, particularly in the heavier rabbit with minimal bedding, especially if housed on wire-mesh floors (Mancinelli *et al.*, 2014). The authors of this study demonstrated a strong breed association, with lop breeds being over-represented with hock pododermatitis. There was also a sex-bias, with females being more prone than males, and a clear bias towards aged individuals. The pressure sores often become secondarily infected with a variety of bacteria and may be difficult to treat when seen at an end stage. Six different grades of lesion have been summarised as follows: 0 (no lesions), 1–2 (alopecia of different sizes and locations), 3–5 (presence of ulcers of different grades of severity) and 6 (deep ulcers and loss of pedal function) (Mancinelli *et al.*, 2014).

Other skin disease

Sebaceous adenitis has been well reported in the domestic rabbit (White *et al.*, 2000). Its cause is unknown but it produces scaling non-pruritic dermatitis starting over the head and neck and progressing to the rest of the body. There have been some associations with other underlying diseases and so may resemble the paraneoplastic syndrome associated with thymomas in domestic cats. In rabbits it has been associated with both thymomas and hepatitis (Florizoone, 2005; Florizoone *et al.*, 2007).

Eosinophilic granulomas have been very occasionally reported in rabbits and are thought to be due to a hypersensitivity reaction to ectoparasites such as fleas or mites. They produce typical ulcerated plaque-like lesions similar to those seen in the domestic cat.

Ehlers–Danlos-like syndrome has been reported in rabbits associated with increased joint laxity and skin hyperextensibility as well as skin fragility. It is believed to be a genetic disorder and has no cure.

Injection site reactions are common with certain medications that can result in skin ulceration or tissue necrosis. Typical examples include many formulations of enrofloxacin and the tetracycline family.

Digestive disease

Oral

Dental disease may present from salivation and anorexia, through jawbone swellings, to full-blown abscesses. Overgrown teeth may be obvious, as with incisor malocclusions, or may be hidden from external view, as with cheek teeth malocclusions. Dental problems may affect other parts of the head, creating abscesses behind the globe of the eye, or the tear duct as it runs over the cheek teeth and maxillary incisor roots, causing pus to appear at the eye or nares.

Causes of dental disease include hereditary defects (Netherland dwarf and lops), due to a shortened rostrocaudal length of skull and abnormal bite, or dietary deficiencies or both. The two most commonly cited dietary deficiencies include a lack of suitable abrasive foodstuffs for dental wear, and a lack of calcium and vitamin D_3 for proper jawbone mineralisation during growth in particular.

Rabbits have evolved to survive on a diet consisting of around 85% grass and 15% leafy herbage. Meadow grass is very high in silicates. These are abrasive and are naturally very wearing. Rabbits' normal dental growth has coevolved to cope with this, and therefore if not fed adequate grass-based diets, teeth will not wear as rapidly and overgrowth will occur. As the rabbit's mandible is narrower than its maxilla, even wear of the cheek teeth occurs by lateral movement of the mandible across the maxilla. In less abrasive, easier-chewed diets, this happens less effectively, and so the outer or buccal edges of the mandibular cheek teeth wear, and the inner or lingual edges of the maxillary cheek teeth wear, causing sharp points to form on the tongue side of the mandibular teeth and the cheek side of the maxillary. These points grow, the angle of the teeth will tilt, and the mandibular teeth then cut into the tongue, and the maxillary teeth into the cheeks leading to deep ulcers, infection, pain and anorexia. All of this may be exacerbated by a low calcium and vitamin D diet which result in poor mineralisation of the jawbones and so allows greater movement of the teeth within the jaw.

The roots of the cheek teeth may also eventually grow back into the jaws as they elongate, due to a lack of space inside the mouth. The

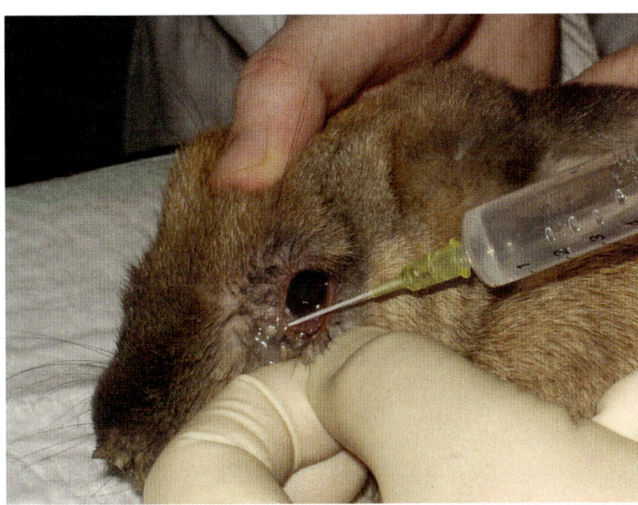

Figure 5.9 Ocular disease may be associated with rabbit snuffles but often starts in the tear duct (dacryocystitis) due to pinching of the duct by overgrown (usually incisor) teeth roots. The single tear duct punctum is being flushed with saline in this image.

roots then push through the ventral aspect of the mandible and may be felt as a series of lumps underneath the angle of the lower jaw. In the maxilla, the roots of the last two cheek teeth can push into the orbit of the eye, causing ocular pain and epiphora.

Incisors may also overgrow. This is associated with the elongation of the molars that result in the mouth being opened wider. The maxillary incisors are tightly curved whereas the mandibular incisors are more gently curving. If the mouth is forced slightly open by the cheek teeth elongating, the maxillary incisors no longer close rostral to the mandibular ones, initially meaning they occlude directly on top of each other. This forces the incisor roots to move back into the jawbones which in the maxilla results in the incisor roots pinching the tear ducts and so causing dacryocystitis with an ocular discharge. This may be misdiagnosed as a primary conjunctivitis (see Figure 5.9).

With progressive mouth opening as the cheek teeth grow further, the maxillary incisors end up caudal to the mandibular ones and so curl back and into the mouth like ram's horns, the mandibular incisors growing up in front of the nose.

Other causes of dental disease include physical trauma to the head and inappropriate 'clipping' of the teeth with nail clippers. Clipping twists and cracks the tooth root causing further deformity and predisposing to infection. Overgrown incisor teeth should only be cut with a high-speed drill or equivalent dental burr.

Radiography of the rabbit head plus close oral examination under anaesthesia is essential for examining the full extent of the dental problem. Positive contrast techniques may be used in the tear ducts to highlight areas of narrowing or blockage (see Chapter 7).

Gastrointestinal

Dietary

Dietary causes, for example a sudden change in diet, will lead to temporary diarrhoea. Other dietary factors include the type of food fed. Spoiled foods and part-fermented grass cuttings will inevitably lead to diarrhoea. In addition, a low level of fibre in the diet will slow caecal and colonic motility and so result in abnormal fermentation by microbial flora causing a lowering of the pH that favours harmful bacteria such as *Clostridium* spp. and *Escherichia coli*. This decrease in caecal pH due to low dietary fibre and a dysbiosis may be one of the causes of so-called mucoid enteritis, a condition typically affecting rabbits between 7 and 14 weeks of age with lethargy, diarrhoea, caecal impaction and the passing of mucus in the faeces.

Iatrogenic

Iatrogenic causes include the oral administration of certain antibiotics, for example penicillin, ampicillin, amoxicillin, cephalosporins, lincomycin, erythromycin and clindamycin. These destroy the normal flora of the gut, leaving bacteria such as *Clostridium spiroforme* or *Clostridium perfringens* (already present in the gut in very small amounts) to flourish. Once these bacteria grow in number and achieve a critical threshold level, they can release toxins which are absorbed into the bloodstream and cause toxaemia and death.

Bacterial

Bacteria, for example *E. coli*, common in young weaner rabbits, are a cause of sudden death, due to the release of enterotoxins, and are present in several strains defined by the term 'enteropathogenic *Escherichia coli*' (EPEC). Death may occur before any signs of diarrhoea. EPEC deaths are most commonly seen between 1 and 14 days of age with yellow-staining diarrhoea. An unknown agent, suspected to be bacterial, is the cause of epizootic rabbit enteropathy (ERE) which is the single biggest cause of mortality in rabbits fattened for the meat industry in Europe. Clinical signs include loss of appetite, over-full stomachs and watery diarrhoea with a high mortality rate. Disease can be stopped by rapid treatment with antibiotics such as tiamulin and bacitracin (Huybens *et al.*, 2008).

Lawsonia intracellularis, which is associated with proliferative enteritis in hamsters, humans, ferrets and pigs, has been associated with a similar condition in weaning rabbits between 2 and 4 months of age.

Clostridium (Bacillus) piliforme has been associated with so-called Tyzzer's disease in rodents and may affect rabbits. Watery diarrhoea with physical depression and a high mortality rate in the presence of overcrowding and high levels of physiological stress are typically seen in young rabbits. Mature rabbits will develop a more prolonged course of the disease with chronic weight loss and organ damage.

Salmonella typhimurium is the *Salmonella* spp. most commonly associated with enteritis in rabbits.

Parasitic

Coccidia, for example *Eimeria* spp., are single-celled protozoal parasites that destroy the lining of the small intestine, causing diarrhoea and death in heavy infestations particularly in young rabbits. In mild cases it may simply cause poor growth and stunting in young rabbits. *Eimeria stiedae* is of particular importance in rabbits as it will also damage the liver, gaining access from the intestines via the hepatic portal vein and damaging the bile duct epithelium, and being commonly recorded in captivity and the wild at rates around 24–31% (Bochynska *et al.*, 2022). Coccidial oocysts may be detected in the faeces but it should be noted that a yeast known as *Cyniclomyces guttulatus*, specific and harmless to rabbits, can be mistaken for a coccidial oocyst (Forsythe and Parker, 1985).

Cryptosporidium parvum, as with many mammals, can cause a transient diarrhoea lasting 3–5 days in rabbit kits around 4–6 weeks of age. Dehydration may be significant and require medical intervention but the infection is often self-resolving otherwise.

The stomach worm *Graphidium strigosum* and the small intestinal worm *Trichostrongylus retortaeformis* are usually only found in rabbits with access to the outside, where they may pick up the eggs of these worms directly from wild rabbits' faeces or indirectly via passive spread from wild birds, etc. A large intestinal pinworm, *Passalurus ambiguus*, is commonly seen, but rarely causes disease. All of these worms' eggs may be detected in the faeces by flotation methods.

A liver worm has been associated with small abscesses in outdoor and wild European rabbits (Bochynska *et al.*, 2022). *Calodium hepaticum* (syn. *Capillaria hepatica*) is a nematode that resides in the liver of rabbits and other small mammals and is passed on when the animal dies or is eaten by another. If the animal dies, the eggs of the worm, deposited in the liver by the adult worm, enter the soil and can infect the next host when it eats the contaminated herbage/soil. It is a potential zoonosis.

Numerous non-pathogenic protozoa (*Entamoeba cuniculi*, *Monocercomonas cuniculi*, *Retortamonas cuniculi*) can be found in the large intestine and caecum of rabbits. *Giardia* may be occasionally found in low numbers in the faeces, residing in the small intestine and rarely causes disease. A tapeworm, *Cittotaenia variabilis*, has been reported in domestic rabbits, although rarely associated with disease.

Viral

Rabbit oral papillomatosis has been reported in laboratory rabbits such as New Zealand whites associated with a suspected viral cause. The papillomas occur on the ventral surface of the tongue.

Rabbit coronaviral disease can affect young rabbits between 3 and 10 weeks old and result in diarrhoea, lethargy, cardiac disease and pericardial effusion with high death rates (DiGiacomo and Mare, 1994).

Rabbit rotavirus infections are generally mild and result in a transient diarrhoea in young kits between 4 and 10 weeks of age. However, some may be more severely affected with anorexia, dehydration and a bile-tinged mucoid diarrhoea.

Viral haemorrhagic disease, a calicivirus, is discussed below under liver diseases.

Neoplasia

Various gastrointestinal and liver neoplasms have been reported, including adenocarcinomas, leiomyomas and leiomyosarcomas of the stomach and intestines; bile duct adenomas and adenocarcinomas of the liver and metastases of uterine adenocarcinomas and lymphoma can also be seen.

Hypomotility disorders

Aetiology and clinical signs: One of the most important factors is the level of indigestible fibre in the diet. A deficiency of fibre results in reduced motility both by a lack of physical stimulation of the colon due to the absence of large fibre particles and a decreased production of volatile fatty acids in the caecum. Other causes include increased adrenergic stimulation due to stress or pain resulting in reduced motility (e.g. dental disease, osteoarthritis) and intestinal infectious diseases, all of which can cause varying effects on gut motility. Most cases in domestic rabbits are due to stress and a long-term dietary deficiency in indigestible fibre.

Stomach impaction seen in cases of hypomotility usually comprises a matt of fur and food material. These trichobezoars in rabbits have been blamed for occlusion of the pylorus so causing gastrointestinal motility disorders. The stomach of the rabbit, however, has been shown to always contain food material and groomed fur (Okerman, 1994). When gastric foreign bodies were artificially created using latex, the rabbits affected showed no reduction in appetite or in weight (Leary *et al.*, 1984). It is now widely assumed that trichobezoar formations are due to reduced gastrointestinal motility rather than the cause of it. Good-quality fibre is essential to good gut health as discussed in Chapter 1. It is believed that the major cause of poor gut health and digestive tract disease in the domestic rabbit is a lack of good-quality fibre in their diet (Davies and Davies, 2003). In a rabbit consuming good-quality fibre, fur consumed naturally during grooming will move out of the stomach into the intestines. When there is a lack of fibre, gut motility decreases and so any fur consumed stays in the stomach for longer and as rabbits cannot vomit, ends up forming a significant trichobezoar.

Intestinal obstructions can occur when material such as fur matts and other indigestible foreign bodies pass into the small intestine and will also lead to stomach distension (see Figure 5.10).

Onset can be rapid or more insidious. The rabbit is often dull, anorexic and lethargic, may show signs of dehydration and is often suffering from hepatic lipidosis and ketoacidosis. Death, when it occurs, is usually due to liver and kidney failure.

Leporine dysautonomia is another cause of hypomotility. Clinical signs include dry mucous membranes, reduced tear production, dilated pupils, bradycardia, urinary retention (with overflow incontinence), caecal and large intestine impaction, loss of anal tone and proprioceptive deficits. Aspiration pneumonia may also be seen due to megaoesophagus.

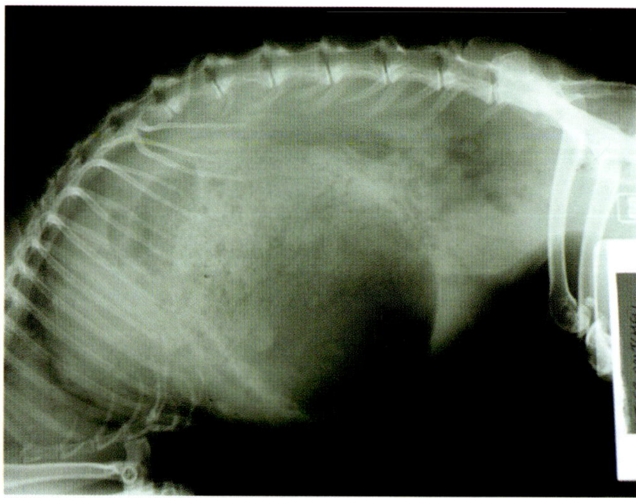

Figure 5.10 Lateral radiograph of a rabbit with a suspected small intestinal obstruction and a massively dilated stomach.

Lower intestine hypomotility has been suggested as the cause of caecolith formation, where inspissated material or dehydrated ingesta result in caecal and then large bowel impactions. Neurological disease such as leporine dysautonomia, encephalitozoonosis and spinal cord and nerve root disease have all been suggested as causes.

Diagnosis: Radiographs of the abdomen may show a distended stomach with food material and an accumulation of gas in stomach and caecum. Blood results show hepatic dysfunction, elevation of hepatic-associated leakage enzymes (aspartate aminotransferase, AST), lipaemia, metabolic acidosis and hyperglycaemia although later cases may show hypoglycaemia, and dehydration as witnessed by an elevated packed cell volume (usually over 45%). Cases where hepatic lipidosis and ketoacidosis are advanced may see damage to the kidneys and resultant elevation in urea, creatinine, phosphate and potassium.

Diagnosis of dysautonomia include absence/reduction of tears on a Schirmer tear test (<3 mm in a minute), dramatic miosis when 0.1% pilocarpine is applied to the eyes, and radiography demonstrating aspiration pneumonia, megaoesophagus, impacted/distended caecum and large intestine and distended urinary bladder. Histopathology reveals chromolytic degeneration of the autonomic neurons similar to that seen in equine grass-sickness cases.

Prevention: Ensure all rabbits are fed on a high-fibre diet, for example freshly grazed grass, good-quality hay or dried grass. In any stressful procedure where significant catecholamine release is likely to occur, for example postoperatively, it is beneficial to use prokinetic drugs such as metoclopramide and ranitidine and to provide adequate analgesia.

Liver disease

Rabbit haemorrhagic disease virus

A calicivirus is known to cause rabbit haemorrhagic disease (RHD) of which there are at least three strains currently recognised. The virus replicates in the liver of rabbits older than 2 months of age (younger rabbits are unaffected by the virus). The virus is transmitted in urine, blood and faeces directly from rabbit to rabbit or via contaminated bedding, food or cage furniture. Incubation period is rapid (1–3 days) and rabbits infected that have not been previously vaccinated against the virus have a high mortality rate (approaching 100%). As its name suggests the virus results in widespread internal haemorrhages, particularly from the liver. Clinically, the rabbit has a fever and may show jaundice, depression and anorexia and, towards the end of the disease course, respiratory nasal foamy discharge, opisthotonus, seizures and other neurological signs may be seen. Diagnosis can be made based on reverse transcriptase polymerase chain reaction (PCR) and clinical signs.

Liver lobe torsion

Liver lobe torsion may produce clinical signs of hypomotility, often with profound depression and cranial abdominal pain. The caudate lobe of the liver may become spontaneously twisted, cutting off the blood supply and this can result in a shock syndrome with clinical anaemia, jaundice, gut stasis, elevation in liver enzymes such as alanine aminotransferase (ALT), AST and gamma-glutamyltransferase (GGT) and, in severe cases, rapid deterioration and death within 12–72 hours. More chronic cases may survive and appear to spontaneously recover after a period of dullness and gut stasis.

Hepatic lipidosis

Aetiology: Hepatic lipidosis is seen most commonly in overweight indoor rabbits that go through a period of anorexia or food withdrawal.

In rabbits we generally assume that increased mobilisation of fat deposits from a period of anorexia/food deprivation/pregnancy is the main cause. However, stress can increase fat mobilisation in overweight rabbits and minor invasive procedures such as saline injections induce an increase in plasma free fatty acid and glycerol levels in obese rabbits (Lafontan and Agid, 1979). A high-fat diet increases the risks of ketonaemia and so ketoacidosis during anorexia (Jean-Blain and Durix, 1985). Pregnant does between days 24 and 30 are insulin resistant, adding to the likelihood they will develop pregnancy ketosis (McLaughlin and Fish, 1994).

The longer the anorexia, the worse the lipid mobilisation and the more the liver is swamped with lipids and free fatty acids. The lipids affect the function of hepatocytes and make them less able to successfully perform the tricarboxylic acid (TCA) cycle which is further exacerbated by an absence of glucose in the bloodstream.

Once the liver has become lipidotic, the kidneys frequently follow.

Clinical signs: The early stages may be imperceptible. Most cases are triggered by a period of anorexia, the main clinical signs being reduction in food intake and faecal output. As the condition progresses, the rabbit becomes comatose, hypoglycaemic and acidotic, and dies of liver and kidney failure. Any rabbit anorexic for 12 hours or more (6–8 hours in pregnant does) should be given assisted feeding.

Diagnosis: There is no liver specific leakage enzyme in the rabbit; therefore, AST, lactate dehydrogenase (LDH) and creatine kinase (CK) are measured together as AST is found in the liver and skeletal muscle, LDH in liver, cardiac and skeletal muscle and CK only in skeletal muscle. GGT elevations are associated with hepatobiliary disease rather than hepatocellular damage, and therefore have been associated with conditions such as hepatic coccidiosis by *E. stiedae*.

Elevations in triglycerides and cholesterol levels will also occur. There may be hypoglycaemia in severe cases, and levels of beta-hydroxybutyrate will be elevated where ketosis is present.

Serum proteins may also be elevated, particularly increases in alpha-2- and beta-2-lipoprotein. Finally, ultrasound and endoscopic biopsy of the liver provides a reliable indication of hepatic lipidosis but obviously gives no indication of the degree of ketoacidosis present.

Respiratory disease

Pasteurellosis

Pasteurella multocida causes 'rabbit snuffles'. It is commonly found in the airways of unaffected rabbits, but it can lead to purulent oculonasal discharge, and wet, matted fur of the forepaws. This can develop into pneumonia. Some strains of *P. multocida* can be more pathogenic than others and may cause septicaemia. Many *P. multocida* can secrete a dermonecrotic toxin similar to that causing atrophic rhinitis in pigs. Hence many rabbits with these infections are left with permanent upper and lower respiratory tract damage. Poor housing with damp ammonia-laden bedding can irritate the airways and allow rapid infection to occur. Dental disease and myxomatosis are other factors. Similarly, overcrowded hutches and concurrent disease elsewhere in the body may lower immunity.

Pasteurella infections may also be found in tooth abscesses and middle ear disease. Infections may result in chronic abscessation of the lungs, mediastinum, pleurae and pericardium.

Other bacterial infections

Bordetella bronchiseptica may be found as a commensal of the upper airways of the rabbit but it can also produce disease. Some strains are cytotoxic and so enhance infections of *Pasteurella multocida*.

Staphylococcus aureus and *Staphylococcus epidermidis* are commonly isolated from the upper respiratory tract of healthy and diseased rabbits. *Staphylococcus aureus* can produce toxins which destroy neutrophils as well as protein A which can bind to immunoglobulins. It has been associated with abscessation of the head, lungs, mediastinum and middle ears.

Pseudomonas aeruginosa has also been associated with respiratory infections, septicaemia and mortalities in rabbits. It is an environmental bacterium and is often associated with damp soiled bedding and environs.

Viral disease

RHD is caused by a calicivirus that has been present in the UK since 1992. It does not cause respiratory disease exclusively, as it will attack all organs within the body, particularly the lungs, digestive system and liver, but can produce a foamy discharge from the nares that may be blood-tinged with tachypnoea and hyperpnoea. See the section on digestive disease for further details.

The myxomatosis virus can also cause respiratory tract discharge and has been associated with a haemorrhagic pneumonia. See the section on skin disease for further details.

Neoplasia

Primary lung carcinomas have been reported but more commonly seen neoplasms of the lungs include secondary metastases from uterine adenocarcinomas, mammary carcinomas, lymphoma or extension of lymphoma from the associated thymus.

Cardiovascular disease

Arterial wall calcification and atherosclerosis

With an excess of dietary calcium/vitamin D_3, calcium becomes deposited in the walls of the major blood vessels, reducing their elasticity and leading to increased blood pressure. This is common in the aorta, and may also occur within the kidney parenchyma itself. Some rabbits may be genetically predisposed to this problem. There is no cure. Prevention is aimed at avoiding oversupplementation with calcium and vitamin D_3. Dietary levels of vitamin D in excess of 2300 IU/kg feed have been shown to be toxic and levels above the recommended range of 800–1200 IU/kg feed have been associated with soft tissue mineralisation (Cheeke, 1987; Zimmerman *et al.*, 1990; Lowe, 2020). Interestingly, one study suggested that vitamin D_3 supplementation may actually help reduce the severity of atherosclerosis (fat deposition) within major arteries such as the aorta by reducing the inflammatory effects such lipids had on the wall of the artery, making its association and effect on vascular disease more complicated (Malek and Shata, 2014). Rabbits are often used as a model for studying human atherosclerosis as they form similar levels of low-density lipoproteins (LDLs) as humans in response to high-fat diets.

Cardiac disease

Overall, cardiac disease is less commonly reported in the domestic rabbit than in pet cats and dogs, with one review of the literature suggesting that the median age of onset was 4.4 years of age, with median weight being 1.7 kg and no sex predisposition (Muller and Mancinelli, 2022). Pericarditis associated with bacteria such as *Pasteurella multocida*, *Streptococcus* spp. and *Staphylococcus* spp. have all been reported.

Cardiomyopathy, atherosclerosis and valvular insufficiency with resultant congestive heart failure are also seen in rabbits. The cause of cardiomyopathy is not always clear and rabbits may be asymptomatic. Dilated cardiomyopathy is more commonly seen than the hypertrophic form but both have been reported. Endocardiosis is seen in older rabbits with the mitral valve being most commonly affected. Alpha-2 drugs such as xylazine and medetomidine have been associated with development of myocardial ischaemia and cardiomyopathy, as has stress. Stress induces catecholamine release resulting in coronary arterial constriction in the rabbit and myocardial ischaemia. End-stage dilated cardiomyopathy and significant valvular insufficiency may present with congestive heart failure with ascites, dyspnoea and tachypnoea.

Arrhythmias

The most commonly seen arrhythmia in rabbits is profound bradycardia associated with a heart block. It may also be a cause of syncope and collapsing bunny syndrome.

Lead poisoning

This has been associated particularly with indoor rabbits that have access to woodwork painted with lead paints or lead water piping. This may lead to anaemia with basophilic stippling of the erythrocytes with Romanowsky stains. Clinically, profound chronic non-regenerative anaemia and neurological signs have been reported. Lead levels above 1.1 μmol/L on heparinised blood are diagnostic.

Lymphoma

Lymphoma has been regularly reported in the domestic rabbit and, as with other species, can affect multiple organs at the same time. Both T- and B-cell lymphomas have been reported, with T-cell lymphoma as one would expect being most commonly identified in the thymus and skin. So-called 'wirehair' rabbits have a recessive gene that makes them highly susceptible to lymphoma (Fox *et al.*, 1970). Thymic neoplasia, both benign and malignant, is common and may result in a number of clinical signs including respiratory difficulties and exophthalmos as the mass enlarges and affects the cranial vena caval return to the heart.

Urinary tract disease

Urolithiasis and cystitis

Cystitis and urolithiasis are common, as rabbits absorb the majority of the calcium present in the intestines, and then excrete any excess into the urine via the kidneys. The commonest urolith is calcium carbonate, which forms readily in the rabbit's alkaline urine, and is

Table 5.1 Urinalysis results for healthy domestic rabbits.

Parameter	Expected values
Urine volume	20–350 mL/kg per day (50–75 mL/kg per day average) (NB: highly dependent on diet)
Urine specific gravity	1.003–1.036
Urine erythrocyte numbers	<5 erythrocytes per high power field
Urine protein levels	Trace to absent (may be more in juveniles and bucks)
Urine colour	Varies from pale yellow to deep red depending on presence/absence of porphyrins
Urine average pH	8.2
Urine crystals	Small volumes of ammonium magnesium phosphate or calcium carbonate are normal

radiodense, often filling the bladder outline on radiographs. Secondary bladder infections are common as the crystals irritate the lining of the bladder. See Table 5.1 for details of urinalysis.

Haematuria

The presence of red-coloured urine in the rabbit does not necessarily indicate haematuria and so urine dipstick tests should not be relied upon for a diagnosis; rather, microscopy to demonstrate erythrocytes with a cut-off of more than five erythrocytes per high-power field is often used for a positive diagnosis. Many red porphyrin pigments from the diet (particularly some leafy greens such as beetroot) will be excreted in the urine. Causes of haematuria include cystitis, uterine tumours, aneurysms, endometrial hyperplasia and kidney disease/infections.

Renal disease

Aetiology

In general, cases of chronic renal failure (CRF) are associated with *Encephalitozoon cuniculi*, pyelonephritis, chronic progressive nephrosis, amyloidosis, renal calcinosis, congenital polycystic kidneys (which tend to produce CRF by 2–3 years of age), neoplasia (kidneys are a common site for lymphoma in rabbits) and renoliths/ureteroliths.

Acute renal failure may be seen associated with *E. cuniculi*, pyelonephritis, drug toxicity, fatty kidney disease and renoliths/ureteroliths causing hydronephrosis.

Clinical signs

Chronic renal failure: This is associated with weight loss, dehydration, loss of appetite, polydipsia and polyuria. In addition, a reduction in gastrointestinal motility with caecal impaction may be observed. Clinical anaemia may be present and other signs associated with specific conditions (e.g. neurological signs with *E. cuniculi* infection) may also be demonstrable.

Acute renal failure: The rabbit is usually in good bodily condition, with a history of recent medication administration (e.g. nephrotoxic drugs such as the aminoglycosides, or non-steroidal anti-inflammatory drugs) or in does in late pregnancy with toxaemia or in obese animals which undergo a period of anorexia where fatty infiltration may occur.

Encephalitozoon cuniculi: This can be a cause of chronic and acute renal failure and, of course, may be associated with neurological signs, for example torticollis, fitting, cataracts and uveitis (often unilateral), muscle tremors, paresis and paralysis of hindlimbs and urinary overflow with urine scalding. Death may occur due to heart failure, renal failure or meningoencephalitis. The organism is a microsporidian parasite found in a wide range of mammals including rabbits and is a potential zoonotic disease in immunocompromised humans. There are different strains of *E. cuniculi*: strain I (found in rabbits and humans), strain II (found in rodents) and strain III (found in dogs and humans). Infection is by ingestion of food contaminated by infected urine, although vertical transmission is possible *in utero*. Replication occurs in the kidneys and spreads to the central nervous system (CNS) as well as the cardiac muscles. The most common renal presentation is chronic renal disease due to a granulomatous interstitial nephritis and tubular degeneration.

Pyelonephritis/renoliths: Rabbits affected may be in severe pain, sometimes vocalising when passing urine. Urine may be obviously turbid with pus, or blood. Individuals may also have gastrointestinal associated signs such as increased borborygmi or gastrointestinal stasis. The patient is often hunched and anorectic. However, some individuals with early renoliths may be clinically unaffected.

Diagnosis

Chronic renal failure: The major acute phase protein in rabbits is C-reactive protein travelling in the beta-globulin fraction. With acute renal failure due to nephritis an increase in alpha-2 globulins is also seen (alpha-2 macroglobulin), as is the case with the nephrotic syndrome. In the nephrotic syndrome (chronic renal disease), there is also an increase in beta-1 globulins (due to transferrin and beta-2 lipoprotein). In CRF, there is often a significant drop in albumin, whereas in acute renal failure there is often elevation (due to dehydration) or normal levels.

In CRF, urea, creatinine and phosphate levels will be raised, and the patient is often anaemic. Urea is often less sensitive than creatinine for detecting renal disease as prerenal azotaemia can be seen with dehydration as well as urea production by endogenous gut bacteria. Only when less than 25% of renal tissue is still functioning will these blood parameters become elevated, so these are not sensitive for detecting early renal disease. A better assessment of glomerular filtration rate (GFR) may be made using endogenous clearance rates for creatine. Weisbroth *et al.* (1974) calculated the normal GFR as 2.2–4.2 mL/kg per minute. This method requires bladder catheterisation and accurate urine output. Urine protein levels should be minimal or absent and therefore presence of protein and casts in the urine is significant and may indicate CRF and/or infection. An assessment of urine protein/creatinine ratio can be made and values in excess of 0.4 are suggestive of kidney disease (Reusch *et al.*, 2009). The presence of increased GGT in the urine has also been linked to renal disease; the normal range is 2.7–96.5 IU/L, with a GGT index (GGT/creatinine ratio, used to remove variations in GGT excretion) of 0.043–1.034 being reported in healthy rabbits (Mancinelli *et al.*, 2012).

Ionised and total calcium levels may be elevated and soft tissue mineralisation seen radiographically, most commonly the aorta and kidneys. Hypermineralisation of the bones may also be seen which is not seen in cats and dogs. Hypermineralisation is exacerbated by diets supplemented with vitamin D as rabbits are sensitive to toxicosis.

Ultrasonographically, the renal outline may be smaller than normal (<3 cm in length craniocaudally and <2 cm ventrodorsally).

Acute renal failure: Blood parameters will be elevated as for CRF, but there is often renal shutdown and anuria. The main difference between acute and chronic failure is the loss of body condition and generally slower onset of debilitation and polydipsia/polyuria in chronic failure.

Ultrasonographically, the renal outline may be larger than normal (>4 cm craniocaudally and <2.5 cm ventrodorsally).

Prerenal azotaemia: This can be differentiated from acute renal failure by the presence of other clinical signs, usually cardiovascular/hypovolaemic shock in conjunction with a urine specific gravity above 1.030. Confirmation occurs with reduction of renal parameters with rehydration and treatment of hypovolaemia.

Encephalitozoon cuniculi: Antibodies are produced 2–3 weeks after infection. There is no correlation between antibody levels and degree of spore shedding, or with the severity of lesions at post-mortem. A rising titre over 3–4 weeks is suggestive of recent infection. An IgG and IgM antibody test and a PCR test to detect spores in urine are available.

Hydronephrosis: This may be diagnosed by intravenous pyelography using an iodine-based radiopaque medium (0.5–1 mL/kg) injected through a peripheral vein. Ultrasonography may be used to determine if there is hydropic degeneration. Doppler flow ultrasound may also help to ascertain renal arterial blood flow.

Renoliths/ureteroliths: These may be easily diagnosed via radiography or ultrasonography. Renoliths are usually bilateral. The prognosis is generally guarded as renal damage is common and may be either acute or more commonly chronic. Pyelonephritis may also be present.

Reproductive tract disease

Female

Uterine adenocarcinoma

This is a common condition seen in does over the age of 4 years with a reported incidence between 50 and 80% (see Figure 5.11). The condition is fatal if not detected early as the tumour metastasises, primarily to the lungs although this may take a year to do so (Weisbroth, 1994). Radiography of the chest is therefore advised if the condition is suspected to determine if spread has occurred. Occurrence of uterine neoplasia is not fully understood in the domestic rabbit as some uterine neoplasms have hormone receptors, suggesting that oestrogen and progesterone exposure may cause them, but some do not, suggesting different aetiologies for cancer development are possible that may have implications when considering ovariectomy versus ovariohysterectomy options (Asakawa *et al.*, 2008).

Venereal spirochaetosis

Rabbit syphilis is caused by the bacterium TPeC. The condition is self-limiting, but produces crusting of the anogenital area, nose and lips. Further information can be found in the section on skin disease.

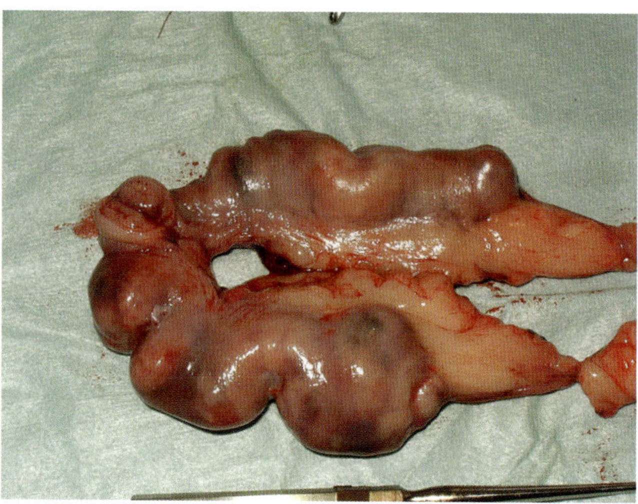

Figure 5.11 Adenocarcinomas in the uterus of a 5-year-old domestic rabbit.

Pyometra, endometritis and endometrial hyperplasia

Pyometras occur in older does and are often due to *E. coli*, *Pasteurella multocida* or *Staphylococcus aureus* infections of hyperplastic endometrial tissues. Endometritis is also commonly seen in older females. Endometrial hyperplasia is commonly seen in older entire does and may result in blood loss from the endometrium with anaemia and haematuria resulting.

Endometrial venous aneurysms

Bleeding from the reproductive tract can be associated with endometritis and open pyometras as well as uterine neoplasia. However, in New Zealand white rabbits and related breeds the venous supply to the uterus can form aneurysms that periodically rupture and so bleed into the lumen.

Pregnancy toxaemia

This is seen usually in the last week of gestation and is associated with a reduction in dietary calorific intake either through inappetence or inadequate food supply. The doe becomes increasingly incoordinated and lethargic and may seizure terminally. Death occurs rapidly within 1–5 days due to the ketoacidosis that develops. Urine becomes acidic and ketones are present. Hyperkalaemia, hyperphosphataemia, hypocalcaemia and ketosis are seen on blood samples.

Mammary gland

Mastitis can occur following pregnancy when the kittens are lost or in phantom pregnancy. Many of the bacteria involved will release endotoxins into the bloodstream causing rapid toxaemia, fever and death of the doe. Others may just cause severe mastitis with abscess formation. As with other reproductive tract diseases, bacteria such as *Pasteurella multocida* and *Staphylococcus aureus* are commonly seen.

Mammary gland neoplasia can be seen in older rabbits and may be benign or malignant. Malignant tumours such as mammary adenocarcinomas may metastasise to other organs including the lungs.

Mammary gland dysplasia has been seen in older New Zealand white does with pituitary prolactin-secreting tumours.

Male

Testicular cancer is reported in male rabbits and, similarly to other species, neoplasms include seminomas, Leydig cell tumours, Sertoli cell tumours, and teratomas.

Musculoskeletal disease

Splay-leg

Splay-leg is an inherited congenital disease wherein the kit cannot position one or more hindlimbs underneath itself. Instead the affected limb sticks out awkwardly. There is often flattening of the femoral head and sometimes hip subluxation with valgus deformity and often patella luxation. There is no treatment for this condition.

Fractured or dislocated spine and disc disease

This is common in indoor-reared, calcium-deficient rabbits. The close confinement leads to weakening of bones and muscles due to disuse atrophy, and dietary calcium deficiency can lead to poorly mineralised vertebrae and limbs making spontaneous fractures more likely, often in the lumbosacral area. Compression fractures and dislocation/subluxation of vertebral bodies are more commonly seen in the thoracolumbar area. There is often a history of the handler picking the rabbit up by the forelimbs without adequately supporting the hindlimbs, with the result that the rabbit kicks out and then fractures the spine.

Disc disease, particularly mineralisation, is common in rabbits and may develop from a few months of age, particularly in giant breeds (Green *et al.*, 1984). This can lead to disc failure and spinal cord trauma.

Other bone fractures

The rabbit skeleton forms a smaller proportion of total body weight than mammals such as dogs, cats or humans. Rabbit long bones also have a thinner, more brittle cortex, and are prone to fissure propagation, shattering with rough handling. Displacement of the superficial flexor tendons in the hind leg may mimic a spinal problem with a shuffling gait and arched back.

In contrast to cats and dogs, in rabbits distal tibial fractures are the most commonly present fracture, followed by metatarsal fractures and then radius/ulna fractures.

Common causes of hindlimb lameness that may be missed are metatarsal and hind feet phalangeal fractures.

Osteoarthritis

This is common in large breeds, even in young animals, and can affect any joint. Most commonly, though, the stifles (due to caudal cruciate damage rather than cranial), hips (often associated with dysplasia) and spine are affected. This may lead to limb disuse, pain, urine staining of the perineum and faecal soiling due to an inability to flex the spine to allow urination and caecotrophy and muscle wasting.

Neurological disease

Encephalitozoonosis

Encephalitozoon cuniculi affects the kidneys and the CNS, and may remain latent for years, producing no clinical signs. Alternatively, paresis/paralysis of the forelimbs and/or hindlimbs, fitting, head tilt or other vestibular symptoms and blindness may be seen along with the previously mentioned renal disease. The most commonly seen clinical signs appear to be vestibular disease and intraocular lesions (uveitis, etc.), with paresis/paralysis also being commonly seen (Harcourt-Brown and Holloway, 2003; Künzel *et al.*, 2008). Diagnosis is as previously described.

Vestibular disease

One very common cause of vestibular disease, as previously mentioned, is encephalitozoonosis. Others include tumours or infarcts of the hindbrain, and more commonly *Pasteurella multocida* or other bacterial infection of the middle and inner ear. Bacteria gain access to the middle ear via the Eustachian canal, or less commonly via a perforated eardrum (e.g. in ear mite infestations). Many rabbits so affected are unable to stand. Prognosis in advanced cases may be poor. Dorsoventral radiography of the middle ear bullae can demonstrate sclerosis of the bullae and loss of trabecular detail indicating infection. Pus is observed in the external ear canal as the disease originating from the middle ear tends to result in tympanic membrane rupture. For this reason ear drops should not be used in rabbits.

Lead poisoning

Lead poisoning may cause anaemia and neurological signs such as fitting, depression and sudden death.

Toxoplasmosis

This is uncommonly seen clinically as most infections tend to produce a subclinical disease course. However, clinical disease has been reported with seizures, ataxia, hindlimb or all four limb paresis and paralysis and so should be considered as a differential diagnosis along with encephalitozoonosis for CNS disease.

Spinal disease

As mentioned under musculoskeletal disease, spinal trauma whether due to vertebral dislocation, compression fractures or disc disease is relatively common, particularly in giant breeds and house rabbits.

Neoplasia

Central nervous system neoplasia is not common, although secondary metastases from primary neoplasia elsewhere, particularly lymphoma and uterine adenocarcinomas, may occur.

Ophthalmic disease

Uveitis

This is commonly seen in rabbits with *Encephalitozoon cuniculi* infections where leakage of the lens contents stimulates a phacoclastic uveitis. This is frequently unilateral. Uveitis can also be seen with bacterial infections, for example *Pasteurella multocida* and of course may lead to glaucoma.

Glaucoma

New Zealand white rabbits have a recessive *bu* gene where intraocular pressures may reach 26–48 mmHg (NB: most tonometers underestimate intraocular pressure in rabbits). Corneal oedema occurs, but the condition does not appear painful and the eye pressure returns to normal as increased pressure results in damage to the ciliary body which produces the intraocular fluid.

Cataracts

These are commonly associated with *E. cuniculi* infection, and often unilateral. However, congenital and spontaneous idiopathic cataracts have been reported.

Conjunctivitis

The milky discharge seen in rabbit eyes is often mistaken for primary conjunctivitis when dacryocystitis due to dental disease pinching the tear duct occurs. Narrowing of the tear duct can be shown by injecting iodine-based dye into the tear duct through the ventral punctum and radiographing the head (see Chapter 7). True conjunctivitis may also be seen, and is one of the clinical signs in myxomatosis.

Aberrant conjunctival overgrowth

This is unique to the rabbit where a fold of conjunctival tissue develops from the limbus of the eye and looks like limbal keratitis. The tissue is not attached to the cornea but overlies it and may be easily removed. The condition is a congenital abnormality with an unknown aetiology.

Exophthalmos

This is seen due to a cranial mediastinal mass surrounding the anterior vena cava that restricts venous drainage from the eyes. The exophthalmos is not permanent but occurs with stress, often disappearing when the stressful incident goes away. Examples include cranial mediastinal abscesses, lymphoma, thymoma and carcinomas.

Retrobulbar abscesses may result in (usually) unilateral exophthalmos and are associated with cheek tooth abscesses.

DISEASES OF THE RAT AND MOUSE

Skin disease

Ectoparasitic

Mites

Myobia musculi tends to affect the head of mice causing intense pruritus that induces self-mutilation. Some mice may be asymptomatic carriers, but equally some may be so severely affected as to die of secondary bacterial infection.

Myocoptes musculinus causes disease over the body of the mouse. It may produce intense pruritus but does not tend to induce the large areas of ulceration which are associated with *Myobia musculi*.

In the rat, the fur mite is *Radfordia ensifera*. The tropical blood-sucking mite *Ornithonyssus (Liponyssus) bacoti* can cause anaemia and general debilitation and has been reported in the USA and Europe.

Notoedres muris is a burrowing mite of rats and causes crusting lesions on the ear tips and tail which may then spread to the rest of the body. It is extremely pruritic in the rat and secondary bacterial infections are common (see Figure 5.12).

Diagnosis of these mites is based on the clinical signs and discovering them on skin scrapings.

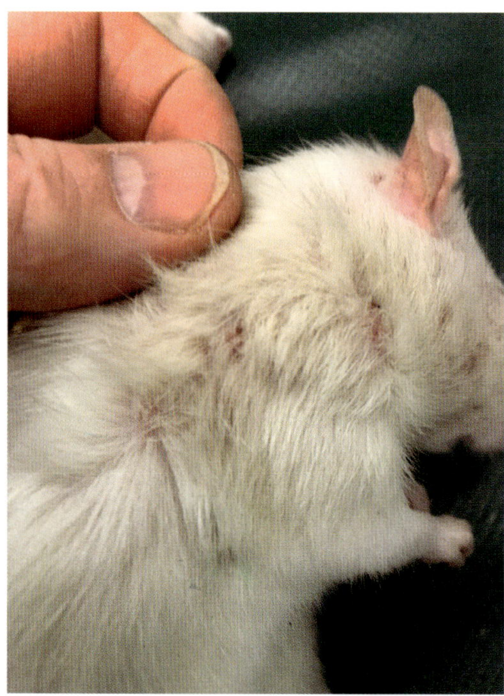

Figure 5.12 Crusting lesions of the body with pruritus can be seen in a number of conditions including *Notoedres muris* infestation.

Lice

The common sucking louse seen in both rats and mice is *Polyplax spinulosa*. This seems to be mildly pruritic, but if present in sufficient numbers (the louse may be seen with the naked eye), it can cause anaemia.

Fleas

In most pet households, infestation of pet rats and mice with either *Ctenocephalides felis* or *Ctenocephalides canis* is possible. These may cause significant anaemia. *Xenopsylla cheopis* is the main vector for the bacterium *Yersinia pestis*, the cause of bubonic plague. It is not found in the UK, but in parts of Africa, China, South America and the western states of the USA.

Viral

Both species may be affected by their own form of poxvirus. These are rare, although the mouse poxvirus (ectromelia) can cause problems in laboratories.

Sialodacryoadenitis virus (rat coronavirus) infection is a disease affecting the tear glands and periorbita of rats and mice. It causes local swelling and epiphora. The tears contain porphyrin pigments making them red (chromodacryorrhea) and mimicking dried blood (see Figure 5.13). The disease is not treatable, but is generally self-limiting, although red tears may reappear in rats at times of stress.

Bacterial

Generalised bacterial skin problems are common as a sequel to any self-induced trauma. Bacteria such as *Staphylococcus aureus* and *Streptococcus* spp. and *Pseudomonas* spp. are seen commonly.

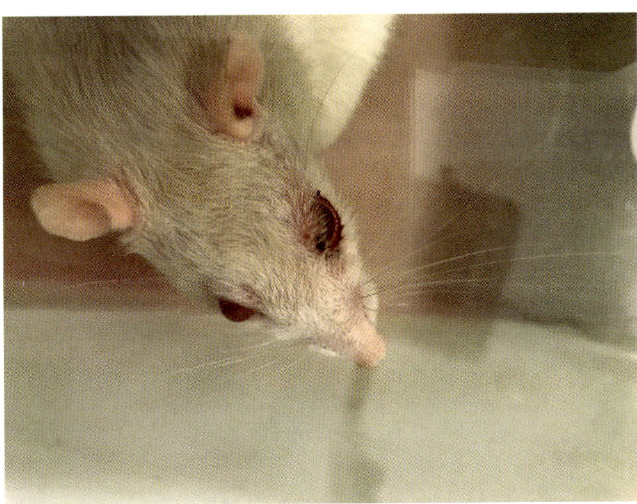

Figure 5.13 Chromodacryorrhea due to a coronavirus in a domestic rat.

Pododermatitis

Sores commonly develop on the hocks of older, overweight rats. They start as pressure sores, allowing secondary infections to occur. Causes include osteoarthritis, excessive weight carriage and poor bedding.

Fungal

In rats and mice dermatophytes such as *Trichophyton mentagrophytes* produce lesions on the head and neck, with a typical scaling and dry crust. The tail may also be affected, and the lesions do not appear to be pruritic. This ringworm does not fluoresce under Wood's lamp.

Miscellaneous

Barbering

Barbering of the whiskers and fur is common, particularly in male mice kept together. The whiskers and fur is chewed short and may proceed to more serious injuries. For this reason male mice should not be kept together.

Ringtail

Ringtail is seen in rats where circular constrictions of the skin covering the tail occur, stopping the blood supply and causing skin sloughing and is predominantly seen in suckling rats between 2 and 19 days of age. It is thought to be due to a reduction in the relative humidity of the environment of the rat. Levels of humidity below 40–50% have been associated with this problem.

Atopy

Atopy is reported in rats. This is an allergic skin condition similar to that seen in dogs and can occur due to contact with any potential allergen in their environment. Classically, the rat is pruritic and is covered in scabs. There is no evidence of mites on skin scrapings, and no response to ivermectin medication.

Progressive necrotising and idiopathic ulcerative dermatitis

Progressive necrotising dermatitis is seen in mice, typically on the ears, and is due to an immune-mediated vasculitis resulting in intense pruritus and self-mutilation. The ear tip sloughs and will heal assuming no secondary infection.

Idiopathic ulcerative dermatitis has been reported in certain strains of black laboratory mouse affecting the head and thorax in particular and again involves a vasculitis. There is some suggestion that dietary deficiencies in essential omega-3 fatty acids may play a role in the disease in these breeds.

Digestive disease

Oral

Dental disease is uncommon in rats and mice. If seen it is usually incisor malocclusion.

Gastrointestinal

Endoparasitic

Pinworms such as *Syphacia obvelata* (chiefly in mice), *Syphacia muris* (chiefly in rats) and *Aspiculuris tetraptera* (chiefly in mice) are common. They may cause no disease at all, but the characteristic asymmetrical eggs may be found in the faeces, or around the anus, where *Syphacia* spp. may cause irritation. Diarrhoea, if present, is generally mild, but severe infestations may cause rectal prolapses. *Rodentolepis (Hymenolepis) nana* is a zoonotic tapeworm that rarely causes clinical disease in mice and rats but has a direct life cycle (infectious from rodent to rodent without an intermediate host) which is unusual for a cestode.

Protozoal

These include *Entamoeba muris*, *Trichomonas muris*, *Spironucleus muris* and *Giardia muris*. All protozoans can cause mild diarrhoea, but many may cause no disease signs at all when present in low numbers and in fully immunocompetent animals.

Bacterial

Salmonellosis: Mice and rats may remain subclinical carriers of the bacteria for years. Diarrhoea is not always seen, and treatment is difficult, as clearing a rat or mouse of *Salmonella* spp. is almost impossible. Euthanasia may be advised due to the human health risk.

Transmissible murine colonic hyperplasia: This is an infection of mice caused by the environmental bacterium *Citrobacter freundii*. It causes progressive thickening of the mucosa of the large intestine, diarrhoea, abdominal pain, anorexia and sometimes rectal prolapse, particularly in young mice 2–4 weeks of age. Death occurs in a small number of cases. The more common outcome is stunting of the mouse. It is highly infectious, and poor cage hygiene allows rapid spread through a colony.

Tyzzer's disease: This is an infection by *Clostridium (Bacillus) piliforme*. It is common in rats, where it can cause sudden death, or watery diarrhoea, perineal staining, and heart and liver disease. It is highly infectious and spread in the faeces.

Viral

Rotavirus: Rotavirus infection is seen before weaning. Chronic infections, yellow diarrhoea and stunted growth are common.

Mouse hepatitis virus: Mouse hepatitis virus (MHV) is a highly pathogenic coronavirus affecting suckling mice. It causes rapid deterioration, a yellow diarrhoea, muscle tremors, fitting and death in infected individuals, and is spread via the respiratory and faecal–oral routes.

Respiratory disease

Mycoplasma pulmonis

The bacterium *Mycoplasma pulmonis* is widespread in rats and mice. It is carried in the upper airways and the reproductive tract. Transmission is by close contact between male and female at mating, mother and young during nursing and by aerosol spread from individual to individual over greater distances. It is highly infectious.

Signs of disease include snuffles, head tilts (inner and middle ear infections), dyspnoea, hyperpnoea and death from advanced bronchopulmonary disease. The course of the infection can be chronic, with repeated bouts of bronchitis and pneumonia (see Figure 5.14). The animals will exhibit poor body condition, a dull staring coat, chromodacryorrhea, anorexia and lethargy. Another presentation includes infertility, reduced fertility and early abortions.

Some factors will encourage onset of the infection and these include other respiratory tract infections (e.g. Sendai virus) and unsanitary conditions. Urine soiling leads to a build-up of ammonia gas which then leads to respiratory tract irritation; infection has also been implicated. Diagnosis is often made on clinical signs but may be confirmed via serology or PCR as the bacterium is difficult to culture.

Other bacterial respiratory infections

Streptococcus pneumoniae (a cause of pneumonia and meningitis in humans and therefore a zoonosis), *Pasteurella pneumotropica*, *Bordetella bronchiseptica*, *Corynebacterium kutscheri*, *Haemophilus* spp. and the cilia-associated respiratory (CAR) bacillus may all occur in rats and mice. Clinical signs are respiratory and reproductive disease. *Chlamydia muridarum* is the mouse pneumonitis (MoPn) agent, but experimentally mice are also susceptible to *Chlamydia psittaci* and *Chlamydia trachomatis*. In all cases infection is via the respiratory route. Severe acute infections produce ruffled fur, hunched stance, laboured breathing and an interstitial pneumonia. Many will die quickly, but more chronic cases will produce cyanosis of the ear and tail tips.

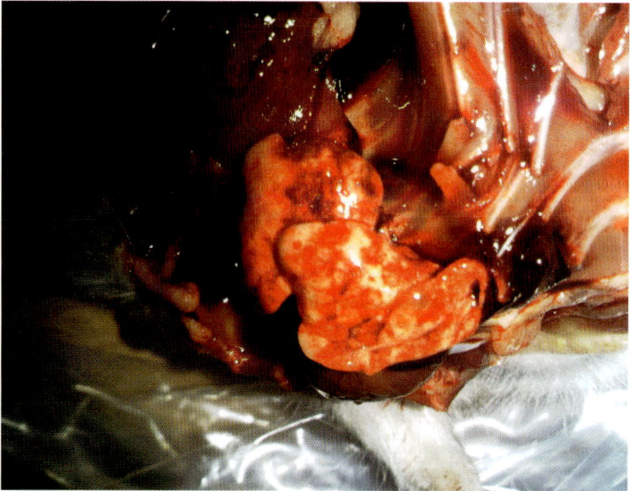

Figure 5.14 Severe bronchopneumonia is common in domestic rats in particular as shown on this post-mortem. Causes can include *Mycoplasma pulmonis*, *Streptococcus pneumoniae* and other bacteria often combined with Sendai virus infections.

Sendai virus

This is a paramyxovirus type 1, transmitted by sneezing, direct contact, and via food bowls or other fomites. It is commonest in recently weaned mice as younger mice are protected by maternal antibodies. Signs of disease include dullness, dyspnoea, chattering of the teeth, weight loss, anorexia and a dull coat. In young mice the mortality rate may be high.

Other viral respiratory diseases

Mouse cytomegalovirus infection

Also known as murid herpesvirus 1 (MuHV-1). Pathology is found in the salivary glands but it can also affect the lungs. Neonates of all mice strains can be affected. Transmission can be via saliva, tears, urine and semen. Clinically apparent disease is rare.

Mouse hepatitis virus

Also known as murine hepatitis virus, MHV is a coronavirus. Natural infections are generally subclinical. The virus can infect nasal mucosa, pulmonary vascular endothelium and the draining lymph nodes. It is highly contagious and spread by aerosol and faeces. It is a problem in laboratories. Elimination of the virus may be achieved by stopping breeding of seropositive animals for 8 weeks plus environmental decontamination.

Pneumonia virus of mice

This can infect mice, rats, hamsters, guinea pigs and gerbils. It is a pneumovirus of the Paramyxoviridae family. In non-immunocompromised rodents it generally produces subclinical infections. In immunodeficient mice it can produce rhinitis, cyanosis, dyspnoea and chronic wasting.

Poxvirus

Cowpox virus can be carried by rodents and may result in disease in other domestic and wild animals (Girling *et al.*, 2011). It is subclinical in rodents. Turkmenian rodent poxvirus has been recorded in laboratory rats in Europe and Russia. Dermal and respiratory lesions with severe respiratory interstitial pneumonia and oedema have been reported.

Hantavirus

Hantaviruses have been reported in pet (and wild) rats and other rodents around the world including the UK. They are a potential zoonosis and rat respiratory virus can cause respiratory signs in pet rats.

Diagnosis of viral respiratory disease in rodents

Many laboratories can offer serological testing for rodent viruses. Virus isolation may also be attempted if fresh tissue or lung washes can be submitted.

Fungal respiratory disease

Pneumocystosis

Pneumocystis carinii is an opportunistic pathogen of the respiratory tract of mice, rats and probably all domestic mammals and humans. Transmission occurs by the inhalation of infective cysts. Mice or rats that are immunosuppressed may develop a fatal pneumonia. Affected mice are hunched and tachypnoeic, with weight loss. Decreased reproductive efficiency is commonly observed in colonies of immunodeficient mice. Histology of the lungs and PCR are used for diagnosis.

***Aspergillus* spp.**

This fungus has been reported as a cause of fatal pneumonia and rhinitis in rats. Corncob bedding was implicated in the source of the fungus.

Other respiratory tract disease

Acidophilic macrophage pneumonia

This can occur in older mice, particularly where there are pulmonary tumours, pneumocystosis or chronic pneumonia. Grossly the lungs appear tan to red in discolouration and do not collapse.

Amyloidosis

This is seen in older mice and hamsters. It can affect any organ and is common in cases of chronic infection and neoplasia. Clinically, the signs depend on the organ affected. It can be more commonly found in male mice, particularly those under stress in overcrowded housing.

Eosinophilic granulomatous pneumonia and asthma

This tends to be a problem in Brown Norwegian rats. It has been associated with asthma, which is common in this breed. However, it has been reported in rats not exposed to allergens and may be associated with an unknown infectious agent. Incidence can be up to 100% at 3–4 months of age.

Neoplasia

This has regularly been reported in older rats and is often due to primary lung tumours. Metastasis from mammary adenocarcinomas is possible in female mice.

Cardiovascular disease

Atrial thrombosis is common in aged mice, usually in the left atrium; it may be accompanied by amyloidosis. Amyloid is deposited in the walls of the great vessels. Cardiac disease is seen clinically as dyspnoea, tachypnoea and abdominal distension.

Cardiomyopathy and myocardial fibrosis are the two most commonly seen cardiac abnormalities. Cardiomyopathy (usually dilated) is particularly common in male rats that are overfed, and can be seen as early as 3 months of age. The incidence of myocardial disease can be reduced by 25–30% by dietary restriction.

Endocardiosis and atrial thrombus formation are common in older rats. Myocardial mineralisation may be seen secondary to chronic renal disease. Congestive heart failure will result.

Myocardial abscesses can be seen with Tyzzer's disease.

Urinary tract disease

Chronic progressive nephrosis

Chronic progressive nephrosis is common in ageing rats and mice. The kidneys become progressively more damaged by protein deposits in the tubular lumens. In certain strains of mice an autoimmune factor is seen. In rats, a high-protein, low-potassium diet has been implicated, with males more susceptible than females. Recurrent disease equally may have a role to play. An increase in thirst and urination may be seen, with weight loss and dehydration. Blood samples demonstrate increased urea and creatinine with low blood albumin.

Urolithiasis and urethral obstruction

Urolithiasis is common in older rats and mice, especially males, where uroliths may block the narrower urethra proximal to the os penis. The composition varies, but is frequently calcium carbonate, ammonium phosphate or calcium oxalate. There is often a secondary cystitis.

Urethral obstruction may occur in male mice due to infections of the bulbourethral glands with *Pasteurella pneumotropica* or the preputial glands with *Staphylococcus* spp. and may result in self-mutilation of the penis.

Nephritis/pyelonephritis

Often seen in older rats and involving bacteria such as *Pseudomonas* spp., *E. coli*, *Proteus mirabilis* and *Klebsiella* spp. Culture and sensitivity testing of samples collected by cystocentesis is advisable.

Interstitial nephritis can occur with *Leptospira* spp. (such as *L. ballum*) in most rodents and this can be a zoonotic disease. Lymphocytic choriomeningitis virus (LCMV) can cause interstitial nephritis and is also zoonotic. Clinically, the rodent presents with anorexia, lethargy, dehydration and abdominal pain. Pet rats if infected may also spread hantavirus via their urine and can be a potential zoonosis.

Renal coccidiosis and bladder worms

Renal coccidian *Klossiella hydromyos* has been reported in rats, sporocysts being found in the urine. Sulfonamides are effective in most cases.

Trichosomoides crassicauda (bladder threadworms) have also been reported in rats (8–12 weeks of age). Clinical signs include poor growth, staring coats and difficulty urinating/cystitis. Worm eggs may be seen in the urine.

Nephrocalcinosis

This can be seen in older rats and is thought to be associated with a high-calcium, low-phosphorus diet, combined with high levels of vitamin D_3. It is believed that oestrogens have a role in causing the disease as it is found more frequently in older females. Radiography is diagnostic.

Hydronephrosis and polycystic disease

Hydronephrosis can occur due to urolithiasis of the ureters. More commonly it is seen as an inherited condition in rats such as the Brown Norway, Sprague Dawley and Gunn breeds.

Reproductive tract disease

Uterine

Dystocias are uncommon in rats and mice. Uterine infections do occur infrequently, with pyometras being seen in rats.

Mammary gland

The mammary glands are commonly affected by cancer in both rats and mice.

In rats, the most frequent is the fibroadenoma. This is a benign but rapidly growing tumour, and can occur in any of the mammary tissue which extends from cranially at the forelimbs to the inguinal region. The masses are well defined and easily removed surgically, although the predisposition appears to be hereditary, and the likelihood of further tumours occurring is high. Many are prolactin sensitive. Fibroadenomas can occur in male rats as well as females. Adenocarcinomas do occur in 10% of cases and may metastasise.

In mice, the mammary cancer most commonly seen is malignant and caused by an RNA virus, the Bittner agent, which, in a susceptible strain of mouse, causes mammary adenocarcinoma. Surgery is often unsuccessful.

Testicular

A form of testicular cancer, a Leydig cell adenoma, is seen in old male rats. It is benign and causes a soft swelling, and may be accompanied by some hair loss.

Musculoskeletal disease

Spondylosis is common in older rats, and may cause incontinence and reduction of function of the hindlimbs. Typically, the lumbosacral area is affected by the osteoarthritis, reducing mobility, causing pain and irritating spinal nerve function.

Neurological disease

Vestibular disease

Head tilts are common in rats. Causes include infections by *Mycoplasma pulmonis* and *Streptococcus pneumoniae*, which can affect the inner ear or hindbrain, thus affecting the vestibular centres. Other causes are tumours, with pituitary tumours reported commonly in older female rats on high-calorie/protein diets.

Lymphocytic choriomeningitis virus

LCMV is mainly seen in wild mice. It is shed in the urine and saliva, and affected mice may show no symptoms, or they may show neurological signs such as head tilts, fitting and death. It is a zoonotic disease and can cause meningitis in humans and other primates.

Degenerative radiculomyelopathy

This is a condition in aged rats similar to that seen in German Shepherd dogs where a progressive, primary, segmental demyelination is seen in rats over 18 months old (Gilmore, 2005).

Ocular disease

Sialodacryoadenitis virus (a coronavirus) causing red tears has been mentioned above, and will infect rats, mice, hamsters and gerbils. Chronic infections may cause permanent reduction in tears, leading to keratoconjunctivitis sicca. Conjunctivitis may occur secondary to this, or to the presence of finely chopped or dusty bedding, creating a foreign body reaction.

Cataracts are often associated with a hereditary deformed eye seen as microphthalmia.

Many young rats and mice have a persistent hyaloid artery which may bleed into the vitreous humour and appear as haemorrhages at the front of the eye.

Albino rats and mice must be given shelter from light, as their retinas are prone to damage. Even normal-coloured rats and mice require a shelter that is light proof.

DISEASES OF THE GERBIL

Skin disease

Ectoparasitic

Demodex merioni rarely causes disease. It has a typical cigar shape under microscopy of skin scrapings. Other mite infestations are rare, although cases of *Notoedres muris* and *Sarcoptes scabiei* have been reported.

Storage mites have been reported as causing irritation to the nose and facial area which is in contact with food.

Bacterial

Staphylococcus aureus infections of the nose and face occur secondary to wet substrate conditions. Sialodacryoadenitis virus infection of the tear glands can also lead to wet dermatitis in the perinasal area, allowing *Staphylococcus aureus* to create a pyoderma.

Fungal

The dermatophyte *Trichophyton mentagrophytes* is the commonest seen, causing areas of hyperkeratosis with grey scaling of the skin, particularly in the head region. Diagnosis is made on microscopy and culture.

Skin tumours

Ventral scent gland adenomas/adenocarcinomas and squamous cell carcinomas, which develop from 2 years of age onwards predominantly in the male gerbil, are significant.

Other skin tumours, such as melanomas, are seen, particularly on the extremities. Squamous cell carcinomas of the ears and nose have been reported.

Endocrine

Cystic ovarian disease (see below) has been associated with symmetrical hair loss over the flanks of female gerbils, along with a swollen abdomen.

Miscellaneous

Tail skin degloving injuries are common in gerbils that have been roughly handled or restrained by the end of the tail. The denuded vertebrae will die off later on, and the tail never regrows.

Digestive disease

Oral

Dental disease is relatively uncommon in the gerbil, although traumatic damage to the incisors leading to fractures and overgrowth may occur.

Gastrointestinal

Bacterial

Tyzzer's disease: This is due to *Clostridium (Bacillus) piliforme* and causes enteritis, but rarely diarrhoea, and often spreads to the liver and heart. The disease lasts for 1–4 days and may produce sudden death or a more lingering disease with dullness, lethargy, a hunched posture, scant or soft faeces and a dull staring coat.

Proliferative ileitis: Due to the intracellular bacterium *Lawsonia intracellularis* which also causes wet-tail in hamsters. It is passed from gerbil to gerbil via the faecal–oral route, and causes thickening of the ileum resulting in maldigestion and malabsorption, producing the classical 'wet tail' of matted damp fur around the rear. The condition is much less common in gerbils than hamsters, but can nonetheless be a serious and fatal condition.

Endoparasitic

The mouse pinworm *Syphacia obvelata* and the rat pinworm *Syphacia muris* rarely cause clinical disease.

The potentially zoonotic cestode *Rodentolepis (Hymenolepis) nana* can be found and is discussed in the following section on hamsters. The gerbil is the definitive host for the pinworm *Dentostomella translucida*, which is considered non-pathogenic.

Respiratory disease

The gerbil is affected by more or less the same respiratory conditions as the rat and mouse, although it is less susceptible.

Cardiovascular disease

Tyzzer's disease may cause myocarditis, otherwise cardiovascular disease is uncommon.

Urinary tract disease

Gerbils are prone to ageing changes involving gradual scarring of renal tissue and the nephrotic syndrome, but the incidence of this is much less than in the rat or mouse.

Reproductive tract disease

Uterine infection

Uterine infections are uncommon in gerbils.

Ovarian cysts

Ovarian cysts are common. The cysts may be quite large and cause distension of the abdomen. The condition is hereditary and bilateral and causes disruption of the oestrus cycle. The cyst secretes low levels of oestrogens which have an effect on fur growth, causing mild alopecia over the flanks.

Uterine and ovarian neoplasia

After cancer of the adrenal gland, cancer of the ovaries (granulosa cell tumours) and the female reproductive tract are the most common tumours in the gerbil. Uterine cancers may cause bleeding from the reproductive tract, or abdominal swelling. Diagnosis may be made on clinical signs or on ultrasound and radiographic examination.

Musculoskeletal disease

Fractures are uncommon in gerbils, as are other musculoskeletal problems, other than the degloving tail injuries mentioned above.

Neurological disease

Vestibular disease

Vestibular disease is common and is usually due to bacterial inner ear disease, often *Mycoplasma pulmonis*, *Pasteurella pneumotropica* or *Streptococcus pneumoniae*, which gain access from the oropharynx via the Eustachian canals and the middle ear. Pus may be observed at the external ear canal in some cases.

Aural cholesteatoma, papilloma and polyp formation with secondary bacterial infection are also common and may result in vestibular disease, particularly in aged gerbils.

Epilepsy

Epilepsy in gerbils appears to be hereditary, and it is advisable not to keep susceptible individuals in rooms with strip lighting, television sets or computer terminals, as these all emit electromagnetic radiation of around 50–60 Hz, which may induce a fit. In addition, handling gerbils from a young age to familiarise them with human contact can reduce the likelihood of seizures in later life.

DISEASES OF THE HAMSTER

Skin disease

Ectoparasitic

Demodex criceti and *Demodex aurati* both infest hamsters and can cause clinical disease. *Demodex criceti* is shorter and rounder, whereas *D. aurati* is longer and more like *D. canis*. The clinical disease is manifested by alopecia over the dorsum caudally and intense white scurf. The mites are easily seen after skin scraping and microscopy (see Figure 5.15). The lesions are mildly pruritic.

Crusting lesions of the ears, face and other extremities have been reported in Syrian hamsters affected by the sarcoptiform mite *Notoedres notoedres*. Diagnosis in all cases is made based on positive skin scrapings.

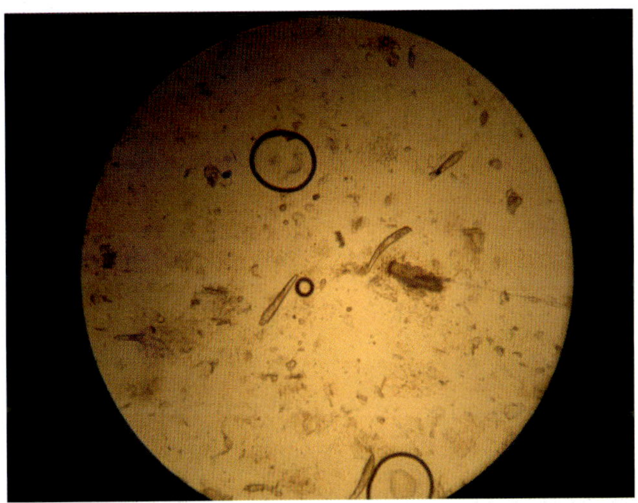

Figure 5.15 *Demodex* spp. mites from a skin scraping in a domestic Syrian hamster.

Fungal

The dermatophyte *Trichophyton mentagrophytes* can be found as a secondary cause of skin disease in hamsters as a sequel to mange or mycosis fungoides.

Bacterial

Primary bacterial skin disease is uncommonly seen in hamsters. The main bacteria isolated from wounds include *Pasteurella pneumotropica* and *Staphylococcus aureus*. Secondary infections of skin ulcers associated with T-cell lymphoma are common.

Skin tumours

The commonest is a form of T-cell lymphoma known as mycosis fungoides. This infiltrates the epidermis, producing chronic thickening of the skin and is pruritic. Alopecia is seen due to the obliteration of the hair follicles. The cancer eventually metastasises.

Melanomas affecting the head, ears and flank scent glands are also seen particularly in Syrian hamsters. These are usually pigmented and fast-growing and occur much more frequently in males than females.

Cutaneous (contagious) lymphoma producing wart-like lesions can be associated with a hamster papovavirus. The virus is host specific and lesions are found in hamsters aged from 3 months to 1 year. The lesions are wart-like and occur most often around the face or perianal area. The virus is highly contagious and is passed through urine. It has a long incubation period and is very resistant. It will also induce lymphoma in other organs. There is no spontaneous resolution.

Endocrine

Hyperadrenocorticism is due to a chromophobe adenoma in the pituitary gland. This secretes excessive levels of adrenocorticotropic hormone (ACTH) which causes bilateral adrenal gland hyperplasia, producing increased levels of cortisol that result in polydipsia, polyuria, symmetrical alopecia, increased appetite and thinning of the skin and coat over the flanks. Plasma cortisol levels should be 13.8–27.6 nmol/L in healthy hamsters. Serum alkaline phosphatase may also be raised in hamsters with hyperadrenocorticism (>40 U/L), normal values being 8–18 U/L. It has been suggested that hamsters may secrete both cortisol and corticosterone; therefore, diagnosis based on blood cortisol levels alone may not be accurate. Ultrasonography of the adrenal gland may show enlargement or abnormalities.

Irritant

Skin irritation has been reported in hamsters kept on cedar pine chips. These are highly resinous and can cause intense skin irritation, particularly over the ventrum and nasal areas. Removal of the hamster from these shavings produces improvement within days.

Digestive disease

Oral

Cheek pouch impaction

Impaction of the cheek pouch may occur because the hamster may have overfilled the pouch or have become ill before emptying it. Because the hamster uses the hindlimb to empty the pouch, losing a hind leg may also lead to impaction on that side.

Cheek pouch prolapse

Prolapse may occur after the hamster has emptied the cheek pouch. The sac, now everted, may not return to normal and protrudes as a pink mass from the mouth. It may also occur due to infection or neoplasia.

Gastrointestinal

Proliferative ileitis ('wet-tail')

The bacterium *Lawsonia intracellularis* produces hypertrophy of the ileum, reducing digestion and absorption which leads to diarrhoea. It can lead to rectal prolapse and intussusceptions. Some hamsters die within 24 hours of contracting the disease without showing any obvious signs.

Bacterial

Tyzzer's disease (*Clostridium piliforme*) can cause serious liver and gastrointestinal disease in hamsters as it does in gerbils.

Salmonellosis is uncommon. The bacterium *Salmonella enteritidis* is the most frequently reported and this is a zoonotic disease. Signs include sudden death, frequently before any diarrhoea is produced. Younger animals seem more susceptible.

Parasitic

Rodentolepis (Hymenolepis) nana is a dwarf tapeworm which is zoonotic, being one of the few cestodes that has a direct life cycle (requires no intermediate host). It appears to cause little or no disease in hamsters. A diagnosis may be made by finding cestode egg sachets in the faeces, or by seeing the cream-coloured, 1–2-mm long egg packet wriggling on the perianal fur.

Iatrogenic

Oral antibiotics such as penicillins and macrolides can lead to an overgrowth of *Clostridium* spp. (often *C. difficile*) that can rapidly result in enterotoxaemia and death of the hamster.

Miscellaneous

Examples of other causes of diarrhoea include rapid diet changes. Certain foods should be avoided altogether, for example those containing lactose and over-sugary fruit such as grapes, kiwi fruit and bananas.

Respiratory disease

Bacteria

Pasteurella pneumotropica

In hamsters it can cause acute or chronic respiratory disease (see section on rats and mice for clinical signs).

Corynebacterium kutscheri

Hamsters may act as carriers but seem not to develop disease from this bacterium.

Viruses

Sendai virus is an RNA paramyxovirus (parainfluenza 1) and affects rats, mice, guinea pigs and hamsters. Hamsters are rarely severely affected by infection.

Severe acute respiratory syndrome coronavirus 2 (SARS-CoV-2) has been shown to easily infect Syrian hamsters and produces a disease pattern similar to that in humans, with older hamsters showing more severe respiratory disease and greater weight loss than young ones (Osterrieder *et al.*, 2020).

Other causes of respiratory disease

Hamsters suffer from pulmonary thromboembolisms due to atrial thrombotic lesions which may prove fatal, and are a cause of sudden death.

Cardiovascular disease

Cardiomyopathy and atrial thromboses

Pathophysiology suggests that cardiomyopathy occurs first followed by left atrial thrombosis and death as a result of coagulopathy. Hypertrophic cardiomyopathy has also been reported as a cause of thrombus formation. In one study the incidence of cardiac disease was assumed to be around 6% (Schmidt and Reavill, 2007). Interestingly, androgens protect the heart from heart disease in hamsters. The age of onset of heart disease in females is therefore younger (around 13.5 months) than that in males (21.5 months). Neutering male hamsters therefore removes this effect and so means that they are more likely to develop heart disease at a younger age.

Diagnosis is based on the signs and the demonstration of an enlarged heart on radiography and ultrasound examination. The latter are often able to show the thrombi in the atria. Cold extremities, tachypnoea and lethargy are commonly reported.

Other causes of cardiovascular disease

Bacterial disease such as Tyzzer's and salmonellosis can lead to myocarditis and heart failure. Amyloidosis is common in all rodents with age and chronic disease and may lead to thickening of arterial walls and organ failure. Lymphoma is commonly seen, with the thymus, skin, spleen, liver and internal lymph nodes all being reported and is common in older hamsters. A contagious lymphoma can be associated with a papovavirus.

Urinary tract disease

Kidney disease

Chronic progressive nephropathy is seen as in mice and rats. Hamsters are also prone to amyloidosis. Clinical signs vary, but may include weight loss, lethargy, polydipsia and polyuria with or without proteinuria.

Polycystic disease is seen in older male hamsters and may also involve the liver. It is congenital in nature and presents as a rapidly enlarging abdomen. Diagnosis is most easily made using ultrasound. Drainage of the cysts can help, but they tend to re-form within 2–4 weeks.

Bladder

Like mice and rats, hamsters can suffer from cystitis and urolithiasis. Calcium oxalate and calcium carbonate are the two commonly seen uroliths.

Endocrine disease

Hyperadrenocorticism

See above under the discussion of skin diseases.

Diabetes mellitus

In the Chinese hamster, diabetes mellitus is a hereditary condition. Clinical signs include polydipsia (drinking often >50 mL of water per day) and polyuria, cystitis, lethargy and weight loss. Glucosuria of 2% is common and blood glucose is often in excess of 25–30 mmol/L.

Reproductive tract disease

Uterus

Pyometra is seen but may be mistaken for the normal reproductive tract discharge found during the oestrus cycle. However, pyometras persist, and smell much worse. Closed pyometras are more difficult to diagnose due to the absence of a discharge, but the hamster is often lethargic, anorectic, polydipsic, dehydrated and has a tender, swollen abdomen.

Ovaries

Cystic ovaries are common in female hamsters over the age of 8 months. The condition is bilateral, and may be accompanied by some mild symmetrical alopecia of the flanks.

Ocular disease

Chinese hamsters are prone to cataract development as a result of diabetes mellitus.

Musculoskeletal disease

Compound fractures of the tibia are the commonest, especially from hamsters falling from the roof or the sides of wire cages up which they have climbed, and leg amputation may be required. Other fractures commonly seen are fractures of spinal vertebrae, or more commonly vertebral subluxations, usually in the lumbar area, again due to falls. These will present as bilateral hindlimb paresis or paralysis.

Neurological disease

Lymphocytic choriomeningitis virus generally produces little or no clinical signs in the hamster. It is excreted in the urine and saliva. It is relatively rare in captive hamsters, being found more commonly in wild mice, but it is a serious zoonotic disease causing meningitis in humans.

DISEASES OF THE GUINEA PIG

Skin disease

Ectoparasitic

Mites

The scabies mite *Trixacarus caviae* causes intense pruritus and distress. The affected individual may scratch itself deeply and may be so severely affected as to cause it to stop eating and even cause abortion in heavily pregnant females. Diagnosis is made on clinical signs and skin scrapings under the microscope.

The fur mite, *Chirodiscoides caviae*, seems to cause less clinical disease.

Cheyletiella parasitovorax occasionally produces pruritus and scaling along the dorsum.

Demodex caviae is commonly found but rarely causes clinical disease. Diagnosis is made by collecting skin scrapings and examining them microscopically.

Lice

Gliricola porcelli and *Gyropus ovalis* are Mallophagan lice and so live off cellular debris, but rarely cause disease.

Bacterial

Cervical lymphadenitis

Cervical lymphadenitis is a disease of the cervical lymph nodes caused by *Streptococcus zooepidemicus*. It is also found in the airways and mouth of the healthy guinea pig, and causes problems when the mucosa of the oropharynx becomes abraded by rough food particles. This leads to local lymphadenitis, with subcutaneous abscessation. The disease may gain access to the bloodstream causing septicaemia which is rapidly fatal.

Pododermatitis

Pododermatitis is commonest in overweight, older guinea pigs, which will spend more time resting, and which will walk on the flat of the hock. It can also be seen in older guinea pigs with osteoarthritis. Bacteria involved include *E. coli*, *Corynebacterium pyogenes*, *Staphylococcus aureus* and *Streptococcus* spp. It is possible to use similar scoring techniques developed in birds and mammals to assess pododermatitis severity in guinea pigs in order to give owners a more accurate prognosis for therapy.

Fungal

Dermatophytosis due to *Microsporum canis* and *Trichophyton mentagrophytes* produces lesions over the head, paws and rear with brittle hairs, grey crusts and some scabs. Diagnosis is as for rats and mice.

Viral

A poxvirus has been detected in association with cheilitis in two guinea pigs with crusting ulcerated lesions around the lips and philtrum.

Neoplasia

Lymphosarcoma affecting the superficial lymph nodes caused by a retrovirus can also produce a blood-borne leukaemia affecting the spleen and liver. The course of the disease is 3–4 weeks, with rapid deterioration, weight loss, secondary infections and organ failure. Treatment with chemotherapeutic agents is frequently unsuccessful.

Benign trichofolliculomas appear as solid cyst-like structures over the lumbosacral area dorsally. Sebaceous adenoma, fibroma, fibrosarcoma, lipoma, liposarcoma and schwannomas have also been reported.

Endocrine

Cystic ovarian disease is extremely common in aged female guinea pigs (a 76% incidence in animals between 1.5 and 5 years old has been reported). The aetiology is unknown, although oestrogenic substances in hay have been implicated. Some are embryological in origin (cystic rete ovarii). Abdominal enlargement and infertility can occur and bilateral non-pruritic alopecia is common. Diagnosis is as for gerbils and hamsters.

Miscellaneous

Guinea pigs may barber each other in the same way as rats and mice. Increasing fibre in the cage and providing more space and tubing or other hides may help to prevent this. Cheilitis is common, and may be due to a lack of vitamin C, although a poxvirus and *Candida* spp. yeasts have also been implicated.

Digestive disease

Oral

Molar overgrowth, most commonly in the mandibular cheek teeth that results in entrapment of the tongue, is common. The normal occlusal plane of the cheek teeth in the guinea pig is actually oblique and slopes from a dorsal position buccally to a ventral position lingually. Causes are similar to those in rabbits, but the need for preformed vitamin C in the diet of guinea pigs is also important as the absence, or deficiency, of vitamin C will result in periodontal disease and dental loosening and loss amongst other more serious conditions. Prevention therefore focuses on a high-fibre diet with vitamin C supplementation and adequate calcium levels in the young growing guinea pig to ensure jawbone and dental mineralisation are adequate.

Gastrointestinal

Hypomotility and gastrointestinal obstruction

As with the domestic rabbit, hypomotility disorders are common where poor-quality, low-fibre diets are fed and where the animal is in pain or discomfort, particularly associated with dental disease. These can lead to slower transit times for indigestible food items such as fur, allowing build-up in the stomach and when this trichobezoar moves intestinal blockages to occur. Gastric dilation, and in some cases volvulus, have also been recorded.

Salmonellosis

Salmonella enteritidis and *Salmonella typhimurium* can both cause enteritis in guinea pigs. The young and debilitated are most at risk. Diarrhoea is uncommon; instead, a dull staring coat, weight loss and abortion are seen.

Other bacterial disease

Yersinia pseudotuberculosis can produce intestinal abscesses, chronic wasting and diarrhoea or acute death. *Mycobacterium tuberculosis*, *Listeria monocytogenes* and *Clostridium perfringens* can also cause intestinal disease. Guinea pigs are also prone to Tyzzer's disease, due to *Clostridium piliforme*.

Endoparasitic

Balantidium coli is a zoonosis and causes large intestinal inflammation and profuse diarrhoea in an immunocompromised guinea pig. A coccidial organism, *Eimeria caviae*, may also cause diarrhoea in piglets.

Cryptosporidium wrairi has been reported as a major cause of small intestinal disease in young guinea pigs resulting in stunting, bloating, diarrhoea and weight loss. Most immunocompetent animals will recover within 4 weeks. Diagnosis is by PCR of faeces or by modified acid-fast stains demonstrating the oocysts.

Faecal impaction

This is seen in older guinea pigs, particularly males. It occurs when excessive folds of loose skin around the anogenital opening trap faecal pellets. This can create serious constipation problems, and localised infection.

Hepatic lipidosis

This condition can develop quickly, particularly in obese guinea pigs that suddenly stop eating. Ketoacidosis can develop and immediate nutritional and fluid support is required. Management is similar to that for rabbits.

Respiratory disease

Bacterial disease

Lung infections are common in guinea pigs housed with rabbits, as the latter often carry the bacterium *Bordetella bronchiseptica* asymptomatically. This bacterium causes a severe bronchopneumonia in guinea pigs. It can also cause otitis media and interna, abscesses and metritis. Other pathogenic bacteria include *Streptococcus pneumoniae*, which is zoonotic and often affects other organs including the heart and reproductive tract; *Klebsiella pneumoniae; Streptobacillus moniliformis; Haemophilus* spp.; *Moraxella* spp.; *Pasteurella pneumotropica* and *Pseudomonas* spp. *Streptococcus zooepidemicus* may also result in bronchopneumonia. *Chlamydia caviae* has been reported in guinea pig breeding colonies and affects guinea pigs between 2 and 8 weeks of age. It is usually asymptomatic although conjunctivitis and rhinitis may be seen, as may abortions and urogenital tract infections. Similarly *Mycoplasma caviae* and *M. cavipharyngis* are known to be present in some guinea pigs but are rarely reported associated with clinical disease.

Diagnosis can be made on history, clinical signs, auscultation of the harsh-sounding chest and, if necessary, radiography showing consolidation of the lungs and bronchioalveolar patterns and culture or PCR testing of respiratory secretions. Serological tests are available to demonstrate an immune system response to many of these pathogens and so may also be used to confirm disease in association with a clinical examination.

Fungal disease

Cryptococcosis has been reported in guinea pigs due to *Cryptococcus neoformans*, a soil-associated yeast. It is generally seen in warm, Mediterranean-style climates and may cause systemic disease, spreading from a primary pneumonia and so may cause chronic weight loss and lymphadenopathy.

Viral disease

Sendai virus has been reported in guinea pigs and may exacerbate bacterial disease. An adenovirus has also been reported in debilitated animals but is generally subclinical.

Guinea pigs have been shown to be able to be infected by SARS-CoV-2. Clinical signs are mild and they are not thought to be significant in its epidemiological spread.

An adenovirus with an incubation period of 5–10 days has been associated with bronchopneumonia in guinea pigs and may have a high mortality rate (Hawkins and Bishop, 2012).

Lung neoplasia

Pulmonary adenoma has been recorded in guinea pigs. The tumour is slow-growing and does not metastasise but causes a reduction in functional lung volume. It may be discovered on radiography or may cause clinical dyspnoea in conjunction with a respiratory pathogen. Lymphoma due to type C cavian leukaemia virus has also been reported.

Avocado toxicity

This has been reported, causing respiratory distress, hydropericardium, generalised congestion, anasarca and death. It appears that the leaves, fruit, bark and seed of avocados are toxic for a number of rodent and avian species.

Cardiovascular disease

Dilated cardiomyopathy, hypertrophic cardiomyopathy and congestive heart failure have all been reported in guinea pigs. Pericardial effusion resulting in tamponade was the most commonly reported significant sequel to heart disease in one survey of cardiac disease in guinea pigs (Muller and Mancinelli, 2022). Hyperthyroidism is commonly seen in guinea pigs and hypertrophic cardiomyopathy may be associated with this as is seen in the domestic cat. Vertebral heart scores for guinea pigs have been determined (see Chapter 7).

Pericarditis has been recorded in conjunction with respiratory tract infection involving *Streptococcus pneumoniae* and may cause heart failure and death. Hypertrophic and dilated cardiomyopathies have been reported. In addition, metastatic and dystrophic mineralisation and pericardial effusions may also be seen. Calcification may be asymptomatic in guinea pigs older than 1 year of age but may equally have been associated with poor growth, muscle stiffness, bone deformities and death. Causes include magnesium deficiency, renal failure and diets high in calcium.

Urinary tract disease

Kidney disease

Chronic progressive interstitial nephritis may be a sequel to diabetes mellitus and staphylococcal pododermatitis and is commonly seen in guinea pigs, particularly those over 3 years of age. Clinically, the guinea pig is polyuric and polydipsic and loses weight. Blood parameters may indicate elevated urea and creatinine levels, often with low blood albumin due to urinary protein losses. Urinalysis may detect cystitis, and commonly reveals proteinuria. Chronic renal amyloidosis is also reported with guinea pigs suffering from diabetes mellitus and *Staphylococcus* spp.-infected skin lesions including pododermatitis.

Bladder

Calcium oxalate or calcium carbonate crystals are commonly found in the urinary bladder. Older boars may experience urethral obstruction due to dried accessory sex gland secretions, as well as being more susceptible to urolith blockage of the urethra at the os penis.

Secondary or primary bacterial cystitis is often seen, the former due to irritation of the bladder by the uroliths, the latter leading to clumps of bacteria around which uroliths form. Clinically the affected guinea pig is dull and lethargic, vocalises and may periodically strain, passing small volumes of blood-stained urine. Diagnosis can be confirmed with examination of the sediment of a centrifuged urine sample. Radiography is also helpful, although calcium oxalate crystals are less radiodense than struvite.

Endocrine disease

Cystic ovarian disease

See the section on reproductive tract disease.

Diabetes mellitus

Spontaneous diabetes mellitus has been reported in guinea pigs. They may present with concurrent scurvy and poor hair coat, as well as polydipsia, polyuria and cataracts. Thickening of the urinary bladder has also been reported. Possible aetiologies include an unclassified infectious agent in Abyssinians (possibly viral in origin), hereditary factors, congenital manganese deficiency in juveniles, and high-sugar, high-carbohydrate diets such as apples and carrots, which exacerbate the problem.

Diagnosis is based on elevated blood glucose levels, often greater than 20 mmol/L (normal values are 3.3–6.9 mmol/L), hyperlipidaemia and results of glucose tolerance tests. For this the guinea pig is fasted for 18 hours. Blood glucose levels are measured, and then a dose of oral glucose is given at 1.75 g/kg body weight. Blood glucose levels 4 hours later are over twice the pre-dose value in diabetic animals and only 1–1.5 times the pre-dose value in normal animals.

Treatment of diabetes in both guinea pigs and hamsters consists of a high-fibre diet. Insulin therapy is rarely indicated and spontaneous recoveries are common. Where insulin is required, NPH insulin at 1 IU every 12 hours has been used.

Reproductive tract disease

Cystic ovarian disease

Cystic ovarian disease is common in female guinea pigs aged over 15 months. It is often bilateral causing a swollen abdomen (see Figure 5.16). There is often bilateral symmetrical fur loss over the flanks where the cysts are follicular and so hormonally productive; however, this may also occur in non-productive cysts where pain and discomfort occurs due to over-grooming, as some cysts can be 5–6 cm or more in diameter. Cystic rete ovarii (non-functional cystic structures of the ovaries that progressively develop) are the most commonly seen and may affect up to 75% of female guinea pigs, most commonly between 2 and 4 years of age (Shi *et al.*, 2002).

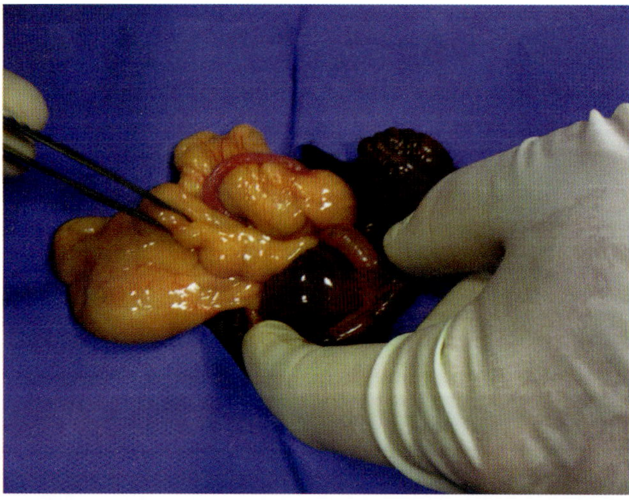

Figure 5.16 Intraoperative view of cystic ovaries and uterus from a guinea pig.

Reproductive tract tumours

In sows ovarian granulosa cell tumours often follow cystic ovaries. Other forms of reproductive tract cancer include uterine adenocarcinomas (which are malignant) and benign leiomyomas. Diagnosis is made on palpation of an enlarged womb, radiographic or ultrasonographic evidence of enlargement of the tract, or presence of reproductive tract discharge, which may be haemorrhagic.

In boars, Leydig cell tumours, Sertoli cell tumours and seminomas are all reported.

Dystocia

If a sow has not given birth before 12 months of age, the fibrocartilaginous ligament which holds the two sides of the pubis and ischium together will become mineralised and fuse. This ligament normally stretches just before parturition under the influence of the hormone relaxin. If it does not, it significantly narrows the birth canal, and this will lead to dystocias. Any maiden sow older than 7–8 months of age should not be mated.

Pyometra and endometritis

These conditions can occur in both breeding and non-breeding sows. *Bordetella* and haemolytic *Streptococcus* spp. bacteria have been commonly isolated but other bacteria such as *E. coli* are also typically seen. A reproductive tract discharge with fever and dullness and inappetence are commonly seen.

Pregnancy toxaemia

This is common in late pregnancy and early lactation in overweight first-time mothers. It is most likely to happen in the presence of concurrent disease (e.g. *Trixacarus caviae* mange), which may reduce the sow's appetite. A rapid mobilisation of body fats occurs, producing ketones. These cause a ketoacidosis that is rapidly fatal. Blood glucose levels are very low (<3 mmol/L) and there is an increase in the acidity of the blood with hyperkalaemia, hyperphosphataemia and hyperlipaemia. The urine becomes acidic. The sow becomes dull, lethargic and hyperpnoeic and then collapses and becomes comatose. Disseminated intravascular coagulation can occur due to the ketoacidosis, significantly worsening the prognosis. Death can occur within 2 days, the sow fitting and convulsing in extremis.

Mammary gland tumours

Mammary gland adenomas are common in older sows. They are slow-growing but may reach appreciable sizes. In 20–30% of cases the tumour may be a malignant adenocarcinoma.

Mastitis

Poor hygiene predisposes the guinea pig to this condition. The bacteria involved (such as *E. coli*) may release endotoxins into the bloodstream which can rapidly cause endotoxic shock.

Musculoskeletal disease

Scurvy

The daily requirement for vitamin C is 10 mg/kg. If this is not met then the animal will develop scurvy typically within 4–5 days. Guinea pigs lack the gene that controls the production of L-gulonolactone oxidase which converts L-gulonolactone to ascorbic acid (vitamin C). Clinical signs include a dull staring coat, dental malocclusions, anorexia, slobbers, diarrhoea and immobility due to painful swollen joints. The guinea pig is in constant pain and clinical signs and history are enough to make a diagnosis. Radiographically, though, it can be seen that the epiphyses of the long bones and the costochondral junctions of the ribs are flared laterally, hence younger, still-growing guinea pigs are more susceptible.

Ulcerative pododermatitis

This is a particularly common condition in guinea pigs that have a more plantigrade stance with non-furred metatarsal areas. This may lead to osteomyelitis. See the section on skin diseases.

Fractures

Fractures of the spine are common in guinea pigs that are housed with rabbits due to trauma. Clinically there is paresis or paralysis of the rear limbs, urinary incontinence, etc. depending on the severity of the lesion. This may be confirmed as a fracture or subluxation on radiography. The prognosis is poor.

Neurological disease

Drug toxicity

Aminoglycosides can induce renal failure; an ascending flaccid paralysis and death in guinea pigs has been reported.

Pregnancy toxaemia

See the section on reproductive diseases for more details.

Spinal trauma

See the section on fractures for details.

Vestibular disease

This has been reported in guinea pigs associated with *Bordetella bronchiseptica*, *Streptococcus zooepidemicus* and *Streptococcus pneumoniae* infections. It is less reported than in the domestic rabbit but has been linked to dental disease. Clinically, head tilts and circling may be seen.

Ocular disease

Hypovitaminosis C can cause flaking of the skin of the eyelids and periocular area, as can dermatophytosis.

Conjunctivitis is often seen in guinea pigs kept on deep shavings or fine-chopped straw due to foreign bodies.

A primary cause of conjunctivitis is *Chlamydia caviae* (formerly known as *Chlamydia psittaci* GPIC isolate), which causes crusting of the lids, reddening of the conjunctiva, increased tear production and a white-green tinged mucous discharge.

Other ocular problems include hereditary and diabetic cataracts, and 'pea eye' – where subconjunctival fat accumulates in the ventral fornix area, making the tissue protrude.

DISEASES OF THE CHINCHILLA

Skin disease

Bacterial

Bacteria are sometimes reported associated with skin abscesses. Most are related to dental disease, but others including abscesses due to *Streptococcus zooepidemicus* and *Pseudomonas aeruginosa* may occur around the head and neck unassociated with tooth infections.

Fur slip

Stress and rough handling will cause clumps of fur to fall out spontaneously. This will regrow, but often not for some time.

Fur ring

In male chinchillas, a ring of fur can become wrapped around the penis inside the prepuce. This must be removed before it causes ischaemia. Males should be checked monthly, but more frequently during the breeding season – every 2–3 days – as it can be caused by mounting behaviour.

Fur matting

This is common if the fur is allowed to become damp. Chinchillas should never be washed, shampooed or allowed to live in damp environmental conditions. Fine pumice sand and Fuller's earth should be provided once or twice daily as a dust bath for fur hygiene and grooming.

Barbering

This is a common problem in chinchillas housed in pairs or groups. The fur of the tail and the whiskers are the most commonly chewed parts, and this increases when environmental stresses such as overcrowding are high, and when the diet is lacking in fibre or when dental disease is present.

Fungal disease

The dermatophyte *Trichophyton mentagrophytes* can cause alopecia in chinchillas, particularly over the nose and pinnae where non-pruritic grey crusts form.

Digestive disease

Oral

Dental disease is very common in chinchillas. Dental (cheek teeth) malocclusion occurs, as with rabbits, usually due to a lack of abrasive foods in the diet, combined with a reduced dietary calcium to phosphorus ratio (less than 1.5 : 1). There is probably a hereditary component to the disease (Crossley and Miguélez, 2001). Elongation of the crowns of the maxillary cheek teeth occurs laterally, so that they penetrate the cheek mucosa, with the crowns of the mandibular cheek teeth flaring medially, impinging on the tongue.

Elongation of the roots of the third and fourth maxillary cheek teeth can cause pain and discomfort, as they penetrate the ocular orbit causing epiphora. The first and second maxillary cheek teeth enter the floor of the nasal passages/sinuses causing sneezing and nasal discharge. The mandibular cheek teeth roots penetrate the ventral aspect of the jaw and can be felt as a series of bumps along its lower border.

When the molars overgrow, gaps form between individual molars. These allow food particles to become wedged between the molars. The food particles then decay, creating periodontal disease and eventually abscesses.

Diagnosis of these problems can be made on clinical signs and radiography. Clinically, the chinchilla is often seen to be drooling saliva (so-called 'slobbers'). It may also be anorectic, have lost weight and started consuming softer fresh foods rather than the harder dry pellets.

Gastrointestinal

Colic

Gas colic is often due to feeding sugary food items such as banana. Clinically there may be teeth grinding, inappetence and a hunched appearance.

Caecocolic disease

Caecocolic disease occurs rarely in chinchillas, but is more likely if the chinchilla is suffering from severe diarrhoea. The caecum or proximal colon may become involved in an intussusception or a torsion. The chinchilla is in severe pain, hunched in posture, often grinding its teeth and drooling saliva, and occasionally rolling around the cage. Loops of bowel in the caudal and ventral portions of the abdomen, grossly swollen with gas, are seen on radiography.

Constipation

Constipation due to ileus is seen most commonly as a sequel to dental disease, obesity, late-stage pregnancy, intestinal or abdominal surgery, and sudden change in diet to a less-fibrous, higher-protein (e.g. all-seed) diet. The chinchilla may produce scant, small faecal pellets for a number of days, and then none at all. Chinchillas so affected are often uncomfortable, and may sit hunched with tucked-in abdomens.

Diarrhoea

Bacterial: Any of the bacteria mentioned in the section on digestive diseases in guinea pigs may cause diarrhoea, with *E. coli* (EPEC strains in particular) and *Salmonella* spp. (particularly *S. arizonae* and *S. enteritidis*) appearing frequently. In addition, *Pseudomonas aeruginosa* has commonly been reported causing diarrhoea, pneumonia and septicaemia. *Clostridium* spp. enterotoxaemia will occur if inappropriate antibiotics are used (e.g. oral penicillin) or large amounts of soluble carbohydrates are offered. *Yersinia enterocolitica* has resulted in enteritis and weight loss with septicaemia in chinchillas, and a chinchilla-specific strain has been identified (Wuthe and Aleksic, 1992). *Yersinia pseudotuberculosis* is less commonly seen but can still cause significant morbidity and mortality similar to that seen in the guinea pig.

Endoparasitic: *Giardia* is a single-celled protozoan parasite found in healthy and sick chinchillas alike, and therefore its role in disease is not fully understood. It is, however, a potential zoonosis. It is currently thought that poor diet, stress or concurrent disease allows the normally present *Giardia* spp. parasite to multiply to sufficient numbers in the large bowel to cause diarrhoea. There is often the presence of soiled fur around the rear, and a general dullness. Diagnosis is by finding the motile, single-celled organisms on microscope examination of fresh faeces samples suspended in isotonic saline or by PCR testing.

Eimeria chinchillae is a coccidial parasite affecting young chinchillas with a transient diarrhoea. However, poor environmental conditions, overcrowding and stress can increase the severity of the disease and mortalities may occasionally be seen.

Rodentolepis (Hymenolepis) nana, a small tapeworm, has also been reported in chinchillas (as well as hamsters, mice, rats and other rodents); unusually for a cestode, it has a direct life cycle and is a potential zoonosis. In low levels of infection the disease is subclinical. In high numbers with concomitant stressors, anorexia, diarrhoea, weight loss and mortalities can occur.

Hepatic lipidosis

Many chinchillas are overweight. They may then go on to develop dental problems or other conditions which may cause anorexia. Fat reserves are mobilised and the liver becomes swamped in fat compounds to the point at which failure may occur, with dullness and anorexia being the two most commonly seen non-specific signs. Diagnosis is made on finding elevated bile acid levels in conjunction with elevated AST and often GGT levels in the blood, and an enlarged liver shadow on radiography.

Respiratory disease

Pneumonia is common in chinchillas housed in damp and drafty conditions, but it may occur in any individual. The pathogens chiefly involved are bacteria such as *Bordetella bronchiseptica*, *Streptococcus pneumoniae*, *Pasteurella pneumotropica* and *Pseudomonas* spp. Diagnosis is as for guinea pigs. *Mycobacterium genavense* has been reported in chinchillas associated with severe granulomatous pneumonia, systemic spread with weight loss and mortality (Huynh *et al.*, 2014).

Cardiovascular disease

Chinchillas are prone to both hypertrophic and dilated cardiomyopathies. In addition, metastatic and dystrophic mineralisation and pericardial effusions may also be seen. Calcification may be asymptomatic and causes are thought to be similar to those in guinea pigs. In chinchillas, ventricular septal defects and tricuspid regurgitation have been reported.

Urinary tract disease

Urinary crystalline deposits have been seen in chinchillas and resemble those found in guinea pigs. Diagnosis is as for guinea pigs.

Reproductive tract disease

Dystocia occurs infrequently. There appears to be no associated significant separation of the pelvis as is seen in the guinea pig, and therefore age at first breeding is not so critical.

Musculoskeletal disease

Fractures are common in chinchillas, and tend to occur in the longer, more slender bones such as the tibia and femur. Chinchilla bones are more brittle than other rodents'.

Neurological disease

Several causes of fitting have been described in chinchillas. These include the virus which causes lymphocytic choriomeningitis (LCMV), as well as the bacterium *Listeria monocytogenes*, which may be spread by wild rodents. Otitis media can be seen with systemic infections with *Pseudomonas aeruginosa*.

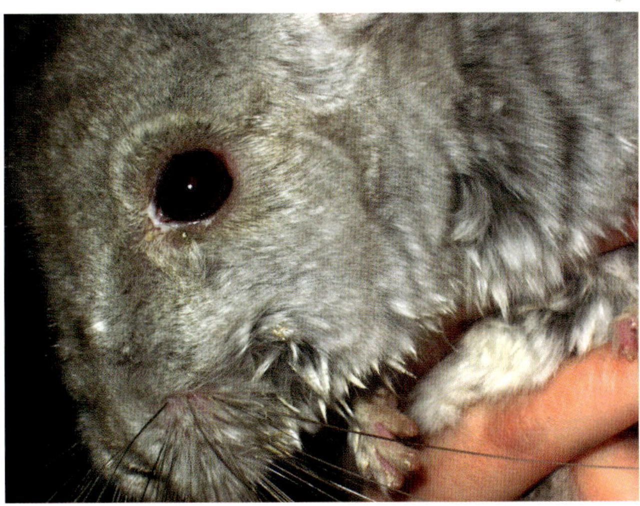

Figure 5.17 Epiphora is commonly associated with cheek tooth dental disease in chinchillas and may be mistaken for a true conjunctivitis.

Ocular disease

Conjunctivitis presents epiphora. It may be due to excessive dust bathing with resultant foreign body irritation, or to the bacteria *Chlamydia* spp. Alternatively, dental disease may be present, so the problem may not be a true conjunctivitis (see Figure 5.17).

DISEASES OF THE DEGU

Skin disease

Neoplasia

Cutaneous fibrosarcomas have been reported as one of the most commonly seen neoplasms in degus. They are more commonly seen in the hindlimbs and in females (Svara *et al.*, 2020).

Managemental

Relatively few skin diseases are reported in degus. One of the most common is self-induced alopecia, associated with a barren environment and lack of social interaction or handling. Areas of alopecia seen in this condition include the medial hindlimbs and forelimbs as well as around the muzzle due to rubbing. Degloving of the skin over the tail can occur in degus similar to that in gerbils and so degus should not be held by the tail.

Digestive disease

Dental disease similar to that seen in chinchillas is commonly seen in degus. Aetiologies are therefore also similar and include a lack of abrasive foodstuffs in the diet and a reduced calcium to phosphorus ratio (less than 1.5 : 1). Pseudo-odontoma has been well reported in degus similar to the situation in prairie dogs (see section on prairie dogs for more information).

Cardiovascular disease

Very few if any cardiovascular diseases are recorded in the literature for degus. A ventricular septal defect was recorded in one case study with a significant holosystolic murmur (4/6) (Sanchez *et al.*, 2019). The case also had cardiomegaly and lung patternation on radiography as would be expected with congestive heart failure.

Thymoma has been reported in a degu causing a cervical ventral subcutaneous mass (Okumura *et al.*, 2022). The same degu later died of a myxosarcoma of the chest with lung metastases and respiratory distress.

Endocrine disease

Diabetes mellitus is a common condition in degus and is associated with damage to the insulin-secreting cells of the islets of Langerhans due to amyloid deposition. A cytomegalovirus, herpesvirus and diets high in soluble carbohydrates (sugars) have all been associated with development of diabetes mellitus in degus (Spear *et al.*, 1984).

Neurological and ocular disease

Ketoacidosis is possible with diabetes mellitus and may result in seizures and coma.

Alzheimer's-like disease has been well reported in degus as they are used as a model for human Alzheimer's disease (Rivera *et al.*, 2016). Clinically it appears around 5 years of age and produces a disease similar to that seen in humans, with an age-related neuropathology and associated with glucose metabolism of the hippocampus similar to that of humans with Alzheimer's disease (Cisternas *et al.*, 2021). However, animals deprived of environmental stimulation and inbred populations may develop disease similar to Alzheimer's at an earlier age (Tan *et al.*, 2022).

Cataracts are commonly seen within a few weeks of the development of diabetes mellitus and retinal macular degeneration, similar to that seen in humans, can occur with age.

DISEASES OF THE CHIPMUNK

Skin disease

Ectoparasitic

Burrowing mites such as *Notoedres muris* as well as *Sarcoptes* spp. have been reported. In addition, chipmunks are susceptible to the harvest mite *Neotrombicula autumnalis*, as well as the avian red mite *Dermanyssus gallinae*. The latter can cause anaemia and is commonly found where birds nest and roost.

Bacterial

Bacteria such as those described for rats and mice are commonly isolated from the skin of chipmunks and their associated abscesses. Abscesses are common in chipmunks housed in groups as they frequently fight.

Neoplasia

Squamous cell carcinomas have been reported in Siberian chipmunks with metastasis to the lungs (Kondo *et al.*, 2018).

Digestive disease

Oral

Overgrown incisors are common due to trauma. Overgrowth or damage of the incisors may cause them to impinge on the floor of the nasal passage. The chipmunk often shows signs of a runny nose with a copious discharge.

Gastrointestinal

Chipmunks suffer diarrhoea from bacteria seen in rats and mice, with *Yersinia pseudotuberculosis* and *Salmonella* spp. being reported. Tyzzer's disease (*Clostridium piliforme*), which may cause liver damage, is also seen.

Respiratory disease

Pneumonia is frequently bacterial, and often occurs after periods of stress such as re-homing and handling. In addition, it is thought that the human influenza virus may be transmissible to chipmunks. Secondary metastasis of skin-associated squamous cell carcinomas have been reported (Kondo *et al.*, 2018).

Cardiovascular disease

Chipmunks are very nervous and care should be taken to handle them carefully and in dimmed lighting. Rough handling and high levels of stress can lead to fitting and cardiac arrest. Endocardiosis has been reported in Siberian chipmunks and congestive heart failure may follow if valvular insufficiency becomes severe enough.

Urinary tract disease

Struvite crystals and calcium oxalate are seen. Bacterial cystitis due to *E. coli* is often associated. Since male chipmunks have a longer urethra and an os penis, urolithiasis causes more problems for males than for females. Haematuria may be seen, and a swollen penis found on close physical examination. The calculi may be demonstrated radiographically and in urine samples.

Reproductive tract disease

Hypocalcaemic paralysis

This can occur soon after parturition, particularly if the chipmunk is on a poor-quality all-seed diet. The female appears lethargic, often is not suckling the young and may become unconscious.

Uterine disease

Uterine infections such as pyometras may be seen. There may be a vulval discharge, sometimes tinged with blood, and the female chipmunk is often anorectic, lethargic and polydipsic. Metritis may be seen shortly after parturition, with the female presenting as collapsed and weakened with a swollen abdomen and signs of peritonitis.

Mammary gland disease

Mastitis is uncommon, but bacteria such as *E. coli*, *Klebsiella* spp. and *Staphylococcus* spp. have been isolated. Mammary gland fibroadenomas and adenocarcinomas have been recorded.

Musculoskeletal disease

Chipmunks are acrobatic and fractures are common and often involve the spine. If a spinal fracture is suspected, radiography may be performed. The prognosis is poor and euthanasia is advised in these cases.

Neurological disease

Fitting is a problem in chipmunks housed in rooms with equipment (some strip lighting and TVs) emitting 50–60 Hz radiation. In addition, some chipmunks may be prone to hereditary epilepsy. Finally, bacteria such as *Listeria monocytogenes* and *Streptococcus pneumoniae*, protozoa such as *Toxoplasma gondii*, and viruses such as LCMV may also cause CNS disease.

DISEASES OF THE PRAIRIE DOG

Skin disease

Ectoparasitic

Mites

Demodicosis has been reported in prairie dogs, resulting in scaling and fur loss over the back and flanks (Jekl, 2006). Sarcoptiform mites such as *Sarcoptes scabiei* and *Notoedres* spp. may all infect prairie dogs when in contact with a source case. Clinical diagnosis for all mites is by skin scraping under anaesthesia.

Fleas

Fleas are commonly seen on wild-caught individuals and due to the ubiquitous nature of dog and cat fleas, prairie dogs may become infested with other species in multi-pet households. Fleas in the wild may transmit the causal agent of bubonic plague, *Yersinia pestis*, from prairie dog to prairie dog.

Lice

Linognathoides cynomyis is a sucking louse specific to the black-tailed prairie dog and although uncommonly seen in captive-bred individuals may cause irritation and mild anaemia.

Bacterial

Bacteria commonly isolated from bite wounds and other skin lesions include *Staphylococcus aureus*, *Pasteurella* spp. and *Streptococcus* spp. Bacterial pododermatitis has been reported as with other rodent species.

Fungal

Ringworm due to *Trichophyton mentagrophytes* and *Microsporum gypseum* may colonise the fur and skin of prairie dogs and may produce clinical disease secondary to conditions such as demodicosis. In young and debilitated animals it may also cause typical scaling and grey scurf with fur loss.

Neoplasia

Neoplasms such as lipomas, squamous cell carcinomas, basal cell carcinomas, lymphoma and adenocarcinomas have all been reported in the skin (Sarvi and Esher, 2023).

Behavioural

Prairie dogs that are housed singly may exhibit behavioural abnormalities including over-grooming and self-mutilation.

Digestive disease

Oral

So-called odontomas are commonly seen around the roots of the upper incisors. These are not often neoplastic in prairie dogs, but rather due to dysplasia of the incisor apical bud associated with impaired tooth eruption caused by repeated trauma and dental fractures and so are often more properly termed 'pseudo-odontomas' or in some cases elodontomas. The apical bud grows and produces new tooth growth in the reserve crown that pushes into the nasal passages and can occlude them causing dyspnoea.

Older prairie dogs may wear down the crowns of the cheek teeth and so be unable to grind food effectively, resulting in progressive weight loss.

Oral squamous cell carcinomas have also been reported in prairie dogs as have salivary gland adenomas and basal cell carcinomas (Ueda *et al.*, 2019).

Gastrointestinal

Bacteria such as *Yersinia pseudotuberculosis* and *Y. pestis* have been associated with prairie dogs in the wild. *Yersinia pestis* is the cause of bubonic plague and prairie dogs in the USA are known to be potential reservoirs of the disease. In captivity, *Y. pseudotuberculosis* may be more commonly seen with clinical signs similar to those reported in other rodents such as the guinea pig. *Salmonella* spp. may cause clinical haemorrhagic diarrhoea and septicaemia in prairie dogs, as with many other species of rodent.

Cestodes such as *Hymenolepis nana* have been reported in prairie dogs, although rarely with clinical disease (Duclos and Richardson, 2000). Its significance is its zoonotic potential. A coccidial parasite, *Eimeria ludoviciani*, has been associated with soft faeces in young prairie dogs and protozoal flagellates such as *Giardia* spp. and trichomonads have been reported, mainly in wild-caught individuals, and may also result in diarrhoea, although many are not clinically affected.

Liver

Hepatocellular carcinomas have been seen in wild and captive prairie dogs, with a suspicion that the tumour may be caused by a viral agent, possible a hepadnavirus (Wright *et al.*, 2017). The tumours appear to metastasise readily and may be associated with hepatitis, lipidosis and cirrhosis (Garner *et al.*, 2004).

Respiratory disease

Bacterial

Bacteria such as *Klebsiella pneumoniae*, *Pseudomonas* spp., *Pasteurella multocida* and *Bordetella* spp. can cause significant respiratory disease in prairie dogs and may be seen secondary to dyspnoea associated with dental disease such as pseudo-odontomas.

Parasitic

Parasitic mites, *Pneumocoptes penrosei*, have been reported causing airway blockage, bronchiectasis and emphysema (Collins, 1988).

Viral

Monkeypox virus has been reported in prairie dogs in the USA that came into contact with animals imported from West Africa in 2003 (DiGiulio and Eckburg, 2004). Monkeypox virus is a significant zoonosis and a legally notifiable disease (must be reported to the relevant government veterinary authority if diagnosed or suspected) in many countries around the world including the UK, European Union and USA. Clinical signs include lymphadenopathy and respiratory disease.

Neoplasia

Primary respiratory tract neoplasia appears uncommon although bronchioloalveolar adenocarcinomas have been reported (Thas and Garner, 2012). Metastasis of carcinomas from the liver and kidneys may occur resulting in dyspnoea. A lipoma of the cranial mediastinum has also been reported causing dyspnoea in a black-tailed prairie dog (Rogers and Chrisp, 1998). Thymomas have also been reported and may do the same (Thas and Garner, 2012).

Cardiovascular disease

Cardiomyopathy

Dilated cardiomyopathy has been reported in prairie dogs. Clinical signs typically appear around 3–4 years of age and can include dyspnoea, lethargy and anorexia. Radiography showing cardiac silhouette enlargement and assessment for vertebral heart scores, and a bronchioalveolar lung pattern have been recorded. Echocardiography can also be used to confirm the diagnosis as with other species.

Neoplasia

Lymphoma, thymoma and splenic haemangiosarcomas have all been reported in prairie dogs (Thas and Garner, 2012).

Urinary tract disease

Kidney

Adenoma and adenocarcinomas of the kidney have been reported in prairie dogs. Chronic progressive nephrosis is also seen in aged prairie dogs.

Reproductive tract disease

Reproductive tract disease is relatively under-reported in prairie dogs. Testicular cancer has been reported, with Leydig cell tumours being most commonly seen. Mammary neoplasia such as adenocarcinomas are also seen from time to time.

Musculoskeletal disease

Metabolic bone disease may be seen in prairie dogs fed a diet low in calcium/vitamin D_3. Clinically, bowing of the long bones, particularly the tibias, as well as dental disease due to osteoporosis of the skull may be seen.

Neurological disease

Neurological diseases specific to prairie dogs are not reported, although similar conditions to other rodents have been seen, for example traumatic spinal disease. Neuronal migration of ascarids such as *Baylisascaris procyonis* (the roundworm commonly seen in raccoons) can result in neurological disease.

DISEASES OF SUGAR GLIDERS AND VIRGINIA OPOSSUMS

Skin disease

Bacterial

Similar pyoderma problems to those seen in eutherian mammals have been reported in marsupials. Fight wounds may be common where stocking densities are high or where sexually mature entire males are housed together and have been reported commonly around the head and eyes. Bacteria such as *Pasteurella multocida*, *Staphylococcus aureus* and *Mycobacterium* spp. have been reported.

Fungal

The dermatophyte *Trichophyton mentagrophytes* has been associated with scaling lesions in Virginia opossums.

Ectoparasites

Specific mites such as *Petauralges rackae* in sugar gliders and *Haemogamasus* spp. in Virginia opossums have been associated with mange. Marsupials also appear susceptible to *Sarcoptes scabiei* mites. Harvest mites (*Neotrombicula autumnalis* and *Guntheria kowanyama*) have also been seen to cause pruritus and self-mutilation.

Common cat and dog fleas are not host specific and so could also infest both species of marsupial.

Neoplasia

Cutaneous lymphoma has been reported in sugar gliders and systemic lymphoma appears common in this species.

Self-trauma

Sugar gliders may self-traumatise digits, genitalia and their tails when stressed, initially just removing the hair and then causing tissue injuries.

Endocrine

Endocrine disease has been reported in older marsupials. Bilateral symmetrical alopecia in older female sugar gliders has been reported and also in Virginia opossums, where it has been associated with prolactin-secreting pituitary tumours (Johnson-Delaney, 2010).

Miscellaneous

Virginia opossums have been reported with scaling of the non-haired portion of the tail. Some cases have been determined as ectoparasite-associated disease and some have resolved when the environmental humidity has been increased.

Digestive disease

Dental disease

Tartar build-up with periodontal disease and abscesses are common in sugar gliders and Virginia opossums and are worsened by sugar-rich soft food diets. Although the teeth of sugar gliders are long, they are not like those of rodents: the teeth do not continuously erupt and so should never be trimmed as exposure of the pulp cavity will occur with concomitant infection.

Bacterial disease

Gastrointestinal infections with bacteria such as *Yersinia pseudotuberculosis*, *Salmonella* spp. and *Clostridium* spp. have been reported in sugar gliders and Virginia opossums. Yersiniosis may result in acute death or a more chronic wasting condition, with granuloma formation in the intestines. Clostridiosis has been associated with acute death, but it and *E. coli* enteritis may also result in diarrhoea, tenesmus and rectal prolapses in sugar gliders. Mycobacterial infections of marsupials have been reported in the wild but are relatively uncommon in captivity.

Parasitic disease

Giardia spp. have been reported in both species and resulted in small intestinal disease with diarrhoea and dehydration.

Cryptosporidium spp. has been reported in neonate sugar gliders, and in immunocompromised individuals has resulted in diarrhoea and a malabsorption maldigestion problem.

Various nematodes have been reported in the gut of the sugar glider, including *Parastrongyloides* spp., *Paraustrostrongylus* spp. and *Paraustroxyuris* spp. In the Virginia opossum, nematodes such as *Capillaria* spp., *Physaloptera* spp., and *Cruzia* spp. have been reported. Intestinal flukes (trematodes) have also been reported in Virginia opossums and may be associated with diarrhoea.

Liver flukes (*Athesmia* spp.) have been reported asymptomatically in sugar gliders but theoretically heavy infestations could result in liver damage.

Toxoplasma gondii, as with other marsupials, may be consumed orally due to contamination of food from felid faeces, although Virginia opossums have been known to eat rodents which can act as an intermediate host. CNS disease with pneumonia and liver failure can occur.

Other disease

Paracloacal glands in sugar gliders can become impacted and infected as a result. The secretions become inspissated and can result in tissue necrosis and cellulitis.

Respiratory disease

Bacterial disease

Infections with *Pasteurella multocida*, *Streptococcus pneumoniae* and *Klebsiella* spp. have all been reported resulting in pneumonia in sugar gliders and Virginia opossums.

Fungal disease

Cryptococcus neoformans, a yeast, has been reported as the cause of pneumonia in sugar gliders. It produces a granulomatous reaction which may be seen radiographically and is difficult to treat. Sources of infection are contaminated feed/environmental plants.

Cardiovascular disease

Cardiomyopathy (dilated) has been reported in both sugar gliders and Virginia opossums and can produce congestive heart failure. Hypertrophic cardiomyopathy may also be seen in Virginia opossums, particularly those over 2 years of age and may present with tachycardia and also renal failure.

Microabscessation of the myocardium and associated heart failure may also be seen in various bacterial infections, particularly those associated with *Clostridium* spp.

Heartworm, *Dirofilaria immitis*, has also been reported as a cause of heart failure in Virginia opossums. It is transmitted principally by mosquitoes and is not currently found in the UK, although it is present in parts of continental Europe and the USA.

Mineralisation of the aorta and main arteries has also been reported in Virginia opossums due to oversupplementation with calcium and vitamin D_3.

Urinary tract disease

Leptospira spp. infections of the urinary tract have been associated with interstitial nephritis, hepatitis and death of marsupials.

Urolithiasis and cystitis have been reported in sugar gliders and may be associated with urinary retention due to a lack of territory (overcrowding). Cystitis may lead to an ascending infection with resultant nephritis. Renoliths are occasionally reported.

Prostatic hypertrophy and prostatitis resulting in dysuria have been reported in Virginia opossums.

Reproductive tract disease

Infections of the pouch can be seen in both species. Bacteria involved include *Pseudomonas* spp., *E. coli* and *Staphylococcus aureus*. Owners should be discouraged from touching the inside of the pouch, especially with bare hands, as the pouch environment is particularly susceptible to infections (similar to the uterus in eutherian mammals).

Infections of the reproductive tract have also been reported as a cause of ill-health and infertility and may result in uterine prolapse in Virginia opossums. Neoplasia of the reproductive tract is also relatively common in older females.

Male sugar gliders are known to self-mutilate the end of the forked penis and also the scrotum when kept on their own.

Infertility may also be seen in individuals that are obese and in situations where there is overcrowding.

Musculoskeletal disease

Nutritional osteodystrophy

Also known as metabolic bone disease, it is common in captive marsupials, particularly in sugar gliders. As with other animals, it is associated with a lack of calcium and vitamin D_3. Clinically, it can present with bowing of long bones, spontaneous fractures and collapse of the spinal column, with resultant paresis/paralysis. Radiographs reveal poor bone mineralisation/density and hypocalcaemia and hypoproteinaemia may be seen on blood biochemistry. Diets that contain large amounts of unsupplemented fruit or meat are common culprits.

Neurological disease

Paresis or paralysis, usually of the hindlimbs, associated with nutritional osteodystrophic collapse of the spinal column resulting in spinal cord damage, is common.

In sugar gliders, seizures associated with hypovitaminosis B_1 have been reported where diets have not been supplemented with this vitamin (home-made sugar/nectar formulas are often deficient in this). Seizures may also be seen with hypoglycaemia and hypocalcaemia so these should also be considered.

In sugar gliders a suggested hypovitaminosis E condition with encephalomalacia has been recorded post mortem as has been seen in other animals with a vitamin E deficiency.

All marsupials are very susceptible to *Toxoplasma* spp. infection which can result in fever, seizures and usually death. Sources are typically contamination of food/environment by the faeces of domestic cats, although the Virginia opossum is known to scavenge dead rodents which can also provide a source.

Migration through the spinal cord of the nematode *Baylisascaris* spp. has also been reported as a cause of paralysis in sugar gliders.

Many aged Virginia opossums will show evidence of fine and intention tremors due to fibrosis of the vasculature within the brain leading to reduced oxygenation.

Ocular disease

Cataracts have been reported in sugar gliders associated with suspected hypovitaminosis A and with diabetes mellitus. Senescent cataracts have been reported in both marsupials. Lipid deposits have been seen in young sugar gliders where the mother has been fed a high lipid-containing diet.

DISEASES OF THE AFRICAN PYGMY HEDGEHOG

Skin disease

Ectoparasitic

Mites

The psoroptiform mite *Caparinia tripilis* and chorioptiform mites *Chorioptes* spp. are a common cause of pruritus and spine loss in hedgehogs including the African pygmy hedgehog (APH). In the wild *Caparinia erinacei* has also been reported. Skin crusting of the nose and limbs with *Notoedres* spp., a sarcoptiform mite, has also been reported. Ear mites such as *Otodectes cynotis* may also be seen, often transferred from a cohabiting pet dog or cat also affected.

Ornithonyssus spp. mites which are blood-sucking have also been reported in APHs and may result in restlessness, loss of appetite and, in heavy infestations, dermatitis and anaemia (see Figures 5.18 and 5.19). Wild birds and rodents are commonly a source of these mites.

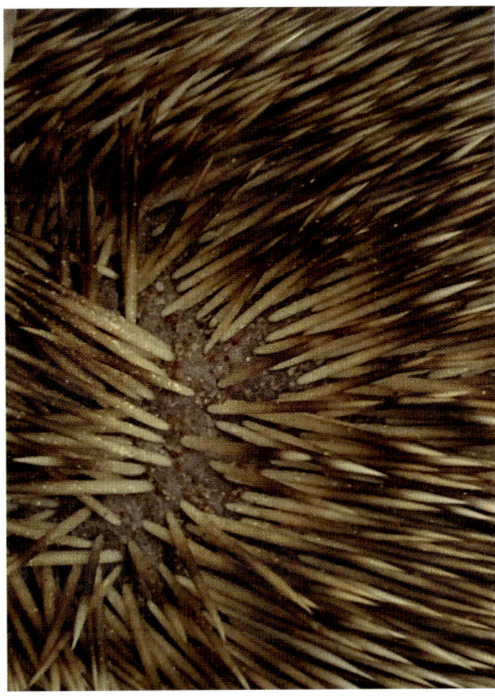

Figure 5.18 *Ornithonyssus* spp. mites appear as small red dots due to their blood-sucking nature and may result in anaemia in a number of species including APHs.

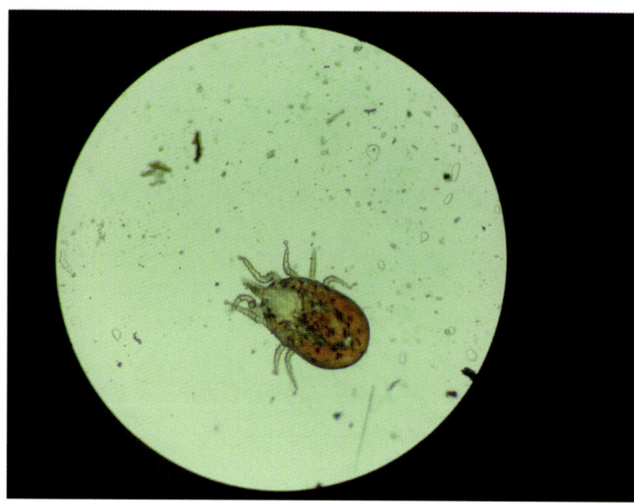

Figure 5.19 *Ornithonyssus* spp. mite under the microscope.

Fleas

In a household setting, fleas may be seen where other pets such as cats and dogs are present and so species such as *Ctenocephalides felis* and *C. canis* are more likely and may result in pruritus and dermatitis.

Bacterial

Secondary bacterial skin infections associated with trauma and mite infestations can be seen in APHs. A variety of bacterial pathogens have been reported, including *Pasteurella* spp., *Streptococcus* spp. and *Corynebacterium* spp. as well as anaerobes such as *Bacteroides* spp. and even mycobacteria.

Fungal

Dermatophytosis associated with *Trichophyton mentagrophytes* var. *erinacei* is the most commonly reported fungal skin disease and is often found secondary to mites (particularly *Caparinia* spp.), although *Microsporum* spp. can also be seen. Grey scaling scurf with spine loss may be seen with heavy infestations.

Autoimmune

A single case of pemphigus foliaceus has been reported with loss of spine, flaking skin, moist erythema and epidermal collarettes (Wack, 2000).

Neoplasia

Skin neoplasia, as with other neoplasms, is common in APHs with sarcomas, sebaceous carcinomas, lipomas, liposarcomas, squamous cell carcinomas, mast cell tumours and mammary gland tumours (usually adenocarcinomas) all being reported.

Digestive disease

Oral

Dental disease including periodontitis and gingivitis is very common. Some therefore recommend feeding some dry food to encourage abrasion and regular dental checks.

Oral neoplasia is common in APHs, with a high incidence of squamous cell carcinomas.

Gastrointestinal

Salmonella spp. enteritis has been reported and may be subclinical or may result in diarrhoea, weight loss, dehydration and death.

Cryptosporidiosis due to *C. parvum* can affect juvenile APHs and, in serious cases, can result in a fatality.

APHs may consume non-food-related material and develop an intestinal obstruction. Clinically, vomiting is rarely seen and signs may be non-specific with lethargy and collapse. Gas distension of the stomach may be seen on radiography but it is a relatively non-specific sign.

Infiltrative lymphoma/lymphosarcomas may affect the digestive tract as well as other body systems

Liver disease

Hepatic lipidosis is common and may be seen in up to half of all sick APHs and so is often a non-specific but nonetheless serious clinical development, similar to the situation in the domestic rabbit.

Primary liver neoplasia, both adenomas and adenocarcinomas, have been reported. An APH administered dexamethasone 2 weeks prior died of the human herpes simplex virus (HSV)-1 associated with liver failure.

Respiratory disease

Bacterial

Pneumonia is the result of infection with the usual bacteria (e.g. *Corynebacterium*, *Pasteurella multocida*, *Bordetella bronchiseptica* and *Mycoplasma* spp.), particularly if associated with low environmental temperatures (<18°C). Diagnosis is based on recovery of the organism from tracheal swabs or bronchoalveolar lavage and supporting radiographic evidence.

Parasitic

Parasitic lung disease is less commonly reported in APHs as most are kept indoors and the source of the lungworms is usually a mollusc that acts as the intermediate host or earthworms that act as paratenic hosts. However, hedgehogs are susceptible to *Capillaria* spp. and *Crenosoma striatum* in particular and so may have a dual verminous with secondary bacterial pneumonia. Faecal screening using Baermann flotation techniques for lungworm, or sampling sputum can aid diagnosis.

Viral

Bronchopneumonia associated with skunk adenovirus-1 infection has been reported in an APH (Needle *et al.*, 2019).

Neoplasia

As with other body organ systems, neoplasia (usually secondary metastases but primary bronchoalveolar carcinomas have been reported) is commonly seen in the lungs.

Cardiovascular disease

Cardiomyopathy

Dilated cardiomyopathy may be seen in up to 40% of older APHs (over 3 years of age) and congestive heart failure associated with atrioventricular valvular defects is also common. Diagnosis has been suggested based on echocardiography of a ventricular fractional shortening less than 25% with a wall thickness minimum of 1.5 mm. Bilateral atrial thrombus formation with thrombotic disease has also been reported as well as valvular endocardiosis with subsequent congestive heart failure. Delk *et al.* (2014) suggested that carnitine deficiency may contribute to cardiac disease in geriatric hedgehogs. Cardiac assessment of APHs has been published in which the mean heart rate was determined as 200 ± 48 beats per minute (Black *et al.*, 2011).

Haematopoietic disease

Haematopoietic disease occurred in 11% of post-mortem lesions in one publication, with lymphoma being the most commonly reported, whether as multicentric disease or associated with the gastrointestinal tract (Raymond and Garner, 2001). Genetic predisposition and a possible retroviral origin for some cases has been suggested. Other forms of haemolymphatic neoplasia reported in APHs include myelogenous leukaemia, eosinophilic leukaemia, intestinal plasmacytoma, multiple myeloma, histiocytic sarcoma, and malignant neuroendocrine carcinoid tumours of the spleen (Johnson, 2020).

Urinary tract disease

Kidney

Nephritis, glomerulosclerosis and tubular necrosis have all been reported histologically in APHs and renal failure is common in APHs over the age of 3 years, although cases as young as 7 months have been reported.

Poorly differentiated renal neoplasia has also been recorded (Harrison and Kitchell, 2017).

Bladder

Urolithiasis is common in APHs and although the composition has not been reported, anecdotally it has been associated with feeding cat food.

Reproductive tract disease

Female

Uterine neoplasia resulting in haemorrhage from the reproductive tract visible at the vulva, metritis and pyometra have been reported frequently in APHs. Numerous neoplasms, including adenoleiomyosarcoma, adenosarcoma, endometrial stromal cell sarcoma, endometrial polyps, adenoleiomyoma, uterine adenocarcinoma, carcinosarcoma and uterine spindle cell tumours, have been reported (Johnson, 2020). Infiltrative lymphosarcoma may also be seen.

Male

Posthitis from substrate entanglement has been reported as common in APHs. There is also a case of accessory sex gland disease in a male APH that caused urethral blockage (Koizumi and Kondo, 2019).

Endocrine disease

Hyperadrenocorticism resulting in 'Cushings-like' disease that causes alopecia, a pendulous abdomen, polydipsia/polyuria and polyphagia has been seen. Blood samples may show an elevated cortisol level.

Carcinomas of the thyroid glands such as thyroid adenocarcinoma, thyroid C-cell carcinoma and thyroid follicular carcinoma have been seen as well as benign thyroid follicular adenomas.

Other endocrine neoplasias reported in APHs include parathyroid adenoma, pancreatic islet cell tumours, pituitary adenoma, pheochromocytoma, adrenal cortical carcinoma, and malignant neuroendocrine tumours. Most are subclinical or present with more general signs such as lethargy, weakness and incoordination.

Musculoskeletal disease

Osteoarthritis and spondylosis sometimes with associated intervertebral disc disease have been reported. Trauma may of course result in fractures, but osteosarcomas are regularly seen in APHs and should be considered where spontaneous fractures, particularly of the limbs, are found.

Neurological disease

Ataxia can be associated with chilling; however, wobbly hedgehog disease/syndrome has also been reported associated with hindlimb ataxia and paresis progressing in an ascending manner to quadriparesis and muscle atrophy. Grossly, the nerves are unaffected but on histopathology the spinal cord and brain are often affected with axonal swelling, degeneration of the spinal cord ventral tracts and axonal and myelin degeneration in the brain white matter. A strong genetic cause is suspected but viral and autoimmune possibilities exist.

CNS neoplasia has also been reported in hedgehogs and includes soft tissue sarcoma, histiocytic sarcoma, ganglioglioma, gemistocytic astrocytoma, oligodendroglioma, anaplastic astrocytoma, microglioma, oligoastrocytoma, meningioma and lymphoma.

Ocular disease

Orbital proptosis is not uncommon and surgical enucleation is often opted for due to the ocular damage caused and difficulty medicating topically.

DISEASES OF THE FERRET

Skin disease

Ectoparasitic

Mites

The ear mite *Otodectes cynotis* causes intense irritation, and the production of copious black wax. This may lead to facial dermatitis, otitis externa, otitis interna and vestibular syndrome. Diagnosis is by finding the typical mites on wax samples (see Figure 5.20).

Less common is *Sarcoptes scabiei* which can cause intense pruritus over the head, ears, paws and tail. Diagnosis is made on skin scrapings.

A fur mite known as *Lynxacarus mustelae* has been reported in young ferret kits associated with ulceration of the head and face (Halck *et al.*, 2023).

Clinical disease associated with *Demodex* spp. has been rarely reported in ferrets.

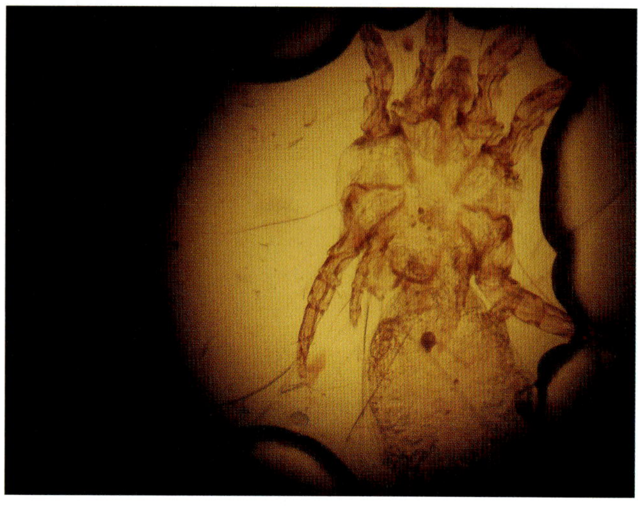

Figure 5.20 Microscopic image of an *Otodectes cynotis* ear mite from a ferret.

Fleas

The domestic cat and dog fleas *Ctenocephalides felis* and *C. canis* may infest ferrets. Many ferrets are used in the UK for hunting, and therefore the rabbit flea *Spilopsyllus cuniculi* or 'stick tight' fleas *Echidnophaga* spp. may also be seen.

Ticks

Ixodes ricinus are commonly found in ferrets used for hunting.

Leishmaniasis

The protozoan parasite *Leishmania infantum* can affect many mammals, including cats dogs and ferrets. It is vectored by sand flies (*Phlebotomus* spp.) and is therefore found in areas such as southern Europe. The disease can present with generalised lymph node enlargement and splenomegaly, but cutaneous lesions include erythema and papules with inflammation that is generally non-pruritic.

Bacterial

Abscesses frequently develop, particularly in the cervical area, due to intraspecific fighting. Bacteria include *Streptococcus* spp., *Staphylococcus* spp., *Trueperella (Arcanobacterium) pyogenes*, *Pasteurella* spp., and *E. coli*. *Trueperella pyogenes* infections often produce copious green-coloured pus, and may be associated with immunosuppressive conditions. *Pseudomonas luteola* has been associated with a pyogranulomatous panniculitis (Baum *et al.*, 2015).

Fungal

Dermatophytosis due to *Microsporum canis* or *Trichophyton mentagrophytes* is relatively uncommon in the ferret. *Malassezia* spp. has occasionally been seen secondary to ear mite infestation causing otitis externa.

Viral

Canine distemper virus (CDV), a paramyxovirus, may affect the skin with a rash over the chin and ventrum followed by brown crusts, particularly around the eyes and chin a week after infection. A nasal discharge may be present. Unless vaccinated, most ferrets will die from canine distemper between 7 and 21 days after contracting the virus.

Neoplasia

Squamous cell carcinomas have been reported occurring on the head, along the nose and ear tips in particular. They are malignant tumours and locally invasive. Sebaceous epitheliomas and basal cell tumours are seen on the head, neck and shoulders and are well-defined benign tumours, but may ulcerate. Fibrosarcomas have been reported in response to injection site reactions, as in cats. Mast cell tumours are very common in ferrets over the age of 4 years but many will spontaneously resolve being generally less aggressive than those seen in dogs and cats. Apocrine gland carcinomas and benign adenomas have also been reported commonly in ferrets. Carcinomas may be associated with anal scent glands, but adenomas may be found over the head and neck as well. Cutaneous (T-cell) lymphoma is occasionally reported but is less commonly seen than other forms of lymphoma in the ferret.

Hormonal

Hyperadrenocorticism is the most commonly seen cause of non-pruritic alopecia in the ferret (although around 40% may be pruritic). Hair loss is mainly over the dorsum and flanks initially. Secondary signs of hyperadrenocortical disease, including pendulous abdomen, thinning of the skin and weight gain, are also seen (see section Endocrine diseases).

In male ferrets, Leydig/interstitial cell tumours can produce excess testosterone and Sertoli cell tumours can produce excess oestrogen resulting in fur loss. In females, granulosa cell tumours of the ovaries have been associated with hair loss, as has the common hyperoestrogenic condition seen in unmated entire females due to persistent exposure to oestrogen.

Digestive disease

Oral

Dental disease is common in ferrets over 18 months of age on wet diets, which cause tartar and periodontal disease.

Oesophageal

Megaoesophagus has been reported in ferrets and results in regurgitation, wasting and aspiration pneumonia. It appears to be an acquired disease rather than congenital but the cause is unknown. Diagnosis is made using positive contrast radiography.

Gastric

Gastric ulceration is a common problem in ferrets and may be associated with *Helicobacter mustelae* infection. Gastric tumours and renal disease may also lead to gastric ulcer development, as will gastric foreign bodies.

The clinical signs vary but include dullness, abdominal guarding, salivation, vomiting, and melaena and weight loss. Further tests involve blood tests for renal disease, radiographs, both plain and barium studies, and ultimately gastric biopsy to demonstrate/culture *Helicobacter mustelae*.

Intestinal

Proliferative ileitis

Proliferative ileitis is similar to the 'wet tail' seen in hamsters and is due to *Lawsonia intracellularis*. Clinically, a green, mucoid, bloody diarrhoea and weight loss are seen. Diagnosis is made on clinical signs primarily and which are unlike almost any other condition. Biopsy can be confirmatory.

Intestinal lymphoma

This is relatively uncommon, but lymphoma of the mesenteric lymph nodes and the liver are seen in older ferrets. This may present with vague gastrointestinal signs, such as constipation, liver disease or even as apparently acute liver failure with jaundice.

Endoparasitic disease

Coccidiosis and giardiasis have both been described as causes of lethargy, diarrhoea and dehydration. Nematode and cestode parasites are rarely seen, although hunting individuals are more likely to be exposed to these parasites, with *Toxocara* spp. and *Toxascaris* spp. being the most commonly seen. Rarely do they cause clinical disease.

Viral disease

A parvovirus known as Aleutian disease is particularly lethal to mink, but in ferrets it produces unpleasant diarrhoea, although it is rarely fatal. It may produce melaenic faeces, fever, loss of weight and a number of other immune system-mediated symptoms.

Ferret epizootic coronaviral enteritis is an alphacoronavirus and results in high morbidity (up to 100%) but low mortality (<5%). Clinical signs include lethargy and anorexia for a period of 48–72 hours after infection, with vomiting initially which then stops. After this profuse green (bile-stained) diarrhoea with mucus is produced (so-called 'green slime disease'). Older ferrets with other diseases may show more severe clinical signs including intestinal ulceration. Younger ferrets have milder disease that resolves in 5–7 days. Some ferrets may be left with a maldigestion/malabsorption syndrome. Clinical tests may show hypoalbuminaemia and increased ALT and alkaline phosphatase with a leukocytosis.

Canine distemper can produce gastrointestinal signs such as diarrhoea. In addition, the influenza virus C may also be responsible for mild diarrhoea.

A member of the rotavirus family can cause diarrhoea in young, unweaned and recently weaned ferrets.

Other bacterial causes of diarrhoea

Salmonellosis due to *Salmonella typhimurium* has been reported and is a potential zoonosis.

Liver disease

The liver is commonly affected by lymphoma, although primary cancer of the liver is uncommon. Hepatic lipidosis has been recorded in persistently anorectic ferrets. In all of these cases the ferret may simply appear to be vaguely unwell, jaundice being an uncommon feature. Blood results may suggest a rise in ALT above 275 IU/L (Hillyer *et al.*, 1997), but it often requires ultrasonographic and biopsy tests to make a diagnosis.

Liver disease associated with copper poisoning has also been reported in ferrets.

Respiratory disease

Bacterial

Bacteria such as *Pasteurella* spp., *Bordetella bronchiseptica*, *Klebsiella pneumoniae*, *Streptococcus pneumoniae*, *Pseudomonas luteola*, *Nocardia* spp., *Mycoplasma* spp. and *Mycobacterium* spp. have all been associated with pneumonia in the domestic ferret (Lennox, 2021). Diagnosis is made on lung radiographs, lung washes and isolation of the bacteria.

Fungal

Cryptococcosis due to *Cryptococcus neoformans* and blastomycosis due to *Blastomyces* spp., two soil-associated yeasts, can cause a fungal pneumonia and sinusitis in any semi-fossorial species such as the domestic ferret. They may spread systemically in immunocompromised patients.

Parasitic

The lungworm *Aelurostrongylus abstrusus* can cause chronic coughing in ferrets. The adult worm sits in the pulmonary vasculature and sheds its eggs into the bloodstream; the eggs then burst into the alveoli and are coughed up, swallowed and passed in the faeces. This parasite uses molluscs (e.g. slugs and snails) as intermediate hosts. The lungworm *Capillaria aerophila* (also known as *Eucoleus aerophilus*) has also been reported in ferrets and will cause coughing. It sits in the actual airways as an adult worm. Again eggs are coughed up and passed in the faeces, where they may be ingested by earthworms or rodents which may act as a paratenic host.

Viral

Canine distemper virus is a paramyxovirus. The virus is spread by aerosol from one infected ferret or canid to another, when they sneeze or breathe. It may also be transmitted on a handler's hands and clothing. The virus gains access through the upper airways and incubates inside the ferret for 7–10 days, spreading throughout the body via the bloodstream.

The first signs of the disease occur on the skin (see section on skin diseases). The ferret is pyrexic and may have a serous oculonasal discharge. Secondary bacterial infections of the lungs on top of widespread immunosuppression often results in the death of an infected ferret. Towards the end of the disease fitting, nystagmus and generalised incoordination are all seen. The condition is fatal in nearly all cases of unvaccinated ferrets. Diagnosis is made on clinical signs, demonstration of viral antigens/antibodies in the bloodstream and/or mucous secretions of the ferret.

Human influenza C virus, an orthomyxovirus, is transmissible from human to ferret and back again. It causes a mainly upper airway disease with a systemic phase, producing pyrexia for 3–4 days.

Infection of ferrets has been widely reported due to SARS-CoV-2 and has been shown to infect ferrets by both direct contact and aerosol (Richard *et al.*, 2020). Currently mild upper respiratory signs have been reported in ferrets and other mustelids such as mink (Molenaar *et al.*, 2020). No evidence thus far has been shown that ferrets are capable of acting as a reservoir or significant source of infection for humans (Csiszar *et al.*, 2020). Recovery has been reported in infected ferrets without treatment.

Cardiovascular disease

Cardiomyopathy

Dilated cardiomyopathy is the most commonly seen, and may lead to congestive cardiac failure with lethargy, fluid respiratory noises, weight loss, polydipsia, ascites and audible systolic murmurs on auscultation of the chest. Diagnosis is made on radiographic signs of lung congestion, occasionally pleural effusion and an enlarged cardiac shadow, ECG changes and ultrasonographic demonstration of heart-wall thinning and valvular incompetence. Hypertrophic cardiomyopathy is rarely seen. Vertebral heart scores have been derived for ferrets to assess the radiographic size of the heart relative to the thoracic vertebrae (see Chapter 7 for further information).

Endocardiosis

Endocardiosis is common in ageing ferrets. The presenting signs are similar to those seen in dogs, with productive coughs, lethargy and, in more serious cases, heart failure with ascites and cyanosed membranes. Diagnosis is by auscultation, clinical signs and ultrasonographic demonstration of valvular incompetence and thickening.

Heartworm

Again, although it is not endemic in the UK, heartworm due to *Dirofilaria immitis* can be seen in ferrets from overseas. The parasite is transmitted by mosquitoes and the adult develops in the right ventricle of the heart. Ferrets affected may present with right-sided heart failure, that is, pleural effusion and ascites. An ELISA test is available but ferrets often produce false-negative results. Right-sided enlargement of the heart may be seen on radiographs and abnormalities may be seen on echocardiographic examination of the heart. In the UK, it is also possible to see the heartworm *Angiostrongylus vasorum*. This nematode uses slugs and snails as the intermediate host. The adult worms live in the right side of the heart and pulmonary vasculature with eggs being shed into the bloodstream, and then entering the airways and being coughed and swallowed and passed in the faeces. Severe cases may show signs of right-sided heart failure.

Lymphoma

Blood-borne leukaemia is uncommon; however, the tissue-associated lymphoma is very common, being the third most frequently seen neoplasia in the ferret after adrenal gland neoplasia and insulinomas. Some authors believe that there are two types of lymphoma: one is a juvenile, aggressive (lymphoblastic) form of lymphoma seen in ferrets under 14 months of age, often found in one site (e.g. thymus or spleen), that develops rapidly and responds well to chemotherapy; the other is a more chronic (lymphocytic) lymphoma typically seen in ferrets over 14 months, which affects more than one site and responds poorly to chemotherapy. Other authors agree that this is what is seen clinically but believe that a staging protocol similar to that used in dogs is more useful (Schoemaker, 2009):

- Stage 1 : a single site is involved (typically but not restricted to the spleen or thymus)
- Stage 2: multiple non-contiguous sites on the same side of the diaphragm
- Stage 3: multiple lymphatic sites on both sides of the diaphragm
- Stage 4: multiple sites on both sides of the diaphragm including non-lymphatic tissue or bone marrow.

Obviously stage 1 has the best prognosis for chemotherapy or surgery and the prognosis steadily worsens to stage 4.

Urinary tract disease

Kidney

Polycystic kidney disease is inherited in ferrets and is rare. Discrete renal cysts are asymptomatic but can be as common as 10–15%.

Pyelonephritis (e.g. *E. coli*) is seen in ferrets. In addition, interstitial nephritis due to *Leptospira* spp. is common in working ferrets coming into contact with wild rodents, which are the reservoir for this disease. Chronic interstitial nephritis is also common in all ferrets and is progressive from 2 years of age resulting in renal failure at 4–5 years of age.

Aleutian disease can produce a strong antibody response and result in circulating antibody–antigen complexes. These can damage the glomerular membranes of the kidneys, and produce membranous glomerulonephritis and tubular interstitial nephritis which may result in renal failure.

Renal function can be assessed using blood levels of urea and creatinine, the latter of which are lower normally than in other mammals (17–46 μmol/L).

Bladder

Urolithiasis is seen in ferrets that are fed protein from a plant source, which creates an alkaline urine pH and allows struvite or magnesium ammonium phosphate salts to precipitate. The provision of solely animal proteins in the diet leads to acidic urine and dissolution of the calculi. Pregnant jills are susceptible, as they are mobilising large volumes of minerals from their bones for fetal development and milk production. Cystine urolithiasis, a genetic condition, has also been reported and is seen in ferrets between 2 and 4 years of age, with males representing the majority of cases (Pacheco, 2020). Male ferrets may experience obstruction at the os penis if large enough calculi form. Clinically they are dull, straining to urinate and sometimes prolapsing the rectum. Often, the prepuce is swollen and the abdomen tense; occasionally crystals may be seen on the hairs around the prepuce. Radiography will confirm the diagnosis.

Stranguria and dysuria may be seen in male ferrets with prostatic hypertrophy and prostatic/paraprostatic cysts which are associated with hyperadrenocorticism.

Endocrine disease

Adrenal

The cause of adrenal disease in ferrets is still not fully understood, but a correlation between neutering and development of the disease has been deduced. The pathophysiology is thought to be due to ferrets (like mice and humans) having luteinising hormone (LH) receptors in their adrenal tissue, and these increase in number as levels of circulating LH increase after gonadectomy. This triggers the production of sex steroid hormones by the adrenal glands and therefore clinical disease (as well as hypertrophy and neoplastic change of the gland). Some suggest that certain genetic lines of ferrets are more predisposed. In ferrets, adrenal gland hyperplasia accounts for 56% of adrenal disease, adrenocortical adenoma for 16% and adenocarcinoma for 26%, all of which can produce sex steroid hormones, particularly oestradiol. In addition, the left adrenal gland seems more likely to develop disease than the right.

Diagnosis of adrenal disease is based on clinical signs, for example polyuria/polydipsia; bilateral hair loss, starting over the tail rump and dorsum and spreading over the flanks and rest of the body; pruritus in 40% of cases; and swelling of the vulva or prepuce in a ferret that has been previously surgically neutered. In male ferrets, prostatic cysts and hyperplasia are seen that may present with dysuria or stranguria. Ultrasound may show enlargement of the adrenal gland, but this can be difficult in early cases. Urinary corticoid/creatinine ratio is often increased and resistant to dexamethasone suppression. The ACTH level is often depressed and an increase in plasma cortisol levels has been observed after injection of human chorionic gonadotropin (Schoemaker *et al.*, 2008). In general a panel of oestradiol, androstenedione, 17-hydroxyprogesterone and dehydroepiandrosterone sulphate with or without cortisol has been recommended by many as effective in detecting adrenocortical disease in ferrets.

Diabetes mellitus

Diabetes mellitus is uncommon in ferrets and usually only seen after pancreatic surgery to remove insulinomas. It presents as a disease similar to that seen in cats.

Insulinoma

Hypoglycaemia may occur due to prolonged fasting (ferrets should not be fasted for more than 4–6 hours due to their high metabolic rates), overdosage with insulin in a diabetic case or due to an insulinoma (an insulin-secreting pancreatic tumour). Insulinomas have been reported as the most commonly seen neoplasm in older ferrets (>4 years) with an incidence varying from 21.7% (Williams and Weis, 2003) to 25% (Li *et al.*, 1998). Tumours secrete insulin continuously and are not altered by the production of hypoglycaemia. Rebound hypoglycaemia can also occur, though, if a brief period of hyperglycaemia has occurred, as the tumours can increase their production of insulin. Metastatic spread of insulinomas is low in ferrets.

Diagnosis of insulinoma is based on clinical signs, which include weakness of hindlimbs, ataxia, collapse, opisthotonus and drooling saliva with pawing at the mouth. Rarely do ferrets exhibit full seizures as is seen in dogs with insulinomas. Blood levels of glucose lower than 3.3 mmol/L are suggestive of insulinoma but not diagnostic. Elevated insulin levels (normal range 35–250 pmol/L; Jenkins, 2000) in the presence of hypoglycaemia are confirmatory. Some ferrets, however, may present with normal glucose levels with elevated insulin due to recent food consumption. These can be very carefully fasted for 3–4 hours to watch for the development of hypoglycaemia in the presence of persistent hyperinsulinaemia.

Hyperoestrogenism

For details, see following section.

Reproductive tract disease

Pregnancy toxaemia

Pregnancy toxaemia is similar to that seen in the guinea pig. It occurs in late gestation, often in a first-time mother, during a period of anorexia. Ketoacidosis develops, leading to dullness, lethargy, vomiting, dehydration, alopecia, neurological signs, abortion and death of the jill.

Dystocia

Dystocia is relatively uncommon in the ferret. It is more common in jills carrying a small litter due to the low levels of fetal corticosteroid produced. If the jill exceeds day 43 of gestation, labour may need to be induced.

Mastitis

Mastitis may occur as an acute illness immediately after parturition. Bacteria commonly present in these cases include *Streptococcus* spp. and *E. coli*. Toxaemia may develop.

A more chronic condition is seen due to the bacterium *Staphylococcus intermedius*. This form of mastitis is highly infectious between jills and destroys much of the mammary tissue, leaving scar tissue and pockets of infection.

Pyometra and metritis

Metritis occurs immediately after parturition and may cause an acute toxic reaction in the jill. The jill may be very dull and pyrexic at this stage, and have no milk production.

Pyometra occurs at any stage, and is manifested by a dark, foul-smelling vulval discharge, polydipsia and sometimes toxaemia. Occasionally, a closed pyometra with no external discharge may occur. Palpation of the abdomen reveals a swollen uterus in the caudal dorsal abdomen. The diagnosis may be confirmed with radiography or ultrasonography.

Hyperoestrogenism

An entire female will remain in oestrus for the whole of the breeding season (March–October), unless she is mated or chemically brought out of oestrus as ferrets are induced ovulators. This chronic long-term exposure to oestrogen results in fatal anaemia from bone marrow suppression. The jill presents as tachypnoeic, with pale, petechiated mucous membranes, lethargic and collapsed. Early signs are a prominently swollen vulva, symmetrical alopecia of the flanks, and often a vulval discharge. Current recommendations are for the jill to be brought out of heat by (1) being mated by an entire or vasectomised male; (2) being injected with proligestone (Delvosteron®, MSD Animal Health), a synthetic progesterone; or (3) implanted with a gonadotropin releasing hormone (GnRH) agonist such as deslorelin (Suprelorin®, Virbac Animal Health). Surgical neutering is not recommended due to adrenal neoplasia.

Prostatic disease

Prostate cysts are particularly common in ferrets with an actively secreting adrenal gland tumour. If enlarged, the prostate will obstruct the urethra, and therefore prevent urination. Large prostatic and paraprostatic cysts are commonly seen with this condition.

Musculoskeletal disease

Fractures

Fractures in ferrets are uncommon, although the spine is the most commonly affected. Posterior paresis or paralysis is often associated with vertebral fractures, but may also be a sign of cardiovascular disease, hypoglycaemia or anaemia. Diagnosis is by radiography and tests already discussed.

Disseminated idiopathic myofasciitis

The cause of this disease is unknown but was reported first in ferrets in 2003 in the USA (Ramsell and Garner, 2010). It is a severe inflammatory condition affecting the muscles and surrounding connective tissues and generally affects ferrets under 18 months of age. Most commonly the ferret has a fever (40–42.2°C), is lethargic, anorexic and dehydrated, with weight loss, loose faeces, lymphadenopathy and often paretic. Occasionally individuals may experience seizures or have oculonasal discharge. Definitive antemortem diagnosis requires biopsy of affected muscle. In advanced cases muscles may also atrophy. Histopathology shows pyogranulomatous inflammation in the fascia between muscle bundles.

Neurological disease

Fitting may be seen towards the end stages of CDV infection, and in hypoglycaemic syndrome and severe anaemia. Posterior paresis may be associated with spinal trauma, cardiovascular disease, hypoglycaemia, anaemia and CDV.

Mild incoordination, posterior ataxia and paresis can be associated with spinal disease due to trauma, abscessation or neoplasia. Aleutian disease can result in antigen–antibody complex-mediated vasculitis that can also produce these clinical signs. Diagnosis of Aleutian disease is often made using serum protein electrophoresis with a gamma globulin level in excess of 20% of the total serum protein level.

Ocular disease

Ophthalmia neonatorum, a failure of the kits' eyes to open, is often due to bacteria from the *Staphylococcus* and *Streptococcus* spp.

Other ocular problems include crusting and weeping associated with CDV, photophobia associated with the influenza virus, and conjunctivitis, night blindness and cataracts associated with hypovitaminosis A. Corneal ulcers due to trauma and local infections are common in ferrets.

Pyogranulomatous panophthalmitis has also been reported associated with systemic ferret alphacoronavirus infection (Lindemann *et al.*, 2015).

References

Asakawa, M.G., Goldschmidt, M.H., Une, Y. and Nomura, Y. (2008) The immunohistochemical evaluation of estrogen receptor-alpha and progesterone receptors of normal, hyperplastic, and neoplastic endometrium in 88 pet rabbits. *Veterinary Pathology*, **45**, 217–225.

Baum, B., Richter, B., Reifinger, M. *et al.* (2015) Pyogranulomatous panniculitis in ferrets (*Mustela putorius furo*) with intralesional demonstration of *Pseudomonas luteola*. *Journal of Comparative Pathology*, **152**(2–3), 114–118.

Black, P.A., Marshall, C., Seyfried, A.W. and Bartin, A.M. (2011) Cardiac assessment of African hedgehogs (*Atelerix albiventris*). *Journal of Zoo and Wildlife Medicine*, **42**(1), 49–53.

Bochynska, D., Lloyd, S., Restif, O. and Hughes, K. (2022) *Eimeria stiedae* causes most of the white-spotted liver lesions in wild European rabbits in Cambridgeshire, United Kingdom. *Journal of Veterinary Diagnostic Investigation*, **34**(2) https://doi.org/10.1177/10406387211066923.

Cheeke, P.R. (1987) Vitamins. In: *Rabbit Feeding and Nutrition Academic Press*, pp. 136–153. London.

Cisternas, P., Gherardelli, C., Salazar, P. and Inestrosa, N.C. (2021) Disruption of glucose metabolism in aged *Octodon degus*: a sporadic model of Alzheimer's disease. *Frontiers of integrative Neuroscience*, **5**, 733007. doi: 10.3389/fnint.2021.733007.

Collins, B.R. (1988) Common diseases and medical management of rodents and lagomorphs. In: *Contemporary Issues in Small Animal Practice: Exotic Animals* (eds E.R.&. Jacobson & G.V. Kollias Jr.), pp. 261–316. Churchill Livingstone, New York.

Crossley, D.A. and Miguélez, M.M. (2001) Skull size and cheek-tooth length in wild-caught and captive-bred chinchillas. *Archives of Oral Biology*, **46**, 919–928.

Csiszar, A., Jakab, F., Valencak, V.G. *et al.* (2020) Companion animals likely do not spread COVID-19 but may get infected themselves. *Geroscience*, **7**, 1–8. doi: 10.1007/s11357-020-00248-3.

Davies, R.R. and Davies, J.A. (2003) Rabbit gastrointestinal physiology. *Veterinary Clinics of North America: Exotic Animal Practice*, **6**, 139–153.

Delk, K.W., Eshar, D., Garcia, E. and Harkin, K. (2014) Diagnosis and treatment of congestive heart failure secondary to dilated cardiomyopathy in a hedgehog. *Journal of Small Animal Practice*, **55**(3), 174–177.

DiGiacomo, R.F. and Mare, C.J. (1994) Viral diseases. *In:* Manning PJ, Ringler DH *&* Newcomer CE, *eds.* The Biology of the Laboratory Rabbit. *2nd ed.* San Diego: Academic Press pp171–204.

DiGiulio, D.B. and Eckburg, P.B. (2004) Human monkeypox: an emerging zoonosis. *Lancet Infectious Diseases*, **4**, 15–25.

Duclos, L.M. and Richardson, D.J. (2000) *Hymenolepis nana* in pet store rodents. *Comparative Parasitology*, **67**, 197–201.

Florizoone, K. (2005) Thymoma-associated exfoliative dermatitis in a rabbit. *Veterinary Dermatology*, **16**, 281–284.

Florizoone, K., van der Luer, R. and van den Ingh, T. (2007) Symmetrical alopecia, scaling and hepatitis in a rabbit. *Veterinary Dermatology*, **18**, 161–164.

Forsythe, S.J. and Parker, D.S. (1985) Nitrogen metabolism by the microbial flora of the rabbit caecum. *Journal of Applied Bacteriology*, **58**, 363–369.

Fox, R.R., Meier, H., Crary, D.D. *et al.* (1970) Lymphosarcoma in the rabbit: genetics and pathology. *Journal of the National Cancer Institute*, **45**, 719–729.

Garner, M.M., Raymond, J.T., Toshkov, I. and Tennant, B.C. (2004) Hepatocellular carcinoma in black-tailed prairie dogs (*Cynomys ludovicianus*): tumor morphology and immunohistochemistry for hepadnavirus core and surface antigens. *Veterinary Pathology*, **41**(4), 353–361. doi: 10.1354/vp.41-4-353.

Gilmore, S.A. (2005) Spinal nerve root degeneration in aging laboratory rats: a light microscopic study. *Anatomical Record*, **174**(2), 251–257.

Girling, S.J., Pizzi, R., Cox, A. and Beard, P. (2011) Fatal cowpox infection in two squirrel monkeys (*Saimiri sciureus*). *Veterinary Record*, **169**(6), 156.

Green, P.W., Fox, R.R. and Sokoloff, L. (1984) Spontaneous degenerative spinal disease in the laboratory rabbit. *Journal of Orthopaedic Research*, **2**, 161–168.

Halck, M.L., Schoemaker, N.J. and van Zeeland, Y.R.A. (2023) Ferret dermatology. *Veterinary Clinics of North America: Exotic Animal Practice*, **26**, 359–382.

Harcourt-Brown, F.M. and Holloway, H.K.R. (2003) *Encephalitozoon cuniculi* in pet rabbits. *Veterinary Record*, **152**, 427–431.

Harrison, T.M. and Kitchell, B.E. (2017) Principles and applications of medical oncology in exotic animals. *Veterinary Clinics of North America Exotic Animal Practice*, **20**(1), 209–234.

Hawkins, M.G. and Bishop, C.R. (2012) Disease problems of guinea pigs. In: *Ferrets, Rabbits and Rodents: Clinical Medicine and Surgery* (eds K.E. Quesenberry & J.W. Carpenter), 3rd edn, pp. 295–310. W.B. Saunders, Philadelphia, St Louis.

Hillyer, E.V., Quesenberry, K.E. and Donnelly, T.M. (1997) Biology, husbandry and clinical techniques. In: *Ferrets, Rabbits and Rodents: Clinical Medicine and Surgery* (eds E.V. Hillyer & K.E. Quesenberry), pp. 243–259. W.B. Saunders, Philadelphia, PA.

Huybens, N., Houeix, J., Szalo, M. *et al.* (2008) Is Epizootic Rabbit Enteropathy (ERE) a Bacterial Disease? In: *Proceedings of the 9th World Rabbit Congress*, pp. 971–975. Verona, Italy.

Huynh, M., Pingret, J.L. and Nicolier, A. (2014) Disseminated *Mycobacterium genavense* infection in a chinchilla (*Chinchilla lanigera*). *Journal of Comparative Pathology*, **151**, 122–125.

Jean-Blain, C. and Durix, A. (1985) Effects of dietary lipid level on ketonemia and other plasma parameters related to glucose and fatty acid metabolism in the rabbit during fasting. *Reproduction Nutrition Developpement*, **25**, 345–354.

Jekl, V. (2006) Demodicosis in nine prairie dogs (*Cynomys ludovicianus*). *Veterinary Dermatology*, **17**(4), 2803.

Jenkins, J.R. (2000) Ferret metabolic testing. In: *Laboratory Medicine: Avian and Exotic Pets* (ed. A.M. Fudge), pp. 305–309. WB Saunders, Philadelphia, PA.

Johnson, D.H. (2020) Geriatric hedgehogs. *Veterinary Clinics of North America: Exotic Animal Practice*, **23**, 615–637.

Johnson-Delaney, C. (2010) Marsupials. In: *Manual of Exotic Pets* (eds A. Meredith & C. Johnson-Delaney), 5th edn, pp. 103–126. BSAVA, Quedgeley, UK.

Koizumi, I. and Kondo, H. (2019) Clinical management and outcome of four-toed hedgehogs (*Atelerix albiventris*) with histiocytic sarcoma. *Journal of Veterinary Medical Science*, **81**(4), 545–550.

Kondo, H., Mitani, S., Suzuki, S. and Shibuya, H. (2018) Squamous cell carcinomas with pulmonary metastasis and endocardiosis in the Siberian chipmunk (*Eutamias sibiricus*): two necropsy cases. *Journal of Zoo and Wildlife Medicine*, **49**(3), 820–823. doi: 10.1638/2018-0023.1.

Künzel, F., Gruber, A., Tichy, A. *et al.* (2008) Clinical symptoms and diagnosis of encephalitozoonosis in pet rabbits. *Veterinary Parasitology*, **151**, 115–124.

Lafontan, M. and Agid, R. (1979) An extra-adrenal action of adrenocorticotrophin: physiological induction of lipolysis by secretion of adrenocorticotrophin in obese rabbits. *Journal of Endocrinology*, **81**, 281–290.

Leary, S.L., Manning, P.J. and Anderson, L.C. (1984) Experimental and naturally occurring gastric foreign bodies in laboratory rabbits. *Laboratory Animal Science*, **34**(1), 58–61.

Lennox, A. (2021) Respiratory disorders of ferrets. *Veterinary Clinics of North America: Exotic Animal Practice*, **24**, 483–493.

Li, X., Fox, J.G. and Padrid, P.A. (1998) Neoplastic diseases in ferrets: 574 cases (1968–1997). *Journal of the American Veterinary Medical Association*, **212**(9), 1402–1406.

Lindemann, D.M., Eshar, D., Schumacher, L.L. *et al.* (2015) Pyogranulomatous panophthalmitis with systemic coronavirus in a domestic ferret (*Mustela putorius furo*). *Veterinary Ophthalmology*, **19**(2), 167–171. doi: 10.1111/vop.12274.

Lowe, J.A. (2020) Pet rabbit feeding and nutrition. In: *The Nutrition of the Rabbit* (eds C. de Blas & J. Wiseman), 3rd edn, pp. 317–366. CABI Publishing, Oxfordshire, UK.

Malek, H.A. and Shata, A. (2014) Effect of a high dose of vitamin D on a rabbit model of atherosclerosis. *International Journal of Immunopathology and Pharmacology*, **27**(2), 195–201. doi: 10.1177/039463201402700206.

Mancinelli, E., Shaw, D.J. and Meredith, A.L. (2012) γ-Glutamyl-transferase (GGT) activity in the urine of clinically healthy domestic rabbits (*Oryctolagus cuniculis*). *Veterinary Record*, **171**, 475.

Mancinelli, E., Keeble, E., Richardson, J. and Headley, J. (2014) Husbandry risk factors associated with hock pododermatitis in UK pet rabbits (*Oryctolagus cuniculus*). *Veterinary Record*, **174**, 429.

McLaughlin, R.M. and Fish, R.E. (1994) Clinical biochemistry and haematology. In: *The Biology of the Laboratory Rabbit* (eds P.J. Manning, D.H. Ringler & C.E. Newcomer), 2nd edn, pp. 111–124. Academic Press, London.

Molenaar, R.J., Vremen, S., Hakze-ven der Honing, R.W., Zwart, R., de Rond, J., Weesendorp, E., Smit, L.A.M., Koopmans, M., Bouwstra, R., Stegeman, A. and van der Poel, W.H.M. (2020) Clinical and pathological findings in SARS-CoV-2 disease outbreaks in farmed mink (*Neovison vison*). *Veterinary Pathology*. 57(5):653–657. doi: 10.1177/0300985820943535.

Muller, K. and Mancinelli, E. (2022) Cardiology in rabbits and rodents: common cardiac diseases, therapeutic options, and limitations. *Veterinary Clinics of North America: Exotic Animal Practice*, **25**, 525–540.

Needle, D.B., Selig, M.K., Jackson, K.A. *et al.* (2019) Fatal bronchopneumonia caused by skunk adenovirus 1 in an African pygmy hedgehog. *Journal of Veterinary Diagnostic Investigation*, **31**(1), 103–106.

Okerman, L. (1994) Inherited conditions and congenital deformities. In: *Diseases of Domestic Rabbits*, 2nd edn, pp. 109–112. Blackwell, Oxford.

Okumura, N., Kondo, H., Suzuki, S. and Shibuya, H. (2022) Thymoma originating from the cervical component of the thymus in a degu. *Journal of Veterinary Diagnostic Investigation*, **34**(1), 126–129. doi: 10.1177/10406387211045643.

Osterrieder, N., Bertzbach, L.D., Dietert, K. *et al.* (2020) Age-dependent progression of SARS-CoV-2 infection in Syrian hamsters. *Viruses*, **12**(7), 779. doi: http://doi.org/10.3390/v12070779.

Pacheco, R. (2020) Cystine urolithiasis in ferrets. *Veterinary Clinics of North America: Exotic Animal Practice*, **23**, 309–319.

Ramsell, K.D. and Garner, M.M. (2010) Disseminated idiopathic myofasciitis in ferrets. *Veterinary Clinics of North America: Exotic Animal Practice*, **13**(3), 561–576.

Raymond, J.T. and Garner, M.M. (2001) Spontaneous tumors in captive African hedgehogs (*Atelerix albiventris*): a retrospective study. *Journal of Comparative Pathology*, **124**, 128–133.

Reusch, B., Murray, J.K., Papasouliotis, K. and Redrobe, S.P. (2009) Urinary protein creatinine ratio in rabbits in relation to their serological status to *Encephalitozoon cuniculi*. *Veterinary Record*, **164**, 293–295.

Richard, M., Kok, A., de Meulder, D. *et al.* (2020) SARS-CoV-2 is transmitted via contact and via the air between ferrets. *Nature Communications*, **11**(1), 3496. doi: 10.1038/s41467-020-17367-2.

Rivera, D.S., Inestrosa, N.C. and Bozinovic, F. (2016) On cognitive ecology and the environmental factors that promote Alzheimer disease: lessons from *Octodon degus* (Rodentia: Octodontidae). *Biological Research*, **20**(49), 10. doi: 10.1186/s40659-016-0074-7.

Rogers, K. and Chrisp, C. (1998) Lipoma in the mediastinum of a prairie dog (*Cynomys ludovicianus*). *Contemporary Topics in Laboratory Animal Science*, **37**(1), 74–76.

Sanchez, J.N., Summa, N.M.E., Visser, L.C. *et al.* (2019) Ventricular septal defect and congestive heart failure in a common degu (*Octodon degus*). *Journal of Exotic Pet Medicine*, **31**, 32–35.

Sarvi, J. and Esher, D. (2023) Rodent dermatology. *Veterinary Clinics of North America: Exotic Animal Practice*, **26**, 383–408.

Schmidt, R.E. and Reavill, D.R. (2007) Cardiovascular disease in hamsters: review and retrospective study. *Journal of Exotic Pet Medicine*, **16**, 49–51.

Schoemaker, N.J. (2009) Endocrine and neoplastic diseases. In: *Manual of Ferrets and Rodents* (eds E. Keeble & A. Meredith), pp. 320–329. BSAVA, Quedgeley, UK.

Schoemaker, N.J., Kuijten, A.M. and Galac, S. (2008) Luteinizing hormone-dependent Cushing's syndrome in a pet ferret (*Mustela putorius furo*). *Domestic Animal Endocrinology*, **34**, 278–283.

Shi, F., Petroff, B.K., Herath, C.B. *et al.* (2002) Serous cysts are a benign component of the cyclic ovary in the guinea pig with an incidence dependent upon inhibin bioactivity. *Journal of Veterinary Medical Science*, **64**, 129–135.

Spear, G.S., Caple, M.V. and Sutherland, L.R. (1984) The pancreas in the degu. *Experimental Molecular Pathology*, **40**, 295–310.

Svara, T., Gombac, M., Poli, A. *et al.* (2020) Spontaneous tumors and non-neoplastic proliferative lesions in pet degus (*Octodon degus*). *Veterinary Science*, **7**(1), 32. doi: 10.3390/vetsci7010032.

Tan, Z., Garduno, B.M., Aburto, P.F. *et al.* (2022) Cognitively impaired aged *Octodon degus* recapitulate major neuropathological features of sporadic Alzheimer's disease. *Acta Neuropathologica Communications*, **10**, 182. doi: 10.1186/s40478-022-01481-x.

Thas, I. and Garner, M.M. (2012) A retrospective study of tumours in black-tailed prairie dogs (*Cynomys ludovicianus*) submitted to a zoological pathology service. *Journal of Comparative Pathology*, **157**, 368–375.

Tokashiki, E.Y., Rahal, S.C., Melchert, A. *et al.* (2019) Retrospective study of conditions grouped by body systems in pet rabbits. *Journal of Exotic Pet Medicine*, **29**, 207–211.

Ueda, K., Ueda, A. and Ozaki, K. (2019) Basal cell adenoma of the salivary gland and possible recurrence as basal cell adenocarcinoma in a black-tailed prairie dog (*Cynomys ludovicianus*). *Journal of Comparative Pathology*, **168**, 13–17. doi: 10.1016/j.jcpa.2019.02.004.

Wack, R. (2000) Pemphigus foliaceus in an African hedgehog. *Proceedings of the North American Veterinary Conference*, p. 1023.

Weisbroth, S.H. (1994) Neoplastic diseases. In: *The Biology of the Laboratory Rabbit* (eds P.J. Manning, D.H. Ringler & C.E. Newcomer), 2nd edn, pp. 259–292. Academic Press, New York.

Weisbroth, S., Flatt, R.E. and Kraus, A.L. (1974) Anatomy, physiology and biochemistry of the rabbit. In: *The Biology of the Laboratory Rabbit* (eds Manning *et al.*), 2nd edn. Academic Press, London p. 65.

White, S.D., Linder, K.E., Schultheiss, P. *et al.* (2000) Sebaceous adenitis in four domestic rabbits (*Oryctolagus cuniculus*). *Veterinary Dermatology*, **11**, 53–60.

Williams, B.H. and Weis, C.A. (2003) Ferret neoplasia. In: *Ferrets, Rabbits and Rodents: Clinical Medicine* (eds K.E. Quesenberry & J.W. Carpenter), 2nd edn, pp. 91–106. WB Saunders, St Louis.

Wright, T.L., Eshar, D., Carpenter, J.W. *et al.* (2017) Suspected Hepadnavirus association with a hepatocellular carcinoma in a black-tailed prairie dog (*Cynomys ludovicianus*). *Journal of Comparative Pathology*, **157**(4), 284–290. doi: 10.1016/j.jcpa.2017.09.004.

Wuthe, H.H. and Aleksic, S. (1992) *Yersinia enterocolitica* serovar 1,2a,3 biovar-3 in chinchillas. *Zentralblatt fur Bakteriologie*, **277**, 403–405.

Zimmerman, T.E., Giddens, W.E., DiGiacomo, R.F. and Ladiges, W.C. (1990) Soft tissue mineralization in rabbits fed a diet containing excess vitamin D. *Laboratory Animal Science*, **40**, 212–215.

Chapter 6 An Overview of Small Mammal Therapeutics

FLUID THERAPY

Maintenance requirements

Insensible fluid loss (that lost through sweat and the respiratory and digestive tracts) is always difficult to assess but in small mammals there is little water lost as sweat, as rodents and lagomorphs have little or no sweat glands, and most do not pant either. However, increased metabolic rates, and their small size, do lead to a large lung surface area in relation to volume and the loss of large amounts of fluids during normal respiration. In addition, glomerular filtration rates are generally higher than those of domestic dogs and cats. This makes their daily maintenance fluid requirement per kilogram nearly double those seen in larger mammals. Some values are given in Table 6.1.

The effect of disease on fluid requirements

Respiratory disease is common in small mammals, especially rabbits, rats and mice. In these animals often chronic levels of lung infection are present, with increased respiratory secretions being the result. Additional fluid loss can therefore be appreciable via this route.

Individuals suffering from diarrhoea will of course experience fluid loss and often metabolic acidosis due to the prolonged loss of bicarbonate ions.

Another route of fluid and electrolyte loss is through skin disease. Rabbits (in particular, those kept in wet or unsanitary conditions) will contract skin infections from environmental bacterial organisms such as *Pseudomonas* spp. These produce lesions that resemble chemical or thermal burns, and leave large areas of weeping, exudative skin causing further fluid loss.

Post-surgical fluid requirements

Surgery may lead to intra-surgical haemorrhaging, necessitating vascular support with isotonic crystalloids or, in more serious blood losses (>10%), colloidal fluids or even blood transfusions. Even if surgery is relatively bloodless, there are inevitable losses via the respiratory route due to the drying nature of the oxygen and anaesthetic gases commonly used.

In addition, many patients are not able or do not want to drink immediately after surgery. Some forms of surgery, such as incisor extraction in rabbits suffering from malocclusion, will lead to inappetence for a period of time. Dehydration may result, as rabbits gain a significant amount of their fluid intake from their diet if they have access to fresh grass, leafy greens and other vegetables.

Electrolyte balance

Electrolyte balance support/management can be necessary in cases of chronic diarrhoea such as in coccidiosis in rabbits or wet tail in hamsters. The main electrolyte losses are bicarbonate and potassium, leading to metabolic acidosis and sodium loss due to organ (usually kidney) disease.

Small herbivores, particularly rabbits, rarely vomit and so electrolyte loss by that route is unlikely to occur. Ferrets can readily vomit particularly with diseases such as stomach ulceration as a result of foreign bodies or bacteria such as *Helicobacter mustelae*. In these cases, metabolic alkalosis may result.

Hyponatraemia (low blood sodium) with a hypotonic plasma represents a true hyponatraemia which requires sodium supplementation to avert cerebral oedema and neurological disease. Causes of true hyponatraemia include acute or chronic renal failure and polydipsia.

Pseudohyponatraemia (hypertonic or isotonic) should not be treated with sodium therapy but treatment directed towards the underlying causative disease. In most animals, pseudohyponatraemia is associated with three main clinical conditions – congestive heart failure, severe liver disease and the nephrotic syndrome – but can also occur in conditions associated with hyperlipidaemia or severe hyperproteinaemia.

Potassium levels may be elevated where haemolysis occurs during sampling, in rhabdomyolysis or where renal failure or urinary obstruction is seen. It is also worth noting that many point-of-care analysers give higher readings for potassium than other biochemistry machines. Hypokalaemia is seen during prolonged diarrhoea, intestinal disease, chronic renal failure, overperfusion with intravenous fluids and where loop diuretics are used.

Fluid types used in small mammal practice

Lactated Ringer's/Hartmann's

Lactated Ringer's solution is useful as a general-purpose rehydration and maintenance fluid. It is particularly helpful for small mammals suffering from metabolic acidosis, such as those with diarrhoea or gut motility issues, but can also be used for fluid therapy after routine surgical procedures.

Glucose/saline combinations

Glucose/saline combinations are useful for small mammals, as they may have been through periods of anorexia prior to treatment, and therefore may well be borderline hypoglycaemic. Glucose/saline

Veterinary Nursing of Exotic Pets and Wildlife, Third Edition. Simon J. Girling.

Table 6.1 Maintenance fluid values for selected small mammals.

Species	Fluid maintenance values (mL/kg per day)
Rabbit	80–100
Guinea pig	100
Chinchilla	100
Other rodent	90–100
Sugar glider	80–100
African pygmy hedgehog	80–100
Ferret	75–100

combinations are also useful for cases of urethral obstruction, such as ferret urolithiasis where a low-potassium but glucose-containing fluid is preferred to counteract the effects of hyperkalaemia.

Hypertonic saline

Although more commonly used in animals in excess of 100 kg body weight, hypertonic saline (7.2% or 7.3%) may be used in small mammals with acute hypovolaemia. When administered intravenously or intraosseously it works by rapidly drawing fluid from the cellular and pericellular space into the circulation to support central venous pressure. See Chapter 8 for further details of its use. It cannot be administered by other routes.

Protein amino acid/B vitamin supplements

Protein and vitamin supplements are useful for nutritional support (e.g. Duphalyte® [Zoetis] at 1 mL/kg per day). These supplements are particularly good in cases where the patient is malnourished or has been suffering from a protein-losing enteropathy or nephropathy. It is also a useful supplement for patients with hepatic disease or severe exudative skin diseases.

Colloidal fluids

Colloids are used when a serious loss of blood occurs in order to support central blood pressure. They can therefore only be used intravenously or intraosseously. Colloids are often a temporary measure, their effects lasting a few hours before they leak out of the vascular system. They can help buy time whilst the cause of hypovolaemia is corrected or a blood donor found. Some of the larger molecule colloids such as hydroxyethyl starch (Hetastarch®) may survive in the bloodstream for 12–24 hours and so may be preferable. Colloids should not be used where acute bleeding or a blood clotting disorder, congestive heart failure or severe kidney disease is present.

Blood transfusions

If the packed cell volume (PCV) drops below 20%, blood transfusions may be required. They must be same species-to-species transfers (i.e. rat to rat, guinea pig to guinea pig). The donor should have a physical health check and routine blood biochemistry and a PCV to ensure it is healthy. A healthy donor may have 1% of their body weight in blood removed for donation. The sample is best taken directly into citrate acid dextrose at a ratio of 1 mL of anticoagulant to 5–6 mL of blood. It is possible in an emergency to instead collect blood into a pre-heparinised syringe but this increases the chances of blood clot formation. Ideally, a blood-giving set should be used to administer the blood to the recipient with a microfilter to remove clots. The administration should be slow, giving 1 mL over a period of 5–6 minutes to ensure no transfusion reactions occur. Therefore sedation and a syringe driver are required. Very little information is currently available about cross-matching blood groups of small mammals, although ferrets, it seems, do not have detectable groups. A very simple 'in-house' cross-matching procedure can be carried out by placing two drops of plasma from the recipient's blood onto a glass microscope slide with a drop of the donor's whole blood and looking for any clots that may form. The absence of macroclots forming at room temperature over 60 seconds suggests (although clearly does not entirely guarantee) compatibility. Intraosseous blood donations may be made if vascular access is not possible. Calculations for volumes of blood required to be collected from the donor are based on those available for cats, that is

$$\text{Vol. of donor blood required}(\text{mL}) = 60 \times \text{BW}(\text{kg}) \times \frac{\text{Desired change in PCV}}{\text{PCV of transfused blood}}$$

where BW is body weight of the recipient (in kilograms).

Oral fluids and electrolytes

Oral fluids may be used in small mammal practice for those patients experiencing mild dehydration, and for home administration where the gastrointestinal tract is functioning normally. The most useful products also contain probiotics/prebiotics which can aid normal digestive function.

Calculation of fluid requirements

Fluid within food is difficult to take into consideration when calculating fluid requirements and therefore it is safer to assume that the debilitated small mammal will not be eating enough for it to matter. Once it is appreciated that maintenance for most small mammals is double that required for the average cat or dog, then deficits may be calculated in a similar manner. Assume that 1% dehydration equates with needing to supply 10 mL/kg fluid replacement, in addition to maintenance requirements. Maintenance requirements are of course daily, and the deficit only needs to be replaced once (although volumes may be split over a few days; see below).

An estimate of the percentage of dehydration of the patient is as follows:

- 3–5% dehydrated: increased thirst, slight lethargy, tacky mucous membranes
- 7–10% dehydrated: increased thirst, anorexia, dullness, tenting of the skin and slow return to normal, dry mucous membranes, dull corneas
- 10–15% dehydrated: dull to comatose, skin remains tented after pinching, desiccating mucous membranes.

Alternatively, if a blood sample may be obtained, a 1% increase in PCV, associated with an increase in total proteins, may be assumed to equate to 10 mL/kg fluid deficit (Table 6.2).

These deficits may be large and difficult to replenish rapidly. Indeed, it may be dangerous to overload the patient's system, particularly

Table 6.2 Comparison of normal PCV and total proteins for selected small mammals.

Species	PCV range (L/L)	Total protein (g/L)
Rabbit	0.36–0.48	54–75
Guinea pig	0.37–0.48	46–62
Chinchilla	0.32–0.46	50–60
Rat	0.36–0.48	56–76
Mouse	0.39–0.49	35–72
Gerbil	0.43–0.49	43–85
Hamster[a]	0.36–0.55	45–75
Sugar glider	0.45–0.53	51–61
Virginia opossum	0.34–0.47	56–78
African pygmy hedgehog	0.35–0.47	51–68
Ferret	0.44–0.60	51–74

[a] The range given for hamsters is an average of Syrian and Russian hamster values.

intravenously or intraosseously, with these fluid levels all in one day. Therefore, the following protocol is worth considering to ensure fluid overload, renal shutdown and pulmonary oedema are avoided.

- Day 1: maintenance fluid levels +50% of calculated dehydration factor
- Day 2: maintenance fluid levels +50% of calculated dehydration factor
- Day 3: maintenance fluid levels.

If the dehydration levels are so severe that volumes are still too large to give at any one time, it may be necessary to take 72 hours rather than 48 hours to replace the calculated deficit.

In addition, in those species such as ferrets which can vomit, the fluid lost in vomitus expelled should be considered, assuming 2 mL/kg per vomit.

In other species such as the small herbivores, where vomiting is rarely seen, it is much more difficult to make estimations, although fluid losses through profuse diarrhoea may approach 100–150 mL/kg per day.

Equipment for fluid administration

Catheters

The blood vessels available for intravenous medication are typically 30–50% smaller than their cat and dog counterparts. Small paediatric butterfly catheters may be used. It is advisable to flush the catheter with heparinised saline, prior to use, to prevent clotting once inserted as many sick small mammals have hypercoagulable blood. Catheters of 25–27 gauge are recommended and are suitable for venous access for rabbits, guinea pigs, chinchillas and ferrets. Occasionally a 28- or 29-gauge catheter may be needed to catheterise a lateral tail vein in a rat or mouse, although 27-gauge catheters often suffice.

Hypodermic or spinal needles

Hypodermic needles are useful for the administration of intraosseous, intraperitoneal and subcutaneous fluids. The intraosseous route may be the only method of giving central venous support in very small patients, or patients where vascular collapse is occurring. The proximal femur, tibia or humerus may be used. Entry can be gained by using hypodermic or spinal needles. Spinal needles may be preferable because they have a central stylet to prevent clogging of the needle lumen with bone fragments after insertion. Spinal needles of 23–25 gauge are generally suitable.

Hypodermic needles may be used for the same purpose, although the risks of blockage are higher. Hypodermic needles may also be used for the administration of intraperitoneal and subcutaneous fluids. Generally, 23–25 gauge hypodermic needles are sufficient for the task.

Nasogastric/oesophageal tubes

Nasogastric tubes are sometimes used in small mammals to provide nutritional support in as stress-free a manner as possible although some prefer naso-oesophageal tubes in species such as rabbits to avoid acid reflux and significant oesophagitis. They are useful as a route for fluid administration assuming the gastrointestinal tract is working normally. It should be noted, though, that in severely dehydrated individuals, there is no way that all of the fluid deficit may be replaced via this route alone. This route is therefore restricted for use in facilitating fluid replacement and is used mainly for nutritional support and rehydrating the gut microflora.

Syringe drivers

For continuous fluid administration, as is required for intravenous and intraosseous fluid administration, syringe drivers are recommended. Their advantage is that small volumes may be administered accurately. An error of 1–2 mL in some of the species dealt with over an hour could be equivalent to an overperfusion of 50–100%! In addition, it is almost impossible to keep gravity-fed drip sets running at these low rates.

Intravenous drip tubing

Fine drip tubing is available for attachment to syringes and syringe-driver units. It is useful if these are luer locking, as this enhances safety and prevents disconnection when the patient moves. It may be necessary to purchase a sheath, such as is available for protecting household electrical cables, to cover drip tubing, as most of the small herbivores are experts at removing or chewing through plastic drip tubing.

Elizabethan collars

It may be necessary to place some of the small herbivores into an Elizabethan-style collar as they are the world's greatest chewers. These can be purchased as cage bird collars and adapted to fit even the smallest of rodents. However, care should be taken in species such as rabbits that exhibit caecotrophy as many will stop this because of the collar. Indeed, many may not eat well and so may require assisted feeding.

Routes of fluid administration

These routes have their advantages and disadvantages, given in Table 6.3.

Table 6.3 The advantages and disadvantages of various fluid therapy routes in small mammals.

Route	Advantages	Disadvantages
Oral	Reduced stress Well accepted Physiological route Minimal tissue trauma Rehydration of gut flora	May increase stress in guinea pigs Risk of aspiration pneumonia in some Not useful in cases of gut disease Slow rates of rehydration Maximum volume is 10 mL/kg (in reality 5 mL/kg is preferred)
Subcutaneous	Large volumes may be given reducing dosing frequency Minimal risk of organ puncture	Guinea pigs react badly to scruff injections and fur slip is common in chinchillas Slow rehydration time May impede respiration due to pressure on chest wall and discomfort Hypotonic or isotonic crystalloid fluids only
Intraperitoneal	Large volumes may be given at one time Uptake faster than subcutaneous if mild dehydration is present Minimal discomfort	Risk of organ puncture Stressful positioning (dorsal recumbency to avoid damaging gastrointestinal tract) Pressure on diaphragm may increase; respiratory effort needed Isotonic or hypotonic crystalloids only and fluids must not contain glucose as this can be irritant and increase the likelihood of peritonitis
Intravenous	Rapid central venous support May be used for continuous perfusion Can be used for colloidal fluids, hypertonic saline, dextrose/glucose and blood transfusions/replacers	Minimal peripheral access in some species (e.g. hamsters, gerbils) Increased vessel fragility due to small patient size Requires increased levels of operator skill
Intraosseous	Rapid support of the central venous system Useful in collapsed and very small patients where vascular access is difficult May still be used for blood transfusions/ replacers Minimal risk of organ damage (puncture)	Not useful in fragile bones or metabolic bone disease Not useful in bone fractures or osteomyelitis Increased risk of infection (osteomyelitis) Painful procedure requiring sedation/analgesia Continuous perfusion required (syringe drivers) otherwise maximum boluses are small (0.25–0.5 mL for myomorph rodents and sugar gliders, 1–2 mL for hystricomorph rodents, prairie dogs and hedgehogs, 2–3 mL for rabbits, Virginia opossums and ferrets)

Oral

Rabbit

The oral route is not good for seriously debilitated rabbits, but it is useful for those with naso-oesophageal feeding tubes in place. It may also be useful for mild cases of dehydration where owners wish to home treat their pet. This route is restricted to small volumes, with a maximum of 10 mL/kg administered at any one time. I prefer a naso-oesophageal tube to a nasogastric to avoid oesophagitis. If a nasogastric tube is inserted, antacids such as omeprazole or ranitidine should be used.

Rat, mouse, gerbil, hamster, chipmunk and prairie dog

Gavage (stomach) tubes or avian straight crop tubes can be used to place fluids directly into the rodent oesophagus. The rodent needs to be firmly scruffed to adequately restrain it with the head and oesophagus in a straight line. This method is often stressful but the alternative is to syringe fluids into the mouth, which may not work as rodents can close off the back of the mouth with their cheek folds. Maximum volumes that can be given via the oral route in rodents vary from 5 to 10 mL/kg. Naso-oesophageal/gastric tubes are not a viable option in rodents due to their small size.

Guinea pig, degu and chinchilla

Naso-oesophageal tubes may be placed and doses of 10 mL/kg may be administered at any one time. Guinea pigs and chinchillas are more likely to regurgitate than rabbits, especially when debilitated, so care is needed.

Marsupial

Gavage (stomach) tubes or avian straight crop tubes can be used to place fluids directly into the marsupial oesophagus. The marsupial needs to be firmly scruffed to adequately restrain it and to keep the head and oesophagus in a straight line. Alternatively, fluids may be drip fed from a syringe or teaspoon into the lip sulcus either side of the mouth and lapped up from there.

African pygmy hedgehog

The oral route is not particularly useful in the majority of hedgehogs due to their tendency to roll up into a ball when stressed.

Ferret

Naso-oesophageal tubes are not well tolerated in ferrets, but many will accept sweet-tasting oral electrolyte solutions from a syringe. Ferrets, especially when debilitated, can regurgitate, so care is needed.

Subcutaneous

The advantages and disadvantages of this method are given in Table 6.3.

Rabbit

The scruff or lateral thorax make ideal sites. This is a good technique to use for postoperative administration of fluids in routine surgical procedures such as surgical neutering. It is possible to give a maximum of 30–60 mL split into two or more sites at one time depending on the size of rabbit.

Rat, mouse, gerbil, hamster, chipmunk and prairie dog

The scruff area is easily utilised for volumes of 3–4 mL of fluids for smaller rodents and up to 10 mL at any one time for rats and 12–15 mL for prairie dogs. The use of a 25-gauge needle is recommended.

Guinea pig, degu and chinchilla

This is an easily used route for postoperative fluids and mild dehydration in these species. The scruff area and lateral thorax are preferred sites (see Figure 6.1). The scruff may however be painful for guinea pigs as it is a site of brown fat deposition and well innervated and so should be avoided in this species. Doses of 25–30 mL may be given at one time, preferably at three or more sites in chinchillas and guinea pigs. Degus, being smaller, tend to have maximum volume of 8–10 mL. Fur slip is a problem in chinchillas.

Marsupial

This is an easily used route for postoperative fluids and mild dehydration in these species. The scruff area and lateral thorax are preferred sites. Volumes of 3-4 mL in sugar gliders and 15–20 mL in adult Virginia opossums may be administered.

African pygmy hedgehog

The 'skirt' or orbicularis area on the edge of the spiny coat may be used for subcutaneous injections, with volumes of 7–8 mL being possible.

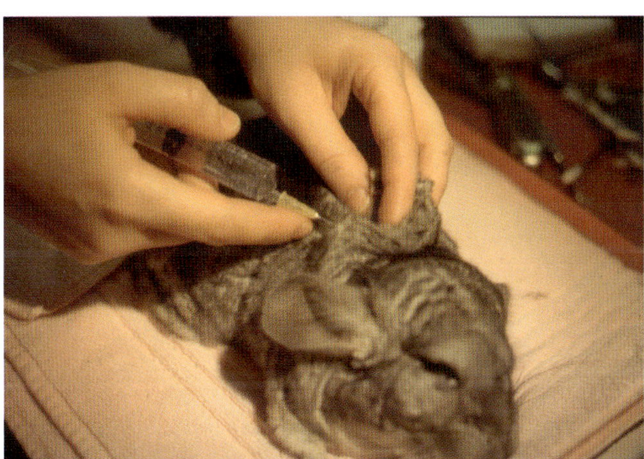

Figure 6.1 Subcutaneous fluids being administered in the scruff region in a chinchilla postoperatively.

Ferret

Volumes of 15–20 mL may be given in two or more sites over the scruff.

Intraperitoneal

The advantages and disadvantages of the intraperitoneal route in small mammals are given in Table 6.3.

Rabbit

The rabbit is placed in dorsal recumbency to allow the gut contents to fall away from the injection zone. The needle is inserted in the lower right quadrant of the ventral abdomen, just through the abdominal wall and the syringe plunger drawn back to ensure that no puncture of the bladder or gut has occurred (see Figure 6.2). A maximum volume of 20–30 mL may be given at one time depending on the size of the rabbit. If cardiovascular or respiratory disease is present then this route may worsen the situation by placing greater pressure on the diaphragm and abdominal vasculature. If positioned correctly, there should be no resistance to injection.

Rat, mouse, gerbil, hamster, chipmunk and prairie dog

The positioning and administration site for rodents is as for rabbits. The needle should be 25 gauge or smaller and maximal volumes of 1–4 mL in smaller rodents, up to 10 mL in large rats and 15 mL in prairie dogs, may be given.

Guinea pig, degu and chinchilla

Similar principles apply for this route as for rabbits and other rodents. Doses of 15–20 mL may be given in guinea pigs and

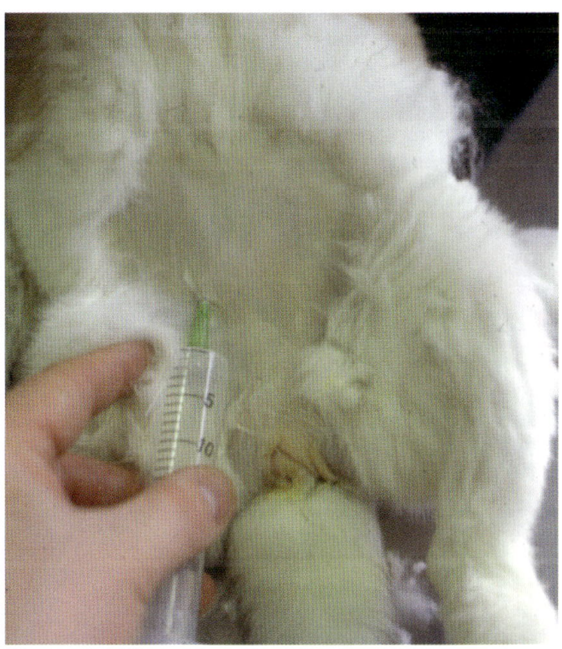

Figure 6.2 Intraperitoneal fluids administered to a rabbit showing positioning required for safe administration to avoid organ and intestinal puncture.

chinchillas and 7–8 mL in degus. This is a good route for mild to moderately dehydrated patients, as intravenous fluids are not so well tolerated.

Marsupial

Similar principles apply for this route as for rabbits and rodents. Doses of 2–4 mL in sugar gliders and 15–20 mL in Virginia opossums may be given.

African pygmy hedgehog

This site is rarely available unless the hedgehog is anaesthetised and so has minimal usefulness in this species.

Ferret

The technique is as for rabbits. Restraint may be difficult in the conscious patient limiting its usefulness. Maximum volumes are 20–25 mL.

Intravenous

The advantages and disadvantages of intravenous fluid therapy in small mammals are given in Table 6.3.

Rabbit

The blood vessel that is best tolerated is the lateral ear vein. The technique for using it is described below.

Lateral ear vein: The following technique should be used (see Figure 6.3):

1. The area should be shaved and surgically prepared. Warm the ear (e.g. with a small hot water bottle/hot hands) and/or apply local anaesthetic cream to dilate the vessel.
2. Use the lateral ear vein. Do not be tempted to use the apparently larger vessel that runs in the midline of the pinna as this is the central ear artery. Catheterisation of this vessel can be performed in an emergency where no other vascular access is available but it may lead to thrombosis followed by ear tip necrosis later.
3. Use a 25–27 gauge butterfly catheter, pre-heparinised. Once in place, tape it in securely and re-flush. Attach the intravenous drip tubing or catheter bung to the end of the butterfly catheter.
4. Fit the rabbit with an Elizabethan collar or apply an intravenous drip guard to the intravenous tubing to prevent chewing, and attach this to the syringe driver. It is possible to tape the butterfly catheter to the back of the rabbit's head if using intermittent intravenous boluses, but it is important to ensure the catheter is regularly flushed with heparinised saline.

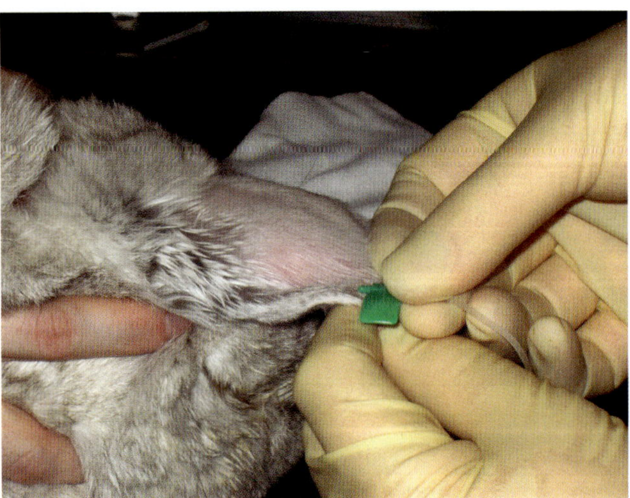

Figure 6.3 Catheterisation of the lateral ear vein in a rabbit using a butterfly catheter.

Cephalic vein: This may be used as for the cat and dog, although this vein may be split in some rabbits. A 25–27 gauge over-the-needle or butterfly catheter may be used for access and taped in as for cats and dogs.

Saphenous vein: For this, it is better to use a 25–27 gauge butterfly catheter as it is relatively fragile. It runs over the lateral aspect of the hock (see Figure 6.4).

All of these routes can be used for intravenous boluses of up to 10 mL for larger rabbits and 5 mL for smaller dwarf breeds; but for continuous therapy, a syringe driver is required.

Rat, mouse, gerbil, hamster, chipmunk and prairie dog

The intravenous route in hamsters and gerbils is extremely difficult, as they have few peripheral veins and the tail veins in gerbils are dangerous to use due to the risk of tail separation. In mice and rats, the lateral tail veins may be used. An intravenous bolus of fluids can be given using a 25–27 gauge insulin needle or by insertion of a butterfly catheter. Warming the tail and applying local anaesthetic cream will help to dilate the vessels and make venepuncture easier. Volumes of 0.2 mL in mice and up to 0.5 mL in rats as a bolus may be given. It is also possible to perform a cut-down jugular catheterisation, but this requires anaesthesia. In prairie dogs, catheters may be inserted, under sedation or preferably anaesthesia, into the cephalic and jugular veins to allow fluid administration. Typically 25–27 gauge are required for the cephalic and 23–25 gauge for the jugular depending on the age of the prairie dog.

Guinea pig, degu and chinchilla

The cephalic and saphenous veins may be used, but generally these are very small and difficult to catheterise. A cut-down technique may be used to access the jugular veins in an emergency.

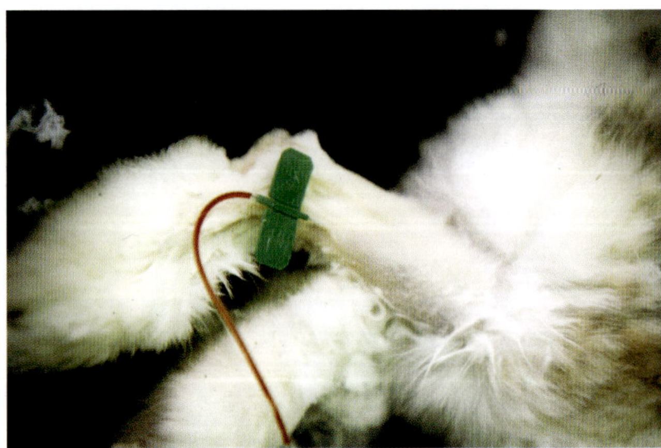

Figure 6.4 Catheterisation of the saphenous vein in a rabbit using a butterfly catheter.

Jugular vein catheterisation: Sedation or anaesthesia is necessary for this procedure, which is as follows:

1. The guinea pig or chinchilla is sedated and placed in dorsal recumbency. The ventral neck is surgically prepared.
2. An incision is made lateral to the midline and parallel to the trachea, through the skin, and the underlying tissues are bluntly dissected to expose the jugular vein.
3. An over-the-needle catheter is preferred, preferably a 25 gauge with wings which can be sutured to the skin after insertion.
4. The catheter is flushed with heparinised saline, a bung is placed over the port and the catheter bandaged in place.

Marsupial

Sugar gliders are difficult to catheterise consciously because of their small size and wriggly nature. The jugular vein is the easiest to catheterise in the sedated/anaesthetised animal for significant fluid administration but tolerance of these catheters is poor. Other peripheral vessels such as the saphenous and cephalic are only accessible with 25–27 gauge needles. In Virginia opossums, the cephalic or saphenous veins are the most accessible. In addition, the lateral tail vein may also be used. However, tolerance of indwelling catheters in the conscious animal is poor and so maintenance is difficult.

African pygmy hedgehog

Venous access is not easy in this species and only possible under sedation or anaesthesia. The cephalic vein is small, as is the lateral saphenous and a 25–27 gauge catheter is required. The jugular vein may be used also requiring a 23–25 gauge needle depending on the size of the hedgehog.

Ferret

Ferrets are well-nigh impossible to catheterise when fully conscious. The cephalic vein may be used with 24–27 gauge over-the-needle catheters; however, movement once consciousness has been regained, frequently dislodges these catheters, and ferrets will often chew the dressings off. Bolus therapy, when unconscious, may be preferable with 5–10 mL given over several minutes.

Intraosseous

The advantages and disadvantages of this route in small mammals are given in Table 6.3.

Rabbit

The proximal femur is the easiest to use. The landmark to aim for is the fossa between the hip joint and the greater trochanter. A 20–23 gauge hypodermic needle or spinal needle is used, and the procedure requires sedation. The area is clipped and surgically prepared and the needle is inserted in the same direction as the long axis of the femur. It may be necessary to cut down through the skin with a sterile scalpel blade in some rabbits. This method will require a syringe-driver perfusion device.

It is possible to use the proximal tibia but this is less well tolerated due to interference with the stifle joint and being more accessible to the patient. There is frequently a need for tubing guards or Elizabethan collars for all intravenous or intraosseous techniques.

Rodents and hedgehogs

The proximal femur may be tolerated, as for rabbits, in larger rats and prairie dogs but smaller species such as hamsters and gerbils often have too small a medullary cavity for needles to be safely inserted.

This is the preferred route for severely dehydrated chinchillas, degus and guinea pigs with the proximal femur being the easiest site. Access is via the natural fossa created by the hip joint and the greater trochanter. Infusion devices such as syringe drivers are advised for this route of administration (see Figure 6.5).

Marsupial

The proximal femur is the easiest bone to use for intraosseous fluid administration. The landmark to aim for is the fossa between the hip joint and the greater trochanter. Insertion is as for rabbits and guinea pigs. In the sugar glider, due to their small size, a 25-gauge needle is required. In Virginia opossums, a 21–23 gauge needle may be used. These are slightly better tolerated than intravenous catheters.

Ferrets

The proximal femur is the easiest bone to use for intraosseous fluid administration. The landmark to aim for is the fossa between the hip joint and the greater trochanter. Insertion is as for rabbits.

Drug toxicities in small mammals

As a general rule, certain antibiotics have a tendency to cause tissue necrosis when injected and these include the tetracycline family as well as many fluoroquinolones (e.g. enrofloxacin) and so these antimicrobials should be used with caution in all small mammals via the parenteral (injection) route. Aminoglycosides such as gentamicin are known to be nephrotoxic and ototoxic and so should also not be used parenterally. Fluoroquinolones should be avoided in young growing animals as they can affect cartilage growth plates and joints resulting in arthropathies.

Lagomorpha

Drugs of the penicillin family should not be used orally due to their ability to cause an enterotoxaemia with *Clostridium* spp. gut overgrowth. The same is true of the cephalosporin and the macrolide

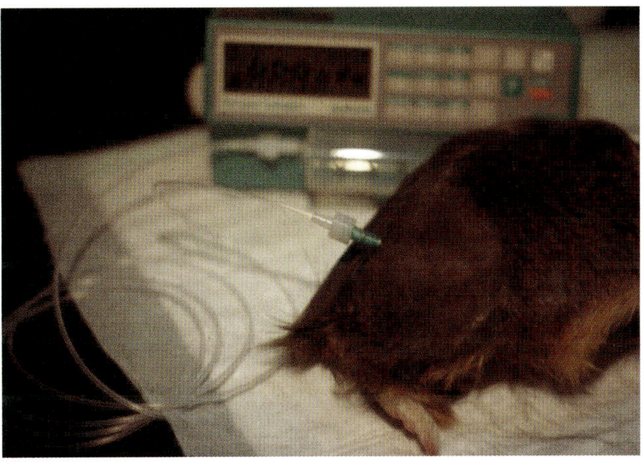

Figure 6.5 Intraosseous catheter placement in a guinea pig using the proximal femur, showing attachment to drip set and infusion device, and before bandaging in place.

family such as erythromycin, clindamycin and lincomycin. Other antimicrobial additives to avoid in rabbits include procaine, which is often added to penicillin preparations and has been shown to be toxic at doses of 0.4 mg/kg and above. Fipronil, a topical ectoparasiticide commonly used in cats, dogs and ferrets, should not be used in rabbits due to its ability to cause neurological disease and in some cases death.

Muridae

Medications containing procaine (such as procaine penicillin) and streptomycin have been reported as causing toxicity in mice and rats.

Gerbils (Cricetidae)

Gerbils are sensitive to harmful side-effects from bacitracin-, streptomycin- and dihydrostreptomycin-containing antimicrobials. They are also adversely affected by potentiated penicillins orally, and these should be used with extreme care. It is not advised to use any macrolides in gerbils (e.g. clindamycin, erythromycin).

Hamsters (Cricetidae)

The following antimicrobials should never be used in hamsters because of their ability to cause a fatal enterotoxaemic condition and in the case of the aminoglycosides because of the risks of renal damage and ototoxicity: bacitracin, all penicillins, all cephalosporins, all macrolides (clindamycin, erythromycin, etc.), and the aminoglycosides (particularly streptomycin, dihydrostreptomycin and oral gentamicin).

Hystricomorpha and prairie dogs

The following antimicrobials should not be used for fear of causing a fatal enterotoxaemic condition particularly when given orally: bacitracin, all penicillins, all cephalosporins and all macrolides. Tetracyclines have been associated with clostridiosis when given orally in guinea pigs. Chloramphenicol can cause ototoxicity in guinea pigs and chinchillas. Metronidazole has been associated with liver failure in chinchillas so caution should be exercised in its use; however, I have used this antimicrobial and not experienced this problem.

Marsupials

Omnivorous marsupials such as the sugar glider and the Virginia opossum seem to be less significantly affected by most antimicrobials, although there is a paucity of data on the safety of many tetracyclines (which generally cause significant tissue damage when injected) and aminoglycosides (which generally are considered to cause kidney and auditory damage).

African pygmy hedgehog

Caution should be used with clindamycin orally, although little other information is available on the toxicity of the other groups of antimicrobials. Penicillins, cephalosporins, fluoroquinolones and sulfonamides have all been used without serious side-effects.

Ferrets

Ferrets are not significantly affected by most antimicrobials although injectable tetracyclines should be avoided due to their ability to cause tissue necrosis.

TREATMENTS FOR DISEASES IN SMALL MAMMALS

The tables in this section are intended to give an overview of the therapies available and are by no means comprehensive. Further resources can be found in the reference list at the end of the chapter.

Lagomorph disease therapies

Tables 6.4–6.8 discuss common treatments for selected diseases of lagomorphs on a system basis.

Table 6.4 Treatment of selected skin diseases in lagomorphs.

Diagnosis	Treatment
Mites, lice, fleas and ticks	Ivermectin/selamectin are the drugs of choice for mites and lice. Note that selamectin only lasts for a short period of time in the rabbit as it is rapidly eliminated (half-life of around 1 day) so higher dosages and more frequent administration in the rabbit (every 7 days) for ectoparasite treatment are recommended at 10–20 mg/kg (Carpenter *et al.*, 2012) Various preparations of ivermectin are available as topical and systemic applications and are typically used at 0.2 mg/kg once every 7 days Imidacloprid has been commonly used topically for treating fleas in rabbits around 10 mg/kg Fipronil has been used to treat and prevent fleas and ticks in species such as ferrets. Fipronil should *not* be used in rabbits and rodents due to serious reported toxicity issues
Blowfly strike	Prevention by removing urine and faecal soiling. Fine mesh to cover outdoor hutch openings. The use of topically applied growth inhibitor cyromazine designed to prevent maggot (larval) maturation to instar L2. Once infected, manually remove maggots and use ivermectin (often at doses of 0.4 mg/kg), covering antimicrobials and fluid therapy but beware of shock associated with tissue damage and maggot death
Bacterial diseases	Based on culture and sensitivity results. Blue fur disease requires a fluoroquinolone (e.g. enrofloxacin) but topical silver sulfadiazine treatments may be needed for more resistant bacterial strains of *Pseudomonas*. spp. Rabbit syphilis (*Treponema paraluisleporidarum* ecovar Cuniculus, TPeC) requires injectable (parenteral) penicillin as may necrobacillosis
Dermatophytosis	Miconazole, enilconazole or clotrimazole topical applications have been used in conjunction with fur clipping. Oral itraconazole may be used at 5 mg/kg once daily although inappetence and liver issues may be a side-effect. Oral griseofulvin can be used, although not in pregnant does due to its teratogenic side-effects
Myxomatosis	No treatment. Prevention is by vaccination (numerous canary pox vectored combined vaccines with or without viral haemorrhagic disease vaccines available commercially)

Table 6.5 Treatment of selected digestive system diseases in lagomorphs.

Diagnosis	Treatment
Dental disease	Prevention by access to good-quality hay, dried grass or fresh grazing ad libitum is essential. When young, a balanced diet with adequate calcium and vitamin D_3 levels to ensure proper jawbone and dental mineralisation. Homogenous pelleted grass-based foods are also useful. Once teeth are overgrown, regular burring to a normal shape must be performed around every 6–8 weeks plus dietary correction
Gastrointestinal foreign body	Digestive lubricants, liquid paraffin, fluid therapy and prokinetic drugs (cisapride, metoclopramide, ranitidine, etc.), if there is no evidence of a complete obstruction. Surgery should be considered if tests indicate a complete obstruction. Maropitant has been used for visceral pain management
Diarrhoea	Fluid therapy. Cause must be determined before treatment If suspect clostridial overgrowth, then use oral colestyramine to bind toxins and prevent absorption plus potentially oral metronidazole (20 mg/kg q12 hours) to kill the clostridia The suspected bacterial cause of epizootic rabbit enteropathy (ERE) has been treated by using tiamulin in feed in commercially reared rabbits Coccidiosis: oral sulfamethoxazole with trimethoprim combinations are licensed for treating coccidiosis in pet rabbits in the UK, generally requiring twice-daily treatment for around 2 weeks. Alternatively oral sulfadimidine at 1 g/L of drinking water for 7 days and then repeated after 7 days. Toltrazuril has been used at 25 ppm in drinking water for 48 hours. In-feed preparations are licensed for commercial rabbits containing diclazuril, monensin, robenidine hydrochloride, lasalocid and decoquinate Nematode infections treated with an ivermectin injection at 0.2 mg/kg or oral fenbendazole at 5–20 mg/kg once daily for 4 days Bacterial enteritis may be treated according to culture and sensitivity results Fluid therapy to correct dehydration and caecolith formation advised
Hypomotility disorder	Dietary management is important. Use of prokinetics, e.g. cisapride (0.5 mg/kg q12 hours), ranitidine (2–5 mg/kg q12 hours) and metoclopramide (0.5 mg/kg q8–12 hours), is required. Fluid therapy is essential with oral prebiotics/probiotics or transfaunation (taking caecotrophs from a healthy rabbit and mixing them with food to administer to the patient) Use of maropitant citrate (2 mg/kg subcutaneously q24 hours) may help where visceral pain or inflammatory conditions are present
Hepatic lipidosis	Prokinetics (if obstructive cause ruled out), e.g. ranitidine, metoclopramide and cisapride. Assisted feeding is important with easily digested foods initially to ensure correct calorie supply but then ensuring correct fibre levels are provided for ongoing support (variety of commercial critical care formulas are available for rabbits and other small herbivores) Transfaunation of caecotrophs from a healthy donor or prebiotics/probiotics are helpful Use of L-carnitine, extract of milk thistle (silymarin) and inositol are helpful in supporting hepatocyte function
Rabbit haemorrhagic disease virus (RHDV)	No treatment. Vaccination is possible using a variety of vaccines, both separate and combined with myxomatosis vaccines. Two strains of RHDV currently available as a vaccine in the UK

Table 6.6 Treatment of selected respiratory and cardiovascular diseases in lagomorphs.

Diagnosis	Treatment
Pasteurellosis	Fluid therapy. Treatment with fluoroquinolone such as enrofloxacin or sulfonamide antimicrobial is advised. In commercial rabbit production, tilmicosin in feed is licensed in some countries Mucolytics (e.g. bromhexine hydrochloride orally or acetylcysteine via nebulisation) and manual cleaning of the nares
Congestive heart failure	This is end-stage heart disease and may have multiple initial causes. Treatment is based on reducing fluid congestion with diuretics, e.g. furosemide (1–4 mg/kg as required) and spironolactone (1–2 mg/kg q24 hours); reducing the afterload the heart has to work against with angiotensin-converting enzyme (ACE) inhibitors but watch for hypotension as rabbits are more sensitive to these drugs than cats and dogs, so usually a lower dose of drugs such as benazepril is advised at 0.1–0.2 mg/kg (Girling, 2003); positive inotropes such as pimobendan (0.25 mg/kg twice daily) If atrial fibrillation is present, then digoxin has been used at 0.005–0.01 mg/kg orally every 24–48 hours. If heart block and bradycardia are seen, then glycopyrrolate at 0.01 mg/kg subcutaneously/intravenously
Lymphoma	Chemotherapeutic regimens involving immunosuppressants such as cyclophosphamide or prednisolone may result in secondary disease where underlying encephalitozoonosis or pasteurellosis is present so care should be taken. Radiotherapy of discrete lesions such as thymic lymphoma or surgical excision where possible are likely to be more successful

Table 6.7 Treatment of selected urogenital tract diseases in lagomorphs.

Diagnosis	Treatment
Urolithiasis	Catheterising and flushing of the urinary bladder and aggressive fluid therapy. Surgery occasionally required to remove discrete larger uroliths or impacted bladders. Reduce dietary calcium (avoid alfalfa/lucerne) and restrict dry food to maximum 25–30 g/day. Antimicrobials and analgesia may be needed, if concurrent cystitis. Radiographs are helpful to look for renoliths, which will worsen the prognosis
Chronic renal failure	Aggressive fluid therapy, initially intravenously or intraosseously but may be supported by subcutaneous fluids once stabilised Urinary bladder flush per urethra and removal of urolithiasis 'silt' where present Treatment of exacerbating conditions, e.g. pyelonephritis, urolithiasis/renolithiasis and encephalitozoonosis ACE inhibitors, e.g. benazepril, have been shown to be helpful in increasing renal perfusion as has been seen in domestic cats, but rabbits are more prone to hypotension and so dosages should be reduced (0.1–0.2 mg/kg q24 hours) (Girling, 2003) Anabolic steroids to prevent catabolism every 3–4 weeks along with multiple B vitamins can help with appetite. Prokinetics, e.g. cisapride, ranitidine or metoclopramide, may also be required to maintain gut motility The reduction of protein in the diet as well as phosphate salts may help preserve renal function – that is, reducing pelleted portion of the diet and increasing leafy greens. The use of phosphate binders such as oral sevelamer has also been tried
Pyometra and endometritis	Surgical neutering with antimicrobial therapy based on culture and sensitivity testing results
Uterine adenocarcinoma	Treatment by surgical neutering before metastasis. Prevention is by surgical neutering when mature enough
Venereal spirochaetosis (*Treponema paraluisleporidarum* ecovar Cuniculus [TPeC])	Penicillin G, single dose, subcutaneously at 40 000 IU/kg. May need to repeat after 7 days. Care should be taken as it can be toxic if given orally resulting in gastrointestinal tract clostridiosis
Pregnancy toxaemia	Fluid therapy to correct acidosis. Intravenous glucose and calcium gluconate may help stabilise. Prognosis often poor by the time clinical signs develop. Prevention is by ensuring adequate food supply and management of any underlying painful or other conditions that may lead to inappetence
Mastitis	Antibiosis based on culture and sensitivity (fluoroquinolones such as enrofloxacin usually effective as bacteria are frequently *E. coli* or *Pasteurella* spp.). Analgesia and anti-inflammatory treatment with non-steroidal anti-inflammatory drugs (NSAIDs) such as meloxicam 0.3–0.6 mg/kg daily (although higher dosages have been safely used) recommended. Fluid therapy and supportive treatment is essential

Table 6.8 Treatment of selected musculoskeletal, nervous system and ocular diseases in lagomorphs.

Diagnosis	Treatment
Osteoarthritis	NSAIDs, e.g. meloxicam, at 0.3–0.6 mg/kg every 24 hours have proved useful. Higher dosages of meloxicam have also been used where safe to do so. More advanced cases may require multimodal analgesia with drugs such as tramadol (10 mg/kg q24 hours) or buprenorphine (0.03 mg/kg q8–12 hours). Gabapentin has also been used where neuropathic pain is observed and low-dose ketamine may also help facilitate analgesia
Fractures	Spinal dislocations and fractures with hindlimb paresis carry poor prognosis. NSAIDs such as meloxicam with opiates such as buprenorphine or fentanyl may be required to control pain Limb fractures carry a better prognosis. Most require external/tie-in fixators as rabbit bones are brittle with large medullary cavities Consider calcium and vitamin D_3 supplementation in cases of metabolic bone disease
Vestibular disease due to otitis media	Fluoroquinolone or sulfonamide antimicrobials are useful where *Pasteurella* or *Streptococcus* spp. infections are present. Anaerobic infections may require injectable penicillins Surgical removal of the lateral wall of the external ear canal can relieve pressure in the short narrow horizontal canal. Bulla osteotomy is difficult and failure rates are high due to the tenacious pus and deep-seated nature of the bullae and their small size. Prognosis is guarded for full recovery, but generally not life-threatening if due to uncomplicated otitis media.
Encephalitozoonosis	Fenbendazole at 20 mg/kg orally once daily for 28 days (Suter *et al.*, 2001). Short-acting corticosteroids have been used in severe cases with neurological disease with some success in addition to fenbendazole (Harcourt-Brown and Holloway, 2003). Management of renal disease may also be required (see Table 6.7) Prognosis guarded once neurological disease is apparent
Lead poisoning	Removal of larger particles by surgery may be possible but frequently the particle size is very small. Treatment with chelating agent, e.g. sodium calcium edetate (27.5 mg/kg q6–8 hours for 5 days), combined with fluid therapy to reduce nephrotoxicity
Anterior uveitis	Test for encephalitozoonosis and treat if positive (see above). Analgesia with systemic NSAIDs plus use of topical tropicamide drops to prevent synechiae formation. Phacoemulsification of the lens and removal may be necessary
Dacryocystitis	Not a true ocular problem but a dental problem with constriction of the tear duct by elongating maxillary incisor root. Treatment is reliant on controlling the dental problem and cannulating and flushing the tear duct
Conjunctivitis	This may occur secondarily to dacryocystitis or as a primary problem. Topical eye drops using fusidic acid or gentamicin is recommended

Muridae disease therapies

Tables 6.9–6.11 discuss common treatments for selected diseases of Muridae (rats and mice, chiefly) on a system basis.

Cricetidae disease therapies

Tables 6.12–6.15 discuss common treatments for selected diseases of Cricetidae (gerbils and hamsters, chiefly) on a system basis.

Hystricomorph disease therapies

Tables 6.16–6.20 discuss common treatments for selected diseases of hystricomorphs on a system basis (chinchillas, degus and guinea pigs).

Sciuromorph disease therapies

Tables 6.21 and 6.22 discuss common treatments for selected diseases of sciuromorphs (chipmunk and prairie dogs) on a system basis.

Marsupial disease therapies

Tables 6.23 and 6.24 discuss common treatments for selected diseases of sugar gliders and Virginia opossums on a system basis.

African pygmy hedgehog disease therapies

Tables 6.25–6.28 discuss common treatments for diseases of African pygmy hedgehogs.

Table 6.9 Treatment of skin diseases in Muridae.

Diagnosis	Treatment
Mites	Ivermectin at 0.2 mg/kg, moxidectin at 0.5 mg/kg or selamectin at 6 mg/kg topically although higher doses around 10–12.5 mg/kg have been used. Ivermectin often requires repeat administration at weekly intervals on three or four occasions
Lice and fleas	Ivermectin or selamectin spot-on
Bacterial disease	Based on culture and sensitivity results. Pododermatitis may require surgical debridement, analgesia (carprofen/meloxicam) and hydrating gels/dressings, as well as improving cage substrate to increase padding. Weight loss also advisable
Dermatophytosis	Topical miconazole, clotrimazole or enilconazole are commonly used. Oral griseofulvin has been used but beware of teratogenicity in pregnant females. Oral itraconazole has also been used (5 mg/kg q24 hours) but beware of hepatotoxicity and anorexia
Atopy and ulcerative dermatitis	Topical soothing canine and feline shampoos and oral essential fatty acids (oil of evening primrose). Oral corticosteroids have been used in acute flare-ups but long-term use has side-effects. Oral antihistamines have also been tried with varying success

Table 6.10 Treatment of selected digestive, respiratory and cardiovascular system diseases in Muridae.

Diagnosis	Treatment
Dental disease	Burring every 3–4 weeks with a low-speed dental burr is advised for incisor malocclusion
Digestive tract parasitic disease	Ivermectin at 0.2 mg/kg once or fenbendazole at 20 mg/kg orally once daily for 5 days for nematodes For coccidiosis, use sulfadimidine in water at 200 mg/L for 7 days. Metronidazole is useful for other protozoa Praziquantel at 5–10 mg/kg orally once for *Rodentolepis (Hymenolepis) nana*; may need to repeat after 10 days to 2 weeks
Digestive tract bacterial disease	Enrofloxacin is effective against a wide range of Gram-negative bacterial infections Oxytetracycline has been used for Tyzzer's disease at 0.1 g/L drinking water. Vancomycin has also been used Other treatments based on culture and sensitivity
Respiratory disease	Culture and sensitivity advised. Oxytetracycline, doxycycline, azithromycin and enrofloxacin are useful against *Mycoplasma* spp., *Streptococcus pneumoniae* and *Klebsiella* spp. infections. Some *S. pneumoniae* infections may be beta-lactamase resistant. Some have suggested doxycycline in combination with enrofloxacin, the doxycycline for its immune-modulatory effects and the enrofloxacin for its antimicrobial effects Consider mucolytics, e.g. bromhexine hydrochloride orally or acetylcysteine by nebulisation. Aerosolised bronchodilators such as albuterol or salmeterol with oral aminophylline may also help. Nebulisation of antimicrobials and ensuring their environment is well ventilated and not ammonia-laden should be considered. Sildenafil citrate has been used as a pulmonary airway protectant in rats with severe mycoplasmosis in conjunction with antimicrobial therapy
Cardiovascular disease	See protocols and drugs for rabbits (Table 6.6)

Table 6.11 Treatment of selected urogenital tract, musculoskeletal, neurological and ocular diseases in Muridae.

Diagnosis	Treatment
Chronic renal failure	Reduce dietary protein but increase the biological value. Reduce phosphate in diet (if necessary, use aluminium hydroxide or sevelamer orally to bind phosphorus in the gut and prevent absorption) Fluid therapy, preferably intravenously/intraosseously initially to stabilise Anabolic steroids and B vitamin supplementation Prevention of chronic progressive nephrosis focuses on a low-calorie, low-protein (4–7%) diet and some advocate soybean protein

(continued)

Table 6.11 (continued)

Diagnosis	Treatment
Urolithiasis	Removal of blockages manually. Reduce calcium content of diet and increase bran levels
	Antimicrobials for preputial gland abscess/cystitis
Mammary neoplasia	Surgical excision may be curative but rapid growth of even benign tumours in rats can mean further development of neoplasia can occur quickly (see Figure 6.6). Prolactin-sensitive mammary tumours (so-called prolactinomas) in rats may be managed with oral cabergoline
Spondylosis	NSAIDs (e.g. meloxicam at 0.5–5 mg/kg orally once/twice daily) and tramadol for pain relief (check for renal disease first before using NSAIDs)
Fractures	Splinting and strict confinement plus analgesia (NSAID); allow rapid callus formation and repair (2–3 weeks)
Vestibular disease	If bacterial, use fluoroquinolone or sulfonamide antimicrobials. If caused by a pituitary tumour, surgery rarely possible
Keratoconjunctivitis sicca	Topical ciclosporin has been used successfully.

Table 6.12 Treatment of skin diseases in gerbils.

Diagnosis	Treatment
Demodicosis	Amitraz washes (1 mL solution to 0.5 L water) once every 2 weeks until negative scrapings. Beware toxicity. Alternatively ivermectin at 0.4 mg/kg once weekly for 6 weeks has been used. Fluralaner orally has been used successfully in hamsters and so may be effective
Bacterial disease	Oral or parenteral antibiosis based on culture and sensitivity results. Enrofloxacin orally or in water, oxytetracycline at 0.8 mg/L water may be useful
Dermatophytosis	Topical miconazole, clotrimazole and enilconazole therapies are often effective. Oral griseofulvin has been used but beware of teratogenicity in pregnant females. Oral itraconazole (5 mg/kg q24 hours) but beware of hepatotoxicity and anorexia
Neoplasia	Surgical excision of ventral scent gland carcinomas or melanomas where possible is advised
Degloving injuries	Fluid therapy. Topical anticoagulants (calcium sprays) or pressure to stem bleeding. Topical/parenteral antimicrobials advised. May need surgery to remove denuded coccygeal vertebrae

Table 6.13 Treatment of selected digestive, respiratory and urogenital system diseases in gerbils.

Diagnosis	Treatment
Proliferative ileitis (wet tail due to *Lawsonia intracellularis* infection)	Difficult, but tetracycline, oxytetracycline and chloramphenicol have been suggested. These however may result in clostridial overgrowth so caution should be taken with case management and probiotics/prebiotics used
Parasitic disease	Ivermectin at 0.2 mg/kg for nematode infestations. Praziquantel at 5–10 mg/kg orally once for *Rodentolepis (Hymenolepis) nana*; may need to repeat after 10 days to 2 weeks
Respiratory disease	Treatment is as for Muridae
Cystic ovarian disease	Surgical ovariectomy/ovariohysterectomy is curative. Alternatively, percutaneous drainage or human chorionic gonadotropin at 100 IU/kg may remove the cysts for a time but they will reoccur. Gonadotropin releasing hormone (GnRH) agonists (e.g. deslorelin) have been used with good effect in some although serous/rete cysts do not respond

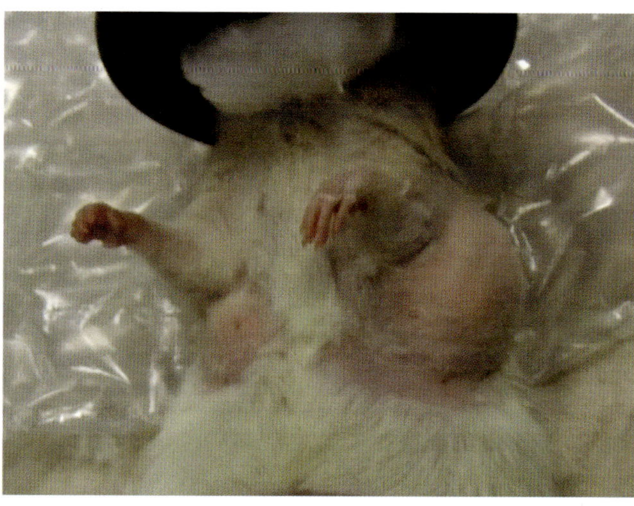

Figure 6.6 Mammary neoplasia in rats is often benign but nonetheless rapidly growing and due to the extensive nature of the mammary tissues may appear anywhere along the ventrum of the torso, pre and post scapula and pre and post thigh.

Table 6.14 Treatment of selected skin and digestive system diseases in hamsters.

Diagnosis	Treatment
Demodicosis	Amitraz has been used but can produce toxic side-effects. Ivermectin may also be used at higher dosages (see Gerbils). More recently fluralaner has been used successfully orally at 25 mg/kg once (Brosseau, 2020). However, the problem is often an underlying immunosuppressive disease that allows the mites to proliferate and so without correcting this, therapy may be unsuccessful
Sarcoptiform mange (*Notoedres notoedri*)	Ivermectin at 0.2 mg/kg once weekly on two to four occasions
Dermatophytosis	See Dermatophytosis in Table 6.12
Hyperadrenocorticism	This is often untreatable. Surgery is generally too complicated with high failure rates. Metyrapone has been used at 8 mg orally once daily, but this is potentially toxic and may result in the death of the hamster
Cheek pouch impactions	Milking the contents manually or with a dampened cotton bud is advised (sedation/anaesthesia may be required). Flushing the pouches with dilute chlorhexidine can remove any superficial infection
Cheek pouch prolapse	Surgical replacement with a cotton bud under anaesthesia. A suture may be placed through the skin into the cheek pouch behind the ear to keep in place
Proliferative ileitis (wet tail due to *Lawsonia intracellularis* infection)	Extremely difficult, see Gerbils (Table 6.13)
Rodentolepis (Hymenolepis) nana	Praziquantel at 5–10 mg/kg orally once; may need to repeat after 10 days to 2 weeks

Table 6.15 Treatment of selected cardiovascular, endocrine, reproductive and musculoskeletal diseases in hamsters.

Diagnosis	Treatment
Aortic thrombosis and cardiomyopathy	Use of furosemide at 0.25–0.5 mg/kg may be useful, as may the ACE inhibitor enalapril at 0.25 mg/kg orally once daily. Beware of hypotensive effects
Hyperadrenocorticism	See Skin Diseases (Table 6.14)
Diabetes mellitus	Protamine zinc insulin therapy at 0.5–1 unit/kg (requires dilution in saline). Aim for 0.25–0.5% glucose in urine and water consumption 10–15 mL/day
	Use glucose/saline intraperitoneally and human glucose oral gels on membranes if evidence of hypoglycaemic overdose
Pyometra	Surgical neutering after fluid therapy and antimicrobial stabilisation
Cystic ovarian disease	Surgical ovariectomy/ovariohysterectomy is curative. Alternatively, percutaneous drainage or human chorionic gonadotropin at 100 IU/kg may remove the cysts for a time but generally they will reoccur
Fractures	Compound fractures of the tibia may require leg amputation. If closed they may heal conservatively with rest and analgesia. Intramedullary pinning with 25–27 gauge needles is possible

Table 6.16 Treatment of selected skin diseases in guinea pigs.

Diagnosis	Treatment
Mites	Ivermectin at 0.2 mg/kg is effective against *Trixacarus caviae* given weekly on three occasions as are selamectin-based compounds given every 2 weeks on three occasions. Analgesics (e.g. meloxicam) and tranquillisers (e.g. diazepam) may be necessary in severe cases
Lice	Pyrethrin powder topically once weekly (use with caution). Ivermectin and spot-on preparations containing imidacloprid with moxidectin may also be useful
Cervical lymphadenitis	Surgical lancing of the abscess and treatment with antimicrobials (e.g. enrofloxacin) is advised
Dermatophytosis	See Dermatophytosis in Table 6.12
Pododermatitis	See Bacterial diseases in Table 6.9

Table 6.17 Treatment of selected digestive, respiratory and urinary system diseases in guinea pigs.

Diagnosis	Treatment
Dental disease	This is similar to rabbits. Change the diet to increase abrasive, grass-based foods. Burr molar spikes every 6–8 weeks under sedation. Treat oral infections based on culture and sensitivity ± information
Bacterial disease	As for hamsters and gerbils, it is based on culture and sensitivity. Enrofloxacin useful for *Salmonella* spp. Chloramphenicol has been used where clostridiosis is suspected, with adsorbents such as colestyramine and of course fluid therapy
Parasitic disease	Nematodes may be treated with 0.2 mg/kg ivermectin. Coccidiosis requires oral sulfadimidine at 40 mg/kg, once daily for 5 days. *Balantidium coli* requires metronidazole orally but use with caution due to risk of liver damage
Faecal impaction	Manual emptying of perianal skin folds daily and flushing with dilute chlorhexidine
Respiratory disease	Enrofloxacin, doxycycline and sulfonamide drugs are useful. Mucolytics, e.g. oral bromhexine hydrochloride and nebulised acetylcysteine, are useful. Nebulised antimicrobials also helpful
	Neoplasia often so advanced by the time diagnosis is made that treatment is not possible
Chronic renal failure	See chronic renal disease of rabbits in Table 6.7
Urolithiasis	Restriction of dry food to 15–20 g/day to reduce dietary calcium levels. Fresh vegetables and fluids to help flush through calcium crystals. Avoid certain forages known to be high in calcium (alfalfa/lucerne). Removal of discrete uroliths (maybe per urethra in females or cystotomy in males). Treat with antimicrobials if cystitis is suspected

Table 6.18 Treatment of selected reproductive, ocular and musculoskeletal diseases in guinea pigs.

Diagnosis	Treatment
Cystic ovarian disease	See hamsters in Table 6.15. Drainage of cysts intraoperatively may make their surgical removal easier (see Figure 6.7)
Pregnancy toxaemia	Oral glucose gel, intravenous or intraperitoneal glucose saline as a 5–7 mL bolus. Dexamethasone 0.2 mg/kg intramuscularly (but will cause abortion). To prevent, do not let sow become overweight prior to pregnancy and ensure any obstruction to eating (dental disease, pain, food restriction) is avoided
Mastitis	Antimicrobials such as enrofloxacin or sulfonamides with fluid therapy and NSAID analgesia. Surgery may be necessary
Hypovitaminosis C (scurvy)	Vitamin C parenterally at 50 mg/kg and 200 mg/L drinking water
Fractures	Splinting with Hexalite material plus cage restriction and analgesia. Surgical fixation with external fixators. Methylprednisolone may be needed if spinal trauma is involved and treatment can be administered within 12 hours. Otherwise NSAID use is preferred
Conjunctivitis	Chlortetracycline eye ointment for *Chlamydia caviae* conjunctivitis. See Scurvy for vitamin C-related problems

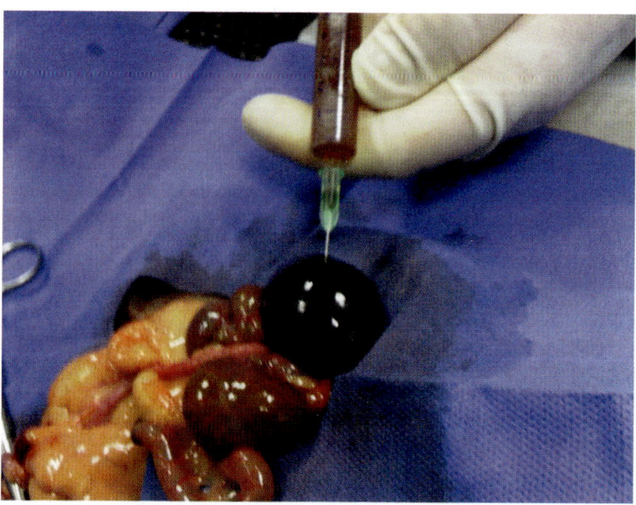

Figure 6.7 Cystic ovaries in a guinea pig being drained intraoperatively to reduce their size and make their removal easier.

Table 6.19 Treatment of selected skin and digestive system diseases in chinchillas and degus.

Diagnosis	Treatment
Dermatophytosis	See Dermatophytosis in Table 6.12
Dental disease	As for rabbits: dental burring under sedation every 6–8 weeks, dietary change to grass-based products Analgesia for root pain using meloxicam ± tramadol orally. Use of prokinetics such as cisapride (0.5 mg/kg q12 hours), ranitidine (2–5 mg/kg q12 hours) and metoclopramide (0.5 mg/kg q8–12 hours) Use of antimicrobials based on culture and sensitivity testing although anaerobes are common and so oral metronidazole at 10–20 mg/kg every 12 hours (some texts suggest metronidazole is hepatotoxic in chinchillas so beware its overuse) Prevention ensuring diets have ad libitum access to good-quality grass hay and a calcium/phosphorus ratio of 1.5 : 1
Hypomotility disorder (colic)	This is generally associated with digestive tract disease or pain and so the cause of the discomfort/disease needs to be determined to ensure proper treatment. Symptomatic treatment of hypomotility can include fluid therapy, analgesia (e.g. meloxicam) and prokinetics as outlined for dental disease
Hepatic lipidosis	Reduce excess fats and soluble carbohydrates in diet. Fluid therapy and assisted nutrition/feeding, e.g. B vitamins, L-carnitine, inositol and milk thistle (silymarin) extract to support hepatocyte function
Bacterial diarrhoea	Antimicrobial treatment is based on culture and sensitivity results. Fluid therapy and analgesia as well as assisted feeding may also be required
Parasitic diarrhoea	Treatment of giardiasis with fenbendazole at 25 mg/kg orally once daily for 3 days Some texts avoid metronidazole due to hepatotoxicity, but I have used it for dental disease and giardiasis at 10–20 mg/kg orally twice daily for 7 days without any side-effects *Eimeria chinchillae* can be treated with oral sulfonamides (see rabbit coccidiosis) *Rodentolepis nana* can be treated with praziquantel (5 mg/kg orally), may require retreatment after 10 days

Table 6.20 Treatment of selected cardiovascular, musculoskeletal, nervous and ocular diseases in chinchillas and degus.

Diagnosis	Treatment
Congestive heart failure associated with dilated cardiomyopathy	Treatment is based on reducing fluid congestion with diuretics such as furosemide (1–4 mg/kg as required) and spironolactone (1–2 mg/kg q24 hours); reducing the afterload the heart has to work against with ACE inhibitors such as enalapril/benazepril; positive inotropes such as pimobendan If atrial fibrillation is present, then digoxin has been used at 0.005–0.01 mg/kg orally every 24–48 hours
Fractures	Long bone fractures are best fixed with external fixation surgically. Smaller fractures may be splinted with human finger splints
Diabetes mellitus and ketoacidosis (degus)	Insulinisation can be attempted based on similar protocols to guinea pigs. Key to stabilisation is to decrease the soluble carbohydrate and increase the complex (fibre) Ketoacidosis can be managed with 40% glucose at 0.5–1 mL/kg by slow intravenous bolus. Bicarbonate supplement to fluids is advised to counteract acidosis
Seizures	Symptomatic treatment with diazepam 1–2 mg/kg intramuscularly. Heat stroke treated with cooled intravenous/peritoneal fluids Listeriosis with oxytetracycline 10 mg/kg twice daily intramuscularly See also ketoacidosis treatment
Conjunctivitis	Use of chlortetracycline eye ointments is recommended for *Chlamydia caviae*. Always check for dental disease in any case of epiphora as molar root elongation pressing on the globe is a common cause of epiphora in chinchillas

Table 6.21 Treatment of selected skin, digestive, respiratory and cardiovascular system diseases in chipmunks and prairie dogs.

Diagnosis	Treatment
Mites	Ivermectin at 0.2 mg/kg is advised. In addition, for *Dermanyssus gallinae*, burn bedding and dust cage with bromcyclen powder
Bacterial skin disease	Antimicrobials based on culture and sensitivity. Generally, enrofloxacin, tetracycline and sulfonamides are safe and effective
Dental disease	Burring of incisor malocclusion with a slow-speed dental drill every 4–6 weeks Pseudo-odontomas may develop in prairie dogs with repeated incisor trauma (e.g. clipping or periodontitis) and may require incisor extraction
Diarrhoea	As for rats and mice
Hymenolepis nana	Oral praziquantel (5–10 mg/kg)
Respiratory disease	Oxytetracycline at 22 mg/kg once daily for 5–7 days is useful for *Mycoplasma* spp. Enrofloxacin and doxycycline may also be used Avermectins such as ivermectin and selamectin have been used for airway mites in prairie dogs
Dilated cardiomyopathy	Use of similar protocols to those in guinea pigs with furosemide diuretics, ACE inhibitors and positive inotropes such as pimobenden

Table 6.22 Treatment of selected urogenital, musculoskeletal and nervous system diseases in chipmunks and prairie dogs.

Diagnosis	Treatment
Urolithiasis	Surgical or manual removal of obstructing uroliths. Give meat-based foods temporarily to acidify urine and dissolve crystals, or increase seeds and fruits and reduce pelleted food
Hypocalcaemic paralysis	Calcium gluconate 100 mg/kg intramuscularly. Prevention based on dietary supplementation. Beware that some cases of paralysis are actually associated with spinal trauma and not hypocalcaemia, so a radiographic assessment is advisable
Uterine infections	Based on culture and sensitivity results. Pyometra may require surgery after fluid stabilisation
Mastitis	Enrofloxacin and oxytetracyclines may be useful with NSAID analgesia. Surgery may be required if abscessation is severe
Fractures	Spinal trauma has a poor prognosis, but methylprednisolone may be used peracutely Minor fractures may respond to cage rest and in-food NSAIDs. Long bone fractures will require fixation preferably with external or tie-in fixators
Seizures	Removal from rooms with 50-Hz electronic equipment such as TV and computer screens. Use of diazepam 0.5–1 mg/kg intramuscularly may help Management of ketoacidosis, see Table 6.20

Table 6.23 Treatment of selected skin, digestive and respiratory system diseases in sugar gliders and Virginia opossums.

Diagnosis	Treatment
Bacterial skin disease	Antimicrobials such as amoxicillin, cefalexin, enrofloxacin and trimethoprim sulfonamides have all been used successfully against bacterial pyodermas in marsupials
Fungal skin disease	See Dermatophytosis in Table 6.12
Parasitic skin disease	Ivermectin at 0.2 mg/kg for mites. Pyrethrin powders have been used against other ectoparasites topically
Dental disease	Extraction of rotten teeth, scaling and polishing and antibiosis with potentiated amoxicillin is recommended
Gastroenteritis	Bacterial disease may be treated with amoxicillin or enrofloxacin Nematodes may be managed with ivermectin (0.2 mg/kg) or fenbendazole (20–50 mg/kg) Giardiasis has been treated with metronidazole and fenbendazole
Paracloacal gland infection/impaction	Antimicrobials such as enrofloxacin, amoxicillin and metronidazole may be required (*E. coli* and anaerobes sometimes seen). Surgery may be required to remove glands
Pneumonia	Bacterial pneumonia has been treated with fluoroquinolones such as enrofloxacin or penicillins

Table 6.24 Treatment of selected cardiovascular, urogenital, musculoskeletal and neurological diseases in sugar gliders and Virginia opossums.

Diagnosis	Treatment
Cardiomyopathy	Treatment is similar to that in ferrets
Heartworm	Treatment and prevention is similar to that in ferrets. Again, beware of anaphylactic shock when treating
Penile trauma	As urethral opening in sugar gliders is at the base of the forked, bifid end of the penis, amputation of the forked ends may be performed if severe trauma is seen, without interfering with urination
Urolithiasis	Catheterisation of the urethra in males to relieve any blockages. Flushing of the bladder or cystotomy to remove larger uroliths
Metabolic bone disease	Correction of the diet to increase calcium and vitamin D_3, provision of ultraviolet light in early stages. Calcitonin has been used once blood levels have been normalised to encourage calcium deposition in the bones. In later stages, the problem is not reversible
Paresis/paralysis	Common sequel to metabolic bone disease, particularly in sugar gliders and so may not be treatable. Radiography to assess severity. Consideration of other nutritional deficiencies such as hypovitaminosis B_1 and E as well as migratory parasites such as *Baylisascaris* spp. and CNS parasites such as *Toxoplasma gondii*
Toxoplasmosis	Therapy can be difficult by the time clinical signs become apparent. However, trimethoprim sulfonamides have been used at 15 mg/kg orally every 12 hours with supportive care (nutrition, fluids, anti-seizure medications)

Table 6.25 Treatment of selected skin diseases in African pygmy hedgehogs.

Diagnosis	Treatment
Mites	Ivermectin at 0.2 mg/kg once and repeated after 14 days I have found success in treating mites using selamectin at 6 mg/kg as a spot-on Fluralaner has been used to treat *Caparinia tripilis* at a single dose of 15 mg/kg (Romero *et al.*, 2017)
Fleas	Products containing imidacloprid as a spot-on can be used to prevent fleas, titrated to the weight of the hedgehog
Bacterial disease	Based on culture and sensitivity with drugs such as enrofloxacin at 5–10 mg/kg, potentiated sulfonamides at 15–30 mg/kg twice daily and potentiated amoxicillin at 10–20 mg/kg twice daily
Dermatophytosis	See Dermatophytosis in Table 6.12
Neoplasia	Surgical excision where possible

Table 6.26 Treatment of selected digestive system diseases in African pygmy hedgehogs.

Diagnosis	Treatment
Dental disease	Extraction of rotten teeth, antibiosis with clindamycin at 5.5 mg/kg twice daily or potentiated amoxicillin is recommended. Encourage dry foods to prevent recurrence
Bacterial disease	This is based on culture and sensitivity results of faeces samples, but fluoroquinolones and potentiated amoxicillin are effective against a range of Gram-negative and anaerobic bacteria
Parasitic disease	Nematode infestations may be treated with ivermectin 0.2 mg/kg or with oral fenbendazole Cryptosporidiosis is generally self-resolving but will often require fluid therapy
Hepatic lipidosis	Assisted feeding with the use of L-carnitine, extract of milk thistle (silymarin) and inositol are helpful in supporting hepatocyte function

Table 6.27 Treatment of selected respiratory, cardiovascular and urinary system diseases in African pygmy hedgehogs.

Diagnosis	Treatment
Bacterial pneumonia	This is based on culture and sensitivity results, but fluoroquinolones and potentiated amoxicillin are effective against a wide range of Gram-negative and Gram-positive respiratory pathogens
Lungworm	Lungworm can be treated using avermectins such as ivermectin, selamectin or moxidectin. Fenbendazole has also been used at 10–30 mg/kg but must be given orally, which may be a challenge in this species When treating cases of patent lungworm infection, massive die-offs of the nematode can result in anaphylaxis. Use of NSAIDs such as meloxicam with fluid therapy may be helpful to counteract this
Congestive heart failure associated with dilated cardiomyopathy	Furosemide at 1–4 mg/kg in acute crisis is useful, intravenously or intramuscularly ACE inhibitor enalapril at 0.5 mg/kg every 48 hours but watch for hypotensive effects. Pimobendan at 0.25 mg/kg every 12 hours may be used as a positive inotrope L-Carnitine (100 mg/kg orally q12 hours) may be helpful
Chronic renal failure	This may be treated as in the domestic cat
Urolithiasis	Surgery may be required to remove obstructions and/or bladder stones. Treatment of any primary or secondary cystitis is based on culture and sensitivity results. Anecdotal evidence of an association with feeding cat-food

Table 6.28 Treatment of selected reproductive diseases in African pygmy hedgehogs.

Diagnosis	Treatment
Uterine neoplasia and uterine infections	Surgical neutering after fluid stabilisation and treatment with broad-spectrum antibiotics until culture and sensitivity results are available

Mustelid disease therapies

Tables 6.29–6.32 discuss common treatments for diseases of mustelids (chiefly the domestic ferret) on a system basis.

Table 6.29 Treatment of selected skin diseases in mustelids.

Diagnosis	Treatment
Mites	Ivermectin at 0.2 mg/kg once and repeated after 14 days
	I have found success in treating ear mites (*Otodectes cynotis*) using spot-on products containing moxidectin, although these products are not specifically licensed for this use in the UK
Fleas	Products containing imidacloprid and moxidectin exist in the UK for treating flea infestation and preventing heartworm disease (*Dirofilaria immitis* infection)
Bacterial disease	Based on culture and sensitivity with drugs such as enrofloxacin at 5–10 mg/kg, potentiated sulfonamides at 15–30 mg/kg twice daily and potentiated amoxicillin at 10–20 mg/kg twice daily
Dermatophytosis	See Dermatophytosis in Table 6.12
Neoplasia	Surgical excision where possible
Hormonal skin disease	Testosterone or oestrogen-dependent alopecia: implantation with a GnRH agonist (e.g. deslorelin). Neutering is no longer recommended due to the development of adrenal gland neoplasia and disease subsequently Hyperadrenocorticism treatment is given in Table 6.32

Table 6.30 Treatment of selected digestive system diseases in mustelids.

Diagnosis	Treatment
Dental disease	Extraction of rotten teeth, antibiosis with clindamycin at 5.5 mg/kg twice daily or potentiated amoxicillin is recommended. Encourage dry foods to prevent recurrence
Gastric ulceration	Remove any gastric foreign bodies as these can result in gastric ulceration Use cytoprotectants: cimetidine (10 mg/kg twice daily), omeprazole (1–4 mg/kg once daily, orally), sucralfate (100 mg/kg daily orally) and bismuth subsalicylate (1 mL/kg three times daily, orally) If *Helicobacter mustelae* is present, combined amoxicillin and metronidazole is advised but enrofloxacin at 4.25 mg/kg every 12 hours with bismuth subcitrate (6 mg/kg q12 hours) for 14 days has also been used successfully (Johnson-Delaney, 2009)
Bacterial disease	This is based on culture and sensitivity results of faeces samples, but fluoroquinolones and potentiated amoxicillin are effective against a range of Gram-negative and anaerobic bacteria. Proliferative ileitis has been successfully treated with chloramphenicol if treated early enough
Parasitic disease	Giardiasis treatment is with metronidazole or fenbendazole Coccidiosis treatment is with sulfadimidine Nematode infestations may be treated with 0.2 mg/kg ivermectin or with oral fenbendazole
Liver disease	Lactulose at 1.5–3 mg/kg orally once daily may help. Supportive therapy with vitamin B supplements and reduced fat/high biological value proteins advised. Use of inositol, L-carnitine and extract of milk thistle (silymarin) may also be useful where hepatic lipidosis is present
Lymphoma	Chemotherapy with drugs such as vincristine, cyclophosphamide and prednisolone has been tried but prognosis is guarded and depends on numerous factors including age, lymphoma grading and type

Table 6.31 Treatment of selected respiratory, cardiovascular and urinary system diseases in mustelids.

Diagnosis	Treatment
Canine distemper virus	There is no treatment. Prevention is by vaccination. No currently licensed ferret vaccine in the UK, although they exist in the USA. In the UK, canine distemper vaccines have been used but care should be taken to choose a vaccine not raised in ferret cell-lines due to increased likelihood of inducing disease. Consultation with the canine vaccine manufacturer is advised for safety and efficacy data
Bacterial pneumonia	This is based on culture and sensitivity results, but fluoroquinolones and potentiated amoxicillin are effective against a wide range of Gram-negative and Gram-positive respiratory pathogens
Congestive heart failure associated with dilated cardiomyopathy	Furosemide at 1–4 mg/kg in acute crisis is useful, intravenously or intramuscularly ACE inhibitor enalapril at 0.5 mg/kg orally every 48 hours or benazepril 0.25–0.5 mg/kg orally every 24 hours but watch for hypotensive effects. Pimobendan at 0.25 mg/kg every 12 hours may be used as a positive inotrope Digoxin may also be used in heart failure where atrial fibrillation occurs
Lungworm and heartworm	These can be treated using avermectins such as ivermectin, selamectin or moxidectin. When treating cases of patent heartworm infection, massive die-offs of the nematode can result in anaphylaxis or vascular blockage. In ferrets, medicines containing moxidectin (with imidacloprid) spot-on have a license in the UK for preventing heartworm
Urolithiasis	Surgery may be required to remove obstructions and/or bladder stones. Feeding an all-meat-based protein diet is essential to prevent formation. Treatment of any primary or secondary cystitis is based on culture and sensitivity results
Acute renal failure	Obstructive urinary disease is the most common cause and typically will be associated with prostatic and paraurethral disease (often linked to adrenal disease) or urolithiasis. Use of intravenous glucose (1–2 mL/kg 50% glucose diluted 1 : 1 with 0.9% saline) to reduce hyperkalaemia which can cause life-threatening cardiac arrhythmias is advised. Intravenous calcium gluconate may also be required to stabilise cardiac electrical activity Removal of the obstruction may require surgery or urethral catheterisation. Management of underlying predisposing factors (e.g. adrenal disease, prostatic infection, urolithiasis) also required
Chronic renal failure	Fluid therapy to correct dehydration. Use of ACE inhibitors such as benazepril (similar to the domestic cat) to improve blood flow to the renal tubules. Phosphate binders such as oral aluminium hydroxide or sevelamer to reduce phosphorus uptake. Use of appetite stimulators, e.g. anabolic steroids and soluble (B) vitamin supplementation

Table 6.32 Treatment of selected endocrine, reproductive and ocular diseases in mustelids.

Diagnosis	Treatment
Diabetes mellitus	Tends to be rare but treatment is based on protamine zinc insulin at 1–2 units per ferret and increasing by 0.5 units until blood glucose falls to 15 mmol/L or urine glucose to 0.5%. Twice-daily dosing may be required
Hyperadrenocorticism	GnRH implants such as deslorelin can help in many cases to reduce tumour size and clinical effects. Typically, a 9.4-mg deslorelin (Suprelorin®) implant will last around 18–24 months (sometimes longer) depending on the time of year implanted. Some adrenal disease does not respond to GnRH (often adenocarcinomas) and may still require surgical resection of the neoplasm if possible
Insulinoma	Surgical excision of pancreatic neoplasm, but may be difficult due to its small size. Management with oral prednisolone (0.25–2 mg/kg q12 hours) with weekly monitoring of blood glucose levels. Diazoxide has been used where resistance to prednisolone is seen
Pregnancy toxaemia	40% glucose at 0.5–1 mL/kg by slow intravenous bolus. Bicarbonate supplement to fluids is advised to counteract acidosis. Dexamethasone may be required in severe cases but abortion will occur
Hyperoestrogenism	Prevention based on implantation of GnRH agonist, e.g. deslorelin at 5 months, or mating with an entire or vasectomised hob, or regular proligestone treatment at the start of the breeding season (50 mg per jill) If disease has developed then treat with blood transfusion if PCV<20%, or in early stages stop oestrus with proligestone or human chorionic gonadotropin and then use GnRH implant
Mastitis	Broad-spectrum antibiotics and NSAIDs with fluid therapy advised. Surgical excision of abscesses may be needed
Pyometra and endometritis	Surgical neutering after fluid stabilisation and treatment with broad-spectrum antibiotics until culture and sensitivity results are available. This may lead to adrenal gland neoplasia in later life

References

Brosseau, G. (2020) Oral fluralaner as a treatment for *Demodex aurati* and *Demodex criceti* in a golden (Syrian) hamster (*Mesocricetus auratus*). *Canadian Veterinary Journal*, **61**(2), 135–137.

Carpenter, J.W., Dryden, M. and KuKanich, B. (2012) Pharmacokinetics, efficacy, and adverse effects of selamectin following topical administration in flea-infested rabbits. *American Journal of Veterinary Research*, **73**(4), 562–566.

Girling, S.J. (2003) Preliminary study into the possible use of benazepril in the management of renal disease in rabbits. *Proceedings of the British Veterinary Zoological Society*, Edinburgh, Scotland, p. 44.

Harcourt-Brown, F.M. and Holloway, H.K.R. (2003) *Encephalitozoon cuniculi* in pet rabbits. *Veterinary Record*, **152**, 427–431.

Johnson-Delaney, C. (2009) Ferrets: anaesthesia and analgesia. In: *Manual of Rodents and Ferrets* (eds E. Keeble & A. Meredith), 1st edn, pp. 245–253. BSAVA, Quedgeley, UK.

Romero, C., Waisburd, G.S., Pineda, J. *et al.* (2017) Fluralaner as a single dose oral treatment for *Caparinia tripilis* in a pygmy African hedgehog. *Veterinary Dermatology*, **28**(6), 622–e152. doi: 10.1111/vde.12465.

Suter, C., Müller-Doblies, U.U., Hatt, J.M. and Deplazes, P. (2001) Prevention and treatment of *Encephalitozoon cuniculi* infection in rabbits with fenbendazole. *Veterinary Record*, **148**, 478–480.

Chapter 7 Small Mammal Diagnostic Imaging

RADIOGRAPHY

Chemical restraint

Health and safety considerations and local laws generally prohibit manual restraint of a patient while ionising radiation is being used. Chemical restraint therefore with drug combinations such as medetomidine/ketamine/butorphanol or sevoflurane/isoflurane is preferred. See Chapter 3 for further details.

Positioning

Lateral and dorsoventral/ventrodorsal views at 90° to each other are routine. Further oblique views may be useful when imaging structures such as the head, where right and left dental arcades may need to be viewed separately. In addition, rostrocaudal (skyline) views of the head may be useful where visualisation of the temporomandibular joint or frontal sinuses is required.

Interpretation of rabbit radiographs

Thorax

The heart sits between the fourth and sixth rib spaces and appears large due to the small size of the thoracic cavity in relation to the overall body (see Figures 7.1 and 7.2). Enlargement of the heart silhouette is common in rabbits and can be due to pericardial fat, cardiomyopathy or disease such as valvular disease resulting in congestive heart failure. Pathological atherosclerosis and mineralisation of the blood vessels can be seen radiographically (Shell and Saunders, 1989). The thymus persists in the adult rabbit and thymic neoplasia can be seen as a precardiac mass (see Figure 7.3). Other causes of a precardiac shadow can include mediastinal abscesses and other forms of neoplasia.

The lungs show similar changes to dogs and cats when affected by infection. They are also one of the main sites of metastasis for certain neoplasms, for example uterine adenocarcinomas. Pleural effusions may also be seen in rabbits, with the characteristic rounding/blunting of the caudal lung lobe border and widened pleural space on dorsoventral views and may be seen in cases of congestive heart failure as may an alveolar pattern suggestive of lung oedema.

Vertebral heart score (VHS) has been determined for a number of pet small mammals. It is measured on lateral thoracic radiographs using the long axis of the heart from heart base at the carina to apex and the short axis perpendicular to the long axis at the heart's widest point. The sum of the long and short axes of the heart are then compared to the animal's vertebral column, measuring from the cranial edge of the body of the fourth thoracic vertebra and measured in increments of a quarter of the vertebral body size. For rabbits under 1.6 kg the VHS range is 6.9–8.1 and for rabbits greater than 1.6 kg 7–8.7 in one study (Onuma *et al.*, 2010).

Abdomen

The caecum should always be full of ingesta, often with small volumes of gas in the healthy rabbit, and is positioned ventrally and to the right side. Excessive gas build-up can be seen in mucoid enteropathy and penicillin toxicity where the whole of the stomach, small intestine, caecum and large intestine may be filled with fluid and gas (see Figure 7.4).

The liver is found completely underneath the caudal ribcage and is a flattened shadow craniocaudally. A number of liver diseases may result in enlargement and extension of the liver beyond the ribcage (e.g. hepatic lipidosis, hepatic coccidiosis due to *Eimeria stiedae* infection, lung lobe torsion).

The stomach should always contain food, but a small gas crescent dorsally may be seen. Excessive gas build-up in the stomach can indicate a blockage or stasis of the bowel. Stomach emptying and intestinal motility are difficult to assess in the rabbit due to the permanently full stomach. However, one contrast study suggested that 32% of a liquid marker should reach the caecum in 1 hour and 80% by 12 hours in the healthy rabbit (Pickard and Stevens, 1972). Solid markers however reached the caecum within 4 hours.

The normal kidney shadow should be 1.4–2.2 times the length of the second lumbar vertebra, with a mean of 1.8 times. Renal calculi are frequently seen, are usually bilateral and may be a cause of intense pain in rabbits (see Figures 7.5 and 7.6). Negative contrast techniques after catheterisation of the bladder using air at 5–8 mL/kg body weight may be used in rabbits to outline the bladder lining. Double contrast techniques can be used with iodine at a rate of 2–3 mL/kg. Excretory urograms may be useful in assessing renal disease using 2 mL/kg of an intravenous iodine-based contrast medium injected into a peripheral vein. In healthy rabbits, the presence of large amounts of calcium 'silt' may lead to a significant outline of the bladder.

The uterus may become enlarged due to neoplasia (e.g. uterine adenocarcinomas), pyometra or gravidity. The vagina may also become enlarged due to venous aneurysms.

In the male rabbit there is no os penis. The testes sit scrotally but can be retracted into the abdomen.

Head

Radiography is essential for assessing dental disease which is common in rabbits (Harrenstein, 1999). Normal lateral, dorsoventral and skyline views of rabbits can be seen in (Figures 7.7–7.9). Root

Veterinary Nursing of Exotic Pets and Wildlife, Third Edition. Simon J. Girling.

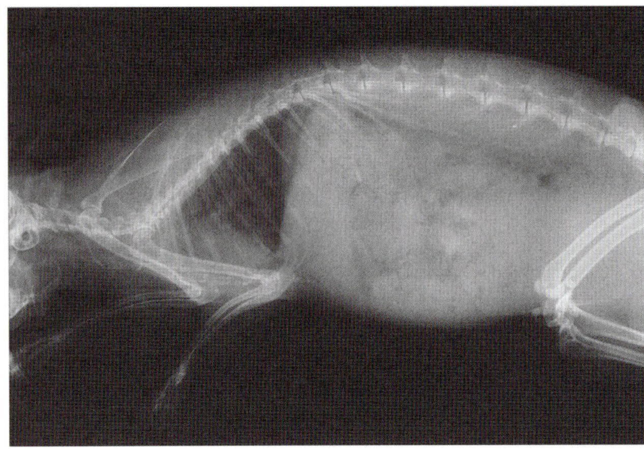

Figure 7.1 Lateral view of a normal rabbit (Fraser and Girling, 2009).

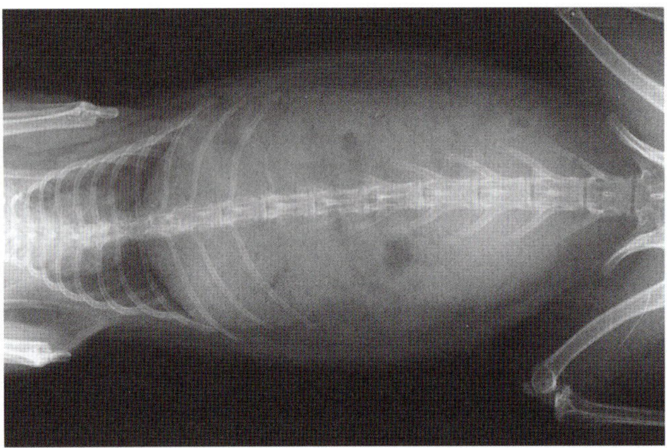

Figure 7.2 Dorsoventral view of a normal rabbit (Fraser and Girling, 2009).

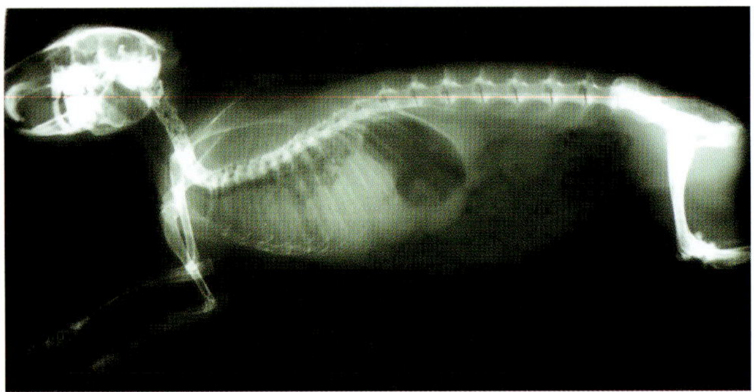

Figure 7.3 Lateral view of a rabbit with a precardiac shadow due to a thymic neoplasm. Note also the dental disease.

elongation and lysis of the alveolar bone is often an early radiographic sign of abnormal dental wear (Redrobe, 2001) (see Figure 7.10). Irregular wear of the teeth and touching of the cheek teeth in the mouth at rest are also indicators of dental disease.

The final stage of dental disease can include abscess formation, dental loss and osteomyelitis (see Figure 7.11). Oblique views of the head may allow the separate examination of one dental arcade from the other to properly image the roots of cheek teeth in particular.

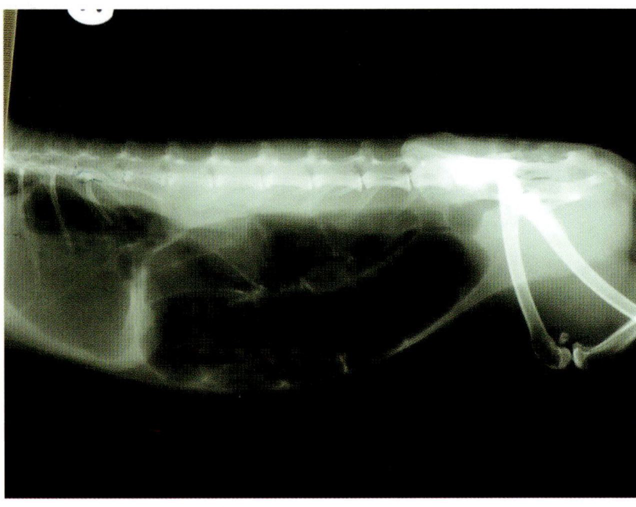

Figure 7.4 Large intestine and caecal gas associated with clostridiosis in a domestic rabbit.

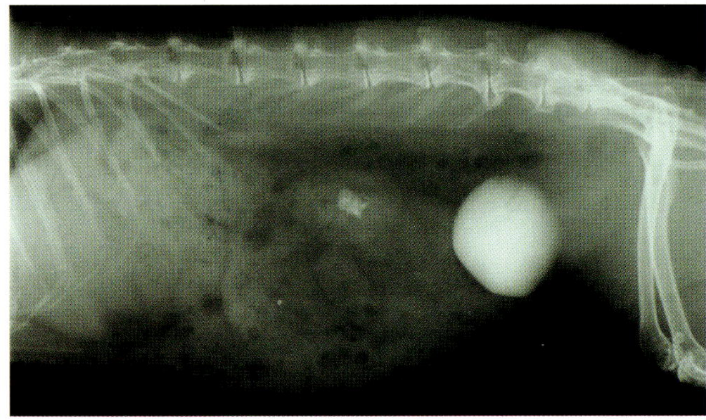

Figure 7.5 Lateral abdomen of a rabbit showing radiodense calculi in left kidney and radiodense silt in bladder. Note also spondylosis lesions in L5–6 and L6–7 (Fraser and Girling, 2009).

Exophthalmos may be due to cheek-tooth abscess, retrobulbar neoplasia and cranial mediastinal masses such as thymic neoplasia; therefore, chest radiographs are also necessary.

Dacryocystitis may be associated with dental disease, often due to maxillary incisor root elongation or infection. Contrast studies of the nasolacrimal ducts may be performed using iodine-based contrast media injected into the ventral tear duct punctum to demonstrate pinching of the duct around the roots of the incisor.

To examine for otitis media resulting in vestibular disease, a dorsoventral square-on view of the skull is necessary. Skull neoplasia has also been recorded in the rabbit (Weisbroth and Hurwitz, 1969).

Appendicular skeleton

Osteoarthritis is common in rabbits, particularly in the stifle joint. Luxation of the elbow has also been observed. Neoplasia of the limb in the form of fibrosarcomas and osteosarcomas are also seen in rabbits. Hypertrophic osteopathy has also been reported associated with an intrathoracic neoplasm (DeSanto, 1997), as has a limb neurofibrosarcoma in association with a thymic neoplasm (Clippinger *et al.*, 1998).

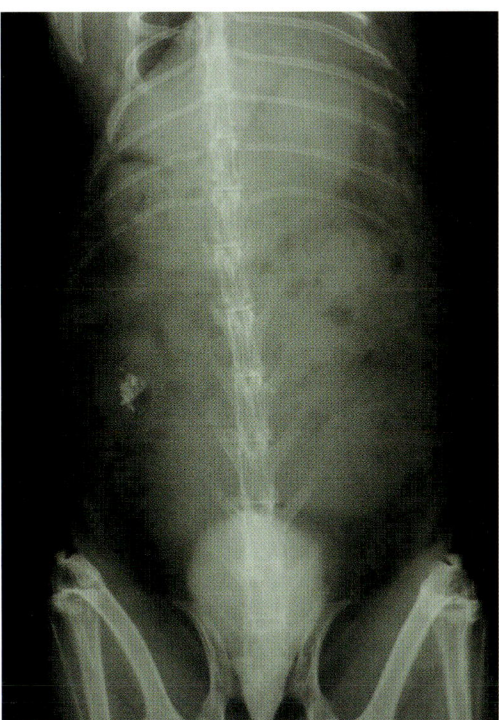

Figure 7.6 Dorsoventral view of the rabbit in Figure 7.5 showing multiple radiodense calculi in left kidney and radiodense silt in urinary bladder (Fraser and Girling, 2009).

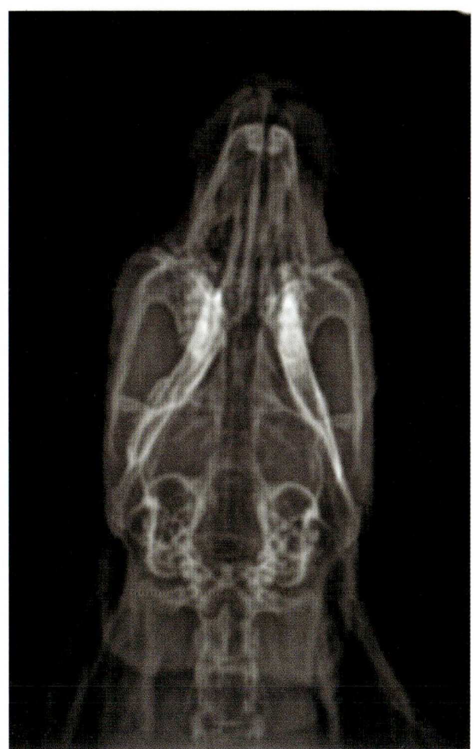

Figure 7.8 Dorsoventral view of a normal rabbit's head.

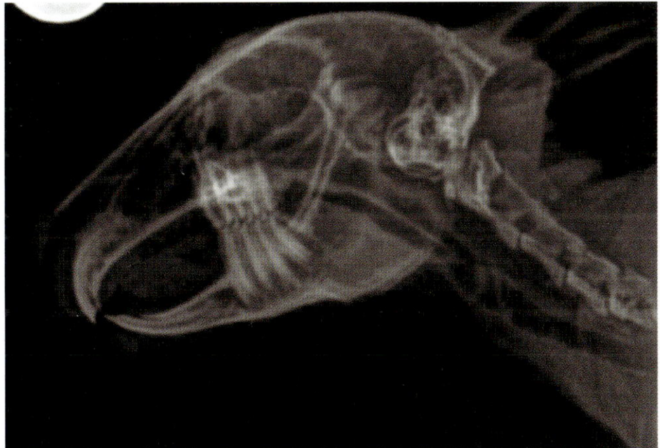

Figure 7.7 Lateral view of a normal rabbit's head.

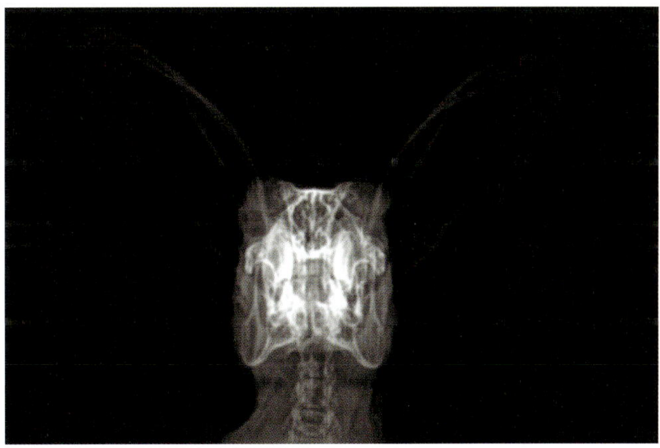

Figure 7.9 Skyline (rostrocaudal) view of a normal rabbit's head.

Axial skeleton and ribs

The spine shows some breed variation in numbers of vertebrae, with some individuals possessing 13 thoracic vertebrae (Kozma *et al.*, 1974). Fractures of the spine, often associated with metabolic bone disease, or luxations/subluxations of the vertebral joints are common.

Arthritis of the spine (spondylosis) and spinous process fractures are also common. In one study, three types of spinal lesions were observed in the rabbit (Green *et al.*, 1984).

1. Change in the nucleus pulposus of the intervertebral discs with chondroid metaplasia, eventually involving the whole spinal column by 2 years of age.
2. Mineralisation with hydroxyapatite deposition in the nucleus pulposus of the discs radiographically, primarily in the thoracic segments (seen as young as 3 months of age).
3. Spondylosis in rabbits over 24 months, chiefly bridging those discs that did not show mineralisation.

Myelography has been described (Longley, 2005). The access point is intervertebral space L5/6 using a 23-gauge, 1¼-inch needle to access the subarachnoid space. Volumes of 0.4 mL/kg of iodine-based contrast medium will extend the media from T2 to L7.

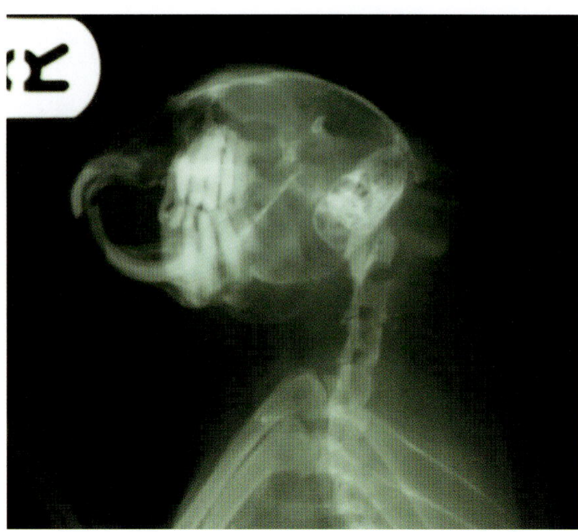

Figure 7.10 Lateral oblique head of a rabbit showing both cheek tooth and incisor malocclusion. Note contact of the occlusal surfaces of cheek teeth and gaps between the teeth that are abnormal. Roots of cheek teeth projecting through ventral mandible and upper/lower incisors meeting end on (Fraser and Girling, 2009).

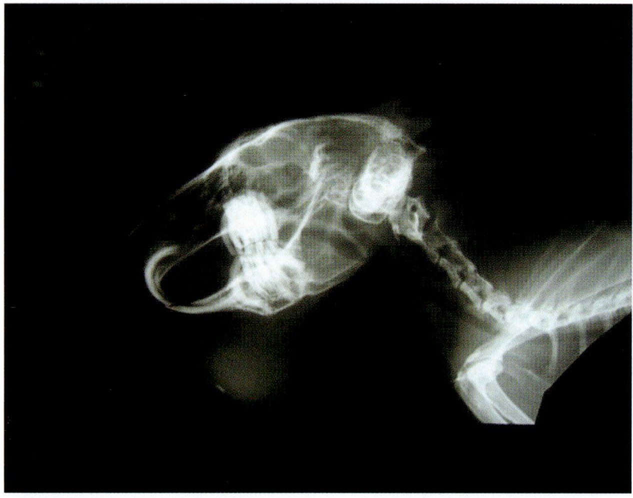

Figure 7.11 Lateral view of a rabbit skull with a mandibular dental abscess. Note the soft tissue swelling (abscess) ventral to the mandible associated with the penetration of the periosteum of the first premolar/cheek tooth root.

Interpretation of rodent, hedgehog and marsupial radiographs

Imaging techniques in rodents and marsupials are the same as for other mammals. Their small size precludes the use of grids. The use of non-screen film may help in examining fine structures. In many cases, short exposure times are required due to the rapid rates of respiration, even when anaesthetised.

Anaesthesia or sedation is required in all cases to allow proper positioning and maintain personnel health and safety. In all cases, several important features of rodents are visible on radiographs. The main problem is that the chest cavity is very small in relation to the abdominal cavity, making examination of the lung fields for minor abnormalities difficult (Girling, 2002) (see Figures 7.12 and 7.13).

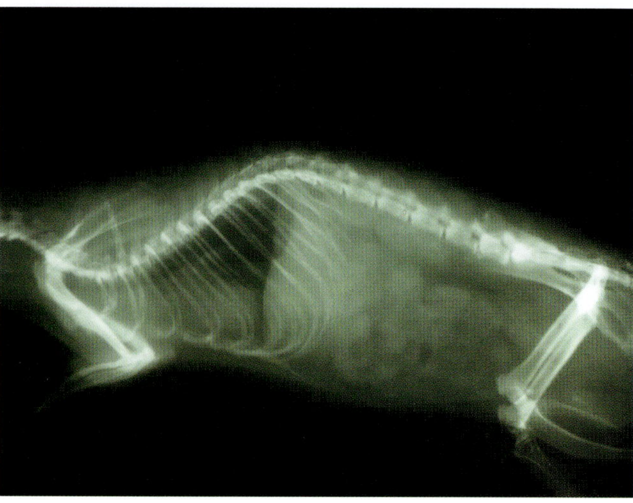

Figure 7.12 Lateral view of a normal healthy adult male rat. Note the small size of the chest, the open growth plates particularly on the proximal tibia and the ischial region of the pelvis and the presence of an os penis.

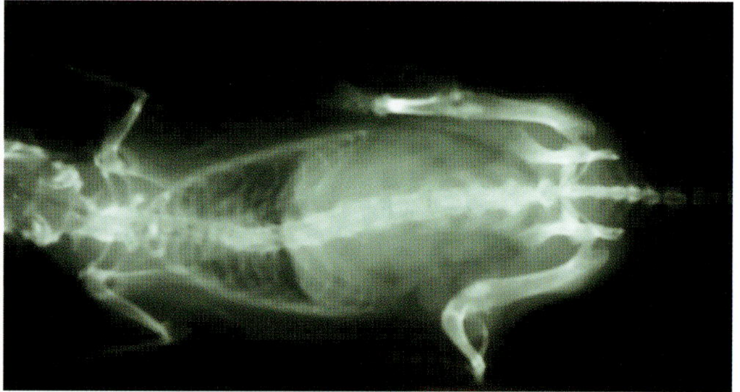

Figure 7.13 Dorsoventral view of a normal healthy adult male rat.

Generally, though, when patients are presented, the pathology is advanced and it may be difficult to see any normal lung tissue. Muridae and hedgehogs are particularly prone to pneumonia, with bronchial and alveolar patterns being seen (see Figure 7.14).

Heart disease is commonly seen in many small mammals (see Figure 7.14). Vertebral heart scores (using the technique described for rabbits) have been derived for a number of small mammals, including chinchillas 7.5–10.2 (Doss *et al.*, 2017); African pygmy hedgehogs, median 8.25 (mean 8.16 ± 0.48) (Black *et al.*, 2011); rats 7–8.5 (Dias *et al.*, 2021); prairie dogs, median 7 (mean 7.12 ± 0.42) (Garcia *et al.*, 2016); and guinea pigs, mean 7.8 ± 0.12 (Masoudifard *et al.*, 2021).

Some species, such as rats, have open growth plates on many long bones, even as adults. Males of most rodents have an os penis, and extensive testicular tissue that, when retracted, may fill the caudal abdomen (see Figure 7.12). In hindgut fermenters, such as the guinea pig and chinchilla, the capacious large intestine and caecum fill the abdomen making discernment of other structures difficult, particularly when filled with gas which can occur through gut stasis associated with pain, clostridiosis and intestinal blockages (see Figures 7.15 and 7.16).

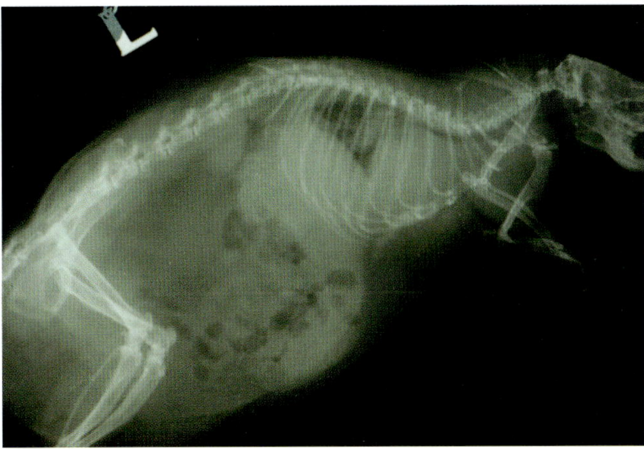

Figure 7.14 Lateral view of an adult (overweight) rat. Note the radiodense masses in the chest typical of mycoplasma pneumonia and lung consolidation. Note also the enlarged heart due to cor pulmonale.

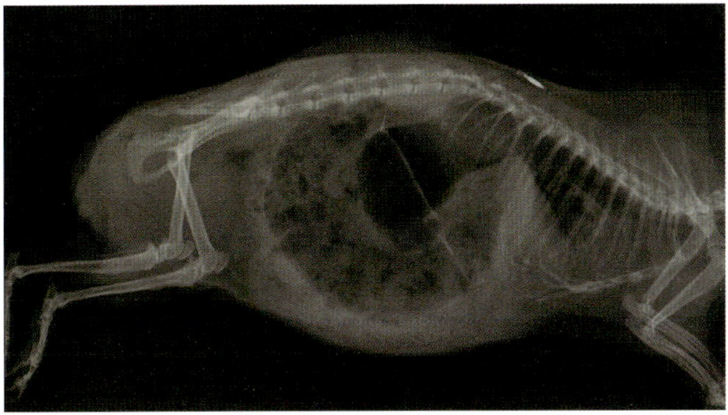

Figure 7.15 Lateral radiograph of a female guinea pig with gas in the stomach, large bowel and caecum associated with pain and discomfort due to cystic ovarian disease.

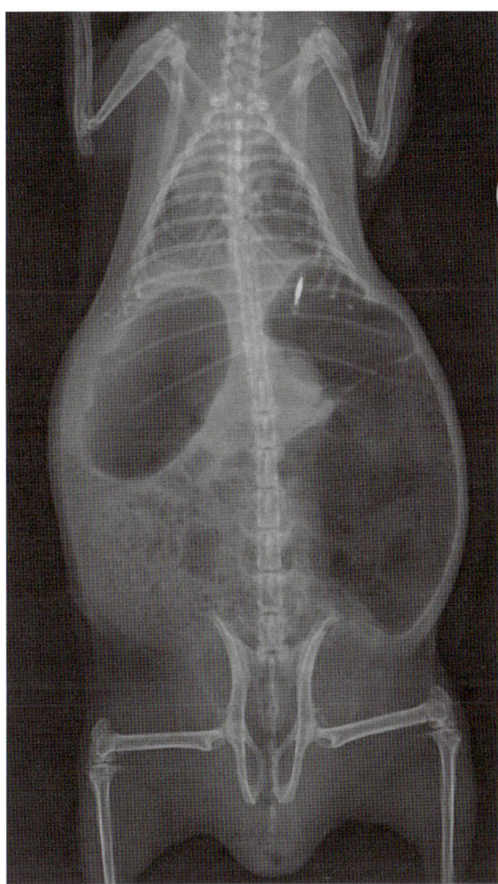

Figure 7.16 Dorsoventral view of the female guinea pig in Figure 7.15 showing gas in the stomach (left side) and large intestine and caecum (right side) associated with discomfort due to cystic ovarian disease. Note the ovaries are difficult to see radiographically despite their size but are faintly visible overlying the bowel either side of midline at the level of the caudal border of the stomach.

Dental disease is particularly common in hystricomorphs such as chinchillas (see Figures 7.17 and 7.18), guinea pigs (Figure 7.19) and degus (Figure 7.20) and radiography is essential in assessing the extent of disease and identifying infection. Similar changes are noted as with rabbits with elongated cheek tooth roots and crowns, apical abscessation, incisor malocclusion and dental loss.

Many marsupials have an epipubic bone projecting cranially from the pubis and thought to support the ventral body wall and pouch. The sugar glider however does not possess this.

Interpretation of ferret radiographs

Thoracic cavity

Heart

The heart is positioned more caudally than in the cat or dog and may be slightly elevated from the sternum due to fat deposition in the pericardiac ligament (Orcutt, 1998).

Cardiac enlargement due to cardiomyopathy and congestive heart failure is common in ferrets (see Figures 7.21 and 7.22). The size of the heart may be assessed using the modified VHS that compares heart length along the long axis against its width on a right lateral plain

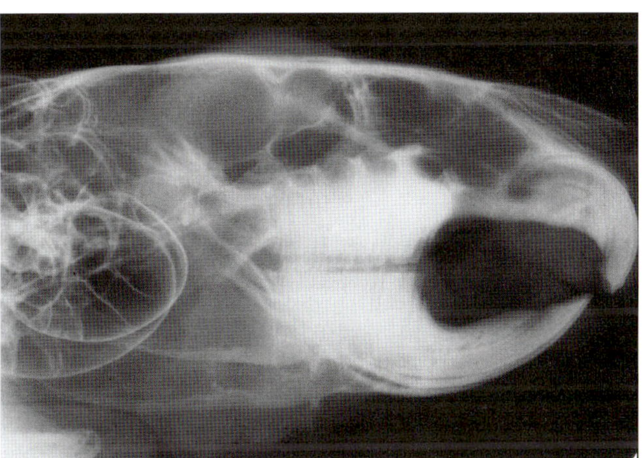

Figure 7.17 Lateral view of a normal chinchilla's skull. Note the radiolucent apices to the cheek teeth, the apical buds where the elodont tooth grows from and the fact that the cheek teeth do not touch at rest and the maxillary incisors close rostral to the mandibular incisors. *Source:* Reproduced with permission from the BSAVA Manual of Exotic Pets, 4th Edition (2002) Figure 01.08 © BSAVA.

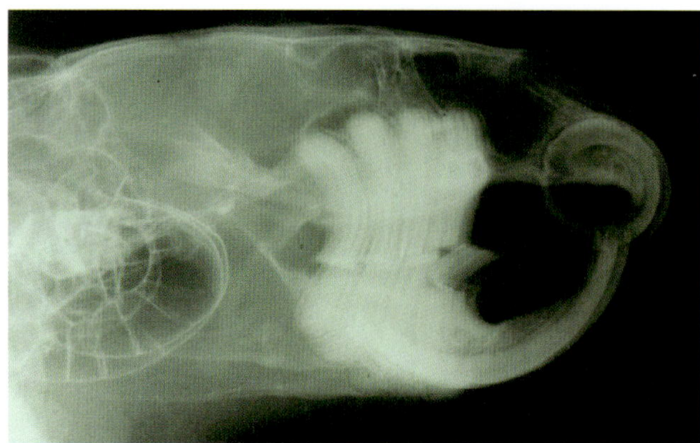

Figure 7.18 Lateral view of an abnormal chinchilla's skull. Note the elongation of the cheek teeth which results in apparent loss of the radiolucent apical buds as these are no overlying the tooth itself due to lateral elongation into the jaws. Note the fractured cheek tooth crown and the incisor malocclusion. *Source:* Reproduced with permission from the BSAVA Manual of Exotic Pets, 4th Edition (2002), Figure 01.09 © BSAVA.

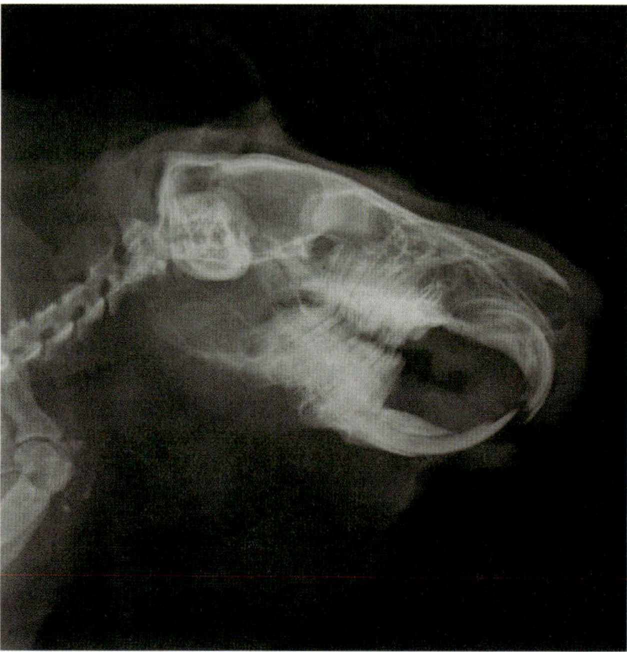

Figure 7.19 Lateral oblique view of an abnormal guinea pig's skull. Note the elongated cheek tooth roots that are starting to migrate through the mandible resulting in palpable 'lumps' on the underside of the jaw as well as the roots in the mandible pushing into the maxillary sinuses and nasal passages causing upper respiratory irritation.

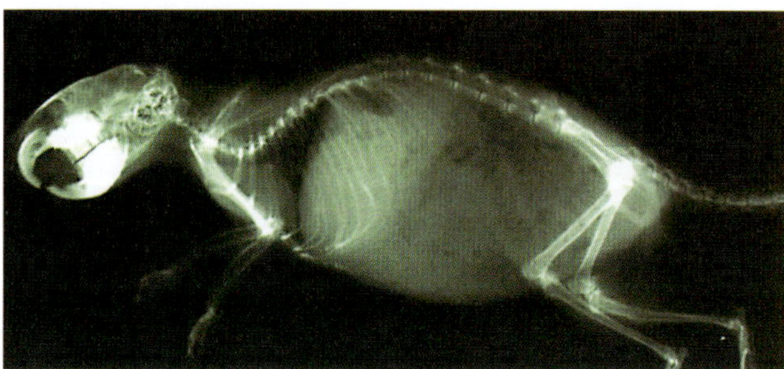

Figure 7.20 Lateral whole-body radiograph of a healthy degu. Note the capacious gastrointestinal tract and the bird-like skeleton similar to the chinchilla's.

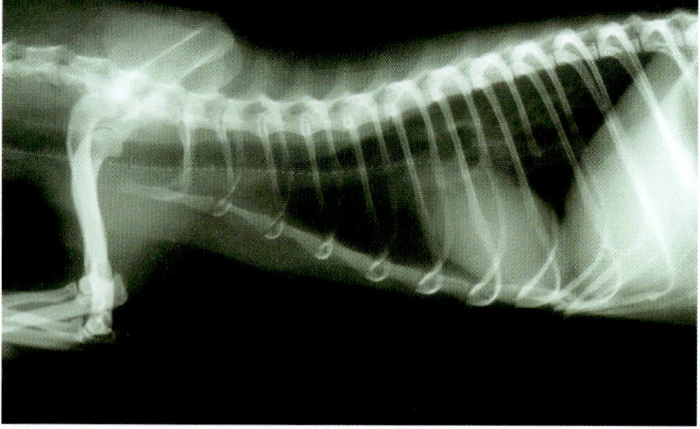

Figure 7.21 Lateral view of the thorax of a normal ferret. Note the apparently more caudal position of the heart and the narrow chest inlet which makes the trachea appear enlarged.

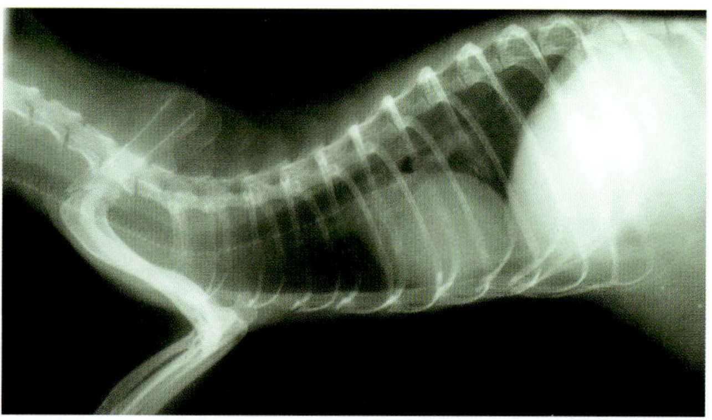

Figure 7.22 Lateral view of the thorax of a ferret with cardiomegaly.

radiograph and relating this to the length of the heart in thoracic vertebral units (a similar calculation seen in the dog and cat). The following formula has been used to assess the heart of both male and female ferrets:

$$\frac{\text{RL LA}(\text{cm})+\text{RL SA}(\text{cm})}{\text{T5}-\text{T8}(\text{cm})}$$

where RL LA indicates right lateral long axis (base of heart to apex), RL SA right lateral short axis (widest part of the heart) and T5–T8 thoracic vertebra 5 to thoracic vertebra 8.

The ratio was 1.35 (standard deviation 0.07) for males and a mean of 1.34 (standard deviation 0.06) for females (Stepien *et al.*, 1999).

Heartworm infestation may show a pleural effusion and cardiomegaly, principally the right side of the heart. In addition, the caudal vena cava is often noticeably dilated (Supakorndej *et al.*, 1995).

Lungs and other organs

Pneumonia produces a typically interstitial and then alveolar pattern similar to that seen in cats and dogs. Lung patterns around the perihilar region suggest lung oedema and congestive heart failure.

Pleural effusions may be seen due to right-sided failure heart failure (e.g. heartworm), neoplasia (e.g. thymic lymphoma), traumatic wounds and pleurisy (see Figures 7.23 and 7.24). Soft tissue

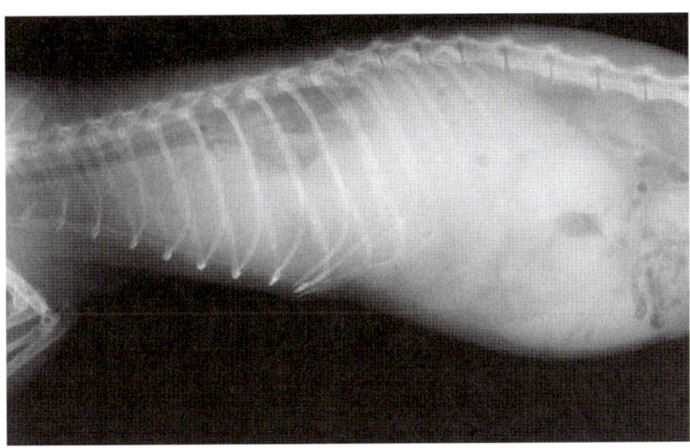

Figure 7.23 Lateral radiograph of a ferret with a pleural effusion prior to drainage. *Source:* Reproduced with permission from the BSAVA Manual of Rodents and Ferrets (2009), Figure 19.07a © BSAVA.

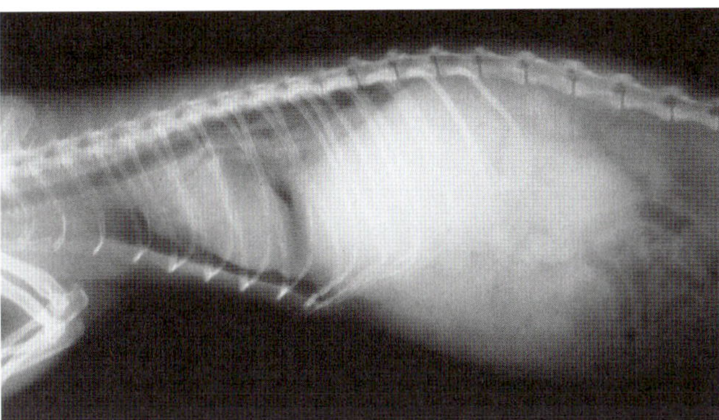

Figure 7.24 Lateral radiograph of the ferret in Figure 7.23 after the pleural effusion has been drained showing a precardiac mass which in this instance was due to a thymic lymphoma. *Source:* Reproduced with permission from the BSAVA Manual of Rodents and Ferrets (2009), Figure 19.07b © BSAVA.

mineralisation due to oversupplementation with calcium and vitamin D_3 can affect the primary vessels, and of course the kidneys.

Oesophagus

Megaoesophagus has been reported, but contrast studies using barium sulphate are often necessary to help define the oesophagus as it is not easily visible. A dose of 10–15 mL/kg orally is recommended and may be made more palatable by mixing it with a meat-based dog/cat food. Pollock (2007), however, describes that strawberry-flavoured barium sulphate is readily accepted by ferrets.

Abdominal cavity

Liver

The liver is normally completely covered by the caudal ribcage. Enlargement of the liver shadow has been associated with neoplasia (such as lymphoma, biliary cystadenoma, cholangiosarcoma and hepatocellular carcinoma), polycystic disease and infectious disease such as mycobacteriosis (Saunders and Thomsen, 2006).

Stomach and intestines

The stomach is on the left side dorsoventrally and immediately behind the dorsal part of the liver shadow on the lateral view. The cranial border of the stomach in a ventrodorsal radiograph extends to the 13th thoracic vertebra (Evans and An, 1998). Normally, the stomach has only small amounts of gas present and no food material (unless the ferret has eaten in the last 1–2 hours). Gastric bloat can be seen in recently weaned ferrets and can produce large amounts of gas (Fox, 1988). Other causes of gas in the stomach are usually due to ulceration of the stomach (e.g. foreign bodies, neoplasia and *Helicobacter mustelae* infections) or small intestinal foreign bodies (see Figure 7.25).

The small intestine is much the same diameter throughout. There is no caecum.

Thickening of the small intestine may be seen due to neoplasia such as malignant lymphoma and to inflammatory disease such as proliferative ileitis caused by the bacterium *Lawsonia intracellularis*. Alternatively, it may be more diffuse as in eosinophilic enteritis and inflammatory bowel disease.

Spleen

As mentioned, the normal spleen may appear relatively large in the ferret and so radiographic interpretation of disease in the spleen may be difficult. Gross splenic enlargement may occur due to neoplasia such as lymphoma (see Figure 7.25) or haemangiosarcomas.

Kidneys

The right kidney is in front of the left as in other mammals. Renal cysts are commonly seen in ferrets, although the genetically inherited polycystic kidney disease is less common (Orcutt, 2003).

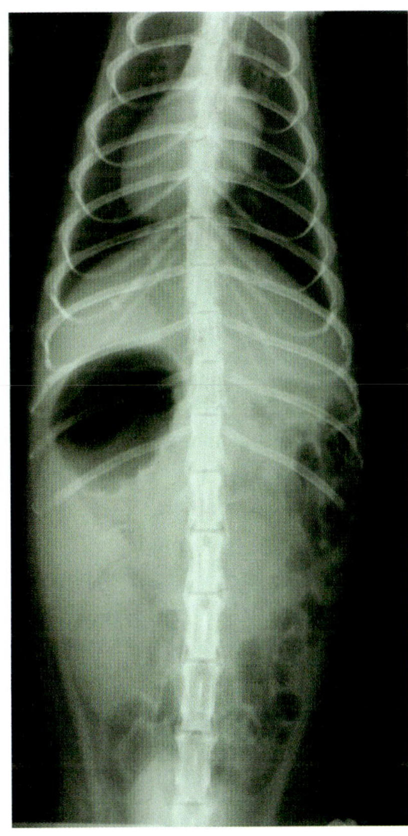

Figure 7.25 Dorsoventral view of the abdomen of a ferret. Note the gas in the stomach and small intestines and the enlarged spleen on the left side immediately caudal to the stomach. This was a case of splenic and gastrointestinal lymphoma.

Urinary bladder

Urolithiasis is common in ferrets and stones may be seen in the distal urethra in males due to the presence of the J-shaped os penis.

Reproductive organs

The male ferret possesses a prostate which is at the neck of the urinary bladder and may be affected by adrenal gland neoplasia with the production of considerable cysts. The os penis is curved in the shape of the letter 'J'.

Radiography may of course be used to detect gravidity in the female – skeletal development occurs around day 29–30.

Contrast radiography of the gastrointestinal tract

The period of fasting for ferrets prior to radiography is around 3–4 hours – longer than this can cause problems, particularly in older ferrets that can be affected by insulinomas. Positive contrast using barium sulphate mixed with meat-based food or strawberry-flavoured barium at 10–15 mL/kg. In cases of stomach/intestine perforation, iodine-based products, for example iohexol, can be used. These should be diluted 1 : 1 with tap water and this mixture then administered at a rate of 10–15 mL/kg orally or by stomach tube (Pollock, 2007).

Complete gastric emptying varies from 75 ± 54 minutes in conscious ferrets to 130 ± 40 minutes in ferrets sedated with ketamine and diazepam (Schwarz *et al.*, 2003). Normally, small intestinal width should not exceed 5–7 mm.

Contrast radiography of the urinary tract

After anaesthesia, catheterisation of the female ferret's bladder is possible but difficult, with the urethral opening positioned approximately 1 cm cranial to the clitoris on the ventral floor of the vestibule. The male ferret is more challenging due to the J-shaped os penis and the small diameter of the urethra. Orcutt (2003) suggests using a 22-gauge, 8-inch jugular catheter to catheterise male ferrets. However, if severe paraurethral/prostatic disease is present, the pressure on the urethra may still prevent passage of a catheter.

Pyelograms may be performed using non-ionic iodine-containing media (e.g. iohexol) at a dose of 720 mg/kg intravenously via a peripheral vein (Orcutt, 2003). Non-ionic iodine medium is preferable to ionic as it does not induce osmotic diuresis so making contrast studies clearer, and it induces less side-effects. The cephalic vein is perhaps the most easily accessed vessel.

Head

Dental disease is common and bisecting angle radiography as used in cats and dogs can help in the detection of periodontal disease and abscess formation.

Benign neoplasia of the skull such as osteomas have been described (Dernell *et al.*, 2001). However, more aggressive neoplasia has also been described, including squamous cell carcinomas of the gums which may invade underlying bone producing radiolucent bony changes on radiography (De Voe *et al.*, 2002).

Axial and appendicular skeleton

The vertebral formula of the adult ferret is C7, T14–15, L5–7, S3, Cd18, and the dental formula is I 3/3 C 1/1 Pm 3/3 M 1/2. The growth plates, particularly in the pelvis and long bones, do not often close until the ferret is more than 7 months of age.

Spinal lesions are frequently reported in ferrets due to traumatic injuries causing vertebral disc collapse. More commonly vertebral body fractures and neoplastic processes are seen (Ritzman and Knapp, 2002).

Chordoma, a tumour of the spinal cord, affects the end of the spine but may also affect the cervical area (Li and Fox, 1998). Other neoplasms affecting the spine in ferrets include lymphoma and plasma cell myeloma, both of which can metastasise and produce lytic bony lesions (Li and Fox, 1998).

ULTRASONOGRAPHY

Physical/chemical restraint and positioning

A right lateral position, using a cut-out imaging window in the table underneath the patient, is useful for the examination of the heart and kidneys, but it can be stressful to some patients and generally requires prior sedation or anaesthesia.

A standing position is often better tolerated in the conscious tractable patient and allows easier access to organs such as the liver which sits underneath the ribcage.

Equipment for small mammals

Ultrasound unit

A sector probe transducer is preferred due to its smaller footprint. This is particularly important if trying to image the heart due to the narrow inter-rib spaces. For imaging structures such as the eye 10-MHz probes may be useful; otherwise 7.5-MHz probes are suitable. B-mode ultrasound is mainly used to provide a two-dimensional real-time image of the organs being examined. M mode is useful when examining the heart to assess its contractility. Pulsed wave Doppler techniques for assessing blood flow direction and the measurement of ejection volumes with continuous wave Doppler techniques are also extremely useful in assessing cardiac disease and may be used in the rabbit as with cats and dogs.

Additional equipment

The patient should be shaved and a coupling gel is applied a few minutes before imaging, as with any species, to allow it to soak into the outer layers of the skin. In some cases, a stand-off is required. Commercial stand-offs are superior to home-made ones as they do not create attenuation, resolution or distortion artefacts.

Rabbit ultrasound interpretation

Thorax

Echocardiography has been described in the rabbit (Tello de Meneses *et al.*, 1989; Marano *et al.*, 1997). Some injectable anaesthetics have an effect on cardiac function, particularly the alpha-2 drugs such as xylazine, medetomidine and dexmedetomidine (Marano *et al.*, 1997). Marini *et al.* (1999) used ultrasonography to demonstrate myocardial fibrosis associated with ketamine/xylazine anaesthesia in rabbits. Also, isoflurane, while having less of an effect on reducing myocardial contractility than halothane, can reduce contractility nonetheless.

Orcutt (2000) used echocardiography to show the problems associated with congestive heart failure. In addition, bacterial endocarditis and atherosclerosis and associated thrombi have also been demonstrated using ultrasound (Snyder *et al.*, 1976).

A prominent thymus and wide cranial mediastinum exist even in the adult rabbit and may be imaged through the heart.

Abdominal cavity

The urinary bladder is often used as an acoustic window to assess many of the caudal abdominal organs, such as the uterus and kidneys. However, calcium carbonate crystals may cause a scintillating snow-storm effect and reduce transmission of the ultrasound beam.

Examination of the liver, just caudal to the xiphoid, is straightforward. Hepatic lipidosis can be diagnosed as an increase in echogenicity. The gall bladder is easily seen.

The normal kidney outline and internal structure is similar to that seen in the cat, although rabbits are unipapillate (see Figure 7.26). A decrease in renal size plus irregular surface is commonly seen in cases of chronic damage caused by *Encephalitozoon cuniculi*.

Adenocarcinomas of the uterus may be demonstrated with ultrasound (see Figure 7.27), which can also be used for pregnancy diagnosis and the presence of pyometra. Venous aneurysms within the vagina may also be seen.

Ocular ultrasound

The eye may be imaged using a 10 MHz probe, preferably with a stand-off. It can be useful to check for lymphoma, ocular abscesses and uveitis lesions caused by lens rupture due to *Encephalitozoon cuniculi*. In addition, retrobulbar masses may be determined using ultrasonography (Redrobe, 2001).

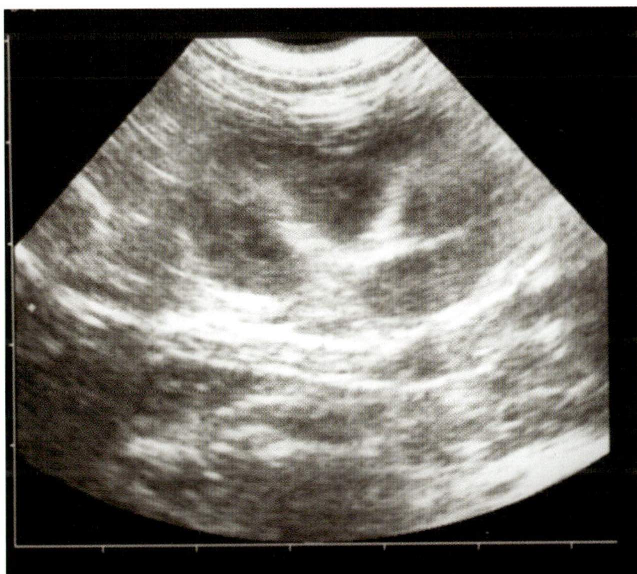

Figure 7.26 A normal rabbit kidney in longitudinal section.

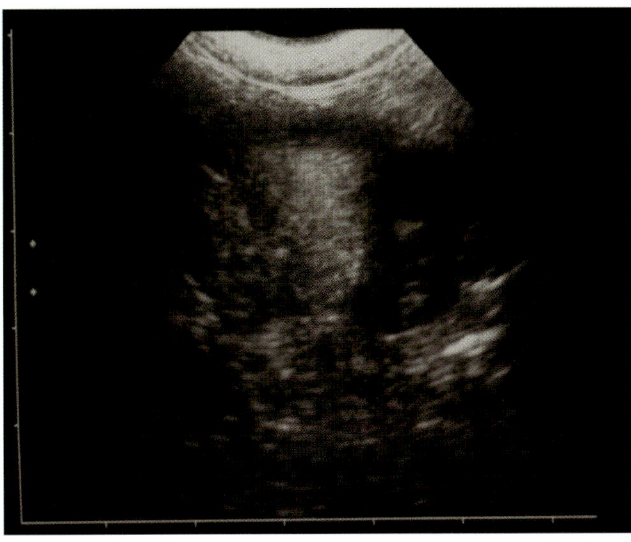

Figure 7.27 Uterine adenocarcinomas in the uterus of a rabbit.

Ferret ultrasound interpretation

Thoracic cavity

Numerous authors have reported M mode and Doppler echocardiography in the ferret (Stepien *et al.*, 2000; Vastenburg *et al.*, 2004). The pulmonary artery (rather than the aorta) was recommended for measurement of volume flow in ferrets due to the difficulty in aligning the aortic outflow tract (Stepien *et al.*, 2000). Vastenburg *et al.* (2004) showed that mitral/pulmonary valve regurgitation was often not significant.

Dilated cardiomyopathy and less commonly hypertrophic cardiomyopathy have been reported in ferrets. Valvular insufficiency is increasingly commonly diagnosed in older ferrets. Aortic regurgitation is a common incidental finding in ferrets with little significance (Petrie and Morrisey, 2004).

Dirofilaria immitis heartworm produces typically a right-sided heart failure with enlargement of the right ventricle, right atrium and caudal vena cava on echocardiography. The adult worms may be seen in the right ventricle, right atrium and pulmonary artery.

Abdominal cavity

Adrenal glands

Adrenal neoplasia has been detected using ultrasound. Average normal adrenal lengths vary from 5 to 13 mm and widths from 2 to 5 mm (Neuwirth *et al.*, 1997) (see Figure 7.28).

Kidneys

About 10–15% of ferrets undergoing a post-mortem report had a coincidental renal cyst (Orcutt, 2003). Polycystic disease including polycystic kidneys is unusual in ferrets and is differentiated from renal cysts by the presence of multiple irregular cysts in the kidneys and often the liver (Puerto *et al.*, 1998).

Spleen

The spleen can be one of the initial sites, along with the thymus and liver, for juvenile lymphoblastic leukaemia and haemangiosarcomas and so may show increased echogenicity and overall size.

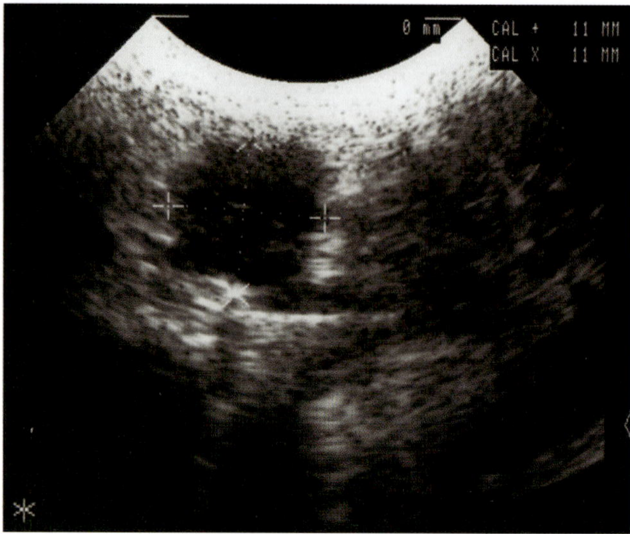

Figure 7.28 Right adrenal gland of a ferret with an adenocarcinoma starting to invade the caudal vena cava.

Liver

Neoplasia of the liver is common in the ferret and includes juvenile lymphoblastic leukaemia, biliary cystadenoma, cholangiosarcoma and hepatocellular carcinoma. The normal liver has six lobes and a gall bladder. Cholecystitis and gallstones have been reported in ferrets (see Figure 7.29).

Pancreas

Insulinomas are very small (1–2 mm) and so are often missed on ultrasound examination.

Intestines

Focal thickening of the ileum caused by the bacterium *Lawsonia intracellularis* and lymphoma which may affect the whole intestine may be seen on ultrasound. *Lawsonia intracellularis* tends to be associated with ileal thickening, while lymphoma can produce patchy focal intestinal thickening. More diffuse areas, as in eosinophilic enteritis and inflammatory bowel disease with hyperechoic areas of gas, may also be seen.

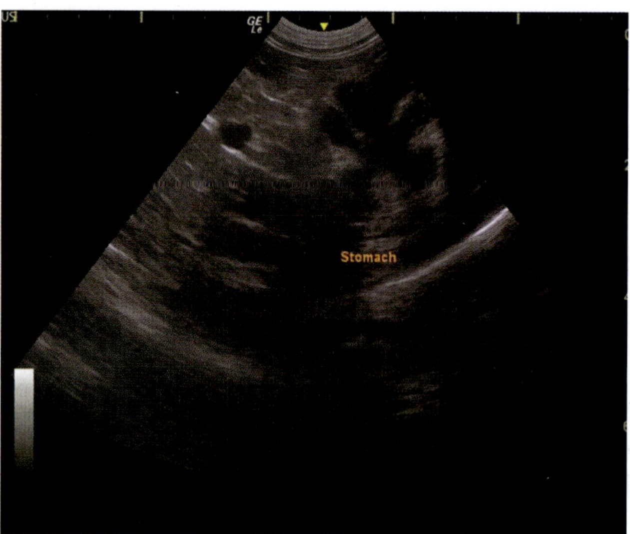

Figure 7.29 Ultrasound image of the liver, stomach and hypoechoic gall bladder of a normal healthy ferret.

Urinary bladder

Urolithiasis is common and may result in cystitis and bladder wall thickening. Paraurethral cysts are common in hyperadrenocorticism (adrenal gland disease) and may be seen in both sexes. Neoplasia is uncommon but has been reported.

Prostate

The prostate is bilobed in the male ferret and sits at the neck of the urinary bladder. Hyperadrenocorticism is associated with the enlargement of the prostate and the development of large cysts, which are easily detectable using ultrasound.

Uterus

The diameter of the non-gravid uterine body has been quoted as 1.1–2.5 mm (An and Evans, 1988). Gravidity, cystic and neoplastic endometrial changes and pyometras may all be diagnosed with ultrasound. It may also be used to detect uterine stump hypertrophy in previously spayed ferrets suffering from hyperadrenocorticism.

Mesenteric lymph node

The mesenteric lymph node, situated at the junction of the cranial and caudal mesenteric veins, may be mistaken for one of the adrenal glands, but its mobile and more ventral position should aid in differentiation. A technique to allow fine-needle aspiration cytology of the mesenteric lymph node as an aid to diagnosing lymphoma has been described in the ferret (Paul-Murphy *et al.*, 1999).

Other organs

Ocular ultrasonography has been recorded. A 10-MHz transducer is required in B mode due to the short focal distances involved. However, despite this, a considerable amount of contact gel is required as a stand-off pad to avoid near-field artefacts. Normal values for the eye have been determined (Hernandez-Guerra *et al.*, 2007).

Other small mammal ultrasound interpretation

A 7.5-MHz probe is usually required. A stand-off may also be useful.

Cardiac disease, common in marsupials, chinchillas and guinea pigs, as well as hamsters and hedgehogs, may be interpreted using ultrasonography using principles described above for rabbits.

Pregnancy diagnosis may be made easily in hystricomorphs using ultrasonography and it is an extremely useful tool for confirming the presence of cystic ovarian disease in guinea pigs, hamsters and gerbils where it is most commonly seen.

Uterine neoplasia is commonly seen in African pygmy hedgehogs and pyometra and endometritis may be observed a variety of rodents, all of which lend themselves to diagnosis by abdominal ultrasound.

In addition, renal structure may be examined where cystic disease of chronic failure and atrophy is suspected. Urolithiasis and cystitis may be assessed by ultrasound in rodents such as guinea pigs and chinchillas.

MRI AND CT SCANNING OF SMALL MAMMALS

These techniques are becoming more commonplace in rabbits and small mammals.

Computed tomography (CT) scanning creates a cross-sectional image of the patient and is particularly good for assessing bony changes such as that seen with advanced dental disease, as has been suggested in chinchillas (Crossley *et al.*, 1998), other rodents and rabbits (see Figure 7.30). In addition, other conditions affecting the head, such as neoplasms, sclerosis of the middle ear and turbinate atrophy and infection, are ideally suited to this modality. Soft tissues can also be imaged by CT and several studies looking at gastrointestinal and liver disease, particularly in rabbits, have been published (Longo *et al.*, 2018; Daggett *et al.*, 2021) (see Figure 7.31). Other radiodense objects that show up well on CT images include uroliths and renoliths (see Figure 7.32). Anaesthesia must be used as the patient must be completely immobile while a rotating X-ray beam images the patient in segments.

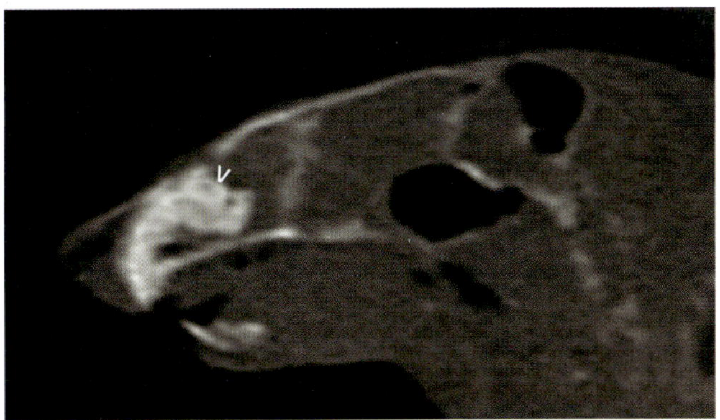

Figure 7.30 Longitudinal CT scan of a gerbil head with a pseudo-odontoma of the maxillary incisor resulting in nasal obstruction identified by the white arrowhead. *Source:* Courtesy of Tobias Schwarz, University of Edinburgh.

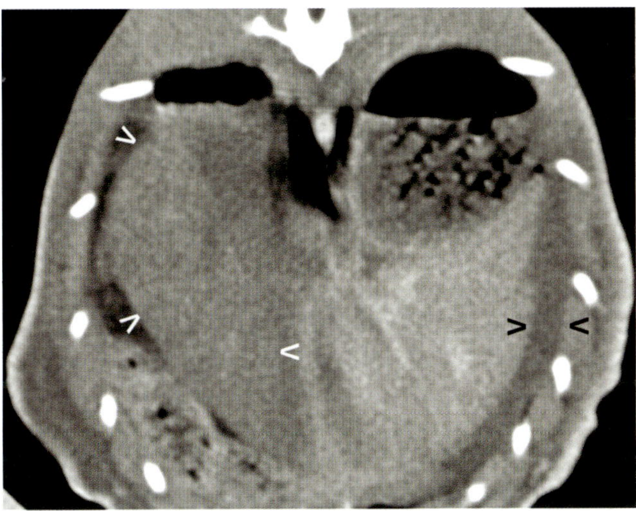

Figure 7.31 Post-intravenous contrast CT image of the liver in a rabbit presenting for anorexia. The right medial liver lobe (white arrowheads) is poorly contrast-enhancing (darker) than the normal left liver lobes and there is perihepatic effusion (black arrowheads). This is a typical feature of liver lobe torsion, a relatively common condition in rabbits. *Source:* Courtesy of Tobias Schwarz, University of Edinburgh.

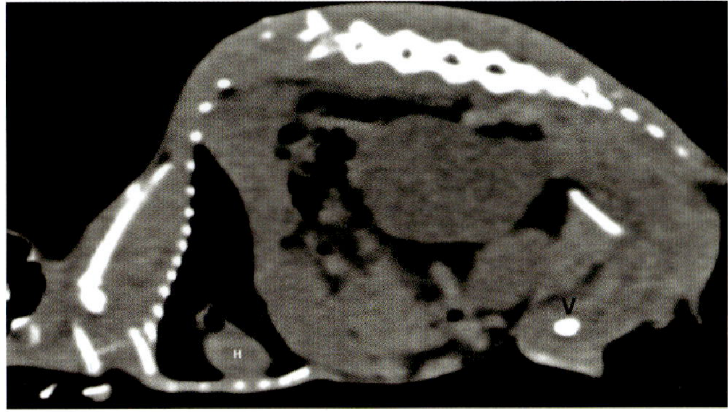

Figure 7.32 Longitudinal CT scan of a chinchilla. The head is to the left and off the image, the heart clearly identified in the radiolucent (black) thorax with a white 'H'. A urethral urolith is identified by the black arrowhead. *Source:* Courtesy of Tobias Schwarz, University of Edinburgh.

Magnetic resonance imaging (MRI) is more useful for assessing soft tissue structures, such as aneurysms, tumours and organ enlargement. It also requires the patient to be anaesthetised and completely immobile. Lesions in organs such as the brain make ideal candidates for MRI, although spinal abscesses (Runge *et al.*, 1998) and pyelonephritis (Runge *et al.*, 1997) have been assessed in the rabbit using MRI.

References

An, N.Q. and Evans, H.E. (1988) Anatomy of the ferret. In: *Biology and Diseases of the Ferret* (ed. G.J. Fox), 1st edn, pp. 15–65. Lea and Febiger, Philadelphia, PA.

Black, P.A., Marshall, C., Seyfried, A.W. and Bartin, A.M. (2011) Cardiac assessment of African hedgehogs (*Atelerix albiventris*). *Journal of Zoo and Wildlife Medicine*, **42**(1), 49–53.

Clippinger, T.L., Bennett, R.A., Alleman, A.R. *et al.* (1998) Removal of a thymoma via median sternotomy in a rabbit with recurrent appendicular neurofibrosarcoma. *Journal of the American Veterinary Medical Association*, **213**, 1140–1143.

Crossley, D.A., Jackson, A., Yates, J. and Boydell, I.P. (1998) Use of computed tomography to investigate cheek tooth abnormalities in chinchillas (*Chinchilla lanigera*). *Journal of Small Animal Practice*, **39**, 385–389.

Daggett, A., Loeber, S., Le Roux, A.B. *et al.* (2021) Computed tomography with Hounsfield unit assessment is useful in the diagnosis of liver lobe torsion in pet rabbits (*Oryctolagus cuniculus*). *Veterinary Radiology and Ultrasound*, **62**(2), 210–217.

De Voe, R.S., Pack, L. and Greenacre, C.B. (2002) Radiographic and CT imaging of a skull associated osteoma in a ferret. *Veterinary Radiology and Ultrasound*, **43**(4), 346–348.

Dernell, W.S., Straw, R.C. and Withrow, S.J. (2001) Tumors of the skeletal system. In: *Small Animal Clinical Oncology* (eds S.J. Withrow & E.G. MacEwen), 3rd edn, pp. 406–454. WB Saunders, Philadelphia, PA.

DeSanto, J. (1997) Hypertrophic osteopathy associated with an intrathoracic neoplasm in a rabbit. *Journal of the American Veterinary Medical Association*, **210**, 1322–1323.

Dias, S., Anselmi, C., Espada, Y. and Martorell, J. (2021) Vertebral heart score to evaluate cardiac size in thoracic radiographs of 124 healthy rats (*Rattus norvegicus*). *Veterinary Radiology and Ultrasound*, **62**(4), 394–401.

Doss, G.A., Mans, C., Hoey, S. *et al.* (2017) Vertebral heart size in chinchillas (*Chinchilla lanigera*) using radiography and CT. *Journal of Small Animal Practice*, **58**(12), 714–719.

Evans, H.E. and An, N.Q. (1998) Anatomy of the ferret. In: *Biology and Diseases of the Ferret* (ed. J.G. Fox), 2nd edn, pp. 19–70. Williams and Wilkins, Baltimore, MD.

Fox, J.G. (1988) Systemic diseases. In: *Biology and Diseases of the Ferret* (ed. J.G. Fox), pp. 258–259. Lea and Febiger, Philadelphia, PA.

Fraser, M.A. and Girling, S.J. (2009) *Rabbit Medicine and Surgery for Veterinary Nurses*. Blackwell-Wiley, Oxford.

Garcia, E.B., Eshar, D., Thomason, J.D. *et al.* (2016) Cardiac assessment of zoo-kept, black-tailed prairie dogs (*Cynomys ludovicianus*) anesthetized with isoflurane. *Journal of Zoo and Wildlife Medicine*, **47**(4), 955–962. doi: 10.1638/2014-0241.1.

Girling, S.J. (2002) Mammalian imaging and anatomy. In: *Manual of Exotic Pets* (eds A. Meredith & S. Redrobe), 4th edn, pp. 1–12. BSAVA, Quedgeley, UK.

Green, P.W., Fox, R.R. and Sokoloff, L. (1984) Spontaneous degenerative spinal disease in the laboratory rabbit. *Journal of Orthopaedic Research*, **2**, 161–168.

Harrenstein, L. (1999) Gastrointestinal diseases of pet rabbits. *Seminars in Avian and Exotic Pet Medicine*, **8**, 83–99.

Hernandez-Guerra, A.M., Rodilla, V. and Lopez-Murcia, M.M. (2007) Ocular biometry in the adult anesthetized ferret (*Mustela putorius furo*). *Veterinary Ophthalmology*, **10**(1), 50–52.

Kozma, C., Macklin, W., Cummins, L.M. and Mauer, R. (1974) The anatomy, physiology and biochemistry of the rabbit. In: *The Biology of the Laboratory Rabbit* (eds S.H. Weisbroth, R.E. Flatt & A.L. Kraus), pp. 50–69. Academic Press, London.

Li, X. and Fox, J.G. (1998) Neoplastic diseases. In: *Biology and Diseases of the Ferret* (ed. J.G. Fox), 2nd edn, pp. 405–447. Williams and Wilkins, Baltimore, MD.

Longley, L. (2005) Epidural catheterisation in rabbits. *Proceedings of the British Veterinary Zoological Society Spring Meeting*, Chester, UK, pp. 56–57.

Longo, M., Thierry, F., Eatwell, K. *et al.* (2018) Ultrasound and computed tomography of sacculitis and appendicitis in a rabbit. *Veterinary Radiology and Ultrasound*, **59**(5), E56–E60.

Marano, G., Formigari, R., Grigioni, M. and Vergari, A. (1997) Effects of isoflurane versus halothane on myocardial contractility in rabbits: assessment with transthoracic two-dimensional echocardiography. *Laboratory Animal Science*, **31**, 144–150.

Marini, R.P., Li, X., Harpster, N.K. and Dangler, C. (1999) Cardiovascular pathology possibly associated with ketamine/xylazine anesthesia in Dutch belted rabbits. *Laboratory Animal Science*, **49**, 153–160.

Masoudifard, M., Rostami, A., Nodolaghi, M.S. *et al.* (2021) Development and evaluation of methods for vertebral heart score determination in guinea pig (*Cavia porcellus*). *Veterinary Research Forum*, **12**(3), 357–360. doi: 10.30466/vrf.2020.108629.2580.

Neuwirth, L., Collins, B. and Calderwood-Mays, M. (1997) Adrenal ultrasonography correlated with histopathology in ferrets. *Veterinary Radiology and Ultrasound*, **38**(1), 69–74.

Onuma, M., Ono, S., Ishida, T. *et al.* (2010) Radiographic measurement of cardiac size in 27 rabbits. *Journal of Veterinary Medical Science*, **72**(4), 529–531.

Orcutt, C.J. (2000) Cardiac and respiratory disease in rabbits. *Proceedings of the British Veterinary Zoological Society Autumn Meeting*, Royal Veterinary College, London, pp. 68–73.

Orcutt, C.J. (2003) Ferret urogenital diseases. *Veterinary Clinics of North America: Exotic Animal Practice*, **6**(1), 113–138.

Orcutt, C.J. (1998) Emergency and critical care of ferrets. *Veterinary Clinics of North America: Exotic Animal Practice*, **1**(1), 99–126.

Paul-Murphy, J., O'Brien, T., Spaeth, A. *et al.* (1999) Ultrasonography and fine needle aspirate cytology of the mesenteric lymph node in normal domestic ferrets (*Mustela putorius furo*). *Veterinary Radiology and Ultrasound*, **40**(3), 308–310.

Petrie, J.-P. and Morrisey, J.K. (2004) Cardiovascular and other diseases. In: *Ferrets, Rabbits and Rodents: Clinical Medicine and Surgery* (eds K.E. Quesenberry & J.W. Carpenter), pp. 58–71. Philadelphia, PA, WB Saunders.

Pickard, D.W. and Stevens, C.E. (1972) Digesta flow through the rabbit large intestine. *American Journal of Physiology*, **222**, 1161–1166.

Pollock, C. (2007) Emergency medicine of the ferret. *Veterinary Clinics of North America: Exotic Animal Practice*, **10**(2), 463–500.

Puerto, D.A., Walker, L.M. and Saunders, M. (1998) Bilateral perinephric pseudocysts and polycystic kidneys in the ferret. *Veterinary Radiology and Ultrasound*, **39**(4), 309–312.

Redrobe, S. (2001) Imaging small mammals. *Seminars in Avian and Exotic Pet Medicine*, **10**, 187–197.

Ritzman, T.K. and Knapp, D. (2002) Ferret orthopedics. *Veterinary Clinics of North America: Exotic Animal Practice*, **5**(1), 129–155.

Runge, V.M., Timoney, J.F. and Williams, N.M. (1997) Magnetic resonance imaging of experimental pyelonephritis in rabbits. *Investigative Radiology*, **32**, 696–701.

Runge, V.M., Williams, N.M., Lee, C. and Timoney, J.F. (1998) MRI imaging in a spinal abscess model: preliminary report. *Investigative Radiology*, **33**, 246–255.

Saunders, G.K. and Thomsen, B.V. (2006) Lymphoma and *Mycobacterium avium* infection in a ferret (*Mustela putorius furo*). *Journal of Veterinary Diagnostic Investigation*, **18**(5), 513–515.

Schwarz, L.A., Solano, M., Manning, A. *et al.* (2003) The normal upper gastrointestinal examination in the ferret. *Veterinary Radiology and Ultrasound*, **44**(2), 165–172.

Shell, L.G. and Saunders, G. (1989) Arteriosclerosis in a rabbit. *Journal of the American Veterinary Medical Association*, **194**, 679–680.

Snyder, S.B., Fox, J.G., Campbell, L.H. and Soave, O.A. (1976) Disseminated staphylococcal disease in laboratory rabbits (*Oryctolagus cuniculus*). *Laboratory Animal Science*, **26**, 86–88.

Stepien, R.L., Benson, K.G. and Forrest, L.J. (1999) Radiographic measurement of cardiac size in normal ferrets. *Veterinary Radiology and Ultrasound*, **40**(6), 606–610.

Stepien, R.L., Benson, K.G. and Wenholz, L.J. (2000) M-mode and Doppler echocardiographic findings in normal ferrets sedated with ketamine hydrochloride and midazolam. *Veterinary Radiology and Ultrasound*, **41**(5), 452–456.

Supakorndej, P., Lewis, R.E. and McCall, J.W. (1995) Radiographic and angiographic evaluations of ferrets experimentally infected with *Dirofilaria immitis*. *Veterinary Radiology and Ultrasound*, **36**(1), 23–29.

Tello de Meneses, R., Mesa, M.D. and Gonzalez, V. (1989) Echocardiographic assessment of cardiac function in the rabbit: a preliminary study. *Annals of Veterinary Research*, **20**, 175–185.

Vastenburg, M.H.A.C., Boroffka, S.A.E.B. and Schoemaker, N.J. (2004) Echocardiographic measurements in clinically healthy ferrets anesthetized with isoflurane. *Veterinary Radiology and Ultrasound*, **45**(3), 228–232.

Weisbroth, S.H. and Hurwitz, A. (1969) Spontaneous osteogenic sarcoma in *Oryctolagus cuniculus* with elevated serum alkaline phosphatase. *Laboratory Animal Care*, **19**, 263–265.

Chapter 8 Small Mammal Emergency and Critical Care Medicine

RABBIT EMERGENCY AND CRITICAL CARE MEDICINE

Introduction

Rabbit emergency and critical care medicine is a rapidly changing discipline, but its need has remained constant. A review of veterinary resuscitation therapy has been carried out for domestic pets such as the cat and dog but so far little review of exotic pets has been done. However, the principles of the RECOVER algorithm, utilised in dog and cat medicine, are broadly applicable to small mammals (Fletcher *et al.*, 2012).

As with other small mammals, emergency therapy in the rabbit should initially follow the 'ABC' (Airway, Breathing and Circulation) protocol already adopted for cats and dogs when the heart is working. However, CAB should be the sequence where cardiac arrest has occurred because the bloodstream in acute cases has sufficient oxygen to keep organs functioning providing the circulation persists. It should be noted that the drugs listed later in this chapter, unless stated otherwise, are not specifically licensed for use in rabbits in the majority of countries worldwide.

Emergency airway access and ventilation (A and B)

Should breathing stop, or hypoxia be detected, then emergency ventilation will be required. This is best achieved by immediate endotracheal (ET) intubation.

Intubation may be achieved blindly, with the rabbit in sternal recumbency. The rabbit's head is lifted and the ET tube is advanced slowly until breathing sounds are heard through the tube. The tube may then be quickly advanced on inspiration. If a transparent tube is used, then condensation from the rabbit's breath when the tube is over the glottis can be seen, aiding intubation. If the rabbit has stopped breathing, then this technique becomes extremely difficult; therefore, a laryngoscope with a Wisconsin 0 paediatric blade or equivalent can be used to visualise the glottis (Heard, 2004). This is best achieved with the rabbit in dorsal recumbency and the tongue pulled laterally. A guide wire may be inserted through the glottis first and the ET tube threaded over the top. Alternatively, a fine endoscope or needlescope may be used as a guide wire instead, threading the ET over the scope prior to intubation. Once through the glottis, the ET tube may be advanced and the scope retracted easily.

An alternative access to the airway in the rabbit is a supraglottal device, also known as a laryngeal mask, a technique used in paediatric human medicine and now adapted for pet small animals such as cats and rabbits. A number of devices are available but one specifically designed for the rabbit is the **v-gel**® Advanced Rabbit (Docsinnovent; www.docsinnovent.com) which comes in six sizes to cope with the wide range of rabbit breeds. The device is similar to an ET tube, having a luer adaptor to connect to an anaesthetic circuit. The distal end, rather than being inserted through the glottis into the trachea, instead sits above the glottis where an inflatable cuff creates a seal and a bung that, when inserted, is distal to the glottis and plugs the oesophagus to prevent air from entering it and inflating the stomach.

Direct intubation or laryngeal masks may be difficult in the rabbit owing to the narrow oral cavity and relatively large size of the tongue caudally or to the presence of an obstruction such as a pharyngeal abscess or foreign body. In an emergency therefore it may be necessary to pass a long through-the-needle catheter into the tracheal lumen between two tracheal rings ventrally. A luer adaptor may be attached to allow connection to an anaesthetic circuit for oxygen administration. A tracheostomy may also be performed in the same way as for a cat or dog. The main difference is that some breeds of rabbit, particularly the doe, have large dew flaps with plentiful subcutaneous fat deposits which may make tracheostomy surgery challenging. Otherwise see the procedure below.

1. The fur is clipped over the ventral neck and the skin quickly prepared with surface antiseptic solution.
2. A longitudinal incision is made in the skin over the trachea caudal to the larynx, followed by blunt dissection through the limited overlying tissues onto the trachea itself.
3. A 180° ventral incision is made between the tracheal rings 3–4 below the larynx.
4. The ET tube is inserted.
5. The ET tube is connected to an anaesthetic circuit (see Figures 8.1 and 8.2).

If intubation is not possible, then either a tight-fitting face mask connected to an anaesthetic circuit may be applied with a high flow rate of oxygen (4–5 L/min), or an Ambu bag can be used to force ventilate the rabbit. Alternatively, moving the rabbit in a see-saw manner may aid ventilation by moving the abdominal viscera backwards and forwards onto the diaphragm thus acting as a pump mechanism (Briscoe and Syring, 2004). This works on the basis that most of the impetus for inspiration comes from the flattening of the diaphragm rather than the outward movement of the ribcage.

Respiration rates typically should be around 10 breaths per minute if resuscitating, and a rough rule of thumb is to assume 10 mL/kg body weight for tidal volume (Fletcher *et al.*, 2012).

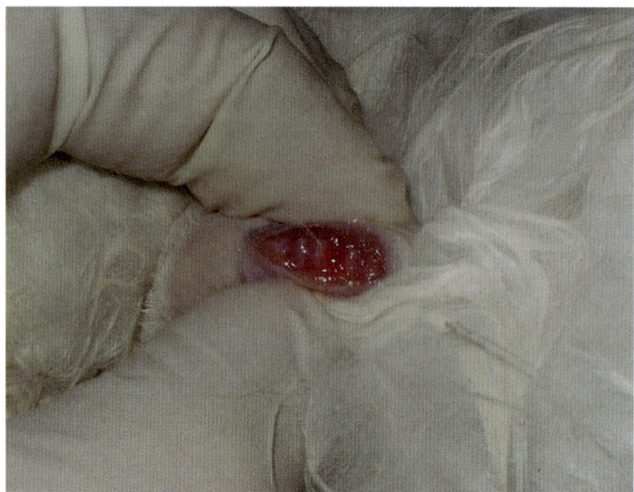

Figure 8.1 Ventral neck of a rabbit with the skin and muscles cut down on to the trachea that has been incised between cartilage rings to allow insertion of the tracheostomy tube.

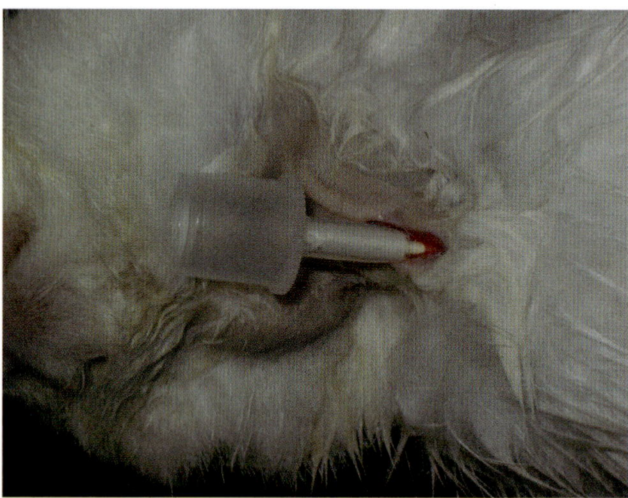

Figure 8.2 Endotracheal tube inserted through the incision created in Figure 8.1 that can now be connected to an anaesthetic circuit and oxygen.

Cardiovascular support (C) and drugs (D)

In mammals under 10 kg, direct cardiac massage by compressing the chest directly over the heart is most effective at increasing thoracic pressure and forcing blood through the arterial vasculature (Henrik, 1992). Heart compression rates of 100 beats per minute need to be achieved in rabbits; the technique recommended for maximising cardiovascular output is circumferential chest compression, as is used in human infants, where the chest is compressed over the heart from both sides at once (Costello, 2004) (see Figure 8.3).

If a cardiac beat is present or a beat is restarted, ECG leads should be applied to discern any dysrhythmias. The type of dysrhythmia reported in rabbits during resuscitation techniques has thus far been different from that reported in cats and dogs. The latter have been associated with electromechanical dissociation, whereas in rabbits profound bradycardia, ventricular asystole and ventricular fibrillation have been reported (Rush and Wingfield, 1992). Adrenaline may be used intratracheally if intubated, or intravenously if no cardiac beat is detected and there is no ECG trace. Adrenaline may be more effective if given by intracardiac injection but the rabbit heart is a small target lying between ribs 4 and 6 and it may be difficult to administer adrenaline directly into the ventricular lumen where it needs to be. In the case of fine ventricular fibrillation, the use of adrenaline has been advocated to convert the electrical activity to coarse ventricular fibrillation which is easier to convert (see Table 8.1 for dosages) (DeFrancesco, 2000).

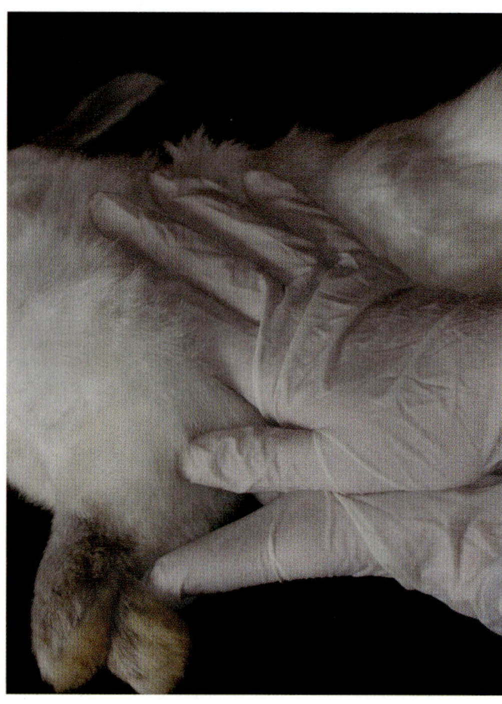

Figure 8.3 Circumferential chest compression is more effective than one-sided chest compression in small mammals.

Table 8.1 Emergency drugs used in rabbits.

Drug	Dosage and route
Adrenaline (1 : 1000 = 1 mg/mL formulation)	0.01 mg/kg IC 0.01–0.1 mg/kg IV, IT, IO NB: dilute to 1 : 10 000 before IV or IC use
Dexamethasone	2 mg/kg IV (use with caution as potentially immunosuppressive)
Diazepam	1–3 mg/kg IV, IM
Doxapram	2–5 mg/kg SC, IV, PO q 15 min
Fluids	100 mL/kg per day maintenance
Furosemide	1–4 mg/kg IV, SC, IM
Glycopyrrolate	0.02–0.1 mg/kg SC, IM 0.01 mg/kg IV
Lidocaine	1–2 mg/kg IV; 2–4 mg/kg IT
Midazolam	0.5–2 mg/kg IV, IM, IN

IV, intravenously; IM, intramuscularly; IO, intraosseously; SC, subcutaneously; IT, intratracheally; IN, intranasally; IC, intracardiac. *Sources:* Kottwitz and Kelleher (2003); Hawkins and Pascoe (2012).

Conversion of coarse fibrillation is based on the use of cardiac massage as described above, or if the clinic has access to defibrillation devices then the use of these externally at 2–10 J/kg (starting at low energies and increasing if no response is achieved) may be performed (Costello, 2004). Greater success is achieved with defibrillation devices if three initial countershocks are applied at low energies.

If severe bradycardia is detected, glycopyrrolate should be used (see Table 8.1) in preference to atropine as 40–60% of domestic rabbits possess serum atropinesterases making atropine ineffective in many cases (Okerman, 1994).

Lidocaine may be administered intratracheally or intravenously if ventricular arrhythmias such as ventricular premature complexes leading to ventricular tachycardia occur (see Table 8.1 for dose). However, lidocaine should not be used in cases of atrioventricular (AV) block or severe bradycardia (DeFrancesco, 2000), which is more commonly seen in rabbits.

Cardiomyopathy and valvular insufficiency with resultant congestive heart failure are also seen in rabbits as is atherosclerosis. Treatment of congestive heart failure initially depends on the use of diuretics such as furosemide at 1–4 mg/kg intravenously, repeated every 4–6 hours as required. Angiotensin converting enzyme (ACE) inhibitors have been used in rabbits but they are more susceptible to hypotensive side-effects than cats or dogs. Therefore, reduced dosages and regular monitoring of the systolic blood pressure using non-invasive techniques devised for cats are advisable (Girling, 2003).

Corticosteroids such as dexamethasone may be used where acute shock or acute central nervous system disease is present, although their usage is increasingly uncommon due to their side-effects (e.g. immunosuppression). However, one study has shown that corticosteroids may improve the chances of success when treating central nervous system disease (torticollis and seizures) in rabbits caused by *Encephalitozoon cuniculi* infection (in conjunction with fenbendazole) (Harcourt-Brown and Holloway, 2003).

It should also be noted that if the rabbit has been given any anaesthetic agents that can be reversed, then this should happen. Examples include atipamezole to reverse medetomidine/dexmedetomidine and naloxone to reverse opiates such as butorphanol and fentanyl.

Other supportive measures

Rabbits with hypothermia are significantly more likely to die on presentation with shock. One study suggested that hypothermic rabbits were three times more likely to die, with the chance of death doubled for each decrease of 1°C below a rabbit's normal temperature (37.9–39.9°C) and so in addition to fluid therapy to support blood pressure and perfusion, warming the patient using warmed fluids, hot air or water circulating blankets is also vital (Di Girolamo *et al.*, 2016).

Diagnostic procedures

ECG (E)

As mentioned above, should cardiac arrest or arrhythmias be detected, ECG leads may be applied as in cats and dogs and the trace assessed. See Table 8.2 for some normal values for rabbits.

Table 8.2 Normal ECG values (lead II) for healthy rabbits.

Parameter	Normal result	Notes
P wave height	0.1–0.15 mV	Deflection is low or negative in lead I and always positive in leads II and III
P wave duration	0.03–0.04 s	
PR interval	0.05–0.1 s	
QRS complex duration	0.015–0.04 s	
R wave amplitude	0.3–0.39 mV	
QT interval	0.08–0.16 s	Change of deflection of the T wave from positive to negative or vice versa indicates myocardial hypoxia as with cats and dogs

Sources: Kozma *et al.* (1974) and Huston and Quesenberry (2004).

Monitoring response to cardiopulmonary resuscitation

Re-evaluation of resuscitation should be made periodically but it is likely that such reassessments should allow at least 2 minutes of therapy to ensure sufficient time is given for a response (Fletcher *et al.*, 2012). Cycles of 2 minutes chest compression followed by reassessment are therefore logical when cardiac arrest has occurred.

Capnography is one of the most useful tools for determining response to cardiopulmonary resuscitation (CPR) and another reason for attempting intubation (or at least ensuring a tight-fitting face mask). End-tidal carbon dioxide ($ETCO_2$) levels may be used to monitor cardiac output during CPR. A steady increase in $ETCO_2$ is more likely to be associated with a successful outcome and, conversely, if the $ETCO_2$ does not increase above 10 mmHg after a resuscitation time of 15–20 minutes, then it is unlikely to be successful (Marino, 1997). In dogs and cats the RECOVER guidelines suggest an $ETCO_2$ capnography of 15 mmHg or more is indicative of good CPR responses (Fletcher *et al.*, 2012).

Blood gas assessment using point-of-care analysers has become commonplace in veterinary practice and can provide helpful physiological information on the critical care and emergency patient. Arterial blood has been used as the mainstay of assessment, although venous blood may be preferable for assessment of blood gases and pH as this more closely represents the status of body organs than arterial blood does. However, one study has cast doubt on the reliability of capnography and pulse oximetry as an assessment of respiratory function in the domestic rabbit, with no significant correlation between SpO_2 and arterial saturation of oxygen (SaO_2) or between $ETCO_2$ and arterial saturation of carbon dioxide $SaCO_2$ (Eatwell *et al.*, 2013). This study suggests that arterial blood gas analysis is more accurate, with ranges of arterial partial pressure of carbon dioxide ($PaCO_2$) of 25.29–40.37 mmHg and arterial partial pressure of oxygen (PaO_2) of 50.3–98.2 mmHg considered normal.

Acidosis is commonly seen in critical care rabbits and can be caused by either respiratory or metabolic reasons, both of which appear to be equally represented in the critical care rabbit (Ardiaca *et al.*, 2013). Compensatory respiratory alkalosis may also be seen in response to pain or initial metabolic acidosis but is uncommon as a primary disease.

HCO_3^- levels indicate the metabolic part of the acid–base balance, with low levels of HCO_3^- correlating with the metabolic acidosis commonly seen in shock scenarios. Elevated HCO_3^- levels suggest metabolic alkalosis, which has been associated with gastrointestinal stasis or blockage (specifically gastric). Loss of HCO_3^- can be seen with gastrointestinal and renal disease.

Blood lactate levels are commonly assessed in emergency situations in dogs and cats and may also be measured in rabbits. Levels above 10 mmol/L are viewed as abnormal, indicating anaerobic respiration associated with shock (Lichtenberger and Ko, 2007). However, lactate levels fluctuate routinely in the healthy rabbit, with elevations occurring normally during production of the hard faecal pellet and falling during caecotroph production, showing alignment with microbe metabolism in the gut. Total lactate levels are typically measured by point-of-care analysers and again may be misleading as total lactate is a combination of both D-lactate (produced by microbes in the gut) and L-lactate (produced by ischaemic muscle and tissue injury). D-Lactate levels can also be elevated with intestinal obstruction. Normal published values of D-lactate in the rabbit are 0.17 ± 0.07 mmol/L (Langlois *et al.*, 2014).

Hyperglycaemia has been shown to be strongly correlated with stress and levels above 25 mmol/L have been associated with obstructive intestinal disease requiring surgical intervention (Harcourt-Brown and Harcourt-Brown, 2012).

Blood sodium levels below 129 mEq/L have been associated with a 2.3 times increase in the rates of mortality in clinically unwell rabbits (Bonvehi *et al.*, 2014). This is, as with other mammals, commonly associated with hyperglycaemia, as glucose and sodium act in synergy to maintain the tonicity of the blood. It is therefore important to measure sodium plasma levels, but measurement of the overall tonicity is also important in order to differentiate true hyponatraemia from pseudohyponatraemia.

Routine haematology and biochemistry measurements will allow assessment of overall body organ function and should not be neglected in the critical care patient.

Radiography

This is essential where acute gastrointestinal signs are present, such as bloat or visceral pain, or where evidence of limb fractures, paresis or paralysis is present and should be performed when clinically safe to do so as part of a full clinical work-up. There is insufficient space in this chapter to go into detail regarding diagnostic imaging but the following conditions may be associated with radiographically visible changes.

Abdominal pain may be associated with a number of conditions, including renal calculi, obstructive and non-obstructive intestinal ileus and peritonitis. Spinal luxations, fractures and dislocations may also be identified radiographically. Gradation of severity may be made as with cats and dogs. Acute treatment with non-steroidal anti-inflammatory drugs (e.g. meloxicam) and other analgesics with immobilisation are advised for spinal trauma with concurrent paresis or paralysis as for other small mammals. Surgery may then be performed for collapsed discs or fractures as for cats and dogs as required.

Ultrasound

This may be of use where renal, bladder, cardiac and hepatic diseases are concerned. Cardiomyopathies (dilated) and atherosclerosis have been reported. Hepatic lipidosis is common in rabbits. Urinary bladders often contain large amounts of calcium salts forming a silt which creates a snow-storm effect on imaging.

Blood testing

Routine haematology and biochemistry assessments should be made – values may be found in standard rabbit textbooks. On a critical care level, blood lactate levels may also be measured in rabbits, with levels above 10 mmol/L being viewed as abnormal (Lichtenberger and Ko, 2007).

Fluid therapy (F)

Hypovolaemic shock

If the rabbit is dehydrated or hypovolaemic, shock doses of fluids should be administered. It should be noted that fluids should be avoided after resuscitation in cases of cardiovascular arrest where there is no hypovolaemia/dehydration prior to the arrest as these fluids may decrease myocardial perfusion pressures and diminish overall nutrient delivery through the cerebral and coronary vasculature (Cole *et al.*, 2002). Rabbits tend to more closely mimic cats in hypovolaemic shock, with the decompensatory stage being seen without compensatory shock, i.e. evidence of bradycardia, hypotension and hypothermia. In these cases a slow intravenous bolus of fluids such as hypertonic saline 7.2–7.5% at 3 mL/kg to draw fluid rapidly into the circulation is advised (Lichtenberger and Lennox, 2010). This can be maintained by follow-up administration of hetastarch (3 mL/kg) over 10 minutes. The patient should be warmed, and crystalloids at 3–4 mL/kg per hour should be administered. It is important to measure systolic blood pressure during this procedure. Once the rabbit has been warmed, the aim is to get the systolic blood pressure above 90 mmHg. This may require further boluses of isotonic crystalloids (10 mL/kg) with hetastarch (5 mL/kg). Once normovolaemia has been achieved, replacement of fluid deficits may be started (remember maintenance values for rabbits are 80–100 mL/kg per day).

Alternatively, a dopamine drip may be used in rabbits. Some studies have suggested that doses of 5–30 μg/kg per minute were not effective in reversing isoflurane-induced hypotension. However, I have used it at 10 μg/kg per minute with good effect in some critical care cases.

General fluid administration

Oral

This is not such a good route for seriously debilitated animals but is useful for those with naso-oesophageal feeding tubes in place, where the gastrointestinal tract is functioning normally. Again, it may be useful for mild cases of dehydration where owners wish to home treat their pet. This route though is restricted to small volumes with a maximum of 10 mL/kg at any one time administered. In practice it may be possible to administer much less than this.

Subcutaneous

The scruff area or lateral thorax make ideal sites. This is a good technique for routine postoperative administration of fluids for longer recovery patients undergoing minor surgical procedures such as neutering. It is possible to give a maximum of 30–60 mL at one time split into two or more sites depending on the size of rabbit.

Intraperitoneal

To perform this it is necessary to tilt the rabbit's head downwards whilst it is in dorsal recumbency to allow the gut contents to fall out of the injection zone. The needle is inserted in the caudal right quadrant of the ventral abdomen. It is inserted just through the abdominal wall and the syringe plunger drawn back to ensure that no puncture of the bladder or gut has occurred. A maximum volume of 20–30 mL may be given at one time depending on rabbit size. Previous notes regarding concurrent respiratory or cardiovascular disease should be considered. If positioned correctly, there should be no resistance to injection.

Intravenous

Venous access is relatively straightforward in the rabbit. The marginal ear vein, jugular vein, cephalic vein and lateral saphenous vein can all be used for intravenous catheter placement. Long-term (>2–3 days) use of the marginal ear vein may, however, cause sloughing of the ear tip, although in my experience this is relatively rare with careful venepuncture technique. Use of a topical local anaesthetic cream is recommended prior to placement. The jugular vein may be difficult to access, particularly in does where there is a pronounced ruff of skin and fat deposits. In addition, it forms the main venous drainage for the eye, and thrombus formation may lead to periocular and ocular swelling with potential for eye damage to occur. An Elizabethan collar can be used to prevent the rabbit from chewing or removing the catheter, although this will prevent caecotrophy and care should be taken to ensure the rabbit is still managing to eat, otherwise assisted feeding (see below) should be instituted.

Intraosseous

Intraosseous catheters may be placed into the proximal femur, in the trochanteric fossa, in a parallel direction to the long axis of the femur. An 18–23 gauge, 1–1.5-inch spinal or hypodermic needle is used. Analgesia should be employed (see Chapter 3) whenever placing an intraosseous catheter and antibiosis may also be required if the catheter site becomes infected.

Intraosseous and intravenous fluid administration should be accurately titrated using syringe drivers rather than relying on drip sets since even a small error in fluid administration may be proportionally more significant considering the small size of many rabbits.

Other medications and supportive nutrition

Many rabbits presented as an acute emergency either already have, or frequently go on to develop, gastrointestinal stasis. Providing obstructive causes have been ruled out, the use of prokinetic medications such as cisapride, metoclopramide and ranitidine is recommended (Table 8.3). Ranitidine also acts to reduce acidity in the stomach, which is beneficial as many rabbits with gastrointestinal stasis have punctate ulceration of the stomach lining. In humans it also has prokinetic effects that encourage emptying of the stomach and some increased motility of the small intestine, which seems to be synergised by metoclopramide; this appears clinically to be the case

Table 8.3 Gut motility-enhancing drugs for rabbits.

Drug	Dose rate	Frequency of dosing and notes
Cisapride	0.5 mg/kg PO	12 hourly
Metoclopramide	0.5 mg/kg SC	8–12 hourly
Ranitidine	2–5 mg/kg PO	12 hourly (in combination with metoclopramide acts to promote motility as well as reducing acidity)

Note that none are licensed for use in rabbits. PO, per os; SC, subcutaneously.

in rabbits in my and others' opinions. It is also important to control pain with adequate analgesia, as stimulation of pain receptors and the sympathetic nervous system will significantly affect gut motility. Some have therefore used drugs such as maropitant citrate (2 mg/kg subcutaneously every 24 hours) where visceral pain is present as well as more traditional analgesics (see Chapter 3 for more information).

Assisted feeding should be carried out in conjunction with the use of prokinetics. This can start off with easily absorbed essential sugars and amino acids either syringed into the mouth or delivered via a naso-oesophageal tube. As the rabbit improves clinically, this should be stepped up to use of proprietary critical feeding formulas. Several such formula foods exist on the market currently, for example Science Selective Recovery® and Science Selective RecoveryPlus® (Supreme Pet-foods); Critical Care for Herbivores® (Oxbow Pet Products); and Emeraid Intensive Care Herbivore® (Lafeber). In an emergency where access to such formulas is not possible, vegetable-based baby foods (lactose-free varieties) can be used. The disadvantage of baby foods is that they do not contain fibre and thus have little or no prokinetic activity, although they do provide nutrients in an easily digestible form.

The levels of energy required for a debilitated rabbit should approach that calculated for growing-to-lactating rabbits using the formula

$$\text{MER} = k \times (\text{body weight}\,[\text{kg}])^{0.75}$$

where $k = 200$ for growth and 300 for lactation (Carpenter and Kolmstetter, 2000). Therefore, for debilitation, the following daily energy requirement may be used:

$$\text{MER} = 250 \times (\text{weight}\,[\text{kg}])^{0.75}$$

To repopulate the intestinal flora, transfaunation of caecotrophs from a healthy rabbit may aid the return of normal bowel function. The use of commercial probiotics designed for rabbits has also been advocated and reduces the risk of transferring potential parasites and other agents to the debilitated patient.

Naso-oesophageal tube in rabbits

A naso-oesophageal tube is preferred by the author as the tubing ends in the distal oeosphagus (rather than a nasogastric tube which ends in the stomach) and so significantly reduces the reflux of acidic stomach contents into the oesophagus, thus reducing the likelihood of oesophagitis. It is placed after first spraying the nose with lidocaine spray and inserting the 3–4 French tube which has been premeasured from the extended nose to the seventh rib. Sterile water should be flushed through the tube before and after feeding to ensure it is correctly placed and does not become blocked. The tube may then be glued, taped or sutured to the dorsal aspect of the head and a bung inserted when not in use. It may be necessary to put an Elizabethan collar on the rabbit to prevent removal.

EMERGENCY CARE OF OTHER SMALL MAMMALS

Emergency airway access and ventilation (A and B)

Providing a direct airway may be very difficult in rodents. In ferrets and omnivorous marsupials, intubation is similar to that in small cats. In small rodents access to the epiglottis may be difficult owing to the nature of rodent anatomy, whereby the soft palate is frequently locked around the epiglottis which is pushed into the nasopharynx making its access via the mouth difficult. It may be possible to intubate using an otoscope or rigid endoscope to visualise the glottal opening.

If the rodent is still breathing, placement in a small container and piping in oxygen may be all that is necessary to ensure better oxygenation.

If the small mammal is not breathing and direct intubation per os is not possible, then any of the following three techniques may be attempted.

1. Massage the chest of the small mammal gently with two fingers on either side of the chest with the rodent in sternal recumbency whilst the head of the rodent is placed into a tight-fitting face mask with 100% oxygen.
2. Place the small mammal in dorsal recumbency, clip the fur over the ventral neck and briefly treat with antiseptic. Grasp the trachea between the fingers of one hand and make a small nick in the skin of over the trachea with a scalpel. Pass a 23–25 gauge over-the-needle catheter between two cartilage rings 1 cm caudal to the larynx. Remove the stylet and leave the catheter in place. This may then be used to administer intermittent positive pressure ventilation (IPPV) and 100% oxygen.
3. Place the small mammal in dorsal recumbency, clip the fur over the ventral neck and briefly treat with antiseptic. Make a skin incision over the trachea caudal to the larynx and bluntly dissect down onto the trachea as with the rabbit. The trachea may then be incised between cartilage rings to insert a tube.

For IPPV, a rate of 20–30 breaths per minute with a pressure of 8–10 cmH_2O may be applied.

Where a significant pleural effusion is present (such as may occur with congestive heart failure or thymic lymphoma in ferrets) a pleural drain may be inserted or a pleural tap carried out as an emergency procedure. This is performed in a similar fashion as with a cat. Sedation with midazolam and ketamine or light anaesthesia with isoflurane or sevoflurane may be required but most tolerate the procedure. Inhalation oxygen should be supplied as flow-by. The lateral chest wall is clipped and surgically prepared. A butterfly needle attached to a three-way tap and a syringe is used and inserted between rib spaces 7 and 9 ventrally and slowly advanced into the pleural space with negative pressure applied to the syringe until fluid flows into the tubing.

Cardiovascular support (C)

As for rabbits, circumferential chest compressions should be instituted, but chest compression rates of 150+ beats per minute should be attempted where possible. The use of thumb and forefinger either side of the chest is usually sufficient.

Drugs (D)

Similar drugs may be used for small mammals as are used for rabbits (Table 8.4). Cardiac disease, particularly dilated cardiomyopathies and associated congestive heart failure, endocardiosis and, in some rarer cases, hypertrophic cardiomyopathies may be seen in ferrets, Virginia opossums, guinea pigs and hamsters. Hamsters are also prone to bacterial endocarditis.

Atropine may be used where bradycardia is seen as none of the species discussed here have serum atropinesterases.

Gerbils are prone to epilepsy which is hereditary. If seizures should occur it may be controlled using midazolam/diazepam.

Diagnostic procedures

ECG (E)

An ECG trace may be difficult to determine due to the animal's small size and fast heart rates. However, it is still often worth applying ECG leads should an arrhythmia be detected on auscultation or where cardiac disease is suspected, preferably using adhesive pads to connect with the patient's feet. Published values for guinea pigs, a species commonly seen with heart disease, are given in Table 8.5.

The type of dysrhythmia reported in ferrets during resuscitation techniques is different from that reported in cats and dogs. The latter have been associated with electromechanical dissociation, whereas in ferrets, as with rabbits, profound bradycardia, ventricular asystole and ventricular fibrillation have been reported (Rush and Wingfield, 1992). Adrenaline may be used, intratracheally if intubated, or intravenously/intracardiac if no cardiac beat is detected and no ECG trace. In the case of fine ventricular fibrillation, the use of adrenaline has been advocated

Table 8.4 Emergency drugs used in small mammals.

Drug	Dosage and route
Adrenaline (1 : 1000 = 1 mg/mL formulation)	0.01–0.1 mg/kg IV, IO, IT NB: dilute to 1 : 10 000 if administering IV
Atropine	0.04–0.1 mg/kg IV, SC, IM, IO, IT
Dexamethasone	0.5–2 mg/kg IV (use with caution as potentially immunosuppressive)
Diazepam	3 mg/kg IV, IM
Doxapram	2–5 mg/kg SC, IV, PO q 15 min
Fluids	100 mL/kg per day maintenance
Furosemide	2–10 mg/kg PO, SC, IM
Glycopyrrolate	0.01–0.05 mg/kg SC, IM, IV
Lidocaine	1–2 mg/kg IV; 2–4 mg/kg IT
Midazolam	0.1–2 mg/kg IV, IM, IN

IV, intravenously; IM, intramuscularly; IO, intraosseously; SC, subcutaneously; IT, intratracheally; IN, intranasally. *Sources:* Kottwitz and Kelleher (2003); Hawkins and Pascoe (2012).

Table 8.5 Normal ECG values in guinea pigs.

Parameter	Normal value
P wave duration	0.015–0.035 s
P wave amplitude	0.01 mV
PR interval	0.048–0.06 s
QRS duration	0.008–0.046 s
QRS amplitude	1.1–1.9 mV
QT interval	0.106–0.144 s
T wave amplitude	0.062 mV
Mean electrical axis	120–180°

Source: Heatley (2009).

to convert the electrical activity to coarse ventricular fibrillation which is easier to convert (DeFrancesco, 2000) (see Table 8.4 for dosages).

Conversion of coarse fibrillation is based on the use of cardiac massage as described above, or if the clinic has access to a defibrillation device, then the use of this externally at 2–10 J/kg (starting at low energies and increasing if no response is achieved) may be performed (Costello, 2004). Greater success is achieved with defibrillation devices if three initial countershocks are applied at low energies.

Monitoring response to CPR

Monitoring rectal temperatures is relatively straightforward in rodents, but assessing capnographic trends to CPR is made more difficult owing to the small size of patients and difficulty intubating. Side-stream capnographs can be used in conjunction with a tight-fitting face mask but clearly the accuracy of any reading depends on how tight fitting the mask is. Trends described for rabbits can be used. Blood pressure assessment using indirect methods is largely constrained by the small size of the patient as cuffs often are not small enough to be a width of only 40% circumference of the limb. For this reason, indirect blood pressure monitoring is not often used in rodents.

Blood lactate levels may be measured in ferrets, with levels above 4 mmol/L (normal range 1–3 mmol/L) being viewed as abnormal and indicating anaerobic respiration associated with shock and poorer prognosis (Lichtenberger, 2007).

Hypoglycaemia has been shown to be strongly correlated with insulinomas in ferrets, with values less than 3 mmol/L being seen along with clinical collapse and prior to this salivation, vomiting and seizuring.

Hypocalcaemia can be seen in young ferrets with metabolic bone disease, lactating jills and primary hypoparathyroidism (De Matos *et al.*, 2014). Hypercalcaemia is common with lymphoma.

Coagulation times in ferrets have been reported as follows: prothrombin time, mean 10.9 (range 10.6–11.6) seconds; partial thromboplastin time, mean 20 (range 18.6–22.1) seconds (Benson *et al.*, 2008). Extended times are occasionally seen with coumerol and warfarin toxicity, but they are uncommon in my experience. Other causes include sepsis, pancreatitis and neoplasia. Management of warfarin derivative poisoning with vitamin K is advised as for dogs and cats should intoxication be suspected.

HCO_3^- levels indicate the metabolic part of the acid–base balance, with low levels correlating to the metabolic acidosis commonly seen in shock scenarios and gastrointestinal and renal disease. Elevated HCO_3^- levels suggest metabolic alkalosis associated with gastrointestinal stasis or blockage (specifically gastric foreign bodies, which are common in ferrets).

Radiography

This is of use where respiratory and cardiovascular diseases are concerned. Lung volumes are small in rodents, and clear lung fields are often difficult to visualise. However, lung tumours are common in rats and guinea pigs, and varying degrees of lung consolidation may be seen in cases of pneumonia, common in rats, mice and guinea pigs. Pleural effusions are seen commonly in ferrets with thymic lymphoma. Cardiomyopathies and heart failure are common in ferrets, guinea pigs and hamsters.

Spinal fractures can be seen in any rodent but are more commonly seen in guinea pigs and chipmunks, and collapsed spinal columns are common with nutritional hyperparathyroidism in sugar gliders.

Urinary bladder stones (calcium oxalate usually) are common in guinea pigs, ferrets and hamsters, and calculi may also be seen in the kidneys.

Gastrointestinal bloat may be seen in chinchillas and guinea pigs associated with severe enteritis or inappropriate antibiotic administration.

Ultrasound

Polycystic ovarian disease is easily diagnosed using ultrasound in guinea pigs, gerbils and hamsters.

Cardiac disease may be diagnosed using the smaller 10 MHz or even 7.5 MHz frequency in larger individuals in the case of ferrets, some hamsters and guinea pigs where cardiac enlargement and valvular disease are common.

Fluid therapy (F)

Hypovolaemic shock

As with rabbits, the rapid support of blood pressure in hypovolaemic shock is essential. A bolus of isotonic fluids is administered (warmed to body temperature) at 10–15 mL/kg intravenously/intraosseously. If severe hypovolaemia is present, then a bolus of hypertonic saline may be administered at 3–4 mL/kg intravenously/intraosseously. This is followed by a bolus of a colloid, preferably hetastarch at 5 mL/kg intravenously (or intraosseously) slowly over 5–10 minutes. Once blood pressure has risen above 50 mmHg or more, then the patient may be warmed and further crystalloid fluids administered. Blood pressure may be measured in larger rodents using the same techniques as in rabbits. In small rodents, such as mice and rats, this may not be possible, so one cycle of crystalloid/colloid fluids should be administered to see if a response to treatment occurs. This may be repeated twice further, leaving an interval of 15–20 minutes between attempts. Warming is essential as the adrenergic receptors do not tend to respond to fluid therapy and catecholamines if the body temperature is less than 36.7°C (Lichtenberger, 2007).

General fluid therapy provision

See the section on fluid therapy in Chapter 6.

Other medications and supportive nutrition

Herbivorous rodents, such as guinea pigs and chinchillas, often benefit from the use of prokinetics as is the case in rabbits. Dosages are similar. Small herbivores should avoid the same antibiotics that are harmful to rabbits. It is possible to safely use fluoroquinolones and trimethoprim sulfonamides in small herbivores at doses similar to those used in rabbits.

For nutritional support the same MER formula for rabbits may be used as for rodents. The value of *k* will change according to the species and has been estimated to be 300–450. Herbivorous rodents can be fed similar formulas to the domestic rabbit. Some manufacturers also produce an omnivore supportive formula (e.g. Lafeber) which may be more appropriate for opossums, chipmunks and even rats and mice.

The maintenance energy requirements for a normal adult ferret are 200–300 kcal (837–1255 kJ) per kilogram body weight daily (Carpenter and Kolmstetter, 2000). The debilitated ferret should approach 1.5–2 times these levels depending on the level of injury or sepsis. Carnivore emergency supportive formulas are available from similar manufacturers as those that supply herbivore formulas, for example Carnivore Intensive Care® (Lafeber) and Critical Care Carnivore® (Oxbow).

General notes on fluid therapy and blood transfusions

If small mammals are dehydrated or hypovolaemic, shock doses of fluids should be administered. It should be noted that fluids should be avoided after resuscitation in cases of cardiovascular arrest where there is no hypovolaemia or dehydration prior to the arrest as these fluids may decrease myocardial perfusion pressures and diminish overall nutrient delivery through the cerebral and coronary vasculature (Cole *et al.*, 2002).

Maintenance values

Maintenance fluid rate for all small mammals is estimated to be 80–100 mL/kg per day, i.e. twice that estimated for cats and dogs. The reason is their generally smaller sizes and higher metabolisms. This leads to greater glomerular filtration rates and insensible losses through the lungs, etc.

Calculation of fluid deficits

These may be calculated as for cats and dogs; however, it is worth noting that much fluid intake is normally consumed as 'food', i.e. in the form of fresh vegetation. This is difficult to take into consideration, and therefore it is safer to assume that the debilitated small mammal will not be eating sufficient amounts for this to matter in the calculation.

As with cats and dogs, assume that 1% dehydration equates with needing to supply 10 mL/kg body weight fluid replacement in addition to the maintenance requirements.

Assumptions then have to be made on the degree of dehydration of the small mammal concerned, and this can be done clinically as follows:

- 3–5% dehydrated: increased thirst, slight lethargy, tacky mucous membranes
- 7–10% dehydrated: increased thirst leading to anorexia, dullness, tenting of the skin and slow return to normal, dry mucous membranes, 'dull corneas'
- 10–15% dehydrated: dull/comatose, skin remains tented after pinching, desiccating mucous membranes.

Alternatively we can rely on the packed cell volume (PCV) and total protein levels to assess dehydration if a blood sample can be taken (see Chapter 5).

- Day 1: maintenance fluid levels +50% of calculated dehydration factor
- Day 2: maintenance fluid levels +50% of calculated dehydration factor
- Day 3: maintenance fluid levels.

If the dehydration levels are so severe that volumes are still too large at any one time, it may be necessary to take 72 hours to replace the calculated deficit rather than 48 hours.

In addition for those species which can vomit, such as ferrets, the levels of vomitus expelled should be considered. As with cats and dogs, assuming 2–4 mL/kg body weight per vomit is an acceptable level.

In other species where diarrhoea only is the norm, such as small herbivores, it is much more difficult to make estimations, although fluid losses may approach 100–150 mL/kg body weight per day.

Fluid types suitable for use

Crystalloids

The main rehydration fluid of choice is likely to be a lactated Ringer's compound. However, species such as guinea pigs are prone to ketosis, and a glucose saline isotonic/hypotonic fluid may be of use. Hypertonic saline is useful where severe hypovolaemia is present as it can rapidly increase blood pressure. However, it should always be followed by isotonic/hypotonic fluids as it does not replace the overall fluid deficit, but rather relies on drawing fluid from the intracellular and extracellular space into the bloodstream.

Colloids

These may be used in small mammals as in cats and dogs.

Additives

Protein amino acid/B vitamin supplements

Additives such as Duphalyte® (Zoetis) are useful for nutritional support, at the rate of 1 mL/kg body weight per day. They are particularly good in cases where the patient is malnourished or has been suffering from a protein-losing enteropathy, such as cases of heavy parasitism, to help replace some of the compounds needed for replenishment. It is also a useful supplement for patients with hepatic diseases or severe exudative skin diseases such as heater burns.

Bicarbonate

This should be considered where metabolic acidosis exists, such as in rabbits with hepatic lipidosis and secondary ketosis and guinea pigs with pregnancy ketosis. Calculations of replacements are same as for cats and dogs.

Electrolytes

Sodium and potassium levels should be monitored and corrected for deficits where found. In practice, potassium levels will often be depressed in cases of long-standing diarrhoea or fluid therapy and elevated in cases of renal disease. The use of calcium gluconate when a patient has a high potassium level can help minimise hyperkalaemia-associated arrhythmias.

Blood transfusions

Blood transfusions are sometimes performed if PCV levels start to drop below 20%. They are best performed by direct, same species-to-species transfers (i.e. a rat to a rat, and a guinea pig to a guinea pig). A healthy donor may have the equivalent of 1% of body weight removed as blood without any deleterious effects. This may be increased to 4% if required, although careful monitoring of the donor after this is needed. The donor should clearly be a healthy animal and in the case of a rabbit one which has tested negative previously for *Encephalitozoon cuniculi* infection.

In rabbits, the volume of donor blood required is calculated by assuming that the domestic rabbit PCV is 30–50%. Aiming for a target of 40% and assuming that the average blood volume of a rabbit is 60 mL/kg body weight leads to the following formula:

$$\text{Millilitres blood required} = \frac{(\text{target PCV\%} - \text{current PCV\%}) \times \text{body weight(kg)} \times 60}{\text{donor PCV\%}}$$

Ferret blood has a short shelf-life at 4°C when collected into citrate phosphate dextrose solution with adenosine and so should not be stored for more than 7 days according to Pignon *et al.* (2014). Depressed PCV and haemoglobin levels with no increase in mean cell volume (MCV) indicative of a non-regenerative anaemia is common in jills not brought out of heat (by mating or contraception) due to bone marrow suppression caused by high circulating oestrogen levels.

Blood sample collection is best taken directly into a collecting bag with citrate acid dextrose at a rate of 1 mL of anticoagulant to 5–6 mL of blood and transferred to the donor via a blood giving set with filters to remove clots. In an emergency, a direct bolus can be given but this increases the risk of clot formation. Intravenous catheters are advised for the transfers as administration should be slow, giving 1 mL over a period of 5–6 minutes if possible, hence sedation or good restraint is required. Very little information is currently available about cross-matching blood groups of small mammals, although it seems that ferrets do not have appreciably detectable groups and so multiple donations may be given. Intraosseous donations may be made if vascular access is not possible.

References

Ardiaca, M., Bonvehi, C. and Montesinos, A. (2013) Point-of care blood gas and electrolyte analysis in rabbits. *Veterinary Clinics of North America: Exotic Animal Practice*, **16**(1), 175–195.

Benson, K.G., Paul-Murphy, J., Hart, A.P. *et al.* (2008) Coagulation values in normal ferrets (*Mustela putorius furo*) using selected methods and reagents. *Veterinary Clinical Pathology*, **37**, 286–288.

Bonvehi, C., Ardiaca, M., Barrera, S. *et al.* (2014) Prevalence and types of hyponatraemia, its relationship with hyperglycaemia and mortality in ill rabbits. *Veterinary Record*, **174**(22), 554.

Briscoe, J.A. and Syring, R. (2004) Techniques for emergency airway and vascular access in special species. *Seminars in Avian and Exotic Pet Medicine*, **13**(3), 118–131.

Carpenter, J.W. and Kolmstetter, C.M. (2000) Feeding small exotic animals. In: *Hill's Nutrition III* (eds L.D. Lewis, M.L. Morris & M.S. Hand), pp. 943–960. Mark Mervis Institute, Marceline, MO.

Cole, S.G., Otto, C.M. and Hughes, D. (2002) Cardiopulmonary cerebral resuscitation in small animals: a clinical practice review. *Journal of Veterinary Emergency Critical Care*, **12**, 261–267.

Costello, M.F. (2004) Principles of cardiopulmonary cerebral resuscitation in special species. *Seminars in Avian and Exotic Pet Medicine*, **13**(3), 132–141.

De Matos, R.E., Connolly, M.J., Starkey, S.R. and Morrisey, J.K. (2014) Suspected primary hypoparathyroidism in a domestic ferret (*Mustela putorius furo*). *Journal of the American Veterinary Medical Association*, **245**(4), 419–424.

DeFrancesco, T.C. (2000) Cardiac emergencies. In: *Kirk and Bistner's Handbook of Veterinary Procedures and Emergency Treatment* (eds S.I. Bistner, R.B. Ford & M.R. Raffe), pp. 54–61. WB Saunders, Philadelphia, PA.

Di Girolamo, N., Toth, G. and Selleri, P. (2016) Prognostic value of rectal temperature at hospital admission in client-owned rabbits. *Journal of the American Veterinary Medical Association*, **248**(3), 288–297.

Eatwell, K., Mancinelli, E., Hedley, J. *et al.* (2013) Use of arterial blood gas analysis as a superior method for evaluating respiratory function in pet rabbits (*Oryctolagus cuniculi*). *Veterinary Record*, **173**(7), 166.

Fletcher, D.J., Boller, M., Brainard, B.M. *et al.* (2012) RECOVER evidence and knowledge gap analysis on veterinary CPR part 7. Clinical guidelines. *Journal of Veterinary Emergency and Critical Care*, **22**(S1), S102–S131. doi: 10.1111/j.1476-4431.2012.00757.x.

Girling, S.J. (2003) Preliminary study into the possible use of benazepril in the management of renal disease in rabbits. *Proceedings of the British Veterinary Zoological Society*, Edinburgh, Scotland, p. 44.

Harcourt-Brown, F.M. and Harcourt-Brown, S.F. (2012) Clinical value of blood glucose measurement in pet rabbits. *Veterinary Record*, **170**(26), 674. doi: 10.1136/vr.100321.

Harcourt-Brown, F.M. and Holloway, H.K.R. (2003) *Encephalitozoon cuniculi* in pet rabbits. *Veterinary Record*, **152**, 427–431.

Hawkins, M.G. and Pascoe, P.J. (2012) Anesthesia, analgesia and sedation of small mammals. In: *Ferrets, Rabbits and Rodents: Clinical Medicine and Surgery* (eds K.E. Quesenberry & J.W. Carpenter), 3rd edn, pp. 429–451. W.B. Saunders, Philadelphia, St Louis.

Heard, D. (2004) Anesthesia, analgesia and sedation of small mammals. In: *Ferrets, Rabbits and Rodents: Clinical Medicine and Surgery* (eds K.E. Quesenberry & J.W. Carpenter), 2nd edn, pp. 356–369. WB Saunders, Philadelphia, PA.

Heatley, J.J. (2009) Cardiovascular anatomy, physiology, and diseases of rodents and small exotic mammals. *Veterinary Clinics of North America: Exotic Animal Practice*, **12**, 99–113.

Henrik, R.A. (1992) Basic life support and external cardiac compression in dogs and cats. *Journal of the American Veterinary Medical Association*, **200**, 1925–1931.

Huston, S.M. and Quesenberry, K.E. (2004) Cardiovascular and lymphoproliferative diseases. In: *Ferrets Rabbits and Rodents: Clinical Medicine and Surgery* (eds K.E. Quesenberry & J.W. Carpenter), 2nd edn, pp. 211–220. WB Saunders, St Louis, MO.

Kottwitz, J. and Kelleher, S. (2003) Emergency drugs: quick reference chart for exotic animals. *Exotic DVM*, **5.5**(November), 23–25.

Kozma, C., Macklin, W., Cummins, L.M. and Mauer, R. (1974) The anatomy, physiology and biochemistry of the rabbit. In: *The Biology of the Laboratory Rabbit* (eds S.H. Weisbroth, R.E. Flatt & A.L. Kraus), pp. 50–69. Academic Press, London.

Langlois, I., Planche, A., Boyson, S.R. *et al.* (2014) Blood concentrations of D and L-lactate in healthy rabbits. *Journal of Small Animal Practice*, **55**(9), 451–456.

Lichtenberger, M. (2007) Shock and CPCR in small mammals and birds. *Veterinary Clinics of North America: Exotic Animal Practice*, **10**(2), 275–291.

Lichtenberger, M. and Ko, J. (2007) Critical care monitoring. *Veterinary Clinics of North America: Exotic Animal Practice*, **10**(2), 317–344.

Lichtenberger, M. and Lennox, A. (2010) Updates and advanced therapies for gastrointestinal stasis in rabbits. *Veterinary Clinics of North America: Exotic Animal Practice*, **13**(3), 525–541.

Marino, P.R. (1997) Cardiac arrest. In: *The ICU Book* (ed. P.L. Marino), pp. 260–298. Lippincott Williams and Williams, Philadelphia, PA.

Okerman, L. (1994) Inherited conditions and congenital deformities. In: *Diseases of Domestic Rabbits*, 2nd edn, pp. 109–112. Blackwell, Oxford.

Pignon, C., Donnelly, T.M., Todeschini, C. *et al.* (2014) Assessment of a blood preservation protocol for use in ferrets before transfusion. *Veterinary Record*, **174**, 277.

Rush, J.E. and Wingfield, W.E. (1992) Recognition and frequency of dysrhythmias during cardiopulmonary arrest. *Journal of the American Veterinary Medical Association*, **200**, 1932–1937.

PART I: SMALL MAMMALS

Part II Avian Species

Chapter 9 Basic Avian Anatomy and Physiology

Classification

Birds are classified into many different family groups according to a number of physical, anatomical and genetic factors. It is useful to know to which group a bird belongs as this can be of some help when faced with a species which you have not seen before.

Table 9.1 contains some of the more commonly encountered family groups of birds seen in general and avian-orientated practices.

The Psittaciformes are among the most colourful and some would say intelligent, of birds kept as pets.

Nervous system

The avian brain is extremely smooth, lacking the many gyri (the ridges in the brain) seen in mammals. Sight appears to be the dominant sense in most birds, but senses of hearing and smell are also significant particularly in specialised hunters (for example the sense of smell in turkey vultures and sense of hearing in many owl species). Two large optic lobes lie between the cerebral hemispheres and the cerebellum, and it is here where the optic nerves communicate and disseminate information. There is no corpus callosum, the cerebral cortex is generally very thin, but the corpus striatum is well developed and is thought to be the site of mental association in birds. An important feature of the bird's brain is the pineal gland/body which sits in the dorsal section of the diencephalon, cranial to the cerebellum in the midline. The pineal body has secretory cells similar to photoreceptors and so will respond to light. They are also linked via the cranial cervical ganglia to the optic nerve. The pineal body is responsible for regulating many seasonal effects such as reproduction and migration as well as circadian rhythms. It has a direct effect via hormone secretion on the hypothalamus.

The avian nervous system has many similarities to its mammalian counterpart. Birds for example possess 12 cranial nerves (CN), the same as in mammals. There are some subtle differences in the anatomy though, for example the olfactory nerve (CN I) passes through the calvarium via a single hole rather than in mammals where it passes through multiple smaller ones in the cribriform plate. In birds, the optic nerve (CN II) is the largest cranial nerve, each one being more than half the diameter of the spinal column and is particularly sizeable in birds of prey such as falcons. Once the optic nerve enters the skull it decussates completely in the majority of birds, meaning a true consensual light reflex is not seen in birds as it is in mammals. The other 10 cranial nerves have the same names and perform similar functions as they do in mammals. One of the more significant is the trigeminal nerve (CN V) that splits into two sensory and one sensory and motor nerve. One of these (the maxillary nerve) often supplies the majority of sensory innervation to the maxillary beak, particularly in waterfowl such as ducks and geese. In contrast in Galliformes, the ophthalmic nerve arising from CN V supplies most of the sensory innervation to the maxillary beak. More information about avian cranial nerves can be found in King and McLelland (1984), Bennett (1994) and König *et al.* (2016).

Each of the wings has a nervous supply from a brachial plexus derived from the spinal nerves from the last four to five cervical vertebrae, although there is considerable species variation with some being supplied by more cranial cervical nerves (e.g. pigeons) and in others an additional accessory brachial plexus is also present composed of again more cranially located cervical nerve roots.

The hindlimbs and caudal body derive many of their nerves from three nerve plexuses in the lumbosacral region: the lumbar, ischiadic (sacral) and pudendal plexuses. The lumbar plexus derives from the last two lumbar and the first one to two sacral spinal nerve roots. Like the other lumbosacral plexuses, it lies in a hollow of the pelvis, dorsal to the cranial kidney area. It supplies the body wall and upper leg muscles and gives rise to the obturator, femoral, cranial gluteal and saphenous nerves. Unlike dogs and cats, birds have an ischiadic (sacral) plexus which is derived from four to seven spinal nerves in the sacral area and which is situated in a hollow of the pelvis dorsal to the mid-kidney structure. It gives rise to the principal nervous supply for the hindlimbs, the ischiadic nerve which is the largest peripheral nerve in the body and the caudal gluteal nerve. Finally, a pudendal plexus forms in a hollow of the pelvis dorsal to the caudal kidney area from five coccygeal spinal nerves and innervates the tail and cloacal area. The location of these plexuses close to the kidneys means that kidney disease often affects the function of nerves supplying the legs and so may manifest as paresis or paralysis of one or both pelvic limbs.

Musculoskeletal system

Most birds have the power of flight. The dense, cumbersome bones of the earthbound mammal would require too much effort to lift into the air. Birds have therefore adapted their skeletal structure, simplifying the number of bones by fusing some together, and generally lightening the whole structure by creating empty spaces within many of the bones. Several of the larger bones, and even some of the vertebrae in the spine, are connected directly or indirectly to the airways, and are referred to as being pneumonised. This replaces the thick medullary cavity or bone marrow present in the centre of mammalian bones, and produces a light trabecular structure. While light, the structure is nevertheless extremely strong.

Veterinary Nursing of Exotic Pets and Wildlife, Third Edition. Simon J. Girling.

Table 9.1 Avian family groups commonly encountered in veterinary practice (note that the list is not exhaustive).

Order	Common species
Accipitriformes	This order includes • Family Cathartidae such as New World vultures • Family Accipitridae such as buzzards, kites, hawks, eagles, Old World vultures and harriers • Family Pandionidae such as ospreys
Anseriformes	This order includes • Family Anatidae which contains most of the commonly seen waterfowl such as the mallard, shoveller, teal, eider ducks, shelducks, geese (e.g. greylags, Canada goose) and swans
Columbiformes	This order includes • Family Columbidae which contains the pigeons and doves
Falconiformes	This order includes • Family Falconidae such as falcons (lanner, gyrfalcon peregrine falcons, etc.), kestrels, caracaras, etc.
Passeriformes	This order is the largest and most diverse and includes • Family Estrildidae such as zebra finches • Family Fringillidae such as greenfinches, goldfinches and chaffinches as well as the canary • Family Passeridae such as the house and tree sparrows
Piciformes	This order includes • Family Rhamphastidae such as toucans and toucanettes • Family Picidae which covers wrynecks, woodpeckers, etc.
Psittaciformes	This order includes those we know as 'parrots' and covers • Family Cacatuidae such as cockatiels, cockatoos, corellas, etc. • Family Psittacidae such as African grey parrots, Amazons, macaws, some parakeets • Family Psittaculidae such as vasa parrots, eclectus parrots, some parakeets (including budgerigars), lorikeets, lorries, lovebirds and rosellas, etc.
Strigiformes	This order includes • Family Tytonidae which contains the barn owls • Family Strigidae which contains the little, saw-whet, pygmy, scops, snowy, eagle, screech, tawny and wood owls

Skull

Beak

The beak, or bill, is the principal feature of the avian skull. It has been modified into a bewildering number of shapes and sizes, depending mainly on the diet to which the bird has become adapted. In all cases it is composed of an upper (maxillary) and lower (mandibular) beak which are covered in a layer of keratin, a tough protein compound similar to that which forms the exoskeleton of insects. This keratin layer is known as the rhamphotheca. It is further classified so that the maxillary layer is referred to as the rhinotheca, and the mandibular layer as the gnatotheca (see Figure 9.1). The rhinotheca and gnatotheca grow from a plate at the base of the respective sides of the beak, the rate of replacement depending upon the type of food eaten and the abrasion the beak receives.

In Psittaciformes (see Table 9.1), the upper beak is powerfully developed and ends in a sharp point overhanging the broader, stouter lower beak. The tremendous power in a parrot's beak is due to a synovial joint or hinge mechanism, known as the (pro)kinetic joint, which joins the maxillary beak to the skull. The parrot's lower beak has a series of well-innervated pressure sensors at its tip, which allow it to test the consistency and structure of objects grasped.

In raptors, the upper beak is sharp and pointed, but lacks the synovial joint attachment so it cannot produce such powerful downward force. Instead, it is used as a ripping instrument.

In Anseriformes (the duck family), the beak is flattened and may have fine serrations at the edges which allow the bird to filter fine particles from the water (see Figure 9.2). Ducks such as mallards and shovellers have this type of beak. These serrations may be further developed to a jagged edge (e.g. in the aptly named sawbill family) which allows the bird to grip slippery food, such as fish. Anseriformes also have nerve endings in a plate at the tips of their maxillary beaks (known as the 'nail') which allow them to find food hidden in mud.

In all birds there is a series of smaller bones behind the lower and upper beaks which allow them to move the beak independently of the

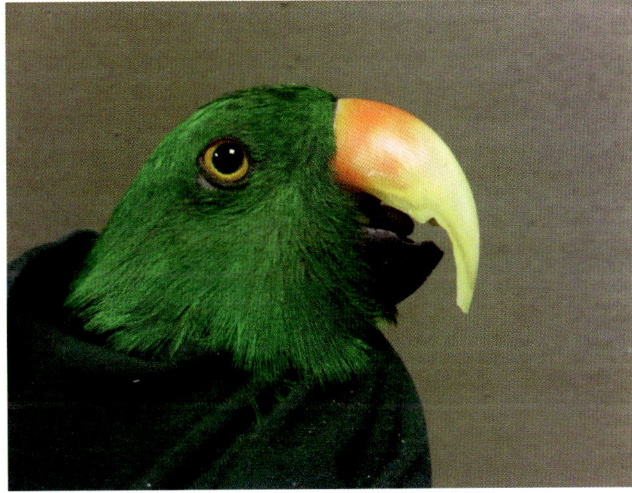

Figure 9.1 The head of a male eclectus parrot showing the yellow-coloured rhinotheca and black-coloured gnatotheca typical of this species and sex.

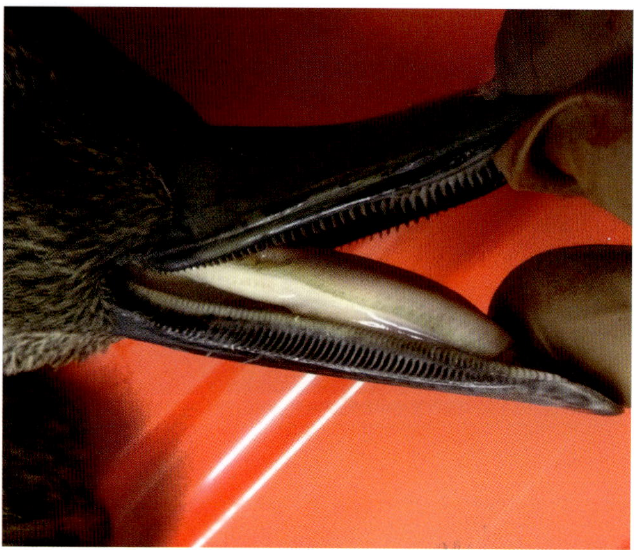

Figure 9.2 Lateral view of the beak of a wild duck at post-mortem showing the fine interlocking serrations used to strain out food particles from the water.

skull. These include the palatine, quadrate and pterygoid bones and the jugal arches. The quadrate bone is perhaps one of the most important, particularly in Psittaciformes, and articulates with the mandible. The quadrate bone slides the jugal bar cranially which pushes the upper beak dorsally. The temporomandibular joint, although present as in mammals, actually has a lesser role in jaw movement in birds. The rest of these bones and their exact movements are beyond this text to describe, but many of the references at the end of this chapter give good accounts of their function.

Nostrils

The nostrils, or nares, lie at the base of the maxillary beak in most birds and are often surrounded by an area of featherless skin known as the cere. This may be highly coloured in some species, such as the budgerigar, where they may be used to identify the sex of the bird. In many Anseriformes the nares lie further distally on the beak and in the case of the kiwi the nares are at the end of the beak. The nares open into the nasal passages and sinus chambers, which in turn connect with a branching network of bony chambers throughout the bird's head. These sinuses vary according to the species, but the majority of avian patients have an infraorbital sinus. This sits below the eyes and is often involved in sinus and ocular infections. It differs from skull sinuses seen in most mammals in that the lateral wall has no bone, being covered by soft tissue only. This means any infraorbital sinus infection often results in swelling on the face of the bird ventral to the eye. These sinuses also communicate with head and neck air sacs. The function of these air sacs is not clear, but they may help with voice resonance. When a bird suffers from sinus infections, the narrow inlets to these sinuses may become partially blocked and act as one-way valves, allowing air into the sacs but not out. The sacs may then overinflate, and soft swellings are then commonly seen over the back or nape of the bird's head.

The sinuses and external nares communicate with the oropharynx via the choanal slit. This is a narrow opening in the midline of the hard palate and is sited immediately over the glottis when the beak is closed, allowing the bird to breathe through its nostrils. The choana is often the area chosen for taking samples when trying to isolate infectious agents for upper airway disease in birds.

The skull of the avian patient connects to the atlas (or first spinal vertebra) via only one occipital condyle at the base of the skull, unlike the mammalian two. There are also a large number of highly mobile cervical vertebrae. These two factors make the avian head extremely agile. However, the atlanto-occipital joint is also a weak point, making dislocation at that site relatively easy.

Vertebral column

Cervical vertebrae

The cervical vertebrae (see Figure 9.3) are independently mobile in the avian patient, as they are in the mammalian patient, and vary in number, depending on the species, between 11 and 25 (swans and ratites having the most). The first cervical vertebra is the atlas and like mammals has no spinous process. The second, the axis, has an elongated body and articulates with the atlas via a cranial projection (the dens as in mammals). The rest of the cervical vertebrae are generally box-like in form and many, particularly caudally, have small vestigial ribs projecting from the ventrolateral surfaces.

Thoracic, lumbar and sacral vertebrae

The majority of thoracic vertebrae (see Figure 9.3) are fused in raptors, pigeons and many other species to form a single bone known as the notarium. In other species such as many waterfowl, they have some limited mobility and are held in place by ossified tendons and ligaments. In many species there are then two intervertebral joints between the notarium and the synsacrum. The synsacrum is composed of fused lumbar, sacral and often last thoracic and first coccygeal vertebrae. The synsacrum fuses with the pelvis itself to form a dorsal shield of bone over the caudal aspect of the bird.

Coccygeal (caudal) vertebrae

There are mobile coccygeal vertebrae caudal to the synsacrum but the majority of the caudal coccygeal vertebrae most distally (see Figure 9.3) are usually fused into a single structure known as the pygostyle – which forms the 'parson's nose' part of the chicken! The pygostyle forms the base for attachment of the tail feathers (rectrices) that are embedded in a fibroadipose tissue (the retrical bulb) ventral to the vertebrae.

Pelvis

The roof of the pelvis is formed by the synsacrum (see Figure 9.3). The two 'sides' of the pelvis are reduced in size compared with mammals but consist of the iliac and ischial bones, with the acetabulum being created where they meet. The acetabulum in birds is not a complete bony socket as it is in mammals, but a fibrous sheet. There is a ridge on the laterodorsal pelvis known as the antitrochanter, which articulates with the greater trochanter of the femur. The function of this ridge is to prevent the pelvic limb from being abducted when perching. The pubic bones of the pelvis do not fuse in the ventral midline as in mammals. Instead, they form fine long bones which extend caudally towards the vent. They provide support for the skin covering the caudal abdomen and not being fused ventrally allows enough space for the passage of eggs in the female bird.

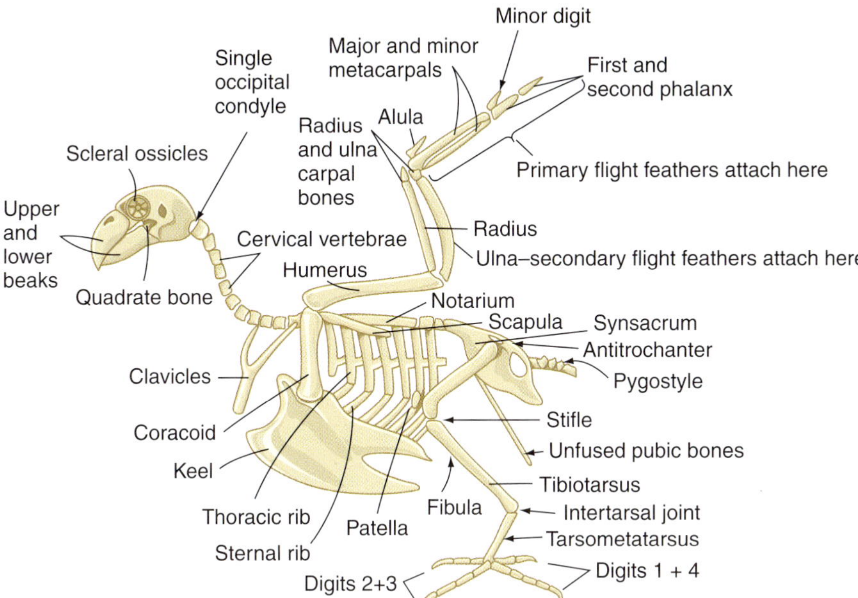

Figure 9.3 Avian (psittacine) skeleton.

Ribcage

Psittaciformes have eight pairs of ribs (see Figure 9.3) and domestic Galliformes and pigeons have seven pairs. Each rib has a dorsal segment known as the thoracic or vertebral rib, and a ventral segment, or sternal rib. These ribs point backwards and rigidly connect the thoracic vertebrae dorsally and the keel, or sternum, ventrally, although in some species the caudal ribs may articulate with other ribs ventrally or even the iliac part of the synsacrum. A caudally projecting process (uncinate process) may be present on some of the vertebral ribs that articulates with the lateral aspect of the rib behind and acts to strengthen the ribcage as well as providing attachment for muscles.

Sternum

The sternal vertebrae are fused in birds to form the body of the sternum. Projecting ventrally from the body of the sternum is the keel (also known as the carina) that provides attachment for the flight (pectoral) muscles. The carina may be a deep structure, as is seen in pigeons, raptors and Psittaciformes, allowing large pectoral muscles to attach for strong flight. Alternatively, the keel may be more flattened, as with Anseriformes, to provide a boat-like structure more suited to floating or almost completely absent in the case of ratites such as the ostrich, emu or rhea. The most cranial portion of the sternum may have a notch to contain the distal coiled trachea in some species of cranes and swans.

Wings

The shoulder joint is formed by the meeting of three bones: the humerus, the scapula (which is smaller and more tubular than the flattened mammalian one) and a third bone known as the coracoid (see Figure 9.3). This latter bone forms a strut propping the shoulder joint against the sternum. The supracoracoid muscle attaches to the sternum and coracoid, and its tendon passes through the triosseal foramen, or opening, formed at the meeting point of the scapula, coracoid and clavicle, and so reaches the dorsal aspect of the humerus where it attaches. Contraction of this muscle, along with some elastic tissues and other smaller muscles present, helps to raise and supinate the wing. The pectoral muscles attach from the keel onto the ventral humerus to pull the wing downwards and pronate the humerus. The clavicles (often referred to as the furcula) articulate with the coracoid bone and provide a degree of spring against the natural tendency for the shoulder joints to move medially and laterally when the bird flaps its wings upwards and downwards. The many bones forming the shoulder joint are pneumonised, including the humerus, which means that it cannot be used for intraosseous fluid therapy. The ulna bone is commonly used for intraosseous fluids in birds as it is not pneumonised, but it should be avoided in some species such as pelicans where it is still connected to the airways. This is also an important point to consider when repairing fractures.

The humerus articulates distally with the radius and ulna at the elbow joint. The radius is the smaller of these two bones and lies cranially. The ulna provides the source of attachment for the secondary flight feathers, which insert directly into the periosteum of this bone (see Figure 9.3). The ulna is often used for intraosseous fluid administration in birds.

The radius and ulna articulate distally with one radial carpal bone and one ulnar carpal bone. These in turn articulate with three metacarpal bones. The first metacarpal bone is the equivalent of the avian 'thumb'. It is known as the alula, or 'bastard wing', and forms a feathery projection from the cranial aspect of the carpometacarpal joint. Its function is to alter the airflow over the wing, so preventing stalling and acting much like the ailerons on the caudal aspect of an airplane wing. The remaining two metacarpal bones are known as the major and minor metacarpal bones and articulate with the first phalanx cranially and the minor digit caudally. The first (or proximal) phalanx then articulates with the second (or distal) phalanx, forming the wing tip. The primary feathers attach to the periosteum of the phalanges and minor metacarpal bones.

The area of the wing is enlarged by thin sheets of elastic tissue which span from one joint surface to another. The largest extends

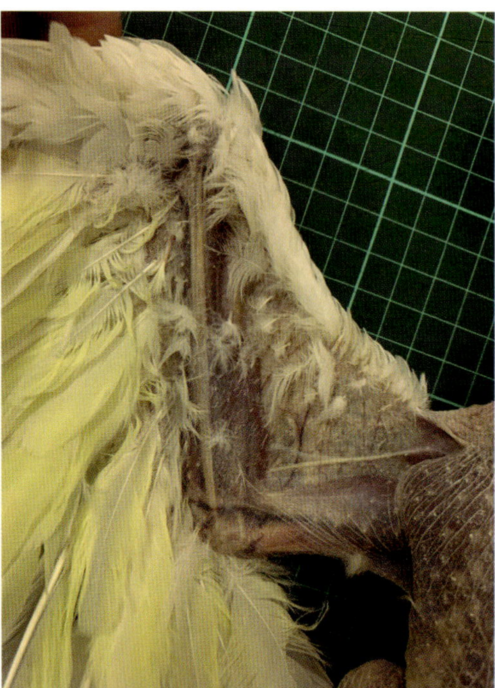

Figure 9.4 Ventral aspect of a cockatoo's wing showing the elastic sheet of the propatagium bridging the elbow joint. Note also the course of the ulnar vein crossing the elbow and becoming the brachial vein on the ventral aspect of the humerus.

from the shoulder to the carpal joint cranially and is known as the propatagium or 'wing web' (see Figure 9.4). This can be used in some species, such as pigeons, for vaccine administration.

Pelvic limb

Nearly all species of bird can walk with the pelvic limbs. There are some though which cannot and if they become grounded may not be able to regain flight. Examples include swifts such as the common swift (*Apus apus*) that has very short pelvic limbs and some waterfowl such as grebe species (e.g. the great crested, *Podiceps cristatus*) due to the very caudal position of the pelvic joints designed for diving and swimming. The acetabulum of the pelvis holds the femoral head (see Figure 9.3). The limb may be locked, and prevented from being abducted, by the greater trochanter of the femur engaging with the antitrochanteric ridge on the pelvis. The femur is pneumonised in many birds. At the stifle joint, the femur articulates with the patella and the tibiotarsal bone. The tibiotarsal bone is so called because it is formed from the fusion of the tibia and the proximal row of tarsal bones and may also be used for intraosseous fluid administration through the cranial cnemial crest or ridge. On the lateral aspect of the proximal tibiotarsus is the much-reduced fibula. The stifle joint has a lateral and medial meniscus and cranial and caudal cruciate ligaments within it similar to mammals.

Distally, the tibiotarsal bone articulates with the tarsometatarsal bone. The tarsometatarsal bone is formed by the fusion of the middle and distal row of tarsal bones and the metatarsal bones II–IV. The joint between the tibiotarsus and the tarsometatarsus is known as the intertarsal, or suffrago, joint and contains a medial and lateral meniscus. Over the caudal aspect of the intertarsal joint is the tibial cartilage which is grooved and allows the tendon of insertion of the gastrocnemius and superficial digital flexor muscles to run over its surface while the deep digital flexor tendons pass through the cartilage. Metatarsal bone V is absent in birds. The tarsometatarsus then articulates with the phalanges. Metatarsal bone I is present in species with four digits and articulates with the distal tarsometatarsus proximally and its proximal phalanx distally. The first digit where present always points caudally and is often referred to as the hallux.

In Psittaciformes, two digits point forwards (the second and third) and two backwards (the first and fourth), creating a zygodactyl limb. The first digit (hallux) has two phalanges, the second digit has three phalanges, the third has four phalanges and the fourth has five phalanges. In many species such as the perching birds (Passeriformes) and raptors, the second, third and fourth digits point forwards and the first points backwards creating an anisodactyl limb. Damage or loss of the first or second digit can be extremely serious for raptors as these two are generally used to grasp and kill prey. Some species, such as the osprey (*Pandion haliaetus*), may move the fourth digit to face forwards or backwards to aid capturing its prey, creating a semi-zygodactyl limb. The ventral aspect of the foot is cushioned with a series of deep and superficial fat pads, the largest one being at the junction of the proximal phalanxes and the distal tarsometatarsus (metatarsal pad) but with smaller ones over each joint between phalanxes.

The main muscles of the pelvic limb are all found proximal to the intertarsal joint, with tendons of insertion and small muscles being found distally.

Special senses

Eye

Visual acuity is generally accepted as being greater in diurnal birds than in mammals. The avian eye differs from the mammalian in that it contains a series of small bones known as the scleral ossicles (see Figure 9.3). They form a ring-shaped structure of overlapping thin sheets of bone that supports the front of the eye at the scleral–corneal junction. The avian eye also differs from the mammalian eye in that it is not a globe, but often pear-shaped, with the narrower end outermost. This is particularly accentuated in owl species and much less so in species such as pigeons where the overall shape is more flattened from rostral to caudal.

The avian eye is large in proportion to the overall size of the skull, with either a paper-thin bony septum separating the right and left orbits or in some cases with no full bony division between the orbits. Birds have a mobile, translucent third eyelid, and upper and lower eyelids, the lower of which is more mobile than the upper, with the exception of Strigiformes (owls) where the upper eyelid is more mobile. Two tear-producing glands commonly exist: the third eyelid, or Harderian gland, which is located at the base of the third eyelid, and the lacrimal gland situated caudolaterally, as in mammals. A nasal gland exists rostrodorsal to the eye and empties into the nasal passages to keep them moist although it is absent in the pigeon. In sea birds, the nasal gland is sometimes referred to as the salt gland as its principal function appears to be to excrete excess sodium chloride in the body. There are two drainage puncta from the internal surface of the upper and lower eyelids rostrally that drain via the nasolacrimal duct into the nasal passages. Penguins, however, only have one lower punctum and no upper.

The colour of the iris may change with age in some species of bird, for example the African grey parrot has a dark grey iris until 4–5 months of age, when it turns yellow-grey, and then silver as it continues to age. The iris of sparrowhawks starts yellow as a juvenile and turns dark orange as they age. In others the iris may be used as an indicator of the sex of the bird: in large cockatoos, for example, the female has a bright red-brown iris, whereas the male's is a dark brown-black. Finally, the avian iris has a mixture of smooth and skeletal muscle fibres within it, unlike mammals which possess only smooth-muscle fibres. This means the avian patient can constrict and dilate its pupil at will. This reduces the value of the pupillary light reflex as a tool in determining ocular function, and healthy surgically anaesthetised birds may actually dilate their pupil when a light is shone into it. Because the two optic nerves are completely separated from each other, the consensual light reflex is also a poor indicator of cerebral function.

The avian retina is thick and possesses no visible surface blood vessels and often has considerably more cones per square millimetre than mammals (around 300 000 for a hawk versus 147 000 for a human) leading to greater acuity. In nocturnal species, while there are not as many cones, a greater number of rods and a large overall globe size all help to increase light sensitivity. Diurnal birds appear to have good colour vision, many being able to see into the ultraviolet spectrum as well.

Due to a lack of surface blood vessels, in order to provide nutrition to the retina birds possess a pleated and folded vascular structure called the pecten oculi, which is found at the point where the optic nerve enters the eye. It contracts intermittently, expelling nutrients into the vitreous humour. It may also have other functions including regulating the pressure and temperature of the eye and protecting the retina.

Ear

There is no pinna in birds, although some species, such as the long- and short-eared owls, have feathers in this area. There is a short, horizontal external canal, covered by feathers, which is located caudolateral to the ocular orbit in the majority of cage birds, domestic fowl and raptors. However, there is significant variation between species and some have an ear canal opening located more ventral and cranial to the eye (e.g. the woodcock, *Scolopax rusticola*). Ear positioning in many carnivorous species is asymmetric (e.g. owls) allowing them to pinpoint prey by sound, even in complete darkness in the case of many owls. Some species have a facial disc of feathers (e.g. many owls) which can also help to reflect sound towards the ears (see Figure 9.5).

On finding the external ear canal, the tympanic membrane may be seen. The middle ear connects to the oropharynx via the Eustachian canal. The mammalian aural ossicles are replaced in the bird by a lateral extra-columella cartilage connected to the tympanum and a medial columella bone which transmit sound waves to the inner ear via the vestibular window.

The inner ear contains the cochlea and the semicircular canals, which fulfil the same functions as in mammals.

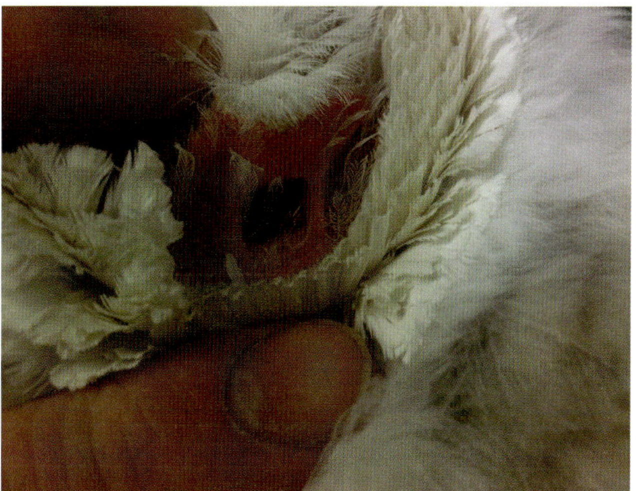

Figure 9.5 External ear canal of an owl. The ears are asymmetrically located behind the facial disc of feathers which can help focus sound in this species.

Respiratory anatomy

Upper respiratory system

The nares open into the nasal passages which contain three nasal conchae (a rostral, middle and caudal), which in turn communicate with the glottis of the larynx via a midline aperture in the hard palate which forms the roof of the caudal mouth. This aperture is called the choanal slit. The sinus system and cervicocephalic air sacs have been previously mentioned.

Larynx

Birds have a reduced laryngeal structure, lacking an epiglottis, the thyroid cartilage, and the vocal folds seen in cats and dogs. The main structure is the glottis, which protects the entrance to the trachea. External muscles pull the glottis and trachea forwards so that it communicates directly with the choanal slit, allowing the bird to breathe through its nostrils when its beak is closed. The glottis is held closed when at rest, only opening on inspiration and expiration.

Trachea

The trachea of avian species differs from the mammalian trachea in that its cartilage rings are complete, signet ring-shaped circles, interlocking one on top of the other, rather than the C-shaped rings of the mammalian trachea. In Psittaciformes and diurnal raptors, the shape of these cartilage rings is slightly flattened in a dorsoventral direction, whereas in most Passeriformes they are round.

In some species, such as the whooper swan, many cranes and the guinea fowl, the trachea forms a series of loops and coils at the thoracic inlet. Other species, such as the emu, have a midline ventral split in the trachea three-quarters of the distance between the head and the thoracic inlet. The tracheal lining mucosa projects through this slit to form a tracheal sac. This improves vocal resonance. Finally, in some species the trachea is partially (e.g. some ducks, many penguins and pelicans) or even fully (e.g. some cranes and storks) divided down the midline into a right and left trachea in the cranial portion which can make intubation for anaesthesia maintenance difficult or complicated.

Syrinx

Before the trachea divides into the two main bronchi, there is a structure known as the syrinx (see Figure 9.6). This is where the bird produces most of its voice. It is composed of a series of muscles and two membranes which can be vibrated, independently of inspiration or expiration. In the male of many breeds and species of ducks, shelducks and sheldgeese a cartilaginous structure known as the syringeal (sometimes called tracheal) bulla sits lateral to the syrinx and is used as a resonance chamber.

Lower respiratory system

Lungs

The lungs of avian species are rigid in structure and do not inflate or deflate significantly. They are flattened in shape and firmly attached to the ventral aspect of the thoracic vertebrae and vertebral ribs. There is no diaphragm in birds, and the common body cavity is referred to as the coelom.

The paired bronchi are supported by C-shaped rings of cartilage, unlike the trachea. The primary bronchi supply each of the two lungs, and rapidly divide into secondary and tertiary bronchi, or parabronchi. There are four main groups of secondary bronchi supplying the lung but their role in gas exchange is minimal. The tertiary bronchi, however, do play a role in gas exchange, as their walls are filled with membranes capable of gaseous exchange. These areas appear as small pits, or atria, to which are connected even finer tubes known as air capillaries. These intertwine with each other to form a three-dimensional mesh interwoven with the blood capillary beds. These air capillaries vary in size but average around 3–5 mm in diameter. This extremely small diameter produces very high forces of attraction between their walls when fluid secretions are present, resulting in rapid blocking of the respiratory surfaces. To stop this from occurring, there are cells within the parabronchi which secrete surfactant, to ensure the airways stay open.

The lung structure may be further classified by the direction of airflow within it into the neopulmonic lung and the paleopulmonic lung. These are mentioned later when discussing respiratory physiology.

Air sacs

The final part of the avian lower respiratory system is composed of the air sacs (see Figure 9.6). These are balloon-like sacs which act as passive receptacles, allowing movement of the air into and out of the rigid avian lungs in response to movements of the body wall and sternum creating negative and positive pressures in relation to atmospheric pressure inside the coelomic cavity. The air-sac walls are very thin and composed of simple squamous epithelium which covers a layer of poorly vascularised elastic connective tissue and do not contribute significantly to gaseous exchange.

In the majority of birds there are nine air sacs. One of these is the separate air sac already mentioned, the cervicocephalic air sac, that does not communicate with the lungs at all. The other eight all communicate with the lungs via a secondary bronchus (except the abdominal air sacs which connect to the primary bronchus on each side). Figure 9.6 shows a schematic of the air sac system of a duck.

In addition to the separate cervicocephalic air sac, the other standard eight air sacs are as follows.

1. A single cervical air sac which lies between the lungs and the dorsal oesophagus and communicates with air spaces within the cervical vertebrae.
2. A single clavicular air sac has two diverticula, one of which involves the heart and, cranial to this, the thorax. The other extends around the bones and muscles of the pectoral girdle and crop. This air sac communicates with the air spaces within the medullary cavity of the humeri, scapulae and sternum.
3. The paired cranial thoracic air sacs lie dorsolaterally in the chest, ventral to the lung field and immediately caudal to the heart.
4. The paired caudal thoracic air sacs lie immediately caudal to the cranial air sacs. These are again positioned dorsolaterally within the chest and tend to be slightly smaller than the cranial ones.
5. The paired abdominal air sacs lie caudal to the caudal thoracic air sacs. They touch the caudal aspect of each lung field before spreading caudally into and around the gut. These communicate with the air spaces in the medullary cavities of the notarium, synsacrum, pelvis and femurs.

Respiratory physiology

Respiratory cycle

The ventral movement of the sternum and the cranial and lateral (outward) movement of the ribs create negative pressure in the coelomic cavity and so inflate the air sacs drawing air down the trachea and through the lungs. There are two portions to the avian lung, known as the neopulmonic and paleopulmonic sections. The neopulmonic part of the lung is caudolateral and is absent in certain species, such as penguins. It differs from the paleopulmonic lung in that air

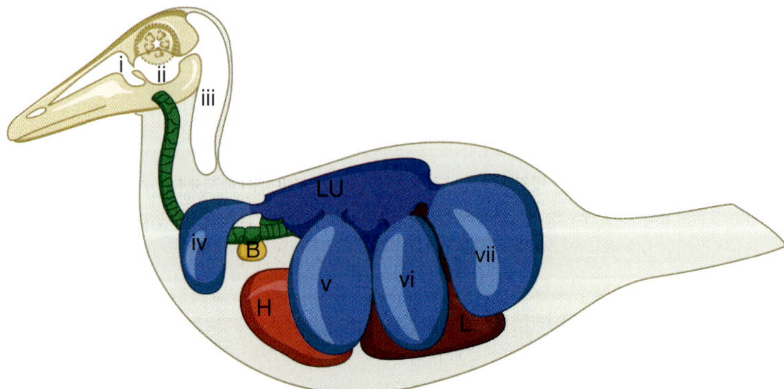

Figure 9.6 Avian air-sac system in a duck: (i) nasal passages; (ii) infraorbital sinus; (iii) cervicocephalic air sacs (single); (iv) clavicular air sacs; (v) cranial thoracic air sacs; (vi) caudal thoracic air sacs; and (vii) abdominal air sacs. H, heart; L, liver; LU, lungs; B, syringeal bulla (male ducks).

Box 9.1 Avian respiratory cycle

Inspiration	Keel moves ventrally and ribcage outwards to create negative pressure inside the body (coelomic) cavity. Fresh air and the air in the dead space of the trachea and the primary bronchi move into the secondary and tertiary bronchi, where gas exchange can begin. In addition some of this air travels through the neopulmonic tertiary bronchi into the caudal thoracic and abdominal air sacs where it takes no part in respiration
Expiration	Keel moves dorsally and ribcage inwards to create positive pressure inside the coelomic cavity. The caudal thoracic and abdominal air sacs contract and expel their air back through the neopulmonic part of the lung and into part of the paleopulmonic lung where gas exchange occurs
Second inspiration	Keel moves ventrally and ribcage outwards to create negative pressure inside the coelomic cavity. The air expelled during expiration through the neopulmonic and paleopulmonic lung continues to move cranially into the cervical, clavicular and cranial thoracic air sacs
Second expiration	Keel moves dorsally and ribcage inwards to create positive pressure inside the coelomic cavity. The air in the clavicular, cervical and cranial thoracic air sacs is expelled through secondary bronchi to the primary bronchi and so out of the body

passes through the paleopulmonic section of the lung in one direction only (from caudal to cranial), whereas the neopulmonic lung allows air movement in both directions through the same parabronchi. The parabronchi in the neopulmonic lung are also arranged haphazardly whereas in the paleopulmonic lung they are stacked parallel to each other. The avian cycle of inspiration and expiration is given in Box 9.1.

It is clear that the avian respiratory system is extremely efficient at extracting oxygen from the air. For one thing, the whole cycle occurs over two inspirations and expirations, allowing oxygen to be extracted on both inspiration and expiration. In addition, the airflow through the parabronchial tubes is at right angles to the accompanying blood flow. This creates a cross-current system, wherein oxygen in the airway is always at a higher concentration than its accompanying blood vessel, so encouraging the movement of oxygen from airway to bloodstream.

Physiological control of respiration

This is, in many ways, similar to mammalian respiratory control. Carotid body chemoreceptors in the carotid arteries monitor the partial pressure of oxygen in the blood, while carbon dioxide-sensitive receptors in the paleopulmonic parabronchi of the airways stimulate respiration once the airway partial pressure of carbon dioxide reaches a critical threshold. Some anaesthetic gases, such as halothane and to a lesser extent isoflurane, can depress the function of these carbon dioxide receptors, creating apnoea in the patient.

Digestive system

Oral cavity

The functions of this part of the digestive system are prehension, mastication and manipulation of food into the oesophagus, just as other mammals use their teeth, lips and tongue. The avian oral cavity differs from the mammalian in that it possesses relatively few taste buds and produces little saliva during the mastication process and the beak (already discussed under the skeletal structure) replaces teeth. Taste buds are supplied predominantly by the glossopharyngeal (IX) cranial nerve with branches from the trigeminal (V) and facial (VII) cranial nerves. Salivary glands tend to produce just mucus but there is evidence that in some species (e.g. the house sparrow) they do produce amylase (King and McLelland, 1984).

Tongue

The avian tongue may be relatively immobile and strap-like, as in Passeriformes (perching birds such as the canary, finch and songbird families), or it may be highly muscular and mobile as in Psittaciformes (parrots, parakeets, etc.), its motor nerve function predominantly supplied by cranial nerves VII (facial) and XII (hypoglossal). Alternatively, it may be extensible and specialised as in the hummingbirds and, to a lesser extent, in the nectar-eating parrots, the lories and lorikeets which have a fringed tongue for pollen and nectar feeding. In fish-eating birds such as penguins it may be covered with backward-pointing papillae and in other fish-eaters such as pelicans it is vestigial in nature.

Oesophagus and crop

The oesophagus is a muscular tube connecting the oral cavity to the first stomach (proventriculus) (see Figure 9.7). As in the lower digestive system, a series of peristaltic waves pass along the oesophagus when food is present, pushing the bolus of food towards the stomach. The oesophagus runs to the right of the trachea in the neck and is lined with many salivary glands. Some fish-eating species of birds have a series of hooks and papillae directed caudally to force slippery food items to travel in one direction only.

Along its route, usually at the thoracic inlet, some species have a diverticulum of the oesophagus, known as the crop (also known as the ingluvies). This is an expansible sac acting as a storage chamber for food. In the majority of birds the crop has no digestive enzyme-secreting properties, although in some species, such as pigeons, a form of lipid 'milk' is produced from the lining, which acts as a source of nutrition for the young. This crop 'milk' is really composed of exfoliated lining cells filled with lipid and which is produced in both sexes under the influence of the pituitary hormone prolactin to feed the young.

Some species, such as a few grain-eating finches, penguins, gulls, toucans, raptors, ducks and geese, do not have a specific crop, but instead have a much more distensible oesophagus, which can be used in the same way to store food, rapidly eaten. The crop, where present, empties into the thoracic portion of the oesophagus, which passes dorsally over the heart before entering the proventriculus or true stomach.

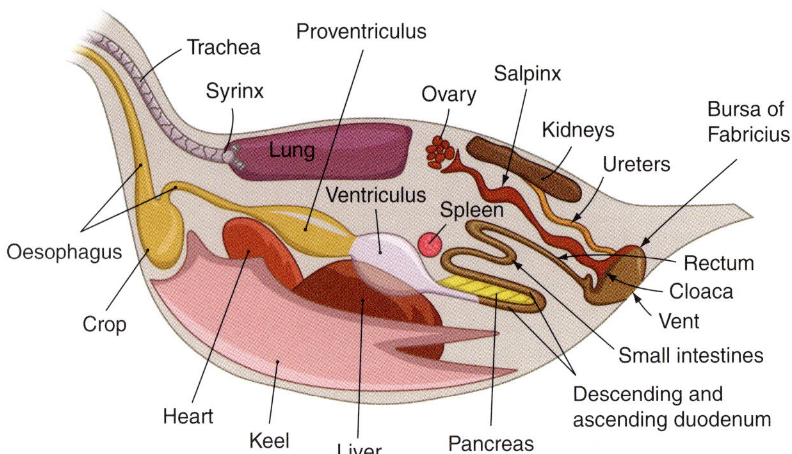

Figure 9.7 Generalised view of the internal organs of a female bird.

Avian 'stomachs'

Birds have two stomachs (see Figure 9.7). The first of these is the 'true' digestive stomach, known as the proventriculus. This organ is responsible for the secretion of the digestive proenzyme pepsinogen and hydrochloric acid. Unlike mammals, the secretion of these two substances occurs from the same compound gland, rather than two separate ones. Other glands exist in the proventriculus secreting hydrogen carbonate-rich fluid and intrinsic factor responsible for the absorption of vitamin B_{12} (cobalamin). In granivorous (seed-eating) birds the sac-like proventriculus empties into the more circular ventriculus, also known as the gizzard or grinding stomach. There is often movement of food backwards and forwards between proventriculus and ventriculus to mix and digest food thoroughly before passing it on to the rest of the gut.

The ventriculus lies on the left side of the avian coelomic cavity, caudally, and empties into the duodenum. Food outflow from it is regulated by a fold-like sphincter. In granivorous species, the ventriculus is larger than the proventriculus and very muscular with two pairs of muscles, one pair of smaller muscles and one larger pair, forming an asymmetric structure (see Figure 9.8). Each muscle bundle is separated from its neighbour by a sheet of tendinous tissue. Grit particles may be consumed by granivorous species and lodge in the ventriculus and act as an abrasive source for grinding seed, aiding in its mechanical breakdown.

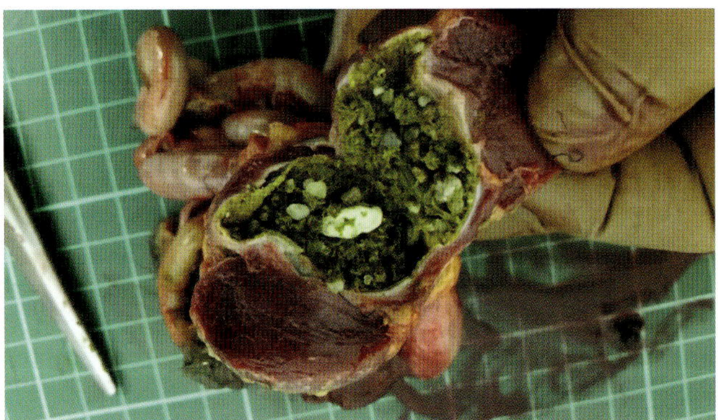

Figure 9.8 View of the opened gizzard (ventriculus) in a granivorous species. Note the asymmetry of the muscles surrounding it and the green bile (biliverdin)-stained food contents and grit particles.

In carnivorous species such as raptors and penguins the ventriculus is more of a simple muscular sac-like organ. The mucosa of the ventriculus is lined with deep tubular glands. In granivorous species in particular these glands secrete a protein substance which, in conjunction with cells shed from the inside of the ventriculus, forms a tough sheet-like layer known as the koilin or cuticle. This layer becomes heavily stained with green bile (biliverdin) refluxing into the ventriculus from the duodenum (see Figure 9.8). Its function appears to be protective and it is periodically replaced. Some species of raptors also produce a koilin and will regurgitate it as a neat package when expelling waste fur and bones from prey which has been consumed.

Small intestine

The first part of the small intestine is the duodenum. It forms a proximal (descending in many species) and then distal (ascending) limb which are adherent to each other forming a 'U' shape, the limbs being separated by the pancreas. The duodenum has separate openings into it from the biliary system of the liver (often two bile ducts) and from the pancreas (often three ducts).

The proximal duodenum contains many mucus-secreting goblet cells which serve to protect its lining from the acidic food mixture leaving the ventriculus. As in the mammalian duodenum, the avian duodenum is covered with a thick carpet of villi, which increases its absorptive area. The small intestinal brush border cells secrete some disaccharidase and monosaccharidase enzymes to further digest food. There is no evidence of the enzyme lactase in birds, so the feeding of milk-sugar or lactose-containing foods is not recommended. Along the intestine are discrete patches of lymphoid tissue, the so-called gut-associated lymphatic tissue (GALT) as seen in mammals. The jejunum and ileum are short in length in most avian pets such as parrots, and are difficult to define from each other although Meckel's diverticulum (the original connection to the yolk sac present as a chick) signifies the end of the jejunum and start of the ileum. It should be noted that Meckel's diverticulum does not persist in all individuals.

Large intestine

The large intestine is frequently referred to as the 'rectum' in birds and is relatively short. It is generally smaller in diameter than the small intestine in cage birds and raptors (see Figure 9.7). The rectum is responsible for the absorption of water and some electrolytes.

At the junction of the ileum and rectum in many species of bird are the (usually) paired caecae. In species such as the duck family or the domestic fowl the caecae may be relatively large. Other examples of species with large caecae are ratites, such as the ostrich or emu, and Galliformes such as the willow grouse and red grouse, which live off twigs and shoots such as heather (see Figure 9.9). The caecae in these species often act as fermenting chambers for the microbial digestion of cellulose and hemicellulose present in these tougher vegetable foods. In some species such as many owls, the caecae are also large but their function is not fully understood. The caecae have significant amounts of lymphoid tissue in all species. However, caecae may be absent in the case of most Psittaciformes or reduced in many Passeriformes to one or two lymphoid deposits. Finally, some species have a single caecum (e.g. herons). Distal to the caecae is the rectum which empties directly into the most cranial part of the cloaca known as the coprodeum.

Cloaca

This is the communal chamber into which the digestive, urinary and reproductive systems empty (see Figures 9.7 and 9.9). The most cranial segment is the coprodeum that receives faeces from the rectum.

The coprodeum is separated by a mucosal fold from the next chamber of the cloaca, the urodeum. The urodeum receives the urinary waste from the ureters, and the reproductive tract opens into it as well. The mucosal fold may be everted or pushed out through the vent, ensuring that the faeces do not contaminate the urodeum and so preventing contamination of the reproductive and urinary system. This fold can also close off the coprodeum from the urodeum completely when the male ejaculates, or when the female is egg laying, so as to prevent faecal contamination of semen or the egg as it passes through the cloaca.

The last chamber of the cloaca before the vent is the proctodeum. The proctodeum is connected to the bursa of Fabricius, which is the germinal centre for the B-lymphocyte line of the immune system (see section on the lymphatic system). The floor of the proctodeum is also where the male phallus is located in those species that possess one (e.g. ratites, many waterfowl and Galliformes).

Gastrointestinal tract innervation

The intestines and avian stomachs are supplied by branches of the tenth cranial nerve (CN X), also known as the vagus, which carries branches of the parasympathetic nervous system. The sympathetic nervous system also contributes to gut innervation, mainly via the intestinal nerve, which is a large plexus of sympathetic nerves that is close to the cranial and caudal mesenteric arteries and supplies the small and large intestines.

Liver

The liver is bilobed and partly covers the heart ventrally and extends caudally, ventral to the proventriculus and cranial to the gizzard (see Figures 9.7 and 9.10). The liver produces bile salts and bile acids,

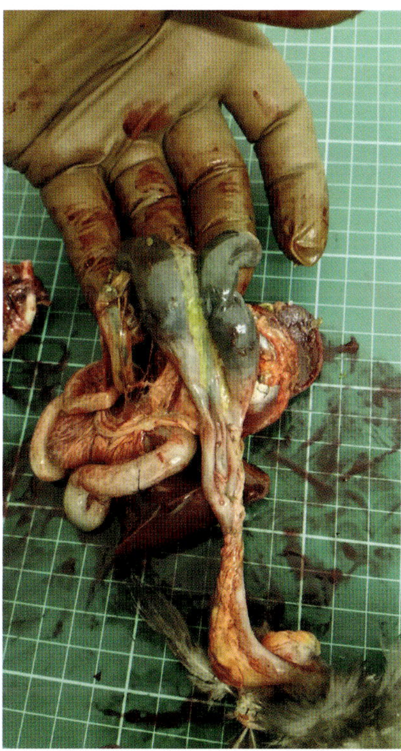

Figure 9.9 Post-mortem view of the prominent paired, in this case grey-green coloured, caecae in a Galliforme lying either side of the large intestine into which they caudally empty just before the rectum enters the cloaca.

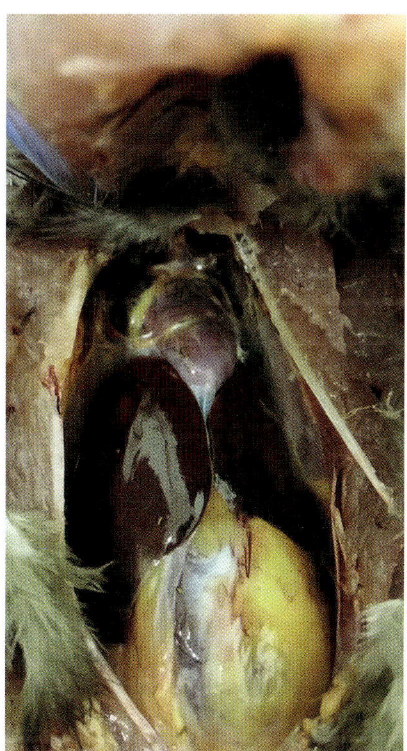

Figure 9.10 Post-mortem ventral view of a typical bird with the keel bone and ventral body wall removed. At the top of the image is the heart, immediately caudal to this are the paired liver lobes. Caudal to them is the intestinal mass and ventriculus covered in yellow fat. Thin membranes can be seen caudal to the heart laterally; these are some of the air sacs.

which are excreted into the duodenum via bile canaliculi and bile ducts and aid in the emulsification of fats in the small intestine.

The blood supply to the liver differs from that of mammals in that there are two hepatic portal veins taking nutrients from the digestive tract and there is both a left and right hepatic artery derived from the coeliac artery.

Some species have a gall bladder, but many parrots and pigeons do not possess one. In those species with a gall bladder, it tends to receive bile only from the right lobe of the liver, the left lobe draining directly into the duodenum.

The main bile pigment in birds is biliverdin. This means that measurement of total bilirubin levels is of limited clinical use in birds for assessing liver disease. It does however mean that liver inflammation and damage may often be indicated by the presence of biliverdin pigments in the urate portion of the droppings. These pigments turn the urates mustard-yellow or lime-green. Blood bile acid levels in starved birds are preferred as indicators of liver function. The predominant liver leakage enzyme (used to assess liver cell damage) in birds is aspartate aminotransferase (AST) rather than alanine aminotransferase (ALT) as is seen in mammals. As AST is also found in muscle cells, when measuring AST in birds it is usual to also measure creatine kinase (CK), which is only found in muscle cells, to help identify the source of any increase in AST detected.

Pancreas

The pancreas lies mainly between the proximal and distal limbs of the duodenum (see Figure 9.7). However, it has three lobes in total: dorsal, ventral and splenic. The gland is tubuloacinar in structure, similar to that of mammals, and is responsible for the secretion of the enzymes amylase, lipase, trypsin, chymotrypsin, carboxypeptidases, ribonucleases, deoxyribonucleases and elastases. As in mammals, it is also responsible for the production of bicarbonate ions which help neutralise the hydrochloric acid from the stomachs. The pancreas empties its exocrine secretions into the duodenum through up to three ducts depending on the species. The pancreas also produces the following hormones: insulin (from B cells), somatostatin (from D cells), glucagon (from A cells) and pancreatic polypeptide (from F cells).

Urinary anatomy

Kidney

The kidneys are paired structures found within the pelvis. They are tightly adhered to the backbone in the lumbosacral area (see Figure 9.7). Each kidney is divided into cranial, middle and caudal lobes (see Figure 9.11). Some of the major nerves supplying the legs pass through/around the kidneys on their way to the pelvic limbs, hence the reason why renal disease, particularly renal neoplasia, may affect the neurological function of a leg. Birds are uricotelic, that is they produce uric acid as the main waste product of protein metabolism as opposed to the urea produced in mammals.

Nephron

The nephron is the functional unit of the kidney, as it is in mammals; however, there are two types of nephron in birds. One is the cortical form that lacks a loop of Henle. It makes up 70–90% of the nephrons, depending on the species, and is found only in the outer cortex of the kidney. It can only produce isotonic urine. The other is known as the medullary nephron, and accounts for the other 10–30%. This does have a loop of Henle, which, like its mammalian counterpart, dips into the inner medullary region of the kidney and can produce hypertonic urine. Irrespective of the type of nephron, both start with a Bowman's capsule and a glomerulus. They then have a proximal tubule as mammals. This is where uric acid, the main waste product of protein metabolism, is actively excreted into the tubule and where glucose, amino acid and electrolyte resorption can occur. The medullary nephron then has a loop of Henle. Following this is the distal tubular component. The distal tubule follows the proximal in the cortical nephron with no loop of Henle. Both types of nephrons ultimately empty into the collecting ducts, with the duct tubes becoming fewer and fewer and their diameter becoming larger and larger until they empty into the ureter.

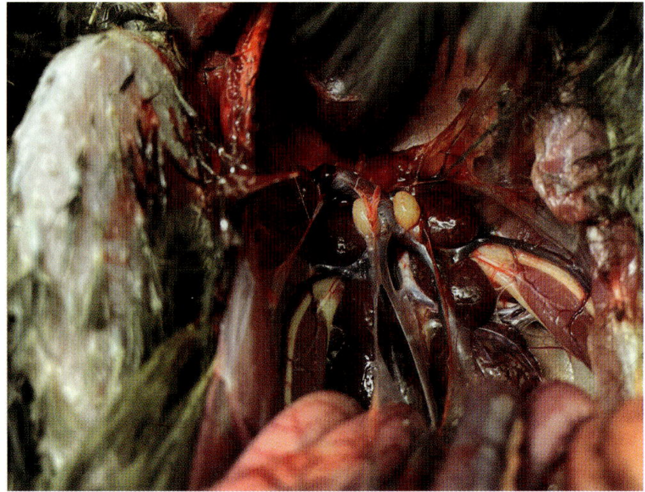

Figure 9.11 Post-mortem ventral view of the kidneys in a parrot. Note the trilobed appearance of each kidney, the complex blood supply and proximity of the nerves supplying the pelvic limbs. This is a male bird as denoted by the paired cream-coloured ovoid testes located medial to the cranial lobes of the kidneys.

Ureters

Each kidney has a ureter that arises from its cranial lobe but often does not emerge from the ventral surface of the kidney until the middle renal division. The ureter passes caudally, on the ventral surface of the middle and caudal renal lobes, receiving branches from the amalgamation of the collecting ducts. Each ureter continues caudally and finally empties into the urodeum segment of the cloaca, on its dorsal surface. Birds do not have a urinary bladder or urethra.

Renal blood supply

Each kidney in the avian patient is supplied by three renal arteries, the cranial, middle and caudal renal arteries, that supply the cranial, middle and caudal renal lobes, respectively.

In addition to this arrangement, the avian kidney also receives blood from the renal portal system. The renal portal veins form a ring of vessels surrounding the kidneys and connect with the vertebral sinus cranially and the caudal mesenteric vein caudally. Within the common iliac vein, draining the hindlimb and anastomosing with the renal portal veins, is a valve. This renal portal valve can divert blood in a number of directions. For instance:

- It can allow blood through from the leg and so on into the caudal vena cava, bypassing the kidneys altogether.
- It could shut and so divert blood from the hindlimb into the kidney tissues. (This is of importance theoretically when administering potentially nephrotoxic drugs or drugs which are excreted by the kidneys into the hindlimbs of birds.)
- The blood could equally be shunted towards the liver via the caudal mesenteric vein or into the internal vertebral venous sinus within the spinal canal. The blood flow is therefore complex and difficult to predict.

Renal physiology and nephron structure

The anatomy of the cortical nephrons is significant because they do not have a loop of Henle, and so there is no countercurrent multiplier system by which the urine may be made more concentrated than the plasma. Therefore, most of the urine produced by birds is isosmotic – it is of the same concentration as the extracellular fluid.

The renin–angiotensin system and juxtaglomerular apparatus present in mammals is also present in birds and functions primarily to control sodium balance and so impacts upon blood pressure. The release of renin in response to falling sodium levels triggers the renin–angiotensin system, producing eventually angiotensin II that itself causes the release of aldosterone from the adrenal glands. Aldosterone, as in mammals, then increases the resorption of sodium from the distal tubules, drawing water with it.

In mammals, when an animal becomes dehydrated, antidiuretic hormone (also known as arginine vasopressin) is released from the posterior pituitary. This causes the opening of channels in the renal collecting ducts for further absorption of water. In birds the hormone released is arginine vasotocin (AVT), which works on several areas of the bird's body as, unlike mammals, birds do not rely solely on the kidneys for water conservation. This is because, as previously mentioned, of their poor ability to produce concentrated hypertonic urine. AVT has more of an effect on the blood flow through the glomeruli rather than on the glomeruli themselves. By reducing this blood flow, it reduces the amount of filtrate produced and so conserves water. It does also have some effect on the collecting ducts of the nephron, increasing water reabsorption.

Uric acid requires little water to be excreted as it is actively excreted by the epithelium of the proximal tubules into the proximal tubular lumen where it binds to serum albumin that has entered the lumen from the glomerular filtration membrane. The albumin binds to the uric acid to form the urates, which is important as it ensures that they do not contribute to the osmolality of the final urine. This albumin–uric acid binding in the proximal tubule lumen also ensures that 'urates' (microspherical smooth structures) are formed rather than the jagged crystalline uric acid, facilitating their easy passage down the nephron and out of the body as does the secretion of mucin material from the tubule itself.

To remove the salts that build up during dehydration, many species of birds have salt glands that excrete concentrated sodium chloride from the body, for example penguins, pelicans, flamingos, and even some species of Falconiformes and Galliformes. They are present in the head and empty into the nostrils and are also influenced, positively this time, by AVT.

Finally, some fluid is reabsorbed in the avian rectum as urine enters the urodeum of the cloaca and may then be refluxed back through the coprodeum and into the rectum.

Cardiovascular system

Heart

The avian heart has four chambers and is larger in proportion to the rest of its body than its mammalian counterpart, averaging 1–1.5% body weight as compared to 0.5% body weight on average in mammals (see Figure 9.12). Birds also have bigger stroke volumes and lower heart rates and overall greater cardiac outputs than a mammal of the same weight (Grubb, 1983). Indeed, the cardiac output is around seven times that of an equivalent-sized mammal with resultant higher blood pressures, around 140–250 mmHg for systolic blood pressure (King and McLelland, 1984).

In the domestic chicken and some other species of bird, the sinus venosus, which forms part of the wall of the right atrium in mammals, is actually a separate, albeit poorly defined, chamber into which the caudal vena cava and the right cranial vena cava empty. The left vena cava empties nearby but is separated from the other two vessels by a septum. Where present the sinus venosus has sinoatrial valves separating the caudal vena cava entrance and the right cranial vena cava from the rest of the right atrium.

The two atria are separated from the ventricles by atrioventricular (AV) valves. The right AV valve has only one muscular flap with no chordae tendineae. The left AV valve has two valves in some species and three in others.

There are two main coronary arteries (a right and left with the right being larger, unlike mammals where the left is larger) supplying blood to the myocardium, and four major coronary veins and one minor vein as opposed to most mammals which have a single major and single minor coronary vein.

Blood vessels

The avian patient differs from the mammalian in that the aorta curves to the right side of the chest rather than the left (see Figure 9.12). It gives off the left and right brachiocephalic trunks shortly after leaving the heart.

The avian 'abdominal' contents are supplied with the same coeliac, cranial and caudal mesenteric arteries as the mammalian. The main difference is that three arteries supply the kidneys. In the case of reproductive organs, the testes are supplied by arteries arising from the cranial renal arteries, while the left ovary is supplied by an artery branching off from the left cranial renal artery. (There is often only one ovary; see the section on the reproductive system.)

The pulmonary artery starts as a single vessel (also known as the pulmonary trunk) from the right side of the heart and then splits into the left and right pulmonary arteries supplying the left and right lungs respectively. The left and right pulmonary veins return blood from the left and right lungs through two separate openings into the left atrium.

The legs are supplied by the femoral artery arising from the external iliac artery. However, the leg is also supplied by a larger vessel than the femoral artery, known as the ischiadic artery. This arises from a

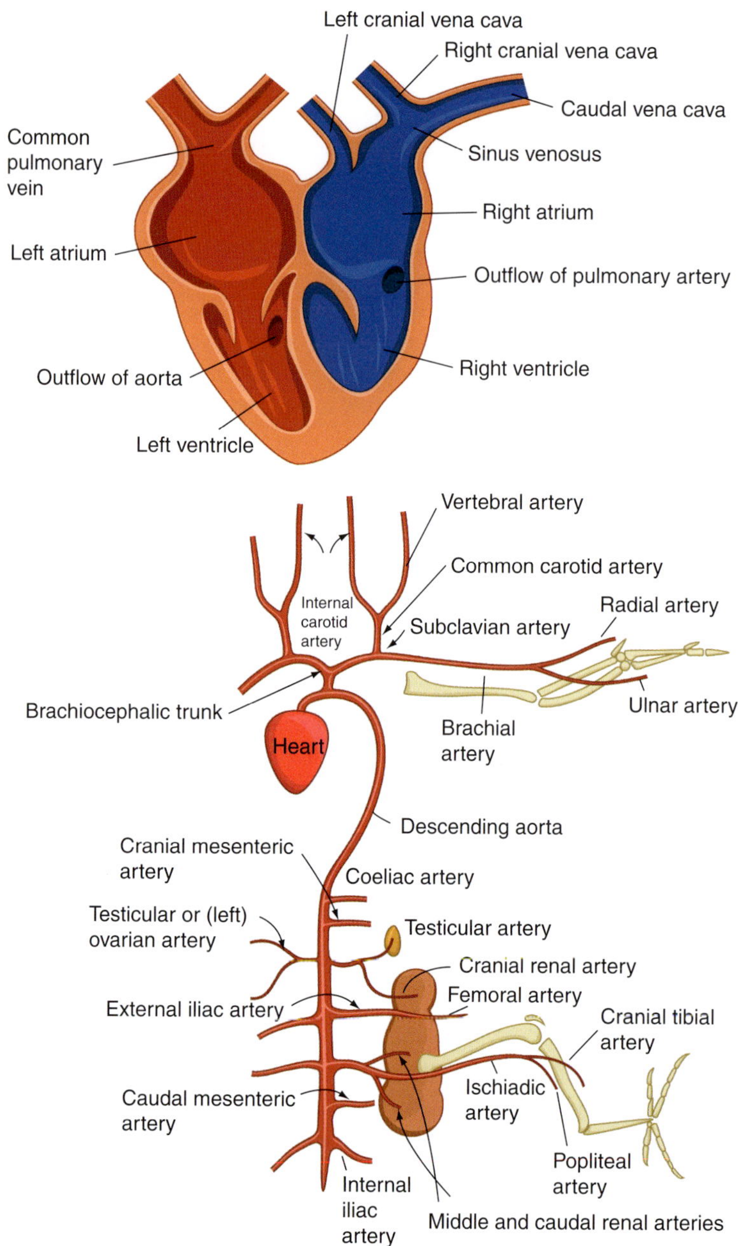

Figure 9.12 Cross-sectional view of the avian heart and dorsal view of the circulation.

common vessel offshoot of the aorta which also creates the middle and caudal renal arteries, and so passes through and over the kidney structure. It continues down the leg, changing into the popliteal and cranial tibial arteries.

The head is supplied with blood chiefly by the left and right carotid arteries that arise as mentioned from the left and right brachiocephalic arteries. The wings are supplied from the subclavian arteries that also arise from the brachiocephalic trunks and which then supply the pectoral muscles (via the axillary artery) that form the breast. The axillary artery then gives rise to the brachial artery that supplies the humeral region. The brachial artery then gives rise to the radial and ulnar arteries to supply the rest of the more distal wing.

Blood is drained from the head chiefly by the right and left external jugular veins. In the majority of avian species, the right jugular vein is much larger than the left and in many receives an anastomosis from the left. These join the right and left subclavian veins to create the right and left cranial venae cavae that empty into the right atrium as mentioned.

The abdominal contents of the bird are drained through a series of vessels: the main vessel returning to the heart is the caudal vena cava which is supplied by two large hepatic veins and many minor ones; the caudal vena cava also receives blood from the common iliac vein and the two testicular or one ovarian vein depending on the sex and species of the bird; the liver is supplied by two hepatic portal veins from the intestines as opposed to the one vessel in the mammalian system.

The common iliac vein receives supplies from the caudal and cranial renal veins and from the structure known as the renal portal circulation.

The majority of the blood from the legs is drained first by the caudal tibial vein, then into the popliteal vein joined by the cranial tibial vein, then ischiadic vein and finally the external iliac vein which itself empties into the common iliac vein.

The wing is drained by the radial and ulnar veins which converge to form the brachial vein. This runs alongside the humerus on its caudoventral aspect and can be used for intravenous injections in many species. The brachial vein runs into the subclavian vein and so on into the left or right cranial vena cava.

Lymphatic system

Spleen

The avian spleen is spherical in many species of Psittaciformes but may be more strap-like in other species, and sits adjacent to the proventriculus. It has white and red pulp areas, as in mammals, and acts to remove old red blood cells, as well as functioning as part of the immune system and in cell production. It is particularly important in systemic infectious diseases, such as psittacosis, where, due to antigenic stimulation, it may increase 10-fold in size.

Thymus

The thymus is composed of a series of islands of lymphoid tissue strung out along the neck and thoracic inlet. It is responsible for the production of T lymphocytes which are necessary for cellular immunity. As with mammals, the thymus decreases in size with age but may still be present in the adult bird, although the presence of a significant thymus in an adult bird has been associated with serious chronic disease such as mycobacteriosis.

Lymph nodes

These do not occur as recognisable organs in birds except in some waterfowl such as ducks and geese. These waterfowl have two main nodes, one near to the gonads and kidneys and one near to the thoracic inlet.

In other species, lymphatic tissue is present in accumulated areas within the internal body organs such as the kidneys, liver, digestive system, pancreas and lungs.

Bursa of Fabricius

This is a structure unique to birds. It is situated in the dorsal wall of the proctodeum segment of the cloaca. It is where the avian B-lymphocyte population, responsible for humoral or antibody immunity, is produced. The bursa, as does the thymus, decreases in size with age and usually disappears altogether in the adult bird.

Endocrine system

Adrenal glands

The paired adrenal glands lie medial to the cranial division of the kidneys. The left adrenal gland is usually larger than the right. The structure of the glands is not consistent between species but tends to have a mixture of chromaffin cells (those secreting adrenaline/epinephrine and noradrenaline/norepinephrine) and adrenocortical cells (those secreting corticosteroids and mineralocorticoids). This means there is often no clear cortex and medulla as in mammals. The predominant corticosteroid in birds is corticosterone and the predominant mineralocorticoid is aldosterone.

Thyroid, parathyroid and ultimobranchial glands

The thyroid glands in birds are paired and sit around the thoracic inlet. They produce triiodothyronine (T3) and thyroxine (T4) as in mammals. These hormones affect metabolic rates, thermoregulation and moulting among other things.

The parathyroid glands are paired and are located caudal to the thyroid glands and produce parathyroid hormone as with mammals that raises blood calcium levels by increasing calcium absorption by the intestines and resorption from bones (important during egg laying in hens).

The ultimobranchial glands are paired and lie caudal to the parathyroid glands although they can sometimes fuse with both thyroids and parathyroids on their respective sides. They produce the hormone calcitonin in response to increased blood calcium levels, leading to a decrease in the mobilisation of calcium from bone and decreased absorption of calcium in the kidneys.

Pancreas

The pancreas is also an endocrine (as well as exocrine) gland and produces principally insulin, glucagon and somatostatin in birds, as with mammals. Broadly speaking, glucagon increases blood glucose levels and insulin decreases it by driving glucose intracellularly. Glucagon is considered more important than insulin in carbohydrate and lipid metabolism in birds and many birds have relatively high circulating levels of blood glucose and are considered relatively resistant to insulin.

Reproductive anatomy

Male

Testes

There are two testes, both of which, unlike most mammals, sit entirely within the abdominal or coelomic cavity. They are positioned craniomedial to the kidneys and are tightly adherent to the dorsum of the body wall either side of the midline (see Figure 9.11).

In species that have set breeding seasons, the testes often enlarge during the reproductive season. This is perhaps most noticeable in species of the pigeon and dove family (Columbiformes), Anseriformes and Galliformes where the testes may enlarge by up to 20 times their out-of-season size. By comparison, in non-seasonal breeders such as many parrots, the testes do not significantly change in size over the course of the year. The testes have a significant surface venous plexus designed to cool them to allow spermatogenesis to occur. In most species the testes are a cream-yellow colour but in some, such as many cockatoos, they may be black due to large amounts of melanin pigmentation. Each testis empties spermatozoa into seminiferous tubules that eventually open through a series of ductules into the epididymis on the dorsomedial surface of the testis. From the epididymis runs a single vas deferens or spermatic cord which traverses the ventral surface of the kidney before entering the urodeum section of the cloaca via an ampulla.

Phallus

There is no phallus in many species of birds. Instead, the semen is transferred by the apposition of the male cloacal vent to female cloacal vent.

Some species do have a phallus, including the Anseriformes, or duck, goose and swan family, as well as the ratite (ostrich, cassowary, emu and rhea) family and the domestic chicken and many other Galliformes. Even within these species there is considerable variation in phallus construction, with some having a protrusible more fibrous phallus, often spiral in shape (e.g. Anseriformes) and others a non-protrusible phallus as is seen in Galliformes such as the domestic chicken.

The phallus lies in its dormant state on the ventral aspect of the cloaca. When aroused it engorges with blood and everts through the vent to curve in a ventral and cranial direction. Along the dorsal surface of the erect phallus runs the seminal groove. The semen drops from the vas deferens openings in the cloaca into the groove, which then guides the sperm into the female cloaca. The phallus therefore plays no part in the process of urination, unlike its mammalian counterpart.

Female

Ovary

There is only one ovary, the left, in most species (see Figures 9.13 and 9.14). One or two species have two ovaries, the kiwi and many hawks (e.g. goshawk) for example. The ovary is cranial to the left kidney, suspended from the dorsal body wall by a mesentery containing numerous short ovarian arteries derived from the aorta. For this reason, when surgically neutering a female avian patient, only the uterus is removed, leaving the ovary intact.

Infundibulum

From this one ovary arises a one-sided reproductive system. Adjacent to the ovary is the fimbria or funnel part of the infundibulum. This 'catches' the oocyst when it is shed into the reproductive tract. Attached immediately to the funnel is the tubular part of the infundibulum, which is also known as the chalaziferous region.

Magnum

Joining onto the infundibulum is the magnum portion of the reproductive system. This is highly coiled and much larger in diameter than the infundibulum, with many folds to its lining. There are multiple ducts leading to the lumen of the magnum, with the most caudal portion containing mucous glands as well.

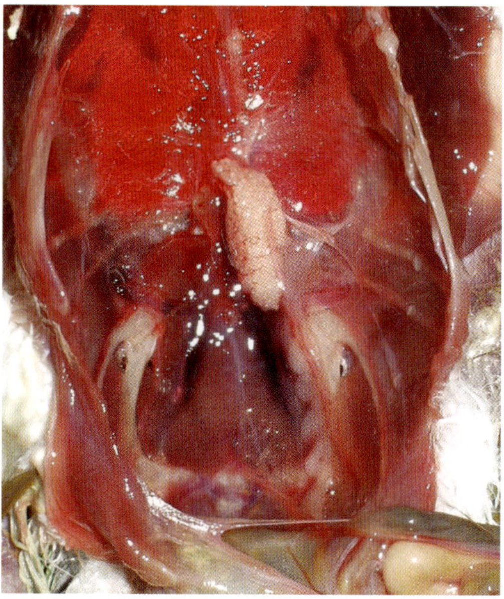

Figure 9.13 Post-mortem ventral view of a female bird showing the single (left) ovary typical of most species and the coiled single oviduct descending to the cloaca. In this image other body organs (except the bright red lungs at the top and the dark red coloured paired kidneys at the bottom) have been removed.

Attached to the caudal portion of the magnum is the isthmus, which is narrower in diameter and less coiled, but with more prominent longitudinal folds.

Uterus

Attached to the caudal portion of the isthmus is the shell gland or uterus. This is a short portion of the tract with many leaf-like folds. It empties into the S-shaped vagina, from which it is separated by a muscular sphincter.

Reproductive physiology

Male

The male avian testes are primarily composed of seminiferous tubules. In between these are the interstitial, or Leydig, cells which are the main source of androgens (male sex hormones) in the male bird. The seminiferous tubules are similar to their mammalian counterparts and contain the Sertoli cells in which the spermatozoa are nourished and the spermatogenic epithelium that produces spermatozoa.

In perching birds (Passeriformes) each vas deferens forms an enlarged area just before entering the urodeum, known as the seminal glomus. The two glomi become so swollen during the breeding

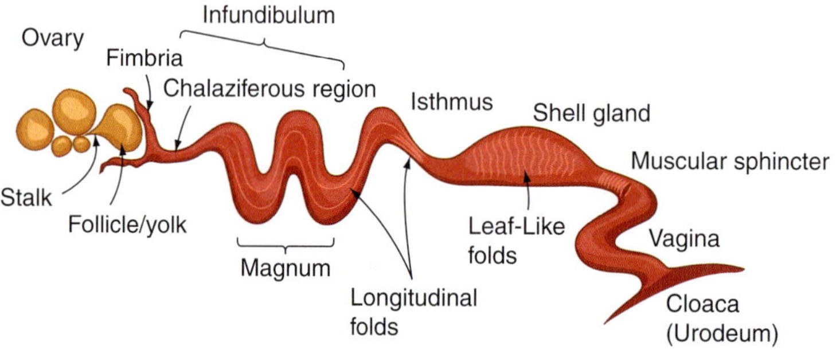

Figure 9.14 Avian female reproductive tract.

season as to form one mass, known as the cloacal promontory, which acts as the storage chamber for sperm. These can be used to sex many species of Passeriformes.

In seasonal breeders, the testes will enlarge during the reproductive season, with sperm production ceasing during the winter months. In many birds the left testis is larger than the right, following a pattern similar to that of the female gonad. The colour of the testes may also change during the breeding season, going from a yellow, or in some instances blackened, colour to a grey or white as they enlarge with spermatozoa.

Female

In the ovary, folliculogenesis (production of the oocyte and its yolk) is similar to that seen in mammals. The cycle is as follows.

1. Each follicle starts with the oocyte. The oocyte obtains its 'yolk' of lipids and proteins from the liver via the bloodstream in response to follicle-stimulating hormone (FSH) which is secreted by the anterior pituitary and causes the thecal cells of the ovary to produce oestrogens.
2. Over the surface of the follicle lies a white band known as the stigma which splits, shedding the oocyst from the follicle into the infundibulum. This occurs following the release of luteinising hormone from the anterior pituitary.
3. The corpus haemorrhagicum and corpus luteum, which are seen in mammals, are absent in birds, although some progesterone hormone production may occur from remaining cells.
4. The ovum is fertilised in the infundibulum (assuming a successful mating) 15–20 minutes after ovulation. The fertilised ovum moves through the tubular portion of the infundibulum (the chalaziferous portion). Here the chalazion, or egg yolk supporting membrane, is deposited around the egg yolk. This is a dense layer of albumen or inner egg white. The ovum moves on into the magnum where the bulk of the egg white (albumen) is deposited. After this the egg moves into the isthmus gaining the tough shell membranes. Finally, it moves into the uterus or shell gland where the mineralised shell and outer cuticle is deposited. It is also here that 'plumping' occurs. This is when the bulk of the water content is added, mainly to the albumen portion of the egg. It is also responsible for the deposition of the outer egg surface (cuticle) providing a microporous, protective breathing membrane on the egg's surface. When the egg is ready, the uterine or vaginal sphincter opens, allowing the egg to move into the vagina.
5. The vagina acts as the main storage site for spermatozoa immediately after copulation and it is where the sperm mature. It is also responsible for expelling the egg when it is ready by muscular contractions.

Incubation

All birds lay eggs and these require incubation for development to occur. In many species the hen bird incubates the eggs, but some take turns between the sexes (e.g. cormorants, Columbiformes, sandpipers) and some it is the responsibility of the male (e.g. cassowaries). Most Psittaciformes require an incubation temperature of 37.3–37.5°C (99.1–99.5°F) (Joyner, 1994). For domestic chickens typically temperature ranges of 37.2–38.9°C (99–102°F) are used. Humidity is also important to avoid dehydration and during incubation this should typically be 50–55% rising to 70% from day 18–21 in domestic chickens. Humidity needs to increase towards the end of incubation to avoid dehydration and consequently difficulty for the chick in exiting the eggshell and membranes. For cockatiels a temperature of 37.5°C (99.5°F) and humidity of 56% for the first 17–18 days followed by a drop in temperature to 36.9°C (98.4F) and an increase in humidity to 67% is required (Cutler and Abbott, 1986). Many raptors are incubated at an average temperature of 37.7°C (99.9°F). Weight loss of the egg due to dehydration is typically 11–16% during the incubation period.

Movement of the egg is also important in birds during incubation and this is typically carried out by the hen or male bird, depending on the species, during the incubation period. If artificially incubating eggs, then it is important that the eggs are rotated to avoid the embryo sticking to the membranes and resulting in a failure to hatch. This movement of the eggs is generally carried out mechanically by artificial brooders as the whole platform the eggs sit on tilts slowly back and forth. However, this should stop a few days prior to expected hatching otherwise it can affect the success of the chick exiting the eggshell. Incubation lengths vary considerably between species (Table 9.2). When a chick hatches its head moves from under its wing and first breaks into the airspace at the blunt end of the egg (known as 'internal pipping'). From there, well-developed muscles in the neck region and the presence of the 'egg tooth', a horn on the tip of the distal rhinotheca, facilitate the neat breaking of the eggshell to allow hatch (see Figures 9.15 and 9.16). Failure to successfully hatch can occur due to many factors, including the following.

1. Early embryonic death due to hypovitaminosis A in the hen.
2. Too much humidity during incubation resulting in a 'wet' chick.
3. Too little humidity during incubation resulting in dehydration and sticky membranes.
4. Lack of rotation of eggs during incubation leading to malpositioning.
5. Malpositioning of the chick (head at wrong end, head not under wing, etc.).

It is generally considered that if an egg is over 80% through incubation, then notochord and central nervous tissue development has occurred and so the unhatched chick is likely to be able to perceive pain. This has significant welfare implications for any decision to cease incubation after 80% of the incubation time has elapsed and

Table 9.2 Typical incubation lengths for selected avian species.

Species	Typical incubation length (days)
African grey parrot	26–28
Amazon parrot	26–28
Barn owl	30–34
Budgerigar	18
Chicken	21
Cockatiel	21
Cockatoo	28–31
Golden eagle	43–45
Harris hawk	32
Peregrine falcon	33–35
Quail	17–23
Scarlet macaw	24–28
Tawny owl	30

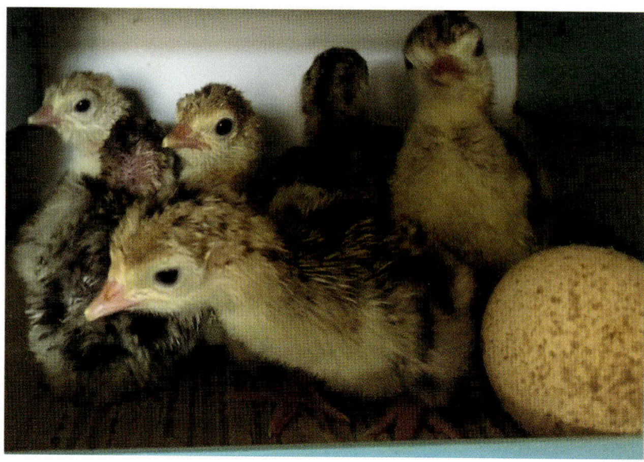

Figure 9.15 Recently hatched domestic turkeys showing the 'egg tooth', a yellow-coloured keratinised horn on the rostrodorsal rhinotheca used to help break out of the shell.

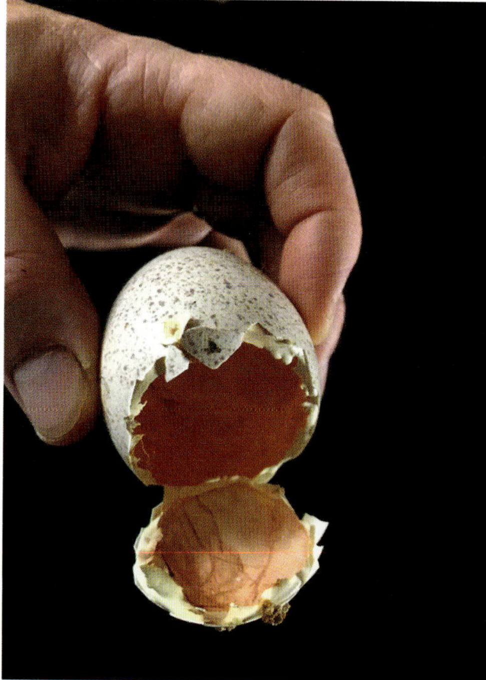

Figure 9.16 Empty eggshell from a successfully hatched chick showing the neat circumferential breaks in the shell and membranes at the 'blunt' end to create a trapdoor allowing the chick to exit.

veterinary advice should be sought as humane euthanasia techniques should be utilised (AVMA, 2020).

Sex determination and identification

In the majority of bird species, sexual identity is chromosomally (i.e. genetically) determined.

Sex identification may be performed in three main ways.

1. Some species show sexual dimorphism. That is, the two sexes appear physically different. For example:
   - When sexually mature, the male budgerigar (in 95% of cases) has a blue cere and the female a brown one.
   - Male cockatiels have a solid-coloured underside to their tails and a vivid orange cheek patch, whereas females have horizontal light and dark bars to the underside of the tail and a paler cheek patch. (Problems do arise in these two species when dilute colour variants [known as lutinos] and albino birds appear as there is often no pigmentation in the cere in these species.)
   - In some species the two sexes have totally different body feather colours. For example, the male eclectus parrot is a vivid green with a yellow beak, whereas the female is red and deep blue with a black beak.
   - Male large species cockatoos have a dark brown or nearly black iris and the females a light or red-brown one.
   - Male canaries will sing during the breeding season.
   - Many male songbirds are more highly coloured than the female. This is also true of many waterfowl, for example many ducks and most Galliformes.
   - In raptors there may be a wide variation in colours and sizes between the sexes. In most raptors, the female is significantly larger than the male bird, often as much as double the size. In some the markings are different (for example the female snowy owl is not only larger but speckled black and white to make her less obvious against the ground where she nests whereas the male is smaller and predominantly white).

   In sexually monomorphic species, such as African grey parrots, many macaws and Amazons, many penguins, flamingo and ibis species, identifying the sex of the bird has to be done by surgical sexing or DNA sexing, as there is no obvious reliable external difference between the sexes.
2. Surgical sexing involves anaesthetising the bird and passing a fine rigid endoscope through the flank/body wall of the patient in order to examine the internal gonad(s) visually. There are risks to such a procedure, which is why the process has been largely replaced by DNA sexing.
3. DNA sexing requires either a sample of the patient's blood or the pulp from a freshly plucked body feather to be genetically examined. This is submitted to the laboratory to determine if the DNA is that of a male or female bird. In birds the female is the heterogametic sex, having sex chromosomes known as ZW; the male is homogametic for the sex chromosomes, being ZZ. This is the reverse of the situation in mammals where females are homogametic and where females are XX and males XY.

Skin and feathers

Skin

Avian skin is much thinner than that of mammals and has little or no hypodermis. This means that in general it is poorly or loosely attached to the underlying structures. However, in regions such as the lower legs, the skin adheres directly to the periosteum of the bone and may be thickened and thrown into scales.

The skin has an outer epidermal layer which is composed of three main layers, from inside to out: the germinatory layer, the maturation layer and the cornified layer.

The dermis is much reduced compared to mammals. It forms very little in the way of a substantial structure but it does give the skin some elasticity, although nowhere near as much as mammalian skin.

There are no sweat glands in avian skin. A bird regulates its temperature by panting, known as gular fluttering, and by altering feather alignment to allow heat either to escape or to be trapped against the body surface.

Claws

The tip of each toe is supplied with a claw, formed of a keratinous material similar to the beak. These may be adapted to form the basic perching claws of the Passeriformes, the multipurpose perching and grasping claws of Psittaciformes or the ripping and prey-capture implements of the raptor family.

The members of the ratite family also have varying numbers of claws on their wing digits, and some falcons, such as the kestrel and peregrine falcon, and many older breeds of domestic chicken have a claw on the first digit or alula of the wing (see Figure 9.17).

Preen (uropygial) gland

The uropygial gland is situated over the synsacrum at the base of the tail (see Figure 9.18). It is a highly developed structure in most waterfowl, as it is responsible for producing oil to waterproof the feathers. The oil produced from the preen gland may also act as a source of vitamin D for the bird. It has a bilobed structure with two tubular exits, one for each lobe. The preen gland is also present in many other species, but is absent in some parrots, Amazons for example, as well as being absent in pigeons and some of the ratites.

Feathers

Feathers are unique to the class Aves (see Figure 9.19). They are arranged in a set pattern over the surface of the body, with some tracts

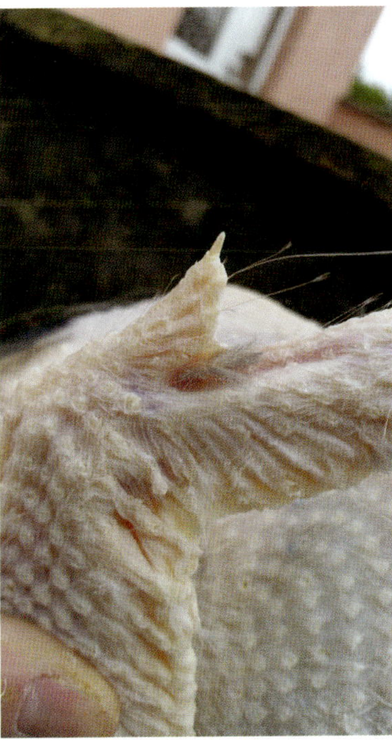

Figure 9.17 Post-mortem view of the ventral carpal and metacarpal area of a Light Sussex chicken. The feathers have been plucked to help demonstrate the first digit (alula) projecting cranial to the wing, the end of which has a rudimentary claw in this breed.

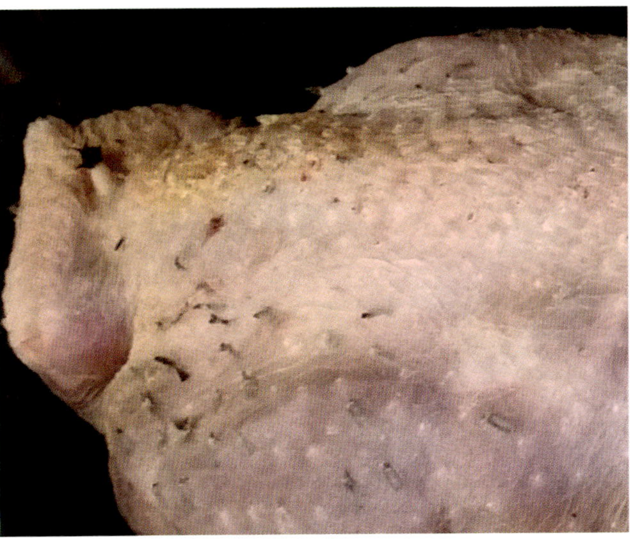

Figure 9.18 Uropygial (preen) gland at the dorsal base of the tail in a domestic turkey. The papilla exiting the gland is often associated with small feathers.

of skin being completely devoid of feather follicles. These areas of skin without follicles are known as apterylae, while other areas have rows of feather tracts known as pterylae.

There are six types of feathers in most species. These are known as:

1. contour or flight feathers
2. down feathers
3. powder feathers
4. semi-plume feathers
5. filo-plume feathers
6. bristle feathers.

Contour feathers

These form the flight feathers on wings and tail, and the main feathers outlining the body. The flight feathers are subdivided into primaries and secondaries, depending on whether they are derived from the 'hand' or manus (the carpus and digits) of the wing (the primaries) or the ulna or antebrachium of the wing (the secondaries). There are also contour feathers forming the tail, known as the rectrices. (The primaries and secondaries combined are referred to as the remiges.)

The remiges attach directly onto the periosteum of the relevant wing bone and so are deeply attached. In addition, they are covered at their bases by smaller feathers on the dorsal aspect of the wing known as covert feathers (see Figure 9.20).

The structure of the contour feather is the classical quill shape. It is supported by the main shaft of the feather which is embedded in the follicle. The part of the shaft to which the vane of the feather is attached is known as the rachis. The vane is formed from parallel side branches set at 45° to the rachis, which are known as barbs. From the barbs arise distal and proximal barbules, each of which has its own smaller hooks known as hamuli. These form interconnections with other barbules, and this allows the feather to form a solid but ultralight structure.

The part of the shaft which is devoid of the feather vane is known as the calamus. This is the part inserted into the follicle and which, in the immature growing feather, is filled with nerves and blood vessels. This is

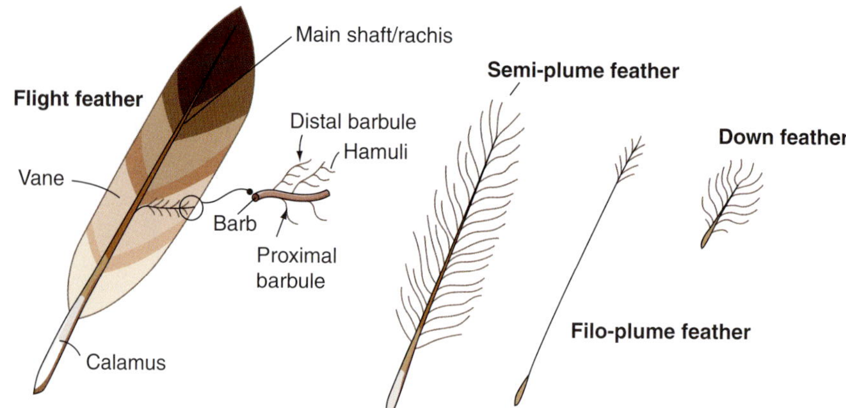

Figure 9.19 Avian plumage: differing types of feathers.

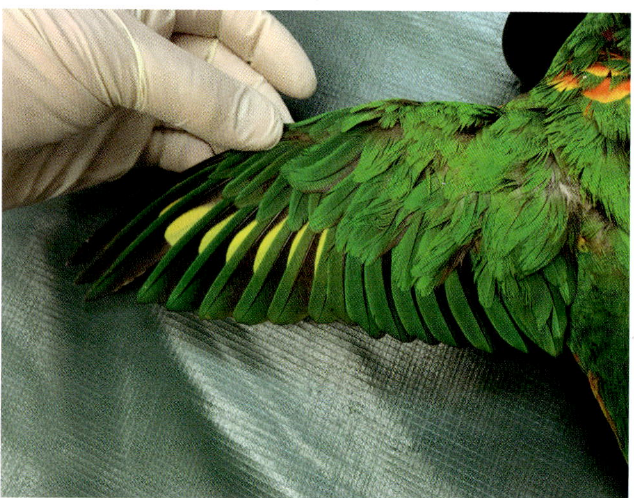

Figure 9.20 Dorsal aspect of a parrot's wing showing the primary, secondary and covert feathers.

known as the feather pulp. It is this area which, when emerging through the skin, is at risk of being damaged by the bird. It can then bleed profusely, giving the young feather its alternative name of 'blood feather'.

Down feathers

The down feathers provide an insulating layer below the contour feathers of the adult bird. They are also the main feather of the chick. They are much shorter in length than the contour feathers and have a 'fluffy' look, as there are no barbules to interlock the vane structure.

Powder feathers

As their name suggests, the powder feathers produce a fine white powder which is shed over the surface of the bird. This appears to act as a semi-waterproof covering. Some species produce more powder than others, African grey parrots and cockatoos for example. This powder may cause irritation to the airways of species which are relatively powder-free, such as Amazon parrots. This is a good reason for not mixing these species together in the same aviary or cage.

Many viral and bacterial agents may infect the powder feathers. The infection is then spread when the powder is shed. Examples of these organisms include *Chlamydia psittaci*, the cause of psittacosis; psittacine beak and feather disease virus (a circovirus); and the gamma herpesvirus which causes Marek's disease. Other feather follicles may also be affected.

Semi-plume feathers

The semi-plume feathers have long shafts but, like the down feathers, they have no barbules. This gives them a 'fluffy' appearance. They are situated below the contour feathers and are thought to provide insulation.

Filo-plume feathers

The filo-plume feathers are situated close to the contour feathers and possess long, fine, bare shafts which end in a clump of barbs. Their roots are surrounded with sensory nerve endings. It is thought that these feathers are responsible for sensing the positions of the adjacent contour feathers. This allows the bird to make accurate alterations of flight and body feather positions.

Bristle feathers

These are similar to the filo-plumes in that they have bare shafts with a few barbs at the tip. They are, however, shorter and found around the beak and eyes, and again seem to have a sensory, tactile function.

Blood feathers and pin feathers

The blood feather is the young immature feather as it emerges from the follicle. It is so named because it possesses a plentiful blood supply.

At this stage, the feather is protected by an outer keratin sheath, which gives it its other name of 'pin' feather. As the feather develops inside this sheath, it is surrounded by a blood supply. As the vane forms, the blood supply retracts to the base of the feather below the skin surface. At this point, the sheath should split and allow the feather to unfurl (see Figures 9.21 and 9.22). If the sheath is damaged prior to retraction of the blood supply, then profuse bleeding will occur.

In some birds the sheath is retained long after the blood supply has regressed, and this gives the appearance of multiple, white, pin-like structures over the plumage. This can be a sign of general debilitation or of a nutritional deficiency.

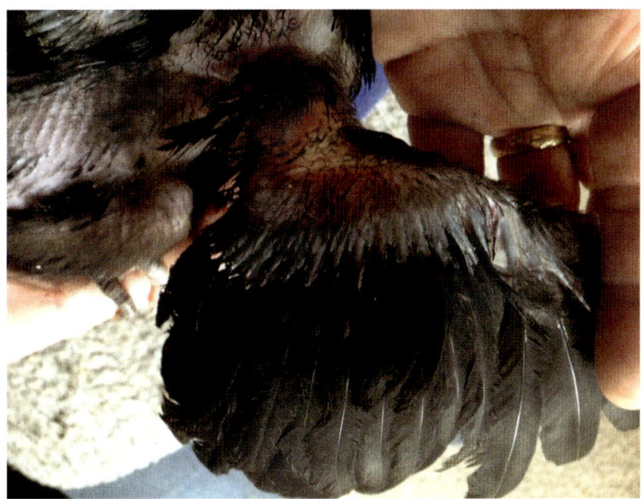

Figure 9.21 Dorsal aspect of the wing of a young chicken showing recently emerged flight feathers with retained feather-sheaths at their base.

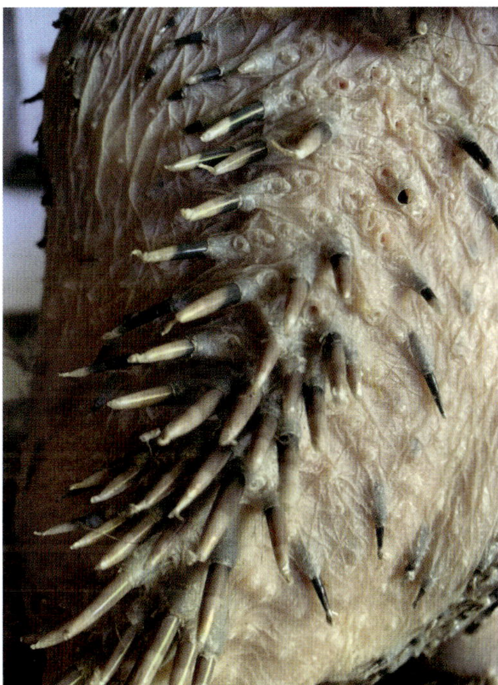

Figure 9.22 Pin or blood feathers newly emerged through the skin are covered in a sheath and surrounded by a blood supply meaning they can bleed profusely if damaged.

Moulting

Moulting occurs most frequently in young birds. Some are hatched without fully developed feathers (altricial species such as parrots) and some with fully developed down feathers (precocial species such as chickens and ducks). The young bird then goes through a series of moults in the first few months to produce juvenile plumage and eventually adult plumage. Moulting occurs in many adult birds once a year, usually just after the breeding season in the late spring/early summer in seasonally breeding species, although a partial prenuptial moult may occur in the spring to change into breeding plumage. Some species will moult more frequently, having a winter and a summer plumage which allows them to blend in with their surroundings, although some feather colour changes can occur through wear of the feathers themselves rather than a replacement of the feather. However, many eagles and large Psittaciformes kept indoors will moult every 2 years.

In general, the stimulus for moulting seems to be a combination of diurnal rhythms and temperature changes and may be mediated through hormones such as prolactin or FSH. Increases in prolactin in many species is associated with broodiness, that is the desire to incubate eggs, and falling levels of prolactin after incubation is completed are associated with moulting. In other species increasing FSH and therefore oestrogen levels are associated with broodiness and decreasing levels with moult.

During moult, the new feather forms at the base of the old and, like a permanent tooth pushing out a deciduous one, it dislodges the existing feather and grows in behind it. Most species do this gradually, taking several weeks to moult all of the feathers fully. Some though, such as some ducks, become completely flightless due to the loss of all of their flight feathers at once.

Haematology: an overview

The cells in a bird's bloodstream are significantly different from those in mammals. There are five main differences.

1. The avian erythrocyte is nucleated and oval in shape. This contrasts with the mammalian anucleate biconcave structure.
2. Heterophils are the equivalent of the mammalian neutrophil. Their function is similar, as the first line of defence against viral and bacterial infections. Heterophils, however, are a rounded cell with a colourless to pale pink cytoplasm and a multilobed nucleus (averaging two to three lobes). They possess brick-red, cigar-shaped to oval granules, and during infection these may appear to disintegrate, with the cytoplasm becoming vacuolated or foamy. This effect is useful in assessing the presence of infection, and these cells are referred to as 'toxic' heterophils. Excessive heterophil counts ($>30 \times 10^9$/L) are associated with diseases such as chlamydiosis/psittacosis, aspergillosis, avian tuberculosis or egg yolk peritonitis.
3. The basophil, lymphocyte and monocyte are basically similar to those in mammals and have broadly the same functions.
4. The eosinophil has a clear blue cytoplasm with a bilobed nucleus which stains more intensely than the heterophil. It has round, bright-red staining granules. It is more commonly seen in increased numbers in parasitic conditions, such as intestinal ascarid (roundworm) infestations. It may appear more basophilic in some species, such as African grey parrots.
5. The thrombocyte (platelet) is nucleated, unlike the mammalian anucleated form, and during severe infections may have some phagocytic functions.

Avian blood samples for haematological analysis may be taken into potassium EDTA tubes except in a few species. Examples of these exceptions are members of the crow, crane, flamingo and penguin families in which the erythrocytes will haemolyse. In these species heparin should be used for haematology. A fresh smear for the differential white cell count should also be made. This is because heparin samples yield inferior staining results, often resulting in excessive basophilic staining with Romanowsky stains.

Biochemistry: an overview

Biochemical parameters may be measured using heparinised blood (plasma) or clotted blood (serum) samples.

Liver biochemical parameters

The most reliable test for liver function in avian species is that for bile acids. Normal ranges vary from species to species, but commonly range from 20 to 80 mmol/L.

Other tests that reflect the level of liver damage in birds include AST rather than the more typically used liver leakage enzyme of mammals, ALT. AST activity is also found in muscle tissue, so often the two other biochemical tests for lactate dehydrogenase (LDH) and CK are performed. This allows some differentiation between liver and muscle damage, as CK is only found in muscles. LDH is released in the early stages of liver disease, but also has some skeletal and cardiac muscle distribution. The enzyme glutamate dehydrogenase (GLDH) is released when liver and kidney cells die or are disrupted. As the renal source of this enzyme goes into the urine directly, and not the bloodstream, blood levels of GLDH reflect any hepatocyte damage. Levels greater than 2 IU/L are considered elevated in psittacines (Hochleithner, 1994). Alkaline phosphatase is too non-specific for liver damage in birds to be of great use.

Kidney biochemical parameters

The only reliable test for renal function is uric acid. Neither urea nor creatinine is useful in avian species. However, uric acid is not a sensitive test, and is only elevated once the majority (>75%) of the renal mass ceases to function. Levels may be falsely elevated in many species particularly carnivores such as raptors immediately after feeding, so samples should be taken in the fasted bird. This may require 24 hours in the case of a large carnivore such as an eagle or penguin. Levels greater than 420 μmol/L in psittacines, 550 μmol/L in fasted raptors and 750 μmol/L in racing pigeons are suggestive of renal damage. Blood tests in chronic renal failure may show a massively elevated uric acid level (>1500 μmol/L) and sometimes potassium levels (>5 mmol/L). Urea levels may also be measured and compared with uric acid levels to ascertain if prerenal azotaemia or renal disease is present, as prerenal azotaemia will cause a predominant rise in urea while leaving uric acid levels within the normal range. The problem is the ratios need to be worked out for each species: the ratio is calculated by multiplying the plasma urea level (in mmol/L) by 1000 and then comparing it with plasma uric acid level (in μmol/L). In peregrine falcons, the ratio is greater than 6.5 (Lumeij, 2000).

Calcium and phosphorus

Levels of calcium and phosphorus depend on nutritional levels and renal function as well as on the presence of vitamin D_3 and functional parathyroid glands. Normal values quoted for total calcium are 2–2.8 mmol/L in most psittacines and 1.9–2.6 mmol/L in pigeons, or 0.96–1.22 mmol/L ionised calcium in African grey parrots. Excessively high levels of calcium (>3 mmol/L) may suggest oversupplementation, providing the bird is not an in-lay hen, when blood levels may raise this high normally due to calcium mobilisation for shell production. Ionised calcium levels represent the biologically active circulating calcium levels and so their measurement is preferred to total calcium levels. Ionised calcium needs to be measured soon after the blood sample is taken, therefore by a point-of-care analyser, as once the blood sample is outside the body of the bird, the metabolism of the blood cells and the exposure to room air will rapidly alter the pH of the blood and so the ionised calcium levels leading to false results.

For phosphorus, 0.9–5 mmol/L in psittacines and 0.57–1.33 mmol/L in pigeons are considered normal. Elevated phosphorus and calcium may suggest renal dysfunction. Low calcium and high or normal phosphorus suggest nutritional deficiency or the hypocalcaemic syndrome seen in African grey parrots. Low phosphorus levels have been associated with intestinal and stomach parasitism, particularly from nematodes such as roundworms (ascarids/parascarids).

Plasma proteins

These are very useful in birds to allow an assessment of nutrition and hepatic function, as well as for assessing the avian patient for the presence, or not, of inflammatory disease. To gain accurate split of the total proteins into albumin and globulins, it is necessary to perform protein electrophoresis. The usual dry chemistry systems present in many veterinary practices and used for mammals are often not accurate enough for this as birds have an additional protein, not present in mammals, called pre-albumin. Pre-albumin and albumin are primarily responsible for oncotic potential and act as carrier proteins for molecules such as hormones. The globulins, as in mammals, are split into acute-phase proteins such as alpha (usually 1 and 2) and beta (often single but occasionally split into 1 and 2) globulins as well as the gamma globulins (the so-called immunoglobulins or antibodies). Analysis of lithium heparin plasma is advised in birds (and reptiles) over serum, as plasma contains fibrinogen, an important acute-phase protein in birds (and reptiles). Analysis of plasma protein electrophoresis can give valuable information on for example the diagnosis of aspergillosis, where elevations in beta globulins are commonly seen (Girling, 2002a,b,c). It may also give valuable information on the likelihood (or not) of survival of birds affected by serious diseases such as aspergillosis by accurate assessment of albumin levels (Naylor *et al.*, 2017).

Blood glucose

Blood glucose measurement is useful in raptors, where the values should range between 17 and 22 mmol/L. If levels fall below 15 mmol/L, hypoglycaemic fitting and coma may develop in small species of raptor. If levels exceed 27 mmol/L, hyperglycaemic fitting can occur. Diabetes mellitus is seen in Psittaciformes such as budgerigars. Here values greater than 30 mmol/L may be observed. It is worth noting though that small elevations in blood glucose commonly occur in stressed birds and should not necessarily be taken to suggest clinical disease.

Sodium and potassium

Sodium and potassium levels in avian species are similar to those in mammals. Sodium deprivation can be an issue in marine species of birds kept in captivity as many are kept in fresh water and are fish-eaters. The process of freezing and defrosting fish leads to a reduction in their sodium levels unless supplementation is given. Elevated potassium levels (often above 5 mmol/L) can be associated with renal failure.

References

AVMA (2020) *AVMA Guidelines for the Euthanasia of Animals, 2020 Edition*. Available at https://www.avma.org/sites/default/files/2020-02/Guidelines-on-Euthanasia-2020.pdf (accessed 16 March 2024).

Bennett, R.A. (1994) Neurology. In: *Avian Medicine: Principles and Application* (eds B.W. Ritchie, G.J. Harrison & L.R. Harrison), 1st edn, pp. 723–747. Wingers Publishing, Lake Worth, FL.

Cutler, B.A. and Abbott, U.K. (1986) Effects of temperature on the hatchability of artificially incubated cockatiel eggs (*Nymphicus hollandicus*). *Proceedings of the 35th West Poultry Diseases Conference*, pp. 104–106.

Girling, S.J. (2002a) *Plasma protein electrophoresis: variations in health and disease in the family Psittaciformes*. Dissertation as part-fulfilment for the RCVS Diploma in Zoological Medicine, RCVS Library, London.

Girling, S.J. (2002b) A fungal granuloma in a corn snake (*Elaphe guttata guttata*) due to *Aspergillus fumigatus* associated with a previously treated abscess. *Bulletin of the British Veterinary Zoological Society*, **2**(1), 27–35.

Girling, S.J. (2002c) Mammalian imaging and anatomy. In: *Manual of Exotic Pets* (eds A. Meredith & S. Redrobe), 4th edn, pp. 1–12. BSAVA, Quedgeley, UK.

Grubb, B.R. (1983) Allometric relations of cardiovascular function in birds. *American Journal of Physiology*, **245**, H567–H572.

Hochleithner, M. (1994) Biochemistries. In: *Avian Medicine: Principles and Applications* (eds B. Ritchie, G. Harrison & L. Harrison), pp. 223–245. W.B. Saunders, Philadelphia, PA.

Joyner, K.L. (1994) Theriogenology. In: *Avian Medicine: Principles and Applications* (eds B. Richie, G. Harrison & L. Harrison), pp. 748–804. Wingers Publishing, Lake Worth, FL.

King, A.S. and McLelland, J. (1984) *Outlines of Avian Anatomy*, 2nd edn, pp. 1–134. Bailliere and Tindall, London.

König, H.E., Misek, I., Liebich, H.G. *et al.* (2016) Nervous system (*systema nervosum*). In: *Avian Anatomy: Textbook and Colour Atlas* (eds H.E. König, R. Korbel & H.-G. Liebich), 2nd edn, pp. 187–209. 5M Publishing, Sheffield, UK.

Lumeij, J.T. (2000) Pathophysiology, diagnosis and treatment of renal disorders in birds of prey. In: *Raptor Biomedicine 3* (eds J.T. Lumeij, J.D. Remple & P.T. Redig), pp. 169–178. Zoological Education Network, Lake Worth, FL.

Naylor, A., Girling, S., Brown, D. *et al.* (2017) Plasma protein electrophoresis as a prognostic indicator in *Aspergillus* species-infected Gentoo penguins (*Pygoscelis papua papua*). *Veterinary Clinical Pathology*, **46**(4), 605–614. doi: 10.1111/vcp.12527.

Chapter 10 Avian Housing and Husbandry

Cage requirements for Psittaciformes and Passeriformes

Cage requirements should ensure that ideal environmental conditions are available at all times to the bird. This not only includes temperature, humidity, ultraviolet light provision but also choice – the bird should have a range of preferred conditions that they can choose to occupy.

Cages to avoid

It is worthwhile avoiding certain cage types.

- 'Hamster' style cages which are wider than they are high. Birds enjoy freedom of movement in a vertical plane and feel more at ease when caged accordingly.
- Tall narrow cages which prevent lateral flight and movement.
- Cages coated in plastic that may be chewed off, as many plastics contain zinc and other compounds which may be toxic.
- Cages that have a poor metallic finish. Many cages are made of zinc alloys and if the finish of the wire surface is poor, the zinc may become orally available to the bird. As parrots in particular use their beaks to manoeuvre themselves around the cage, the tendency is to swallow the zinc dust coating the wire. The zinc builds up in the bird's body over a number of weeks and can lead to kidney and liver damage and, in severe cases, death – a condition referred to in texts as 'new wire-cage disease'.
- Cages with very small doors on them, which makes catching the bird difficult.

The preferred construction material for cages for Psittaciformes and Passeriformes is stainless steel. This is non-toxic and easy to keep clean.

Cage 'furniture'

Various items are important for providing basic needs and improving welfare. Consideration should be given to the type and position of perches, food and water bowls, floor coverings and toys.

Perches

Perches should be made of various different diameters, in order to provide exercise for the bird's feet and to prevent pressure sores from forming. The presence of single-diameter-sized perches will lead to pressure being applied to the same parts of the bird's feet continuously. This causes reduced blood circulation and results in corns and ulcers. If not corrected, it will ultimately lead to deep foot infections, referred to as bumblefoot or pododermatitis. The perches are best made of hardwood branches, such as beech, mahogany, and witch-hazel, which are relatively smooth and non-toxic. It is important to avoid using branches from trees such as ornamental cherries and laburnum, which are found in many gardens, as these are poisonous. If using branches collected from hedgerows, it is important to clean them with an avian-friendly disinfectant first to prevent contamination and disease transmission from wild birds. Concrete perches should be avoided as some parrots have been known to eat these, causing gastrointestinal problems or mineral oversupplementation leading to kidney problems.

Perches should never be covered with sandpaper. This does not keep their nails short, which is often the reasoning behind their use, but does lead to foot abrasions that can become seriously infected, resulting in conditions such as bumblefoot.

Perches should be positioned so as not to allow the bird to foul the food and water bowls and should not be stacked on top of one another as this allows any other bird in the cage to defecate onto the one below!

Food and water bowls

Food and water bowls should not be made of metal alloys as some are galvanised with zinc or have soldered edges that contain lead. Both lead and zinc are highly toxic to any cage bird. Plastic or ceramic bowls are therefore preferred. Alternatively, single-pressed (i.e. no soldered seams) stainless steel food bowls can be used instead.

Floor coverings

Sawdust, shavings and bark chips should be avoided for pet cage birds as these are difficult to keep clean and are often consumed. Newspaper, kitchen towel paper, and the sandpaper sold in many pet shops are better options for cage birds. However, certain ground-dwelling species, such as quail, may benefit from bark chippings or shavings as a floor covering because it allows natural foraging activity. Whatever the floor covering used, it should be changed regularly, at least twice-weekly. Newspaper or other paper coverings have the advantage that they are easy to remove, so it is easier to maintain hygiene standards, and the droppings may be observed for any changes from normal.

Toys

Passeriformes, the perching birds such as canaries, finches and mynah birds, are generally less interested in toys, although providing their food in novel forms can improve environmental enrichment. Psittaciformes, on the other hand, are considered more intelligent. On average the larger parrots have a mental ability of the typical 2-year-old human, and so benefit from toys and mental stimulation. Toys offered should of course be safe, attractive, and of a size and number appropriate to the number of birds and space allowed.

Veterinary Nursing of Exotic Pets and Wildlife, Third Edition. Simon J. Girling.

Some toys are harmful and should be avoided. These include the following.

- *Open chain links*: a bird's foot can easily become caught in one of these, particularly if the bird has an identification ring on its leg.
- *Bells with clappers in them*: birds, particularly parrots, will remove and often swallow these. The clappers are often made of a lead alloy, which is potentially dangerous as birds are very susceptible to lead and other heavy metal poisons.
- *Human mirrors*: these have various lead oxides as their backing and so present another source of lead poisoning. Polished, stainless steel mirrors are better.
- *Plastic children's toys*: the plastics are often too soft, and so are easily broken up and swallowed, sometimes leading to gut impaction. Some toys contain zinc, which is toxic.
- *Toxic plants*: many tropical houseplants, such as spider plants and cheese plants for example, are poisonous.

Some 'toys' that may be safely offered include:

- Whole vegetables, such as apples, pears, broccoli, beetroot or carrots.
- Pine-cones and clean hardwood branches such as beech or mahogany (cockatoos and macaws particularly love to strip bark from these). Edible fruit trees such as apple trees and grape vines may also be used. It is essential that these are well cleaned and have not been sprayed with fertilisers/pesticides/fungicides first.
- Ryegrass (not treated with arsenic to prevent fungal growth) and sprouted beans growing in a shallow dish may be particularly well accepted by smaller Psittaciformes and many Passeriformes, such as canaries.
- Placing favourite food items inside hollowed-out pieces of wood – so the bird has to pick the food out – can keep a bird occupied for hours.
- Thick ropes and closed chains may be used to suspend toys. However, no bird should be left unattended with these as they can easily become entangled.

Positioning of the cage

Correct positioning of the cage is vitally important. Wrong positioning can lead to a permanently stressed bird. Severe illness or even death may result from an incorrectly placed cage.

Birds of the Psittaciformes and Passeriformes families are typically prey animals rather than predators and are therefore constantly on the lookout for potential predators. If left to their own devices, they will position themselves in such a way as to minimise risk. This means achieving some height (to avoid ground-based predators) and getting themselves into a position where a predator can only approach from one or two sides.

Therefore, some perches should be at eye level to achieve a little height. It is important not to place the bird too far above this as the bird may then start to feel dominant to its owner and may become increasingly difficult to catch. To minimise fear of predator attack, the cage should be placed in a corner of the room, rather than in its centre. For greater security, three of the four sides may be 'blocked off', for example by a wall or with a towel.

The positioning should also allow, preferably direct, sunlight to fall on the cage for some part of the day, although the bird should not be in sunlight continuously as this will lead to heat stress. Day length should mimic that of the bird's native habitat, which often means a 12- to 14-hour day followed by a 10- to 12-hour period of darkness, and cages may be covered to provide the correct number of hours of darkness. Towels are often used to cover the cage for this purpose, but it is important to ensure that ventilation remains adequate.

Room temperature is also important. Smaller cage birds have a large body surface area in relation to their size and therefore lose heat rapidly. A comfortable room temperature should be maintained day and night for most species. This should be 16–20°C for most commonly kept Psittaciformes and Passeriformes. It is especially important to maintain room temperature for young birds and those that have lost feathers, for example through feather plucking.

The room chosen for the bird is also important. For example, the bird should not be placed in the kitchen. Many birds are potential carriers of zoonotic diseases that are more easily transmitted by close proximity to food preparation areas. In addition, many fumes produced by cooking can be life-threatening to birds. Some of these toxic fumes include:

- Fumes from overheated Teflon-coated pans. These are lethal to birds within minutes but are completely undetectable to the human sense of smell.
- Fumes from frying fats can cause serious lung oedema and death within minutes.

With no antidote to even mild exposure to these hazards, they must simply be avoided. Supportive therapy is discussed in Chapters 14 and 16.

Birds should also not be kept in bedrooms because the owner may be exposed to dander and faecal matter. This can cause allergic or anaphylactic reactions and pose a risk of zoonotic diseases which many birds carry. In addition, bedrooms are often the coldest rooms in the house and so often not suitable for a bird. If a bird is to be housed indoors, choose the living room or assign it a special room of its own.

Outdoor enclosures: aviary flights

One problem that occurs with indoor housing of cage birds is often the lack of exposure to ultraviolet radiation as well as visual stimulation. Ultraviolet light is required for vitamin D synthesis and is blocked by standard glass windows. Some evidence also suggests that ultraviolet light exposure is necessary for normal circadian rhythms to be set and to reduce stress and mental health problems which may lead to feather plucking and generalised illness. Specific ultraviolet lamps are now being sold for birds that are kept indoors. However, it is becoming increasingly common to encourage owners to provide some form of outdoor enclosure for their pet birds for all or part of the year.

Exposure to the changing day lengths is required for setting the diurnal and seasonal body clock of the bird, particularly for temperate species. Another advantage of an outdoor enclosure is that it can be made sufficiently large to allow the bird(s) room to fly and exhibit other natural display activities. These outdoor enclosures are often referred to as aviary flights and may be used to house several members of the same species or even mixed species depending on the species concerned.

Aviary flight construction

Construction

Aviary flights are frequently constructed of wood and stainless steel. The flight flooring is often made of concrete. This is preferable to a soil covering that can allow the build-up of pathogens and can be extremely difficult to clean. The rest of the flight is usually based on stainless steel mesh sides supported by a hardwood or stainless-steel frame. The roof is also of wire mesh, or clear corrugated plastic, and some form of nest box or enclosed roosting area, for breeding and extra protection during bad weather, is provided. Many of these flights are attached to the sides of houses, providing a solid wall to one side and the additional protection that the heat and eaves of the house offer. Additional heating may be advisable and indeed required in certain climates.

Any wire mesh used to form the sides of the aviary flight should ideally be made from stainless steel, rather than a galvanised alloy to avoid the risk of zinc poisoning. The size of the mesh depends on the size of the species kept.

If wood is used, it should preferably be hardwood and must not have been treated with any potentially avian-harmful wood preservatives, such as creosote.

It is sensible to provide a double-door system to gain entry to the aviary flight. Usually one door gives access to a corridor, from which each aviary flight has a door branching off. This helps to minimise the risk of a bird escaping during entering or exiting.

Another potential hazard of outdoor flights is the risk of rodent and wild bird access to the system. This can cause fouling of food and water bowl contents as well as the transmission of diseases including yersiniosis and avian influenza. Care should be taken to ensure that the wire mesh is regularly inspected for signs of damage and that the food and water bowls are placed in a part of the cage with a solid roof over them to minimise faecal contamination by wild birds.

Positioning

Protection from the prevailing wind direction is important to prevent chilling. Equally important is to ensure that the nest or roosting box is not in direct sunlight all day. Temperatures in wooden constructed buildings will soar during the summer, leading to hyperthermia of adults and chicks alike. It is also useful to provide an area in the flight that protects from wind in the winter and provides shade in the summer. This allows the bird to alter its own microclimate at will, minimising environmental stresses.

Nest box

The nest or roosting box should be large enough to accommodate all birds housed in the flight and should be cleaned out regularly during the non-breeding season. During the breeding season, if breeding pairs are kept, the box should not be disturbed at all to avoid stress and mismothering of the eggs or young. It is also important to provide additional nest boxes if multiple pairs of breeding adults are kept together to reduce intra- and inter-species aggression. The nest boxes should be waterproofed and positioned out of the prevailing wind and direct sunlight. They are generally constructed of marine plywood. This can lead to chewing of the boxes by the larger parrot species, and so some breeders coat the inside and outside of the box with stainless steel wire. Care should be taken of the material used for this, and the wire should not have sharp edges that may harm chicks inside the box.

Perches

Within the flight, perches made of hardwood should be provided. These should be of differing diameters, as discussed earlier, and be sufficient to provide all flight occupants with a perch. Food bowls may be clipped to the mesh sides of the flight or placed in an alcove recessed into one of the walls. Food and water bowls should not be placed in the roost or nest boxes, as fouling of the water and fights are much more likely to occur. Again, multiple tiering of perches, especially over food and water bowls, is to be avoided as it may lead to widespread contamination of food and water.

Substrate

If mixed-species aviary flights are used, ground-dwelling species, such as quail, are often included. In these cases some form of substrate is required, with bark chips or peat being the most popular. Care should be taken in these cases to ensure that the flooring is kept very clean and that any Psittaciformes present do not start eating large quantities of substrate.

Raptors

Cage requirements

The cage requirements for raptors may be different from those for Psittaciformes and Passeriformes. This is due to both the different environmental requirements of raptors and the reasons for which they are being kept. For example, many trained raptors are kept tethered for a part of their lives, although good welfare principles suggest that, once trained to tethering, they should be kept loose in an outside aviary system for the majority of their lives in order to allow the individual choice, the main principle of positive animal welfare.

The tethering restraint device commonly used in raptors is the jess, a leather strap that is attached to each leg via an anklet at the tarsometatarsal area just above the foot (see Figure 10.1). Each jess is the same length and comes in two types. A restraint jess has a slit in the distal end and is attached to a metallic swivel that allows rotation. This swivel is

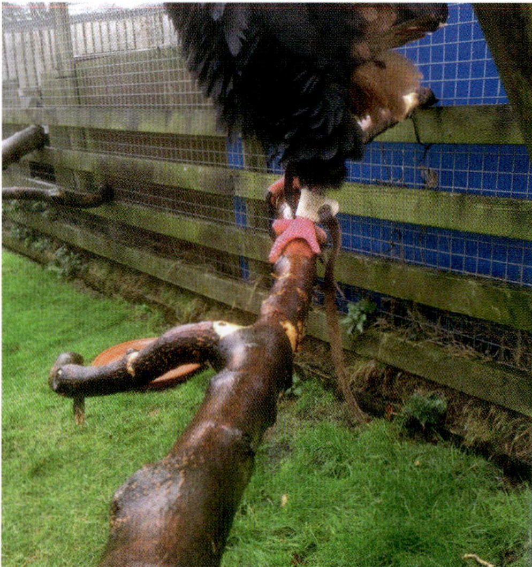

Figure 10.1 Eagle with anklets and flight jesses attached. Note the absence of a slit in the distal end of the flight jess to avoid possible entanglement should the bird fly off into a tree or bush.

then attached to a leash. The leash may then be used to tether the bird to a perch, which is usually positioned close to the ground. It is important to keep the leash relatively short to prevent the bird reaching sufficient flight velocity before the leash becomes taut as this can seriously damage its legs. A flight jess is used for holding the bird on a gloved hand and does not have a slit in the distal end as this can increase the chances of the raptor becoming entangled in any tree should it fly up into one.

Cage or shelter designs

Cages are generally sited outdoors and vary to suit the particular raptor and the presence or absence of tethering.

As with Psittaciformes and Passeriformes, the cage design should provide protection from the weather as well as from rodents and other potential pests and predators.

Tethered raptors

Historically during the summer months, a weathering – a three-sided, solid wooden construction with a solid roof and open at the front – has been used (see Figure 10.2). The perch is placed centrally on a floor covered with sand or gravel. Recommended minimum dimensions for these shelters are 2.5 × 2.0 m for Falconidae and 3.5 × 2.5 m for hawks and eagles (Forbes and Parry-Jones, 1996). Current best practice suggests that use of tethering and therefore weatherings for prolonged periods of time are not welfare friendly as they do not allow the raptor choice and so should be phased out in favour of access to aviary flight systems for the majority of the time.

The weathering form of shelter is also prone to three major problems.

1. During the summer, the weathering may become extremely hot, and so adequate shade must be provided to prevent heat stroke. Dehydration may also be a problem as most raptors obtain their water from their food and will not drink free water.
2. Another problem is the risk of predation due to the open housing and the restrained, low position of the bird.
3. During cold weather spells the birds, being tethered close to the ground, are prone to frost damage with wing tip oedema and loss of the wing extremities as a consequence (see Figure 10.3).

Aviary flights

These are often built along similar designs to the Psittaciformes and Passeriformes styles already mentioned. There is a major difference, though, in that raptors do not socialise well with other raptors, and so aviaries tend to contain individuals or a breeding pair and no others.

One of the more successful designs is a pattern similar to the weathering, except the front is covered with a wire mesh rather than being open and the birds are not tethered (free-lofted). Roofing materials that have been found to minimise overheating during the summer, but are waterproof, include the compound Eternit®, which is a type of concrete matting (Forbes and Parry-Jones, 1996).

As with the aviary flights already mentioned, it is advisable to have a double-door system so as to avoid escapees. Food is often provided on a feeding block mounted on one side of the aviary, off the ground. It is accessed either directly from inside the aviary or from outside the aviary via an access hatch. Feeding frequency is generally geared to the appetite of the individual bird, but care must be taken as overfeeding non-working raptors with fatty prey such as laboratory rats can lead to atherosclerosis and obesity.

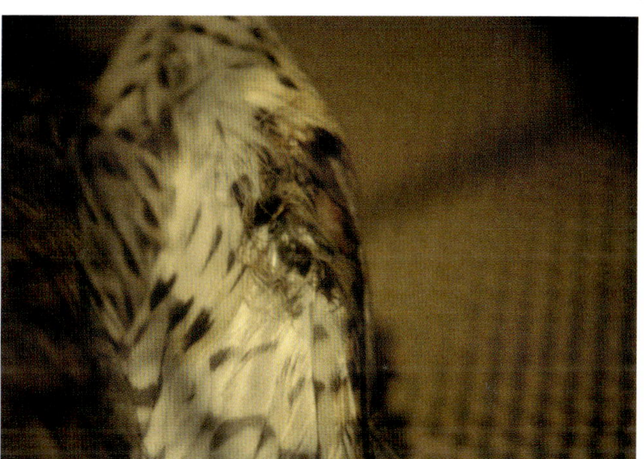

Figure 10.3 Wing tip oedema in a bird of prey associated with frost damage.

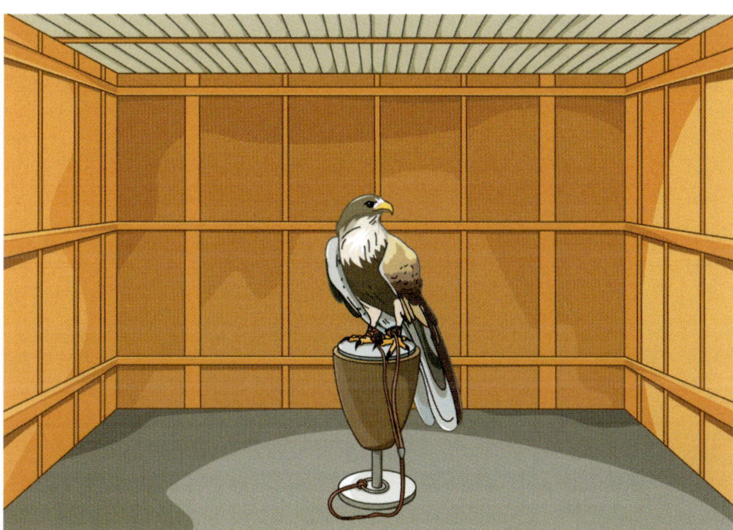

Figure 10.2 Basic layout of a weathering for raptors: a three-sided and roofed building, usually of wood, with a gravel floor and open at the front. The bird is tethered to a perch in the centre.

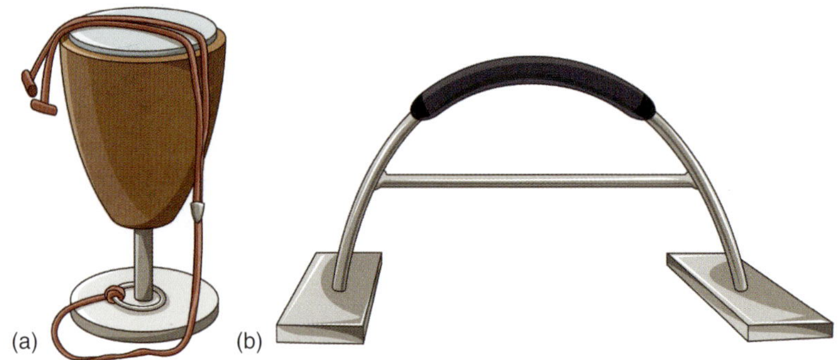

Figure 10.4 (a) A block perch for falcons, with tether, metal swivel and jesses. (b) A bow perch for hawks with padding to prevent bumblefoot.

Water should be provided fresh each day, even for those species which do not routinely drink. Many free flight aviaries also provide some form of shallow bathing area, which should be kept scrupulously clean on a daily basis.

The floor should be of solid concrete, with excellent drainage to minimise the build-up of potential pathogens.

Perches

These depend on whether the bird is tethered or free flying. In tethered situations there are two types of perches (see Figure 10.4).

The first is the block perch, which is mainly used for falcons. As its name suggests, it comprises a block of flat wood, mounted on a short pole (usually 30–60 cm long). The block is often padded with a material such as Astroturf® to provide cushioning for the feet. This is to prevent bumblefoot or deep-seated foot infections. Raptors, particularly falcons, will remain motionless on block perches for hours at a time, putting continuous pressure on the same parts of the sole of the feet. This causes reduced blood supply and necrosis of small areas of skin which may become secondarily infected leading to bumblefoot (see Figure 10.5). This is another reason for not persistently tethering such birds.

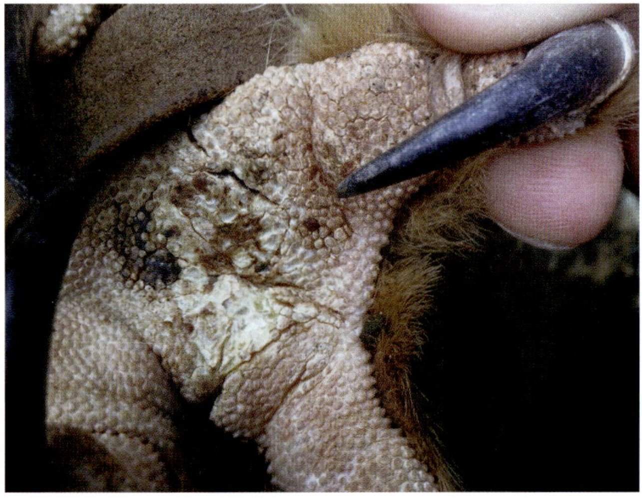

Figure 10.5 Bumblefoot (pododermatitis) in an eagle owl (*Bubo bubo*).

The second type of perch for tethered raptors is the bow perch. This is a curved rod, usually of tubular iron or steel with padding wound around the highest point of the curve for the bird to grasp. This is the commonest perch offered to the larger raptors such as hawks and eagles.

In both cases the length of the leash should not be so long as to allow the bird sufficient speed off the perch to be violently jerked backwards when it becomes taut but neither should it be so short that if the bird should lose its footing, it becomes suspended in mid-air by its legs.

Hacking boxes

These are carry boxes to move birds of prey around from place to place. They have a simple design and are often made of wood or plastic, with a perch and a front opening door. The raptor is placed into the box, and the jesses are attached to a swivel and leash that then exits the box so the falconer can control the bird by grasping this leash before the door is opened (see Figure 10.6).

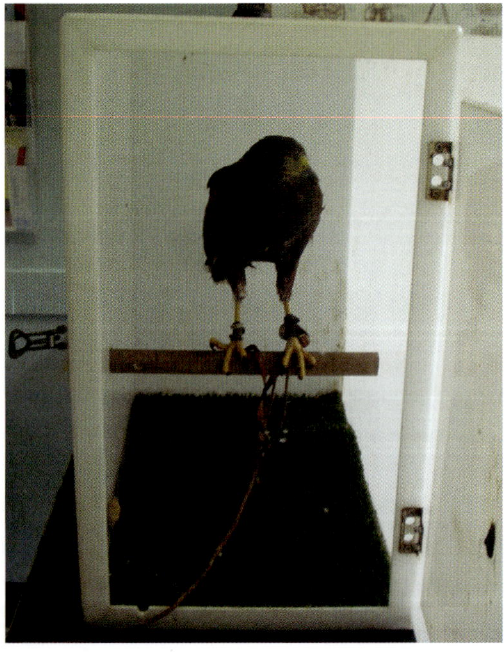

Figure 10.6 A hacking box containing a Harris hawk (*Parabuteo unicinctus*). Note the leash attached to the jesses that trails outside the box and the Astroturf® covering the floor of the box.

Columbiformes

Shelter requirements

There is huge variation in the forms of housing offered to doves and pigeons in the UK. To a large extent, it depends on the reason for which the bird is being kept. Ornamental doves and pigeons are often kept in dovecotes or dove lofts, many of which are hundreds of years old. Conversely, the more athletic racing pigeons are housed mostly in lofts specifically designed for the purpose and divided into breeding quarters, roosting areas and traps for racing.

The RSPCA (2011) recommends that the flooring of pigeon enclosures is solid to encourage foraging behaviours and that box perches approximately 30 cm square and 15 cm deep are located in blocks along one wall simulate as much as possible a more natural environment. The Universities Federation of Animal Welfare (UFAW) handbook recommends that minimum perching space is 20 cm per dove and 30 cm per pigeon (McGregor and Haselgrove, 2010). The Joint Working Group on Refinement (JWGR, 2001) recommends pens (7 m long × 3 m wide × 3 m high) or tunnel aviaries (20 m long × 7 m wide × 3.5 m high).

Racing pigeons

A loft design will depend largely on the individual owner's preference and space available. It is recommended that the minimum space requirement in the loft area is 0.25 m^2 per bird with headroom of around 2 m for the younger stock. This requirement should be doubled for adult individuals (Harper, 1996).

The provision of wooden doweling perches is standard. It is recommended that 20–25% more perching space than there are birds be provided to avoid overcrowding stresses (Harper, 1996). The perches should be arranged side by side rather than stacked vertically. This is because, as with all birds, the dominant individuals take the highest perches leading to soiling of birds below.

Within the loft system, an owner may house his or her pigeons in several different ways.

Racing loft – natural loft system: In the natural loft system, both male and female pigeons are housed together during the reproductive season. Each pair has its own nest box and perch but can mix with the other pairs in a communal area. As its name suggests, this system is the most natural, but it may be more stressful for the birds, demanding that they race and rear their young at the same time.

Racing loft – widowhood loft system: The widowhood loft houses only the males. The hen birds are housed in an adjacent loft, and this provides an additional incentive for the males to race back! To reduce fighting, it is necessary to provide more room per bird, and each bird often has a double-sized nest box as well as individual feeding stations. The racing season in the UK is from April to July for the older birds and July to September for the younger ones. The females are allowed into the widowhood loft just before the males to allow rearing of a single chick. After this the hens are removed and the males fed to fitness for racing.

Young loft: The young loft is used to house that year's young and so will have differing populations of pigeons throughout the year. Depending on the breeding success of the year, overcrowding can occur and the diseases and stress that go with it.

Anseriformes

Shelter requirements

The order Anseriformes is a large one but there is a common requirement for all the species and that is the need for open water. The form in which it is presented, however, depends on the species. The swan family will benefit from deeper water in which they can swim and dabble, whereas the duck family can cope with shallower water requirements.

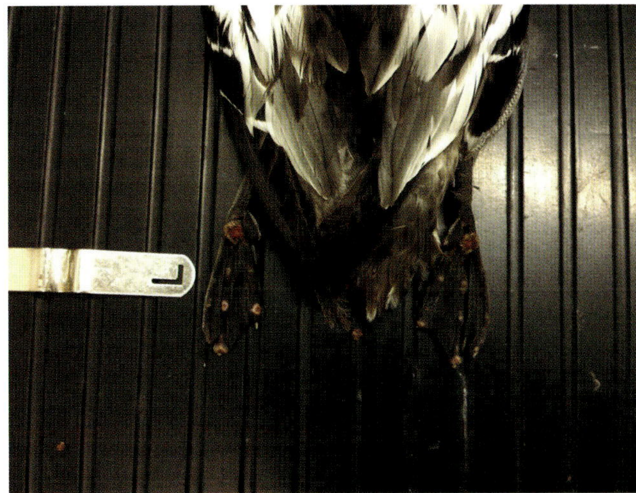

Figure 10.7 Pododermatitis (bumblefoot) in a duck associated with inappropriate substrate and pond margins.

The type of species kept also determines the nature of the enclosure. For example, geese enjoy areas of open grassland to graze. However, they are inclined to turn grass around a pond into a mud-bath. This can lead to the rapid spread of pathogens, such as avian tuberculosis (*Mycobacterium avium*). Because of this, many waterfowl keepers will concrete the edges of ponds or place obstacles around them to prevent such damage occurring.

Other factors must be taken into account when providing ponds. One is the high incidence of bumblefoot or pedal dermatitis and abscessation, which is made worse if the standing surfaces surrounding the pond are rough and muddy (see Figure 10.7). A smooth concrete finish is therefore preferred.

Any open unfenced pond should also contain an island at its centre. This is useful to encourage nesting, and prevent predation from terrestrial carnivores such as foxes.

Maintenance of water quality

Maintaining good water quality can be one of the most difficult aspects of keeping waterfowl. With large stocking densities or with muddied margins to the water area, the water itself can be rapidly turned into a murky breeding ground for bacteria and parasites. It is important to prevent stagnation of the water, which means the standing water must move out of the pond, to be replaced by fresh water. Ideally this should be achieved by using natural resources such as local streams, but in some cases water has to be piped in and out to achieve it.

Other methods of water purification include the planting of certain marginal bog plants, which can also provide cover for waterfowl and enhance the look of a pond. A specific reed type (*Phragmites australis*) has been used for this.

Mixing species

Many waterfowl keepers will wish to keep several different species together. There are some species which cannot be kept in the same water. Examples include mixing freshwater species and salt-water species. Salt-water birds can be kept on fresh water, but they do need very deep water levels to enable them to dive properly.

Other combinations to avoid include:

- Mixing together more than one pair of trumpeter swans
- Mixing of Hawaiian geese with Canada geese
- Mixing of a pair of Bewick's swans with a pair of whistling swans (Forbes and Richardson, 1996).

It is generally advisable to keep any swan or shelduck as a single pair on smaller ponds as multiple pairs will always fight in the nesting season.

Other considerations

One of the main concerns of any waterfowl keeper is the loss of birds to wild predators, such as foxes, cats, weasels, stoats and mink. The provision of an island in the centre of an expanse of water is one of the most useful preventive measures. Other measures include the erection of fox-proof fencing (fencing with an external overhang to the top edge of 30–50 cm to prevent climbing and staking the mesh for 30–50 cm along the ground out from the vertical fence line to prevent digging) or the setting of live traps for mink, weasels and stoats. In the UK, it is worthwhile noting that if non-native species of birds are allowed to escape, the owner could be in contravention of the Wildlife and Countryside Act 1981, which expressly forbids the release of non-native species into the wild.

Quarantine

Birds are highly susceptible to viral diseases, and many small Psittaciformes may carry *Chlamydia psittaci* without showing clinical signs. For this reason it is important to consider quarantining any new bird addition before adding it to your collection. Periods of quarantine suggested have varied from 4 weeks to 6 months. Testing for important diseases should be undertaken within this period.

The new bird(s) should be housed preferably not only in a separate cage/aviary but in a separate airspace as many diseases such as psittacosis and bornavirus may spread through the aerosol route. Separate utensils and bowls should be used, and the quarantined birds should be cleaned out and fed last to avoid cross-contamination. Ideally, outer clothing such as a boiler suit should be worn as an added precaution and foot-dips used. Disinfection of all utensils and surfaces is important to avoid potential spread of diseases. Disinfectants suitable for birds should be both safe and effective against pathogens such as *Chlamydia psittaci*, avian influenza and in some cases avian tuberculosis.

Hospitalised birds

The guidelines given above should be applied as much as possible for any hospitalised bird. Raptors may be brought in on their mobile block or bow perch and tethered inside a standard veterinary kennel unit which is sufficiently large enough to allow them to stretch their wings in all three dimensions (assuming they are trained to be tethered). Parrot minimum cage sizes should be similarly assessed, but often they can be housed in their own cages within the veterinary practice to maintain some degree of familiarity. Such temporary housing should be exactly that, for short periods only. For longer periods of treatment, larger spaces such as aviary flights should be provided to encourage exercise and this may be difficult to achieve in many veterinary practices.

In hospital settings it is important to site birds away from areas of noise and from potential predators (e.g. cats, dogs and ferrets) that may stress the patient. If the bird is presented with a condition such as feather plucking, uncommon in raptors but occasionally seen in Harris hawks and common in parrot species, then every attempt should be made to maintain environmental temperatures above 20°C to avoid chilling. Dimming lights may also help reduce stress as may providing some low-level background noise such as a radio, particularly for prey species such as Psittaciformes and most Passeriformes.

Waterfowl may be kept out of water for a few days, but if longer periods are anticipated then attempts should be made to provide water for swimming and to encourage preening and dabbling behaviour, assuming wounds and illness allow.

It is vitally important that any practice-owned bird-cage is cleansed thoroughly between patients to avoid spread of diseases. Again, the use of suitable avian-friendly disinfectants that are effective against avian influenza and, in susceptible species, *Chlamydia psittaci* and avian tuberculosis is recommended.

References

Forbes, N.A. and Parry-Jones, J. (1996) Management and husbandry (raptors). In: *Manual of Raptors, Pigeons and Waterfowl* (eds P.H. Benyon, N.A. Forbes & N.H. Harcourt-Brown), pp. 116–128. BSAVA, Cheltenham, UK.

Forbes, N.A. and Richardson, T. (1996) Husbandry and nutrition (waterfowl). In: *Manual of Raptors, Pigeons and Waterfowl* (eds P.H. Benyon, N.A. Forbes & N.H. Harcourt-Brown), pp. 289–298. BSAVA, Cheltenham, UK.

Harper, F.D.W. (1996) Husbandry and nutrition (pigeons). In: *Manual of Raptors, Pigeons and Waterfowl* (eds P.H. Benyon, N.A. Forbes & N.H. Harcourt-Brown), pp. 233–236. BSAVA, Cheltenham, UK.

JWGR (Joint Working Group on Refinement) (2001) Laboratory birds: Refinements in husbandry and procedures. Fifth Report of the BVAAWF/FRAME/RSPCA/UFAW Joint Working Group on Refinement. *Laboratory Animals*, **35**(Suppl. 1), S1–S163.

McGregor, A. and Haselgrove, M. (2010) Pigeons and doves. In: *The UFAW Handbook on the Care and Management of Laboratory and Other Research Animals* (eds R. Hubrecht & J. Kirkwood), pp. 686–696. Wiley Blackwell, Oxford https://doi.org/10.1002/9781444318777.ch44.

RSPCA (2011) Pigeons: Good practice for housing and care. Available at https://www.rspca.org.uk/documents/1494935/9042554/Pigeons+%282011%29+%28PDF+395KB%29.pdf/d7728207-861f-a78b-df91-5c61e76c93bf?t=1557664523069#:~:text=Pigeons%20should%20be%20housed%20in%20pens%20that%20permit,pens%20are%20best%20because%20they%20permit%20short%20flights (accessed 13 October 2023).

PART II: AVIAN SPECIES

Chapter 11 Avian Handling and Chemical Restraint

Handling the avian patient

Is there a need to restrain the avian patient?

This may seem a basic point, but it is sometimes necessary to be sure that restraint is required. A decision on whether the bird in question is safe to restrain has to be made.

Points that need to be considered include the following.

- Is the bird in respiratory distress, and is the stress of handling going to exacerbate this?
- Is the bird easily accessible, allowing quick, stress-free and safe capture?
- Does the bird require medication via the oral or injectable route, or can it be medicated via nebulisation, food or drinking water?
- Does the bird require an in-depth physical examination at close quarters, or is cage observation enough?

If the decision is reached that restraint is necessary, it should be remembered that many avian patients are prey species and as such can be highly stressed individuals in unusual surroundings, so any restraint should involve minimal periods of handling and captivity.

Techniques useful in handling avian patients

The majority of avian patients seen in practice (with the exception of many of the owl family, Strigiformes) are diurnal, so reduced or dimmed lighting usually has a calming effect. This can be used to the handler's advantage when catching a flighty or stressed bird.

In the case of Passeriformes and Psittaciformes, turning down the room lights or drawing the curtains or blinds in order to dim the room is enough. Use of red lights can also be helpful in diurnal species as many do not see as well in dimmed red lighting. For birds of prey such as falcons and some hawks, there may well be access to the practice's or the bird's own hoods. These are leather caps which slot over the head and draw tight around the neck, leaving the beak free but completely covering the eyes. They are used to calm some raptors when on the wrist or during handling or transporting; however, a bird not accustomed/trained to the hood should not be subjected to it.

It is also advisable to keep noise levels down when handling avian patients as their sense of hearing is often their next best sense after sight. With these two factors borne in mind, stress and time for capture can be greatly reduced.

Prior to approaching the capture of the avian patient, all items of cage furniture or other obstacles, such as toys, water bowls, food bowls and perches, should be removed from the cage or box. This helps to avoid self-trauma and reduces the time needed to capture the patient.

Once you have made these initial arrangements, you can then confidently approach the avian patient.

Equipment used in avian handling

Birds of prey

The majority of captive birds of prey are trained to be restrained by jesses. In any case leather gauntlets are a must for restraint of all birds of prey as their talons, and the power of the grasp of each foot, can be extremely strong. The feet of birds of prey and not the beak (unless dealing with the larger species such as eagles where the beak is also a formidable weapon) represent the major danger to the handler. It is important to note that when the bird of prey is positioned on the gauntleted hand, the wrist of this hand (traditionally the left hand in European falconers) is kept above the height of the elbow. If not, the bird has a tendency to walk up the arm of the handler with potentially serious and painful results. The type of gauntlet should be either ideally a specific falconer's gauntlet or one of the heavy-duty leather pruning gauntlets available from garden centres. The larger the bird of prey, generally the larger and thicker and more extensive the gauntlet required; many have added sections protecting the forearm as well as the hand. To handle a bird of prey in a veterinary hospital setting, the following steps should be taken.

- First, place the gauntleted hand into the cage or box beside the bird's perch.
- Grasp the jesses (these are the leather straps which are attached to the anklets) with the thumb and forefinger of the gauntleted hand and encourage the bird to step up onto the glove. Most birds prefer to step up, so always position your hand slightly above the perch.
- Once the bird is on the hand, retain hold of the jesses between thumb and forefinger close to the bird's leg and loop the end of the jesses through the third and fourth fingers. In birds where a hood can be used, such as many of the falcons, then slip the hood over the bird's head assuming it is trained to accept the hood.

The bird of prey may then be safely examined 'on the hand' and frequently is docile enough to allow manipulation of wings and beak, for small injections to be administered or for oral dosing.

If the bird of prey does not have jesses on but is trained to perch on the hand, it may well step up onto the gauntlet of its own accord. If not, then it is advisable to have the room darkened for Falconiformes. Alternatively, a blue or red light source could be used. This allows the handler to see the bird but prevents the bird of prey seeing normally as their sight is limited in these light spectra.

You must then 'cast' the bird by grasping it from behind, ensuring that you are aware of where its head and feet are.

In order to cast the bird of prey for a closer examination, the bird may be approached, once on the fist, by a second handler from behind with a thick towel, ensuring that you are aware of where the bird's head is. The towel is draped quickly over the wings and the handler's hands

Veterinary Nursing of Exotic Pets and Wildlife, Third Edition. Simon J. Girling.

are rapidly moved down to grasp the legs just above the feet to prevent the bird footing (grasping) either itself or the handler. The bird's dorsum may then be brought against the handler's ventrum and another person can then examine the bird more closely. It is vitally important that the handler keeps the feet separated from each other to prevent the raptor grasping one foot with its other foot and so avoiding puncture wounds and infection that can have serious consequences. If the raptor is loose in its aviary, then it is advisable to use nets and towels.

Finally, it is important to remember that the majority of birds of prey are regularly flown, so it is vital to preserve the integrity of their flight and tail feathers. A falconer may not thank you for saving his or her bird's life if they then cannot fly that bird until after the feathers have been replaced at the next moult which in most cases happens only once a year.

Parrots and other cage birds

All of these birds will benefit from the use of subdued or blue or red light to calm the bird and to allow it to be restrained with minimal fuss.

The main weapon of the Psittaciformes, due to the kinetic hinge joint in the upper bill, is its beak and powerful bite. (The hyacinth macaw, the largest in the family, can easily crack the largest Brazil nuts and even sever a finger.)

The main weapon of the Passeriformes may be the beak, although this is less damaging as a biting weapon. It may still be a sharp stabbing weapon in the case of starlings and mynahs.

Heavy gauntlets are not recommended for restraint of either family group as they do not allow for accurate judgement of grip on the patient. They may be used with extreme caution in larger more aggressive parrots where there are legitimate concerns over being seriously bitten. In the majority of Psittaciformes, though, dish or bath towels for the larger species and paper towels for the smaller ones are advised. These provide some protection from being bitten without masking the true strength of the handler's grasp. This is very important because, as you will remember from the previous chapter, birds do not have a diaphragm and so rely solely on the outward movement of their ribcage and keel for inspiration. Restriction of this with too tight a grip can be fatal.

Before attempting to restrain the patient, its cage should be cleared of all obstacles which may hinder capture or result in injury of the patient. The towel and hand are then introduced into the cage, and the bird is firmly but gently grasped from behind. First grasp the head. Position the thumb and forefinger beneath the lower beak, pushing it upwards and preventing the bird from biting. Then use the rest of the towel to wrap around the bird, gently restraining its wing movements. This will avoid excessive struggling and wing trauma (see Figure 11.1). The patient may then be cocooned in the towel with the head still held extended from behind through the towel and the rest loosely wrapped around the bird's body. Individual limbs may then be drawn from the towel one at a time for examination, or the body accessed for examination or drug administration.

The towel technique is also better than gloves alone because the towel presents a larger surface area for the bird to try to evade when being initially caught. The bird is then less likely to try to bolt for freedom, whereas a bare hand is a much smaller target and encourages escape attempts.

For smaller cage birds, a piece of paper towel may be used and the bird transferred to a latex gloved hand. For these smaller birds the neck of the bird should be held between the index and middle fingers.

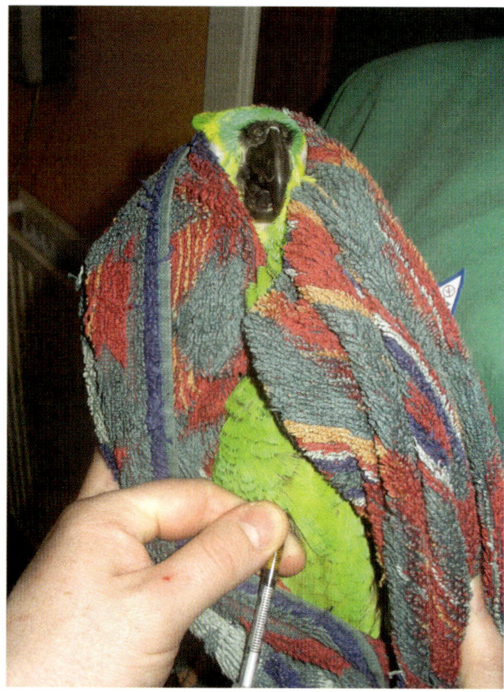

Figure 11.1 Restraint of larger parrots may be easily performed with a towel as with this Amazon parrot receiving an intramuscular injection.

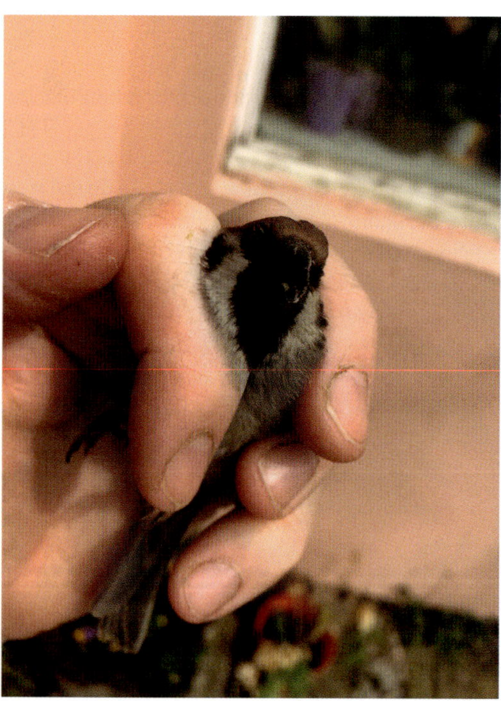

Figure 11.2 Smaller birds such as this sparrow may be restrained with one hand with the head held between forefinger and middle finger and the hand gently surrounding the bird to prevent wing-flapping.

You can then use your thumb and forefinger to manipulate the legs or wings. The rest of the hand should gently cup the bird's body to discourage struggling (see Figure 11.2). It is still necessary to be cautious with this approach to prevent over-constraining the patient as this could cause physical harm.

Other avian species

Toucans and hornbills: These have an impressive beak, with a serrated edge to the upper bill. Providing the head is initially controlled using the towel technique previously described for parrots, an elastic band or tape may be fastened around the bill to prevent biting. The handler still needs to be careful of stabbing manoeuvres, and it is a good idea to work with a second handler who is solely responsible for containing the beak. Otherwise, restraint is the same as for the Passeriformes.

Columbiformes: These can be restrained in a manner similar to the Psittaciformes. When holding the bird once caught, a modified grip may be used where the bird's wings and feet are cupped in one hand from the dorsum, whilst resting the sternum of the bird in the other hand.

Waterfowl: Restraint of these species is relatively straightforward but may become hazardous with the larger species particularly swans and geese. The first priority is capturing the head. This can be done by grasping the waterfowl around the upper neck from behind. It is important to ensure that the handler's fingers curl around the neck and under the bill, while the thumb supports the back of the neck and the potentially weak area of the atlanto-occipital joint. Failing this, a swan's or shepherd's crook, or other smooth metal, or a wooden pole with a hook attached, can be used to catch the neck, again high up under the bill. Care should be exercised with these 'swan hooks' as overzealous handling can lead to neck trauma.

Having restrained the head and beak, it is essential that you rapidly control the powerful wings by using a towel, thrown or draped over the patient's back and loosely wrapped under the sternum. Many institutions have access to more specialised goose or swan cradle bags that can wrap around the body, containing the wings but allowing the feet, head and neck to remain free.

The waterfowl may now be safely carried or restrained by tucking its body (contained within the towel or restraint bag) under one arm and holding this close to the torso. With the other hand, the handler may hold the neck loosely from behind, just below the beak.

Raptors: These can be restrained on the gloved hand using jesses for visual examinations. Some birds of prey such as many falcons will also accept a hood which acts to calm the bird further and reduce its likelihood of flapping/bating (see Figure 11.3). However, for closer inspection and to induce gaseous anaesthesia it is often necessary to cast the bird from the glove by grabbing the wings and legs from behind. A towel draped over the wings may help prevent the bird from flapping and injuring itself but it is important to ensure that the feet are controlled to stop the bird from grabbing the handler and itself, both of which can lead to significant damage (see Figure 11.4).

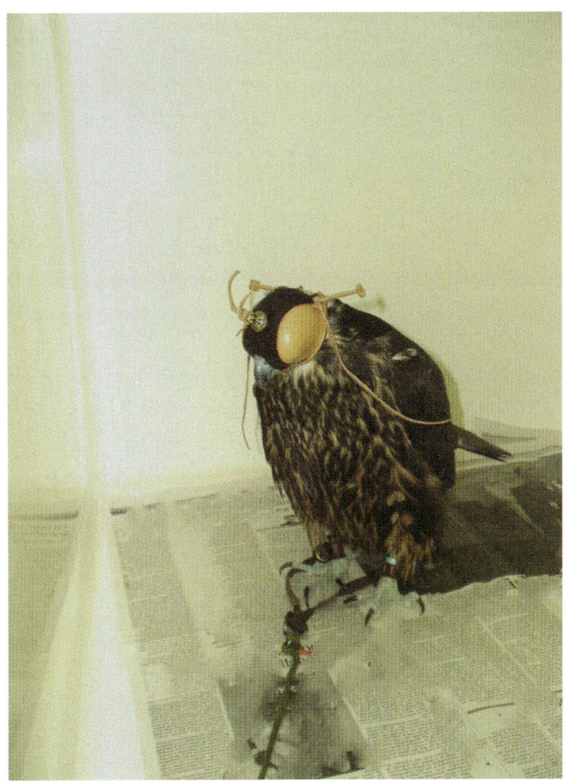

Figure 11.3 Falcon with a hood on as well as restraint jesses attached to a swivel and leash to allow easier handling.

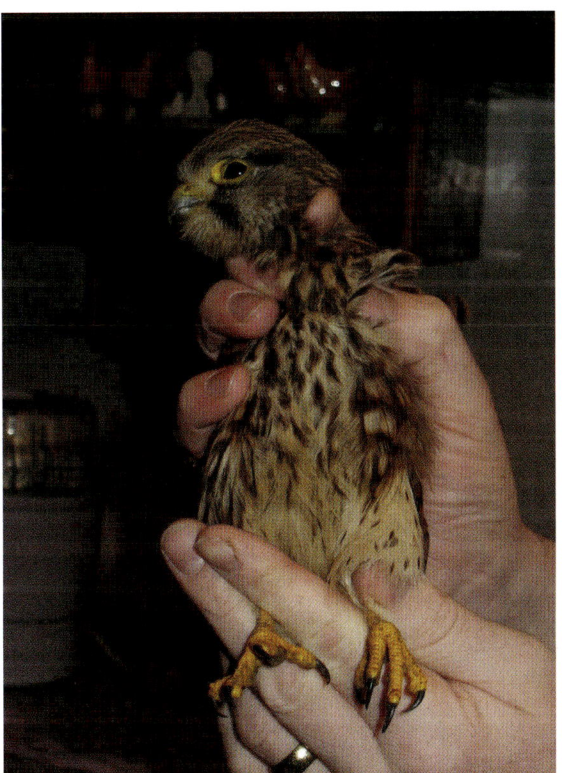

Figure 11.4 Kestrel being restrained for closer examination. Note the handler's control of the feet to prevent the raptor from grabbing itself or the handler and so causing harm.

Capturing escaped avian patients

Where a bird is loose, a number of methods can be used to capture it. Darkening the room and reducing its area, if possible, are both helpful to calm and confine the bird.

In the case of larger parrots, the use of a heavy bath towel thrown over the bird can confine it long enough to allow the handler to restrain the head from behind and then wrap the patient in the towel.

For smaller birds, a fine aviary or butterfly net is extremely useful for catching the bird safely either in mid-flight or against the side of the cage or room. The mesh should be fine enough to ensure that no limbs or feathers will become entangled within it. The mesh is best made of a dark or black material to restrict light and calm the bird.

It is important to ensure that the patient is rapidly transferred from the net into the handler's hands or a container as this is the most stressful period of the capture, and the inability to see whether the patient is in respiratory distress can lead to fatalities.

To recapture escaped raptors, a lure, baited with prey, can be used. Most raptors will remain within the area of their release for several days, and many captive-reared birds will not be able to kill prey for themselves. They will then become hungry and will often look for their handler to offer prey, either on the glove if they are trained birds, or within the vicinity of their cage if they are non-trained exhibit or breeding birds. Use of radio tracking and telemetry is commonplace when flying raptors and can aid recovery in fly-off cases. Patience and persistence are two essential virtues when trying to recapture escaped raptors!

Aspects of chemical restraint

Assessment of the patient's status

All methods of chemical restraint require that the patient is first restrained manually, even though it may be for a short period, while the medication is being administered. The aim is to keep the period of manual restraint to a minimum in order to reduce stress.

Before any form of chemical immobilisation can be used, an assessment of the patient's status must be made. The following points need to be considered.

- Is the procedure to be performed necessary for life-saving medication or treatment, or can it be postponed if the patient's health is suboptimal?
- Is the patient's condition likely to be worsened by the anaesthetic drugs used?

Implications of avian respiratory anatomy and physiology

There are several differences between avian and mammalian anatomy and physiology that are important to note when considering restraint and anaesthesia.

1. Some species do not possess nostrils (nares) and instead breathe through gaps in the angle of the beak. These are often diving species such as gannets and pelicans. It is important when restraining these species therefore not to completely close the beak aperture or asphyxiation can occur.
2. Absence of a complete larynx. The bird does have a glottis, but there are no vocal cords or epiglottis to worry about on intubation. The majority of the vocal sounds a bird makes come from the syrinx, which lies at the bifurcation of the trachea into the bronchi.
3. Presence of complete cartilaginous rings supporting the trachea. This is important for two reasons:
   - On the plus side, it is difficult to suffocate the bird by constricting the neck when restraining the bird.
   - However, there is no 'give' to the trachea, and so inflatable cuffs on endotracheal (ET) tubes should not, if at all possible, be inflated as this will cause pressure necrosis in the lining of the trachea. In some cases, such as when flushing out the crop or proventriculus of the bird to remove foreign bodies, it may be necessary to inflate the cuff in order to prevent inhalation pneumonia when flushing. This must be performed with great care and the tube deflated as soon as possible after flushing.
4. Avian lungs are semi-rigid structures. It is the air sac system that is responsible for the movement of air through the lungs, in combination with the lateral movement of the chest wall and ventral movement of the keel. Therefore, if there is any form of restriction to the outward movement of chest and keel, ventilation will be reduced, leading to hypoxia.
5. In some species such as penguins, storks and cranes, the presence of a partial or complete vertical division of the trachea into a left and right side, immediately caudal to the glottis (the so-called crista ventralis), may make intubation more difficult. Either a short ET tube is required or, in some extreme cases, two ET tubes, one for each side (and so two anaesthetic circuits) may be required.
6. Some species have other adaptations to the trachea, such as a very long trachea coiled in the caudal cervical/cranial sternal region (e.g. storks), which can predispose to fluid build-up and blockage in this area as well as increasing the dead space. Others may have a tracheal pouch (e.g. emus) in the cervical region ventrally which can inflate when attempting intermittent positive pressure ventilation (IPPV), resulting in poor lung ventilation and so requiring the neck to be bandaged to prevent this.

Pre-anaesthetic preparation

Blood testing

It may be advisable to run biochemistry and haematology tests on avian patients prior to administering anaesthetics, particularly in older and obviously unwell individuals. Blood may be taken from the following vessels.

- The right jugular vein in nearly all species (it is significantly larger than the left in many birds) (see Figure 11.5).
- In the larger species the brachial vein, which runs cranially on the ventral aspect of the humerus (see Figure 11.6).
- In many waterfowl, long-legged birds and raptors, the medial metatarsal vein, which runs, as its name suggests, along the medial aspect of the metatarsal area (see Figure 11.7).

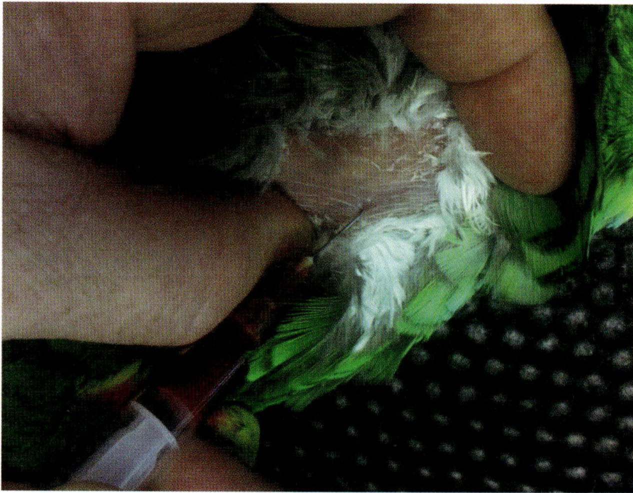

Figure 11.5 The right jugular vein is the largest accessible vein in most cagebirds such as this Amazon parrot.

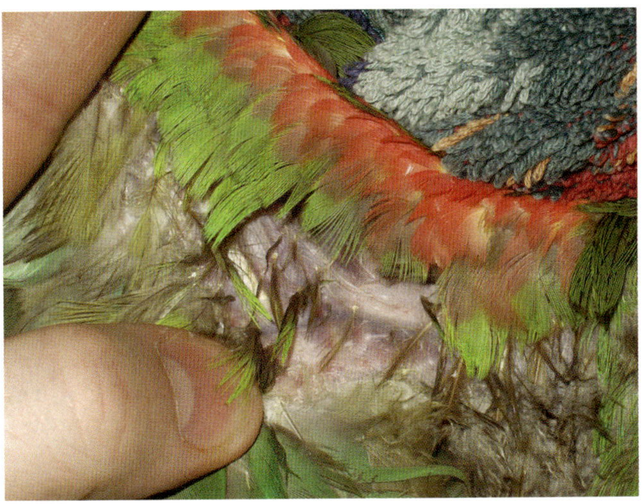

Figure 11.6 The brachial vein is easy to see but it is fragile and 'blows' easily.

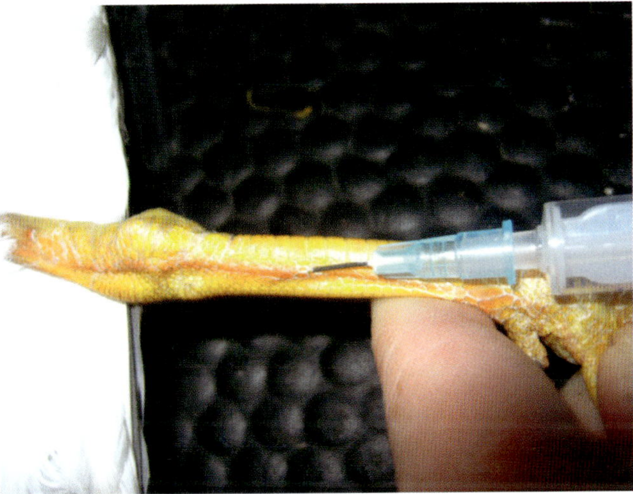

Figure 11.7 The medial metatarsal vein is easy to access in waterfowl and long-legged birds.

However, it is also worth noting that physical restraint, as previously mentioned, increases the bird's stress levels and oxygen consumption and it may be safer for the patient to be anaesthetised with a volatile gas in 100% oxygen for the blood sample to be taken.

Fasting

Because of the high metabolic rate of many small cage birds, extended fasting may be detrimental to their health and their ability to recover from anaesthesia. This is because hepatic glycogen stores, which provide the most rapid form of stored energy, can be quickly depleted. Birds larger than 300 g body weight, that have larger glycogen stores, are less likely to become hypoglycaemic with fasting.

The purpose of fasting is to ensure emptying of the crop (where present) and stomach(s) (particularly the proventriculus in granivorous species). Fasting prevents passive reflux of fluid or food material during the anaesthetic which may then be inhaled, obstructing the airway or causing pneumonia.

Ideally, most small birds are fasted for between 1 and 3 hours depending on their body size. The smallest have the shortest period of fasting, often amounting to just 1–2 hours at most. Birds weighing over 300 g may be able to tolerate an overnight fast of 8–10 hours, assuming good health and body condition, and this may be necessary particularly if surgery on the gastrointestinal system or crop is intended. Large carnivores such as eagles or penguins may require a longer period of starvation, particularly if they have had a recent large meal (24 hours or so in many cases).

In birds of prey, it is also standard to avoid feeding 'casting' material in the 24–48 hours prior to a planned anaesthetic. Casting material is the indigestible parts of prey (fur, feathers, bone) that would normally be regurgitated (cast) 12–24 hours after being consumed. If fed less than 24 hours prior to an anaesthetic, this casting may not have occurred, and the material can lead to bacterial fermentation in the stomachs as well as pressing on the lungs and air sacs making anaesthesia more complicated and difficult.

In neonate birds, the crop can be extensive and liquid or semi-liquid food can be retained in significant quantities in the stomachs. These individuals should be managed with extreme care as passive reflux and regurgitation is common. Flushing out the crop and maintaining the patient with its head and cranial body elevated can help reduce these risks. Intubation is always recommended to reduce aspiration of food and maintain the airway.

Whatever the period of fasting, water should only be withheld for 1 hour or so prior to anaesthesia.

Pre-anaesthetic medications

Pre-anaesthetic medications are infrequently used in birds. Of those used, fluid therapy is perhaps the most important and often neglected. Preoperative, as well as intraoperative and postoperative, fluids can make the difference between successful surgery and failure. Fluid therapy is covered in more detail in Chapter 14.

Antimuscarinic premedicants

Atropine and glycopyrrolate have been used as pre-anaesthetic medicants to reduce vagally induced bradycardia and oral secretions which may block ET tubes. They both, however, may have unwanted side-effects. The two main side-effects are:

- Causing unacceptably high heart rates, increasing myocardial oxygen demand and so increasing the risk of cardiac hypoxia and arrest.
- Making oral or respiratory secretions so thick and tenacious that they make ET tube blockage even more likely.

However, they are an important component of the crash trolley to counteract the heart block which may occur during anaesthesia. Doses of atropine 0.01–0.02 mg/kg or glycopyrrolate 0.01 mg/kg, both administered intramuscularly or intravenously, have been used.

Benzodiazepine premedicants

Diazepam or midazolam may be used in some species such as waterfowl, pelicans and penguins as these in particular may exhibit periods of apnoea during mask induction of anaesthesia and it may be difficult to administer gaseous anaesthesia due to their beak shape and size. The apnoea seen in these species is thought to be a stress response (often referred to as a 'diving response') mediated by the trigeminal receptors in the beak and nares. When this response is triggered, the breath is held and the blood flow is preferentially diverted to the kidneys, heart and brain making induction with gaseous anaesthetics, such as isoflurane, difficult. Benzodiazepines seem to increase the threshold for triggering this response and so can allow gaseous anaesthetic induction in these species.

Dosages of midazolam as a premedicant vary from 2 to 6 mg/kg intramuscularly. It has also been used intranasally from 0.5 mg/kg in Psittaciformes to allow minor procedures such as claw trimming, or as a premedication at dosages varying from 3 to 7.3 mg/kg (Vesal and Eskandari, 2006; Doss *et al.*, 2018). In canaries, intranasal diazepam and midazolam (a 5 mg/mL solution of each drug with 25 μg applied to each nostril) also produced sedation, with diazepam producing longer effects (up to 38 minutes versus 17 minutes for midazolam) (Vesal and Zare, 2006). Interestingly, the reversal agent used for benzodiazepines (flumazenil) may also be successfully used when administered intranasally with doses of 2.5 μg per nostril being used in canaries (Vesal and Eskandari, 2006; Vesal and Zare, 2006). Reversal can be important as midazolam has a longer half-life than diazepam and may cause prolonged recoveries, which may not be helpful in species of waterfowl such as geese as they will need to be kept away from water for several hours after recovery to be safe (Valverde *et al.*, 1990). Addition of butorphanol to a benzodiazepine significantly increases sedation and has been used in pelicans administered intramuscularly at doses of 1 mg/kg midazolam and 0.5 mg/kg butorphanol (Horowitz *et al.*, 2014). However, recovery can take several hours with this combination unless reversal agents are used.

Butorphanol

The partial opiate butorphanol has been used as a premedicant in cage birds and dosages of 1–3 mg/kg have been used in psittacine birds. It has been shown to have isoflurane-sparing effects in cockatoos (*Cacatua* spp.), that is it allows a lower dosage of isoflurane to be administered and yet still maintain surgical anaesthesia (Curro *et al.*, 1994).

Induction of anaesthesia

Anaesthesia, as with mammals, may be induced with two main categories of drugs: injectable anaesthetics and inhalational anaesthetics.

Injectable agents

Advantages of injectable anaesthetics include:

- Ease of administration (most birds have a good pectoral muscle mass for intramuscular injections)
- Rapid induction
- Low cost
- Good availability.

Disadvantages include:

- Recovery is more dependent on successful organ metabolism.
- Reversal of medications in emergency situations is more difficult.
- Prolonged and sometimes traumatic recovery periods may ensue (e.g. ketamine).
- Muscle necrosis at injection sites and lack of adequate muscle relaxation may occur with some medications (e.g. ketamine).

In alphabetical order the following are some of the injectable anaesthetics more commonly used in avian practice.

Alfaxalone: This has been used and published in a number of species including pigeons, parrots (budgerigars and lovebirds), finches and flamingos. It has been used at dosages of 4–12.6 mg/kg intramuscularly, or 2 mg/kg intravenously as an induction agent and appears to be effective (Villaverde-Morcillo *et al.*, 2014; Balko *et al.*, 2019; Greunz *et al.*, 2021). It does produce more significant cardiorespiratory effects than isoflurane-induced anaesthesia alone and has been associated with loss of thermoregulation when used at higher sedative dosages of 15–20 mg/kg in budgerigars (Romano *et al.*, 2020). In addition it has been associated with rough inductions and recoveries in lovebirds (Greunz *et al.*, 2021) and is not favoured in birds by myself.

Ketamine and ketamine combination anaesthesia: When used alone, ketamine produces inadequate anaesthesia and recoveries are often traumatic, with the patient flapping wildly. Doses of 20–50 mg/kg are quoted (Forbes and Lawton, 1996). However, combining it with the benzodiazepines diazepam (0.5–2 mg/kg) or midazolam (0.2 mg/kg) helps with muscle relaxation and sedation, reduces flapping on recovery and allows the dose of ketamine to be reduced to around 10–20 mg/kg (Curro, 1998). To speed recovery, benzodiazepines such as midazolam or diazepam may be reversed using flumazenil (0.04–0.05 mg/kg intramuscularly).

Ketamine may also be combined with xylazine (1–2.2 mg/kg) (Forbes and Lawton, 1996) or medetomidine (60–85 μg/kg) (Forbes and Lawton, 1996). Xylazine is generally not now recommended due to its moderate to severe depression of respiration with a high incidence of cardiac arrhythmias due to atrioventricular (AV) blockade. Dexmedetomidine has also been used at half the dosages (in μg/kg) of medetomidine. Use of medetomidine and dexmedetomidine improves the quality of sedation and allows reduction of the ketamine dosage to 10–20 mg/kg depending on the species and procedure. Medetomidine and dexmedetomidine may also be reversed with atipamezole, so speeding up recovery. However, such alpha-2 drugs can have severe cardiopulmonary depressive effects and may compromise blood flow to the kidneys, risking renal damage and so should not be used where cardiovascular or renal disease is present. Sun-conures have been noted to be particularly intolerant of ketamine/alpha-2 combinations and they are not recommended for this species (Rosskopf *et al.*, 1989).

The ketamine and ketamine-combined medications are usually given intramuscularly via the pectoral muscles. Induction will take on average 5–10 minutes. Recovery times vary, as mentioned, and are ketamine dose-dependent, but can be hastened when an alpha-2 antidote, such as atipamezole, is used.

It is also worth noting that ketamine is actively excreted from the proximal tubule of the kidneys, and so any kidney damage can lead to a prolonged recovery when using this drug.

Propofol: Propofol is given intravenously, depending on the species via a jugular, medial metatarsal or brachial vein catheter. It has been used at 5–10 mg/kg to induce anaesthesia in a range of avian species but it produces profound apnoea and often central nervous system excitation on recovery and so is less commonly used as an induction or anaesthetic agent in birds. In addition, cardiac electrical disturbance with runs of ventricular complexes has been recorded in birds given this drug (Lukasik *et al.*, 1997).

Tiletamine/zolazepam: This drug combination is composed of a dissociative anaesthetic similar to ketamine (tiletamine) and a benozodiazepine (zolazepam). It is currently marketed as Telazol® in North America and Zoletil® in Europe and has been used in avian species at doses of 5–10 mg/kg intramuscularly. It produces reliable immobilisation but can have prolonged recovery periods and there is no specific antidote/reversal agent, although flumazenil has been used to try to reverse the benzodiazepine component.

Inhalation agents

To induce anaesthesia using inhalation agents, face masks are used and generally well tolerated. For smaller species, in order to minimise gas escaping into the room, the entrance hole to the mask may be reduced using a nitrile glove stretched across the entrance and a small slit cut in it just slightly larger than the bird's head. For long-beaked species it may be possible to adapt plastic drinks bottles to fit over the beak, allowing delivery to the nares with minimal gas leakage.

Nitrous oxide: This is uncommonly used in routine avian anaesthesia. It has good analgesic properties, but accumulates in large hollow organs. There is some thought that it may therefore accumulate in the air sacs and appears to prolong anaesthetic recovery times. Some recent evidence disputes this, but it cannot be used on its own for anaesthesia. It must be used in combination with halothane or isoflurane to allow a surgical plane of anaesthesia to be reached.

Isoflurane: Isoflurane is still one of the commonest anaesthetics used in the avian patient. It is also specifically licensed for use in avian species in several countries including the UK. Induction may be achieved by face mask at 4–5% concentration, reducing to 1.25–2% for maintenance, preferably via ET tubing inserted into the trachea or an air sac. If using a mask for maintenance, an increase in gas concentration of 25–30% is required.

Advantages of isoflurane include:

- Low blood solubility and minimal organ metabolism of the drug by the bird (<0.2%). This means that the drug does not accumulate in the bloodstream and is rapidly excreted by the patient, allowing rapid changes in anaesthetic depth.
- Minimal cardiopulmonary effects at sedative or light anaesthesia levels, although a dose-dependent cardiopulmonary depression does occur.
- Little tendency to cause cardiac arrhythmia (although they can still occur).
- Unlike halothane, isoflurane does not require significant metabolism in the liver, making it suitable for the majority of sick avian cases.
- Cardiovascular arrest does not occur at the same time as respiratory arrest, allowing time for resuscitation should it occur.
- Isoflurane has a minimum alveolar concentration (MAC) – the concentration that produces no response in 50% of cases when subsequently exposed to a noxious stimulus – of 1.44% in cockatoos and 1.32% in ducks (Ludders *et al.*, 1990; Curro *et al.*, 1994). However, considerable species variation exists, with a lower MAC of 1.07% being recorded in thick-billed parrots (*Rhynchopsitta pachyrhyncha*) and 1.06% in cinereous vultures (*Aegypius monachus*) (Mercado *et al.*, 2008; Kim *et al.*, 2011).

It should be noted that arrhythmias have been reported in isoflurane-anaesthetised birds, although at a low level but particularly during induction and recovery and maybe more so than in sevoflurane anaesthesia. Second-degree heart block seems to be the most commonly reported arrhythmia (Aguilar *et al.*, 1995; Joyner *et al.*, 2008). Dose-dependent respiratory depression does occur in birds.

Sevoflurane: Like isoflurane, it requires little or no organ metabolism and is considered safe in a wide range of birds. Slightly higher percentages are required to induce and maintain the patient compared with isoflurane and are in the region of 5–8% sevoflurane, but low blood solubility does allow rapid changes in anaesthesia levels (Greenacre, 1997). This is because it is less soluble in avian blood than isoflurane (blood gas partition coefficient of 0.69 versus 1.41 for isoflurane), although it is considered less potent with an overall MAC of 2–3%. MAC values have been specifically determined for thick-billed parrots at 2.35% (Phair *et al.*, 2012). Dose-dependent cardiopulmonary depression does still occur as with isoflurane.

Maintenance of anaesthesia

For prolonged anaesthetic procedures, gaseous maintenance is required and considered safest. Isoflurane and sevoflurane are currently the agents of choice.

It is advisable to intubate the bird for more effective control of rate and depth of anaesthesia wherever possible. Gaseous anaesthetics such as isoflurane have respiratory depressive effects that are dose dependent. This means that with prolonged procedures, the patient may become apnoeic and require either manual or positive pressure ventilation. This can be more of a risk with some species, such as the African grey parrot, than with others.

Endotracheal intubation

The beak must be held open manually or by using an avian gag or attaching short lengths of bandage to the upper and lower beaks. One handler can then hold the beak open, while a second intubates the bird (see Figure 11.8). The glottis will be easily visible at the base of the tongue, in the midline. Intubation can be made easier in parrots if the fleshy tongue is grasped with atraumatic forceps, enabling the tongue and the glottis to be pulled forward. Sizes of ET tube vary but would be typically 3–3.5 mm internal diameter for an African grey parrot and up to 4–5 mm internal diameter for a larger macaw. The smaller tubes will block more easily with respiratory secretions, and the use of parasympatholytics generally does not prevent this. Indications of tube blockage include apnoea that may be preceded by an increased expiratory phase of respiration. Such cases should be extubated and the tube checked for mucous plugs followed by reintubation with a clean tube.

As mentioned in Chapter 9, some species have a complete or partial division of the trachea into right and left sides and this can sometimes make intubation difficult (see Figure 11.9).

It is better not to routinely inflate the cuff on ET tubes because of the risk of causing severe damage to the lining of the rigid avian trachea. It is therefore important to use a well-fitting tube. Cuffs can be inflated for short periods if carrying out stomach washes to remove foreign bodies, where the risks of inhalation are increased, but they

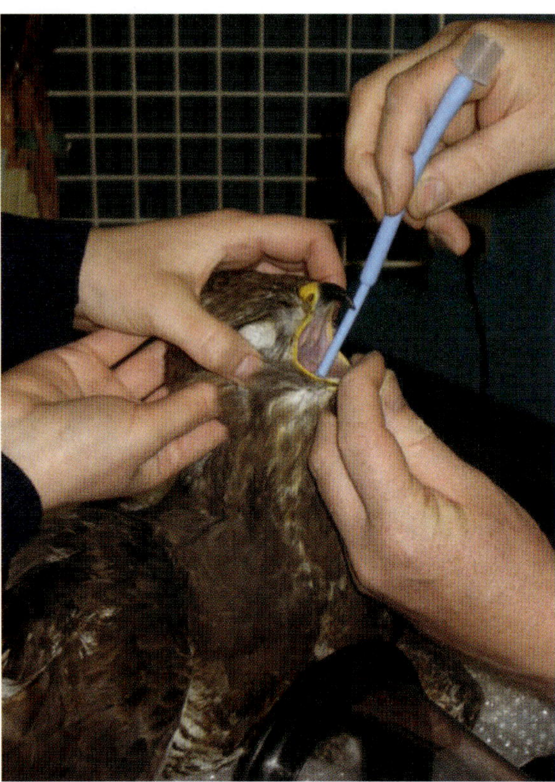

Figure 11.8 Intubation of a buzzard using a 'Coles' endotracheal tube which is tapered at the tip to make intubation easier.

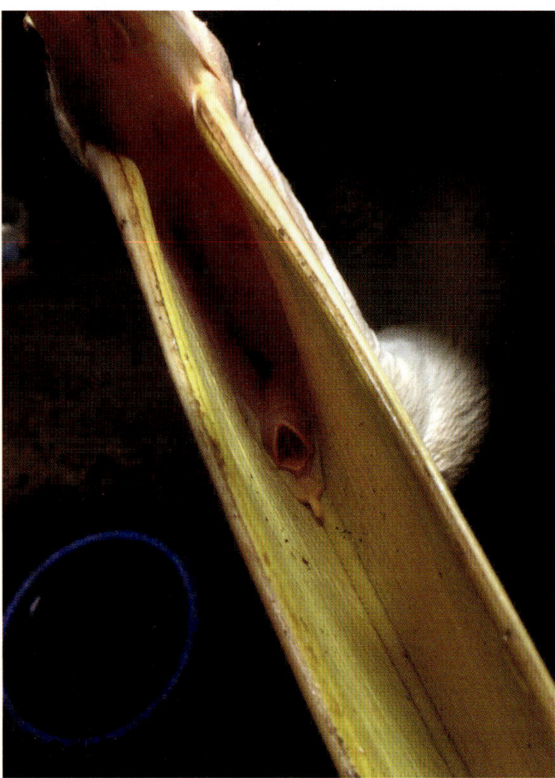

Figure 11.9 Intubation of some species such as penguins, cranes, storks and in this case a pelican, can be complicated by the presence of a ventral or complete septum dividing the trachea into a right and left side.

should be deflated as soon as possible. The consequences of tracheal damage due to ET tube cuffs include tracheal strictures which can develop several weeks after the anaesthetic and result in a narrowing of the trachea and subsequent severe dyspnoea (Sykes *et al.*, 2013).

Once intubated it is usual to tape the tube to the lower beak to ensure it does not become dislodged during the anaesthetic.

Anaesthetic circuits

Anaesthetic circuits used must be non-rebreathing and minimise dead space as the commonly seen avian patients are often less than 1 kg in weight and so have small lung/air-sac volumes. The use of non-rebreathing circuits also means that changes to the percentage of gaseous anaesthetic supplied on the vaporiser are reflected quickly in the levels supplied to the patient. Oxygen flow rates are often in the region of 100–200 mL/kg per minute. Modified Bain circuits or Mapleson C circuits are useful for these reasons. The Ayres T-piece may be used for larger parrots, larger birds of prey and waterfowl. In any instance, a 0.25–0.5 L rebreathing bag is frequently necessary.

Air sac catheterisation

In an airway obstruction, or if head or oral surgery is required, it may be necessary to deliver the inhalant gases via a tube placed directly into one of the air sacs. This is possible because many of the avian air sacs are very close to the skin surface. These structures take no part in gaseous exchange, simply allowing the shunting of the air back and forth through the rigid lung structure; however, as birds extract oxygen from the air on expiration as well as inspiration, it does not matter which direction the oxygen and gases are introduced into the lungs.

Air sacs that may be catheterised include the clavicular air sacs and more commonly the abdominal or caudal thoracic air sacs. A small stab incision is made in the skin over the air sac. The underlying body wall muscle is bluntly dissected with a pair of haemostats, and the ET tube may then be inserted to a depth of 4–5 mm and sutured in place. The clavicular air sacs lie at the thoracic inlet, just dorsal to the clavicles. The caudal thoracic air sacs may be entered between the sixth and seventh ribs in Psittaciformes. The abdominal air sacs may be entered by pulling the leg cranially so that the femur crosses the last ribs, incising just caudal to the stifle.

Monitoring of anaesthesia

Accurate monitoring of anaesthesia is clearly crucial for patient safety. The depth of anaesthesia should be adequate enough for the procedure required, while cardiovascular and respiratory parameters should remain constant. The following points should be considered.

- During the initial stages of anaesthesia (stages 1 and 2), the respiratory rate will be shallow and erratic. The patient will be lethargic and have drooping eyelids, a lowered head and ruffled feathers.
- As the depth increases, palpebral, corneal, pedal and cere reflexes will remain, but all voluntary movement ceases.
- As the next stage of anaesthesia (stage 3) is reached, the respiration rate becomes regular, and the depth of breathing is increased. The corneal and pedal reflexes are slow and the palpebral reflex disappears. This is the light plane of anaesthesia required for minor procedures. The depth at which the pedal reflex is lost but the corneal reflex is retained will allow most surgical procedures to be performed.

- As anaesthesia is allowed to deepen, respiratory rate and tidal volume will continue to decrease until, if allowed, respiratory arrest will occur. Therefore, monitoring of the rebreathing bag, for rate and depth of respiration, can provide valuable information.

One study indicated that the ideal anaesthetic depth occurred when the patient's eyelids were completely closed, pupils were mydriatic, pupillary light reflex was delayed, corneal reflex resulted in slow movement of the third eyelid across the eye, all muscles were relaxed and all pain reflexes were absent (Korbel *et al.*, 1993). It should therefore be noted that it is normal for three neurological reflexes to still be present during a surgical plane of anaesthesia according to König *et al.* (2016):

1. A slow but complete corneal reflex
2. Partial pupillary dilation and
3. A reduced pupillary light reflex.

It is worth noting that many birds will respond more adversely to having a feather plucked than a sharp surgical incision of the skin.

Equipment used for monitoring anaesthesia

The following are some of the useful modalities for monitoring anaesthesia in avian patients listed in alphabetical order.

Blood gases: Point-of-care analysers can be helpful in assessing ventilation of the avian patient. Normal mean arterial values for non-anaesthetised pigeons have been published and vary from 95 mmHg for PaO_2 and 34 mmHg for $PaCO_2$ (Bouverot, 1978) to 87 mmHg for PaO_2 and 29.2 mmHg for $PaCO_2$ (Piiper *et al.*, 1970). Normal non-anaesthetised venous values for Quaker parrots have been reported as 28.4–46 mmHg for PO_2 and 27.3–29.9 mmHg for PCO_2 (Rettenmund *et al.*, 2014). In African grey parrots anaesthetised with isoflurane there appears to be a strong correlation between side-stream capnography and $PaCO_2$, with the acknowledgement that the capnograph consistently overestimated $PaCO_2$ by around 5 mmHg (Edling *et al.*, 2001).

Blood pressure: Blood pressure may be difficult to assess indirectly due to the small diameter of the distal pelvic limb of birds which makes it problematic to find a suitably sized cuff. However, direct blood pressure assessment in birds has been carried out and mean published values during isoflurane or sevoflurane anaesthesia vary as follows.

1. Systolic arterial blood pressures: 88–93 mmHg in Columbiformes (Touzot-Jourde *et al.*, 2005); 99 mmHg in chickens (Naganobu *et al.*, 2000); and 163 mmHg in Amazons (Acierno *et al.*, 2008).
2. Mean arterial blood pressures: 75–82 mmHg in Columbiformes (Touzot-Jourde *et al.*, 2005); 84 mmHg in chickens (Naganobu *et al.*, 2000); 143 mmHg in cockatoos (Curro *et al.*, 1994); and 155 mmHg in Amazons (Acierno *et al.*, 2008).
3. Diastolic arterial blood pressures: 60–72 mmHg in Columbiformes (Touzot-Jourde *et al.*, 2005); 69 mmHg in chickens (Naganobu *et al.*, 2000); and 148 mmHg in Amazons (Acierno *et al.*, 2008).

Capnography: Capnography may be used in birds. Side stream tends to be preferred owing to many patients' small size. An end-tidal CO_2 level of 30–45 mmHg indicates adequate ventilation in an African grey parrot (Edling *et al.*, 2001). The advantage of capnography is that it can then be used to indicate the rate and depth of respiration required when performing IPPV. It can also provide advanced warning of blocked tubes and other ventilatory problems as well as providing valuable information on the success of resuscitation techniques should they be required.

Cardiac auscultation: A stethoscope may be used to monitor the heart rate externally, or, during anaesthesia, an oesophageal stethoscope may be inserted assuming the patient is large enough. An allometric scaling formula to calculate the expected heart rate of a bird has been developed (Schmidt-Nielsen, 1984):

$$\text{Heart rate}\left(\text{beats per minute}\right) = 155.8 \times \left(\text{body weight}\left[\text{kg}\right]\right)^{-0.23}$$

Doppler: Doppler flow recorders can be useful for assessing peripheral perfusion and rate and rhythm of pulse. The medial metatarsal vessels (which as their name suggests run up the medial aspect of the lower leg) can be readily used for this technique in most birds, although they are small in psittacines and more difficult to locate.

Electrocardiogram: ECG leads may be attached to the avian skin using adhesive pads or fine needles rather than the more cumbersome and traumatic alligator clips. These leads may be attached to the wing web (propatagium) and the folds of skin connecting the thigh area to the body wall cranially. In larger birds, an oesophageal ECG probe may also be successfully used as with mammals. The avian ECG differs somewhat from its mammalian counterpart due to a much larger RS wave than Q. Readers are advised to consult standard texts for further information on the ECG trace for avian patients (Lumeij and Richie, 1994; Oglesbee *et al.*, 2001). An example of a lead II normal ECG trace in a bird is shown in Chapter 16.

Pulse oximetry: Pulse oximeters may also be used to measure the relative saturation of haemoglobin with oxygen. Reflector probe attachments are the best and may be used cloacally or orally. However, care should be taken in interpreting results due to the difference in haemoglobin structure between birds and mammals, and the fact that commercially available oximeters are calibrated for mammalian haemoglobin. This means that the actual values in birds using these analysers cannot be relied on, although changes/trends may still be helpful. In addition, many birds can be hypercapnic despite being well oxygenated, so monitoring end-tidal CO_2 is suggested as more accurate for assessing avian ventilation (Edling *et al.*, 2001).

Again, it is important to find an oximeter that can read the higher heart rates of birds as these will be greater than those of cats or dogs.

Respiratory flow monitors: Respiratory flow monitors can be used if ET tubes are involved, although the very low flow rates of some smaller avian species may not register on machines designed with cats and dogs in mind due to the lower tidal volume.

Additional supportive therapy

Recumbency

It is important that the ribcage and sternum are unrestricted, otherwise hypoxia will develop. Common positions for surgery include lateral or dorsal recumbency. Dorsal recumbency may however cause apnoea as organs such as the liver, heart and gastrointestinal tract may press on the dorsally located lungs and air sacs. This is exacerbated in birds because of the lack of a diaphragm and the fact that the air sacs are thin-walled. Some of the larger species also have a problem with ventral recumbency due to the weight of the bird pressing on the keel or sternum, preventing their movement. However, the smaller species generally do not suffer as severely from this problem and may be positioned according to need. It is important in any species of bird though to be prepared to carry out IPPV due to these anatomical features and the likelihood of respiratory depression occurring during anything but the shortest anaesthetic procedure.

Intermittent positive pressure ventilation and resuscitation techniques

If a bird's respiratory rate becomes depressed below 3–4 breaths per minute, then it should be given respiratory assistance (IPPV). This is commonly required during prolonged anaesthetic procedures, recumbency issues as noted above, where deep anaesthesia is required (e.g. orthopaedic surgery), or where an air sac or pneumonised bone such as the humerus and sometimes femur is breached as occurs during endoscopy, some coeliotomies and orthopaedic surgery as this evacuates the carbon dioxide reserve that is the stimulus for inspiration (see Figure 11.10). IPPV in these circumstances should be performed throughout the anaesthetic. This is best done with a mechanical ventilator unit, operating at around 10–15 cmH_2O (see Figure 11.11). If using manual 'bagging' techniques, then the gentlest of touches on the rebreathing bag – enough just to allow the bird's ribcage to rise – should be used. If the bird is totally apnoeic, then a rate of 6–10 breaths per minute should be started.

If there are concerns regarding the bird's breathing then the usual anaesthetic checklist should be reviewed, for example checking flow rates, patency of ET tubing, anaesthetic gas levels and capnography readings, and the emergency ABC (Airway, Breathing, Cardiovascular) protocol initiated if signs confirm instability. In general, where apnoea is combined with evidence of reducing heart rates and other

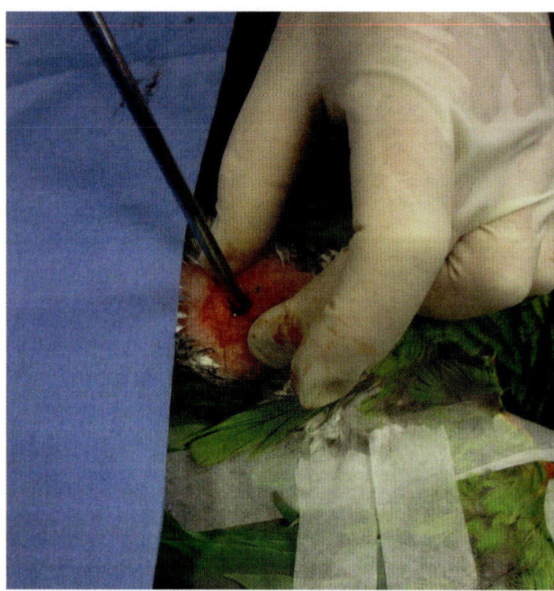

Figure 11.10 Endoscopy or any breach of an air sac or pneumonised bone is likely to result in apnoea through the evacuation of the carbon dioxide reserve.

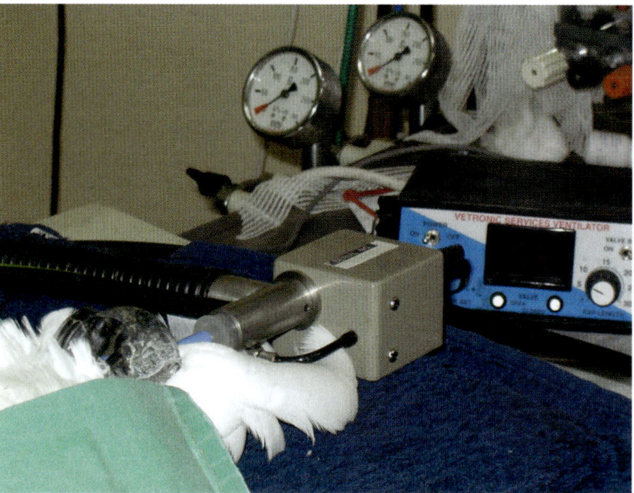

Figure 11.11 A cockatoo attached to a small animal ventilator after intubation.

clinical signs noted above, the percentage of anaesthetic gas delivered should be reduced or the anaesthetic ceased and respiratory support started.

If resuscitation is required and the avian patient is still breathing, even sporadically, then IPPV with 100% oxygen should be used.

Doxapram has been used orally or by injection to stimulate the central nervous system respiration centres at dosages of 10 mg/kg by injection or 0.5 mg orally. However, increasing evidence suggests that doxapram may be harmful where airways are blocked and oxygenation is reduced, as the drug works by stimulating the central nervous system breathing centre, thereby increasing its oxygen demand and consequently, if combined with hypoxia, may hasten cell death. If circulation and oxygenation are adequate, doxapram may still be helpful.

If the bird is being maintained on a mask and it is not possible to intubate it, it is possible to carry out assisted ventilation by grasping the uppermost wing at the carpus and gently but firmly moving it in and out at 90° to the chest wall. This will simulate muscular movement of the ribcage and so allow air to move back and forth through the air sacs and lungs. Alternatively, the sternum may be pushed towards the spine. Sternal compression can also be useful for cardiac massage in cases of cardiac arrest as direct cardiac massage is rarely possible due to the heart's position behind the solid keel. In any case, intubation and connection to an anaesthetic circuit with 100% oxygen will increase the chances of survival.

Cardiac arrest frequently and rapidly follows apnoea, and it is then extremely difficult to revive an avian patient. Adrenaline may be given at 1000 units/kg body weight, preferably via ET tubing or directly through the glottis into the trachea. Alternatively, it may be administered intravenously via either the right jugular vein or the brachial wing vein, but generally there is a poor success rate. The heart is protected by the sternum and ribs and so intracardiac injection of adrenaline, as can be performed in mammals, is rarely possible in birds.

The likelihood of apnoea occurring depends on the type of anaesthetic used. Xylazine is notorious as a deep respiratory depressant (Curro, 1998). Isoflurane will also produce respiratory depression in African grey parrots, even at the lowest surgical levels and so IPPV is routinely used in avian anaesthesia (Forbes and Lawton, 1996).

Maintenance of body temperature

Maintaining the body temperature is important for the successful outcome of any anaesthetic procedure. The large body surface to volume ratio of many birds results in loss of body heat at a faster rate than dogs and cats.

Minimising the risk of hypothermia: To minimise hypothermia a series of procedures can be used.

- The surgical field should receive minimal plucking of feathers and minimal soaking with surgical antiseptic solutions. Avian skin has low levels of bacteria and fungi in comparison to mammals and so facilitates a reduced surgical preparation protocol.
- The patient should be covered with surgical drapes, preferably clear drapes to allow visualisation of the patient whilst retaining heat.
- The patient may be placed onto a circulating warm water pad or under a hot air blanket, but the size of the patient may be so small as to reduce their usefulness.
- Warm water-filled nitrile gloves may be placed close to the patient. These should not be allowed to come into direct contact with the bird, as when too hot they may scald, and as they cool they may actually draw heat away from the patient.

Although it is important to prevent hypothermia, care should also be taken not to induce hyperthermia, particularly in those cold-adapted species that have significant insulation (e.g. penguins). During the operation, cloacal temperature can be measured directly and some probes are available that can be inserted into the oesophagus depending on the bird's size. It is preferable to use an electronic probe as most mercury-based medical thermometers do not register temperatures as high as the core body temperature of birds (typically 41–43°C).

Fluid therapy and blood transfusions

Healthy anaesthetised birds should receive replacement fluids at 10 mL/kg per hour for the first 2 hours, and then 5–8 mL/kg per hour thereafter to prevent overhydration (Curro, 1998).

If blood loss occurs during surgery, then the replacement volume of crystalloid fluid should be three times the blood loss volume. However, if the volume of blood lost is greater than 30% of the normal total blood volume, then a blood transfusion should be considered. Other indicators for blood transfusions are a total plasma protein level below 25 g/L and/or a packed cell volume (PCV) below 15% (0.15 L/L).

Blood donors should at least be of the same avian family, for instance parrot to parrot, and preferably the same species, for example one budgerigar to another budgerigar, as success rates are improved by ensuring the transfusion is from the same species. Care should be given to ensuring the health status of the donor is fully known including not only its physical health but also its disease status. Diseases such as *Chlamydia psittaci*, psittacine beak and feather disease and psittacine bornaviral disease are commonplace and may not show clinically in birds for many weeks or months and yet the bird can still be infectious. It is useful to remember that on average one drop of blood is roughly equivalent to 0.05 mL in volume, and that the estimated blood volume of an avian patient is 10% of its body weight in grams. This means, for instance, that a healthy 500-g African grey parrot would have roughly 50 mL of blood circulating in its body. However, it is equally worrying to note that a 40-g budgerigar will only have 4 mL of blood, and thus the loss of 25% of its blood volume will occur with just 20 drops of blood (1 mL).

Routes of administration of fluids will depend on the surgical procedure and the health status of the patient. Subcutaneous routes are frequently used for healthy birds undergoing minor or routine surgery. Areas that can be used for this purpose include the interscapular area, the axillae, and the fold of inguinal skin which lies cranial to each thigh.

For more serious dehydrated cases and of course for blood transfusions, the intraosseous and intravenous routes should be used (see Chapter 14).

Postoperative recovery

Recovery should always involve ventilation with 100% oxygen. The ET tube should be removed once the bird starts to cough or swallow. It is important to note that practically all avian patients will appear disorientated and will attempt to flap their wings during recovery. Every attempt should be made to constrain them gently (without restricting respiration) to ensure that they do not damage their wings or feathers. This can best be achieved by lightly wrapping them in a towel or cloth.

With isoflurane anaesthesia, recovery is complete in 5–10 minutes, and the patient is often then able to perch. However, if ketamine and certain premedications are used, recovery may take much longer, anything up to 3–4 hours, especially if there is no antidote or reversal agent administered or available. During any recovery the environmental temperature should be kept between 25 and 30°C to prevent hypothermia developing. It also helps to keep the recovery area quiet and dimly lit to ensure minimal adverse stimulation.

The patient should be encouraged to take food as soon as it is able. This is to minimise the deleterious effects of hypoglycaemia seen in many smaller avian species that have high metabolic rates.

Analgesia

Pain assessment in birds

Pain assessment in many birds is difficult as many are prey species and so, like small herbivores, will not demonstrate pain and often become immobile when watched. Clearly some procedures such as orthopaedic surgery (see Figure 11.12) are always going to be painful. Feather grooming may cease with mild pain, but will increase and move to feather chewing or plucking with more serious pain, particularly if localised to one spot. In social species of birds, pain will often result in that individual isolating itself from the group. Others may sleep more and become less interactive with their owners, or become more aggressive or demonstrate inappropriate aggression towards cage mates, owners or handlers. Very localised pain, such as in a pelvic limb, may result in very obvious levels of pain response with lack of weight-bearing, but it is nonetheless helpful to create simple pain scales from 0 to 5 or 0 to 10 to grade the levels of abnormal behaviours observed to allow assessment in response to analgesia (Desmarchelier *et al.*, 2012a).

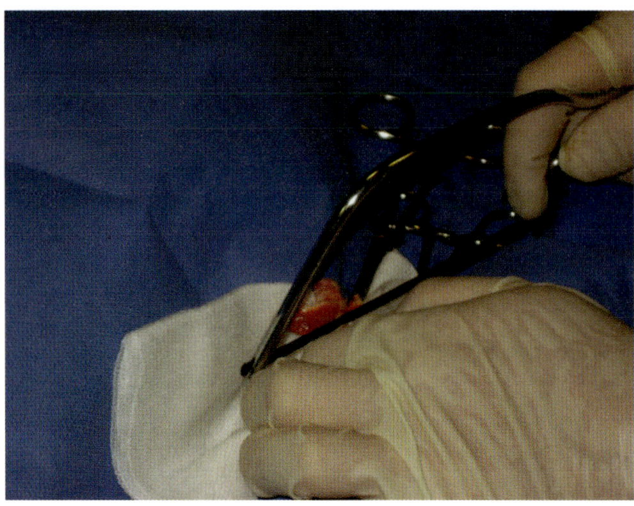

Figure 11.12 Orthopaedic surgery clearly requires good analgesia and birds will often obviously demonstrate pain associated with the procedure. However more subtle indicators of pain can be difficult to discern in avian patients, particularly potential prey species such as many cage birds.

Opioid analgesics used in birds

Butorphanol: Butorphanol, at a dose of 1–3 mg/kg intramuscularly or 0.02–0.04 mg/kg intravenously, reduces the amount of isoflurane required during anaesthesia. Species variation may exist as cockatoos and African grey parrots, but not blue-fronted Amazon parrots, showed anaesthetic-sparing effects at doses of 1 mg/kg (Curro, 1994; Curro *et al.,* 1994). Butorphanol has been used at 2 mg/kg intramuscularly as a single injection in Hispaniolan Amazon parrots as pre-emptive preoperative analgesia, where sevoflurane has been used for endoscopy, and shown to be both safe and effective (Klaphke *et al.*, 2006). Butorphanol has been shown to have less than 10% bioavailability when given orally at 5 mg/kg in Hispaniolan Amazon parrots, and so the oral route is not recommended (Sanchez-Migallon *et al.*, 2008). Adverse effects such as dysphoria have not been reported in birds. Dosage frequency appears to be as frequent as 2 hours in birds.

Butorphanol does, however, cause some respiratory depression. It also requires metabolism by the liver for excretion. However, these disadvantages are much reduced in comparison with many other opioid analgesics.

Buprenorphine: Work in pigeons has shown predominantly kappa opioid receptors in the central nervous system and butorphanol is a mu receptor agonist (Mansour *et al.*, 1988) so may not be effective in some species. Buprenorphine does not appear to be effective at 0.1 mg/kg in African grey parrots, and it has been shown that the drug does not reach plasma levels known to be effective in humans at this dosage (Paul-Murphy *et al.*, 1999, 2004). However, dosages of 0.25–0.5 mg/kg in pigeons increased the latency period for withdrawal from noxious electrical stimuli from 2 to 5 hours (Gaggermeier *et al.*, 2003). It is postulated that birds may not possess distinct mu and kappa receptors or that the two receptors have similar functions in birds.

Opioids do, however, have some respiratory suppression side-effects and will require some liver metabolism to excrete, but these are much reduced in comparison with other opioid analgesics.

Morphine and hydromorphone: In Galliformes such as the chicken and quail, morphine appears to be a sedative and so makes it difficult to assess whether it has analgesic effects (Singh *et al.*, 2017; Khalilzadeh *et al.*, 2022). Hydromorphone in cockatiels appeared to have little effects in one study and in Amazon parrots appeared to be an effective analgesic but resulted in ataxia, agitation and signs of nausea (Houck *et al.*, 2018; Guzman *et al.*, 2020).

Nalbuphine hydrochloride: This predominantly kappa receptor-active opioid (some partial mu activity) has been shown to have little respiratory depression, good bioavailability after intramuscular dosage and few sedative effects, but it did increase threshold values of thermal foot withdrawal in Hispaniolan Amazon parrots for up to 3 hours when dosed at 12.5 mg/kg (Keller *et al.*, 2009). Increased dosage of nalbuphine did not increase analgesia.

Non-steroidal anti-inflammatory drug analgesics used in birds

Cyclooxygenase (COX) has been demonstrated in chickens (Mathonnet *et al.*, 2001). Therefore, it is assumed that COX receptors are present in other birds. The distribution of COX-1 and COX-2 enzymes varies between species, and both enzymes appear important in pain pathways.

As with all non-steroidal anti-inflammatory drugs (NSAIDs), particular care should be taken with patients with gastrointestinal or renal disease just as you would with mammalian patients. Avian patients, due to their kidney structure, are more sensitive to some of these side-effects. The recent mass mortalities due to use of the NSAID diclofenac acid in Indian white backed vultures (*Gyps bengalensis*), which has seen a 95% population decline, are an example of the potential toxic effects of some NSAIDs in birds. Concurrent fluid therapy is therefore often advised when using NSAIDs, with or without gastrointestinal protectants such as sucralfate and ranitidine, and NSAIDs such as diclofenac acid should not be used.

Carprofen: Carprofen has also been widely used but its dosage is difficult to elucidate. Extremely high doses (30 mg/kg) had to be administered to provide analgesia in chickens with experimentally induced arthritis (Hocking *et al.*, 2005). In a study in Hispaniolan Amazon parrots, a dose of 3 mg/kg produced an improvement in lameness of an arthritic limb within 2 hours but the effect wore off before the 12-hour dosage interval used in mammals (Paul-Murphy *et al.*, 2009).

Celocoxib: This has been used to manage cases of proventricular dilatation disease at doses of 10–20 mg/kg orally every 24 hours, but theoretically is also likely to provide analgesia (Dahlhausen *et al.*, 2002; Clubb, 2006).

Meloxicam: There appears to be a wide variation in dosage within birds for meloxicam with budgerigars receiving 0.1 mg/kg every 24 hours for 7 days showing signs of glomerular congestion (Pereira and Werther, 2007) and Hispaniolan Amazon parrots showing improved weight-bearing on an arthritic limb at 1 mg/kg intramuscularly every 12 hours (Cole *et al.*, 2009). A pharmacokinetic study carried out by Wilson *et al.* (2005) suggested that 0.5 mg/kg orally every 12 hours was required to maintain serum levels in ring-necked parakeets (*Psittacula krameri*). In Hispaniolan Amazon parrots, dosages of 1 mg/kg given intravenously, intramuscularly and orally maintained therapeutic levels for around 16 hours via all three routes (Molter *et al.*, 2013). In zebra finches, dosages of 1–2 mg/kg needed to be administered every 12 hours to be effective in one study (Miller *et al.*, 2019). In pigeons doses of 0.5 mg/kg were considered ineffective as an analgesic for orthopaedic pain, dosages of 2 mg/kg every 12 hours orally being needed to control the pain adequately (Desmarchelier *et al.*, 2012b). It is therefore apparent that birds often metabolise NSAIDs rapidly but there is considerable species variation and so caution should be used when faced with a new species. For example, brown pelicans appear to have a longer metabolic handling of meloxicam and dosages of once every 24 hours resulted in toxicity levels being achieved within a few days, implying that the appropriate dosage interval in this species was nearer once every 36 hours (Horgan *et al.*, 2020).

Other analgesics used in birds

Gabapentin: Gabapentin (a gamma-aminobutyric acid analogue) has been used in multimodal analgesia in birds. It is believed to work via N-type calcium ion voltage-gated channels. It has been shown to relieve self-mutilation in three studies (Doneley, 2007; Siperstein, 2007; Shaver *et al.*, 2009). Doses of 10 mg/kg every 12 hours in a little corella has been used to treat self-mutilation with no adverse effects noted over 90 days (Doneley, 2007) and doses of 15 mg/kg every 8 hours have been used in a pharmacokinetic study in Hispaniolan Amazon parrots that enabled serum levels to be maintained above that considered to provide analgesia in humans (Baine *et al.*, 2015).

It is worth remembering that drugs such as ketamine and the alpha-2 adrenergic drugs have analgesic properties as well.

Local anaesthesia: Local anaesthetics such as lidocaine (lignocaine) may be used as ring blocks around amputations to reduce the chances of postoperative self-mutilation (the preparations without adrenaline are preferred to avoid cardiac disturbances). Doses of lidocaine should not exceed 4 mg/kg and should be diluted to at least 1 : 10. Typically dosages of 2–3 mg/kg are used safely in healthy birds.

Bupivacaine has also been used, but there are concerns that its toxic effects take longer to resolve in birds than in mammals. In ducks (*Anas platyrhynchos*) a dose of 2 mg/kg subcutaneously showed a faster uptake versus elimination rate, but evidence of sequestration and redistribution of bupivacaine suggested by increases in plasma concentrations 6 and 12 hours after dosing suggests that toxicity may be delayed (Machin and Livingstone, 2001). Bupivacaine has also been used as intra-articular injections in chickens with osteoarthritis and showed improved analgesia (Hocking *et al.*, 1997) and has been mixed 1 : 1 with dimethyl sulfoxide and applied to beak amputations in chickens where an increase in feed consumption was observed (Glatz *et al.*, 1992).

Tramadol: Tramadol has been suggested for use in bald eagles at 5 mg/kg every 12 hours and achieved plasma concentrations equivalent to that required in humans for analgesia. Its oral bioavailability in birds is higher than that observed in humans or dogs (mean 97.94%) and its half-life in bald eagles was two times that reported in dogs but half as long as that in humans (Souza *et al.*, 2009). In Hispaniolan Amazon parrots, oral dosage of 30 mg/kg was required to provide serum levels that resulted in analgesia but only for a period of 6 hours post administration (Souza *et al.*, 2012). Dosages of 10 mg/kg once daily in African penguins (*Spheniscus demersus*) appear to provide pharmacokinetic therapeutic levels (Kilburn *et al.*, 2014); however, doses of 5–10 mg/kg twice daily in king penguins (*Aptenodytes patagonicus*) resulted in sedation in my experience, similar to that observed with multiple dosing in bald eagles, indicating that ongoing monitoring for side-effects of long-term medicated birds needs to occur (Souza *et al.*, 2009).

References

Acierno, M.J., da Cunha, A., Smith, J. *et al.* (2008) Agreement between direct and indirect blood pressure measurements obtained from anesthetized Hispaniolan Amazon parrots. *Journal of the American Veterinary Medical Association*, **233**(10), 1587–1590.

Aguilar, R.F., Smith, V.E., Ogburn, P. and Redig, P.T. (1995) Arrhythmias associated with isoflurane anesthesia in bald eagles. *Journal of Zoo and Wildlife Medicine*, **26**(4), 508–516.

Baine, K., Jones, M.P., Cox, S. and Martin-Jiminez, T. (2015) Pharmacokinetics of compounded intravenous and oral gabapentin in Hispaniolan Amazon parrots (*Amazona ventralis*). *Journal of Avian Medicine and Surgery*, **29**, 165–173.

Balko, J.A., Lindemann, D.M., Allender, M.C. and Chinnadurai, S.K. (2019) Evaluation of the anesthetic and cardiorespiratory effects of intramuscular alfaxalone administration and isoflurane in budgerigars (*Melopsittacus undulatus*) and comparison with manual restraint. *Journal of the American Veterinary Medical Association*, **254**(12), 1427–1435. doi: 10.2460/javma.254.12.1427.

Bouverot, P. (1978) Control of breathing in birds compared with mammals. *Physiological Reviews*, **58**(3), 604–655.

Clubb, S.L. (2006) Clinical management of psittacine birds affected with proventricular dilation disease. *Proceedings of the Annual Conference of the Association of Avian Veterinarians*, pp. 85–90.

Cole, G.A., Paul-Murphy, J., Krugner-Higby, L. *et al.* (2009) Analgesic effects of intramuscular administration of meloxicam in Hispaniolan Amazon parrots (*Amazona ventralis*) with experimentally induced arthritis. *American Journal of Veterinary Research*, **70**, 1471–1476.

Curro, T.G. (1994) Evaluation of the isoflurane-sparing effects of butorphanol and flunixin in Psittaciformes. *Proceedings of the Annual Conference of the Association of Avian Veterinarians*, pp. 17–19.

Curro, T.G. (1998) Anaesthesia of pet birds. *Seminars in Avian and Exotic Pet Medicine*, **7**(1), 10–21.

Curro, T.G., Brunson, D.B. and Paul-Murphy, J. (1994) Determination of the ED50 of isoflurane and evaluation of the isoflurane-sparing effect of butorphanol in cockatoos (*Cacatua* spp). *Veterinary Surgery*, **23**(5), 429–433.

Dahlhausen, B., Aldred, S. and Colaizzi, E. (2002) Resolution of clinical proventricular dilatation disease by cyclooxygenase 2 inhibition. *Proceedings of the Annual Conference of the Association of Avian Veterinarians*, pp. 9–12.

Desmarchelier, M., Troncy, E., Beauchamp, G. *et al.* (2012a) Evaluation of a fracture pain model in the domestic pigeon (*Columba livia*). *American Journal of Veterinary Research*, **73**(3), 353–360.

Desmarchelier, M., Troncy, E., Fitzgerald, G. and Lair, S. (2012b) Analgesic effects of meloxicam administration on postoperative orthopedic pain in domestic pigeons (*Columba livia*). *American Journal of Veterinary Research*, **73**(3), 361–367.

Doneley, B. (2007) The use of gabapentin to treat presumed neuralgia in a little corella (*Cacatua sanguinea*). *Proceedings of the Australian Association of Avian Veterinarians Conference*, pp. 169–172.

Doss, G.A., Fink, D.M. and Mans, C. (2018) Assessment of sedation after intranasal administration of midazolam and midazolam–butorphanol in cockatiels (*Nymphicus hollandicus*). *American Journal of Veterinary Research*, **79**(12), 1246–1252. doi: 10.2460/ajvr.79.12.1246.

Edling, T.M., Degernes, L., Flammer, K. and Horne, W.B. (2001) Capnographic monitoring of African Grey parrots during positive pressure ventilation. *Journal of the American Veterinary Medical Association*, **219**, 1714–1717.

Forbes, N.A. and Lawton, M.P.C. (1996) Formulary. In: *Manual of Psittacine Birds* (eds P.H. Benyon, N.A. Forbes & N.H. Harcourt-Brown). BSAVA, Cheltenham, UK.

Gaggermeier, B., Henke, J. and Schatzmann, U. (2003) Investigations on analgesia in domestic pigeons (*C. livia*, Gmel., 1789, var *dom.*) using buprenorphine and butorphanol. *Proceedings of the European Association of Avian Veterinarians*, pp. 70–73.

Glatz, P.C., Murphy, L.B. and Preston, A.P. (1992) Analgesic therapy in beak-trimmed chickens. *Australian Veterinary Journal*, **69**, 18.

Greenacre, C.B. (1997) Comparison of sevoflurane to isoflurane in Psittaciformes. *Proceedings of the Annual Conference of the Association of Avian Veterinarians*, pp. 123–124.

Greunz, E.M., Limon, D. and Bertelsen, M.F. (2021) Alfaxalone sedation in black-cheeked lovebirds (*Agapornis nigrigenis*) for non-invasive procedures. *Journal of Avian Medicine and Surgery*, **35**(2), 161–166. doi: 10.1647/19-00015.

Guzman, D.S.-M., Douglas, J.M., Beaufrere, H. and Paul-Murphy, J.R. (2020) Evaluation of the thermal antinociceptive effects of hydromorphone hydrochloride after intramuscular administration to orange-winged Amazon parrots (*Amazona amazonica*). *American Journal of Veterinary Research*, **81**(10), 775–782. doi: 10.2460/ajvr.81.10.775.

Hocking, P.M., Gentle, M.J., Bernard, R. and Dunn, L.N. (1997) Evaluation of a protocol for determining the effectiveness of pretreatment with local analgesics for reducing experimentally induced articular pain in domestic fowl. *Research in Veterinary Science*, **63**(3), 263–267.

Hocking, P.M., Robertson, G.W. and Gentle, M.J. (2005) Effects of non-steroidal anti-inflammatory drugs on pain-related behaviour in a model of articular pain in the domestic fowl. *Research in Veterinary Science*, **78**, 69–75.

Horgan, M.D., Knych, H.K., Siksay, S.E. and Duerr, R.S. (2020) Pharmacokinetics of a single dose of oral meloxicam in rehabilitated wild brown pelicans (*Pelecanus occidentalis*). *Journal of Avian Medicine and Surgery*, **34**(4), 329–337. doi: 10.1647/1082-6742-34.4.329.

Horowitz, I.H., Vaadia, G., Landau, S. *et al.* (2014) Butorphanol–midazolam combination injection for sedation of great white pelicans (*Pelicanus onocrotalus*). *Israel Journal of Veterinary Medicine*, **69**, 35–39.

Houck, E.L., Guzman, D.S.-M., Beaufrere, H. *et al.* (2018) Evaluation of the thermal antinociceptive effects and pharmacokinetics of hydromorphone hydrochloride after intramuscular administration to cockatiels (*Nymphicus hollandicus*). *American Journal of Veterinary Research*, **79**(8), 820–827. doi: 10.2460/ajvr.79.8.820.

Joyner, P.H., Jones, M.P., Ward, D. *et al.* (2008) Induction and recovery characteristics and cardiopulmonary effects of sevoflurane and isoflurane in bald eagles. *American Journal of Veterinary Research*, **69**, 13–22.

Keller, D., Sanchez-Migallon, G.D., Klauer, J., et al. (2009) Pharmacokinetics of nalbuphine HCl in Hispaniolan Amazon parrots (*Amazona ventralis*). *Proceedings of the American Association of Zoo Veterinarians Conference*, p. 106.

Khalilzadeh, E., Mousavi, S., Dolatyarieslami, M. *et al.* (2022) Effect of morphine and ibuprofen on nociceptive behavior, preening and motor activity following tonic chemical pain in the Japanese quail (*Coturnix japonica*). *Veterinary Anaesthesia and Analgesia*, **49**(5), 499–509. doi: 10.1016/j.vaa.2022.07.001.

Kilburn, J.J., Cox, S.K., Kottyan, J. *et al.* (2014) Pharmacokinetics of tramadol and its primary metabolite O-desmethyltramadol in African penguins (*Spheniscus demersus*). *Journal of Zoo and Wildlife Medicine*, **45**(1), 93–99. doi: 10.1638/2013-0190R.1.

Kim, Y.K., Lee, S.S., Suh, E.H. *et al.* (2011) Minimum anesthetic concentration and cardiovascular dose–response relationship of isoflurane in cinereous vultures (*Aegyptius monachus*). *Journal of Zoo and Wildlife Medicine*, **42**, 499–503.

Klaphke, E., Schumacher, J., Greenacre, C. *et al.* (2006) Comparative anesthetic and cardiopulmonary effects of pre- versus postoperative butorphanol administration in Hispaniolan Amazon Parrots (*Amazona ventralis*) anesthetized with sevoflurane. *Journal of Avian Medicine and Surgery*, **20**, 2–7.

König, H.E., Misek, I., Liebich, H.G. *et al.* (2016) Nervous system (*systema nervosum*). In: *Avian Anatomy: Textbook and Colour Atlas* (eds H.E. König, R. Korbel & H.-G. Liebich), 2nd edn, pp. 187–209. 5M Publishing, Sheffield, UK.

Korbel, R., Milovanovic, A., Erhardt, W., et al. (1993) Aerosacular perfusion with isoflurane: an anesthetic procedure for head surgery in birds. *Proceedings of the 2nd Annual Conference of the European Association of Avian Veterinarians*, pp. 9–37.

Ludders, J.W., Mitchell, G.S. and Rode, J. (1990) Minimal anesthetic concentration and cardiopulmonary dose response of isoflurane in ducks. *Veterinary Surgery*, **19**, 304–307.

Lukasik, V.M., Gentz, E.J., Erb, H.N. *et al.* (1997) Cardiopulmonary effects of propofol anesthesia in chickens (*Gallus gallus domestica*). *Journal of Avian Medicine and Surgery*, **11**, 93–97.

Lumeij, J.T. and Richie, B. (1994) Cardiology. In: *Avian Medicine: Principles and Applications* (eds B. Richie, G. Harrison & L. Harrison), pp. 697–711. Wingers Publishing, Lake Worth, FL.

Machin, K.L and Livingstone, A. (2001) Plasma bupivacaine levels in mallard ducks (*Anas platyrhynchos*) following a single subcutaneous dose. *Proceedings of the American Association of Zoo Veterinarians Conference*, pp. 159–163.

Mansour, A., Khachaturian, L.M.E., Akil, H. and Watson, S.J. (1988) Anatomy of CNS opioid receptors. *Trends in Neuroscience*, **11**, 301–314.

Mathonnet, M., Lalloue, F., Danty, E. *et al.* (2001) Cyclooxygenase 2 tissue distribution and developmental pattern of expression in the chicken. *Clinical and Experimental Pharmacology and Physiology*, **28**, 425–432.

Mercado, J.A., Larsen, R.S., Wack, R.F. and Pypendop, B.H. (2008) Minimum anesthetic concentration of isoflurane in captive thick-billed parrots (*Rhynchopsitta pachyrhyncha*). *American Journal of Veterinary Research*, **69**, 189–194.

Miller, K.A., Hill, N.J., Carrasco, S.E. and Patterson, M.M. (2019) Pharmacokinetics and safety of intramuscular meloxicam in zebra finches (*Taeniopygia guttata*). *Journal of the American Association for Laboratory Animal Science*, **58**(5), 589–593. doi: 10.30802/AALAS-JAALAS-19-000032.

Molter, C.M., Court, M.H., Cole, G.A. *et al.* (2013) Pharmacokinetics of meloxicam after intravenous, intramuscular, and oral administration of a single dose to Hispaniolan Amazon parrots (*Amazona ventralis*). *American Journal of Veterinary Research*, **74**(3), 375–380. doi: 10.2460/ajvr.74.3.375.

Naganobu, K., Fujisawa, Y., Ohde, H. *et al.* (2000) Determination of the minimum anesthetic concentration and cardiovascular dose response for sevoflurane in chickens during controlled ventilation. *Veterinary Surgery*, **29**(1), 102–105.

Oglesbee, B.L., Hamlin, R.L. and Hartman, S.P. (2001) Electrocardiographic reference values for macaws (*Ara* species) and cockatoos (*Cacatua* species). *Journal of Avian Medicine and Surgery*, **15**(1), 17–22.

Paul-Murphy, J., Brunson, D.B. and Miletic, V. (1999) Analgesic effects of butorphanol and buprenorphine in conscious African grey parrots (*Psittacus erithacus erithacus* and *Psittacus erithacus timneh*). *American Journal of Veterinary Research*, **60**, 1218–1221.

Paul-Murphy, J., Hess, J. and Fialkowski, J.P. (2004) Pharmacokinetic properties of a single intramuscular dose of buprenorphine in African grey parrots (*Psittacus erithacus erithacus*). *Journal of Avian Medicine and Surgery*, **18**, 224–228.

Paul-Murphy, J.R., Sladky, K.K., Krugner-Higby, L.A. *et al.* (2009) Analgesic effects of carprofen and liposome-encapsulated butorphanol tartrate in Hispaniolan parrots (*Amazona ventralis*) with experimentally induced arthritis. *American Journal of Veterinary Research*, **70**(10), 1201–1210.

Pereira, M.E. and Werther, K. (2007) Evaluation of the renal effects of flunixin meglumine, ketoprofen and meloxicam in budgerigars (*Melospittacus undulatus*). *Veterinary Record*, **160**, 844–846.

Phair, K.A., Larsen, R.S., Wack, R.F. *et al.* (2012) Determination of the minimum anesthetic concentration of sevoflurane in thick-billed parrots (*Rhynchopsitta pachyrhyncha*). *American Journal of Veterinary Research*, **73**(9), 1350–1355. doi: 10.2460/ajvr.73.9.1350.

Piiper, J., Drees, F. and Scheid, P. (1970) Gas exchange in the domestic fowl during spontaneous breathing and artificial ventilation. *Respiration Physiology*, **9**(2), 234–245.

Rettenmund, C.L., Heatley, J.J. and Russell, K.E. (2014) Comparison of two analyzers to determine selected venous blood analytes of Quaker parrots (*Myiopsitta monachus*). *Journal of Zoo and Wildlife Medicine*, **45**(2), 256–262.

Romano, J., Hasse, K. and Jonston, M. (2020) Sedative, cardiorespiratory and thermoregulatory effects of alfaxalone on budgerigars (*Melopsittacus undulatus*). *Journal of Zoo and Wildlife Medicine*, **51**(1), 96–101. doi: 10.1638/2019-0059.

Rosskopf, W.J., Woerpel, R.W. and Reed, S. (1989) Avian anaesthesia administration. Proceedings of the American Animal Hospital Association, pp. 449–457.

Sanchez-Migallon, G.D., Paul-Murphy, J., Barker, S., et al. (2008) Plasma concentrations of butorphanol in Hispaniolan Amazon parrots (*Amazona ventralis*) after intravenous and oral administration. *Proceedings of the Annual Conference of the Association of Avian Veterinarians*, pp. 23–24.

Schmidt-Nielsen, K. (1984) *Scaling: Why Is Animal Size So Important?* Cambridge University Press, Cambridge.

Shaver, S.L., Robinson, N.G., Wright, B.D. *et al.* (2009) A multimodal approach to management of suspected neuropathic pain in a prairie falcon (*Falco mexicanus*). *Journal of Avian Medicine and Surgery*, **23**, 209–213.

Singh, P.M., Johnson, C.B., Gartrell, B. *et al.* (2017) Analgesic effects of morphine and butorphanol in broiler chickens. *Veterinary Anaesthesia and Analgesia*, **44**(3), 538–545. doi: 10.1016/j.vaa.2016.05.006.

Siperstein, L.J. (2007) Use of Neurontin (gabapentin) to treat leg twitching/foot mutilation in a Senegal parrot. *Proceedings of the Association of Avian Veterinarians Conference*, p. 335.

Souza, M.J., Martin-Jiminez, T., Jones, M.P. and Cox, S.K. (2009) Pharmacokinetics of intravenous and oral tramadol in the bald eagle (*Haliaeetus leucocephalus*). *Journal of Avian Medicine and Surgery*, **23**, 247–252.

Souza, M.J., Guzman, D.S.-M., Paul-Murphy, J.R. and Cox, S.K. (2012) Pharmacokinetics after oral and intravenous administration of a single dose of tramadol hydrochloride to Hispaniolan Amazon parrots (*Amazona ventralis*). *American Journal of Veterinary Research*, **73**(8), 1142–1147. doi: 10.2460/ajvr.73.8.1142.

Sykes, J.M., Neiffer, D., Terrell, S. *et al.* (2013) Review of 23 cases of postintubation tracheal obstructions in birds. *Journal of Zoo and Wildlife Medicine*, **44**(3), 700–713.

Touzot-Jourde, G., Hernandez-Divers, S.J. and Trim, C.M. (2005) Cardiopulmonary effects of controlled versus spontaneous ventilation in pigeons anesthetized for coelioscopy. *Journal of the American Veterinary Medical Association*, **227**(9), 1424–1428.

Valverde, A., Honeyman, V.L., Dyson, D.H. and Valliant, A.E. (1990) Determination of a sedative dose and influence of midazolam on cardiopulmonary function in Canada geese. *American Journal of Veterinary Research*, **51**(7), 1071–1074.

Vesal, N. and Eskandari, M.H. (2006) Sedative effects of midazolam and xylazine with or without ketamine and detomidine alone following intranasal administration in ring-necked parakeets. *Journal of the American Veterinary Medical Association*, **228**(3), 383–388. doi: 10.2460/javma.228.3.383.

Vesal, N. and Zare, P. (2006) Clinical evaluation of intranasal benzodiazepines, alpha-agonists and their antagonists in canaries. *Veterinary Anaesthesia and Analgesia*, **33**, 143–148.

Villaverde-Morcillo, S., Benito, J., Garcia-Sanchez, R. *et al.* (2014) Comparison of isoflurane and alfaxalone (Alfaxan) for the induction of anesthesia in flamingos (*Phoenicopterus roseus*) undergoing orthopedic surgery. *Journal of Zoo and Wildlife Medicine*, **45**(2), 361–366. doi: 10.1638/2012-0283R2.1.

Wilson, G.H., Hernandez-Divers, S., Budsberg, S.C., Latimer, S., Grant, K. and Perthel, M. (2005) Pharmacokinetics and use of meloxicam in psittacine birds. *Proceedings of the 8th European Association of Avian Veterinarians, Arles*, pp. 230–232.

Chapter 12 Avian Nutrition

Classification of birds according to diet

The dietary preferences of bird species may be used to help classify them into groups that often possess similar physical characteristics dictated by these preferences.

There are two main categories of cage and aviary birds which are defined in a non-scientific manner into hardbills (sometimes referred to as hooked-bills) and softbills.

- Hardbills are predominantly members of the parrot and finch families. They will eat a variety of foods, both fruit and vegetable, and also seeds and nuts. To cope with these, the parrot family for example has developed a powerful crushing beak, the upper part of which has a synovial joint at its connection with the skull that allows even greater pressures to be generated as well as tough keratin covering the substantial beak, hence the term 'hardbill'.
- Softbills come from a variety of species, from the insectivorous birds, such as wild blackbirds and starlings, to the nectivorous hummingbirds and the omnivorous toucans. Most genuinely have a soft beak that is easily deformable, but some do not so the term 'softbill' is confusing.

Raptors, or birds of prey, including owls, falcons, eagles and buzzards, all possess a sharp hooked beak used as a ripping tool for tearing prey.

In all these cases, the individual species have become highly evolved to handle certain types of food. We also know that many of these creatures in the wild have a changing food supply throughout the year, so what may form a staple diet in the summer does not necessarily apply in the winter.

General nutritional requirements

Water

Water is a necessity. However, just as important as providing it is maintaining its quality. Many birds will dunk their food in water, and indeed if the water feeders are poorly situated, may defecate in the water bowls. This can lead to massive bacterial population explosions and gastroenteritis, sour crop and other health problems.

The quality of water that comes from the tap is also important. Many older buildings may still have lead pipes supplying their water source. In England and Wales, it is estimated that around 8.9 million homes (34%) at the end of the twentieth century still had lead water pipes (Potter, 1997). This can leach into the water and then the lead can build up in a bird's body over a period of weeks or months, leading to poisoning. Birds are much more sensitive to lead poisoning than humans. It is an insidious disease and results in chronic bone marrow and immune system suppression as well as liver and kidney damage. Safe levels have previously been reported for humans of less than 50 µg/L of water but there is increasing evidence that any level of lead may be harmful to bird and human alike and modern UK guidelines now suggest maximum levels of 10–25 µg/L as being advisable.

Problems can also arise when mineral and vitamin supplements are administered in the drinking water. The nutrient-enriched water can encourage bacterial growth over a few hours, requiring owners to be rigorous about bowl hygiene if they are giving their bird any of these 'tonics'. Therefore in general it is not advisable to administer minerals and vitamin supplements via the drinking water. Instead, it is recommended to supplement the food as required.

The amount of water consumed by individual birds will depend on the diet being offered. On dry biscuit or seed-based diets, water consumption will be higher than for birds which consume large amounts of fruit and vegetables – even so, a budgerigar, for example, may only consume as little as 5 mL of water in a 24-hour period.

Maintenance energy requirements

It is extremely difficult to determine the basal metabolic rate (BMR) (sometimes referred to as the resting energy requirement or RER) of avian patients, as this term covers the energy expenditure when at complete rest in a thermoneutral environment after a period of sleep. Therefore, the more useful concept of maintenance energy requirement (MER) is used in birds. MER is the energy usage in a moderately active adult bird in a thermoneutral environment. This can still be difficult to calculate with accuracy; however, studies of the adult budgerigar for example have suggested that current MER levels are 30 kJ/day (around 7.2 kcal/day) and for a canary around 62 kJ/day (14.9 kcal/day) are adequate (Harper and Turner, 2000). The dietary energy levels of most Psittaciformes are considered adequate at a range of 3200–4200 kcal/kg and Passeriformes at 3500–4500 kcal/kg of dry matter fed (Pollock, 2007).

Formulas have been devised to calculate BMR and MER which can be used to calculate energy requirements in species where published values are not available. BMR in kilocalories per day (kcal/day) may be calculated using the formula:

$$\mathrm{BMR} = k \times \left[\mathrm{weight}(\mathrm{kg})\right]^{0.75}$$

The constant, k, varies with family groups, and has been estimated at 78 for non-passerine (i.e. non-perching birds such as parrots) and 129 for passerines (perching birds such as finches, canaries, thrushes, etc.).

MER is dependent on the BMR and may be calculated from it by the following formula:

$$\mathrm{MER} = 1.5 \times \mathrm{BMR}$$

Veterinary Nursing of Exotic Pets and Wildlife, Third Edition. Simon J. Girling.

MER values may increase as mentioned with other high-energy demand conditions, for example a young growing bird may need its MER multiplied by a factor of two to three, infections may require its MER to be multiplied by a factor of 1.5 and a bird suffering from a severe traumatic injury such as a fracture may require its MER to be multiplied by a factor of two. It should be noted however that not only is there considerable species variation but variation during the lifetime of an individual species. An example in monk (Quaker) parakeets (*Myiopsitta monachus*) showed that assuming a two-times increase in MER during their growth phase was inaccurate, with a significant boost required during feather production (period of 18–23 days post hatch) (Petzinger *et al.*, 2015). Moulting is also a time of high-energy demand, being particularly acute in those species that moult all their flight feathers in one go (many waterfowl, penguins and birds of prey for example). In some passerines, energy requirements may increase by 52% at peak moult (Murphy and King, 1992). Even parrots, which tend to moult a few feathers at a time rather than all of them at once, may see a spike in energy demand when flight feathers are replaced.

Clearly if a bird's MER is significant and yet the foods offered are so low in energy content that the bird has to eat more of it than will fit into its digestive system in 24 hours, the bird will rapidly lose body condition. Many pet birds, however, have the opposite problem in that they are often offered high-energy foods such as oil-based seeds and will continue to eat until their digestive tracts are full, leading to excessive calorific intake and obesity. For example, oilseeds, such as rapeseed or sunflower seeds, have an energy content of 25 MJ/kg, as opposed to carbohydrate-based seeds such as millet that have a lower energy density of 17 MJ/kg. If the diet of a parrot is then based on oilseeds, obesity is much more likely to occur (Harper and Skinner, 1998).

Protein and amino acids

Total protein levels between 12 and 15% as crude protein (CP) are considered acceptable for most cage birds (typically kept Psittaciformes and Passeriformes). Proteins are assembled from groups of up to 22 amino acids. In general terms, it seems that for humans and most cage birds, 10 amino acids are essential and therefore must be provided in the diet. The others may be manufactured from these 10. The essential amino acids are:

- arginine
- histidine
- isoleucine
- leucine
- lysine
- methionine
- phenylalanine
- threonine
- tryptophan
- valine.

In addition, it is known that if a diet is low in the amino acids methionine or arginine, an extra supplement of the amino acid glycine is required. Glycine is also very important in young growing, particularly psittacine, birds as they are often unable to synthesise it in their livers (Taylor *et al.*, 1994; Koutsos *et al.*, 2001). Serine and proline have also been indicated as important for young avian species, and so while not essential in adult birds as they can manufacture it, they are nonetheless important in the diet for growth (Scott *et al.*, 1982; Murphy, 1996; Klasing, 1998).

Cysteine levels as a minimum percentage of 0.203% are needed for adequate feather strength (Tsiagbe *et al.*, 1987). Deficiencies in methionine can cause dark horizontal lines to appear on developing feathers, but excesses of methionine in the diet may also result in softer and weaker feathers (Tsiagbe *et al.*, 1987). Lysine values of 0.8–1.5% of diet fed are quoted as necessary for adult psittacine birds (McDonald, 2006). Levels of methionine, cysteine and lysine are important during breeding as in one study with budgerigars, adequate overall protein levels were provided but because of a deficiency in these three amino acids, due to a diet of millet, oats and canary seed, reproduction failed (Angel and Ballam, 1995). The requirements for adult budgerigars was considered around 2% in another study (Earle and Clarke, 1991).

Proteins are assessed on their ability to provide these essential amino acids, with poor proteins supplying only non-essential ones. This is quantified by the term 'biological value'. Foodstuff of high biological value contains more of the essential amino acids. For adult companion cage birds, assuming a high biological value, overall levels of 10–15% protein content in the diet have been shown to be adequate, with evidence suggesting that larger granivorous species require a higher percentage protein (Kamphues *et al.*, 1997; Harper and Skinner, 1998; McDonald, 2006). In young growing blue-fronted Amazon parrots, an optimal overall protein level of 24.4% for maximum weight gain was reported in one publication which also suggested a minimum level of 18% (Carciofi *et al.*, 2008). Much of this protein in psittacines often, rightly or wrongly, comes from seeds. Some seeds are very high providers of certain amino acids. Sunflower seeds, white millet and rapeseed for example provide high levels of the sulphur-containing amino acids methionine and cystine/cysteine. These amino acids are important during moulting when new feathers are being produced rapidly and a deficiency can lead to feather stunting and abnormal structure. Species variations of course exist within the Psittaciformes, with nectivorous species such as lorikeets and lories requiring lower dietary proteins as they are able to cope with a level as low as 2.9% assuming good biological value (Frankel and Avram, 2001).

However, deficiencies in certain amino acids have been shown to cause disease (see Figure 12.1). For example, a deficiency in lysine causes depigmentation of feathers and a lack of arginine is associated with feather picking. In some species of birds, for example raptors, a deficiency in essential amino acids is extremely rare due to their high animal protein-based diet – it is naturally of a high biological value. However, strict carnivores such as raptors and penguins need more than the usual 10 essential amino acids in their diet (for example requiring taurine similar to mammalian carnivores such as cats and ferrets), so if poor-quality meat or vegetable proteins are fed to these species, deficiencies may occur.

Fats and essential fatty acids

Fats provide high concentrations of energy as well as supplying the bird with essential fatty acids (EFAs). The latter are required for cellular integrity and are used as the building blocks for internal chemicals. These internal chemicals, such as prostaglandins, play an important part in reproduction and inflammation. Fats also provide

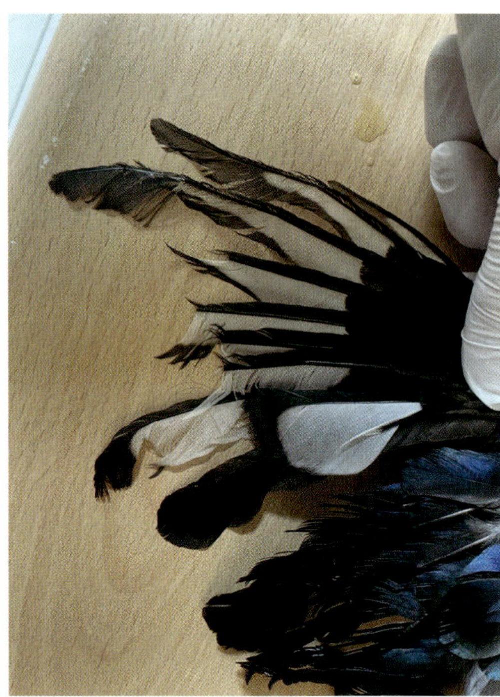

Figure 12.1 Amino acid deficiencies may lead to feather growth abnormalities.

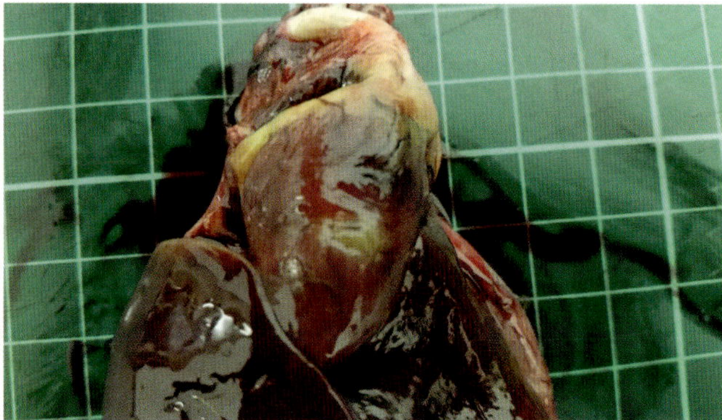

Figure 12.2 Excessive amounts of high-oil-based seeds can lead to atherosclerosis in cage birds causing heart disease among other things.

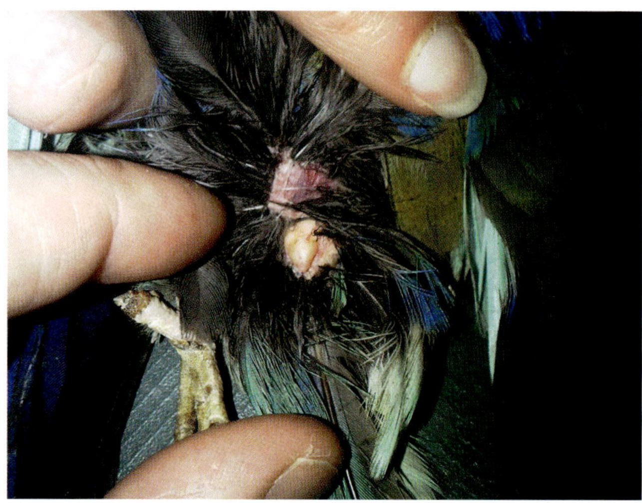

Figure 12.3 Preen gland impaction has been associated with a deficiency in essential fatty acids and vitamins A and E.

a carrier mechanism for the absorption of fat-soluble vitamins, such as vitamins A, D, E and K.

The primary EFA for cage birds is linoleic acid, as it is for mammals (Brue, 1994). The absolute (minimum) dietary requirement of this fatty acid is 1% of the diet. If the diet becomes deficient in this EFA, there will be a rapid decline in cell structure. This is shown clinically by the skin becoming flaky, dry and prone to recurrent infection. Linoleic acid deficiency also leads to fluid loss through the skin, which in turn leads to polydipsia. It is, however, unlikely that any seed-eating bird will be deficient in linoleic acid, as it is widely found in sunflower seeds and safflower seeds among others.

Another EFA which is thought to be important for birds is alpha-linolenic acid, which is necessary for some prostaglandin and eicosanoid production.

The problem of overconsumption of fats in cage birds which are not exercising regularly is well known, and leads to hypercholesterolaemia and atherosclerosis. High-fat oilseeds are prime culprits for this (see Figure 12.2). The same applies to underworked raptors fed overweight laboratory rats. Female raptors are particularly prone to this after the breeding season, when large amounts of cholesterol are mobilised for yolk production. Hypercholesterolaemia can also be hereditary as well as dietary in raptors, but it can be reduced by regular exercising and feeding of lean, low-fat prey. Saturated animal fats are particularly bad for seed and fruit eaters, causing rapid atherosclerosis. In raptors and other strict carnivores such as penguins, additional EFAs are required such as arachidonic acid, which is found in animal fats but not plant or seed-based fats.

Preen gland impactions have many causes but may also be associated with a deficiency in EFAs and vitamins A and E (see Figure 12.3).

Carbohydrates

Carbohydrates are mainly used for rapid energy production. This is particularly important in many small cage birds, because they are in constant demand of rapid supplies of energy for their often hyperactive and high-metabolism lives. Birds that are debilitated in some way will particularly benefit from the supply of high-carbohydrate foods.

Fibre

Dietary fibre does not seem to be important for commonly kept cage and aviary birds. As raptors and penguins are carnivorous, they do not have a dietary fibre requirement either. Only a few wild birds, such as the ratites (ostriches, emus, rheas and cassowaries) and Galliformes such as grouse require fibre and have large fermenting caeca. The red grouse (*Lagopus lagopus scotica*) and other members of the *Lagopus* genus, including ptarmigan and willow grouse for example, live predominantly on heather shoots, willow, aspen and birch for certain times of the year. Life-stage can also be important as many of these species will consume more insects than leaves and twigs as juvenile birds because their undeveloped caecal digestion cannot cope with a high-fibre diet.

Apart from these general dietary requirements, birds, like all animals, require a variety of vitamins and minerals for a healthy diet.

Vitamins

Vitamins are broadly categorised into:

- Fat-soluble vitamins A, D, E and K
- Water-soluble vitamins such as the B vitamin complex and vitamin C.

Fat-soluble vitamins

Vitamin A: In cage birds and waterfowl the diet frequently contains vitamin A precursors, which are present as plant carotenoids. In many birds, the most important version of these, in terms of how much vitamin A can be produced from it, is beta-carotene (Harper and Skinner, 1998). Terminology can be confusing when it comes to dietary levels as many mention vitamin A levels as international units per kilogram of food (IU/kg) and others as micrograms per kilogram of food (μg/kg) and it is not easy to convert from one to another as it depends upon the proportions of differing carotenes (of which there are many) or whether the vitamin A is preformed within the food source. Vitamin A must be provided in its preformed state in carnivores such as raptors and penguins as they cannot synthesise it from precursors such as beta-carotene or other carotenes.

Vitamin A is needed for a number of functions, the best known of which is maintenance of the light-sensitive pigment in the retina of the eye. It is also important in epithelial cell turnover and keratinisation, innate skin and epithelial surface immunity (IgA production) as well as the integrity and function of the gastrointestinal, respiratory and urinary tracts. It is also important for phagocytic activity in the immune system (macrophages and heterophils) and deficiencies can cause depletion of lymphocytes. In many birds such as some Passeriformes (perching birds such as canaries) and Phoenicopteriformes (flamingos) carotenoids are important for feather pigmentation particularly reds and pinks.

Hypovitaminosis A is a commonly seen problem in companion birds, particularly parrots. This is mainly due to the very low levels of beta-carotenes present in seeds, especially in the often-fed sunflower seeds, millet and peanuts. The minimum requirement for vitamin A is quoted as 40 IU per budgerigar (Harper and Skinner, 1998). This may be met by as little as 0.4 g of carrot per day but would require 200 g of millet seed to provide the same amount – five times a budgerigar's average weight!

If a deficiency in vitamin A occurs, then cellular turnover of epithelial surfaces are affected and one such change is that mucous membranes become thickened. Oral and respiratory secretions dry up because of damage to salivary and mucous glands that occurs with the squamous metaplasia changes to the epithelium. This is compounded in the respiratory tract by failure of the ciliary mechanisms that have a role in removing foreign particles. This, combined with vitamin A's role in immune system function, leads to an increased incidence of respiratory and digestive tract infections (see Figure 12.4). One of the most frequently seen infections, particularly in parrots fed an all-seed diet, is the fungal respiratory disease aspergillosis. Sterile pustules and cornified plaques inside the mouth are also commonly seen, with enlargement of the sublingual salivary glands. In carnivorous species, deficiencies produce similar clinical signs as for cage birds with increased predisposition to

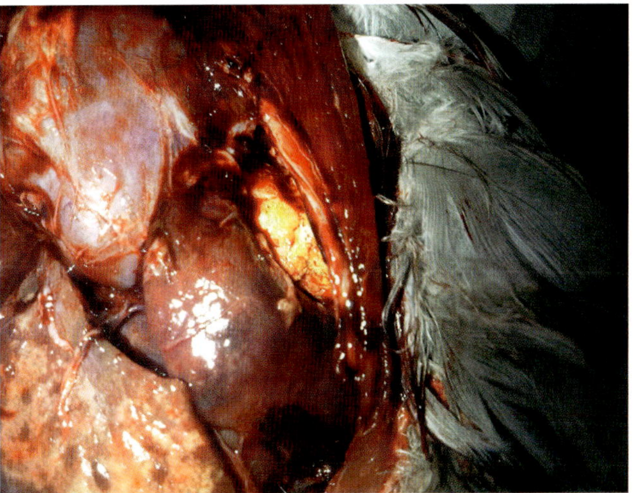

Figure 12.4 Hypovitaminosis A may lead to decreased respiratory system function and immunity leading to aspergillosis as seen in the post-mortem of this African grey parrot.

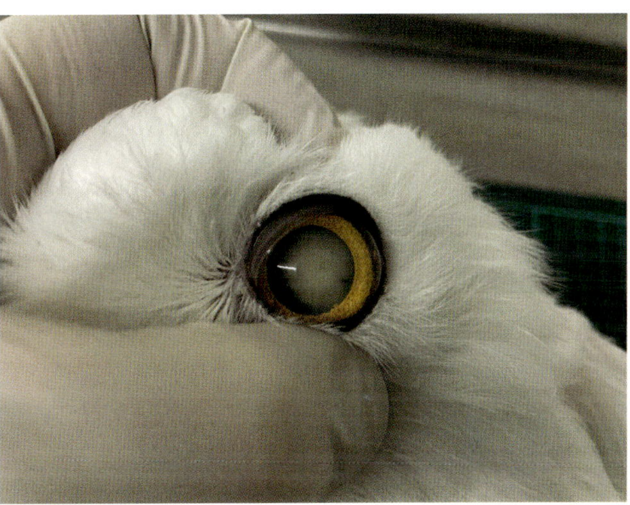

Figure 12.5 Cataract development can occur of course with age but has also been associated with hypovitaminosis A in carnivorous species in particular.

aspergillosis in particular as well as conditions unique to the species concerned, such as salt gland adenitis in penguins (Naylor *et al.*, 2018). Deficiencies in vitamin A have also been associated in birds with nuclear cataract development (see Figure 12.5).

Vitamin A is also required for bone growth, for the normal function of secretory glands such as the adrenals and for normal reproductive function. On another level, coloured plumage, particularly the reds and yellows, are often derived from vitamin A in Passeriformes. Therefore, birds such as red-factor canaries will become paler in colour if they are fed a diet deficient in the beta-carotenes required to produce vitamin A.

Because it is fat soluble, vitamin A can be stored in the body, primarily in the liver and so any dietary changes may take time to produce clinical signs due to this tissue reserve. The recommended dietary levels vary quite considerably depending on the species and also text. For example, ranges of dietary vitamin A from a minimum of 8000 to a maximum of 11 000 IU/kg of food offered for

Passeriformes and Psittaciformes has been recommended (Scott, 1996; Kollias and Kollias, 2000; Orosz, 2014), although the National Research Council suggests lower levels of 2500–5000 IU/kg food fed with toxicity occurring at 20–30 times this level (Brue, 1994). In adult cockatiels, a species that is reported as being more commonly affected by vitamin A toxicity than deficiency, maintenance values for vitamin A were considered adequate in one study at 2000–4000 IU/kg food fed (Koutsos and Klasing, 2002). In penguins suggested levels are 1700–5600 IU/kg dry matter of food fed as preformed vitamin A and it is common to supplement species being fed previously frozen and then defrosted fish as vitamin A levels deplete with time during frozen storage (Crissey *et al.*, 2002).

Hypervitaminosis A can occur particularly in granivorous and nectivorous species that can easily convert beta-carotenes to vitamin A, especially if they are then fed commercially prepared diets or supplements with vitamin A. Examples of toxicity have been reported particularly in cockatiels (granivorous) and lorikeets (nectivorous) where clinical signs associated with this oversupplementation included recurrent digestive yeast infections, conjunctivitis and mortalities (Koutsos *et al.*, 2003; Park, 2006). In these publications, evidence of ill health occurred where vitamin A levels in excess of 3000 μg/kg of diet fed in the case of cockatiels and in excess of 1000 IU/kg of diet fed in nectivorous species, evidence supported also by McDonald (2004). There is also evidence in those species which are susceptible to iron storage disease (including lories and lorikeets) that excessive vitamin A (as well as excessive vitamin C) can increase liver iron uptake and liver deposition and so hasten disease (McDonald, 2003).

Vitamin D: This vitamin is primarily concerned with calcium metabolism, and vitamin D_3 is the most active in calcium homeostasis. Plants are not effective as suppliers of this compound as they can only provide ergocalciferol.

Cholecalciferol is manufactured in the bird's skin in a process enhanced by ultraviolet (UV)-B light. Indoor-kept birds without artificial UV-B provision produce much less of this compound and this can lead to deficiencies. Exposure to just 11–45 minutes of unfiltered sunshine has been shown to prevent rickets in growing chickens (Heuser and Norris, 1929). It is important to note that traditionally used glass for domestic windows filters out the important UV-B spectrum. Cholecalciferol must then be activated, first in the liver (to become 25-hydroxycholecalciferol) and then by the kidneys (to become 1,25-dihydroxycholecalciferol), before it becomes fully functional as a hormone important for calcium metabolism. It works with parathyroid hormone to increase reabsorption of calcium at the expense of phosphorus from the kidneys. It also increases absorption of calcium from the intestines and mobilises calcium from the bone, increasing blood calcium levels.

Hypovitaminosis D_3 can lead to clinical disease of the bones (rickets). This is exacerbated by diets low in calcium. Commonly affected species typically include indoor-kept cage birds fed all-seed diets and raptors fed all-skeletal meat diets with no calcium supplementation. These situations typically produce well-muscled, heavy birds that have poorly mineralised bones. Radiographic evidence of deficiency shows flaring of the epiphyseal plates at the ends of the long bones. The long bones then deform, particularly the tibiotarsal bones in long-legged birds, but any bone can be affected, especially weight-bearing ones in the wing or leg. One study carried out by Nightengale *et al.* (2022) showed that Hispaniolan Amazon parrots housed indoors without UV light had significantly lower vitamin D and blood ionised calcium (the biologically active portion of blood calcium) levels than Hispaniolan Amazon parrots housed outdoors. Use of unfiltered sunlight in another study of South American parrots significantly increased the ionised calcium and 25-hydroxycholecalciferol levels in the blood and the same study showed significant increases in ionised calcium and 25-hydroxycholecalciferol in African grey parrots exposed to artificial UV-B radiation (Stanford, 2006). Another suggested that deficiencies in vitamin D led to an increased incidence of feather plucking (West *et al.*, 2019). Low levels of vitamin D_3, specifically 25-hydroxycholecalciferol, have been associated with hypocalcaemia (particularly low blood ionised calcium) in African grey parrots (Stanford, 2007). Where skeletal deformities are reported due to a deficiency many bones can be affected, but in one study the tibiotarsus, one of the major weight-bearing bones of the bird's body, was most affected (Harcourt-Brown, 2003). The recommended minimum levels are 500 IU/kg of food offered for Psittaciformes and 1000 IU/kg for Passeriformes (Kollias and Kollias, 2000; Orosz, 2014). Levels of 200 IU/kg food fed in domestic poultry, 900 IU/kg in domestic turkeys and 1200 IU/kg in quail are considered adequate, showing that even within one order (Galliformes) there is considerable species variation (McDonald, 2006). Blood levels of 25-hydroxycholecalciferol above 50 nmol/L have been quoted as normal in the domestic chicken (Dacke, 2000).

Hypervitaminosis D_3 is caused by oversupplementation with vitamin D_3 and calcium, and leads to calcification of soft tissues, such as the medial walls of the arteries, and the kidneys. This leads to hypertension and organ failure. The recommended maximum levels are 2000 IU/kg of food offered for Psittaciformes and 2500 IU/kg for Passeriformes (Kollias and Kollias, 2000; Orosz, 2014). Metastatic calcification of soft tissues and mortalities were seen in budgerigars in one report with excessive dietary levels of vitamin D of 40 520 IU/kg of food fed (Olds *et al.*, 2015).

Vitamin E: Vitamin E compounds are found in several active forms in plants. Vitamin E comprises a range of compounds, principally tocopherols and tocotrienols in four forms, alpha, beta, gamma and delta. Alpha-tocopherol has the highest biological activity followed by beta, delta and gamma (McDonald, 2006). Vitamin E has an important role in immune system function, particularly lymphocyte cell activity, as well as reproductive activity. Vitamin E is combined with selenium in the metalloenzyme glutathione peroxidase. This enzyme mops up the free radicals that are produced in the metabolism of dietary polyunsaturated fats, which could otherwise cause cellular damage. Vitamin B_2 (riboflavin) is also important in the synthesis of glutathione peroxidase and so may complicate the issue. At appropriate dietary levels vitamin E is viewed as an antioxidant, but in excess it can act as an oxidant (see below).

Hypovitaminosis E produces a condition known as 'white muscle disease' in which damage occurs to the muscle bundles and their myoglobin content, leading to pale-coloured muscles and muscle weakness. This may become clinically apparent in vitamin E-deficient long-legged birds in particular when they undergo periods of intense activity (running), for example ratites such as ostrich, rhea and emu. This can result in muscle damage, including cardiac damage, release of intracellular potassium and cardiac arrhythmias, muscle rupture and even death (so-called capture myopathy; see also Chapter 29). In addition, birds such as cockatiels deficient in vitamin E may be more susceptible to gastrointestinal diseases, such as infection with the protozoal gut parasite *Giardia* spp. and this may result in the passage of undigested whole seeds in their droppings. Vitamin E deficiency can also lead to decreased fertility by failing to protect spermatozoa and oocytes from oxidative damage (Rangaraj and Hong, 2015).

Hypovitaminosis E may occur due to a reduction in fat metabolism or absorption, as can occur with small intestinal, pancreatic or biliary diseases. It may also occur in herbivores because of a lack of green plant material in the diet, as this is the main source of tocopherols. Excessive amounts of dietary zinc can also lead to alpha-tocopherol depletion in young chicks so care should be taken to ensure the diet is properly balanced (Lu and Coombs, 1988). Vitamin E deficiency may also occur in carnivorous birds fed on diets high in polyunsaturated fatty acids, such as fish-eating raptors, pelicans, penguins and other species fed on fish that has been previously frozen. These oily fish diets rapidly deplete vitamin E reserves used up in metabolising the polyunsaturated fats. Over time the freezing storage process increases the numbers of free radicals that again increase vitamin E requirements. Supplementation of such diets in these species with vitamin E is therefore commonplace in zoological collections.

Meat source can also be important for terrestrial carnivores. For example, day-old chicks, a common dietary source for raptors, provide a higher level of vitamin E (alpha-tocopherols) than turkey breast meat, highlighting the issues of appropriate meat selection for raptors (Schinck *et al.*, 2008). The recommended minimum level is 50 ppm for both Passeriformes and Psittaciformes (Kollias and Kollias, 2000; Orosz, 2014).

Hypervitaminosis E is uncommon. Hypervitaminosis may occur with oversupplementation of diets in semi-aquatic fish-eating species. As noted above, supplementation with vitamin E in fish-eating birds is commonplace. This may lead to an oversupplementation of vitamin E particularly where non-oily fish (e.g. whiting) are fed, but it also depends on the species of bird as some have higher requirements than others. Vitamin E, when oversupplemented (levels in excess of 500–1000 IU/kg of food fed), can paradoxically become a toxic oxidant as the process by which vitamin E interacts with tissues is a so-called redox reaction (it can act both as an oxidant and reductant depending upon its levels) and so excesses can lead to medical issues, possibly through its ability to counteract vitamin K and reduce the absorption of vitamins A and D (Nichols *et al.*, 1989; McDonald, 2006; Nijboer, 2022). In one study in pelicans, a decrease in growth rates and coagulopathies were observed with such oversupplementation (Nichols *et al.*, 1989).

Vitamin K: Vitamin K (menadione) is an important vitamin in the blood clotting process. It also increases bone quality through the management of osteocalcin and so ensures calcification of bones. Because vitamin K is produced by bacteria normally present in the gut, a true deficiency is rare in the majority of birds, although absorption will be reduced when fat digestion/absorption is reduced as in, for example, biliary or pancreatic disease. One exception is perhaps an unusual species of parrot, the fig parrots (*Psittaculirostris*, *Opopsitta* and *Cyclopsitta* spp.) that eat a significant amount of termites in the wild and so is thought to be dependent on the vitamin K produced in the gut of the insect. Dietary supplementation of this genus of parrot in captivity with 300 µg of vitamin K (phytomenadione) is recommended to avoid early haemorrhagic disease and mortalities (Jordan and Silva, 1991).

The consumption of warfarin- and coumarin-derived compounds (such as those found in plants like sweet clovers) can increase the demand for clotting factors. It can also be a problem for raptors that have eaten prey that has been killed by coumarin and related rodenticides. This is clearly a significant issue for wild raptors, with one study in France suggesting that 50% of all dead birds of prey sampled were positive for anti-vitamin K rodenticides (Moriceau *et al.*, 2022). The deficiency produced causes internal and external haemorrhage, but vitamin K also functions in calcium/phosphorus metabolism in the bones as mentioned above and this may also be affected. The recommended minimum level for raptors, Passeriformes and Psittaciformes is 1 ppm (Wallach and Cooper, 1982). In domestic Galliformes, the optimal levels varied with the age of the chickens: 8 mg/kg feed for very young chicks (starters less than 5 weeks), 2 mg/kg for growers and 2 mg/kg for finishers in the broiler industry to ensure adequate bone density (Zhang *et al.*, 2003).

Water-soluble vitamins

Vitamin B_1 (thiamine): Thiamine is found widely in plant and animal tissues alike. It is concerned with a number of cellular functions, one of which involves the integrity of the central nervous system.

Hypovitaminosis B_1 is uncommon in cage birds but may occur in zoological species. The most likely cause is the presence of enzymes called thiaminases in the diet, which destroy thiamine. A common source of thiaminases is frozen then defrosted fish, which may be fed to some raptors such as sea eagles and ospreys and of course to captive penguins, pelicans, etc. However, thiamine antagonists are present in foods such as blackberries, beetroot, coffee, chocolate and tea. When a deficiency occurs, neurological signs such as seizures, opisthotonus, weakness and head tremors appear. It is common for foot tapping to be seen in penguins. In addition, the fungal infection aspergillosis is a common sequel to B_1 deficiency in many carnivores. The recommended minimum dietary level for raptors, Psittaciformes and Passeriformes is 4 ppm (Kollias and Kollias, 2000) or 5 g of usable vitamin B_1 per day for raptors (Wallach and Cooper, 1982). For penguins the typical levels recommended are 25–30 mg/kg food fed on a wet matter basis and 100–120 mg/kg food fed on a dry matter basis (Crissey *et al.*, 2002). It is routine to supplement birds fed previously frozen then defrosted fish with vitamin B_1 on a daily or every other day basis.

Vitamin B_2 (riboflavin): Vitamin B_2 is present in particularly small amounts in seeds, and so deficiency is primarily seen in seed-eating birds. Hypovitaminosis B_2 causes growth retardation and curled toe paralysis in chicks. This is due to its function in cartilage, collagenous and nerve cell tissue growth. In domestic chickens, vitamin B_2 deficiency reliably causes reversible demyelination of peripheral nerves and so could be expected to cause peripheral neurological disease (paresis and paralysis) in other species (Cai *et al.*, 2023). Vitamin B_2 deficiency has also been associated with nuclear cataracts and white muscle disease as it is important for the production of glutathione peroxidase. Birds can be supplemented using commercial powder supplements or simple brewer's yeast. The recommended minimum levels are 6 ppm for Psittaciformes and Passeriformes (Kollias and Kollias, 2000), 3.6 mg/kg for game birds (Austic and Cole, 1971) and 4 mg/kg of feed offered for waterfowl (Scott and Norris, 1965).

Vitamin B_3 *(niacin)*: Niacin is found widely in many foods, but the form that occurs in plants has a low availability to the bird. It is used in many cellular metabolic processes.

Birds fed a high proportion of one type of seed, such as waterfowl overfed on sweetcorn, can become deficient. This results in retarded growth, poor feather quality and scaly dermatitis on the legs and feet. Intertarsal joint deformities can occur in the larger waterfowl. The recommended minimum requirements are 50 ppm for Passeriformes and Psittaciformes (Kollias and Kollias, 2000) or 55–70 mg/kg of feed in general (Wallach and Cooper, 1982).

Vitamin B_5 *(pantothenic acid)*: Pantothenic acid is found widely in plants and animals and so deficiency rarely occurs. When it does occur in birds, signs include crusting of the feet, eyelids and commissures of the beak, poor feather growth and general epidermal desquamation. The recommended minimum levels are 20 ppm for Passeriformes and Psittaciformes (Kollias and Kollias, 2000) or 35.2 mg/kg of feed in ducks (Scott and Norris, 1965).

Vitamin B_6 *(pyridoxine)*: Any deficiency of pyridoxine will result in retarded growth, hyperexcitability, convulsions, twisted neck and polyneuritis, although a deficiency is rarely seen. Recommended minimum levels are 6 ppm in Passeriformes and Psittaciformes (Kollias and Kollias, 2000) or 2.6–3 mg/kg of feed for game birds (Scott and Norris, 1965).

Vitamin B_9 *(folic acid/folate)*: Folic acid deficiency leads to severely impaired cell division. This can lead to a number of problems, such as failure of reproductive tract development in hen birds, a macrocytic anaemia due to failure of red blood cell maturation and immune system cellular dysfunction.

Folic acid is needed to form uric acid, the waste product of protein metabolism in birds. Therefore, a relative deficiency of folic acid may occur in some individuals fed a very high protein diet. In addition, some foods, such as cabbage and other brassicas, as well as oranges, beans and peas, contain folic acid inhibitors. The use of trimethoprim sulfonamide drugs may also reduce gut bacterial folic acid production. The recommended minimum requirements are 1.5 ppm for Passeriformes and Psittaciformes (Kollias and Kollias, 2000) or 1.25 mg/kg of feed (Scott and Norris, 1965).

Biotin: True deficiencies are rare due to gut bacterial production. Deficiencies produce a range of signs, including exfoliative dermatitis and gangrenous toes. The recommended minimum requirements are 0.25 ppm for Passeriformes and Psittaciformes (Kollias and Kollias, 2000) or 0.09–0.15 mg/kg of feed in waterfowl (Wallach and Cooper, 1982).

Vitamin B_{12}: Vitamin B_{12} is produced by intestinal bacteria so deficiency is uncommon, although it may occur after prolonged antibiotic medication. Vitamin B_{12} is required for many metabolic pathways and neurological function and a deficiency may cause a knock-on deficiency in folic acid. It will cause slow growth, muscular dystrophy in the legs, poor hatching rates and high mortality rates in young birds, as well as hatching deformities. The recommended minimum requirements are 0.01 ppm in Passeriformes and Psittaciformes (Kollias and Kollias, 2000) or 0.009–0.25 mg/kg of feed offered (Wallach and Cooper, 1982).

Choline: Choline may be synthesised in the body, but not in sufficient quantities for the growing bird. Because of their interactions, the need for choline is dependent on levels of folic acid and vitamin B_{12}. Excess dietary protein increases choline requirements, as does a diet high in fats. Deficiencies cause retarded growth, disrupted fat metabolism, fatty liver damage and perosis (slipping of the Achilles tendon off the intertarsal joint groove). The recommended minimum requirements are 1500 ppm for Passeriformes and Psittaciformes (Kollias and Kollias, 2000) or 1300–1900 mg/kg of feed offered (Wallach and Cooper, 1982).

Vitamin C: There are only a few wild birds that have a direct need for dietary vitamin C as most species can manufacture it themselves in their kidneys or liver. The species requiring dietary vitamin C include the red-vented bulbul (*Pycnonotus cafer*) and the willow ptarmigan/red grouse (*Lagopus lagopus* sp.) as well as the crimson sun-conure. Birds in general do not need vitamin C in their diets as it can be produced from glucose in the liver due to the presence of the enzyme L-gulonolactone oxidase. If a bird is suffering from moderate to severe liver disease, even though it may not normally require vitamin C in its diet, it may then require a dietary source of vitamin C.

Vitamin C is needed for the formation of elastic fibres and connective tissues and is an excellent antioxidant similar to vitamin E. Deficiency leads to scurvy in which there is poor wound healing, increased bleeding due to capillary wall fragility and bone weakness.

Vitamin C also increases gut absorption of some minerals, such as iron. This may be important for chronically anaemic patients, but can be a danger for some softbills, such as the mynah, hornbill and toucan families, as well as hardbills that are nectivorous (e.g. lories and lorikeets) as these birds are prone to liver damage from excessive dietary uptake of iron. They are also prone to an increased risk of yersiniosis (infection with the bacterium *Yersinia pseudotuberculosis*) as this bacterium is ferrophilic (loves iron) and so can lead to a peracute septicaemia and death.

L-Carnitine: This is a quaternary ammonium compound that is water soluble and viewed to act like a vitamin. It is synthesised by the liver (and so with severe liver disease a deficiency can occur) and is found in large amounts in muscle tissue. It is important for good cardiac function and so deficiencies can result in cardiac disease. Deficiency of L-carnitine may also play a role in the development of abnormal fat deposition (e.g. lipomas) in obese birds as suggested in one study (De Voe *et al.*, 2004).

Minerals

There are two main groups of minerals: macrominerals and microminerals.

Macrominerals (such as calcium and phosphorus) are present in large amounts in the body. Microminerals or trace elements (such as manganese, iron and cobalt) are all necessary for normal bodily function but are needed in far lower quantities.

Macrominerals

Calcium: The active form of calcium in the body is the ionic, double-charged molecule Ca^{2+}. Lowered levels of this form lead to hyperexcitability, fitting and death. This can occur even though the overall body reserves of calcium are normal.

Calcium levels in the body are controlled by vitamin D_3, parathyroid hormone and calcitonin, all balancing each other. The ratio of calcium to phosphorus is particularly important – as one increases, the other decreases and vice versa. A ratio of 2:1 calcium to phosphorus is desirable in food for growing birds and 1.5:1 for adults. In periods of high egg-laying, though, to keep pace with the output of calcium into the shells, a ratio of 10:1 may be needed (Brue, 1994). A known deficiency problem occurs in many birds fed an all-seed diet due not only to the lack of calcium in such a diet but also the presence of phytates (phosphorus-containing compounds) that bind calcium in the gut and prevent absorption. This is particularly a problem in African grey parrots (*Psittacus erithacus erithacus*), which may present with collapse or seizures due to low blood calcium levels if fed such diets (Stanford, 2007). Excessive calcium in the diet (>1%), however, reduces the use of proteins, fats, phosphorus, manganese, zinc, iron and iodine and, combined with a high level of vitamin D_3, may lead to calcification of soft tissue structures such as blood vessels.

Phosphorus: Phosphorus, like calcium, is used in bones. It is also used in the storage of energy as adenosine triphosphate (ATP), and as a part of the structure of cell membranes. Levels of phosphorus are controlled in the body as for calcium, the two being in equal and opposite equilibrium with each other. Nutritional secondary hyperparathyroidism may occur when dietary phosphorus exceeds calcium, and this can lead to progressive bone demineralisation and renal damage due to high circulating levels of parathyroid hormone.

High dietary phosphorus, particularly as phytates, will reduce the amount of calcium which can be absorbed from the gut, as it forms complexes with the calcium present there. This can be a big problem in cage birds which are predominantly seed eaters, as cereals are high in phosphorus and low in calcium. It may also be a problem for raptors fed pure meat with no calcium/bone supplement.

Magnesium: Most of the magnesium in the body is found in the bone matrix. However, it is also essential for phosphorus transfer in the formation of ATP, and for cell membranes in soft tissues such as the liver. Most magnesium is absorbed in the small intestine, but large amounts of calcium in the diet will reduce magnesium absorption. The recommended minimum levels are 600 ppm (Kollias and Kollias, 2000) or 475–550 mg/kg of feed (Wallach and Cooper, 1982).

Sodium: Sodium is the main extracellular positive ion and regulates the body's acid–base balance and osmotic potential. Along with potassium, it is responsible for nerve signals and impulses.

A true dietary deficiency (hyponatraemia) is rare, but may occur due to chronic diarrhoea or renal disease. These disrupt the osmotic potential gradient in the kidneys leading to further water loss and dehydration. Excessive levels of sodium in the diet (greater than 10 times recommended levels) lead to poor feathering, polyuria, hypertension, oedema and death. Minimum levels are quoted as 5–10 mg/kg of feed offered (Wallach and Cooper, 1982) or around 0.12% of the diet offered (Kollias and Kollias, 2000).

Potassium: As with mammals, potassium is the major intracellular positive ion. It is essential in maintaining membrane potentials and it is the principal intracellular cation affecting acid–base reactions and osmotic pressure. Rarely is there a dietary deficiency, but severe stress may cause potassium deficiency (hypokalaemia). This is caused by increased kidney excretion of potassium due to an elevation in plasma proteins, which is often seen at times of stress. In addition, prolonged fluid therapy, use of potassium-wasting diuretics such as furosemide and chronic diarrhoea may all lead to a low blood potassium level. This can lead to cardiac dysrhythmias, muscle spasticity and neurological dysfunction.

Potassium is present in high amounts in certain fruits such as bananas. It is controlled in the body in equilibrium with sodium under the influence of the adrenal hormone aldosterone, which promotes sodium retention and potassium excretion. The recommended minimal level is 0.4–1.1 mg/kg (Scott and Norris, 1965).

Chlorine: This mineral is the major extracellular negative ion. It is responsible for maintaining acid–base balance in conjunction with sodium and potassium. Deficiencies are rare due to its combination with sodium in the diet as salt.

Microminerals (trace elements)

Iron: Iron is required for the formation of the oxygen-binding centre of the haemoglobin molecule. Absorption from the gut is normally relatively poor as the body is very good at recycling iron from old red blood cells.

Certain species have a greater ability to absorb iron from the small intestine. The mynah, hornbill and toucan/toucanet families are examples. This ability may become a problem when diets rich in iron are presented to these species. For example, rodents and day-old chicks may be fed to toucans, and so occasionally are various brands of dog or monkey biscuits. In addition, vitamin C increases iron absorption by converting the iron into the more easily absorbed ferrous (Fe^{2+}) state. This can lead to a condition known as haemochromatosis, where the liver becomes fatally overloaded with absorbed iron. The recommended minimum iron requirement for Passeriformes and Psittaciformes is 80 ppm, but for toucans a maximum of 60 ppm, or less than 160 mg/kg of feed, is recommended (Worrell, 1991) based on a wild-type diet containing 150 mg/kg (Otten *et al.*, 2001). In mynahs such as the hill mynah (*Gracula religiosa*) a much lower range of 19–25 mg/kg (7–9 ppm) of feed fed is recommended (Dorrestein *et al.*, 2000). For nectivorous species prone to iron storage disease such as the lorikeets, even lower levels are recommended with 80 mg/kg of feed being typical (McDonald, 2003). It is also interesting to note that the same species that are prone to haemochromatosis are also more susceptible to disease when exposed to the bacterium *Yersinia pseudotuberculosis* as this bacterium is ferrophilic. Sudden mortalities may therefore be seen in these species if they have iron overload, associated with a peracute yersiniosis. Dietary deficiencies rarely occur. However, ground-foraging species reared on impervious surfaces such as wire or concrete have suffered iron deficiency. This is because soil consumption, which occurs during ground feeding, is another source of iron.

Copper: Copper is used for haemoglobin synthesis, collagen synthesis and the maintenance of the nervous system.

Deficiencies occur, as with iron, in some ground-feeding species like pheasants and other game birds, reared on surfaces such as concrete where soil consumption during the foraging process does not occur. Signs include chronic anaemia with general weakness, limb deformities and hyperexcitability. The recommended minimum requirements are 8 ppm for Passeriformes and Psittaciformes, and 4 ppm for Galliformes (Wallach and Cooper, 1982).

Zinc: This is a vital trace element involved in wound healing and tissue formation, forming part of a number of enzymes.

Deficiencies can occur in young, rapidly growing birds fed on plant material high in phytates such as cabbage, wheat bran and beans. This is because, as with calcium, the phytates bind zinc and prevent its absorption from the gut. In addition, high dietary calcium itself decreases zinc uptake. Deficiencies cause retarded growth, poor feathering, enlarged intertarsal joints and slipped Achilles tendon (perosis). The minimum recommended requirement is 50 ppm for Passeriformes and Psittaciformes (Kollias and Kollias, 2000).

Manganese: Manganese is primarily found in plant materials but is often present in unavailable forms. Efficient bile salt production is required for its absorption, so birds with hepatic and biliary dysfunction are most at risk of a deficiency.

Manganese is necessary for normal bone structure and hence deficiencies are most commonly manifested by the swelling and flattening of the lateral condyles of the intertarsal joint, allowing the Achilles tendon to slip out of the groove created for it (perosis). In addition, the tibiotarsus and tarsometatarsus may exhibit lateral rotation. Young may be born with retracted beaks and shortened long bones. The recommended minimum requirement is 55–60 mg/kg of feed (Wallach and Cooper, 1982).

Iodine: The sole function of iodine is the synthesis of thyroid hormones. Deficiencies cause goitre, and produce effects such as reduced growth, stunting and neurological problems. It is a relatively common finding in budgerigars fed an all-seed diet without additional supplementation. They adopt a classic hunched posture on the perch and make audible breathing noises because the enlarged thyroid gland constricts the tracheal lumen. They may also be seen to regurgitate seed from the crop. Goitre is one of the differential diagnoses in a vomiting budgerigar. Levels of 4 mg per budgerigar per week prevent goitre from developing (Blackmore, 1963).

Selenium: Its functions are similar to those of vitamin E, as it is found in the enzyme glutathione peroxidase. If there is a general deficiency of both selenium and vitamin E, a condition known as exudative diathesis will occur. This is when the smaller, subcutaneous blood vessels become damaged and leakier. Fluid then moves rapidly out into the subcutaneous spaces and oedema forms over the neck, wings and breast. This is often followed by stunted growth, limb weakness and death. Riboflavin (vitamin B_2) is also used in the production of glutathione peroxidase, so deficiencies in this water-soluble vitamin may also result in similar clinical signs.

The selenium content of plants is dependent on where they were grown and the levels of selenium in the soil. The recommended minimum requirement is 0.1 ppm for Passeriformes and Psittaciformes (Kollias and Kollias, 2000).

Selenium toxicity has been reported in birds and results in clinical signs such as fracture of nails and beak as well as feather damage often dorsally all due to keratin damage. Levels greater than 10 mg/kg of food fed have been recorded as causing toxicosis in waterfowl (O'Toole and Raisbeck, 1997).

Examples of food types for Psittaciformes and Passeriformes

Some of the more commonly offered food types for Psittaciformes and Passeriformes are listed below.

Seeds

Rape seed, millet, canary seed, hemp and linseed are useful for smaller species such as finches, canaries, budgerigars and cockatiels.

Safflower, sunflower and pumpkin seeds are useful for larger parrots but beware of addiction to sunflower seeds.

Nuts

Almonds, walnuts, Brazil nuts, pine nuts and hazel nuts are useful for larger parrots, but be careful of addiction to peanuts as they are high in fat and may be associated with *Aspergillus* spp. toxin poisoning. Nuts are high in calories and fats and in excess may lead to hepatic lipidosis and atherosclerosis.

Fruits

A wide variety of fruits are useful foods. Examples include apple, pear, melon, mango, papaya, pomegranate, guava, apricot, peach, nectarine, oranges and bananas. Grapes and kiwi fruit should be fed sparingly due to their high sugar content, which can cause diarrhoea. Oranges should also only be fed in small amounts, since excess can cause gastric upset, and they should not be fed to nectar feeders such as lorikeets and species such as toucans and mynah birds due to their high vitamin C content and iron absorption facilitation. In addition, fruits such as strawberries and papaya not only are high in vitamin C but also have moderate to high iron content and so should not be fed to species that have problems with iron storage disease (lorikeets, toucans, mynahs, etc.).

Vegetables

Broccoli, watercress and wild rocket are good sources of beta-carotenes and calcium. Other good vegetables include Swiss chard, kale, sweet pepper, carrot, beetroot, pea shoots, mung beans (particularly sprouted ones), cauliflower, tomato and sweetcorn.

Do not feed avocados as these cause severe fatty liver damage in birds. Lories, lorikeets and hummingbirds are all nectar feeders and so require a specialised artificial syrup food. Many are commercially produced. They may also take very ripe fruits, and enjoy eating the pollen from flowers and can be converted to a parrot biscuited/pelleted diet.

Pellets

There are a number of commercially available pelleted diets for cage birds, particularly Psittaciformes. They vary in their compositions between species, life-stage as well as biscuit/kibble size and therefore the correct type of pellet should be selected for the species and life-stage concerned. Parrots have good colour vision and therefore care should be taken to avoid pelleted foods that are not homogeneous (i.e. where there is nutritional variation between different-coloured biscuits in the same diet) as this can lead to an imbalance. In the majority of cases a pelleted diet is not fed exclusively, rather it should form around one-third to half the daily ration, with fruit, seeds, pulses and vegetables making up the rest.

Specific nutritional requirements

Nutritional requirements for growth

Embryonic growth

The egg is a perfect capsule of nutrients providing all that is needed for the developing embryo. The hen must be fed a balanced diet to ensure that she has the nutrients available to instil into the egg. If she is fed a poor or deficient diet, then the egg may not be fertile. It could also undergo the following.

- Early embryonic death; this is often signalled by a blood ring left in the yolk, which suggests a vitamin A deficiency.
- Retarded embryonic development, often associated with vitamin B deficiencies.
- Embryonic deformities, which may be seen with manganese, zinc or other trace element deficiencies.

Post-hatch growth

Hatching occurs after the developing chick has absorbed the external yolk sac, and the chick must then be supplied within 3–4 days with high levels of energy and protein for the growth phase. The remaining internal yolk sac supply will last that long.

When feathers are produced, a huge demand for protein occurs, as feathers are made of keratin, a protein, and will eventually make up one-tenth of the bird's weight. In addition, there will be several feather changes during the first 2 years of life, as juvenile down plumage is replaced by adult plumage. As an adult bird, a minimum dietary requirement of 0.203% cysteine is required to ensure adequate feather strength or fractures can occur (Tsiagbe *et al.*, 1987).

Young birds also have a much larger requirement for calcium and vitamin D_3 for developing bones. On average, sexual maturity for the larger parrots, such as African grey parrots, macaws and cockatoos, is not reached until 2–4 years of age, so this growth phase may be prolonged.

If, during this growth phase, disease or low environmental temperatures are introduced, energy is diverted to immune system function and heat supply. This results in less energy for growth and in slowing of the growth rate. This may be reversed in later periods of growth, assuming no permanent damage has been caused. The obvious side-effect of this, though, is that adult weights are achieved at a later age. If a retarded bird is supplied with excess nutritional levels after this period of leanness, a compensatory growth spurt may occur and the chick appears to grow more rapidly than other birds of that age group.

For all of this growth to occur, it has been estimated that minimum energy requirements for small Psittaciformes and Passeriformes are five times that of adults. Young chicks nearly double their weights over 48 hours and require a protein level of 15–20%, as opposed to an adult's protein need of 10–14% (Harper and Skinner, 1998). Commercial and home-prepared diets for chicks are usually pre-formulated mashes containing protein, eggs and dairy products which have a good broad spectrum of amino acid supplementation and 20% protein levels. It is vital that the amino acid lysine is present at dietary levels of 0.8–1.5% for adequate growth to occur (Roudybush and Grau, 1985, 1986). Deficiencies in cystine/cysteine can also result in weakening of feathers when they are being produced, allowing them to fracture easily.

Excessive protein supplementation may be equally damaging. Levels greater than 25% of the diet have been shown to lead to behavioural problems, and claw, beak and skeletal deformities, particularly if combined with a lack of calcium. Levels of 0.6–1.2% of the diet as calcium have been quoted for chick growth (Brue, 1994) with a calcium/phosphorus ratio of 2 : 1 maintained.

It should also be noted that lack of access to sufficient water in the first few days post hatch can lead to significantly increased mortality rates (Koutsos *et al.*, 2001).

Nutritional requirements for breeding

These requirements include those needed for egg production as well as for courtship behaviour. The requirements for egg production are high, with large volumes of fats needed for the yolk, calcium for the shell and proteins for the albumen (egg white). As egg production commences, the hen bird will increase the volume of food consumed, so removing the need to increase the energy concentration of the diet being offered. It is, however, essential that the diet offered is a balanced one, with increased protein content, particularly from methionine and cystine/cysteine (the sulphur-containing amino acids) and lysine. Protein levels in budgerigars must be above 13.2% of the diet, assuming all essential amino acids are provided for in the diet (Angel and Ballam, 1995).

In addition, a moderate increase in the amount of calcium and vitamin D_3 offered (an increase of 0.35% of the adult maintenance requirement for calcium) is needed, so that levels approach 1% of diet (Harper and Skinner, 1998). This not only helps to ensure proper calcification of eggshells and the developing embryo, but also helps prevent egg-binding in the hen. This is when poor calcium reserves lead to low calcium blood levels, weakness, uterine muscular paresis, egg retention, shock and death.

Other compounds that, if supplied above the minimum daily requirements mentioned earlier, help with egg production include vitamins A, B_{12}, riboflavin and the mineral zinc. In addition, it is useful for improved hatching rate to increase the levels of the B vitamins biotin, folic acid, pantothenic acid, riboflavin (B_2) and pyridoxine (B_6), as well as vitamin E, iron, copper, zinc and manganese, to above the minimum daily requirements.

Nutritional requirements for the older bird

As with cats and dogs, the aim is to provide a diet of high digestibility whilst reducing slightly the protein, sodium and phosphorus levels. This preserves renal function and prevents hypertension.

In addition, lowering cholesterol and unsaturated fat levels is important, as atherosclerosis is common in older birds. The levels of vitamins A, E, thiamine (B_1), B_{12}, and pyridoxine (B_6), the mineral zinc, amino acid lysine and fatty acid linoleic acid should also be slightly increased to ensure that any decrease in digestive function and age-related cellular damage is contained.

Special nutritional requirements for debilitated birds

Extra nutritional support for debilitated and diseased birds is vital and plays an essential role in ensuring recovery of the avian patient after disease or debility. Enteral nutrition is currently the most usual method of supporting the debilitated patient, with parenteral (intravenous) nutrition still being in its infancy in avian therapeutics.

First, fluid requirements should be assessed, as any animal will succumb to dehydration long before starvation. The reader is referred to Chapter 14 for a more detailed discussion of this topic.

Second, energy requirements should be estimated. These can be calculated roughly from the MER by multiplication as follows:

Starvation = $0.5 \times$ MER

Trauma = $1.5 \times$ MER

Sepsis = $2.5 \times$ MER

Burns = $3\text{–}4 \times$ MER

From these crude estimations, a rough idea of the levels of nutrition demanded and the energy concentration of the diet can be derived.

Third, protein requirements should be evaluated, as debilitation will increase amino acid and protein turnover. This may be through the increased use of proteins in the immune system response, or for repair of damaged tissue or simply after using tissue proteins as an energy source.

Birds with liver disease

Birds affected by hepatic dysfunction should be fed a diet which reduces liver use by decreasing its need to convert body tissues into blood glucose and decreasing its need to break down the waste products of excess protein metabolism. Therefore, birds should be fed a diet high in digestible carbohydrates, such as boiled rice, pasta or potatoes, for energy and sugars. Protein sources should be of high biological value (high in essential amino acids) such as those found in whole eggs. This is in an attempt to keep to a minimum the overall amount of protein fed, particularly purine-producing proteins such as are found in fish, meat, etc. These protein sources lead to the greater build-up of waste products of protein digestion, which the liver then has to detoxify and eliminate via the kidneys. The feeding of frequent, small meals is also advisable for liver disease patients, as is the addition of vitamin B supplements to the diet. Use of L-carnitine supplementation should also be considered where hepatic dysfunction occurs as the liver is often unable to synthesise this important cardiac muscle protectant.

Birds with renal disease

Like the liver, the kidney is responsible for eliminating the waste products of protein metabolism (see Figure 12.6). It is therefore important in renal disease to reduce overall protein levels whilst ensuring that the protein sources provided have a high biological value.

In addition, restricting phosphorus in the diet is helpful, as excess may lead to demineralisation of the bone, increased levels of parathyroid hormone and further renal damage.

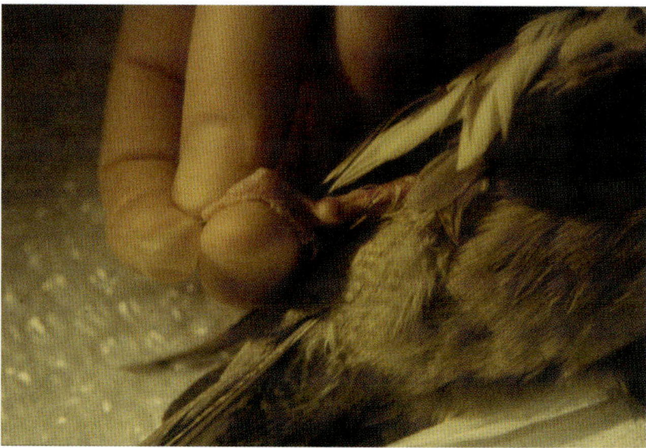

Figure 12.6 Gout crystals may form in joints (articular gout) as in this cockatiel (*Nymphicus hollandicus*) with renal disease.

Finally, restricting sodium is important to reduce fluid retention and decrease hypertension. Vitamin B supplementation can help as an appetite stimulant. It is advisable to supplement it in any case as being a water-soluble vitamin, it can be flushed out of the body where polyuria occurs, leading to deficiency.

Birds with heart disease

Heart disease is commonly seen in older parrots and some raptors, particularly females. It is also seen as a sequel to iron storage disease (haemochromatosis) in lorikeets, toucans and mynahs. Reduction of sodium in the diet to reduce hypertension due to fluid retention is helpful where possible. So too is lowering cholesterol levels by removing saturated fats, such as dairy products and overly fatty prey for raptors (e.g. removing the yolk sac if feeding day-old chicks). Avoiding meat in general for granivorous/herbivorous birds such as parrots is advised. For toucans, mynah birds, lorikeets and related species, the avoidance of high iron-containing diets and foods that facilitate iron absorption (e.g. excess vitamin C) is essential to prevent haemochromatosis and the cardiac damage which can ensue. Offering L-carnitine supplements may also be helpful in preserving cardiac muscle integrity.

Birds suffering from maldigestion and malabsorption syndromes

Cage birds suffering from maldigestion and malabsorption syndromes such as pancreatic disease should be fed highly digestible carbohydrate foods such as rice, potatoes and pasta, whilst reducing all fats in the diet such as seeds, meat, etc. High biological value proteins should also be fed for balance. The addition of pancreatic enzyme supplementation is to be considered, along with B-vitamin supplementation.

Birds suffering from anaemia

Anaemic patients should have the cause of their anaemia investigated, as common causes include heavy-metal poisoning and chronic disease processes. Other aids to increasing red blood cell production (erythropoiesis) are supplementation with iron and with smaller increases in copper and cobalt levels. Vitamin B_{12}, niacin and folic acid levels should be six times the normal minimal values to ensure that the extra demands caused by increased red cell production are met. Supplementation of vitamin K levels should also be considered where prolonged clotting times are suspected.

Other dietary factors and conditions

Hypocalcaemic tetany

A specific disease of African grey parrots commonly between the ages of 2 and 4 years is hypocalcaemic tetany. This is due to a failure to mobilise calcium into the bloodstream. The afflicted parrot will become weak, collapse and start fitting which may progress to coma and death. It appears to be a hereditary condition and birds often grow out of it if carefully managed. Afflicted birds appear to have plenty of calcium in their bones, but seem unable to mobilise it. Management therefore consists of providing sufficient dietary calcium (as well as vitamin D and UV-B radiation exposure) so that blood levels remain normal.

Obesity

In overweight or obese birds, particularly where a fatty liver syndrome is suspected, strict management of the diet is indicated.

Correcting dietary deficiencies

Attempting to encourage new food consumption

Many species of bird are highly intelligent, particularly members of the order Psittaciformes. This means that the introduction of new foods, in an attempt to correct dietary deficiencies, can be a significant problem. The following techniques may be employed to tempt a cage bird to accept new food items.

Overcoming unfamiliarity

Just because the bird was not interested in the food item today is no reason to suspect that it may not try the food tomorrow. Just like children, birds may view a new or unfamiliar food with suspicion and reject it purely for that. The key is to keep re-presenting the food, preferably on the top of its food bowl, so that the bird has to remove it to get to the usual food underneath. The bird may eventually become used to its sight, smell and taste, and may therefore start to eat it.

Tempting the bird with food

Many birds want to eat what their owners are eating, as obviously it must be better than the rubbish in their own food bowl! This can be used to our advantage, as the owner can sample the food in front of the bird and then offer it to the bird. This can trigger acceptance.

Fooling the bird with food

Covering the food item that you wish the bird to eat in the flavour or colour of a food item it already likes can work well. An example would be honey- or peanut butter-coated broccoli or carrot.

Pelleted commercial diets

Many pelleted avian diets are available for a wide range of species, from flamingos to toucans, parrots to ducks and other poultry. Their main advantage is homogeneity – the bird cannot pick and choose what it wishes to eat, but is rather forced to eat a balanced preprepared diet.

The disadvantages include the problem of selection. Some of these diets are multicoloured and birds have good colour vision and may pick out one coloured biscuit to eat only. This is fine if all the biscuits are of the same composition no matter what the colour but does lead to wastage. In addition, palatability can be a problem, so getting a bird to eat some of these diets can be difficult.

Fresh water must be available at all times, as these diets are dry pellets and chronic dehydration can occur.

Avian mineral and vitamin supplements

These are important, particularly for species fed a home-prepared diet that may be imbalanced. They are produced by many companies and cover all varying aspects of supplementation. Some are put in the food itself, some in water. The latter may be problematic as the taste may prevent water consumption or the vitamins may encourage bacterial growth in the water bowl. Multivitamin and mineral preparations may be used as a general supplement to a diet where the individual bird will not take a wide variety of food types; an example is the seed-obsessed parrot. They should be used, though, not as an excuse to give up on offering other food types, but more to ensure nutritional balance whilst trying to encourage the bird onto a more stable diet. They may also be used, even when a balanced diet is being fed and eaten, to supplement a bird at certain times of its life when requirements for minerals and vitamins increase, such as during egg-laying, growth, moulting and old age.

Dietary requirements peculiar to specific families

Larger members of the Psittaciformes

Larger members of the parrot family, such as cockatoos, macaws, Amazons and African grey parrots, have slightly different requirements from the smaller members of the family, such as the conures and parakeets. Many of the larger parrots require slightly more fats in their diets (particularly any macaws), to increase their calorific density, than their smaller cousins. This is not so surprising considering that the normal wild diets of these parrots involve a moderate amount of oil-based nuts and seeds. It is advisable therefore that larger nuts, such as hazel nuts, Brazil nuts and cashews, should be included in the diet of these species.

An example of the MER required by some of the larger species of parrot includes 452 kJ/day for the scarlet macaw (*Ara macao*) as opposed to 200 kJ/day for the lesser sulphur-crested cockatoo (*Cacatua sulphurea*) (Nott and Taylor, 1993). Therefore, to maintain calorific intake, a scarlet macaw will have to eat far more of a sunflower seed, which has an energy content of approximately 24 kJ/g dry matter (18 g dry matter or nearly 22.5 g fresh), as opposed to a cashew nut which has an energy content of 32 kJ/g dry matter (14 g dry matter or nearly 17 g fresh).

However, many of the larger parrots, especially the Amazons and African grey parrots, are also prone to atherosclerosis, or hardening of the major arteries, due to cholesterol deposition in their walls which often becomes calcified. This happens if their diets are persistently high in saturated fats, such as meat and dairy products, but may also occur with chronic overconsumption of high-fat nuts and seeds. Hepatic lipidosis, or the obliteration of liver cells with fat, is also a common sequel to oversupplementation of the diet with high-fat nuts and seeds in parrots. So it is important to get the balance right.

In formulating these diets it is also important that attention is paid to calcium and mineral levels, as seeds and nuts are extremely poor suppliers of these. Nuts (particularly peanuts/groundnuts) may also be a potential source of fungal growths of *Aspergillus* spp. These can not only produce spores which may cause respiratory disease, but can also produce highly poisonous toxins, known as aflatoxins and gliatoxins, which may cause sudden death, neurological damage or chronic hepatic damage, depending on the dose consumed.

The most commonly seen deficiencies in the larger psittacines occur with vitamin A, vitamin D_3 and the mineral calcium. This is particularly the case with African grey parrots because of hypocalcaemic tetany, an inherited condition of 2–4-year-old birds, where blood calcium levels cannot be maintained. This can lead to hypocalcaemic fits. In addition, African grey parrots fed an all-seed diet are very prone to respiratory infections, especially aspergillosis (the air sac and lung infestation with the fungus *Aspergillus fumigatus*). This is often associated with hypovitaminosis A.

However, as with so many nutrients, too much is as bad as too little. Excessive levels of vitamin D_3 commonly cause toxicosis in African grey parrots and macaws, leading to soft tissue calcification and renal damage. Excessive vitamin A can also cause problems in the large parrots and in hand-reared chicks, causing liver damage, kidney damage and haemorrhage. Excessive vitamin E can result in increased blood clotting times and can act as an oxidising agent leading to increased free-radical production that may increase morbidity and decrease fertility.

Raptors

Raptors are carnivorous. They therefore require regular fresh rodent or avian prey. If fed whole, these usually provide a balanced diet. To determine the amounts of prey to be fed, a rough rule of thumb is that the larger the raptor, the smaller the food consumption is as a percentage of that bird's weight. A golden eagle, for example, may consume 5–7% of its body weight per day, whereas a sparrowhawk would perhaps consume 25% body weight per day.

For raptors in training, the main aim is to keep the birds lean and slightly hungry to make it easier to hand-train them. If underfed, however, the consequence is starvation; if overfed the bird will become obese, and atherosclerosis is a major problem in overfed raptors. To try to prevent under- or over-feeding it is important to weigh the raptor on a daily basis to ensure constant weight levels. However, this is not always possible, for example when breeding or moulting raptors must not be handled, and so at certain times of the year it may be difficult to assess their condition. Nevertheless, during this period it is useful, as with any animal, to increase the levels of nutrition to ensure healthy egg production or feather growth. Care should be taken with egg-laying female raptors, though, to ensure they are not fed obese prey items, as the presence of cholesterol and lipids for yolk production in their bloodstream makes them very prone to atherosclerosis at this time.

Water consumption

Water consumption is of course vital. Dehydration may occur due to the feeding of previously frozen and then thawed prey, only because the freezing process causes dehydration of the carcass. Therefore, when defrosting the rodent or avian prey item, it is advisable to soak it in water.

Food composition

Protein levels are at 15–20% and this is desirable for full fitness (Cooper, 1991). However, excessive levels of protein (>30%) should be avoided, as this can lead to increased blood levels of protein degradation products such as purines, which are converted into uric acid for renal excretion. However, if purine levels are excessive, the uric acid concentration will exceed that which can be dissolved in the blood, leading to the precipitation of uric acid and causing gout.

Optimum fat levels in prey offered to raptors have been estimated at 20–25% (Cooper, 1991). Prey such as some laboratory rats and mice, as mentioned, can cause hypercholesterolaemia and atherosclerosis in underworked raptors.

Mineral supplementation may be necessary. This is especially so in chicks which are often fed small pieces of meat, rather than whole prey. This can result in calcium deficiencies, as muscle tissue is low in calcium and high in phosphorus. A ratio of calcium to phosphorus of 2 : 1 for growth and 1.5 : 1 for maintenance should be achieved.

Prey

The feeding of certain types of prey should be done with care. For example, pigeons fed to larger birds of prey can be a source of *Trichomonas gallinae* infestation. This is a protozoan parasite which invades the crop and digestive system, causing regurgitation, vomiting and weight loss in the affected raptor. Therefore, it is recommended that if pigeon is to be fed, it is deep frozen and then thoroughly defrosted to kill any *Trichomonas* spp. organisms present in the carcass. Some raptors are more tolerant of *T. gallinae* exposure (e.g. peregrine falcons, *Falco peregrinus*) due to their natural preferred diet of Columbiformes. Other parasites such as the worm *Capillaria* spp. can also be transmitted from prey bird to raptor.

In other avian and mammalian prey, the presence of lead shot is again a potential hazard and a cause of lead poisoning in raptors, resulting in neurological disease, renal and liver failure and death. It is therefore important to avoid feeding wild, lead-shot/lead bullet-shot animals to captive birds of prey.

Other problems due to poisoning from prey offered are pesticides and herbicides, particularly the organochlorines and organophosphates. These concentrate in animal fats and so pass up through the food chain, producing the highest concentrations in top predators such as raptors.

In addition, there are compounds such as the polychlorinated biphenyls (PCBs). These are used for a number of purposes, including insulation and electrical circuitry, and may enter the food chain through small rodents. These also concentrate in animal fats, so concentrating their levels in the tissues of animals as one moves up the food chain. They cause problems similar to those caused by the pesticides: reproductive problems, chick mortalities and neurological tremors which can lead to death.

Day-old chicks are a common food source for captive raptors. They are not a balanced diet, being low in calcium and high in calories and fat. Some recommend the removal of the yolk sac (still retained in a day-old chick) before feeding to reduce the fat and calorie levels but this does not alter the low calcium to phosphorus ratio.

Food management for racing pigeons

The day-to-day feeding of racing pigeons includes the provision of a grain- and pulse-based diet once or twice daily. For racing pigeons, one trend is the feeding of carbohydrate-based foods, such as grains, early on in the course of a week, and then increasing the protein levels with supplements and pulses as the racing day, often a Saturday, approaches. Many companies now produce homogenous pelleted feeds for racing pigeons, containing differing levels of protein depending on whether they are actively training or rearing young. Grit can be given freely. It is insoluble and aids in the grinding of grain in the gizzard. This is important in species such as pigeons, which do not de-husk seed before swallowing it. Water is offered, as with game birds, from communal feeders, and pigeon owners will often add multivitamins, minerals and medicants to these fountain feeders.

Food management for fish-eating birds

Fish-eating captive species of bird such as pelicans, penguins and some raptors are often fed fish that have been frozen and then defrosted. Freezers for storage should ideally be at −18°C maximum – basically the colder the better. The freezing of fish leads to an increase in thiaminase production (resulting in a relative deficiency in vitamin B_1) and a slow deterioration of vitamin A and increase in free-radical production (resulting in a relative deficiency in vitamin E). Supplementation of fish-eating species with vitamins B_1, A and E is therefore commonplace in captivity. Sodium levels may also become depleted with freezing and thawing and so again may require supplementation. Defrosting of fish should be controlled and temperatures not allowed to exceed 7°C (preferably below 4°C but of course above 0°C) to avoid spoiling of the fish due to bacteria present in their digestive tracts (often *Clostridium* spp.) that may cause serious disease. Fish should not be defrosted in running warm water as this leads to rapid depletion of nutrients.

Waterfowl

Nutrition of waterfowl receives less attention, as many geese and ducks are kept in outdoor smallholding settings and so live predominantly on grass and other herbage. Geese in particular need ample grass for grazing. It is essential to ensure that access to poisonous plants or trees, such as laburnum and foxgloves, is restricted, as these birds will eat almost anything. In poor weather, or with limited grass production, commercial pelleted food should be given. There are now commercial duck and geese pellets available. Alternatively, the use of poultry 'layer' pellets can be tried.

Commercial pellets come in four main categories:

- Pellets designed for the brooding, egg-laying female, which are higher in calcium and protein
- Pellets for the very young waterfowl chick up to 2–3 weeks of age (known as 'starter pellets' or 'crumbs')
- Pellets for the juvenile growing waterfowl (up to 4–6 months)
- Adult non-breeding maintenance pellets.

The differences lie in the provision of proteins and calcium, with the highest being in the starter pellets (at around 20% protein) through to the lower end as adult pellets (14% protein). There are now companies which also produce special diets for other ornamental waterfowl such as sea duck and flamingos. (Flamingos require more protein and a selection of salts to encourage plumage colouration.)

Duck and geese enclosures in particular need to be routinely examined for evidence of foreign objects, such as lead shot, barbed wire fragments, and so on. This is because of these birds' desire to consume any and every loose potential food item they can find when foraging.

References

Angel, R. and Ballam, G (1995) Dietary protein effect on parakeet reproduction, growth and plasma uric acid. *Proceedings of the First Annual Conference Nutrition Advisory Group*, Toronto, p. 91.

Austic, R.E. and Cole, R.K. (1971) Impaired uric acid excretion in chickens selected for uricemia and articular gout. *Proceedings of the 1971 Cornell Nutritional Conference*, 2–3 November, Buffalo, Colarado.

Blackmore, D.K. (1963) The incidence and aetiology of thyroid dysplasia in budgerigars (*Melopsittacus undulatus*). *Veterinary Record*, **75**, 1068–1072.

Brue, R.N. (1994) Nutrition. In: *Avian Medicine: Principles and Application* (eds B. Ritchie, G. Harrison & L. Harrison), pp. 63–95. WB Saunders, Philadelphia, PA.

Cai, Z., Finnie, J., Manavis, J. and Blumbergs, P. (2023) Avian riboflavin deficiency causes reliably reproducible peripheral nerve demyelination and, with vitamin supplementation, rapid remyelination. *Human and Experimental Toxicology*, **42**, 9603271231188970. doi: 10.1177/09603271231188970.

Carciofi, A.C., Sanfilippo, L.F., de Oliveira, L.D. *et al.* (2008) Protein requirements for Blue-fronted Amazon (*Amazona aestiva*) growth. *Journal of Animal Physiology and Animal Nutrition (Berlin)*, **92**(3), 363–368. doi: 10.1111/j.1439-0396.2007.00800.x.

Cooper, J.E. (1991) Nutritional diseases including poisons. In: *Veterinary Aspects of Captive Birds of Prey*, pp. 124–142. Standfast Press, Glos.

Crissey, S.D., McGill, P. and Slifka, K.A. (2002) Penguins: nutrition and dietary husbandry. Fact sheet 012. In: *Nutrition Advisory Group Handbook*, pp. 1–19. Association of Zoos and Aquariums (AZA) Nutrition Advisory Group.

Dacke, G.C. (2000) Parathyroids, calcitonin and vitamin D. In: *Sturkie's Avian Physiology* (ed. G.C. Whittow), 5th edn, pp. 472–485. Academic Press, London.

De Voe, R.S., Trogdon, M. and Flammer, K. (2004) Preliminary assessment of the effect of diet and L-carnitine supplementation on lipoma size and bodyweight in budgerigars (*Melopsittacus undulatus*). *Journal of Avian Medicine and Surgery*, **18**(1), 12–18.

Dorrestein, G.M., Mete, A., Lemmens, I. and Beynen, A.C. (2000) Hemochromatosis/iron storage: new developments. *Proceedings of the Annual Conference of the Association of Avian Veterinarians*, 233–238.

Earle and Clarke (1991) The nutrition of the budgerigar (*Melopsittacus undulatus*). *Journal of Nutrition*, **121**, S186–S192.

Frankel, T.L. and Avram, D.S. (2001) Protein requirements of rainbow lorikeets, *Trichoglossus haematodus*. *Australian Journal of Zoology*, **49**, 435–443.

Harcourt-Brown, N. (2003) Incidence of juvenile osteodystrophy in hand-reared grey parrots (*Psittacus e. erithacus*). *Veterinary Record*, **152**, 438–439.

Harper, E.J. and Skinner, N.D. (1998) Clinical nutrition of small psittacines and passerines. *Seminars in Avian and Exotic Pet Medicine*, **7**(3), 116–127.

Harper, E.J. and Turner, C.L. (2000) Nutrition and energetics of the canary (*Serinus canarius*). *Comparative Biochemistry and Physiology B Biochemistry and Molecular Biology*, **126**(3), 271–281. doi: 10.1016/s0305-0491(00)00210-8.

Heuser, G.F. and Norris, L.C. (1929) Rickets in chicks III: the effectiveness of mid-summer sunshine and irradiation from a quartz mercury vapour arc in preventing rickets in chickens. *Poultry Science*, **8**, 89–98.

Jordan, R. and Silva, T. (1991) Breeding and rearing Salvadori's fig parrot at Loro Parque, Tenerife *Psittaculirostris salvadorii*. *International Zoo Yearbook*, **30**, 173–177.

Kamphues, J., Otte, W. and Wolf, P. (1997) Effects of increasing protein intake on various parameters of nitrogen metabolism in grey parrots (*Psittacus erithacus erithacus*). *First International Symosium on Pet Bird Nutrition* (eds J. Kamphues, P. Wolf and N. Rabehl), p. 118.

Klasing, K. (1998) *Comparative Avian Nutrition*. CABI Publishing, Wallingford.

Kollias, G.V. and Kollias, H.W. (2000) Feeding passerine and psittacine birds. In: *Small Animal Clinical Nutrition* (eds M.S. Hand, C.D. Thatcher, R.L. Remillard & P. Roudebush), 4th edn, pp. 979–991. Mark Mervis Institute, Marceline, Missouri.

Koutsos, E.A. and Klasing, K.C. (2002) Vitamin A nutrition of cockatiels. *Proceedings of the Joint Nutrition Symposium*, Antwerp, Belgium, p. 141.

Koutsos, E.A., Matson, K.D. and Klasing, K.C. (2001) Nutrition of birds in the order Psittaciformes: a review. *Journal of Avian Medicine and Surgery*, **15**(4), 257–275.

Koutsos, E.A., Tell, L.A., Woods, L.W. and Klasing, L.C. (2003) Adult cockatiels at maintenance are more sensitive to diets containing excess vitamin A than to vitamin A deficient diets. *Journal of Nutrition*, **43**(4), 26–30.

Lu, J. and Coombs, G.F.J. (1988) Excess dietary zinc decreases tissue α-tocopherol in chicks. *Journal of Nutrition*, **118**, 1349–1359.

McDonald, D. (2003) Feeding ecology and nutrition of Australian lorikeets. *Seminars in Avian and Exotic Pet Medicine*, **12**(4), 195–204.

McDonald, D. (2004) Dietary vitamin A requirements of lorikeets. In: *Annual Conference Proceedings of the Association of Avian Veterinarians Australian Committee* (ed. G.M. Cross), pp. 83–86. Kakadu, Australia, Association of Avian Veterinarians Australian Committee.

McDonald, D. (2006) Nutrition and dietary supplementation. In: *Clinical Avian Medicine* (eds G.J. Harrison & T.L. Lightfoot), pp. 86–107. Spix Publishing Inc, Palm Beach, Florida.

Moriceau, M.-A., Lefebvre, S., Fourel, I. *et al.* (2022) Exposure of predatory and scavenging birds to anticoagulant rodenticides in France: exploration of data from French surveillance programs. *Science of the Total Environment*. doi: 10.1016/j.scitotenv.2021.151291.

Murphy, M.E. (1996) Nutrition and metabolism. In: *Avian Energetics and Nutritional Ecology* (ed. C. Carey), pp. 31–60. Chapman and Hall, New York.

Murphy, M.E. and King, J.R. (1992) Energy and nutrient use during moult by white-crowned sparrows, *Zonotrichia leucophrys gambelii*. *Ornis Scandinavica*, **23**, 304–313.

Naylor, A., Pizzi, R., Cole, G. *et al.* (2018) Suspected hypovitaminosis A-associated salt gland adenitis in northern rockhopper penguins (*Eudyptes moseleyi*). *Journal of Zoo and Wildlife Medicine*, **49**(2), 420–428.

Nichols, D.K., Wolff, M.J., Phillips, L.G. and Montali, R.J. (1989) Coagulopathy in pink-backed pelicans, *Pelecanus refescens*, associated with hypervitaminosis E. *Journal of Zoo and Wildlife Medicine*, **20**, 57–61.

Nightengale, M., Stout, R.W. and Tully, T.N. (2022) Plasma vitamin D (25-hydroxyvitamin D) levels in Hispaniolan Amazon parrots (*Amazona ventralis*) housed indoors over time. *Avian Diseases*, **66**, 148–154.

Nijboer, J. (2022) Nutrition in piscivorous (fish-eating) birds, MSD Veterinary Manual. Available at https://www.msdvetmanual.com/management-and-nutrition/nutrition-exotic-and-zoo-animals/nutrition-in-piscivorous-fish-eating-birds (accessed 19 December 2023).

Nott, H.M.R. and Taylor, F.J. (1993) The energy requirements of pet birds. *Proceedings of the Annual Conference of the Association of Avian Veterinarians*, pp. 233–239.

Olds, J.E., Burrough, E., Madson, D. *et al.* (2015) Clinical investigation into feed-related hypervitaminosis D in a captive flock of budgerigars (*Melopsittacus* undulatus): morbidity, mortalities and pathologic lesions. *Journal of Zoo and Wildlife Medicine*, **46**(1), 9–17.

O'Toole, D. and Raisbeck, M.F. (1997) Experimentally induced selenosis of adult mallard ducks: clinical signs, lesions, and toxicology. *Veterinary Pathology*, **34**(4), 330–340.

Orosz, S.E. (2014) Clinical avian nutrition. *Veterinary Clinics of North America: Exotic Animal Practice*, **17**, 397–413. doi: 10.1016/j.cvex.2014.05.003.

Otten, B.A., Orosz, S.E., Auge, S. and Frazier, D.L. (2001) Mineral content of food items commonly ingested by keel billed toucans (*Ramphastos sulfuratus*). *Journal of Avian Medicine and Surgery*, **15**(3), 194–196.

Park, F. (2006) Vitamin A toxicosis in a lorikeet flock. *Veterinary Clinics of North America: Exotic Animal Practice*, **9**(3), 495–502.

Petzinger, C., Heatly, J.J. and Bauer, J.E. (2015) Growth curves and their implications in hand-fed Monk parrots (*Myiopsitta monachus*). *Veterinary Medicine (Auckland)*, **15**(6), 321–327. doi: 10.2147/VMRR.S73804.

Pollock, C. (2007) Expert panel on companion bird nutrition. 12 December 2007, LafeberVet Website. Available at https://lafeber.com/vet/expert-panel-on-companion-bird-nutrition (accessed 30 Decembe 2023).

Potter, S. (1997) Lead in Drinking Water. Research paper 97/65. https://researchbriefings.files.parliament.uk/documents/RP97-65/RP97-65.pdf (accessed 11 November 2023).

Rangaraj, D. and Hong, Y.H. (2015) Effects of dietary vitamin E on fertility functions in poultry species. *International Journal of Molecular Science*, **16**(5), 9910–9921. doi: 10.3390/ijms16059910.

Roudybush, T.E. and Grau, C.R. (1985) Lysine requirements of cockatiel chicks. *Proceedings of the 34th Western Poultry Diseases Conference*, **34**, 113–115.

Roudybush, T.E. and Grau, C.R. (1986) Food and water interrelations and the protein requirement for growth of an altricial bird, the cockatiel (*Nymphicus hollandicus*). *Journal of Nutrition*, **116**, 552–559.

Schinck, B., Hafez, H.M. and Lierz, M. (2008) Alpha-tocopherol in captive falcons: reference values and dietary impact. *Journal of Avian Medicine and Surgery*, **22**(2), 99–102.

Scott, M.L. and Norris, L.C. (1965) Vitamins and vitamin deficiencies. In: *Diseases of Poultry* (eds H.E. Biester & L.H. Schwarte), 5th edn. Iowa State University Press, Ames, Iowa.

Scott, M.L., Nesheim, M.C. and Young, R.J. (1982) *Nutrition of the Chicken*. M.L. Scott and Associates, Ithaca, NY, USA.

Scott, P.W. (1996) Nutrition. In: *Manual of Psittacine Birds* (eds P.H. Beynon, N.A. Forbes & M.P.C. Lawton), pp. 17–26. BSAVA, Cheltenham, Gloucester.

Stanford, M. (2006) Effects of UVB radiation on calcium metabolism in psittacine birds. *Veterinary Record*, **159**, 236–241.

Stanford, M. (2007) Clinical pathology of hypocalcaemia in adult grey parrots (*Psittacus e. erithacus*). *Veterinary Record*, **161**, 456–457.

Taylor, E.J., Nott, H.M. and Earle, K.E. (1994) Dietary glycine: its importance in growth and development of the budgerigar (*Melopsittacus undulatus*). *Journal of Nutrition*, **124**(12 Suppl), 2555S–2558S. doi: 10.1093/jn/124.suppl_12.2555S.

Tsiagbe, V.K., Kraus, R.J., Benevenga, N.J. *et al.* (1987) Identification of volatile sulfur derivatives released from feathers of chicks fed diets with various levels of sulfur-containing amino acids. *Journal of Nutrition*, **117**, 1859–1865. doi: 10.1093/jn/117.11.1859.

Wallach, J.D. and Cooper, J.E. (1982) Nutritional diseases of wild birds. In: *Non-infectious Diseases of Wildlife* (eds G.L. Hoff & J.W. Davis), pp. 113–126. Iowa State University Press, Ames, IA.

West, J.A., Tully, T.N., Nevarez, J.G. and Stout, R.W. (2019) Effects of fluorescent lighting versus sunlight exposure on calcium, magnesium, vitamin D, and feather destructive behavior in Hispaniolan Amazon parrots (*Amazona ventralis*). *Journal of Avian Medicine and Surgery*, **33**(3), 235–244. doi: 10.1647/2018-378.

Worrell, A. (1991) Serum iron levels in rhamphastids. *Proceedings of the Annual Conference of the Association of Avian Veterinarians*, 120–130.

Zhang, C., Li, D., Wang, F. and Dong, T. (2003) Effects of dietary vitamin K levels on bone quality in broilers. *Archiv für Tierernährung*, **57**(3), 197–206. doi: 10.1080/0003942031000136620.

Chapter 13 Common Avian Diseases

Skin and feather disease

Feather plucking

Feather plucking is predominantly seen in the Psittaciformes, members of the parrot order. It can be one of the most complicated conditions in avian medicine to diagnose the underlying cause and even more difficult to treat. The causes of feather plucking can vary tremendously. For examples, see below (see Figure 13.1).

1. Ectoparasites
2. Endoparasites
3. Skin infections/dermatitis (bacterial, viral and fungal)
4. Iatrogenic (e.g. poor wing clip)
5. Behavioural
6. Organopathy
7. Heavy metal poisoning (lead, zinc)
8. Psittacosis (*Chlamydia psittaci* infection)
9. Salmonellosis
10. Hormonal
11. Environmental contaminant (e.g. nicotine-tainted feathers)
12. Viral diseases affecting other organs (e.g. bornavirus, the causal agent of proventricular dilatation disease)
13. Pain
14. Hepatitis/hepatomegaly (e.g. hepatic lipidosis)
15. Atopy/allergic skin disease

Diagnosis requires a full, detailed history to be taken as well as a full health examination. A diagnosis of a behavioural condition can only be made accurate by extensive history-taking and elimination of medical conditions from the picture. This may include an array of test modalities, including blood analysis, polymerase chain reaction (PCR) testing, skin biopsy, microbial culture and diagnostic imaging.

Behavioural feather plucking

The most basic classification is to divide feather pluckers into two types. The first is the true feather plucker which removes the whole feather. The second is the feather chewer which just mutilates the feather but leaves it embedded in the skin. In addition, some species of psittacine bird such as cockatoos may also exhibit a more advanced condition with self-mutilation of the body as well as feather plucking.

Feather plucking, as previously mentioned, is mainly seen in Psittaciformes, although some of the hawk family such as the Harris hawk (*Parabuteo uncinatus*) are also susceptible.

Behavioural feather plucking may be diagnosed often only after the ruling out of infectious/pain causes.

Ectoparasites

Ectoparasites are not as commonly seen in cage birds as might be expected. There are, however, many important skin and feather parasites of raptors, game birds and waterfowl kept in captivity.

Mites

Cnemidocoptes: They are seen mainly in the budgerigar, canary and domestic poultry. The mites burrow into the outer layers of skin which increases cornification in response, leading to conditions known as 'scaly beak' and 'tassle foot'. The presenting signs are crusting and enlargement of the cere at the base of the beak (most commonly in budgerigars) and thickening and proliferation of the skin of the legs (more commonly in passerines and poultry). Another mite peculiar to pigeons is the depluming mite (*Cnemidocoptes laevis*). This mite causes disintegration of the feather quill, causing it to break off close to the skin and producing bald areas.

Sarcoptes: Scabies mites (*Sarcoptes* spp.) are uncommonly seen, but have been reported in macaws, particularly on the unfeathered part of the face where the clinical signs are more obviously seen. Advanced disease can produce clinical signs of feather loss and widespread self-trauma as it is intensely pruritic.

Dermanyssus: The red feather mite (*Dermanyssus gallinae*) has been reported in poultry, raptor flights, pigeon lofts and, in some cases, cage and aviary birds such as parrots, particularly those in outside flights. This mite does not live on the bird permanently. It hides in the cracks and crevices of the cage or shelter during the day and crawls out to attack the bird when it is roosting at night making it difficult to eradicate (see Figure 13.2). It is a blood-sucking mite and can cause anaemia and weakness in heavily parasitised birds as well as generally poor feather quality.

Ornithonyssus: Another blood-sucking mite is the northern fowl mite (*Ornithonyssus sylviarum*). This mite inhabits the host continuously, so it is easier to detect and to treat. Other species of *Ornithonyssus* may be seen causing pruritus and feather loss associated with wild bird exposure, particularly in birds housed in outdoor aviary flights (see Figure 13.3).

Other mites, such as skin mites *Backericheyla* spp. and *Neocheyletiella media* in passerine birds such as finches, and *Epidermoptes bilobatus* and *Michrolichus avus* in a variety of species, may also cause pruritus. Quill mites such as *Dermatoglyphus* spp. and *Syringophylus* spp. may also cause pruritus, feather picking and loss.

Veterinary Nursing of Exotic Pets and Wildlife, Third Edition. Simon J. Girling.

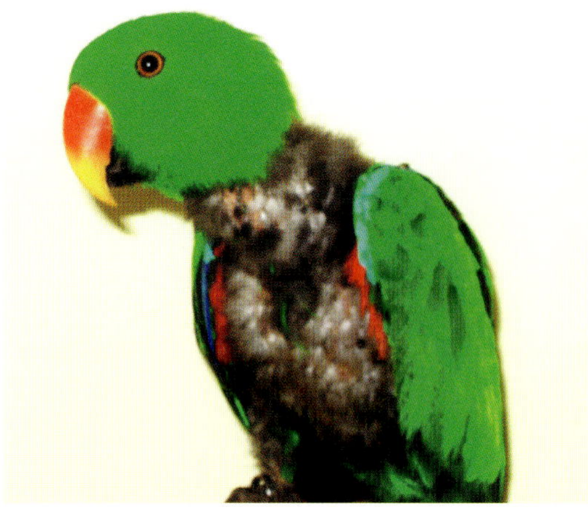

Figure 13.1 Feather plucking may have many causes.

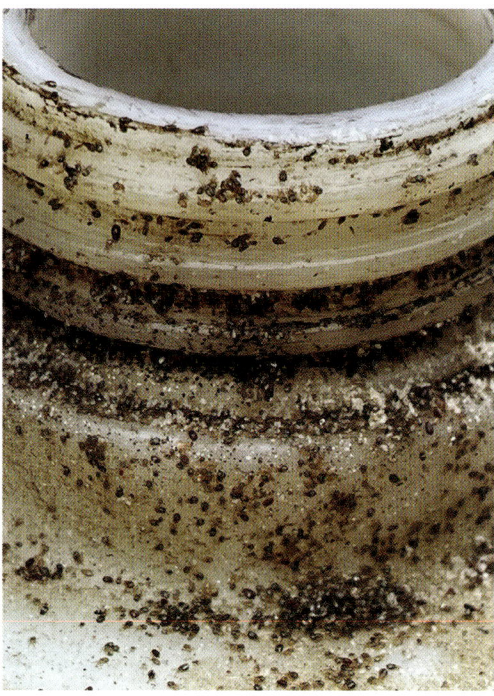

Figure 13.2 Red mite (*Dermanyssus gallinae*) around the top of a water feeder with the filler-cap removed. This mite hides in such places out of the daylight and feeds on birds overnight and may result in significant anaemia.

Lice

All avian lice belong to the Mallophaga, and so cause their damage by chewing and biting the feathers. They are generally elongated, squeezing in between the barbs of the feathers. They are more commonly seen in outdoor-housed birds and the main route for infestation for captive birds is from wild birds.

The most significant waterfowl louse genus is *Holomenopon* spp. but others commonly reported include *Anaticola* spp. and *Trinoton* spp. (see Figures 13.4 and 13.5). Related genera of mites (*Menopon* spp., *Menacanthus* spp., *Psittacobrosus* spp.) have also been found in Galliformes, Struthioniformes, Gruiformes, Ciconiiformes, Falconiformes and Psittaciformes among others, both in the wild and in captivity. *Menacanthus stramineus* is an extremely common louse

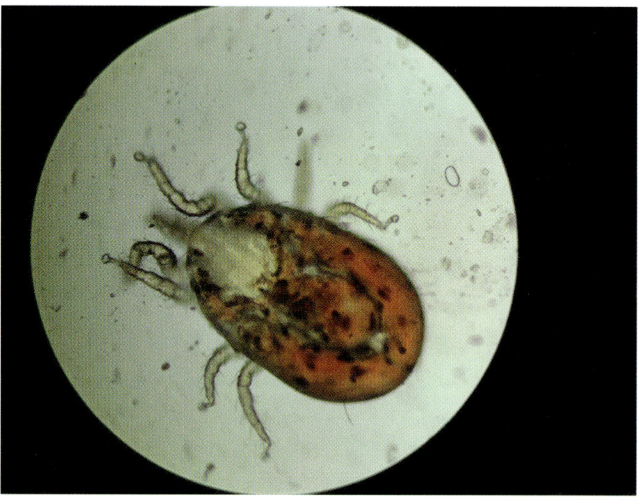

Figure 13.3 *Ornithonynssus* spp. is a blood-sucking mite, but unlike *D. gallinae* is often found on the bird during the day.

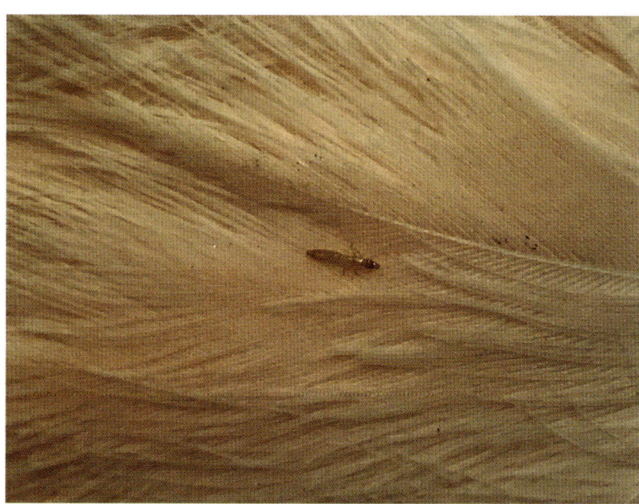

Figure 13.4 Image of *Anaticola* spp. louse on a flamingo.

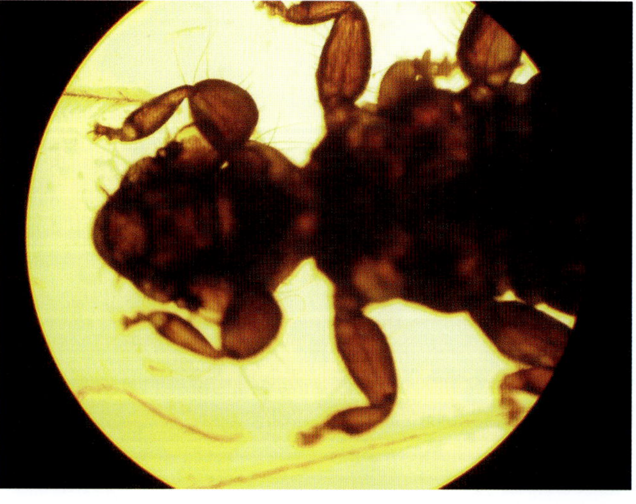

Figure 13.5 Microscope image of a *Holomenopon* spp. louse from a mute swan.

of captive chickens and turkeys and may result in significant feather damage if present in high enough numbers. *Holomenopon* spp. has been associated with damage of feathers, leading to a lack of normal structure and so loss of waterproofing in waterfowl. This causes the feathers to look bedraggled and soggy and is often referred to as 'wet feather disease'.

In pigeons, two main types of louse are seen: the body louse (*Hohorstiella lata*) which is haematophagous and the slender louse (*Columbicola columbae*) which is seen on the wings. The former may result in anaemia and lethargy. The latter causes damage to the structure of the feather, destroying the interlocking of the barbs which keep the feather's shape intact, and so give the pigeon a somewhat ragged appearance.

Flies

The blowfly family (Calliphoridae), such as the blue, black and green bottles, may be drawn to birds with diarrhoea or with wounds. The maggots (second larval stage or L2) of these species then eat their way through the skin and into the bird with devastating results, and allow the colonisation of the wounds by smaller species of fly maggot such as the housefly.

The Hippoboscidae family contains such species as the sheep and horse keds, which are however capable of infesting aviary birds. They are also common in free-flown birds such as raptors as wild birds often act as the source. The juvenile form of the fly is flightless and so spends large amounts of time living on its host. These species will often create infection and anaemia. They can also transmit blood-borne parasites, for example avian malaria (*Plasmodium* spp.), *Haemoproteus* spp. and *Leucocytozoon* spp., which may cause anaemia and immunosuppression. The pigeon louse-fly (*Pseudolynchia canariensis*) has been associated with transmission of *Haemoproteus* spp. as well as pigeon adenovirus 1 and possibly pigeon poxvirus.

Mosquitoes

Female mosquitos (*Aedes*, *Anopheles* and *Culex* spp.) can be haematophagous parasites to birds and as such they can cause irritation and act as a vector for avian malaria (*Plasmodium* spp.), as well as causing the spread of other blood parasites (*Haemoproteus*, *Leucocytozoon* spp.) and viruses, such as West Nile fever, eastern and western encephalitis viruses and the transfer of avian poxvirus. Mosquito presence is increasing in more northerly countries such as the UK with global warming and so this problem is likely to become more significant with time in these regions.

Gnats

Gnats such as blackflies (Simuliidae) and midges (Ceratopogonidae) are blood-sucking flying insects and in birds can transmit blood-borne parasites such as *Leucocytozoon* and *Haemoproteus* spp.

Ticks

In the northern hemisphere these are predominantly *Ixodes* spp. but in semi-equatorial regions, soft-bodied ticks of the family Argasidae are also commonly found. *Ixodes* spp. can rapidly be fatal to birds, possibly due to the presence of a toxin in the saliva of the tick. They are seen relatively uncommonly, but can occur in raptors being used for ground quarry hunting, as ticks are ground dwellers. They are also common in aviary-kept birds where surrounding trees overhang the aviary. The ticks may be carried on wild birds and so drop off roosts and nests into an aviary beneath. All ticks may transmit bacteria, such as members of the *Rickettsia* genus, as well as the majority of blood-borne parasites and viruses. The soft-bodied tick *Argas persicus* found in equatorial/tropical regions is a significant vector in the domestic poultry industry as it transmits the blood-borne parasite *Borrelia anserina* that causes avian spirochaetosis, a severe disease of poultry with high mortality levels.

Endoparasites

The parasite *Giardia* spp. can infest many species of birds but has been commonly reported in cockatiels. It causes a small intestinal disease and seems to result in coelomic discomfort that causes the affected bird to pluck the feathers over its flanks and ventrum. In addition, severe ascarid nematode infections have been associated with feather plucking in psittacine birds often in the region caudal to the keel bone.

Viral diseases affecting the skin

Circoviral disease

Psittacine beak and feather disease (PBFD) is caused by a member of the circovirus family often referred to as beak and feather disease virus. There is evidence for the presence of different strains of the virus in different species, but the current thinking is that this is one virus affecting psittacine birds and that the virus originated in Australasian psittacine birds (Bassami *et al.*, 2001; Varsani *et al.*, 2010). However, separate new strains of circovirus in budgerigars have been identified (Varsani *et al.*, 2010). In the majority of species, circoviral disease is a terminal infection after a chronic disease course. Some species may nevertheless recover from infection, such as many lorikeets and lories and even budgerigars and fig parrots, but these species may therefore act as carriers and transmitters of the disease to other species (Raidal, 2016). African grey parrots (*Psittacus erithacus* subsp.) are an example where two main forms of the disease are commonly seen: an acute form seen in juvenile birds that presents with clinical anaemia and immunosuppression (and frequently secondary aspergillosis), and a chronic form seen in adult birds which causes increasing feather, nail and beak dystrophia, death finally occurring due to dysphagia and inanition (see Figure 13.6). In many birds, the first feathers to be affected are the powder feathers – this is more obvious in cockatoos which normally produce lots of powder down and so normally have a very dusty beak. Those cockatoos infected with circovirus often have a shiny beak free of dust.

In eclectus parrots (*Eclectus* spp.) and lovebirds (*Agapornis* spp.), early circoviral disease can present with self-mutilation making circoviral infection a differential in feather plucking. In budgerigars, the disease is known as 'French moult', with birds from 4 to 5 weeks becoming depressed then showing necrosis of developing feathers. Some may die after 1–2 weeks with diarrhoea and crop stasis.

Transmission of circovirus in psittacine birds is by feather dander, oral and faecal routes. There is a suggestion it may be transferred vertically through the egg, although this has yet to be definitively proved. The virus is highly resilient in the environment and can remain viable for months outside the bird (Raidal and Cross, 1994).

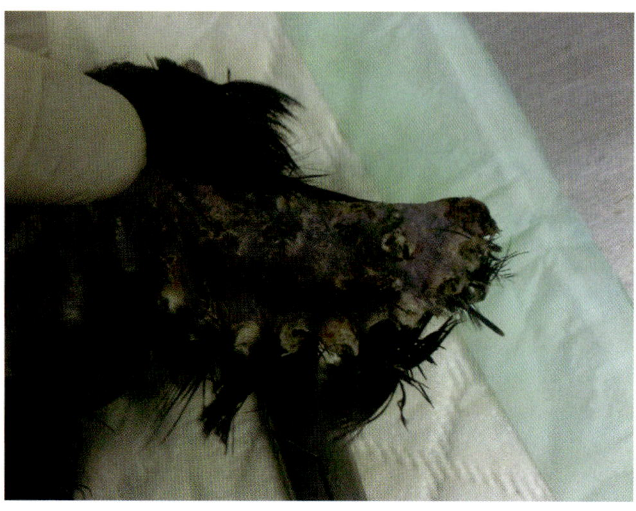

Figure 13.6 PBFD infection leading to abnormal feather development. Loss of the beak and nails often accompanies this leading to inanition.

In Columbiformes, a separate circovirus disease causes a typical disease pattern in young squabs aged between 2 months and 1 year and is known as pigeon circovirus. Incubation period is 2 weeks. Transmission is via the faecal–oral, oral, dander and vertical (through the egg) routes (Silva *et al.*, 2022). Clinical signs include anorexia, diarrhoea, weight loss, respiratory disease and lethargy. Death commonly occurs within 3–5 days. The disease produces immunosuppression and therefore concurrent infections are common – most, typically *Chlamydia psittaci*, *Aspergillus* spp., pigeon adenovirus, *Spironucleus columbae* and *Escherichia coli* infections, contributing to the so-called young pigeon disease syndrome (YPDS) (Silva *et al.*, 2022).

Diagnosis of circoviral disease is based on PCR demonstration of the viral antigen in blood or feather pulp – it is advised that both are submitted as frequently one or other can be negative depending on the stage of the disease. Others have suggested liver biopsy in grey parrots as this appears to be the target organ (Grund *et al.*, 2005). Alternatively, histopathology of skin biopsies can demonstrate viral inclusions and at post-mortem in young birds, depletion of B lymphocytes from the bursa of Fabricius with viral inclusions in the bursa, thymus and bone marrow. Antibody tests have also been developed with haemagglutination inhibition tests and can give an indication of exposure to the virus.

There is no treatment for the virus although avian gamma-interferon therapy has been tried with varying degrees of success. Vaccination has been attempted, but if the bird is already infected, then vaccination has been shown to actually deteriorate the bird's condition. Management of the environment with peroxide disinfectants (e.g. Virkon-S®, Antec International Ltd. at 1% concentration) has been shown to help in reducing contamination in one report (Cross, 2004).

Polyomavirus

Avian polyomavirus (APV) infection is common and causes systemic disease in various species of psittacine, gallinaceous, passerine and raptor birds. In budgerigars (*Melopsittacus undulatus*), it is the cause of budgerigar fledgling disease/feather duster disease. In this condition, neonates in infected flocks may die suddenly at around 10–15 days. Others may develop abdominal distension, reduced feathering and haemorrhages under the skin. Some may show neurological signs such as ataxia and tremors of the head. If infected after 15 days of age, they will often survive but develop feather abnormalities preventing flying. In juvenile finches (primarily Gouldian finches), a different strain of polyomavirus is seen with clinical signs that include weight loss, fluffed appearance, diarrhoea and dehydration with internal haemorrhages and a high mortality rate. A separate polyomavirus has also been identified in canaries (*Serinus canaria*) with similar signs plus loss of feathers and some neurological signs. Many of these had secondary infections.

Diagnosis is based on clinical signs and PCR testing of cloacal swabs or tissues at post-mortem. Testing indicates that the canary and finch strain are different (Shivaprasad *et al.*, 2009). Clinical gross post-mortem signs and basophilic intranuclear inclusion bodies on histopathology are suggestive.

There is no treatment for this condition, although there is a vaccine in the USA (Psittimune APV®, Biomune Co.).

Avipoxviruses

These can occur in all avian species, although none have so far been recorded in Strigiformes. Signs include pox-like proliferative lesions (so-called 'dry' form of the disease), occurring predominantly on the face, particularly around the eyelids, and also the feet and cere. These become secondarily infected and may lead to more extensive lesions. Respiratory tract disease may also be seen (so-called 'wet' form of the disease) and may result in the sloughing of the lining of the trachea and smaller airways, causing asphyxiation. Transmission may occur directly from bird to bird, and by flying biting-insect vectors. The poxvirus affecting canaries is particularly virulent and may cause serious mortality in canary flocks and has also been associated with lung neoplasia/pathological proliferative lesions.

Diagnosis is based on demonstrating the classical Bollinger bodies, seen due to virus particles inside infected cells, as well as the clinical signs described and PCR testing for genetic nuclear material (DNA).

Papillomavirus

This may lead to proliferative skin masses on the feet and legs of passerine birds and they are considered enzootic in some populations of waterfowl, Gruiformes and Ciconiiformes and may mimic mite infestations. Rarely in psittacine birds, proliferative lesions on the face and around the beak may be seen. Papillomas of the digestive tract are now thought not to be caused by a papillomavirus but rather by a herpesvirus. Diagnosis is by histopathological demonstration of intranuclear inclusion bodies. There is no treatment at present other than surgical excision of papillomas when they are causing irritation. Their regrowth though is common. Herpesvirus infections in psittacine birds are also associated with internal papillomatosis (see section on digestive tract diseases).

Bacterial disease affecting the skin

Examples include *Salmonella typhimurium* var. Copenhagen joint infection of pigeons, which may then erupt as a boil visible on wing joints such as the elbow; and *Staphylococcus* spp. and *E. coli* infections of the feet of many species, which cause bumblefoot.

'Bumblefoot' (pododermatitis)

In raptors, it is more frequently seen in falcons. Persistent pressure on the same parts of the sole of the foot when perching restricts the blood flow to these areas. This will ultimately lead to hypoxia and death of tissues, followed by open sores and deep pedal infections. Bacteria most commonly seen are *E. coli* and *Staphylococcus* spp., but yeasts such as *Candida* spp. may also be seen in cases that have been on antibiotics for prolonged periods of time. Many categorisations for the differing stages of bumblefoot have been described, the most basic being proposed by Cooper (1985), which divides the lesions into three types: type 1, which only involves the epidermis; type II, which involves soft tissues that become infected with typically *Staphylococcus aureus*, *E. coli*, *Pseudomonas* spp. and occasionally yeasts; and type III, which involves bones, ligaments, etc. and has the worst prognosis. Images of pododermatitis can be found in Chapter 10.

Another more detailed breakdown of the staging of bumblefoot further refines classification into five main classes/categories (Oaks, 1993; Remple, 1993).

- Class I: devitalisation of the skin of the plantar foot without a breach of the skin itself. This class has the best chance of success with treatment as infection is not present and husbandry changes to management, perch design and topical emollient creams/ointments can be successfully used. This can be further divided into two categories:
  - A: evidence of a bruise or ischaemia
  - B: evidence of a callus.
- Class II: evidence of inflammation/infection of the deeper tissues beneath the skin lesion with no signs of swelling. This class has a good prognosis but is likely to require surgical debridement and/or antimicrobial usage. This can be further divided into two categories both involved in allowing microbial invasion of soft tissues:
  - A: puncture wound
  - B: ischaemic necrosis of the epithelium.
- Class III: a more generalised infection with inflammation and swelling of the underlying soft tissues. This class carries a good to guarded prognosis, with surgical intervention, antimicrobial usage and support dressings being required. This can be further divided into three categories:
  - A: an acute insult with serous discharge and oedema and hyperaemia of the tissues
  - B: a more chronic insult with a fibrotic reaction in an attempt to wall off the lesion/infection
  - C: a caseous response due to a build-up of necrotic tissue.
- Class IV: a deeper and well-established infection with a chronic tenosynovitis (infection of the tendons and their protective sheath) and occasional arthritis and osteomyelitis. This category always carries a guarded to poor prognosis for successful treatment which always requires surgery, the use of antimicrobials (including antibiotic-impregnated polymethylmethacrylate beads). Radiography is recommended for any foot lesion and is helpful in differentiating class III from class IV. This can be further divided into two categories:
  - A: a fibrotic reaction
  - B: a caseous reaction (common for a purulent exudate to occur when synovial structures are involved).
- Class V: a further development of class IV with osteomyelitis, chronic tenosynovitis and loss of the use of the foot. This carries a grave prognosis and generally euthanasia of the patient is advised.

Fungal diseases affecting the skin

These tend to be secondary to other injuries, or skin mutilation. *Candida albicans* has been reported in lorikeets and associated with hypovitaminosis A. It has also been seen in lovebirds with feather loss around the eyes, beak and neck with scaling and has been reported to be associated with pododermatitis.

Malessezia spp. have been associated with pruritus in galahs, eclectus parrots, mynah birds and cockatiels (Reavill *et al.*, 1990).

Dermatophytosis ('ringworm'), due usually to *Trichophyton schoenleinii*, has been recorded in Galliformes such as the chicken where it is also known as 'favus', Latin for honeycomb due to its circular to hexagonal proliferations similar to a honeycomb shape. It is generally seen most commonly around the wattles and comb but can spread to the rest of the body and result in feather loss.

Allergic skin conditions

There is evidence that allergic skin disease occurs in birds including Psittaciformes (Colombini *et al.*, 2000). Serological tests do not seem to be reliable in birds, but intradermal skin testing has been shown to be useful in determining allergens and has been shown to give significantly different results in feather plucking and normal birds (MacWhirter *et al.*, 1999). Codeine phosphate is used as the positive control as it gives more consistent results than histamine (Colombini *et al.*, 2000). The intradermal skin test is carried out using the skin either side of the keel over the pectoral muscles, which limits the amount of allergens that can be tested for in one go; in addition, due to the thin nature of the avian skin, the bird requires to be anaesthetised with isoflurane. However, the results indicate that some feather plucking parrots do have an allergic response to allergens, such as sunflower seeds, house dust mites and *Aspergillus* spp. Hypovaccination has not been tried on any major scale but I have had some positive effects with hypovaccines.

Miscellaneous diseases affecting the skin

Split keel

Split keel is commonly seen in young, overweight, hand-reared birds, particularly those which have been carelessly wing clipped. It occurs when the bird attempts to fly off a high perch, and due either to poor wing muscling or lack of flight feathers, drops like a stone and hits the ground with force. This often splits the thin skin covering the prominent keel area and this split may become secondarily infected. This delays healing, and may necessitate the use of antimicrobials or even surgery to achieve wound healing.

Ulcerative skin disease

Ulcerative skin disease can be due to bacterial infections, for example *Staphylococcus* spp., or may be due to fungal infections such as with *Aspergillus* spp. Birds most commonly affected are species such as lovebirds, cockatoos and cockatiels.

The bird traumatises the skin underneath each wing, leading to a weeping ulcerative dermatitis. The infections may be primary or secondary. Little is known about the true initial causes of this condition, although some suggestions recently have included allergic skin conditions similar to those seen in dogs.

Psittacosis/chlamydiosis

Systemic infection with *Chlamydia psittaci* has been implicated in some parrots with feather plucking and generally poor feather quality.

Changes in feather colouration and structure

This may occur due to a lack of one nutrient, such as the paler colour seen in some canary breeds (e.g. red factors) when deprived of vitamin A. Vitamin A in particular is required for the production of the yellow and red colouration of feathers in some species. Other colour changes which can be seen include the following.

- Vasa parrots will develop white feathers rather than their normal grey, when they are infected with PBFD virus.
- Red colouration of the grey feathers in African grey parrots may also be seen with hepatic disease and with PBFD virus.
- Black feathers appearing in green-coloured birds such as Amazons can suggest liver disease.

Fret marks

Fret marks are another common feather abnormality seen in birds with a history of illness. These are breaks in the integrity of the feathers due to poor production of the interlocking barbs. This produces a noticeable band on all those feathers which were growing at this time and which appears different in structure and often colour. The presence of fret marks suggests some systemic disease or malnutrition at the time the feathers were being produced and can be a useful external indicator of a bird's recent past health, although they say nothing about its current health status.

Hormonal skin disease

Hypothyroidism has been recorded in chickens and African grey parrots. Clinical signs include slow growth and poorly coloured feathers, which often lack the interlocking barbules and so appear ragged. Diagnosis is based on the thyroid stimulating hormone (TSH) test where 1 IU/kg of TSH is administered intramuscularly after measurement of basal thyroxine (T4) levels. T4 levels are then measured 24 hours later, over which time a 2.5 times increase in T4 should have occurred. Failure to do so suggests hypothyroidism. It has been suggested that an underlying cause of hypothyroidism may be a dietary deficiency of iodine.

Tumours and feather cysts

The more common skin tumours include subcutaneous lipomas, and the so-called xanthoma seen particularly along the distal wings of birds (e.g. budgerigars). This is more an accumulation of fat deposits within the cells, producing a thickening of the area, and a characteristic yellow colouring of the skin.

Feather cysts are seen commonly in budgerigars and canaries. The condition occurs when a new growing feather fails to find its way through the skin surface, and so continues to grow while trapped under the skin. The feather cyst becomes an enlarging caseous nodule, which can ulcerate and become secondarily infected. It is thought that the condition is hereditary and the affected birds should be removed from breeding stock.

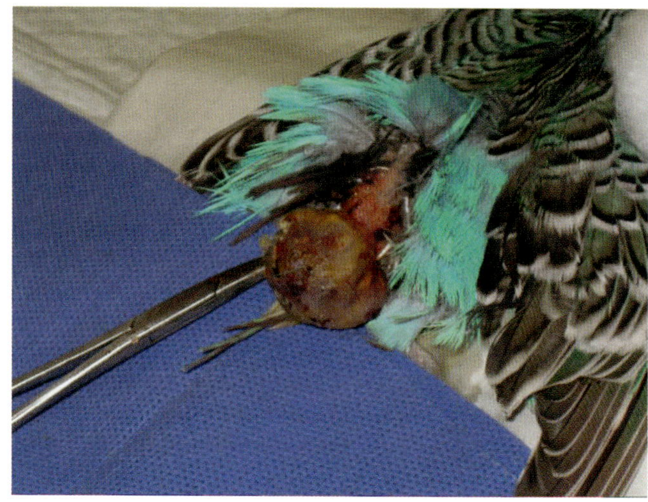

Figure 13.7 A large benign adenoma of the preen gland in a budgerigar.

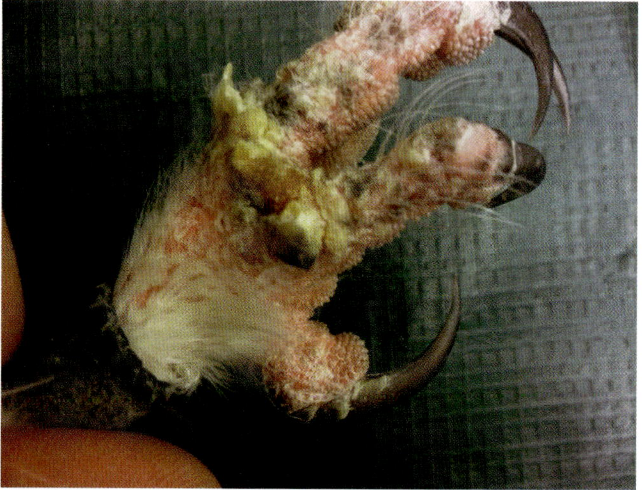

Figure 13.8 Squamous cell carcinoma development on the feet of a barn owl (*Tyto alba*).

Tumours of the preen gland are relatively common particularly in budgerigars and may reach significant sizes (see Figure 13.7). Many are benign adenomas, although adenocarcinomas with ulceration can also be seen.

Tumours such as squamous cell carcinomas, melanomas and adenocarcinomas are also occasionally reported on exposed areas of skin such as the feet and lower legs or sometimes the face (see Figure 13.8)

Oil spills

Seabirds and shore birds alike become coated with crude oil, making them flightless and removing their waterproofing. Many also succumb to the toxic and irritant effects of the oil itself including anaemia due to red blood cell haemolysis and stomach ulceration, which is more commonly seen with the lighter crude oils.

Treatment is based on a number of principles which include stabilisation of the often dehydrated and malnourished bird, followed by prevention of further irritation and absorption of oil across mucous membranes (including activated charcoal), and finally removal of the oil from the pelage (feathers and skin) (see Chapter 14).

Heavy metal toxicosis

Acute heavy metal (principally lead and zinc) toxicosis has been associated with neurological and renal disease in birds. However, chronic lead toxicosis in particular is also implicated in feather plucking. Older houses often have wooden surfaces that have been painted with decades of lead-based paints, which parrots are adept at chewing off. Kitchen units may use lead in the 'leading' of glass doors. Solder and many pewter items contain lead including foil on bottles of wine. Diagnosis is via blood testing; the cut-off level for lead is greater than 0.2 ppm (20 μg/dL or 1.25 μmol/dL) measured in lithium heparin whole blood (not EDTA as this chelates heavy metals and so gives a falsely low reading). Levels greater than 0.5 ppm (50 μg/dL or 2.6 μmol/dL) are diagnostic. Some argue that as lead is not required for any bodily system function and therefore the presence of any lead in an animal's body is significant.

Wing tip oedema

This, as its name suggests, is seen clinically as swelling and oedema of the wing tips (carpus distally) and is most commonly associated with frostbite in raptors. It will often lead to avascular necrosis of the wing tips once the oedema has subsided if not treated quickly.

Digestive disease

Crop

Ingluvitis

Ingluvitis is inflammation of the crop. It can be caused by an overgrowth of the yeast *Candida albicans* or bacteria such as *E. coli* and other Gram-negative bacteria. *Candida albicans* infection tends to be confined to the crop and gastrointestinal tract. It is often a sequel to prolonged antibiotic therapy such as tetracycline treatment of chlamydiosis/psittacosis or in neonate psittacine birds. Clinical signs usually involve regurgitation and delayed crop emptying. Diagnosis is by visualising the thickened crop lining, which has been likened to a thick towel surface and by demonstration of typical peanut-shaped budding yeasts on cytology. Presence of pseudohyphae (extensions from the yeast capsule) on cytology often indicates deeper tissue involvement and worsens the prognosis.

Ingluvitis can also be due to parasites such as *Trichomonas* spp., which are a common cause of regurgitation of seed in budgerigars and cockatiels. In pigeons and raptors, *Trichomonas* spp. cause a condition known as 'canker' or 'frounce', respectively, which results in caseous yellow nodules at the corners of the oropharynx and the proximal oesophagus. It can however spread throughout the body and result in high levels of mortality, particularly in some species of raptor. The feeding of wild-caught pigeons to raptors is a prime means of transmitting this particular pathogen. If a raptor owner is to feed wild-caught pigeon, then it should first be frozen for 3–4 weeks and then thoroughly defrosted before being fed, so as to kill off any *Trichomonas* spp. present. Diagnosis of the causal agent is by crop wash (in cage birds) or direct sampling of any lesion. The volume of saline used to carry out the crop wash varies from 0.5 mL in a budgerigar up to 10 mL in a large macaw. The sample can be examined in a drop of saline and using polarised light it may be possible to see the motile *Trichomonas* spp. organism. It can also be examined using both Gram stain and Diff-Quik-style dichrome/Romanowsky stains. However, *Trichomonas* spp. may be difficult to pick up using both methods as it is often in the lining of the crop. Willette *et al.* (2009) describe trichomoniasis as the most clinically significant parasitic disease in birds of prey. Certain species, however, seem more susceptible, for example peregrine falcons (*Falco peregrinus*) which naturally feed on wild Columbiformes are less likely to suffer from trichomoniasis. Conversely, northern goshawks (*Accipiter gentilis*), gyrfalcons (*Falco rusticolus*) and barn owls (*Tyto alba*) are much more susceptible. In addition, young birds seem more susceptible.

Bacterial infections causing ingluvitis due to *E. coli*, *Pseudomonas* spp. and *Aeromonas* spp. are also not uncommon, particularly in juvenile birds and neonates.

Sour crop

Sour crop in Psittaciformes is associated most commonly with juvenile birds. It occurs when the contents of the crop ferment, producing a foul-smelling acidic environment. This condition may be life-threatening. In raptors, although they do not have a true crop, oesophagitis may be associated with overconsumption of food that results in food sitting in the distensible oesophagus for prolonged periods of time. The crop and oesophagus in Galliformes and Psittaciformes has a near-neutral pH and so if food is present for too long a period of time it can ferment and lead to sour crop.

Crop impaction

Crop impaction occurs in juvenile cage birds such as Psittaciformes that may overeat. The condition may be due to poor motility associated with neurological conditions such as lead poisoning or proventricular dilatation disease. Alternatively, impaction may occur if a floor covering composed of shavings or sawdust is eaten by the birds (this is particularly common in Galliformes such as chickens, pheasants and other young game birds).

Capillariasis

Capillariasis is the name given to infestation of the crop lining with the nematode *Capillaria* spp. This is mainly a problem for pigeons and raptors, but is also seen from time to time in Passeriformes (e.g. finches and canaries) as well as species of Galliformes (e.g. pheasants and grouse). It is much rarer in Psittaciformes.

Clinically, raptors flick their head from side to side when eating and will regurgitate. In pigeons, acute infections are associated with high mortality because of intense vomiting. In cases of capillariasis, characteristic bipolar eggs may be seen in the faeces and mucus from the oral cavity (see Figure 13.9). The life cycle of *Capillaria* spp. is often indirect and may involve earthworms. Different species of *Capillaria* spp. can affect different parts of the digestive tract. For example, in chickens, turkeys, ducks and quail *C. contorta* affects the mouth, oesophagus and crop, whilst *C. caudinflata* affects the small intestine.

The parasite *Streptocara* spp. has been associated with oesophageal damage in waterfowl similar to that caused by *Capillaria* spp. in other birds.

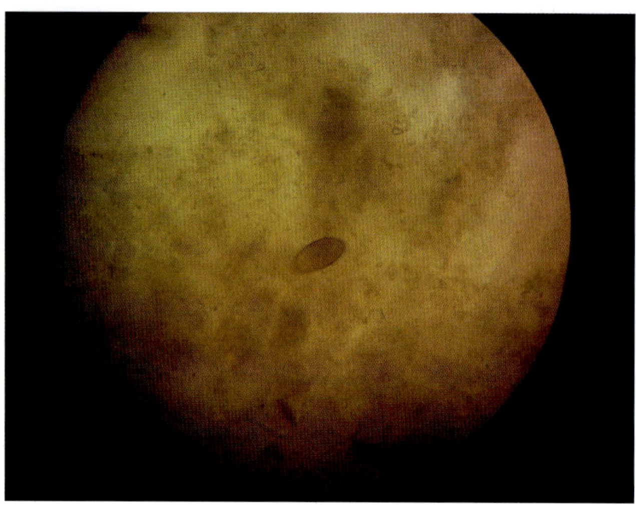

Figure 13.9 Microscope view of *Capillaria* spp. egg in an avian faecal sample.

Crop burns

These are frequently seen in hand-reared Psittaciformes. They generally occur when the owner has fed the juvenile bird a rearing formula porridge that has been microwaved and not thoroughly stirred and allowed to stand, resulting in 'hot spots' within the mixture that will cause local burns. These can be full thickness, causing the crop, subcutis and skin to slough after 7–10 days.

Foreign bodies

Many larger Psittaciformes may consume foreign objects, which become lodged in the crop and may cause irritation and retching, and may lacerate the thin crop lining. Retrieval of the object via endoscopic examination under anaesthesia is advised, with repair of any lacerations.

Associated crop disorders

The lack of iodine in an all-seed diet will cause thyroid gland enlargement (goitre). This enlarged gland will press on the crop and proximal oesophagus, so limiting its ability to empty and fill. Often seen in budgerigars, they will adopt a horizontal posture, lying across the perch with the head slightly raised. There is frequent intermittent regurgitation of seed.

Proventriculus

Proventriculitis

Inflammation of the true stomach (proventriculus) can be caused by the yeasts *Candida* spp. and *Macrorhabdus ornithogaster* (formerly known as *Megabacterium*). Signs can include the vomiting of food, the passing of undigested seed in the faeces and, in the case of Psittaciformes, anorexia, diarrhoea and weight loss.

In budgerigars and many finches, the incidence of *Macrorhabdus ornithogaster* infection is relatively high. Many birds are carriers with no clinical signs, but a percentage of a flock will show a 'going light' syndrome. They will eat voraciously, but lose weight, often passing undigested food/seed in their faeces which are often loose. They may also vomit. Diagnosis is by finding the typical bacillus-like Gram-positive chains of the yeast in faeces. This is made easier by suspending faeces in 20 times the volume of physiological (0.9%) saline and then examining the suspension after 10–15 seconds as the organism takes longer than most of the faecal material to settle with gravity. PCR tests are also available.

'Megabacteriosis' is seen in a wide host of other species, including canaries, parrotlets, cockatiels, galahs, corellas, lovebirds, ostriches and even domestic poultry (ducks, chickens, turkeys, guinea-fowl, partridges, quail and geese).

Proventricular dilatation disease

Proventricular dilatation disease (PDD) has been reported in over 60 species of predominantly psittacine but also some non-psittacine birds. It was first reported in macaws (giving it the alternative name 'Macaw wasting disease') and its current name is derived from the lymphoplasmacytic ganglioneuritis, which damages the nerves supplying the proventriculus and resulting in progressive muscular flaccidity leading to a maldigestion syndrome, starvation and eventually death. Passage of part-digested food and often undigested seed in the faeces of Psittaciformes is commonly reported. The disease affects all the nerves associated with the digestive system but it also affects the central nervous system (CNS) and even the cardiac electrical conduction system and so affected birds may show non-digestive tract signs such as ataxia, nervous tremors, central blindness, fitting, torticollis and sudden death (Berhane *et al.*, 2001; Steinmetz *et al.*, 2008). The virus may also affect other tissues of non-neural origin. The median age of onset appears to be 3–4 years but has been reported as early as 5 weeks of age and as old as 17 years (Phalen, 2006; Smith, 2009). Secondary infections with *Candida* spp. and *Macrorhabdus ornithogaster* are common.

The virus causing the disease is an avian bornavirus of which there are many recorded genotypes (Gancz *et al.*, 2009; Gray *et al.*, 2009; Shivaprasad *et al.*, 2009). Avian bornavirus 2 and 4 (ABV-2 and ABV-4) are most frequently detected, with ABV-4 being most commonly seen in psittacines and evidence suggests that specific genotypes of the virus affect only specific related species of bird (Hoppes *et al.*, 2010; Staeheli *et al.*, 2010). In canaries, a series of three bornaviruses (*Orthobornavirus serini*) have all been associated with a similar proventricular dilatation disease (Rinder *et al.*, 2022).

Koch's postulates have been fulfilled in the cockatiel (*Nymphicus hollandicus*) (Hoppes *et al.*, 2010) and Patagonian conures (Gray *et al.*, 2010) – in other words, the virus has been taken from infected birds showing classical clinical signs and deliberately introduced into an unaffected bird which then resulted in the production of the same clinical signs and recovery of the virus so confirming it as the causal agent. Bornaviruses cause most of the clinical signs by stimulating the body's immune system to attack its own nerves (hence the lymphocytic/plasmacytic infiltrates around the nerves themselves). Multi-bird households have a significantly higher incidence of infection with avian bornavirus than single-bird households (71.4% versus 51.3%). Infection may be associated with higher incidences of feather plucking, with 76% of positive cases showing plucking behaviour in one study (Zantop, 2010). Transmission is suspected to be faecal–oral but respiratory transmission is also suspected and vertical transmission (through the egg) has been proved although appears uncommon (Perpinan *et al.*, 2007; Lierz, 2016). Incubation period may be rapid as witnessed by the young age of some cases but may also take up to 7 years to manifest itself.

Definitive diagnosis is difficult. Clinically, the disease has been diagnosed based on detection of antigen in faeces by reverse transcription (RT)-PCR but again showing further discrepancies. Serology to detect antibodies against bornavirus infection is also commonly used, as mentioned, but frequently does not correlate with the severity of clinical signs as is typical with serological tests. Histopathology to demonstrate a lymphocytic/plasmacytic infiltrate to nerves in body organs, particularly the crop and proventriculus, has also been used to diagnose the disease.

Proventricular/ventricular impaction

If insoluble grit is fed, the grit builds up and can block the gizzard. Other causes of impaction are seen in juvenile cockatoos (*Cacatua* spp.) and African grey parrots (*Psittacus erithacus*), which often compulsively ingest items in their environment such as fragments of wood and plastic. These birds present as vaguely unwell, losing condition, rarely with vomiting although recurrent bacterial enteritis has been reported (Speer, 1998). Gizzard impaction may also be seen in Galliformes and Struthioniformes (ostriches, rheas, emus) fed long fibrous plant-based foods such as long grass or hay, particularly when young.

Endoparasites

Helminths

Ascaridia spp.: Ascarids are commonly seen in cage and aviary birds, particularly those that have a deep litter or earth floor to their aviary, as this allows maturation of any worm eggs that are passed in the faeces. Species seen include *Ascaridia platycerci* (psittacine birds), *A. hermaphrodita* (in a hyacinth macaw), *A. columbae* (found in psittacine birds and Columbiformes), *A. columbae* (found in Columbiformes but also reported aberrantly in Psittaciformes such as budgerigars) and *A. galli* (found in Galliformes and psittacine birds).

Infected individuals may show no external signs, but if parasitised heavily enough they may lose weight, have diarrhoea or, in severe cases, may experience intestinal blockage and death. In addition, damage to the liver may occur due to the migration of the larval worm and is well reported in the case of *A. columbae* in both pigeons and budgerigars (Wehr and Shalkop, 1963; Mines and Green, 1983). Ascarids have a direct life cycle. This means that the eggs passed in the faeces of an infected bird, after a few days or weeks, can be directly infectious to another bird without having to be taken up by an intermediate host, although paratenic hosts such as earthworms can also be implicated in their transmission. Diagnosis is made by finding the thick-walled eggs in the faeces of the affected bird (see Figure 13.10).

Capillaria spp.: In pigeons, *Capillaria obsignata* burrows into the lining of the intestine where it can cause severe diarrhoea and regurgitation, often with fatal consequences. Other *Capillaria* spp., as previously mentioned, can infect the small intestine and stomachs of birds, for example *C. caudinflata* can infect the small intestine of Galliformes such as chickens, turkeys and quail as well as waterfowl such as ducks. Diagnosis is by demonstrating the presence of the bioperculate eggs in the faeces or regurgitated material produced by the infected bird (see Figure 13.9). Its life cycle is direct, as with the ascarid family.

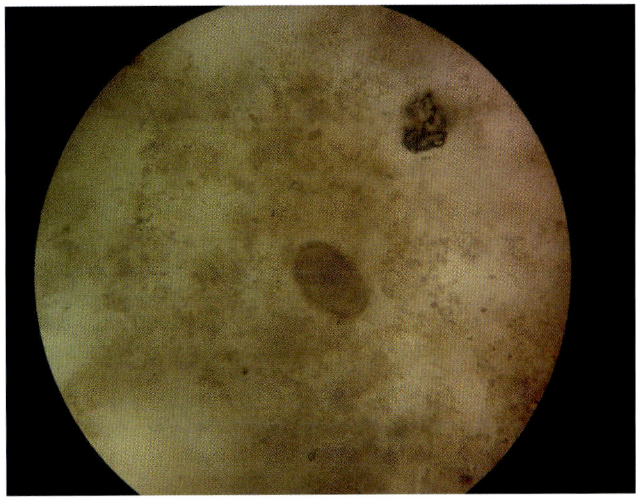

Figure 13.10 Typical thick-walled egg of *Ascaridia* spp. nematode in the faeces of a bird.

Other digestive system worms seen in birds

Other species of worm found in the digestive system are largely nematodes and include *Ornithostrongylus quadriradiatus* which is found in the intestine of pigeons. It is a blood-sucking worm, similar to the hookworms. It causes severe damage and leads to bile-stained greenish vomitus and green mucoid faeces along with progressive emaciation and death. Its eggs are thin-walled and more spherical than the *Capillaria* spp. eggs.

Waterfowl: There are many different species of nematode worms affecting waterfowl. *Echinuria* spp. cause a high mortality rate in young ducks and swans (often *E. uncinata*). It is often found at the proventricular–ventricular junction. It is transmitted via the intermediate host *Daphnia* spp., the water flea. It can produce tumour-like lumps in the lining of the proventriculus and gizzard, which may lead to partial blockage of these organs. In addition it may result in perforation of the stomachs and lead occasionally to coelomitis and death.

Epomidostomum and *Amidostomum* spp. can infest the gizzard of geese and ducks, causing bleeding into the lumen, diarrhoea, enteritis and weight loss. In young birds, it causes growth retardation and even death. *Epomidostomum uncinatum* has been regularly recovered from a range of wild ducks including wigeon, mallards, pintail and teal in Great Britain (Beverley-Burton, 1972).

Game birds: *Heterakis isolonche* is a significant cause of mortality in young pheasants, causing severe damage to the caecal lining. In many Galliformes, such as turkeys and chickens, this worm carries another pathogen with it, *Histomonas meleagridis*, a single-celled protozoan parasite that can cause significant focal liver necrosis, particularly in turkeys, giving the disease its name of black spot as it causes black circular necrotic lesions in the liver.

Corvids and thrushes: *Porrocaecum* spp. have been associated with weight loss and intestinal/stomach granulomas.

Non-helminth digestive system parasites

Motile protozoan parasites: *Giardia psittaci* is commonly found in cockatiels and budgerigars. Signs of the disease vary, and in the case of the cockatiel it has been associated with a deficiency in vitamin E, producing feather plucking.

Diagnosis is by finding the parasites on faecal smears. The sample is suspended in saline and examined using the ×400 microscope lens. The sample must be fresh, as the parasite disintegrates rapidly once the faeces dry. When fresh, movement of the organism, which has eight flagellae, can be observed.

Hexamita (Spironucleus) columbae infection is commonly found in pigeons. It produces weight loss and diarrhoea. It is seen in young birds towards the end of the breeding season when environmental contamination is high. Coinfection with pigeon circovirus has resulted in YPDS with poor-doing young birds. Diagnosis is by finding large numbers of the motile, eight-flagellae-bearing, elongated protozoa using the ×400 microscope lens on a slide of fresh faeces suspended in saline.

Trichomonas spp. may affect the intestines as well as the crop.

Cochlosoma spp. are flagellate single-celled protozoan parasites, which have been associated with widespread mortalities in Australian finches. *Cochlosoma anatis* has also been commonly reported in turkeys, ducks and geese. It causes diarrhoea, dehydration and moulting abnormalities particularly in birds between 10 days and 6 weeks of age.

Coccidiosis: *Eimeria* spp. infest many species, from pigeons and cage birds to Galliformes and waterfowl. They shed oocysts in the faeces that have four sporocysts each with two sporozoites. They principally affect the intestines but some species can affect the kidneys and some can be systemic. The intestinal *Eimeria* spp. typically contribute to the 'going light' syndrome where the bird loses condition. In pigeons, heavy burdens of *E. columbarum* and *E. labbeana* may affect racing performance but they are most typically associated with mortalities in young pigeons between 3 and 4 months of life (Krautwald-Junghanns *et al.*, 2009). Clinical signs may appear before oocysts are detected in the faeces. *Eimeria* spp. in cranes (*E. gruis* and *E. reichenowi*) can become rapidly disseminated throughout the body via mononuclear white blood cells and the liver and lungs may be particularly badly affected with mortalities being commonly reported. In hill mynah birds, *Eimeria* spp. have been associated with haemorrhagic enteritis.

Isospora spp. may affect the intestines or become disseminated systemically. They shed oocysts in the faeces that have two sporocysts each with four sporozoites. In canaries, *Isospora canaria* affects canaries of 2 months of age and older producing diarrhoea and emaciation, primarily damaging the duodenum which may be oedematous at post-mortem. In canaries and many other Passeriformes, *Atoxoplasma* spp. (now considered a form of *Isospora* spp.) may also be found. It is transmitted via the faecal–oral route and initially infects the epithelium of the intestines but then spreads from the gut into the mononuclear white blood cells and is carried through the bloodstream affecting organs such as the liver and spleen, resulting in organ enlargement and bile duct proliferation but has also been found in the lungs in canaries (Sanchez-Cordon *et al.*, 2007). The liver enlargement gives the disease its other name, 'black spot', because the large dark liver is visible through the thin skin of the canary's ventral abdomen (see Figure 13.11). Diarrhoea or sudden death may be seen, but the disease may be asymptomatic.

Atoxoplasmosis is a significant disease of a range of Passeriformes particularly the Bali starling or Bali mynah (*Leucopsar rothschildi*) and many thrush species. Diagnosis of atoxoplasmosis is by finding the oval to round oocysts in the bird's faeces using sugar flotation methods, or by direct smear of the liver or by examining the white blood (mononuclear) cells from a blood sample for evidence of the parasite.

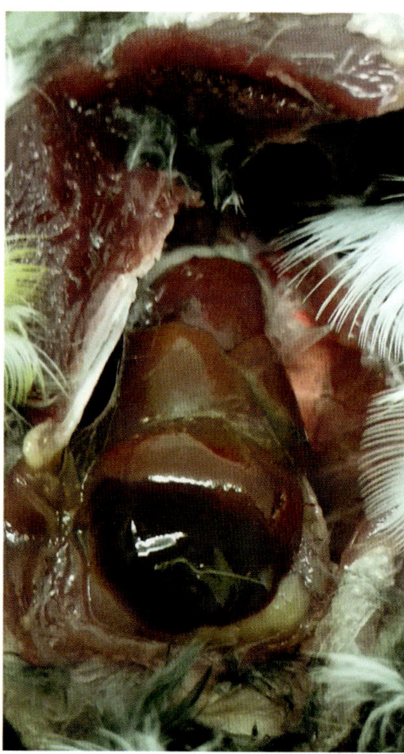

Figure 13.11 Post-mortem of a case of atoxoplasmosis. Note the enlarged liver which is distended and discoloured caudally.

Caryospora spp. cause crop and intestinal damage predominantly in carnivorous species of bird. There is often high mortality in young birds, with adults exhibiting abdominal discomfort. There are over seven species of *Caryospora* known to affect birds of prey, the two most commonly seen in captivity being *C. falconis* and *C. neofalconis* although species have also been identified in kingfishers such as kookaburra (Forbes and Simpson, 1997; Heidenreich, 1997; Yang *et al.*, 2014). Transmission is by direct means although there is evidence that rodent prey can act as a heteroxenous host. Clinical signs include general debility, diarrhoea, weight loss and anorexia and are most commonly seen in young raptors between 3 and 6 months of age. The parasite sexually reproduces in the gut, but encysted forms can be found in the muscle and CNS, and result in an encephalitis with neurological signs such as torticollis. Merlins (*Falco columbarius*) appear particularly susceptible with sudden death occurring. Diagnosis can be made on clinical signs and the presence of huge numbers of oocysts in the faeces with a typical single sporocyst with eight sporozoites within it.

Cryptosporidium spp.: This coccidian organism appears to be able to infect any epithelial surface and so has been reported in the gastrointestinal, respiratory and urinary tracts. It has a direct life cycle and the transmission route is faecal–oral, in food (other avian prey) or by respiratory aerosol. In psittacine birds, the proventricular form is the most commonly observed, with birds coinfected with *Macrorhabdus ornithogaster* being most likely to die (Messenger and Garner, 2010). In turkeys, *C. meleagridis* has a predilection for the intestines and can cause diarrhoea and weight loss but it has also been reported in a wide range of other species as well (Ravich *et al.*, 2014). Species of *Cryptosporidium* have however also caused renal disease and failure.

Sarcocystidae: The family Sarcocystidae contains the following genera relevant to birds: *Sarcocystis*, *Toxoplasma* and *Neospora*. They typically have indirect life cycles, requiring an intermediate host or hosts. *Sarcocystis* spp. typically affect carnivorous and omnivorous birds, the intermediate hosts being their vertebrate prey. They infect the intestines and may be asymptomatic or may result in diarrhoea and weight loss. Oocysts are like those of *Isospora* (two sporocysts each with four sporozoites). *Sarcocystis* spp. are more likely to cause significant disease in intermediate hosts and these can be birds. Species such as *S. falcatula* whose final/definitive host is the Virginia opossum can cause mortalities in birds which act as an intermediate host. *Sarcocystis calchasi* that uses birds of prey such as hawks as definitive hosts can cause mortalities in other species of birds such as psittacines, which become infected via the faecal–oral route (Rimoldi *et al.*, 2013).

Toxoplasma and *Neospora* spp. have a mammalian carnivore as their definitive host (felids and canids, respectively) but birds may become infected from their faeces and in the case of *Toxoplasma gondii* through consumption of infected intermediate hosts (usually rodents). Both can cause systemic disease in aberrant intermediate avian hosts with encephalitis, pneumonitis, hepatitis and death being reported (Dubey, 2002).

Bacterial gastrointestinal disease

Bacteria such as *E. coli*, *Campylobacter* spp., *Clostridium* spp., *Pseudomonas* spp., *Salmonella* spp., *Yersinia* spp. and *Chlamydia psittaci* may all cause diarrhoea and even toxaemia, septicaemia and death. *Salmonella* spp. may result in a persistent infected state in birds that recover and these then can act as sources of infection to other animals. The most serious salmonellae seen in birds are *Salmonella typhimurium*, *S. enteritidis* and *S. arizonae*. Clinical signs resemble those seen in yersiniosis but are generally more chronic. However, significant mortality can occur, particularly in finches and other small passerine birds. In pigeons, *S. typhimurium* var. Copenhagen typically produces swollen joints, especially on the wings, referred to as 'boils' by pigeon racers and fanciers. In addition, weakness, lethargy, green urates, diarrhoea and death of young hatchlings may all point to a salmonella problem. In pigeons, after paramyxovirus (PMV)-1, salmonellosis is the next most common cause of neurological signs and may also mimic mycobacterial disease when infecting bones. Culture and sensitivity testing using specific *Salmonella* spp. culture medium should always be performed on avian faecal samples in cases of diarrhoea and weight loss.

Escherichia coli is generally absent from the intestines of passerine and psittacine birds (Dorrestein, 2009), but is typically found in 97% of all pigeon intestinal tracts (Harlin and Wade, 2009). Clinical signs of *E. coli* infection include diarrhoea and sudden death and may be associated with epizootic mortalities in imported finches.

Clostridium spp. have been associated with gastrointestinal disease and death of a wide range of birds. They may be found in the gastrointestinal tract of many species notably raptors. *Clostridium perfringens* is considered a normal part of the flora of a raptor's digestive system. However, as with clostridial bacteria in rabbits, overgrowth may occur in poorly conditioned birds resulting in enterotoxaemia. In addition, food spoiled by clostridial toxins will result in rapid death of the raptor. Cage birds such as parrots may be affected by clostridiosis where food has become spoiled. It is more commonly seen in nectar feeding species such as lories and lorikeets.

Yersinia pseudotuberculosis is an environmental bacterium that can cause significant disease and peracute mortalities in susceptible species. It is a bacterium that requires iron, and so in cases of susceptible species exposed to high iron-containing diets, infection is common. Such species include, but not exclusively, toucans, toucanettes, hornbills, lories, lorikeets and many starlings. The condition is made more likely where diets contain high levels of iron, or by diets that are acidic in nature (e.g. those containing increased vitamin C levels through feeding citrus fruits) as acidity increases the ferrous (Fe^{2+}) nature of foods and so increases iron absorption.

In addition, the mycobacterium *Mycobacterium avium* subspecies *avium*, the cause of avian tuberculosis, is often seen in waterfowl and raptors, but can affect any species of bird. It inhabits the gut and associated organs and is thus spread via the faecal–oral route. The majority of pathology is therefore in the gastrointestinal tract including the liver before then spreading throughout the body via the bloodstream. It is often implicated in chronic wasting disease and produces classical caseous nodules throughout the gut and liver. Other species of *Mycobacterium* have also been commonly reported, particularly in Psittaciformes, and include *M. genavense* and less commonly *M. kansasii*, although the latter has been more associated with skin lesions than a more systemic infection (Palmieri *et al.*, 2013; Duvall *et al.*, 2021). Diagnosis is made on Ziehl–Neelsen stains demonstrating the acid-fast bacteria, PCR and bacterial culture of the faeces. Mycobacterial disease is frequently not treatable and as it is a zoonotic disease, consideration should be given to euthanasing affected birds.

Viral gastrointestinal disease

Duck plague virus

The duck plague virus is a member of the alpha herpesvirus family (Anatid alphaherpesvirus 1). It affects ducks, swans and geese. It is spread in the faeces and oral secretions and is also believed to be transmitted vertically through the egg and may be carried latently with no clinical disease. Alternatively, it may cause violent diarrhoea, anorexia and neurological tremors, inability to fly and swimming in circles or death with no premonitory clinical signs. The virus damages B and T lymphocytes in particular, causing immunosuppression. It can be associated with mass outbreaks in waterfowl. Blue-winged teal (*Spatula discors*) appear particularly susceptible and mallards (*Anas platyrhynchos*) appear moderately resistant which is important as mallards are commonly carriers and may spread the virus to more susceptible species (Hansen and Gough, 2007). Death usually occurs within 3–12 days of infection, and 1–10 days after developing clinical signs. The virus can remain viable in water in ponds for several months at low environmental temperatures (around 2 months at 4°C). Diagnosis is made on the clinical signs and isolation of the virus from faeces or PCR, or on demonstration of intranuclear inclusion bodies in the gut wall on post-mortem.

Avian papillomatosis

This condition in Psittaciformes is thought to be due to a herpesvirus. It causes papillomas throughout the digestive system and frequently in the cloaca. In the cloaca, it often leads to irritation and eversion or even prolapse due to repeated straining. Other clinical signs include regurgitation, recurrent bouts of enteritis, passage of blood in the faeces and infertility. Papillomatosis is also linked with a high incidence of liver, biliary tree and pancreatic cancer in affected birds.

Diagnosis is made in the live bird by PCR, diagnostic imaging and, in the case of the cloaca, visualising the papillomas aided by applying 5% acetic acid to the lesion, which will cause the papillomas to turn white while normal mucosal folds will remain pink.

Avian adenovirus

Avian adenoviruses have been reported in pigeons, Psittaciformes, Galliformes, waterfowl and raptors. The virus is spread through the faecal–oral route and possibly by aerosol/inhalation as well as being passed vertically through the egg. Disease is often associated with the gastrointestinal tract, with hepatitis, pancreatitis and catarrhal enteritis being seen, often with splenitis. One avian adenovirus specifically targets the spleen in pheasants (so-called marble spleen disease) although lung lesions are also commonly seen. However, lesions have also been reported in the trachea (particularly in quail and ducks), kidneys (reported in lovebirds) and CNS (reported in raptors and Psittaciformes). Other symptoms include a reduction in egg production and hatchability and, in peracute cases, hydropericardium. Diagnosis is based on PCR testing of faeces/cloacal swabs.

Goose parvovirus

Goose parvovirus is the cause of Derzsy's disease and is a highly infectious disease of domestic geese, although Canada geese, snow geese and Muscovy ducks are also reported as being susceptible. The virus is spread via the faecal–oral, nasal and vertical (egg) routes. Goslings between 1 and 21 days of age are most susceptible and the virus rapidly spreads to multiple organs including the liver, spleen, heart, adrenal, thyroid glands and thymus producing high mortality rates with diarrhoea and sloughing of the mucosa of the tongue. Older birds may have feather abnormalities (particularly down feather loss) and skin hyperaemia as well as growth retardation and neurological disease. Birds over 4–6 weeks of age appear to have an innate immunity and are not susceptible to infection.

Newcastle disease/PMV-1 and avian influenza virus

These viruses are discussed in more detail in the section on respiratory tract diseases as their main clinical signs tend to be more respiratory and sometimes neurological. They can however both cause watery diarrhoea that may be associated with biliverdinuria (yellow-green coloured urates) and they are legally notifiable diseases in the UK, European Union and many other countries due to their significant economic impacts on domestic poultry.

Liver disease

Haemochromatosis

Haemochromatosis is where excessive amounts of iron are deposited in the liver. Birds affected are commonly members of the toucan, toucanette, mynah, hornbill and starling families, although it has also been reported in Psittaciformes (particularly lories and lorikeets). In the wild, these species often live in areas with iron-poor soil, and their digestive systems are therefore adapted to absorb as much iron as possible. When presented with an iron-rich diet and high levels of vitamin C (which encourages iron absorption from the gut), too much iron is absorbed. This iron is then deposited in the liver, eventually leading to damage and failure. Iron storage also increases the risk of developing infections associated with ferrophilic bacteria such as *Yersinia pseudotuberculosis*.

Clinical signs include ascites, dullness, dyspnoea (due to the ascites pressing on the air sacs), abdominal swelling and sudden death. Diagnosis is based on clinical signs, a knowledge of susceptible species and liver biopsy to assess iron levels. Liver biopsy can be a dangerous procedure, particularly if the bird has ascites. There is then a real danger of rupturing air sacs and drowning the bird.

Avian tuberculosis (*Mycobacterium avium* infection)

Avian tuberculosis may produce liver disease, causing classical caseous nodules throughout the structure, and is also associated with intestinal disease. It is often seen in waterfowl, cranes and storks but can occur in any avian species (see Figure 13.12).

Other liver bacterial diseases

Any bacteria, such as *Salmonella* spp., *E. coli* and *Pseudomonas* spp., which breaches the gut wall may affect the liver directly via the enterohepatic circulation. In addition, the pansystemic infection of *Chlamydia psittaci* will cause hepatitis manifested clinically, as with so many hepatic disorders, by green-to-yellow coloured urates due to biliverdinuria. Diagnosis is based on clinical signs, biochemistry and isolation of the bacteria from the gastrointestinal tract and, if possible, from hepatic swabs.

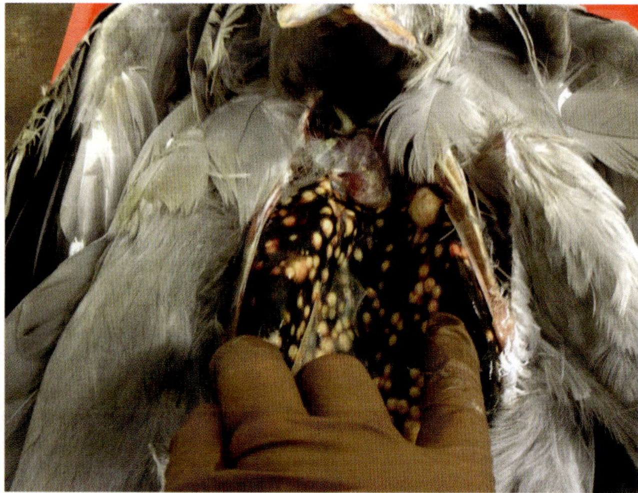

Figure 13.12 Post-mortem of the liver of a crane with widespread avian tuberculosis.

Viral liver diseases

Psittacid herpesvirus isolates 1, 2 and 3 have been recorded, all of which can cause Pacheco's disease in psittacine birds. Old World psittacine birds appear more resistant to infection than New World ones, with Amazon parrots, macaws and conures being considered the most susceptible. Clinical signs may be sudden death for New World birds, or a more prolonged course of depression, anorexia, regurgitation and green diarrhoea before death in more resistant species. Occasionally, haemorrhagic diarrhoea may be seen. Some cockatoos have been reported as surviving infection (although probably remain persistently infected). Carrier birds may start to shed the virus and so infect others during periods of physiological stress. Transmission appears to be via oropharyngeal secretions and faeces. At post-mortem, the liver is often bronze in colour and enlarged. The kidneys may also be enlarged and the intestines and brain congested. Intranuclear inclusion bodies (Cowdry type A) with hepatocellular necrosis are suggestive. Diagnosis can also be made using PCR technology on cloacal or oropharyngeal swabs. A vaccine is available in the USA. A separate budgerigar herpesvirus also exists and evidence suggests that this virus can pass through the egg to the chick. This virus can result in a decreased hatching rate.

Raptor herpesviruses: Currently raptors have three distinct isolates: Falconid herpesvirus 1 (FHV1), Strigid (owl) herpesvirus 1 (SHV1) and Accipitrid (eagle) herpesvirus 1 (AHV1). All cause hepatitis and splenitis with typical herpesvirus inclusion bodies. Wernery and Kinne (2004) suggest that transmission is via the ocular/intranasal route in falcons. It is worth noting that the Falconid herpesvirus has around 99.4% genetic similarity with Columbid herpesvirus 1 and some authors believe they are the same virus (Raghav and Samour, 2019).

Falconid herpesvirus: This virus affects Falconidae and occurs mainly in Europe and the Middle East. It is usually fatal, particularly in gyrfalcons and causes liver and spleen swelling and necrosis, bone marrow necrosis and gut inflammation with haemorrhage. It is transmitted directly from bird to bird and via prey items.

Strigid (owl) herpesvirus: This virus causes liver, spleen and bone marrow necrosis and is specific to the owl family. It is invariably fatal within 3–9 days. Yellow nodules may be found in the gut and the pharyngeal mucosa and secondary *Trichomonas* spp. infections are common. Necrotic lesions are seen in the liver, spleen and bone marrow. It is spread in urine and faeces, as well as oral secretions. Some birds that survive will remain latently infected. There is no treatment or vaccine available.

Pigeon herpesvirus (Columbid herpesvirus 1): This can cause a mild pharyngitis/oesophagitis with cellular necrosis in young birds. Older birds are frequently immune but remain persistent carriers. Anorexia, regurgitation and sometimes neurological signs in conjunction with green urates are suggestive. Inclusion body hepatitis can be seen on biopsy of affected livers. Pigeons often have recurring *Trichomonas* spp. infections in affected flocks.

Duck viral hepatitis: Duck viral hepatitis affects chiefly young ducklings under 3 weeks of age and is caused by a member of the *Picornaviridae*. It is rapidly fatal and produces severe liver damage and haemorrhage from the liver surface.

Avian reovirus: Not all are pathogenic but some can cause significant disease particularly in budgerigars and African grey parrots. Reoviruses are also reported in Galliformes, waterfowl, finches and pigeons. Transmission is faecal–oral, but also vertical (through the egg) in poultry. High mortalities have been reported in the UK in budgerigar flocks (Manvell *et al.*, 2004; Pennycott, 2004). Clinical signs in budgerigars include anorexia, fluffed-up appearance, dyspnoea, nasal discharge, diarrhoea and sudden death. Post-mortem reveals hepatitis, nephritis, serositis with ascites, pneumonia and splenitis with subcutaneous haemorrhages. There are often lymphoplasmacytic infiltrates of various organs, haemosiderosis, haemorrhage and fibrin deposition. Infections are commonly associated with other pathogens such as *C. psittaci*, adenovirus and *M. ornithogaster* infections.

Avian leukosis/sarcoma virus: This family group of viruses is known to induce a tissue-borne leukaemia (lymphoid leukosis) in Psittaciformes, Galliformes and Passeriformes (such as the canary). It destroys the liver and kidneys, which become infiltrated by rapidly dividing lymphocytes. Hen birds seem more susceptible than cock birds, and it is shed in the faeces, oral/respiratory secretions and semen. It is also passed in genetic material from mother to young in the egg. Clinical signs include hepatomegaly and renomegaly, ascites, respiratory distress, weight loss, green-coloured urates, polydipsia and polyuria. There is no treatment. Other neoplasms have also been associated with avian leukosis/sarcoma virus and include fibrosarcomas, osteochondrosarcomas, adenocarcinomas, granulosa cell tumours and seminomas.

Hepatic lipidosis

Hepatic lipidosis is usually diet related. High-fat diets (such as the all-seed diets so beloved of Psittaciformes) and lack of exercise lead to obesity and fat deposition in the liver cells or hepatocytes. Liver function suffers as a consequence. This condition may also be seen in raptors that are not working but are still being well fed. Affected birds are often sleek plump birds, which then become dull and lethargic, and may exhibit signs varying from ascites to respiratory distress and clotting defects.

Toxic liver conditions

Toxins from a number of sources may cause hepatic damage in the avian patient. These include the heavy metal toxicoses such as lead and zinc poisoning. It may also include other metals such as copper, chromium and mercury.

Lead poisoning: Lead poisoning is frequently seen in waterfowl which have inadvertently eaten environmental lead shot from hunting or fishing. Psittaciformes may also be affected, as they will consume or destroy many household items that contain lead (see section on skin diseases) and birds of prey/raptors fed wild-caught, lead-shot prey.

Clinical signs of lead toxicosis can include:

- Weakness (S-shaped neck of the swan, slumped stance in raptors frequently resting on the intertarsal joints)
- Lethargy, vomiting, passage of blood in the faeces (very common in Psittaciformes)
- Passage of lime green faeces (very common in raptors due to biliverdinuria)
- Chronic non-regenerative anaemia

- Seizures
- Kidney and liver damage
- Death.

Diagnosis is by finding blood lead levels in excess of 0.2 ppm (12.5 μmol/L), with those in excess of 0.4–0.6 ppm (25–37.5 μmol/L) being diagnostic. In addition, radiography will often show lead particles as radiodense areas in the proventriculus and ventriculus.

Zinc poisoning: It is mainly seen in Psittaciformes shortly after they have been moved into a new cage (giving its alternative name 'new wire cage disease'). Occasionally, the finish of these cages is of poor quality and a fine powder of zinc oxide forms the surface of the wires. The parrot manoeuvres itself around the cage with feet and beak and takes in small volumes of this powder on a daily basis. After 4–6 weeks, liver and kidney damage with bone marrow suppression will occur, and the bird may present weak, lethargic, having seizures and with anaemia. Other sources of zinc include some forms of coin, some plastics and other alloys. Diagnosis is made on clinical signs, history and finding zinc blood levels above 1.5–2 ppm (1500–2000 μg/L).

Other poisons affecting the liver: Aflatoxins released by *Aspergillus* spp. are known to be hepatotoxic and carcinogenic, as are the organic poisons found in rapeseed, ragwort and the castor bean. Treatment is rarely possible.

Pancreatic disease

Diabetes mellitus is a common condition in budgerigars and cockatiels. It may be hereditary. Pancreatitis can result in the development of this disease.

Clinical signs include polydipsia and polyuria, often with dramatic weight loss despite a healthy appetite.

Diagnosis is made on the clinical signs in conjunction with persistently raised blood glucose (often above 25 mmol/L up to 44 mmol/L). Some glucose may be found in the urine normally, but high levels (>1%) are strongly suggestive of disease.

Pancreatitis can be seen in birds. It has been linked with infections due to PMV-3 (e.g. cockatiels). The passage of partially digested seed or pasty tan-coloured faeces may be seen combined with weight loss.

Respiratory disease

Upper respiratory tract

Nostrils

Clinically often feathers are stained just above the nares, and there may be sneezing and head flicking due to the discharge.

Rhinoliths, concretions of dried secretions that form a ball of solid material blocking the entrance to the nasal passages, may be caused by dietary insufficiencies such as hypovitaminosis A, and/or may involve local or deeper infections due to bacteria such as *Mycoplasma* spp. (e.g. pigeons and chickens) or *Chlamydia psittaci* (e.g. Psittaciformes).

Fungi, such as *Aspergillus* spp., or viruses, such as the avipoxvirus group, are also common causes of upper respiratory (as well as lower respiratory) tract disease. The mite *Cnemidocoptes* spp. may also contribute to blockage of the nostrils (e.g. Psittaciformes and raptors).

Some species of parrot, such as Amazons, are susceptible to nasal irritation in dry environments, and in the presence of feather dander, produced by African grey parrots and cockatoos.

A congenital defect is the absence of a patent internal choanal slit. This prevents the normal nasal secretions from draining ventrally into the oropharynx. The secretions then present as a clear nasal discharge.

Theromyzon tessulatum is the duck nasal leech and is a common parasite. It may lead to secondary infections of the nasal passages.

Pigeon herpesvirus (PHV) affects young (<6 months) pigeons. It causes a nasal discharge, sneezing and necrotic plaques to form inside the mouth and upper airways. It may also cause the cere to become discoloured and crusty. In severe cases death associated with liver and neurological disease may occur (see section on digestive disease). There is no specific treatment or vaccine available, although many will survive.

Sinusitis may be seen in conjunction with rhinoliths and nasal discharges. It may be visible as a swelling on the face, often ventral to the eye in the area of the infraorbital sinus.

Lower respiratory tract

Trachea

Gapeworm infection: *Syngamus trachea* is found in a wide range of birds including many Galliformes, pigeons and raptors. This parasite has a direct life cycle but uses the earthworm (and sometimes snails, slugs and arthropods) as a paratenic host in which numbers can become very high. It finally matures in the windpipe of the final host bird. There it causes irritation and secondary infection and may be present in sufficient numbers to kill the bird through obstruction of the windpipe. Diagnosis is made by finding the characteristic Y-shaped red-coloured worms (the male and female worms are permanently joined in copulation) in the mucus of the mouth and trachea.

Cyathostoma bronchialis is a gapeworm that affects geese and ducks and also has a direct life cycle but is more commonly consumed through paratenic hosts such as the earthworm as with *S. trachea*. It is also found in the trachea, but also the bronchi and lungs.

Avipoxvirus: In Amazon parrots, a severe form of avipoxvirus may cause the sloughing of the lining of the windpipe, resulting in dyspnoea, pneumonia and even death from secondary infection. All avipoxviruses typically cause pox lesions on the face, particularly around the eyes and mouth, the pharynx and trachea, but may also produce lesions on the feet. Secondary infections are common. In pigeons there are vaccines available. Diagnosis is confirmed by finding the characteristic Bollinger bodies that are the reproductive centres of virus replication within the host cells.

Aspergillosis: The fungus *Aspergillus* spp. can grow anywhere in the respiratory system including the windpipe, particularly around the syrinx. This can produce a lesion that blocks the windpipe in a matter of days. This condition is particularly common in raptors and many Psittaciformes such as African grey parrots. Diagnosis is discussed below.

Air sac mites: The air sac mite *Sternostoma tracheacolum* is common in Passeriformes such as canaries, Lady Gouldian finches and goldfinches where they prefer the trachea and bronchi, and cause dyspnoea. The mites may be seen if the feathers of the neck region are wetted and a bright, cold light is shone from behind the bird. The mites are silhouetted as dark pinheads moving within the trachea.

Another form of air sac mite, *Cytodites nudus*, is seen in waterfowl, and produces dyspnoea often with a cough.

Avian cholera: This is a disease of waterfowl caused by the bacterium *Pasteurella multocida*. It causes a thick mucoid discharge from the mouth and trachea, dyspnoea and often death in young birds. A related bacterium, *Reimerella* (*Pasteurella*) *anatipestifer*, will cause tracheal and upper airway discharge in ducklings and a condition known as duck septicaemia. It is a common cause of mortality.

Lungs and air sacs

The absence of a diaphragm in avian species means that any disease causing fluid retention or production, such as liver damage, has the potential to affect breathing. This is particularly so when a thin-walled air sac ruptures and allows fluid to access the respiratory system. The bird may then become suddenly severely dyspnoeic.

Chlamydia psittaci infection: This bacterium produces the condition chlamydiosis, also known as ornithosis and psittacosis and is a serious zoonosis.

Psittacosis refers to the condition in Psittaciformes, ornithosis to the condition in other avian species and chlamydiosis may be applied to both. The bacterium is of great significance, first because of its widespread presence, particularly in the smaller species such as cockatiels and budgerigars, and second because birds may act as carriers of the bacteria for months to years without necessarily showing any signs of disease. They may shed the bacterium intermittently, which can make detection of carriers difficult. Infection rates in one recent study of Psittaciformes suggested that 12.6% of birds were infected (Nemeth *et al.*, 2016).

The disease is spread via faecal, oral and respiratory secretions and feather dander and evidence shows it may also be transferred from the hen bird through the egg to her offspring. Different strains of the bacteria affect different species of bird. Not all strains are as potent, either to the bird or to humans. The strain of *C. psittaci* seen in Psittaciformes for example is more virulent and more zoonotic than the strains seen in pigeons, waterfowl and other species.

Pigeons are commonly affected by chlamydiosis, showing persistent conjunctivitis and sneezing, and the conjunctivitis may affect only one eye (so-called 'one-eye cold'). Conversely, in species such as the macaw family, the first sign of psittacosis may be sudden death.

Chlamydia psittaci can infect almost every internal organ, including the spleen, the liver and the kidneys. It has also been reported as a cause of otitis media, meningoencephalitis and bursitis. It would be more accurate therefore, in species such as the Psittaciformes, to consider chlamydiosis as a systemic disease often with respiratory symptoms.

Diagnosis of chlamydiosis: Because of the intermittent shedding of the bacteria that frequently occurs in carriers, no one diagnostic technique is 100% accurate (sensitive). Radiography and white blood cell counts are useful, as infected Psittaciformes often have markedly enlarged spleens on radiography and white blood cell counts in excess of 30×10^9/L with a significant heterophilia. Liver leakage enzymes (e.g. aspartate aminotransferase, AST) are also often elevated and the faeces may be loose with the uric acid (white) portion of the dropping turning mustard yellow to lime green (due to biliverdinuria).

The standard test is a PCR used to detect the bacteria in droppings, respiratory secretions or, on post-mortem, from internal organs. Because of intermittent shedding, faecal testing may not detect all cases but collecting droppings over 3–5 days helps to minimise false negatives. Alternatively, a single swab taken from the conjunctiva, choana (slit in the hard palate that communicates with the nasal passages and sinuses) and cloaca (in that order) can also be submitted for PCR testing and has been shown to be more sensitive in smaller psittacine species such as cockatiels (Balsamo *et al.*, 2017).

Commercial antibody tests detect antibodies (IgY) produced by the bird's immune system, and so may be beneficial in testing birds that are carriers of the disease but not shedding it into the environment. The disadvantage of any antibody test is that the bird may test positive, even though it may not currently be infected, due to historic disease and also may test negative and yet be infected if it is immunosuppressed or in the early stages of the disease before antibody production occurs.

Chlamydiosis is a significant zoonosis: all humans are susceptible, but those most at risk include:

- The very young
- The very old
- Those on immunosuppressive medication (e.g. corticosteroids, chemotherapy)
- Those with immunosuppressive diseases (e.g. diabetes mellitus, AIDS).

If the owner falls into one of these categories, then serious thought should be given to rehoming or even euthanasing the bird.

In a pet shop situation, where the public are at risk, the affected livestock must be removed from public areas into a specific quarantined area. All handlers of birds during the treatment period should wear suitable face masks and protective clothing when in the same airspace as the birds. Faeces should be incinerated.

The owner should also be informed of the symptoms of chlamydiosis in humans, and advised to contact their medical doctor immediately to receive testing and/or medication if any of these occur.

The symptoms of chlamydiosis in humans include all or some of the following:

- A dry, non-productive cough
- Flu-like muscle pains and fever
- Migraines
- Kidney and liver damage
- Dyspnoea
- Heart damage
- Occasionally death.

Despite all of these problems, chlamydiosis is not a notifiable disease in the UK unless it is diagnosed in domestic poultry or is found on a zoo premises that is approved under so-called 'Balai' (Directive EC 92/65) legislation. This does not, however, diminish the employer's responsibilities under health and safety guidelines to ensure that all staff, as well as owners, are aware of the risks and health hazards, and that all precautions are taken to ensure adequate protection of staff dealing with the infected birds.

Veterinary nurses and technicians are equally obliged to follow practice protocols and health and safety procedures when dealing with positive cases. Protective personal equipment (PPE), particularly appropriate face masks, gloves and disposable outer clothing, are an important part of this.

Aspergillosis: This is the fungal condition caused by *Aspergillus* spp., usually *Aspergillus fumigatus* (although *A. flavus* and *A. niger* have also been reported). This pathogen is found widely in the environment and so any bird may be affected. It has previously been considered as non-infectious from one bird to another, although sporulation can occur inside the avian body and these spores exhaled, so in my opinion spread from bird to bird may occur. Certain environments will contain more airborne microscopic spores of this fungus. These include environments with decomposing vegetation, including the bottom of a parrot cage that has not been cleaned recently. Dietary deficiencies such as hypovitaminosis A and hypovitaminosis B_1 have also been associated with an increased risk of disease. In addition, the presence of mycotoxins from *Aspergillus* spp. in food fed to cage birds can increase their susceptibility to infection (Li *et al.*, 2015).

Certain species are very susceptible, including most raptors (e.g. gyrfalcons, golden eagles, northern goshawks and snowy owls) and many penguins (e.g. gentoo and king penguins). In Psittaciformes, all species can suffer from this condition, but African grey parrots are most commonly reported.

Younger birds are more commonly affected than adults. Aspergillosis may also be seen in birds that are immunosuppressed due to concurrent illness (e.g. PBFD in young African grey parrots) or immunosuppressive medication (e.g. corticosteroids).

The fungal spores settle out on the surface of the respiratory tract, particularly in the region of the syrinx, the abdominal air sacs and the lung structure itself. In penguins an orientation towards the cranial air sacs and lungs is more commonly seen and may be related to their differing lungs that have more paleopulmonic structure than neopulmonic (see Chapter 9). This can lead to blockage of an airway or, in the case of the syrinx, may obstruct the windpipe leading to an acute crisis. In any case it can lead to the production of large balls of fungus, or fungal granulomas that are commonly seen particularly within the air sacs and lungs (see Figure 13.13).

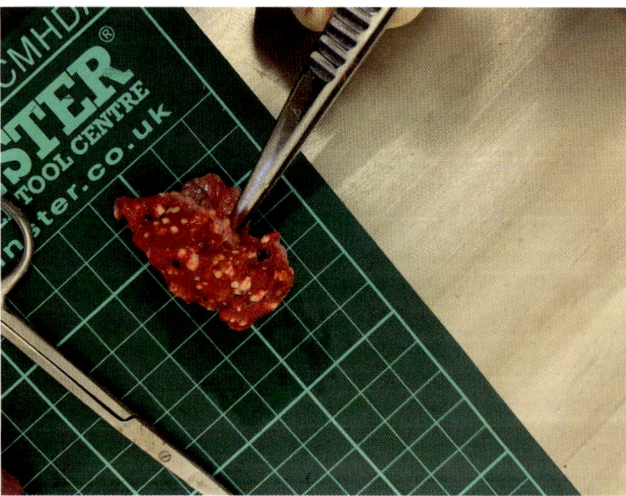

Figure 13.13 Post-mortem of a bird lung with aspergillosis showing the fungal growth as a series of caseous granulomas.

The fungus can also invade the bloodstream and be transported to other organs, such as the liver, kidneys and CNS, resulting in other signs relevant to the organ affected. In addition, it may invade adjacent organs or structures such as the spinal cord in the case of the caudal thoracic and abdominal air sac infections, leading to pelvic limb dysfunction.

Aspergillus spp. can also produce toxins such as aflatoxin. This is highly toxic to birds and rapidly causes liver damage, failure and death. In addition, a gliotoxin may also be released causing CNS damage with paresis, fitting and other neurological signs being observed.

Diagnosis of aspergillosis: Full blood cell counts are useful as the condition will often cause a markedly elevated white blood cell count ($>30 \times 10^9$/L) with a significant heterophilia and often monocytosis (see Figure 13.14). Radiographs are useful for showing thickening of the air sacs, and any fungal granulomas within them. Computed tomography (CT) scans are also extremely helpful in showing spread of the fungus through the lung structure and other organs.

Rigid endoscopy is frequently essential to examine the syrinx and the internal air sacs, allowing sampling for culture and potential debulking of any fungal granulomas.

Tracheal and lung washes may be performed with sterile saline (0.5–1 mL/kg of bird) flushed into the trachea of the anaesthetised bird, and then immediately aspirated.

Recent work has confirmed the difficulty in diagnosing aspergillosis:

1. Antibody results can be positive in birds not currently infected with aspergillosis and negative due to anergic responses.
2. *Aspergillus* galactomannan tests used in humans for invasive aspergillosis can also produce positive results in non-infected birds although confirmed cases had 2.6 times the levels than presumptive healthy birds.

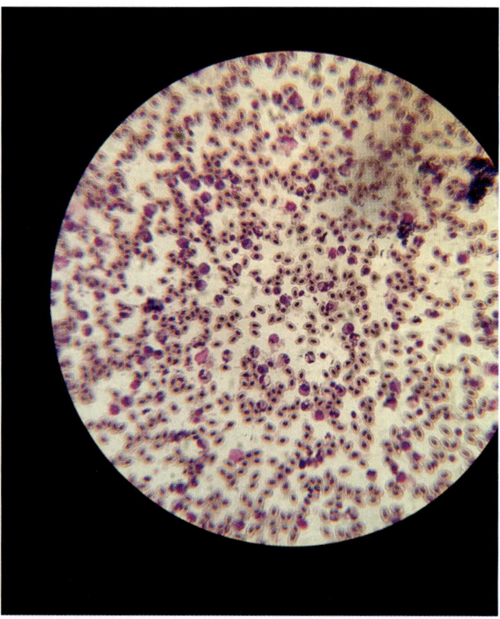

Figure 13.14 Romanowsky-stained blood smear from a bird with aspergillosis. Note the heterophilia and monocytosis.

3. Derangements in the plasma protein electrophoresis trace were 2.4 times more likely in positive cases than healthy ones, with specific elevations of beta- and gamma-globulins (Cray *et al.*, 2009, 2010). Girling (2002) describes typical plasma protein electrophoresis responses to aspergillosis in a number of psittacine species. Variations in response which are dependent on species and sexual maturity include the following: *Ara* spp. produced a significantly higher alpha-1 globulin level when infected compared with other psittacines, whereas *Psittacus* spp. and *Amazona* spp. produced a higher alpha-2 globulin response; elevations in beta-globulins were significant in cases of aspergillosis, and across the species elevations above 3.5 times normal were considered significant indicators of aspergillosis. Work by Naylor *et al.* (2017) showed that plasma protein electrophoresis was helpful in predicting survivability of gentoo penguins affected by aspergillosis as those with a total plasma albumin (pre-albumin plus albumin) of less than 26 g/L generally did not survive treatment.
4. Use of lateral flow devices to sample respiratory mucus from the glottis and blood samples for *Aspergillus* spp. antigens have been shown to be effective in gentoo penguins (Mota *et al.*, 2023).

Paramyxovirus/Newcastle disease: This is a condition seen primarily in domestic poultry and pigeons and is important, as Newcastle disease (PMV-1) and pigeon paramyxovirus 1 are both notifiable due to their ability to cause mortality and debility in commercial poultry. This means suspicion or confirmation of the disease must be reported to the relevant government veterinary authority; in the UK, this is currently the Animal and Plant Health Agency (APHA) which is part of the Department of the Environment, Farming and Rural Affairs (DEFRA).

Symptoms of paramyxovirus disease may include:

- Dyspnoea
- Tachypnoea
- Periocular oedema
- Listlessness and neurological signs, e.g. wing drooping
- Head tilt and circling (torticollis)
- Diarrhoea with biliverdinuria (yellow/green urates)
- In chickens, a drop in egg production and eggs produced with soft shells
- Sudden death.

The virus is thought to be transmitted via droppings, but this can be disseminated on the feet of carers and wheels of vehicles so good biosecurity and the use of appropriate disinfectant foot-dips is important to prevent spread. Diagnosis is based on the symptoms and confirmation is made by both serology using viral haemagglutination inhibition tests and demonstration of the viral antigen by PCR tests.

Other paramyxoviruses have been recorded in birds and are not notifiable. Serotype 5 (PMV-5) was seen in the 1970s in budgerigars, manifested by depression, diarrhoea and high mortality. Serotype 3 (PMV-3) has been reported in small psittacines more recently causing torticollis and circling and has been associated with pancreatitis in cockatiels (Jung *et al.*, 2009).

Influenza virus disease: Avian influenza (AI) viruses are all of type A, enveloped single-stranded RNA viruses belonging to the *Orthomyxoviridae* family and have high genetic variability. They are classified in a number of ways, including the properties of the outer envelope haemagglutinin (HA) and neuraminidase (NA) glycoproteins. These give rise to the commonly used 'H' and 'N' classification for AI viruses, for example strain H5N1. AI viruses are also classified according to their pathogenicity, for example high pathogenic AI (HPAI) and low pathogenic AI (LPAI), with LPAI often producing few clinical signs in infected birds. All known HPAI are of the H5 or H7 haemagglutinin subtype (although confusingly not all H5 and H7 strains are HPAI). In HPAI virus infection (e.g. H5N1), widespread mortality with peracute deaths in domestic poultry and many wild and exotic species of bird is reported. Significant declines in wild species of seabird in particular have been reported in the UK and elsewhere, with the UK and Irish northern gannet (*Morus bassanus*) population for example being significantly reduced in 2022 by up to 30% (Paradell *et al.*, 2023; Scottish Seabird Centre, 2024). Interestingly, in gannets surviving infection, changes in the colour of the iris (from pale blue to navy blue or black), with pupil shape alterations were noted, suggestive of a previous iritis and corneal oedema (Hodgkinson and Chamberlain, 2023).

Other clinical signs in captive and wild birds can include:

- Cyanosis of mucous membranes with severe respiratory disease
- Haemorrhages under the skin
- Neurological disease (wing drooping, leg weakness/paralysis and torticollis)
- Diarrhoea with biliverdinuria (yellow/green urates)
- Cessation or significant drop in egg production.

However, it is possible for certain species of birds, such as waterfowl and gulls, to carry the virus asymptomatically and so introduce the virus to new areas. In pigeons infected experimentally with HPAI, gross pathological findings were mild and confined to the nervous system with lymphohistiocytic meningoencephalitis (Klopfleisch *et al.*, 2006).

If certain strains are isolated or suspected due to the severity of clinical signs (H5 and H7) they are, like Newcastle disease, notifiable to government authorities (again in the UK to APHA) and compulsory culling of birds will be enforced in the UK, European Union and many countries around the world.

Prevention of infection should involve the use of virucidal footbaths (in the UK these ideally should be DEFRA approved and used at the correct dilution), careful storage of feed to prevent spoiling by wildlife and avoiding wearing the same clothing outside the aviary system. Indoor or at least under-netting housing of birds is also considered important to reduce contact with wild species, and recently national housing orders have become commonplace in the UK during times of high AI prevalence. Commercial quarantine aviaries should have completely separate airspaces for separate consignments. Negative pressure ventilation systems are also advised. New arrivals should be quarantined for a minimum of 30 days before being introduced to the rest of the collection. In the face of an outbreak, it may be possible in some countries to vaccinate valuable and genetically rare avian species to prevent infection (in the European Union and UK under EU Decision 2006/474) but if a bird still becomes infected then currently management still involves the culling of these birds.

It is worth noting that AI viruses are zoonotic and while serious disease in humans is uncommon, mortalities have been reported. Mortalities have also been reported in other mammals, most recently in October 2023 when H5N1 caused significant mortalities in southern elephant seal (*Mirounga leonina*) pups in Argentina (Campagna *et al.*, 2023).

Bacterial pneumonias and air sacculitis: Psittacosis has already been mentioned and may result in bacterial pneumonia and air sacculitis.

Mycoplasmosis: *Mycoplasma* spp. have been isolated from most species of bird. In many pigeons and small passerine and psittacine birds, clinical signs include conjunctivitis and upper respiratory disease. *Mycoplasma. gallisepticum* has been implicated in many of these outbreaks.

Others are due to secondary bacterial infections such as those occurring in raptors after infestation by the raptor air-sac mite *Serratospiculum* spp.

Diagnosis is made on clinical signs, full blood cell counts, full body radiographs and the use of PCR and in some cases serological tests to show exposure to *Mycoplasma* spp.

Pasteurellosis: *Pasteurella multocida* is the cause of avian cholera, with *P. multocida* serotypes 1 and 3 seen most commonly. In passerine birds, the disease is usually spread via aerosol or contaminated equipment. In raptors, it often gains access to the body via infected prey, causing an oesophagitis and pharyngitis and can lead to septicaemia. For falconry birds, vaccination has been recommended using commercial polyvalent killed *Pasteurella* vaccines (Willette *et al.*, 2009).

Other bacteria: *Aeromonas* spp. and *Pseudomonas* spp. have been reported in cases of upper respiratory tract and gastrointestinal disease (the former may present as a septicaemic syndrome as well). *Bordetella avium* can cause an upper respiratory tract infection and has been associated with the lockjaw syndrome in cockatiels where the beak becomes fixed and cannot open. *Klebsiella pneumoniae*, *K. ozaenae* and *K. oxytoca* have all been associated with contaminated water whether for drinking or in incubators. They tend to colonise the gut first and then spread via the bloodstream to the respiratory tract.

Enterococcus faecalis has been linked to chronic tracheitis, air sacculitis and pneumonia in canaries.

Diagnosis is made on clinical signs, full blood cell counts, full body radiographs and of course culture and identification of the bacteria where possible.

Respiratory toxins: Birds are extremely sensitive to the odourless fumes given off by overheated Teflon-coated pans. The consequence can be a reaction causing pulmonary oedema with severe dyspnoea and often death before treatment can be initiated. A similar situation is seen with poisoning due to the toxic fumes from smoke or cooking fat inhalation. Birds should never be kept in a room where cooking occurs.

Cardiovascular disease

Heart disease

Cardiac neoplasia

Tumours of the heart are not common but fibrosarcoma, haemangioma, haemangiosarcoma, lymphosarcoma, melanosarcoma, rhabdomyoma and rhabdomyosarcomas have been reported (Fitzgerald and Beaufrere, 2016).

Cardiomyopathy

Dilated cardiomyopathy has been reported in birds and is associated with rapid growth, hypoxia, high altitude, furazolidone, monensin and sodium toxicities, vitamin E and selenium deficiencies, rancid fat in the diet and inbreeding (Strunk and Wilson, 2005). It is common in poultry, particularly young turkey poults. Diagnosis ante-mortem can be challenging as many cases are clinically 'silent' with first presentation being the sudden death of the bird. Diagnostic radiography has suggested that the cardiac width (CW) in psittacine birds such as African grey parrots, orange-winged Amazons and Senegal parrots on a ventrodorsal view should be between 51 and 61% of the width of the body at the level of the widest part of the body/thorax (usually the fifth pair of ribs) (Straub *et al.*, 2002). In raptors various formulas have been derived but, as in mammals, these are species-specific. For example, in the peregrine falcon (*Falco peregrinus*), Lumeij *et al.* (2011) calculated expected CW in millimetres as follows:

$$\text{CW} = 0.83 \times \text{sternal width} \\ \left(\text{at the level of widest cardiac width}\right) + 0.83$$

Hypertrophic cardiomyopathy has also been reported and the mechanism by which this develops appears to be the same as for mammals, namely atherosclerosis and pulmonary hypertension. Examples include an excess of salt (NaCl) in the diet of young birds leading to hypertension that leads to left ventricular hypertrophy. Right ventricular hypertrophy is commonly seen where pulmonary fibrosis (e.g. secondary to *Mycoplasma* and viral pneumonia and also allergic pneumonitis) occurs.

Congenital heart defects

With the success of breeding programmes to produce colour variants, the incidence of congenital heart defects has increased. Congenital cardiac and left ventricular aneurysms have been identified in cockatiels and blue and gold macaws (Schmidt *et al.*, 2003). Congenital aortic hypoplasia has also been reported in a Moluccan cockatoo and a ventricular septal defect with persistent truncus arteriosus in an umbrella cockatoo (Evans *et al.*, 2001).

Endocardiosis

This has been reported in birds particularly in the left AV valve, resulting in insufficiency as with mammals. It is more commonly seen in older birds (see Figure 13.15).

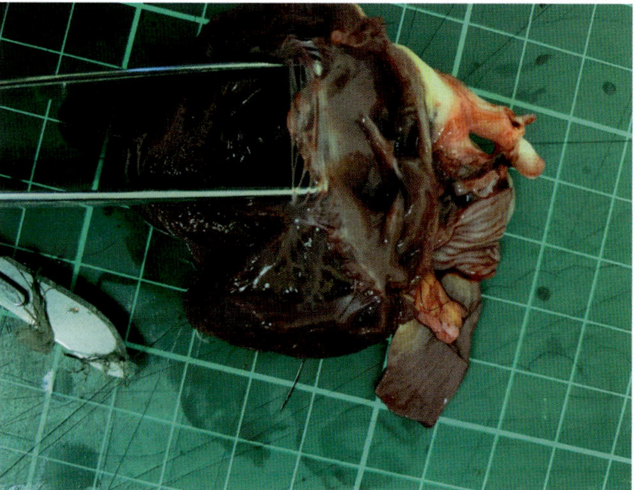

Figure 13.15 Endocardiosis with secondary heart failure is also seen in older pet birds.

Vegetative endocarditis and myocarditis

Chlamydiosis can lead to myocardial damage, as can a number of septicaemic and bacteraemic conditions. It can also lead to vegetative endocarditis.

Streptococcus gallolyticus (formerly known as *S. bovis*) has resulted in acute/peracute death of pigeons. Initial clinical signs include inability to fly and drooping wings followed by anorexia, polyuria/polydipsia, green urates and ascites. Peracute cases have evidence of septicaemia with pericarditis.

Many Gram-negative bacteria such as *E. coli*, *Klebsiella* spp. and *Pseudomonas* spp. can also lead to syndromes such as vegetative endocarditis.

Mycobacterial disease has also been associated with myocarditis and pericarditis.

Parasites such as those causing toxoplasmosis and sarcocystosis have been reported in birds as a cause of myocarditis, heart failure and death.

Viruses such as psittacine polyomavirus and bornavirus (the cause of gastric dilatation disease) can lead to heart nerve damage, arrhythmias and sudden death, with 79% of all positive birds showing cardiac lesions (Gancz *et al.*, 2012). In addition in North America, West Nile virus infection is commonly reported associated with cardiovascular disease in psittacines and wild birds of prey (Saito *et al.*, 2002; Palmieri *et al.*, 2011).

Vascular disease

Arterial calcification

Oversupplementation of calcium and vitamin D_3 may lead to loss of elasticity and increased blood pressure, heart failure and organ damage.

Atherosclerosis

This is often due to lack of exercise and inappropriate, high-fat diets. The major arteries become thickened with cholesterol deposits, their lumen diameter decreases and they become less elastic, so blood pressure increases. Calcification of the plaques often occurs, particularly if excessive amounts of vitamin D_3 and calcium are consumed. This can all lead to cardiac failure and aneurysm development both of which can lead to sudden death.

Serum cholesterol and very low-density lipoprotein levels have been used as a risk indicator for atherosclerosis in psittacine birds (as well as humans). Diet is therefore an important risk factor, with excess dietary cholesterol leading quickly to atherosclerosis. For example, in one study where budgerigars were fed a diet containing 2% cholesterol they developed atherosclerosis within 3 months that progressed to significant pathology by 6 months (Finlayson and Hirchinson, 1961).

Other factors have also been identified in psittacines, including age (birds between 20 and 30 years), female sex (thought to be due to the high circulating lipid levels during breeding) and certain genera (*Psittacus*, grey parrots; *Amazona*, Amazon parrots; *Nymphicus* spp., cockatiels) (Beaufrere *et al.*, 2013). In raptors and psittacine birds, the vessels most likely to be affected include the ascending aorta and the brachiocephalic trunk (Oster and Pariaut, 2021).

Haematological disease

Anaemia may be due to poisoning by heavy metals (e.g. lead or zinc), debilitation or haemoparasites. *Leucocytozoon* spp. inhabit red and white blood cells and cause intravascular haemolysis leading to anaemia, and spleen and liver damage where the parasite multiplies. It is transmitted by blackflies and is known to cause serious problems in young Galliformes, raptors and Anseriformes.

Other significant blood parasites include the malarial parasite *Plasmodium* spp., which can cause severe anaemia, lethargy, vomiting, seizures and death, particularly in penguin species, snowy owls and gyrfalcons and their hybrids. *Plasmodium* spp. are transmitted by *Anopheles* spp. mosquitoes or by direct blood-to-blood transfer during fighting. Clinical signs include mucous membrane pallor, lethargy, haemoglobinuria and death. A common haemoparasite, *Haemoproteus* spp., which inhabits the avian red blood cell, generally does not cause disease. It is transmitted via biting flies (Hippoboscids).

Atoxoplasmosis caused by *Isospora* (*Atoxoplasma*) *serini* in canaries can multiply in the liver resulting in massive liver enlargement (black spot disease) due to the projection of the liver beyond the caudal sternum ventrally. It tends to occur in juvenile canaries aged 2–9 months with clinical signs of general debilitation, diarrhoea and, in around one-fifth of cases, neurological signs. It has been implicated in the 'going-light' syndrome of greenfinches (Cooper *et al.*, 1989). Mortality can be significant, around 80%. Impression smears of the cut surface of the liver and spleen will show the intracellular coccidian in the cytoplasm of monocytes indenting the monocyte nucleus into a crescent shape. Faecal examination is often unrewarding due to the low number of oocysts shed after the initial acute phase of the disease.

Blood-borne leukaemia is uncommon in birds. Much more commonly seen are the tissue-associated lymphomas. Avian type C retrovirus group (avian leukosis-related viruses) includes avian leukosis and sarcoma virus (ALSV). Transmission is both horizontal (faeces and saliva) and vertical via gonadal cells. Female birds are more susceptible than males and the incubation period can be many months. It may result in immunosuppression and has been associated with discrete renal tumours in budgerigars resulting in unilateral leg paralysis.

A type C retrovirus unrelated to ALSV is the cause of lymphoma in turkeys. Marek's disease is a gamma herpesvirus affecting Galliformes, inducing lymphomatous changes in peripheral nerves, bursa, thymus and visceral organs.

Urinary tract

Acute renal disease

Aetiology

Acute renal disease is often due to bacterial causes. It may also be caused by poisons such as zinc antifreeze and chocolate or due to non-steroidal ant-inflammatory drugs (NSAIDs), such as diclofenac that has caused the precipitous decline of white-backed vultures (*Gyps bengalensis*) in India. Viruses such as APV in Psittaciformes and infectious bronchitis virus in Galliformes and bacteria such as *E. coli* and *Chlamydia psittaci* infections have also been implicated (see Figure 13.16). Another cause in geese is the coccidial parasite *Eimeria truncata*, which produces lethargy, rapid weight loss and

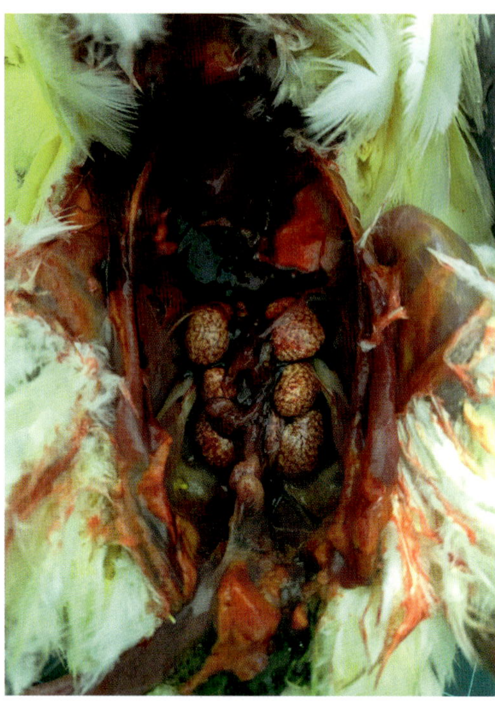

Figure 13.16 Nephritis with renal failure in a parrot. Note the swollen nature of the kidneys and the multiple white streaks of uric acid (gout) throughout the kidneys.

diarrhoea with high mortality rates. An acute syndrome in adult merlins (*Falco columbarius*) exists where the kidneys become damaged by fatty degeneration, the bird often dying in good body condition. Its exact aetiology is unknown. Acute renal failure may also be due to shock – cardiogenic or, more commonly, hypovolaemic.

Diagnosis

PCR tests are available for many viral diseases such as polyomavirus and bacteria such as *Chlamydia* spp. Otherwise, it is based on clinical signs such as anuria or oliguria, and extreme depression, with a history of exposure to the relevant poison. Blood tests may show a massively elevated uric acid level (>1500 µmol/L) and sometimes potassium levels (>5 mmol/L). It should be noted that a moderate rise in uric acid levels will occur, particularly in raptors, for several hours after a meal. Urea levels may also be measured and compared with uric acid levels to ascertain if prerenal azotaemia or renal disease is present, as prerenal azotaemia will cause a predominant rise in urea. The problem is the ratios need to be worked out for each species – the ratio is calculated by multiplying the plasma urea level (in mmol/L) by 1000 and then comparing it with plasma uric acid level (in µmol/L). In peregrine falcons, the ratio is greater than 6.5 (Lumeij, 2000). Birds are often anuric with acute renal failure and so urinalysis is not possible.

Chronic renal disease

Aetiology

As with acute nephritis, this has a number of causes.

1. Toxicity/poisonings (e.g. lead, use of nephrotoxic drugs such as some NSAIDs and aminoglycosides)
2. Chronic infection
   a. Bacterial (e.g. *Pseudomonas* spp.)
   b. Viral (e.g. infectious bronchitis, pigeon herpesvirus, psittacine herpes and reovirus and psittacine polyomavirus)
   c. Fungal (e.g. aspergillosis)
   d. Parasitic (e.g. microsporidia such as *Encephalitozoon hellum* and some coccidia, e.g. *Eimeria truncata* in geese)
3. Excessive levels of calcium and vitamin D_3 in the diet
4. Long-term excessive levels of protein in the diets of Psittaciformes
5. Neoplasia (e.g. ALSV in budgerigars which can be associated with adenocarcinomas and nephroblastomas, but also lymphoma)
6. Chronic dehydration (e.g. in hens incubating eggs)
7. Renal lipidosis (e.g. Galliform chicks, adult merlins correlated with a high-fat/low-protein diet, starvation, biotin deficiency and chronic liver disease)
8. Amyloidosis (e.g. aged waterfowl)
9. Hypovitaminosis A as this vitamin controls epithelial turnover including proximal tubular epithelium and a deficiency leads to squamous metaplasia and dysfunction.

Bacteria may enter the kidneys either via reflux or via the ureters from the cloaca, or via the bloodstream directly from the intestinal tract due to the renal portal system that exists in birds.

Excessive supplementation of calcium and vitamin D_3 can lead to calcification of soft tissue structures, leading to renal calcinosis and failure.

In laying hens, renal urolithiasis, which can lead to post-renal failure due to blockage of the renal tubules, occurs due to the high circulating calcium levels present during egg-laying, some of which overspill into the urine. This may be exacerbated if the bird becomes egg-bound due to pressure on the kidneys, so restricting renal blood flow and creating ischaemia.

ALSV infection in budgerigars results in renal tumours in birds of 3–6 years old. Clinically, this may present as unilateral limb paresis/paralysis due to pressure on the ischiatic nerve that passes through the kidney, or with coelomic distension and no other clinical signs. Other suspected ALSV infections have been reported in psittacine birds, Galliformes, Columbiformes and passerine birds resulting in lymphoid neoplasia often in the liver, spleen or kidneys.

Diagnosis

Diagnosis of chronic renal disease in birds is based on a number of tests.

1. Uric acid measurement exceeding 500 µmol/L. This test should be performed in a fasting bird, as (particularly in the meat-eating raptors and penguins) a recent meal can elevate the levels falsely and fasting in larger species may require 24 hours.
2. Elevations in plasma/serum potassium levels above 5 mmol/L may be seen in terminal renal failure and this is often associated with cardiac arrhythmias such as heart block.
3. Excessively high levels of total calcium (>3 mmol/L) suggesting oversupplementation, providing the bird is not an in-lay hen, when blood levels may rise high normally due to calcium mobilisation for shell production.
4. Radiography may show kidney enlargement in the case of nephritis and tumours. It will also show increased radiodensity in cases of calcinosis. Normally, the avian kidney is difficult to see as it is located in the roof of the synsacrum, but with renomegaly it often

projects cranially in front of the ilium on a lateral view. Urography may be used to assess renal excretion. The ulnar vein is typically used and iodine-based contrast is injected at 2 mL/kg with the first view being taken after 30 seconds. The dye should have reached the ureters by 1 minute post injection.

5. Ultrasound examination is difficult owing to the presence of air sacs. However, it may be of use in some species where the probe can be placed on the lateral body wall without coming up against the ribcage (e.g. Galliformes and Columbiformes) and where large neoplasms are present.
6. Urinalysis: green urates indicate biliverdinuria and liver disease. Normal urine specific gravity in birds tends to be 1.005–1.020. The pH is variable but is between 6 and 8 depending on species and diet fed (more acidic in laying hens and carnivores and more alkaline in bacterial nephritis cases and herbivores/frugivores). Ketones may be found in cases of beta-oxidation of fats, which can occur in disease but also during migration stress. An examination for protein or fat casts should be made. Small numbers of red cells and bacteria (from faecal contamination) and uric acid crystals are normal. Large amounts of blood may indicate heavy metal toxicosis or neoplasia. Protein levels up to 2 g/L are normal. Glucose levels should be low. High levels of glutamate dehydrogenase (GLDH) indicate severe kidney cell damage. The presence of coccidia or cryptosporidia is of course also significant. Rosskopf *et al.* (1986) describes the change from granular/cellular casts to haemoglobin casts as resolution of an inflammatory process. Finally, early work on measurement of *N*-acetyl-beta-D-glucosaminidase (NAG) in the urine of birds has shown that its levels increase when tubular damage occurs, but normal values are not currently available for birds.
7. Blood pressure monitoring may show hypertension with systolic blood pressures in excess of 200 mmHg with chronic renal failure (see also Chapter 16).

Renal biopsy can be used to ascertain definitive diagnoses of the condition. This can be performed through a left or right flank approach using rigid endoscopy.

Renal failure will lead to a build-up of uric acid, which rapidly reaches its saturation point. After this, crystals of uric acid form in the bloodstream and adhere to vital structures. This causes encasement of these structures in the hard, white crystalline uric acid, further damaging them.

Sites initially and preferentially found with uric acid deposits (visceral gout) include the kidneys themselves (see Figure 13.16), the heart, pericardial sac, liver and of course the joints.

Renal urolithiasis

Renal urolithiasis is common in laying hens. It can lead to renal failure due to blockage of the renal tubules. It occurs because of the high levels of calcium that circulate during egg-laying, some of which spills over into the urine. The situation may be exacerbated if the bird becomes egg-bound, pressing on the kidneys, restricting renal blood flow and creating renal ischaemia.

Renal tumours

Renal tumours are common (e.g. budgerigars) often due to ALSV as described earlier.

Reproductive tract disease

Egg binding

This is the most common complaint of the avian reproductive system. There is a history of compulsive egg-laying and poor diet, in the case of indoor psittacine birds one high in seeds without supplementation and therefore low in calcium and vitamin D_3. The hen bird becomes lethargic and dull and sits on the floor of its cage. Egg abnormalities or uterine rupture may also contribute, with increased incidence in chickens associated with environmental conditions that are too cold.

Diagnosis of egg binding: Clinical signs plus palpation of the egg if it is situated in the lower reproductive tract, just caudal to the sternum. Radiography is useful for more cranially situated eggs.

Egg yolk coelomitis

This is a life-threatening condition where internal laying of yolks and their rupture occurs. If the yolk ruptures, the lipids it contains cause an intense inflammatory reaction and coelomitis. This may then become secondarily infected. In any case, it often generates an inflammatory response including a raised white cell count (often $>30 \times 10^9$/L). There is often a history of regular egg-laying followed by a cessation and then lethargy and collapse. It is more regularly seen in cockatiels, budgerigars, macaws and of course domestic Galliformes such as the chicken. Diagnosis can be confirmed with ultrasound and needle aspiration, although care should be taken to avoid puncture of air sacs.

Hyperoestrogenism

This is commonly seen in compulsive egg-laying hen birds which may enter a state of consistent egg production and hyperoestrogenism. Increased medullary bone deposition is one of the most obvious clinical signs, easily observed radiographically with increased bone density particularly in the tibiotarsus and femur bones, although some believe it can occur in any part of the skeleton but with a predilection for those two sites (Canoville *et al.*, 2019). Because of increased oestrogen levels, other problems such as progressive non-regenerative anaemia and ventral body wall ('abdominal') midline herniation are commonly seen and may lead to serious consequences.

Neoplasia

Ovarian tumours are the most commonly seen female reproductive tract tumour. They can enlarge dramatically and so cause dyspnoea and may be associated with abdominal distension, increased medullary bone deposition in long bones (due to hyperoestrogenism) and ventral abdominal hernias. Adenocarcinomas, adenomas and granulosa cell tumours are the most commonly reported. They may be associated with leg paresis in the same way as kidney neoplasia.

A similar problem is seen in males as testicular neoplasia, involving one or both testes, is also commonly seen in budgerigars. These tumours may metastasise to the liver. Most are inoperable due to their size and vascularity. Some testicular tumours produce oestrogens and so may result in medullary bone deposition, as may be seen in compulsive egg-laying female birds, and may also be associated with changes in secondary sexual characteristics, such as the colour of the cere of male budgerigars changing from blue to the more typically female brown (Hoggard and Craig, 2022). They may also be associated with abdominal herniation.

Prolapsed oviduct

This may be a sequel to egg binding and often involves prolapse of the cloaca as well. Tissues become rapidly desiccated and infected if outside of the body.

Salpingitis

Salpingitis is also known by the name of vent gleet because of the discharge from the cloaca which accompanies it. It is due to infection of the uterus, the more caudal portion of the reproductive tract or salpinx. Signs may vary from non-specific malaise, with a bird becoming intermittently dull and lethargic, to an obvious purulent discharge. Egg-laying may produce malformed eggs or may cease altogether.

Musculoskeletal disease

Articular gout

Articular gout is seen commonly in older cage and aviary birds and can occur with chronic renal disease. It may also occur in joints and tendon sheaths in birds where there is hyperuricaemia, whether that is due to renal failure or dehydration. Uric acid crystals in gout deposits are needle-like in shape and are believed to be the reason why increased pain occurs, unlike the urates produced normally through the urinary tract which have been bound with proteins and so are spherical in shape. Suspected articular gout deposits obtained by aspiration from affected joints can be used to positively identify uric acid using the murexide test: a drop of nitric acid is added to the aspiration, which is then flame-dried and a drop of concentrated ammonia is added that results in a purple/mauve colouration.

Carpometacarpal luxation

This condition is often known by its colloquial name of 'angel wing' and is seen commonly in budgerigars, macaws, chickens, geese and many other waterfowl. It describes a condition where the carpometacarpal joints in either wing rotate and subluxate so that the distal primary feathers point dorsally giving a fan-like (angel) appearance. It is thought that the condition may have a connection with calcium/vitamin D_3 deficiency (rickets) combined with an excess of dietary protein levels, and so is viewed as a developmental or growth deformity. The condition is often seen around the time of the emergence of the primary feathers as when they emerge these are heavy due to being filled with blood within their protective developmental sheaths. This extra weight on the distal wing causes lateral rotation of the distal wing and so carpometacarpal luxation.

Fractures

The assessment of injuries is essential to triage patients. Fractures occur commonly in many cage and aviary birds. The fractures which occur are often open fractures due to the brittle nature of the bones, which produce very sharp fragments. Any bird that has injuries so bad that a leg needs to be amputated should be considered for euthanasia as no bird manages well on one leg, particularly if they weigh over 150 g. Wing amputations will likely mean the refusal to release wild birds due to their inability to either escape predation or search for food or both. In addition there is likely to be no breeding potential for males as they usually cannot mount the female successfully to mate without the balancing force of two wings. Chapter 14 details the prognosis and management of a variety of avian bone fractures.

Nutritional osteodystrophy/metabolic bone disease

Nutritional osteodystrophy is due to a deficiency in vitamin D_3 and calcium. Several syndromes are seen. The most common is bowing of the tibiotarsal and tarsometatarsal bones. This is because the weight of the growing bird cannot be properly supported by the poorly mineralised bones. In addition, angel wing can be seen when the primary feathers emerge leading to carpometacarpal subluxations and unless corrected permanent inability to fly. Often the diets of the birds have high levels of protein as well as low calcium and vitamin D_3, promoting rapid growth and further exacerbating the situation.

Perosis

Perosis is a developmental condition and so seen in younger chicks, particularly Galliformes, and affects the intertarsal joint. The groove in which the Achilles tendon runs over the intertarsal joint is too shallow, so allowing the tendon to slip laterally or medially resulting in an inability to extend the intertarsal joint and lower limb. It is thought this may be associated with a deficiency in manganese, choline and zinc (see Figure 13.17.

Pinwheel

Pinwheel is a developmental deformity of the stifle (knee) joint of young pigeons. It occurs typically around 2–4 weeks of age. The squab cannot flex its stifle, and since only one leg is usually affected, it leads to the circling or pinwheeling, which gives the condition its name. It seems to occur in well-fed chicks reared in flat-bottomed nests with little nesting material and is exacerbated by a poor calcium and vitamin D_3 diet. Prevention is the key to success. Treatment is usually ineffective.

Neurological disease

Fitting/seizures

This condition has many aetiologies, including:

- Trauma (flying into glass windows, etc.)
- Nutrition (hypoglycaemia, hypocalcaemia, hypovitaminosis B_1)
- Heavy metal poisoning (lead and zinc primarily)

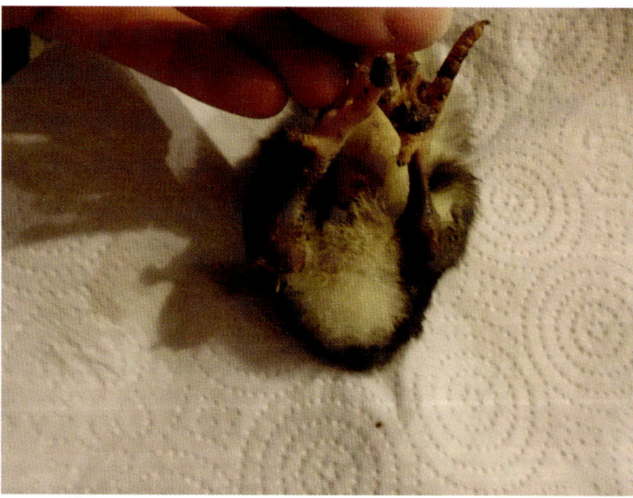

Figure 13.17 Perosis resulting in slipping of the Achilles tendon in the right leg of a domestic chicken.

- Plant and pesticide poisons
- Meningoencephalitis (bacterial, fungal, viral or protozoal)
- Organopathy (particularly hepatic disease)
- Idiopathic epilepsy (reported in red-lored Amazons)
- Vestibular disease (again typically viral, bacterial or fungal in aetiology)
- Cardiovascular disease (fat emboli during egg production, atherosclerosis)
- Neoplasia
- Congenital CNS disease (cerebellar hypoplasia seen in lutino colour birds)
- Metabolic (hypocalcaemia, hypoglycaemia, etc.).

The breed of bird may suggest a condition, for example a fitting African grey parrot between the ages of 2 and 4 years may well have hypocalcaemia syndrome, and waterfowl are prone to lead poisoning from consumption of lead shot and fishing tackle weights.

Heavy metal toxicosis

Heavy metal toxicosis is common in Psittaciformes, waterfowl and raptors. In raptors, it is often due to feeding wild lead-shot prey. In waterfowl, it is often due to their consumption of environmental abandoned lead fishing weights or spent lead shot from shotgun discharges. In Psittaciformes, it may be due to lead paints on woodwork of old buildings, lead strips on windows/kitchen units, pewter ware/wine tops, etc.

Zinc poisoning is generally a disease of Psittaciformes and may be associated with housing in zinc-galvanised cages. The parrot manoeuvres itself around the cage using beak and feet and so will take in small amounts of zinc oxide; after 4–6 weeks enough may have been consumed to cause toxicity.

In all cases of heavy metal poisoning, a range of clinical signs can be seen that include weakness, paresis (raptors often rock back onto their intertarsal joints with one foot holding the other, waterfowl have serpentine necks and are unable to fly), liver problems (diarrhoea and biliverdinuria), regurgitation/ileus, kidney failure (polydipsia/polyuria), anaemia and fitting. Diagnosis is made on clinical signs and confirmed by radiography, which demonstrates metal particles in the gizzard, and blood levels of lead greater than 0.2 ppm or zinc greater than 2 ppm (see section on digestive disease for more details).

Other causes of neurological disease

Egg binding

Egg binding is a common cause of bilateral hindlimb paresis and paralysis in hen birds. The egg becomes stuck in the pelvic inlet, placing pressure on the nerves in the roof of the pelvis/synsacrum that innervate the legs. Radiography will aid in diagnosing this condition.

Hyperglycaemia

One or two species of raptor (e.g. northern goshawk) are prone to hyperglycaemia that may result in seizures. In this species hyperglycaemia is more likely when retraining at the start of the season occurs and the bird is overweight. Blood glucose levels often exceed 30 mmol/L (normal range 12–17 mmol/L).

Hypocalcaemic syndrome of African grey parrots

This is commonly seen in African grey parrots between the ages of 2 and 4 years. It occurs where, although bone calcium quality is adequate, the parrot is unable to mobilise calcium reserves to maintain blood calcium levels. This is often compounded by a low calcium and vitamin D_3 diet commonly associated with feeding unsupplemented seeds such as sunflower and peanuts. This leads to hypocalcaemia, muscular weakness, tremors, collapse, fits and death. Ionised calcium is the biologically active form of the mineral and so is preferred over total calcium when measuring blood levels. Blood ionised calcium levels should be 0.96–1.22 mmol/L in healthy African grey parrots (Stanford, 2003).

Hypoglycaemia seizure/collapse

In the case of small raptors, such as kestrels, sparrowhawks, etc., that have a high metabolic rate, the condition of hypoglycaemia is seen in malnourished or highly stressed birds. There is often a history of being flown in poor weather and failure to monitor body weight regularly during the flying season.

Kidney disease

Any form of kidney disease which results in swelling of the renal parenchyma can theoretically place pressure on the leg nerves and so produce varying signs of paresis and paralysis of the pelvic limbs.

Kidney tumours

Unilateral leg paralysis is a common peripheral neuropathy in budgerigars. It is often due to tumours of the kidneys induced by ALSV infection (see above).

Paramyxovirus/Newcastle disease

Paramyxovirus is frequently isolated from pigeons. The condition is preventable by vaccination, which is compulsory in pigeons presented at races and shows under the Disease of Poultry Order 1994 (SI 1994/3141). In addition to respiratory problems, the virus can also cause neurological diseases. Signs of this include wing drooping, circling, torticollis and opisthotonus.

Spinal abscesses and fungal infection

Spinal abscesses and fungal infection can occur in birds. Spinal abscesses may occur from bacteria, which have spread there via the bloodstream, particularly after spinal trauma, such as bruising after a flying injury. Fungal granulomas are common in cases of aspergillosis, and may invade the spinal cord as many vertebrae are pneumonised and so connected to the air sac system.

Wing paralysis

Wing paralysis is common after flying injuries or fracture of the humerus. This fracture results in rotation laterally of the distal fragment, resulting in the bone often lacerating the radial nerve.

References

Balsamo, G., Maxted, A.M., Midla, J.W. *et al.* (2017) Compendium of measures to control *Chlamydia psittaci* infection among humans (psittacosis) and pet birds (avian chlamydiosis). *Journal of Avian Medicine and Surgery*, **31**(3), 262–282. doi: 10.1647/217-265.

Bassami, M.R., Ypeleaar, I., Berryman, D. *et al.* (2001) Genetic diversity of beak and feather disease virus detected in psittacine species in Australia. *Virology*, **279**(2), 392–400.

Beaufrere, H., Ammersbach, M., Reavill, D.R. *et al.* (2013) Prevalence of and risk factors associated with atherosclerosis in psittacine birds. *Journal of the American Veterinary Medical Association*, **242**(12), 1696–1704.

Berhane, Y., Smith, D.-A., Newman, S. *et al.* (2001) Peripheral neuritis in psittacine birds with proventricular dilatation disease. *Avian Pathology*, **30**(5), 563–570.

Beverley-Burton, M. (1972) Helminths from wild anatids in Great Britain. *Journal of Helminthology*, **46**(4), 345–355.

Campagna, C., Uhart, M., Falabella, V. *et al.* (2023) Catastrophic mortality of southern elephant seals caused by H5N1 avian influenza. *Marine Mammal Science*, **40**(1), 322–325. doi: 10.1111/mms.13101.

Canoville, A., Schweitzer, M.H. and Zanno, L.E. (2019) Systemic distribution of medullary bone in the avian skeleton: ground truthing criteria for the identification of reproductive tissues in extinct Avemetatarsalia. *BMC Evolutionary Biology*, **19**, 71. doi: 10.1186/s12862-019-1402-7.

Colombini, S., Foil, C.S., Hosgood, G. and Tully, T.N. (2000) Intradermal skin testing in Hispaniolan parrots (*Amazona ventralis*). *Veterinary Dermatology*, **11**, 271–276.

Cooper, J.E. (1985) Foot conditions. In: *Veterinary Aspects of Captive Birds of Prey*, 2nd edn, pp. 97–111. Standfast Press, UK.

Cooper, J.E., Gschmeissner, S. and Greenwood, A. (1989) Atoxoplasma in greenfinches (*Carduelis chloris*) as a possible cause of 'going light'. *Veterinary Record*, **124**, 343–344.

Cray, C., Reavill, D., Romagnano, A. *et al.* (2009) Galactomannan assay and plasma protein electrophoresis findings in psittacine birds with aspergillosis. *Journal of Avian Medicine and Surgery*, **23**, 125–135.

Cray, C., Watson, T., Rodriguez, M. and Arheart, K. (2010) Serodiagnostic testing options for avian aspergillosis. *Proceedings of the Annual Conference of the Association of Avian Veterinarians*, pp. 371–372.

Cross, G.M. (2004) *Draft Threat Abatement Plan for Psittacine Circoviral (Beak and Feather) Disease Affecting Endangered Psittacine Species.* Department of the Environment and Heritage, Commonwealth of Australia, Canberra, Australia.

Dorrestein, G.M. (2009) Bacterial and parasitic diseases of passerines. *Veterinary Clinics of North America: Exotic Animal Practice*, **12**(3), 433–451.

Dubey, J.P. (2002) A review of toxoplasmosis in wild birds. *Veterinary Parasitology*, **106**, 121–153.

Duvall, A., Greenacre, C., Grunkemeyer, V. and Craig, L. (2021) Cutaneous mycobacteriosis caused by *Mycobacterium kansasii* in a yellow-naped Amazon parrot (*Amazona auropalliata*). *Journal of Avian Medicine and Surgery*, **35**(2), 227–234. doi: 10.1647/20-00036.

Evans, D., Tully, T., Strickland, K. *et al.* (2001) Congenital cardiovascular anomalies, including ventricular septal defects in 2 cockatoos. *Journal of Avian Medicine and Surgery*, **15**(2), 101–106.

Finlayson, R. and Hirchinson, V. (1961) Experimental atheroma in budgerigars. *Nature*, **192**, 369–370.

Fitzgerald, B.C. and Beaufrere, H. (2016) Cardiology. In: *Current Therapy in Avian Medicine and Surgery* (ed. B.L. Speer), pp. 252–328. Elsevier, St Louis, Missouri.

Forbes, N.A. and Simpson, G.N. (1997) *Caryospora neofalconis*: an emerging threat to captive-bred raptors in the United Kingdom. *Journal of Avian Medicine and Surgery*, **11**, 110–114.

Gancz, A.Y., Kistler, A.L., Greninger, A., et al. (2009) Avian Bornaviruses and proventricular dilatation disease. *Proceedings of the Annual Conference of the Association of Avian Veterinarians*, p. 5.

Gancz, A.Y., Clubb, S. and Shivaprasad, H. (2012) Advanced diagnostic approaches and current management of proventricular dilatation disease. *Veterinary Clinics of North America: Exotic Animal Practice*, **13**(3), 471–494.

Girling, S.J. (2002) *Plasma protein electrophoresis: variations in health and disease in the family Psittaciformes.* Dissertation as part-fulfilment for the RCVS Diploma in Zoological Medicine. RCVS Library, London.

Gray, P., Villaneuva, I., Mirhosseini, N., Hoppes, S., Payne, S. and Tizard, I. (2009) Experimental infection of birds with avian Bornavirus. *Proceedings of the Annual Conference of the Association of Avian Veterinarians*, p. 7.

Gray, P., Hoppes, S., Suchodolski, P. *et al.* (2010) Use of avian Bornavirus isolates to induce proventricular dilatation disease in conures. *Emerging Infectious Diseases*, **16**, 473–479.

Grund, C.H., Kohler, B. and Korbel, R.T. (2005) Evaluation of various tissues for diagnosis of psittacine beak and feather disease (PBFD). *Proceedings of the 8th European Association of Avian Veterinarians Conference and 6th Scientific European College of Avian Medicine and Surgery Meeting*, Arles, France, 24–30 April 2005.

Hansen, W.R. and Gough, R.E. (2007) Duck plague virus. In: *Infectious Diseases of Wild Birds* (eds N.J. Thomas, B. Hunter & C.T. Atkinson), pp. 87–107. Blackwell Publ, Ames, Iowa.

Harlin, R. and Wade, L. (2009) Bacterial and parasitic diseases of Columbiformes. *Veterinary Clinics of North America: Exotic Animal Practice*, **12**(3), 453–473.

Heidenreich, M. (1997) Parasites. In: *Birds of Prey: Medicine and Management*, p. 133. Blackwell Science, Oxford.

Hodgkinson, G. and Chamberlain, D. (2023) Iritis in gannets as a consequence of avian influenza. *Veterinary Record*, **192**(6), 257. doi: 10.1002/vetr.2866.

Hoggard, N.K. and Craig, L.E. (2022) Medullary bone in male budgerigars (*Melopsittacus undulatus*) with testicular neoplasms. *Veterinary Pathology*, **59**(2), 333–339. doi: 10.1177/03009858211069126.

Hoppes, S., Gray, P.L., Payne, S. and Shivaprasad, H.L. (2010) The isolation, pathogenesis, diagnosis, transmission and control of avian Bornavirus and proventricular dilatation disease. *Veterinary Clinics of North America: Exotic Animal Practice*, **13**, 495–508.

Jung, A., Grund, C., Muller, I. and Rautenschlein, S. (2009) Avian paramyxovirus serotype 3 infection in *Neopsephotus*, *Cyanoramphus* and *Neophema* species. *Journal of Avian Medicine and Surgery*, **23**, 205–208.

Klopfleisch, R., Werner, O., Mundt, E. *et al.* (2006) Neurotropism of highly pathogenic avian influenza virus a/chicken/Indonesia/2003 (H5N1) in experimentally infected pigeons (*Columba livia f. domestica*). *Veterinary Pathology*, **43**, 463–470.

Krautwald-Junghanns, M.-E., Zebisch, R. and Schmidt, V. (2009) Relevance and treatment of coccidiosis in domestic pigeons (*Columba livia* forma *domestica*) with particular emphasis on toltrazuril. *Journal of Avian Medicine and Surgery*, **23**(1), 1–5. doi: 10.1647/2007-049R.1.

Li, S., Dhaenens, M., Garmyn, A. *et al.* (2015) Exposure of *Aspergillus fumigatus* to T-2 toxin results in a stress response associated with exacerbation of aspergillosis in poultry. *World Mycotoxin Journal*, **8**(3), 323–333. doi: 10.3920/WMJ2014.1765.

Lierz, M. (2016) Avian bornavirus and proventricular dilation disease. In: *Current Therapy in Avian Medicine and Surgery* (ed. B.L. Speer), pp. 28–46. Elsevier, St Louis, Missouri.

Lumeij, J.T. (2000) Pathophysiology, diagnosis and treatment of renal disorders in birds of prey. In: *Raptor Biomedicine 3* (eds J.T. Lumeij, J.D. Remple & P.T. Redig), pp. 169–178. Zoological Education Network, Lake Worth, FL.

Lumeij, J.T., Shaik, M.A.S. and Ali, M. (2011) Radiographic reference limits for cardiac width in peregrine falcons (*Falco peregrinus*). *Journal of the American Veterinary Medical Association*, **238**(11), 1459–1463.

MacWhirter, P., Mueller, R. and Gill, J. (1999) Ongoing research report: allergen testing as part of diagnostic protocol in self-mutilating psittaciformes. *Proceedings of the Annual Conference of the Association of Avian Veterinarians*, p. 125.

Manvell, R., Gough, D., Major, N. and Fouchier, R.A. (2004) Mortality in budgerigars associated with a reovirus-like agent. *Veterinary Record*, **154**, 539–540.

Messenger, G.A. and Garner, M.M. (2010) Proventricular cryptosporidiosis in small psittacines. *Proceedings of the Annual Conference of the Association of Avian Veterinarians*, pp. 55–58.

Mines, J.J. and Green, P.E. (1983) Experimental *Ascaridia columbae* infections in budgerigars. *Australian Veterinary Journal*, **60**(9), 279–280.

Mota, S.M., Girling, S.J., Cole, G. *et al.* (2023) Application of a novel *Aspergillus* lateral-flow device in the diagnosis of aspergillosis in captive gentoo penguins (*Pygoscelis papua papua*). *Journal of Zoo and Wildlife Medicine*, **54**(2), 360–366.

Naylor, A., Girling, S., Brown, D. *et al.* (2017) Plasma protein electrophoresis as a prognostic indicator in *Aspergillus* species-infected gentoo penguins

(*Pygoscelis papua papua*). *Veterinary Clinical Pathology*, **46**(4), 605–614. doi: 10.1111/vcp.12527.

Nemeth, N.M., Gonzalez-Astudillo, V., Oesterle, P.T. and Howerth, E.W. (2016) A 5-year retrospective review of avian diseases diagnosed at the Department of Pathology, University of Georgia. *Journal of Comparative Pathology*, **155**, 105–120.

Oaks, J.L. (1993) Immune and inflammatory responses in falcon staphylococcal pododermatitis. In: *Raptor Biomedicine* (eds P.T. Redig, J.E. Cooper, J.D. Remple & D.B. Hunter), pp. 72–87. University of Minnesota Press, Minneapolis, MN.

Oster, S.C. and Pariaut, R. (2021) Cardiac disease of raptors. *Journal of Avian Medicine and Surgery*, **35**(4), 382–389.

Palmieri, C., Franca, M., Uzall, F. *et al.* (2011) Pathology and immunohistochemical findings of West Nile virus infection in Psittaciformes. *Veterinary Pathology*, **48**(5), 975–984.

Palmieri, C., Roy, P., Dhillon, A.S. and Shivaprasad, H.L. (2013) Avian mycobacteriosis in psittacines: a retrospective study of 123 cases. *Journal of Comparative Pathology*, **148**(2–3), 126–138. doi: 10.1016/j.jcpa.2012.06.005.

Paradell, O.G., Goh, T., Popov, D. *et al.* (2023) Estimated mortality of the highly pathogenic avian influenza pandemic on northern gannets (*Morus bassanus*) in Southwest Ireland. *Biology Letters*, **19**(6), 20230090. doi: 10.1098/rsbl.2023.0090.

Pennycott, T. (2004) Mortality in budgerigars in Scotland: pathological findings. *Veterinary Record*, **154**, 538–539.

Perpinan, D., Fernandez-Bellon, H., Lopez, C. and Ramis, A. (2007) Lymphoplasmacytic myenteric, subepicardial and pulmonary ganglioneuritis in four nonpsittacine birds. *Journal of Avian Medicine and Surgery*, **21**, 210–214.

Phalen, D. (2006) Implications of viruses in clinical disorders. In: *Clinical Avian Medicine* (eds G. Harrison & T. Lightfoot), pp. 721–760. Spix Publishing Inc., Palm Beach, FL.

Raghav, R. and Samour, J. (2019) Inclusion body herpesvirus hepatitis in captive falcons in the Middle East: a review of clinical and pathologic findings. *Journal of Avian Medicine and Surgery*, **33**(1), 1–6.

Raidal, S. (2016) Psittacine beak and feather disease. In: *Current Therapy in Avian Medicine and Surgery* (ed. B.L. Speer), 1st edn, pp. 51–59. Elsevier, St Louis, Missouri.

Raidal, S. and Cross, G.M. (1994) The hemaglutination spectrum of psittacine beak and feather disease virus. *Avian Pathology*, **234**, 621–630.

Ravich, M.L., Reavill, D.R., Hess, L. *et al.* (2014) Gastrointestinal cryptosporidiosis in captive psittacine birds in the United States. *Journal of Avian Medicine and Surgery*, **28**, 297–303.

Reavill, D.R., Schmidt, R.E. and Fudge, A.M. (1990) Avian skin and feather disorders: a retrospective study. *Proceedings of the Annual Conference of the Association of Avian Veterinarians*, Phoenix, Arizona, pp. 248–254.

Remple, J.D. (1993) Raptor bumblefoot: a new treatment technique. In: *Raptor Biomedicine* (eds P.T. Redig, J.E. Cooper, J.D. Remple & D.B. Hunter), pp. 154–160. University of Minnesota Press, Minneapolis, MN.

Rimoldi, G., Speer, B., Wellehan Jnr, J.F.X. *et al.* (2013) An outbreak of *Sarcocystis calchasi* encephalitis in multiple psittacine species within an enclosed zoological aviary. *Journal of Veterinary Diagnostic Investigation*, **25**, 775–781.

Rinder, M., Baas, N., Hagen, E. *et al.* (2022) Canary Bornavirus (*Orthobornavirus serini*) infections are associated with clinical symptoms in common canaries (*Serinus canaria dom.*). *Viruses*, **14**(10), 2187. doi: 10.3390/v14102187.

Rosskopf, W.J., Woerpel, R.W. and Lane, R.A. (1986) The practical use and limitations of the urinalysis in diagnostic pet avian medicine: with emphasis on the differential diagnosis of polyuria, the importance of cast formation in the avian urinalysis and case reports. *Proceedings of the Annual Conference of the Association of Avian Veterinarians*, Miami, Florida, pp. 61–73.

Saito, E.K., Sileo, L., Green, D.E. *et al.* (2002) Raptor mortality due to West Nile virus in the United States. *Journal of Wildlife Diseases*, **43**(2), 206–213.

Sanchez-Cordon, P.J., Gomez-Villamandos, J.C., Gutierrez, J. *et al.* (2007) *Atoxoplasma* spp. infection in captive canaries (*Serinus canaria*). *Journal of Veterinary Medicine*, **54**, 23–26.

Schmidt, R.E., Reavill, D.R. and Phalen, D.N. (2003) Cardiovascular system. In: *Pathology of Pet and Aviary Birds* (eds R.E. Schmidt, D.R. Reavill & D.N. Phalen), pp. 3–16. Iowa State Press, Ames, Iowa.

Scottish Seabird Centre (2024) Bass Rock gannet count. https://www.seabird.org/press-releases/new-technologies-help-researchers-to-quantify-the-impact-of-avian-flu-on-the-world-s-largest-northern-gannet-colony (accessed 4 February 2024).

Shivaprasad, H.L., Franca, M., Honkavuori, K., Briese, T. and Lipkin, W.I. (2009) Proventricular dilatation disease associated with bornavirus in psittacines. *Proceedings of the Annual Conference of the Association of Avian Veterinarians*, pp. 3–4.

Silva, B.B.I., Urzo, M.L.R., Encabo, J.R. *et al.* (2022) Pigeon circovirus over three decades of research: bibliometrics, scoping review, and perspectives. *Viruses*, **14**(7), 1498. doi: 10.3390/v14071498.

Smith, J. (2009) Unusual outbreak of PDD in a psittacine nursery. *Proceedings of the Annual Conference of the Association of Avian Veterinarians*, pp. 9–13.

Speer, B.L. (1998) Chronic partial proventricular obstruction caused by multiple gastrointestinal foreign bodies in a juvenile umbrella cockatoo (*Cacatua alba*). *Journal of Avian Medicine and Surgery*, **12**(4), 271–275.

Staeheli, P., Rinder, M. and Kaspers, B. (2010) Avian bornavirus associated with fatal disease in psittacine birds. *Journal of Virology*, **84**(13), 6269–6275.

Stanford, M. (2003) The significance of serum ionized calcium and 25-hydroxycholecalciferol (vitamin D3) assays in African Grey parrots. *Exotic DVM*, **5**(3), 1–6.

Steinmetz, A., Pees, M., Schmidt, V. *et al.* (2008) Blindness as a sign of proventricular dilatation disease in a grey parrot (*Psittacus erithacus erithacus*). *Journal of Small Animal Practice*, **49**, 660–662.

Straub, J., Pees, M. and Krautwald-Junghanns, M.E. (2002) Measurement of the cardiac silhouette in psittacines. *Journal of the American Veterinary Medical Association*, **221**, 76–79.

Strunk, A. and Wilson, G.H. (2005) Avian cardiology. *Veterinary Clinics of North America: Exotic Animal Practice*, **6**(1), 1–28. doi: 10.1016/s1094-9194(02)00031-2.

Varsani, A., Regnard, G.L. and Bragg, R. (2010) Global genetic diversity and geographical and host-species distribution of beak and feather disease virus isolates. *Journal of Genetic Virology*, **92**(pt4), 752–767.

Wehr, E.E. and Shalkop, W.T. (1963) *Ascaridia columbae* infection in pigeons: a histopathologic study of liver lesions. *Avian Diseases*, **7**(2), 206–211.

Wernery, U. and Kinne, J. (2004) How do falcons contract a herpesvirus infection? Preliminary findings. *Falco*, **23**, 16–17.

Willette, M., Ponder, J., Cruz-Martinez, L. *et al.* (2009) Management of select bacterial and parasitic conditions of raptors. *Veterinary Clinics of North America: Exotic Animal Practice*, **12**(3), 491–517.

Yang, R., Brice, B. and Ryan, U. (2014) A new *Caryospora* coccidian species (Apicomplexa: Eimeriidae) from the laughing kookaburra (*Dacelo novaeguineae*). *Experimental Parasitology*, **145**, 68–73.

Zantop, D.W. (2010) Bornavirus: background levels in 'well' birds and links to non-PDD illness. *Proceedings of the Annual Conference of the Association of Avian Veterinarians*, pp. 305–310.

Chapter 14 An Overview of Avian Therapeutics

FLUID THERAPY

Maintenance requirements

In birds there is almost no water lost as sweat as they have no proper skin sweat glands. However, there are greater losses compared with cats and dogs, due to their increased metabolic rates and because of their high body surface and lung area to body weight ratio. This means that proportionately large amounts of fluids are lost through respiration.

To compensate, birds can conserve water more efficiently than mammals. Unlike urea, their waste protein excretory product, uric acid, requires very little water to be excreted. However, the losses and gains equal out, so that maintenance levels in companion birds have been estimated as 50 mL/kg per day, which is similar to cats and dogs.

The effect of disease on fluid requirements

With any disease the need for fluids increases, even if no obvious fluid loss has occurred. The disease process may affect the kidneys causing increases in the glomerular filtration rate or reduction in water reabsorption by the collecting ducts, leading to increased urine output, or there may be a loss of absorption of water from the small or large intestine. For example, the endotoxins produced in cases of *Escherichia coli* septicaemia or enteritis cause a reduction in the response of the renal collecting ducts to arginine vasotocin (AVT), the avian equivalent of antidiuretic hormone (ADH) released from the pituitary. This will lead to less concentration of the urine, more fluid loss and dehydration.

Respiratory disease is common in avian patients, especially in cases of chlamydiosis, hypovitaminosis A and aspergillosis, all of which may lead to fluid loss.

Individuals suffering from diarrhoea will experience fluid loss and often metabolic acidosis due to prolonged loss of bicarbonate. There may also be chronic losses of potassium.

Most avian patients have the potential to regurgitate. Fluid loss by this route is therefore not uncommon. The secretions of the crop are mainly neutral to alkali, and so losses are more likely to give straightforward neutral water loss. However, more severe true vomiting will occur in birds with proventricular disease, such as proventricular dilatation disease (PDD) and 'megabacteriosis', and metabolic alkalosis due to loss of hydrogen ions will ensue.

Another route of fluid and electrolyte loss is through skin disease. Lovebirds and cockatiels in particular are prone to ulcerating skin conditions, particularly under the wings. These produce lesions which resemble chemical or thermal burns, and leave large areas of weeping exudative skin which allow fluid and electrolyte loss.

Post-surgical fluid requirements

Surgical procedures bring their own requirements for fluid therapy. There is the possibility of haemorrhage during surgery, necessitating vascular support with an aqueous electrolyte solution or, in more serious blood losses (>10%), colloidal fluids or even blood transfusions (see Figure 14.1).

Even if surgery is relatively bloodless, there are inevitable losses via the respiratory route because of the drying nature of the gases used to deliver the anaesthetics commonly used in avian surgery. Smaller birds have larger surface areas in relation to volume, and this applies to the lung fields as well as the skin. Avian patients also have an air sac system, which increases the surface area for fluid loss even further.

Many patients are not able to drink immediately after surgery. The period without food or water intake may stretch to a few hours, enough time for any avian to start to dehydrate. Finally, some forms of surgery, such as prosthetic beak repair procedures, will lead to inappetence for a period.

Electrolyte replacement

In cases of chronic fluid loss, electrolytes as well as fluids will often need replacing. Chronic diarrhoea, such as in coccidiosis or *Giardia* infestations, will cause loss of food, water and electrolytes to waste. The main electrolyte losses involve bicarbonate and potassium.

Because many birds have a crop between the mouth and the true stomach, birds may well regurgitate rather than vomit. The crop contents are alkaline to neutral, and so metabolic alkalosis is unlikely to occur with regurgitation or crop problems, indeed metabolic acidosis is more likely. However, in serious proventricular disease, such as the viral condition 'macaw wasting syndrome', stomach megabacteriosis or ulcers, loss of hydrogen ions will occur and metabolic alkalosis can ensue. True vomiting is more commonly seen in carnivorous species that generally do not have a crop.

Fluids used in avian practice

Lactated Ringer's/Hartmann's

This is useful for rehydration and to supply maintenance needs. It is useful for avian patients suffering from metabolic acidosis, for example those with chronic gastrointestinal disease and bicarbonate loss, but it can also be used for fluid therapy after routine surgical procedures. The quantity of potassium present in lactated Ringer's solution is unlikely to cause a problem in birds with hyperkalaemia (such as those suffering from rapid weight loss or with serious skin or tissue trauma). Should hyperkalaemia be present the use of calcium gluconate (5 mg/kg) or the addition of a glucose-containing fluid will help drive the potassium ions into the cells and so reduce the hyperkalaemic threat.

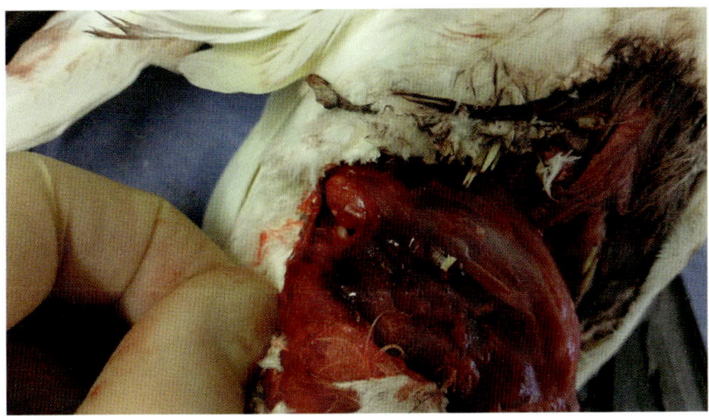

Figure 14.1 Trauma such as limb fractures may result in shock and significant blood loss and require fluid therapy and blood transfusions.

In hypokalaemic birds (such as those suffering from chronic diarrhoea, vomiting or burns or on long-term glucose/saline fluids), the addition of potassium to the fluids at rates of 0.1–0.3 mEq/kg body weight may help stimulate appetite and reduce the risk of cardiac arrhythmias.

In cases of metabolic acidosis, an assessment of bicarbonate ion loss can be made from a blood sample using a point-of-care analyser. However, in some cases it may not be possible in practice to measure it. Therefore, if persistent vomiting or chronic weight loss or trauma occurs and metabolic acidosis is suspected, a rough approximation may be made. Give a sodium bicarbonate supplement at 1 mEq/kg at 15–30-minute intervals until clinical improvement of signs or a maximum of 4 mEq/kg has been reached. (This supplement must not be given with the lactated Ringer's solution as it will precipitate out.)

Hypertonic saline

This is typically a product containing 7.2% saline and may be used in birds with acute hypovolaemia. It works by rapidly drawing fluid from the cellular and pericellular space into the circulation to support central venous pressure. It must be administered intravenously or intraosseously. See Chapter 16 for further details of its use.

Glucose/saline combinations

Glucose/saline solutions are useful for small avian patients. These may well have been through periods of anorexia prior to treatment and therefore may be borderline hypoglycaemic. The concentration to start with when dehydration is present is 5% glucose/0.9% saline. Once dehydration has been reversed, the avian patient may be moved on to the 4% glucose/0.18% saline concentration for maintenance purposes. It is worth noting however that subcutaneous use of dextrose-containing solutions may actually be counterproductive in birds as one study in pigeons suggested that the dextrose administered was not absorbed quickly, but rather acted as an osmotic draw, pulling water from the circulation and further dehydrating the bird (Martin and Kollias, 1989).

Protein amino acid/B vitamin supplements

Protein and B vitamin supplements can be useful for nutritional support. They are particularly useful for replacing nutrients in cases where the patient is malnourished or has been suffering from a protein-losing enteropathy or nephropathy. They are also good supplements for patients with hepatic disease or severe exudative skin disease such as thermal burns. However, they may have some serious side-effects in certain species; for example, those products containing vitamin B_6 (pyridoxine) should not be used in many birds of prey as they have been shown to be toxic and resulted in deaths of gyrfalcons (*Falco rusticolus*) and peregrine falcons (*Falco peregrinus*) when dosed above 5 mg/kg intramuscularly (Samour *et al.*, 2016).

Colloidal fluids

Colloidal fluids are used less frequently as they can have serious side-effects and should not be used where underlying blood clotting issues occur or internal bleeding is present as they prolong clotting times. See Chapter 16 for shock fluid therapy.

Blood transfusions

Blood transfusion should be considered if the packed cell volume (PCV) drops below 15% (0.15 L/L). Birds are more tolerant of blood loss than mammals as the oxygenation of their blood is more efficient. Donors should be from the same species (e.g. African grey parrot to African grey parrot, or budgerigar to budgerigar). Pre-transfusion cross-matching using a slide technique may be helpful but in reality few if any blood groups have been identified in cage birds. A major cross-match is performed by adding a drop of donor's blood to the serum or plasma of the recipient and watching for red cell clumping or haemolysis that may indicate an immune system response. Blood can be collected from the donor into a container or syringe with acid citrate dextrose anticoagulant or, in an emergency, a heparinised syringe may be used. Ideally, a blood filter should be used before blood is transfused into the recipient bird, but frequently this is not possible in general practice, and so collection and administration should be done with care to reduce haemolysis and clumping.

It is useful to remember that one drop of blood is roughly equal to 0.05 mL and that the estimated blood volume of an avian patient is 10% of its body weight in grams. However, birds are capable of coping with blood loss better than an equivalent-sized mammal and this may be associated with their ability to mobilise interstitial fluid as well as a rapid erythrocyte production rate (Parkinson, 2023). Volumes of blood that can be transfused range from 0.25 mL in a budgerigar to 5 mL in an African grey parrot.

Oral fluids and electrolytes

Oral fluids may be used in avian practice for those patients experiencing mild dehydration, and for 'home' administration. Many products are commercially available for avian species, although domestic dog and cat products can be used but those containing vitamin B_6 should be avoided in birds of prey as even the oral route can prove toxic in species such as gyrfalcons and peregrine falcons, as previously mentioned (Samour *et al.*, 2016).

Calculation of fluid requirements

Fluid therapy is likely to be necessary in any sick bird with perhaps the exception of one in cardiogenic shock which is often associated with heart murmurs or a coelomic effusion. A critically ill avian patient is assumed to be at least 5% dehydrated. As with cats and dogs, you should assume that 1% dehydration is equal to the need to supply 10 mL/kg body weight of fluid in addition to maintenance requirements. Rough assumptions then have to be made on the degree of dehydration of the bird concerned:

- 3–5% dehydrated: increased thirst, slight lethargy, tacky mucous membranes, increased heart rate
- 7–10% dehydrated: increased thirst, anorexia, dullness, tenting of the skin and slower return to normal over eyelid or foot, dry mucous membranes, dull corneas, red or wrinkled skin in chicks
- 12–18% dehydrated: dull to comatose, skin remains tented after pinching, desiccating mucous membranes, sunken eyes.

These deficits may be large and the volume required for replacement will be difficult to administer rapidly. Indeed, it may be dangerous to overload the patient's system with these fluid levels all in one go. To spread the deficit evenly, it is advised that the following protocol be used.

- Day 1: maintenance fluid levels +50% of calculated dehydration factor
- Day 2: maintenance fluid levels +50% of calculated dehydration factor
- Day 3: maintenance fluid levels.

If the dehydration levels are so severe that volumes are still too large to be given at any one time, it may be necessary to take 72 hours rather than 48 hours to replace the calculated deficit.

To add to the problem, debilitated avian patients may also be anaemic, and therefore PCVs may appear misleadingly normal, so total protein levels are an additional parameter to look at when assessing dehydration. Uric acid levels may also be measured, as these will often increase in cases of moderate to severe dehydration. Other useful parameters include weight measurement and of course fluid intake and urine output. Table 14.1 gives some normal PCV and total protein values.

Table 14.1 Normal packed cell volume (PCV) and total blood protein for selected avian species.

Species	PCV (L/L)	Total protein (g/L)
African grey parrot	0.45–0.53	32–52
Amazon parrot	0.41–0.53	30–52
Budgerigar	0.44–0.58	20–30
Cockatiel	0.43–0.57	24–48
Cockatoo	0.40–0.54	30–50
Macaw	0.42–0.56	26–50
Canada goose	0.35–0.49	37–56
Mallard duck	0.42–0.56	32–45
Mute swan	0.32–0.5	36–55
Chicken	0.24–0.43	33–55
Pheasant	0.28–0.42	42–72
Pigeon	0.36–0.48	21–35
Barn owl	0.41–0.57	24–46
Tawny owl	0.36–0.47	27–46
Peregrine falcon	0.37–0.53	25–40

Equipment for fluid administration

The equipment required to administer fluids to birds is often very small in size. For example, the blood vessels available for intravenous medication are often 30–50% smaller than their cat or dog counterparts and tend to be highly mobile and much more fragile and prone to rupture.

Crop tubes

These are useful as a route for fluid and nutrition administration. Crop tubes come either as straight or curved metal tubes, both with blunt ends. To insert a crop tube, extend the bird's head. Starting from the left side of the inside of the lower beak, pass the tube down the proximal oesophagus into the crop at the right side of the thoracic inlet. Mouth gags may need to be used in the larger species. Maximal volumes which may be given vary from 0.5 mL in a budgerigar to 15 mL in a large macaw (see Figures 14.2 and 14.3).

Catheters

Because they have a length of tubing attached to the needle, butterfly catheters are extremely useful for the small and fragile avian vessels. If the syringe or drip set is connected to this piece of flexible tubing rather than directly to the catheter, there is less chance of the catheter becoming dislodged, should the bird draw back after the catheter is inserted. Also, the piece of clear tubing on the catheter allows you to see when venous access has been achieved, as blood will flow back into this area without having to draw back on the syringe (which would collapse the fragile veins anyway).

It is advised to flush any catheter with heparinised saline prior to use to prevent clots forming. Catheters of 25–27 gauge are recommended and will cope with venous access for budgerigars through to small conures; 23–25 gauge will suffice for larger parrots and some of the bigger waterfowl and raptors.

Ordinary over-the-needle catheters may also be used for catheterisation of jugular veins. The latex catheter is useful for long-term

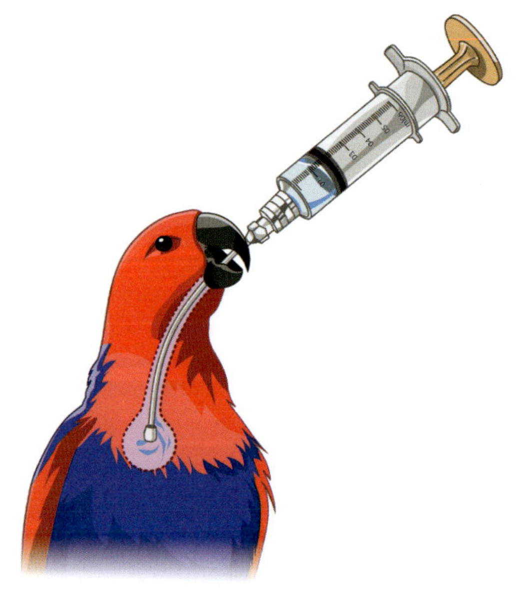

Figure 14.2 Diagram of the method of inserting a crop tube. Approach from left side of beak and aim towards the lower right neck region.

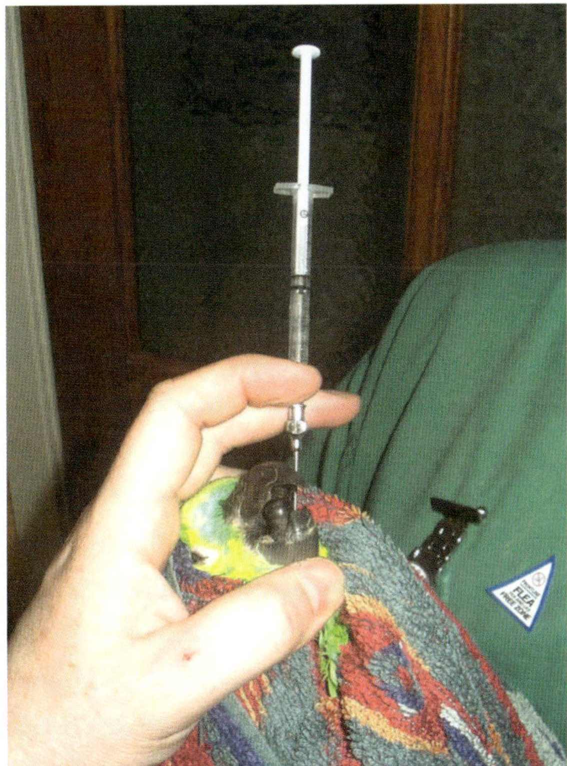

Figure 14.3 Crop tubing an Amazon parrot.

maintenance of venous access, as butterfly catheters tend to rupture the vessels if left in for long periods. It is better to use an over-the-needle catheter, which has plastic flanges so that it can be sutured to the skin at the site of insertion to prevent removal.

Hypodermic or spinal needles

Spinal needles have a central stylet to prevent clogging of the lumen of the needle with bone fragments after insertion and are therefore useful for intraosseous catheterisation. Spinal needles of 21–25 gauge are usually sufficient for most cage birds. Straightforward hypodermic needles may also be used for the same purpose, although the risks of blockage are higher. Hypodermic needles may also be used, of course, for the administration of subcutaneous fluids. Generally, 21–25 gauge hypodermic needles are sufficient for cage birds.

Syringe drivers

For continuous fluid administration, such as is required for intravenous and intraosseous fluid administration during anaesthesia, syringe drivers may be used. They are however less useful in the conscious bird due to poor tolerance of drip tubing; hence bolus fluid therapy is more commonly used in avian practice in the conscious hospitalised bird for ongoing fluid therapy.

Collars

It may be necessary to apply an Elizabethan-style collar to psittacine birds as they are inclined to remove intraosseous and intravenous catheters if they can reach them. There is also a selection of lightweight Perspex neck braces which may be better tolerated. However, these are not so useful when jugular vein catheters are used.

Routes of fluid administration

There are four main routes available for administration of fluids to birds:

- Oral
- Subcutaneous
- Intravenous
- Intraosseous.

The advantages and disadvantages of the four routes are given in Table 14.2. The intraperitoneal (more accurately intracoelomic) route used in mammals is not available for use in birds due to the lack of a diaphragm and the presence of air sacs. This means that any injection into the body cavity (or coelom) may inadvertently enter an air sac and thence on to the bird's airways, resulting in drowning.

Oral

Lactated Ringer's solution, probiotic or oral electrolyte solutions or 5% dextrose solutions may be used. Commonly used volumes that may be administered via crop tube are given below and may be repeated two to three times per day if the bird is handleable:

- Budgerigar: 0.5–1 mL
- Cockatiel: 2.5–5 mL
- Conure: 5–7 mL
- Cockatoo: 10 mL
- African grey: 8–10 mL
- Macaw: 10–25 mL.

Subcutaneous

Table 14.2 gives the advantages and disadvantages of subcutaneous fluid therapy. The sites for subcutaneous fluid administration are located in the inguinal web of skin which attaches the leg to the body cranially, the axillary region immediately under each wing, and the dorsal interscapular area.

Intravenous

Table 14.2 gives the advantages and disadvantages of intravenous fluid therapy in avian species.

Blood vessels used for intravenous therapy

In larger species of bird, veins which may be used for intravenous therapy include the basilic and ulnar veins, which run on the underside of the wing. The right jugular vein may be used for bolus injections in all species down to the size of a canary. In some birds, a jugular vein catheter may be tolerated for repeated bolus injections, although it should be cranially located to reduce the likelihood of self-removal (see Figure 14.4). In waterfowl, such as swans and ducks, raptors and some larger parrots, the medial metatarsal vein, which runs along the medial aspect of the lower leg, can be used. Avian species will tolerate catheterisation of this vessel extremely well for several days.

Volumes of fluid which may be administered intravenously

Isotonic solutions may be given at 10–15 mL/kg per bolus. Care should be taken to ensure that the patient does not have cardiogenic

Table 14.2 Advantages and disadvantages of various avian fluid therapy routes.

Route	Advantages	Disadvantages
Oral	Reduced stress (if competent handler) Physiological route Less trauma Home therapy possible	Increased stress (if inexperienced) Not useful in cases of digestive tract dysfunction or disease Risk of aspiration pneumonia if regurgitation Slow rate of rehydration (not good for serious hypovolaemia) Inaccurate method of dosing (unless crop tubing)
Subcutaneous	Faster uptake of fluids than oral route Volumes given may be large, reducing dosing frequency Birds often absorb subcutaneous fluids more rapidly than mammals	Reduced uptake in severe dehydration or peripheral vasoconstriction May be painful in smaller species Only hypotonic or isotonic fluids may be used
Intravenous	Rapid rehydration and support of central venous pressure Use of hypertonic colloidal fluids and blood transfusions possible Good for waterfowl where medial metatarsal veins can take indwelling catheters or multiple venepuncture	Venous access may be difficult in some species Veins may be fragile Some species will not tolerate permanent indwelling intravenous catheters
Intraosseous	Rapid rehydration and support of central venous pressure Useful in smaller species where venous access is difficult May be better tolerated for indwelling catheters than intravenous routes Use of hypertonic colloidal fluids and blood transfusions possible	Potentially painful procedure requiring analgesia and local or general anaesthetic Risk of bone fracture or osteomyelitis Bolus of fluids takes longer to administer due to rigid confines of bone cortices Avoid use of pneumonised bones (e.g. humerus and femur and, in unusual species such as the pelican family [*Pelecanus* spp.], even the ulnar bone which is preferentially used for intraosseous fluid therapy in other species) as will cause drowning

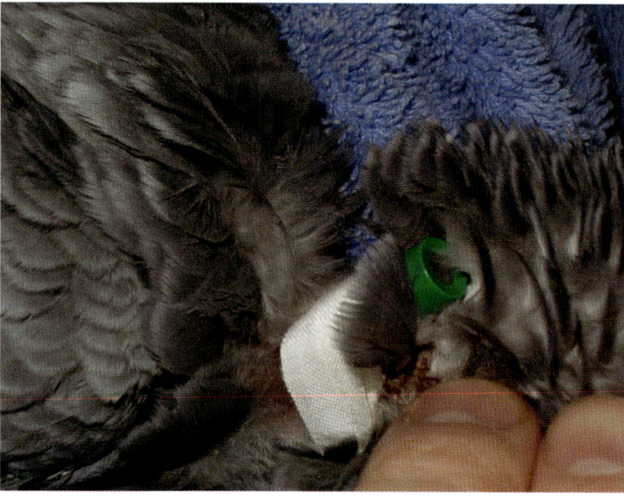

Figure 14.4 A jugular catheter placed in the right jugular of a parrot. Note the silk tape which is then sutured to the bird's skin to hold the catheter in place. Note also the bung as intravenous fluids in birds are generally given as boluses rather than continuous rate infusion due to the intolerance of drip sets, etc.

shock as intravenous fluids are contraindicated. Maximum intravenous bolus volumes are given below:

- Finch: 0.5 mL
- Budgerigar: 1 mL
- Cockatiels: 2 mL
- Conure: 6 mL
- Amazon parrot: 8 mL
- Owl: 10 mL
- Cockatoo: 14 mL
- Buzzard: 12–14 mL
- Macaw: 14 mL
- Swan: 25–30 mL.

Placement of intravenous catheters

Right jugular vein catheterisation

1. Sedate or lightly anaesthetise the avian patient, preferably with isoflurane, to ensure no trauma occurs and to minimise stress.
2. The feathers overlying the area should be wetted and parted. An area of no feather growth (known as apterylae) lies over the immediate area of the right jugular vein in cage birds and some raptors.
3. Raise the vein at the base of the neck with a thumb and swab the area lightly with surgical spirit.
4. Use a 23–25 gauge over-the-needle catheter, pre-flushed with heparinised saline. Insert it in a caudal direction, as these are often better tolerated than cranially pointing ones, particularly when administering fluids.
5. Once in place, suture the catheter securely to the skin on either side with fine nylon and re-flush to ensure it is properly in the vein. Then attach the intravenous drip tubing or catheter bung to the end of the catheter.
6. Sometimes a light bandage may be necessary to protect the catheter. In severe cases, an Elizabethan bird collar may be used (although the latter may catch on the catheter so is generally best avoided). Many avian patients will tolerate a catheter unprotected at this site for 24–48 hours.

Medial metatarsal catheterisation for waterfowl: This procedure may be used for larger Psittaciformes and raptors. It may also be performed with the bird conscious, particularly in waterfowl, as the blood vessel is less mobile and so less likely to rupture.

1. Wipe the inside of the lower leg with surgical spirit or povidone-iodine just below the intertarsal joint.
2. The vessel runs from the anterior aspect distally to a more medial aspect proximally and is obvious without digital pressure.

3. Use a 23–25 gauge over-the-needle catheter inserted in a proximal direction (i.e. in the direction of blood flow up the leg).
4. Tape the catheter in place using zinc oxide tape and apply a catheter bung after flushing with more heparin saline.

Intraosseous

Table 14.2 gives the advantages and disadvantages of intraosseous fluid therapy in avians.

Bones used for intraosseous fluid therapy

The two bones most commonly used for intraosseous fluid therapy are the ulna and the tibiotarsus. The ulna may be accessed from a distal or proximal aspect, and the tibiotarsus is accessed from a cranial proximal aspect through the crest just distal to the stifle joint.

Placement of intraosseous catheters

Proximal tibiotarsus: This is the procedure for placing a tibiotarsal intraosseous catheter.

1. Sedation or anaesthesia is needed for conscious animals. In all cases good analgesia must be administered.
2. Pluck the area overlying the cranial aspect of the tibial crest and surgically prepare this with dilute povidone-iodine.
3. Insert a 21–25-gauge needle through the tibial crest (depending on the size of the patient), screwing it into the bone in the direction of the long axis of the tibiotarsus distally.
4. Flush the needle with heparinised saline. The advantage of using a spinal needle is that it has a central stylet, which helps prevent it from becoming plugged with bone fragments.
5. Tape the needle securely in place and apply an antibiotic cream around the site. Radiography of the area to ensure correct intramedullary placement of the needle is advised.
6. Once correct placement has been assured, attach the needle to intravenous tubing and a syringe driver and bandage this securely in by wrapping bandage material around the limb. If the catheter has merely been placed for use later, insert a catheter bung and bandage in place.
7. Finally, fit an Elizabethan collar or avian neck brace if the patient shows signs of trying to remove the catheter.

Distal ulna in all species (except pelicans where it is pneumonised) (see Figures 14.5 and 14.6): Sedation or isoflurane/sevoflurane anaesthesia is often required.

1. Pluck the feathers over the distal aspect of the carpal joint of the wing to be used.
2. Surgically prepare the site with povidone-iodine or surgical spirit and flex the distal tip of the wing caudally. This flexure exposes the distal aspect of the radius and ulna bones within the carpal joint. The ulna is the larger of the two bones, unlike in mammals, but as with mammals it lies caudal to the radius.
3. Palpate the end of the ulna with the carpal joint maximally flexed, and insert a 23–25 gauge hypodermic or spinal needle, screwing it into the medullary cavity of the bone along the long axis of the ulna from a distal to proximal direction.
4. Flush the catheter with heparinised saline and place a catheter bung over the end. Radiographs may be taken to ensure accurate placement, and antibiotic cream can be used at the site of insertion.

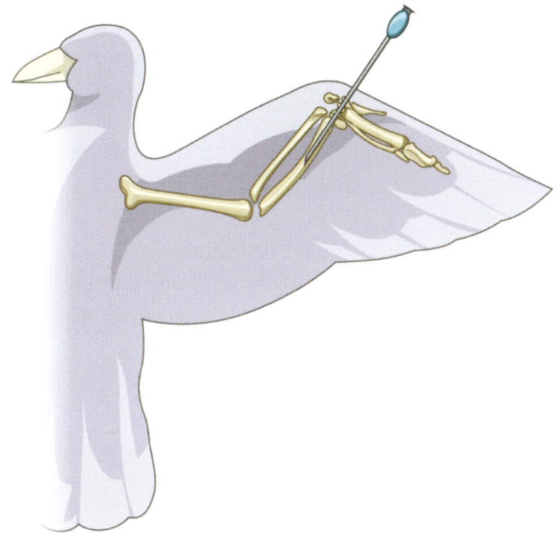

Figure 14.5 Method of inserting an intraosseous catheter into the distal ulna. Note the flexed carpal joint and that the ulna runs caudal to the radius.

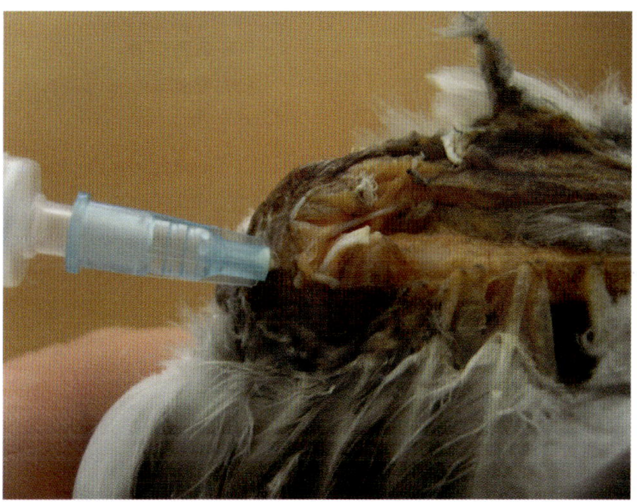

Figure 14.6 Simple method of giving a bolus of fluids via the distal ulna in a cadaver using a hypodermic needle and syringe.

5. Bandage the wing to the side of the bird to immobilise it. Encircle the thorax and pass both cranial and caudal to the opposite wing's attachment at the chest wall, otherwise the bird may flap wildly and loosen the catheter or traumatise itself.
6. The catheter may then be used for either intermittent slow bolus injections or for attachment to a syringe driver for continuous perfusion.

TREATMENT OF AVIAN DISEASES

As this text is aimed at the veterinary technical nurse, it is not intended to give exhaustive lists of treatments or drug dosages, but rather to give an idea of the treatments possible and the techniques useful to aid recovery. For drug dosages, the reader is referred to one of the many excellent texts listed in the additional reading list at the end of this book.

Avian dermatological disease therapy

Table 14.3 highlights some of the treatments and therapies commonly used for the management of avian skin diseases. In addition, the management of the bacterial pododermatitis condition known as 'bumblefoot' as well as behavioural feather plucking is also discussed.

Treatment and prevention of bumblefoot

This condition is seen in almost any species, and prevention is better than cure. Some methods to prevent bumblefoot from developing include the following.

- Provide a variety of different-diameter natural wood perches for cage and aviary birds. These will allow the feet of the bird to expand and contract as they grip the differing perches allowing blood to be pumped through the foot, preventing devitalisation, and also applying pressure to different areas, preventing corns.
- For falcons and raptors, perches should be covered in padding such as Astroturf®, particularly if they are tethered for days at a time. This cushions the foot and prevents the excessive pressure that causes ischaemia.
- A good-quality diet is vital. Vitamin A is particularly important for skin integrity and local immunity, as well as vitamin B_1 and minerals such as calcium. Preventing obesity is also important as this will lead to increased pressure on the feet.

In the case of existing pododermatitis:

- For type I–II lesions (Oaks, 1993), padding the perches and increasing flying time is a simple solution. In the case of raptors, increasing the time spent flying helps, and the use of antibiotics has been recommended where inflammation is present. Use of propentofylline can help with blood circulation to the feet.
- If a scab exists, it should be debrided under anaesthesia with dilute antiseptic such as povidone-iodine and followed, if on the plantar surface, by padding of the foot. The padding is formed from a non-adherent dressing such as Coflex®/Vetband®, which is wound in small strips around the base of each digit. This lifts the plantar aspect of the foot off the perch, thus allowing increased circulation.
- For type III–IV lesions (Oaks, 1993), it is recommended that a culture of the lesion is taken in order to choose the correct antimicrobial. The wounds should be repeatedly debrided with dilute povidone-iodine and the toes bandaged. In more severe cases, the application of a ball bandage (where a wad of padding is placed in the grip of the foot and the foot bandaged to this ball) may be necessary (see Figure 14.7). Alternatively, casting materials may be used to create a large but lightweight 'corn plaster', which removes pressure from the affected area of the foot. It is usually necessary to do this to both feet to avoid putting pressure on the non-affected foot. If bones are involved or deep-seated soft tissue infections, then antibiotic-impregnated polymethylmethacrylate (AIPMMA) beads have been shown to improve healing and recovery rates. These beads are implanted and sewn into the wounds where they release antibiotic slowly at the site of the infection over a period of weeks. Alternatively, drains may be placed in the affected foot, exiting proximally on the caudal aspect of the tarsometatarsus. This allows the wounds to be flushed with antibiotics for a number of days. The foot should be placed into a ball bandage dressing, which should be changed after each flush.
- For type V lesions the prognosis is grave and euthanasia is commonly carried out (Oaks, 1993).

Table 14.3 Treatment of avian skin diseases.

Diagnosis	Treatment
Avipoxvirus	No specific treatment. Antibiosis and topical treatment with dilute povidone-iodine are useful
Broken flight feathers	May result in poor flight which can be important in birds of prey amongst others. Technique known as 'imping' can be carried out using feathers from previous year's moult. The moulted feather can be cut to length and glued to the broken flight feather shaft using a small piece of bamboo or wood as an insert. Try and match the feather for shape and size (and of course it must be from the correct wing) to give best results
Ectoparasites	**Mites** (e.g. *Cnemidocoptes* spp.): ivermectin 0.2 mg/kg once orally, topically or by injection. Repeat after 10–14 days. Other drugs such as moxidectin and selamectin have also been used successfully and safely. *Dermanyssus gallinae* will require treatment of cage/aviary environment as they only live on the host at night. Predatory mites have also been used to control *D. gallinae* **Lice**: Commercial louse powders are available containing *cis*-permethrin or piperonyl butoxide. Pyrethrin-based powders have been used in poultry. Diatomaceous earth has also been used in poultry but tends to be less successful
Neoplasia and feather cysts	Surgical excision in the case of neoplasia. For cysts, excision or marsupialisation (opening the cyst and sewing the capsule to the skin surface) may be required. Radiosurgery is helpful to reduce haemorrhage
Psittacine circovirus/ Psittacine beak and feather disease (PBFD)	Avian gamma-interferon (not commercially available) has been used with success at 1×10^6 IU injected once daily for 90 days (Stanford, 2004) Historically, prevention was possible by live vaccine (produced in Australia), but this must not be given to already infected birds as it accelerates the course of the disease. This vaccine is not available at the time of publication
Psittacine polyomavirus	No treatment is available. Prevention may be attempted using a commercial vaccine from the USA (Biomune II Psittimmune®)
Pigeon poxvirus	Vaccines may be available, although no longer in the UK
Ulcerative dermatitis	Appropriate antibacterial and antifungal medication. Behavioural aspects, e.g. environmental enrichment or exposure to UV light, need to be considered. Possibility of allergic skin disease

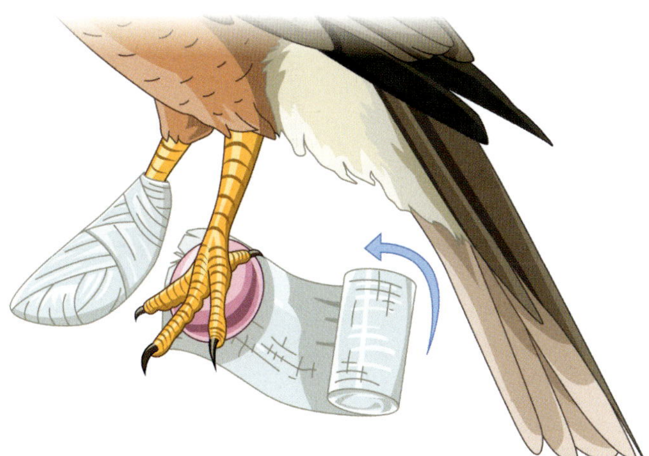

Figure 14.7 Application of a ball bandage to the feet of a raptor with bumblefoot. Note gauze packing to support the foot before using elasticated bandage material.

Treatment of behavioural feather plucking

This can be extremely difficult and it cannot be stressed enough that a full work-up to rule out infection, nutrition or uncontrolled pain as the cause of feather plucking/mutilation should be carried out. For example, subclinical PDD or chlamydial or circoviral disease can result in self-mutilation.

If the cause is sexual frustration due to the keeping of a single sexually mature parrot, these cases may improve by the pairing with a suitable mate. Alternatively, the reproductive hormone axis may be blocked temporarily by reducing daylight to less than 10 hours to mimic the non-breeding season in seasonal breeders. Gonadotropin releasing hormone (GnRH) agonists such as leuprolide acetate (100 μg/kg intramuscularly which lasts for 3–4 weeks) or deslorelin (4.7 mg implant lasts 6–10 months) have been used to inhibit the pituitary–gonadal axis. Deslorelin is more readily available in a long-acting implant form in the UK and is implanted subcutaneously over the back of the head where it cannot be removed by the parrot. Remember that this drug works by initially stimulating the sex hormone axis and therefore the condition may initially worsen until the axis is shut down.

Many larger parrots develop feather plucking disorders often due to a lack of socialisation as they have been hand-reared. They would typically spend many years with their parents in the wild and so hand-reared birds often do not have normal avian social interactive skills and are human focused and this may manifest in self-destructive behaviours, particularly if they become bonded to an owner and then are deprived of their company for long periods regularly. These birds can be more difficult to manage but training these individuals to accept basic commands along with environmental enrichment such as puzzle toys can help. Training parrots to simple commands such as 'up' to step up onto a hand or proffered perch, 'down' to step back onto its own perch, 'no' when an undesirable action has occurred and vocal praise plus a treat when the parrot does what you want are good places to start this.

Environmental enrichment is essential to take the bird's mind off self-destructive behaviours. Food puzzles, toys and regular changing of these to reduce boredom and provide novelty are important. Background noise, such as a low level of radio sound, is also important as very quiet environments can be stressful to prey species as this would often indicate the presence of a predator in the wild. Access out of the cage is important, but they should have free access back into it as the cage should be seen as a safe zone.

A reassessment of the diet of the parrot should always be undertaken as so many are either being offered an unbalanced diet or eating a deficient diet despite being offered the correct nutrition because it is offered in a form that allows too much choice. Favourite food items should be used to encourage foraging behaviours and as rewards when the bird does what the owner wishes it to do.

Physical prevention of self-mutilation may be necessary in the form of Elizabethan collars or neck braces, particularly for cockatoos which can be prone to tissue damage. These collars and braces should not be used on their own without correction of the underlying psychological problem.

Psychotropic drugs similarly should not be used without attempting to alter the underlying cause. Diazepam has been used at 0.5 mg/kg for short-term control of self-mutilation in cockatoos with anxiety and hysteria. Haloperidol has been used in those where skin mutilation has occurred and appears to be the most successful in the more extreme self-mutilation cases at 0.1–0.9 mg/kg orally every 24 hours, although severe extrapyramidal effects have been reported in macaws (Lennox and van der Heyden, 1993; Starkey *et al.*, 2008). Clomipramine has also been used but seems less successful if behavioural modification therapy is not included and has been associated with deaths (possibly due to its arrhythmogenic effects), and amitriptyline has also been found to be effective but similarly has resulted in severe extrapyramidal effects in macaws and toxicity in African grey parrots (Starkey *et al.*, 2008). Fluoxetine has been used successfully at a low starting dose of 0.5–1 mg/kg orally every 24 hours building up to 1–5 mg/kg orally every 24 hours for feather damaging behaviours in parrots (Desmarchelier, 2021).

Avian digestive tract disease therapy

Table 14.4 highlights some of the treatments and therapies commonly used for the management of avian digestive tract diseases.

Avian respiratory tract disease therapy

Table 14.5 highlights some of the treatments and therapies commonly used for the management of avian respiratory tract diseases. Avian nasal sinus flushing is described, which is useful in the treatment of upper respiratory tract disease. Air sac tube placement may be necessary during surgery or treatment of tracheal/syringeal disease, or when a tracheal/syringeal obstruction occurs.

Performing a sinus flush

Apply the hub of a syringe (minus its hypodermic needle) to one external nostril. To make a snug fit between syringe and nostril it is often helpful to remove the rubber stopper of a 2-mL syringe, pierce a hole through its centre and attach this to the hub of the syringe containing the medication. The bird is held inverted and the contents of the syringe (0.5 mL for a budgerigar, up to 5–7 mL for a large macaw or raptor) are expelled into the nostril. The mixture should

Table 14.4 Treatment of avian diseases of the digestive system.

Diagnosis	Treatment
Bacterial/fungal infections	Bacterial infections recommended to be based on culture and sensitivity results, although *Salmonella* spp. infections often require fluoroquinolones such as enrofloxacin *Macrorhabdus ornithogaster*: amphotericin B for 3–5 days (e.g. in water 2% preparation at 5 g/L for 5–14 days; or 25–100 mg/kg dosed orally twice daily for 14 days). Cider vinegar added to drinking water at 60–120 mL/L to acidify water and reduce spread in the flock may also be helpful *Candida albicans*: nystatin 300 000 units/kg orally twice daily. Alternatively, itraconazole 10 mg/kg orally twice daily (NB: has toxicity issues in African grey parrots and in my experience also turkey vultures, barn owls and king penguins, so used at 5 mg/kg orally twice daily in these species). Associated with a lack of dietary vitamin A
Cloacal papillomas	Surgical removal using caustic silver nitrate under anaesthesia
Coccidiosis	*Caryospora* spp.: clazuril 5–10 mg/kg orally every other day for three doses or 5–10 mg/kg daily for two doses *Eimeria* and *Isospora* (intestinal phase): sulfadimethoxine in water for 5 days – beware use in birds with renal disease or during the laying period Toltrazuril has also been used but some preparations in water must be diluted before administering as it is a highly alkaline drug. Dosages of 7 mg/kg orally for 1–2 days have been recommended. However, for the pigeon coccidia *Eimeria columbarum* and *E. labbeana* higher dosages of 20 mg/kg in drinking water for 2 days have been recommended (Krautwald-Junghanns *et al*., 2009) Diclazuril is also routinely used for coccidiosis in racing pigeons Monensin, a coccidiostat, has been used in pelleted feed, often with nicarbazin to prevent coccidial (*Eimeria* spp.) infection in poultry (chickens). It should be noted that this product (and lasalocid) are highly toxic to many mammals such as horses, primates and pigs as well as some species of birds such as ratites (e.g. rheas, emus and ostriches) and so should be used with caution *Cryptosporidium* spp. has been treated with paromomycin 100 mg/kg orally twice daily for 7 days (Guzman *et al*., 2023)
Crop impaction	Crop wash under anaesthetic with warm water. Milk the contents out. Make sure the bird is intubated with a snug fitting tube or lightly inflate the cuff to avoid inhalational pneumonia whilst flushing, then immediately deflate to avoid a stricture formation
Crop burns	Leave until full extent of skin slough develops (often 5–7 days) and treat with covering antimicrobials and pain relief ± fluid therapy. Surgically debride the necrotic skin and underlying tissues and close in separate layers using monofilament dissolving suture material. Large deficits may require flaps or skin grafts
Sour crop	Food should leave crop after 3–4 hours. If not crop, wash and remove manually. May need antimicrobials plus sodium bicarbonate (antacid) plus metoclopramide
Diabetes mellitus	Protamine zinc insulin 0.1–1 unit/kg. Dilute in saline to allow accurate dosing. Rarely controls blood glucose, so aim is rather to stop weight loss. Twice-daily dosing often required
Duck plague	No treatments. Vaccines are available in many countries for prevention
Haemochromatosis	Iron chelation agent, e.g. deferoxamine 100 mg/kg once daily. Phlebotomy (1–2 mL/kg of blood removed once weekly). Diet should contain <60 ppm iron to prevent haemochromatosis for susceptible species and have low vitamin C, which facilitates iron uptake. A diet of 32 ppm was suggested in starlings as an adjunct to treating haemochromatosis (Olsen *et al*., 2009) Inositol has been used to prevent further iron build-up in the liver in starlings at 20 g/kg of food fed (Olsen *et al*., 2009)
Hepatic lipidosis	Reduce fats and proteins in diet but maintain biological value of proteins. Vitamin B and K supplements are advisable. Use of hepatic-supporting drugs such as silymarin (milk thistle), inositol and L-carnitine, or *Spirulina* as dietary supplements. Lactulose syrup (0.3 mL/kg, i.e. 200 mg/kg) orally once to twice daily can reduce ammonia levels and chances of hepatic encephalopathy
Lead/zinc poisoning	Heavy metal chelation agent, e.g. sodium calcium edetate 20–50 mg/kg twice daily by injection for 5 days minimum. D-Penicillamine 50–55 mg/kg orally twice daily may also be used. Beware of renal toxicity so fluid therapy is essential. Flushing out proventriculus/ventriculus to remove all metal particles is also advisable
Nematodes (e.g. *Capillaria* spp.)	Fenbendazole 15–20 mg/kg daily orally for 3–5 days for *Capillaria* spp. and other nematodes – care during moult as can damage growing feathers. Radiomimetic effects reported and suppression of white blood cell counts have been seen. For ascarids, dosing once with 20 mg/kg and then repeating in 2 weeks for heavier burdens may be sufficient Flubendazole available as an in-feed wormer for poultry and game birds Ivermectin 0.2 mg/kg orally or by injection once. May repeat 10–14 days later
Pacheco's disease and other herpesvirus infections	Limited success if caught early in the course of the disease with the use of aciclovir 80 mg/kg orally every 8–12 hours
Protozoa (e.g. *Trichomonas* spp., *Hexamita* spp., *Giardia* spp., *Cochlosoma* spp.)	Metronidazole 10–30 mg/kg orally twice daily for 3–5 days. May need 50 mg/kg orally for *Hexamita* spp. in pigeons for 7 days. Watch for toxicity Carnidazole for pigeons with *Trichomonas* infections but can be used in other birds as well at 20–25 mg/kg orally once. Some more serious infections require up to 5 days of treatment Ronidazole 100–400 mg/L as drinking water for 5 days for pigeons and passerines with *Trichomonas* infections (higher doses may be required in resistant strains). Same dose for cochlosomiasis
Proventricular dilatation disease	No guaranteed treatment although interferon alpha-2 may produce some temporary improvement (Guzman *et al*., 2023). The gastrointestinal effects may be managed with dietary changes (switch to rearing formulas that are more easily swallowed and digested) plus the use of NSAIDs such as celecoxib (10 mg/kg orally once daily). Gabapentin can be used to control neuropathic pain (although not the virus itself) at doses of 10–25 mg/kg orally every 12 hours (Rossi *et al*., 2018)

Table 14.5 Treatment of avian respiratory system disease.

Diagnosis	Treatment
Aspergillosis	Treatment is difficult and prolonged. Surgical debridement of granulomas, possible air sac tube placement (see below) Nebulisation with amphotericin B/suitably diluted F10® (Health and Hygiene Pty Ltd., South Africa) three to four times daily particularly for the first 1–2 weeks is useful Intravenous amphotericin B 1.5 mg/kg for 3–5 days has been described but it is nephrotoxic, so care should be used and hydration ensured Oral itraconazole 10 mg/kg twice daily is effective but this drug can cause toxicity issues in African grey parrots at this dosage and so a lower dose of 5 mg/kg twice daily is recommended. I have also seen toxicity issues in other species such as barn owls, king penguins and turkey vultures with dosages of 10 mg/kg twice daily and so use the African grey parrot dosage for these species as well Voriconazole has been used in a wide range of species and is very effective at 10–15 mg/kg orally every 12 hours. Toxicity with voriconazole use in penguins has been reported as the metabolites of the drug can cause neurological disease and so dosages of 5 mg/kg orally twice daily have been used but 'rest days' (i.e. days without medication) may still be required to avoid side-effects (Hyatt *et al.*, 2015, 2017). Terbinafine 10–15 mg/kg orally twice daily may be used instead but resistance to this drug from *Aspergillus* spp. is common Treatment periods for itraconazole, voriconazole and terbinafine are often 3–12 months due to the resilience of the fungus and difficulty of getting the drug to some of the sites of infection (air sacs) due to their poor blood supply
Bacterial lower respiratory tract disease	This depends on bacterial culture and sensitivity testing. However, mycoplasmosis tends to respond to fluoroquinolones (e.g. enrofloxacin) and tetracyclines (e.g. doxycycline), and pasteurellosis will respond to fluoroquinolones and sometimes potentiated pencillins
Ornithosis/psittacosis/ infection with *Chlamydia psittaci*	Use of doxycycline advised. Preparations in water have been used but many larger parrots will not take these medications in water so injections of human doxycycline hyclate 75–100 mg/kg intravenously once weekly may be used. Periods of 42 days plus are advised (the lifespan of the alveolar macrophage in which the organism often resides). A recent publication suggests 21 days of doxycycline at 35 mg/kg orally once every 24 hours or 21 days of azithromycin 40 mg/kg orally once every 48 hours is effective in clearing *C. psittaci* infection in cockatiels (Guzman *et al.*, 2010) NB: *Candida* spp. overgrowth of the gut is a common sequel to prolonged antibiotic therapy such as doxycycline and so may also require treatment
Respiratory parasites (e.g. *Syngamus trachea* and air-sac mites)	Ivermectin 0.2 mg/kg once. May be repeated in 10–14 days to catch the recently hatched eggs
Paramyxovirus	No treatment. Prevention is via vaccination in pigeons (e.g. Colombovac PMV Suspension for subcutaneous injection, Zoetis; Nobilis Paramyxo P201®, MSD Animal Health). Essential for racing pigeons in UK by law (Disease of Poultry Order 1994 (SI 1994/3141))
Smoke inhalation toxicity	Supportive therapy. Furosemide 1–4 mg/kg intravenously/intramuscularly (beware of nephrotoxicity). Oxygen-enriched atmosphere is advised, and in severe cases methylprednisolone 10–20 mg/kg or prednisolone 6 mg/kg for lung oedema may be given. Beware of corticosteroids and other immunosuppressive drugs as side-effects such as aspergillosis and bacterial infections may appear
Upper respiratory tract disease	Antimicrobial therapy based on culture/sensitivity. Swab from the choanal slit. Surgical removal of rhinoliths, sinus flushes (see below), parenteral antimicrobials

exit through the infraorbital sinus and out through the eye, and through the internal choanal slit and out of the mouth. Holding the bird upside down minimises aspiration of this mixture.

Repeat the procedure for the other nostril.

Air-sac tube placement

In many cases of syringeal aspergillosis or when performing tracheal washes in a dyspnoeic bird, the placement of an air-sac tube may be vital to keep a patent airway. This is further discussed in Chapter 16.

Nebulisation

A nebulisation circuit may be used to administer oxygen or drugs in aerosol form to avians with respiratory disease. Antibiotics such as gentamicin that are effective against Gram-negative bacteria, but which if given intravenously can be nephrotoxic and ototoxic, may be administered by nebulisation as they will not cross the air–blood barrier.

Avian reproductive tract disease therapy

Egg binding

Supplementation with calcium 100 mg/kg by slow intravenous injection, or intramuscularly, is the first step where there is suspicion of hypocalcaemic flaccidity.

The hen should then be placed in a warm humid environment and kept in a quiet situation. Fluid therapy is also advisable, as the reproductive tract frequently becomes dry and friable due to the pressure of the retained egg.

Historically, oxytocin has been used (a hormone absent in birds, vasotocin being produced instead) and in reality it results in some significant cardiovascular side-effects and can be painful as well as providing poor smooth muscle contractions.

Prostaglandin E_2 gel at 0.02–0.1 mg/kg topically at the entrance of the reproductive tract to the cloaca to allow dilation of the vaginal sphincter has also been used. It may be necessary to lubricate the exit of the reproductive tract with a sterile water-based gel.

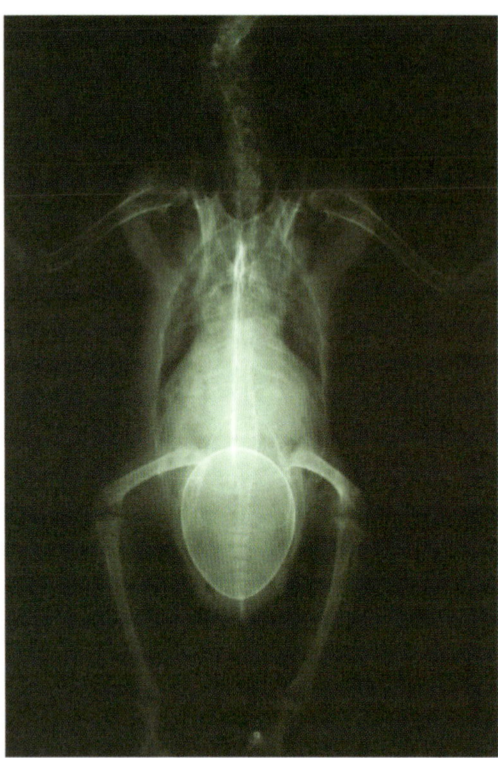

Figure 14.8 Radiograph of an egg-bound parrot. Note the significant size of the egg in relation to the body that leads to issues of organ and blood supply constriction, which can become rapidly life-threatening if not alleviated.

If none of these methods work, then collapse the egg within the bird in order to reduce the pressure which causes the ischaemia of the intestines and kidneys (see Figure 14.8). This may be done by passing a 23-gauge hypodermic needle attached to a 2-mL syringe through the body wall midline and into the egg; alternatively, if the egg can be seen via the cloaca, then a 20-gauge needle attached to a 2-mL syringe can be passed through the cloaca and into the end of the egg. The contents of the egg are then aspirated to collapse it. It is generally not necessary to go in after the shell fragments, as these will usually be passed over the next 24 hours.

Covering antibiotics and analgesia should also be considered, particularly if collapse of the egg has been carried out.

Prevention

First, it is important to provide a well-balanced diet, which is correctly supplemented in calcium and vitamin D_3 with preferably access to ultraviolet (UV) light.

Second, if the hen has started to lay eggs, or has a history of problems, a few environmental changes may be performed to reduce further stimulus to lay. In long-day breeding birds, the first of these is to reduce daylight to a maximum of 10 hours daily. This tries to mimic the conditions found in midwinter and should help to discourage reproductive activity in the hen.

It is also useful to remove nest boxes from the cage to reduce the visual stimulus to nest and reproduce.

The use of plastic commercial egg replacers to fool the hen into thinking she has produced a full clutch of eggs is useful with indeterminate egg layers such as cockatiels which will keep laying eggs until they reach a certain clutch size. If egg replacers are not available then do not remove eggs that have been laid. With budgerigars, it does not matter as they are determinate egg layers – they will lay a set number of eggs irrespective of whether they are removed or not.

If egg-laying persists, then hormonal therapy may be tried to suppress the reproductive cycle. Injections of progesterone, such as medroxyprogesterone acetate, have been the mainstay of hormonal modulation. The downside to this medication is the damaging effect the progesterone has on liver function, as well as the risk of iatrogenic diabetes mellitus. Progesterones are therefore no longer recommended in birds. Human chorionic gonadotropin has been used at 500–1000 IU/kg on days 1, 3 and 5. This has fewer side-effects and can stop egg-laying for up to 6 weeks. More recently, GnRH agonists have been used, specifically deslorelin implants that can last for many months. These cause the GnRH–pituitary–ovarian axis to become refractory by hyperstimulation, so causing it to shut down.

The last resort is spaying of the bird (salpingectomy). This is a risky operation and involves the removal of the salpinx. The ovary is left, due to its multiple arterial blood supply that makes removal dangerous.

Table 14.6 highlights some of the other treatments and therapies commonly used for the management of avian reproductive tract diseases.

Table 14.6 Treatment of reproductive system diseases.

Diagnosis	Treatment
Egg yolk coelomitis	Abdominocentesis may be necessary to relieve pressure from the air sacs but should be performed cautiously via midline ventrally under anaesthesia. Antibiotics are also often required effective against Gram-negative bacteria (particularly coliforms) as secondary infection is common. Supportive therapy for shock may also be required. Short-term shutdown of the reproductive tract with GnRH agonist implants should be considered to prevent further episodes, but long-term treatment may require laparotomy and debridement of granulation tissue, lipids and a salpingectomy. The prognosis is guarded
Prolapsed oviduct	May be a sequel to egg binding and often involves prolapse of the cloaca. Uterus is the most commonly prolapsed part of the oviduct. Tissues become rapidly desiccated and infected if outside of the body. If the tissues are not too devitalised, they may be pushed back with a moistened cotton bud under general anaesthetic. Two simple interrupted sutures may be placed, one either side of the vent, to try to reduce the aperture and prevent recurrence. If the oviduct is devitalised, then removal may be necessary. The cloaca may need to be sutured in place if it repeatedly prolapses via a midline coeliotomy
Salpingitis	Microbial culture and sensitivity testing is recommended to allow correct choice of antimicrobial from a swab of the reproductive tract. However, even when the correct antibiotic is chosen for the bacteria isolated, the infection may not be fully cleared. This may be due to the area affected which walls off the infection from the body and results in the need to consider spaying the bird

Avian urinary tract disease therapy

Table 14.7 highlights some of the treatments and therapies for avian urinary tract diseases.

Avian musculoskeletal system disease therapy

Table 14.8 highlights some of the treatments and therapies commonly used for the management of avian musculoskeletal system diseases. The process for splinting a fractured wing is also described.

Temporary wing splinting

Splinting of wing fractures may be performed with bandage material. It should be noted, though, that when a bird's joint is kept immobilised for a few days it starts to stiffen. This can be disastrous for raptors and wild birds. Bandaging techniques are therefore more suitable for cage and aviary birds and for emergency first-aid support dressings, or where it is possible to maintain joint movement.

The technique for humeral, radial or ulnar fractures is described below.

- Flex the wing using Coflex/Vet Wrap.
- Starting from the point of the elbow, take the bandage over the dorsal aspect of the wing to a point just distal to the point of the carpus.
- Place the bandage over the ventral aspect of the wing, heading back to the point of the elbow.
- Cover the dorsal aspect of the wing to a point just proximal to the carpus.
- Put the bandage onto the ventral aspect of the wing towards the digits.
- Roll it over the leading edge of the wing and the dorsal aspect once more and back to the elbow.

This 'figure-of-eight' technique bunches the primary feathers together and so uses their structure as a splint.

Avian neurological system disease therapy

Table 14.9 highlights some of the treatments and therapies commonly used for the management of avian neurological system diseases.

Miscellaneous conditions

Oil spills

Stabilisation

This involves fluid therapy to correct the dehydration that is commonly present due to diarrhoea. Birds are also often hypothermic due to plumage damage which destroys its insulative properties. Gentle warming in warm air, such as that from a hair dryer, can be used to bring body temperature to near normal as well as using warmed fluids. Heated cages with dimmed lighting to reduce further stress are also advisable. As these birds may have been unable to feed for days, readily digestible liquid food should be provided, if necessary by crop tube.

Initial treatment

Oral administration of adsorbents, such as activated charcoal, can help prevent further absorption of oil. Stomach and intestinal protectants, such as ranitidine, omeprazole or sucralfate, may be required as ulceration may be seen particularly with the more refined oils. Covering antibiotics and further fluid and nutritional support may also be necessary. Because of the extreme stress of the situation, many birds succumb to systemic fungal diseases such as secondary aspergillosis and this may necessitate additional treatment. It is worth noting that many birds are also anaemic as a result of haemolysis caused by absorbed oils and through loss of blood from gastrointestinal ulceration; consequently, blood transfusions should be considered for those with a PCV less than 15% (0.15 L/L).

Table 14.7 Treatment of avian urinary tract disease.

Disease	Treatment
Acute renal disease	Fluid therapy (see above and also Chapter 16) and diuretics, particularly if shock is present, to restart urine production. The diuretic used is principally furosemide 1–4 mg/kg intravenously or intramuscularly Specific therapy for heavy metal poisoning is based on the chelating agent, e.g. sodium calcium edetate 10–30 mg/kg twice daily intramuscularly for 5 days. Alternatives can include D-penicillamine 30–50 mg/kg orally once or twice daily but this can cause vomiting For renal coccidiosis, the use of clazuril 5–10 mg/kg orally every third day on three occasions, or sulfadimidine 25 mg/kg orally twice daily for 3 days, resting for 2 days and repeating for 3 days For chlamydiosis, doxycycline is the antibiotic of choice (see respiratory tract section), but for Gram-negative bacteria fluoroquinolones or third-generation cephalosporins are advised
Chronic renal disease	Even once the causative agent is removed/treated, management of chronic renal failure is challenging Fluid therapy is required in the early stages of treatment (see above and Chapter 16). Supplementation of water-soluble vitamins (B vitamins but avoid B_6 in raptors) and the use of anabolic steroids (to reverse catabolism and bone marrow suppression) have also been advocated The use of allopurinol 10–30 mg/kg orally every 12–24 hours is advised when uric acid levels are high, but in some species (e.g. red-tailed hawk) this has been associated with an increase in uric acid levels (Lumeij and Redig, 1992). Colchicine is used in humans to reduce uric acid and can be used in birds at 0.02–0.04 mg/kg orally every 12–24 hours Many birds are too ill to stabilise and euthanasia should be considered where uric acid levels remain persistently above 1200–1500 μmol/L Surgery may be performed to remove gout crystals in joints and alleviate some of the pain and discomfort. However, the underlying renal disease needs to be rectified. Diet of a high bioavailability but lower protein source is sensible. Omega-3 fatty acids have been suggested as useful (Pollock, 2006)

Table 14.8 Treatment of avian musculoskeletal system diseases.

Diagnosis	Treatment
Carpometacarpal luxation	Bandage wings to the body wall for 4–6 weeks if early on in the condition. Once rotation has occurred, the only option is surgical. Poor prognosis for wild release
Fracture management	In all cases it is important, particularly for wild birds, to obtain as near a 100% successful repair otherwise there could be a welfare issue releasing such a bird into the wild *Coracoid, furcula* These usually recover with rest alone – occasionally, they may require an intramedullary pin *Humerus* This is the most common fracture in raptors (especially hawks). The bone is pneumonised and mid-shaft fractures often result in trauma to the radial nerve and carry a poor prognosis. A tie-in external fixator is often required *Elbow dislocation* Poor prognosis as transarticular fixation is needed so a return to full flight is unlikely *Ulna and radius* If only the ulna is fractured and there is no displacement, cage rest is generally effective with restricted wing movement for 2–3 weeks. If the radius is fractured then intramedullary pin fixation is required. NB: Watch for synostosis between ulna and radius as this can result in reduced pronation and supination which is important for flight manoeuvrability and particularly important for birds that hover *Femur* This is uncommon but may be seen in heavier birds. The bone is pneumonised in raptors but often not in Psittaciformes. A tie-in external fixator will be required *Tibiotarsus and tarsometatarsus* Often associated with trapping or jess injuries in raptors. If a crushing injury occurs then there is a poor prognosis. If it is a clean break but still viable then generally a good prognosis. An external fixator with a tie-in is needed unless it involves small species in which case an 'Altman splint' may be used with two pieces of zinc oxide tape applied on either side of a reduced fracture *Digit injuries* These may be dressed with a ball bandage (see Figure 14.7) or if amputation is necessary, a light padded elasticated support (see Figure 14.9)
Nutritional osteodystrophy	Once bones are deformed and mineralised the only options are surgical. Prevention is geared to adequate diet, calcium supplementation, etc., and not providing excess proteins which generate too rapid growth rates
Wing tip oedema	Prevention by avoiding tethering birds low to the ground in cold weather. Treatment using circulation-enhancing medications such as propentofylline 5 mg/kg orally twice daily or isoxsuprine 5–10 mg/kg orally once daily

Table 14.9 Treatment of avian nervous system diseases.

Diagnosis	Treatment
Fitting/seizuring	Treatment is based on diagnosis of the cause For heavy metal toxicity see Table 14.4 For hypocalcaemic syndrome, see above; also seen in young raptors Symptomatic treatment: dimmed lighting, reduced noise levels, careful handling. Use of diazepam 0.2–1 mg/kg intravenously/intramuscularly (can also be used intracloacally) or midazolam 1–2 mg/kg If the condition occurs in a small raptor, it may be hypoglycaemic, therefore administer 0.25–1 mL 40% glucose/dextrose w/v diluted with the same volume of 0.9% saline, intravenously and slowly and to effect Northern goshawks are also prone to hyperglycaemia at the start of the training season. Diagnosis based on a blood glucose >30 mmol/L. To treat use protamine zinc insulin 0.1 unit and repeat until glucose levels fall below 15 mmol/L (Forbes, 1996) Lories and lorikeets fed on home-prepared nectar formulations may experience hypovitaminosis B_1 and seizures. Injections of 3 mg/kg once followed by dietary supplementation at 35 mg/kg food are successful if the bird is treated quickly Penguins and other fish-eating birds may also suffer from hypovitaminosis B_1 due to the presence of thiaminases in previously frozen fish. Daily supplementation with vitamin B_1 is therefore commonly performed to prevent neurological signs at a rate of 35 mg/kg food fed
Hypocalcaemic syndrome of African grey parrots	Acute collapse: slow intravenous/intramuscular injection of 50–100 mg/kg calcium gluconate. Diazepam (0.2–0.5 mg/kg) or midazolam (1–2 mg/kg) intramuscularly to control fitting Prevention requires adequate dietary calcium and vitamin D_3. This can be achieved through nutritional supplements, UV light provision (UV strip lamps if indoors or obviously access to unfiltered natural sunshine) and access to vegetables and some dairy products (e.g. bio-yoghurts and cottage cheese). Most birds grow out of the condition by 5–6 years of age but appropriate nutrition is still important
Newcastle disease/PMV-1	Treatment is not possible but vaccination for pigeon paramyxovirus (PMV)-1 is compulsory in racing pigeons in the UK and European Union. Vaccines include Colombovac® (Zoetis) and Nobilis Paramyxo P201® (MSD Animal Health). Pigeon PMV-1 is a notifiable disease in the UK and so if suspected or diagnosed should be reported to the local Animal and Plant Health Agency (APHA) office
Proventricular dilatation disease	This may result in central nervous system (CNS) disease such as torticollis, circling, central blindness and fitting. See Table 14.4 for management of proventricular atony. See Seizuring above for control of fitting. Prognosis is poor with CNS signs
Spinal disease	Fractures of lumbar spine are common sequels to window/car strike incidents. Surgery to stabilise can be attempted with postoperative use of anti-inflammatories such as meloxicam 0.2–1 mg/kg once daily and physiotherapy of the pelvic limbs. Prognosis is frequently poor Aspergillomas may also invade the spinal canal from the underlying lung or air sacs. Treatment is as for aspergillosis in Table 14.5. Prognosis is again poor

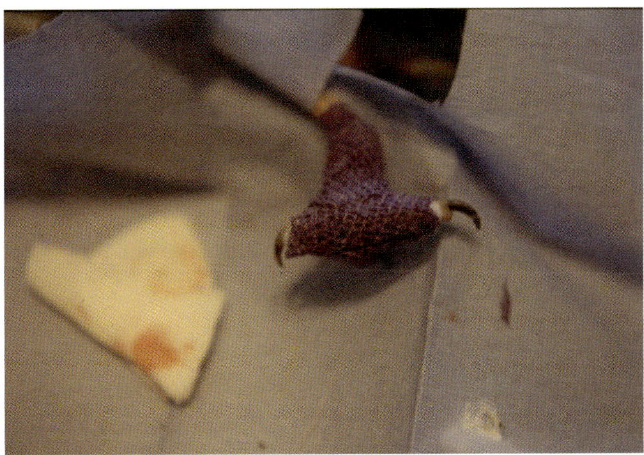

Figure 14.9 A light padding and elasticated bandage support for a toe amputation.

Cleaning

The best cleaning agent for removal of oil is washing-up liquid, which should be diluted 1 part to 50 parts water. This should be lathered into the oil and sprayed off using a shower head attachment. The water supply should be kept at around the bird's own body temperature (40–45°C) to reduce further loss of body heat. This is important as it may take up to an hour to clean some birds. Attention must be paid to thoroughly cleaning all of the feathers, so a cleaning pattern or routine should be used. Washing can stop when the water starts to form small bead-like droplets on the feathers indicating a return to waterproofing.

Once the oil has all been removed, the feathers should be dried initially using a hair dryer, and then by placing the bird in a heated cage. After cleaning and ensuring that the birds are feeding properly and maintaining condition, it is often necessary to retain waterfowl in captivity for a few days to ensure that they are regularly preening to waterproof their feathers.

Lead and zinc poisoning

Treatment with sodium calcium edetate at 20–50 mg/kg twice daily intramuscularly is recommended as a chelating agent; fluid therapy should also be administered as both the heavy metal and the drug are nephrotoxic. Treatment should continue until a return to 'normal' blood levels of lead (<0.2 ppm) or zinc (<2 ppm) are seen assuming all radiodense material has been removed from the gut. The latter may be facilitated by a proventriculus wash with warmed saline under anaesthetic. A tube may be passed with care through the oesophagus and past the crop into the proventriculus. This is then flushed out by tilting the bird's head down. It is essential that an endotracheal tube is used in this process, and that it is snug fitting or the cuff has been lightly inflated with air. If the particulate matter has moved on, the use of peanut butter on bread for Psittaciformes or waterfowl has been suggested as a means of 'sticking' heavy metal particles and allowing passage out of the ventriculus and gut.

References

Desmarchelier, M. (2021) Clinical psychopharmacology for the exotic animal practitioner. *Veterinary Clinics of North America: Exotic Animal Practice*, **24**, 17–35.

Forbes, N.A. (1996) Fits and incoordination. In: *Manual of Raptors, Pigeons and Waterfowl* (eds P.H. Beynon, N.A. Forbes & N.H. Harcourt-Brown), pp. 197–207. BSAVA, Cheltenham, UK.

Guzman, D.S.-M., Beaufrere, H., Welle, K.R. *et al.* (2023) Birds. In: *Exotic Animal Formulary* (eds J.W. Carpenter & C.A. Harms), 6th edn, pp. 222–443. Elsevier, St Louis, Missouri.

Guzman, D.S-M., Diaz-Figueroa, O., Tully Jnr, T. et al. (2010) Evaluating 21-day doxycycline and azithromycin treatments for experimental Chlamydophila psittaci infection in cockatiels (Nymphicus hollandicus). *Journal of Avian Medicine and Surgery*, **24**(1), 35–45. doi: 10.1647/2009-009R.1.

Hyatt, M.W., Georoff, G.A., Nollens, H.H. *et al.* (2015) Voriconazole toxicity in multiple penguin species. *Journal of Zoo and Wildlife Medicine*, **46**(4), 880–888. doi: 10.1638/2015-0128.1.

Hyatt, M.W., Wiederhold, N.P., Hope, W.W. and Stott, K.E. (2017) Pharmacokinetics of orally administered voriconazole in African penguins (*Spheniscus demersus*) after single and multiple doses. *Journal of Zoo and Wildlife Medicine*, **48**, 352–362.

Krautwald-Junghanns, M.-E., Zebisch, R. and Schmidt, V. (2009) Relevance and treatment of coccidiosis in domestic pigeons (*Columba livia* forma *domestica*) with particular emphasis on toltrazuril. *Journal of Avian Medicine and Surgery*, **23**(1), 1–5. doi: 10.1647/2007-049R.1.

Lennox, A.M. and Van Der Heyden N. (1993) Haloperidol for use in treatment of psittacine self-mutilation and feather plucking. *Proceedings of the Annual Conference of the Association of Avian Veterinarians*, pp. 119–120.

Lumeij, J. and Redig, P. (1992) Hyperuricaemia and visceral gout induced by allopurinol in red-tailed hawks (*Buteo jamaicensis*). *Proceedings VIII Tagung der Fachgruppe Gefugelkrankheiten. Deutsche Veterinärmedizinische Gesellschaft*, pp. 265–269.

Martin, H. and Kollias, G.V. (1989) Evaluation of water deprivation and fluid therapy in pigeons. *Journal of Zoo and Wildlife Medicine*, **20**(2), 173–177.

Oaks, J.L. (1993) Immune and inflammatory responses in falcon staphylococcal pododermatitis. In: *Raptor Biomedicine* (eds P.T. Redig, J.E. Cooper, J.D. Remple & D.B. Hunter), pp. 72–87. University of Minnesota Press, Minneapolis, MN.

Olsen, G.P., Russell, K.E., Dierenfield, E. *et al.* (2009) Impact of supplements on iron absorption from diets containing high and low iron concentrations in the European starling (*Sturnus vulgaris*). *Journal of Avian Medicine and Surgery*, **20**(2), 67–73.

Parkinson, L. (2023) Fluid therapy in exotic animal emergency and critical care. *Veterinary Clinics of North America: Exotic Animal Practice*, **26**, 623–645.

Pollock, C. (2006) Diagnosis and treatment of avian renal disease. *Veterinary Clinics of North America: Exotic Animal Practice*, **9**, 107–128.

Rossi, G., Dahlhausen, R. and Orosz, S. (2018) Avian ganglioneuritis in clinical practice. *Veterinary Clinics of North America: Exotic Animal Practice*, **21**, 33–67.

Samour, J., Perlman, J., Kinne, J. *et al.* (2016) Vitamin B6 (pyridoxine hydrochloride) toxicosis in falcons. *Journal of Zoo and Wildlife Medicine*, **47**(2), 601–608. doi: 10.1638/2015-0172.1.

Stanford, M. (2004) Interferon treatment of circovirus infection in grey parrots (*Psittacus e. erithacus*). *Veterinary Record*, **154**, 435–436.

Starkey, S.R., Morrisey, J.K., Hickam, J.D. *et al.* (2008) Extrapyramidal side effects in a blue and gold macaw (*Ara arauana*) treated with haloperidol and clomipramine. *Journal of Avian Medicine and Surgery*, **22**, 234–239.

Chapter 15 Avian Diagnostic Imaging

Physical restraint

Purpose-built Perspex restraint boards may be purchased. The basic design is a flat sheet of Perspex with at one end a neck vice which constrains the head. A couple of attached fine ropes can be applied to the legs, and a strap will restrain the wings in a dorsal extended position.

However, I prefer to use general anaesthesia when radiographing avian species and not to use restraint boards in order to minimise stress.

The only occasions where the use of general anaesthesia can complicate matters are in the use of positive contrast digestive system studies, where transit times are important and anaesthesia will of course alter these; and in the case of horizontal beam radiography, which may be used to determine fluid lines in an ascitic patient, as the avian patient needs to be vertical on a perch.

Chemical restraint

In general, the method of chemical restraint preferred by the author is isoflurane or sevoflurane gaseous anaesthetic in 100% oxygen to both induce the patient (at 3–4% for isoflurane and 4–6% for sevoflurane) and to maintain (at 1.5–2% for isoflurane and 2–3% for sevoflurane) preferably after intubation. For more information on chemical restraint, see Chapter 11.

Avian patient radiography

As with other species, the traditional two views at 90° to each other are required to provide a three-dimensional perspective. The legs should be pulled caudally to avoid excessive overlying of the caudal coelom (see Figures 15.1 and 15.2). The wings of the bird in a lateral view are pulled dorsally to avoid them overlying the body. In a ventrodorsal view, the wings are extended laterally. This means that the views of the wings in both a lateral and ventrodorsal image are actually the same (ventrodorsal) which can make imaging wing lesions at 90° very difficult although not impossible (see Figures 15.3 and 15.4).

Positive contrast techniques

Barium

This is routinely used to highlight foreign bodies in the gastrointestinal tract, and to differentiate opacities in the caudal coelom, such as retained eggs, from the rest of the coelomic contents. Usually, it is only performed in stabilised patients as it requires 1–4 hours fasting to empty the gut, and it requires that the patient be conscious for serial radiographs, which is stressful (although it may be performed using horizontal beam radiography with the bird on a perch). For smaller birds such as cockatiels and budgerigars, 3–5 mL of a 25–30% barium mixture should be crop tubed. For larger birds such as African grey parrots and Amazons, 12–15 mL may be used, and for the larger macaws, 20–30 mL. Serial radiographs are taken at 30 minutes and then hourly until 2 hours post administration, then at 4, 8 and 24 hours post administration.

Transit times vary with species: an African grey parrot's proventriculus will empty around 10–30 minutes after administration of barium sulphate into the crop, reaching the small intestines around 30–60 minutes, the large intestine at 60–120 minutes and the cloaca at 120–130 minutes (see Figure 15.5). Many hawks on the other hand will show proventriculus emptying times around 5–15 minutes post crop tubing, reaching the small intestine around 15–30 minutes, the large intestine around 30–90 minutes and the cloaca around 90–360 minutes (McMillan, 1994).

Barium will also highlight dilations of the crop and proventriculus as can occur in some neuropathies (both toxic and infectious), or parasitic diseases, as well as swellings, growths, ulcers, etc.

Iodine

Aqueous-based iodine contrast techniques may be used for intravenous excretory urography examinations when examining the kidney structures for the presence of abnormalities, or for angiography, often using fluoroscopy.

Iodine may also be used for gastrointestinal studies where intestinal surgery may be required as barium is contraindicated in this scenario. Fewer published studies are available to determine expected transit times of what is a less viscous liquid and this can make motility studies difficult to interpret. However, it may be helpful to determine the presence of foreign bodies, filling defects and proventricular enlargement.

Iodine of course is commonly used in computed tomography (CT) to increase the radiodensity of organs, tissues and vascular systems, which can help highlight abnormal vascularisation associated with neoplasia and inflammatory disease. It has also been used for angiography to demonstrate, amongst other things, the extent of atherosclerotic lesions in the major blood vessels (Hein *et al.*, 2022).

In addition, conditions such as choanal atresia, which is a common cause of a permanent clear sinus discharge, may be elucidated by iodine-based contrast techniques, where iodine is injected into the nasal sinuses and is significantly less irritant in this area than barium.

Normal radiographic findings

The avian skeleton is significantly different from its mammalian cousin. Many bones have become fused, for example no tarsal bones survive, with the proximal row having fused to the distal end of the

Veterinary Nursing of Exotic Pets and Wildlife, Third Edition. Simon J. Girling.

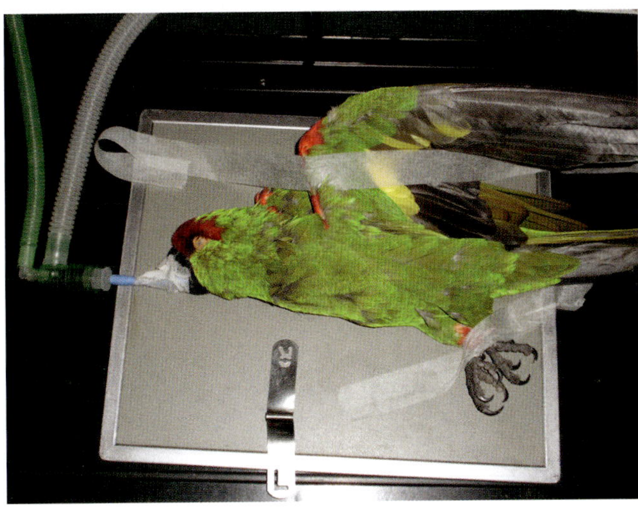

Figure 15.1 Positioning for a right lateral view radiograph in a bird.

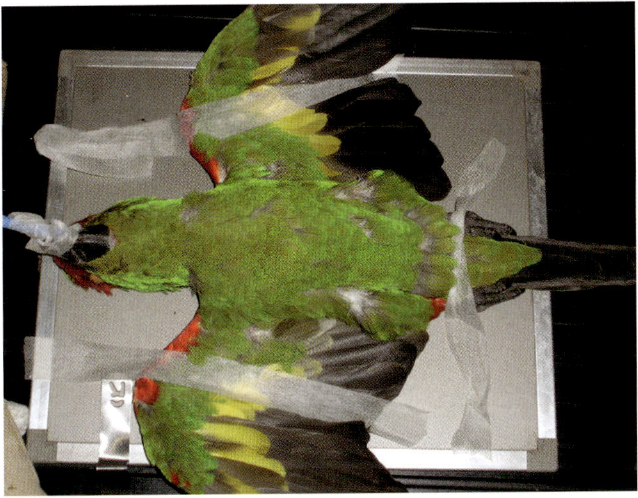

Figure 15.2 Positioning for a standard ventrodorsal view radiograph in a bird.

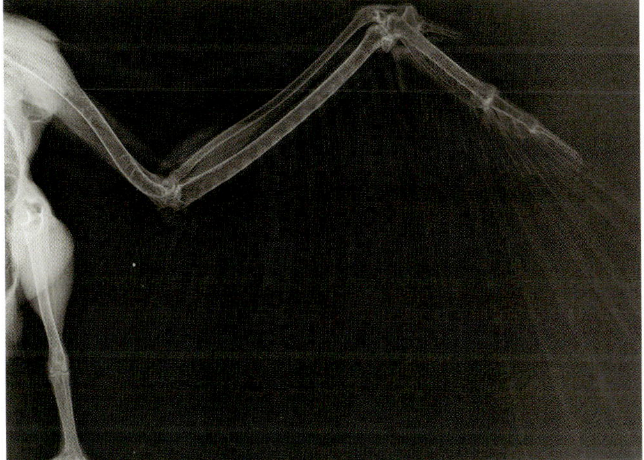

Figure 15.3 Ventrodorsal view of a bird's wing. Note the pneumonised humerus and the attachment of the flight feathers to the periosteum of the ulna (secondary flight feathers) and 'hand' of the bird (primary flight feathers). Some feathers are more radiodense than others and these are typically newly emerged feathers that still have a sheath and/or blood supply to them. Note also the delicate nature of the propatagium and the presence of the alula or 'thumb' of the bird wing projecting cranially from the carpus.

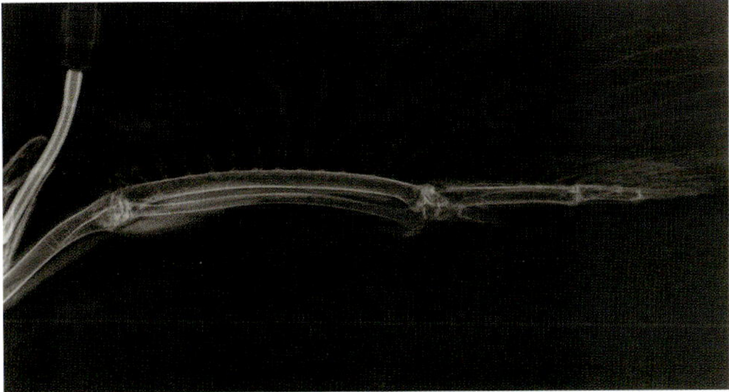

Figure 15.4 Craniocaudal view of the wing of the bird in Figure 15.3 demonstrating the curve of the wing bones, particularly the radius and ulna, to create a greater surface area on the dorsal wing than the ventral, which gives natural lift in flight.

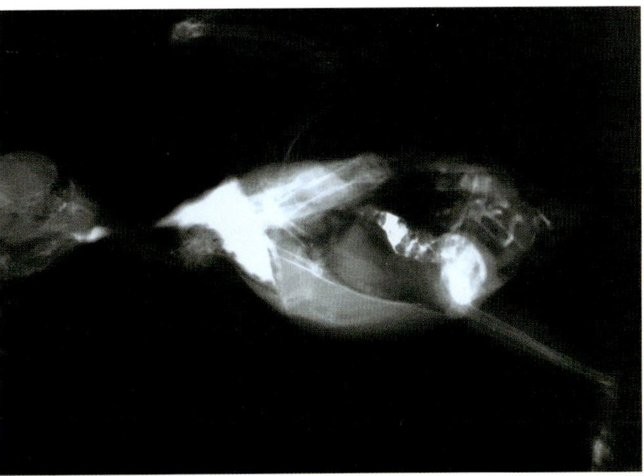

Figure 15.5 Lateral barium digestive tract study in an African grey parrot 1 hour post administration. Note the presence of contrast media in the crop, the proventriculus, the ventriculus and the intestines indicating a normal but rapid gastrointestinal transit time.

tibia forming the tibiotarsus, and the distal row fusing with the proximal metatarsals forming the tarsometatarsus. Birds possess a prominent keel in many species, including the Psittaciformes, formed from the fusion and extension of the sternal vertebrae and this has been used as a yardstick by which the size of other body organs can be assessed (see Figures 15.6 and 15.7).

However, some species such as the ratite family and many waterfowl have a flattened, more boat-shaped sternum without the prominent midline crest. Indeed the term 'ratite' (which covers ostrich, rhea, emu, cassowary and kiwi) comes from the Latin *ratis* meaning 'raft' alluding to their lack of a keel (see Figure 15.8).

Many bones are pneumonised (i.e. connected to the air-sac system and therefore have an air-filled medullary cavity rather than bone marrow); common examples include the femur and the humerus, although individual variation between species occurs.

The pelvis is not fused ventrally, having two separate slender pubic bones projecting caudal to the femur from the main body of the pelvis. The dorsal aspect of the pelvis creates a protective dome fusing with the sacral bones and forming the synsacrum. The thoracic vertebrae and sacral vertebrae are both largely fused and

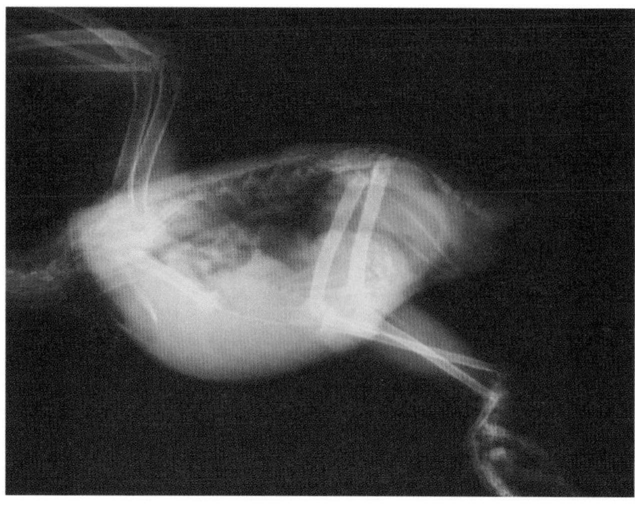

Figure 15.6 Right lateral view of a normal African grey parrot.

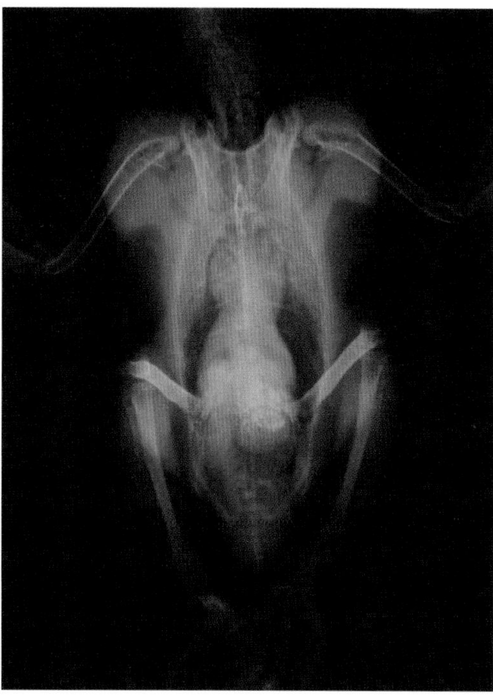

Figure 15.7 Ventrodorsal view of a normal African grey parrot.

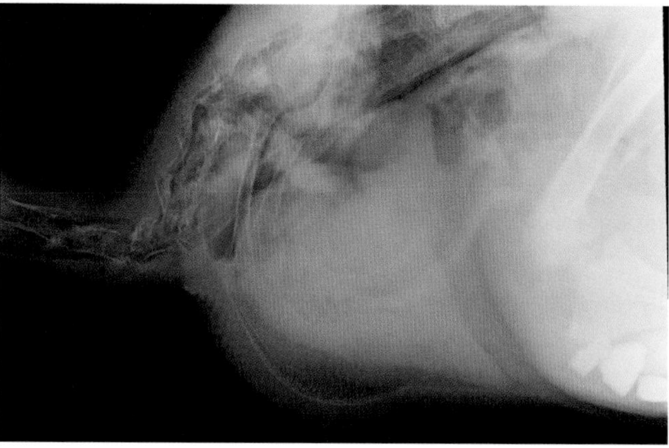

Figure 15.8 Lateral view of a rhea showing the lack of a keel to the sternum. Note the stones present in the stomachs, a common finding in many ratites.

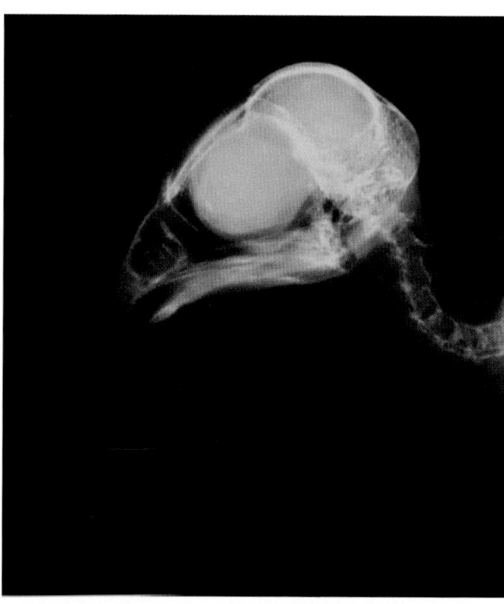

Figure 15.9 Lateral view of a kestrel's skull showing the prominent hooked beak and caudal to that the large eye sockets with scleral ossicles, the small bones that support the structure of the eye around the scleral junction, and caudal to that the small calvarium containing the brain.

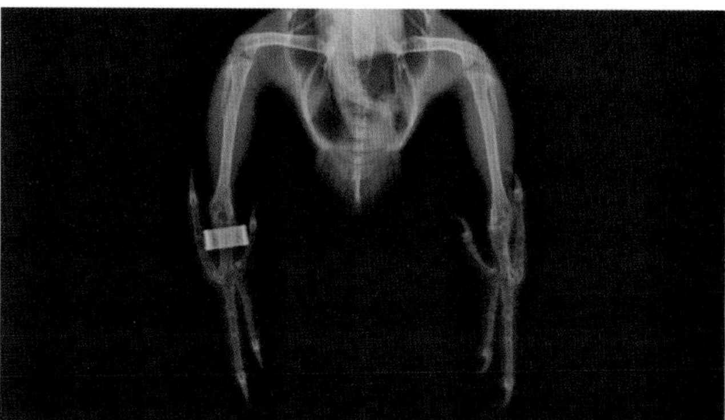

Figure 15.10 Dorsoventral view of a parrot's feet (ventrodorsal view of the body) showing the zygodactyl limb with two digits pointing cranially (1 and 4) and two pointing caudally (2 and 3). Note also the short tarsometatarsus immediately proximal to the digits which is common in the Psittaciformes.

immobile. In contrast the cervical vertebrae are highly mobile and so radiographically the radiolucent intervertebral disc spaces can be seen.

Considerable species variation exists in the skeletal structure, perhaps most notably in the head, neck and feet. Raptors have notable adaptations of the head (see Figure 15.9) and feet, with the majority having an anisodactyl limb (one toe pointing backwards and three forwards). Parrots and some species such as kingfishers have a zygodactyl limb (two toes pointing forwards and two backwards; see Figure 15.10). Many cranes, herons, storks, waterfowl and other wading birds have long and mobile cervical vertebrae (and often long solid beaks) (see Figure 15.11). A ring of bones (scleral ossicles) supporting the eye globe

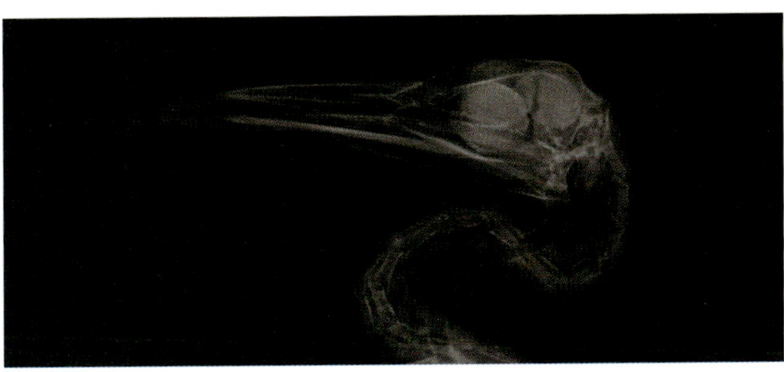

Figure 15.11 Lateral view of a heron showing the numerous and mobile cervical vertebrae and the long beak but note that the bones of the maxilla and mandible do not extend to the end of the beak, the tip being composed of keratinised tissues. Note also the large eye globes supported by a ring of scleral ossicles.

at the corneal–scleral junction are commonly seen in all birds although they are poorly mineralised in many (see Figures 15.9 and 15.11).

As mentioned many longer-legged species of bird have significant elongation of the tibiotarsus and tarsometatarsus bones whereas the Psittaciformes for example have a very short tarsometatarsus (see Figure 15.10). Many of the cranes, storks, Strigiformes and Galliformes have significant ossification of the tendons in the tibiotarsal and tarsometatarsal area and this is a normal finding (see Figure 15.12).

The body cavity, as with reptiles, is not divided into a thorax and abdomen as there is no diaphragm. In addition, the avian lungs are a rigid structure, paired and closely adherent to the dorsal body wall in the cranial coelom and appear homogeneously mottled on lateral radiographs. The air sacs which fill the coelom appear as marked radiolucent areas, and allow clear definition of many internal organs. The trachea is mobile and elongated, and may have many coils in certain species of waterfowl such as the trumpeter swans and cranes and storks. In many male ducks, such as the common mallard, the trachea may have a swelling at its base formed by a bulla, which is a perfectly normal finding (see Figure 15.19).

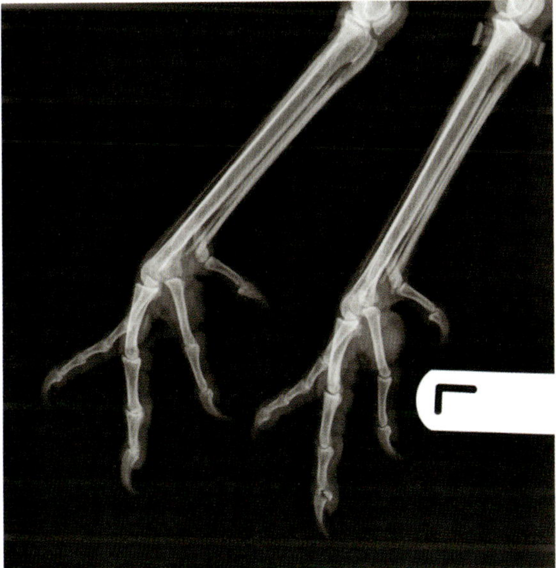

Figure 15.12 Lateral view of the lower limb of a Galliformes bird showing the ossified tendons, in this case caudal to the tarsometatarsus, which are a normal feature of this family of birds. The intertarsal joint is at the top of the image and note the increased soft tissue density on the main pad of the left leg associated with pododermatitis.

On lateral radiographs, the heart may be clearly seen at the dorsal cranial edge of the sternum with the major arterial and venous trunks leaving and entering it. The caudal border of the heart merges with the liver shadow. Dorsal to the liver on the lateral view lies the spleen, which is spherical in many Psittaciformes and Sphenisciformes (penguins), and enlarges markedly during infectious diseases such as chlamydiosis and malaria respectively. It may be more strap-like in Passeriformes and raptors. In this region also lies the 'true' acid-secreting stomach or proventriculus, slightly dorsal to the liver on a lateral view. Immediately caudal to this lies the often grit-filled, in granivorous species, ventriculus, also known as the gizzard or second stomach and this is often located just caudal to the sternum. In carnivores and omnivores the change from proventriculus to ventriculus is not clear and one large stomach is apparent. Caudal to the stomachs lie the intestinal mass. The kidneys lie on the dorsal body wall within the shadow of the pelvis and may be seen to project cranially when enlarged due to inflammatory disease or tumours. Just cranial to the pelvis and caudal to the lung field on the lateral view also sit the gonads. In the case of male Columbiformes and Passeriformes, the testes may enlarge considerably during the breeding season and appear as large radiodense structures in this area.

The ventrodorsal view is useful for comparing the thoracic and abdominal air sacs, which are prime sites for fungal granuloma formation in diseases such as aspergillosis in cage birds and birds of prey. The heart shadow is clearly outlined on the ventrodorsal view, and in Psittaciformes it forms the upper part of an hourglass shape, with the lower chamber being produced by the shadow of the liver. Some species such as the larger cockatoos and macaws may have a small heart shadow and/or a small liver shadow, accentuating the 'waist' of the hourglass shape, which may be a normal radiographic finding (see Figures 15.6 and 15.7). In many carnivores and Passeriformes, the heart shadow merges with the liver shadow and does not form an hourglass shape (see Figure 15.13). The width of the heart at its widest point on a ventrodorsal view may be compared with the width of the ribcage at its widest (often around the 5th pair of ribs) and in medium-sized psittacine birds (200–500 g) it should be 51–61% of the thoracic width. Alternatively, the width of the heart may be compared with the length of the sternum, and for medium-sized parrots this should be 36–41% of the sternal length (Straub *et al.*, 2002).

The gizzard or ventriculus is often clearly seen in Psittaciformes, Galliformes and other predominantly granivorous species due to grit consumed which is radiodense. In the ventrodorsal view it lies to slightly to the left of midline in the caudal coelomic region.

The ventrodorsal view can make identification of the kidneys and gonads difficult and contrast media such as intravenous techniques may help highlight them.

Abnormal radiographic findings

Skeletal

Evidence of fractures may be obvious as with most long bone fractures, or slightly less blatant, as with femoral head fractures and spinal injuries. Radiography is also essential to ensure correct alignment of bones and siting of pins and external fixators (see Figure 15.13).

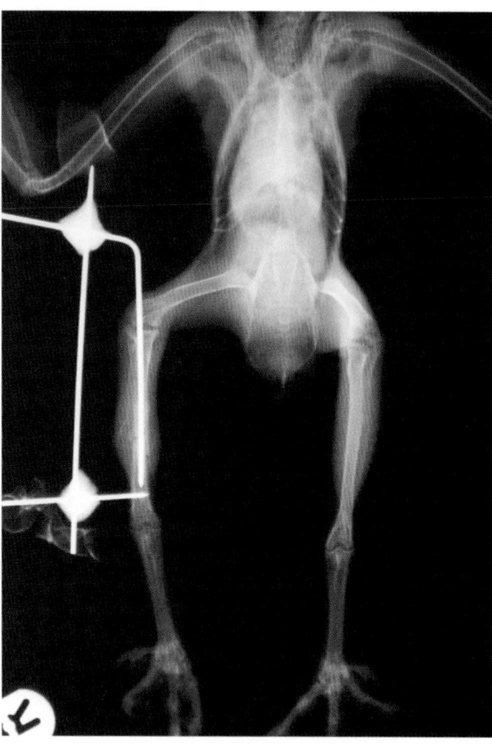

Figure 15.13 Ventrodorsal view of an owl with a tibiotarsal fracture with an external fixator applied to realign the bones. Note also how the heart and liver shadow merge unlike in Psittaciformes where their combined shadows create an hourglass shape.

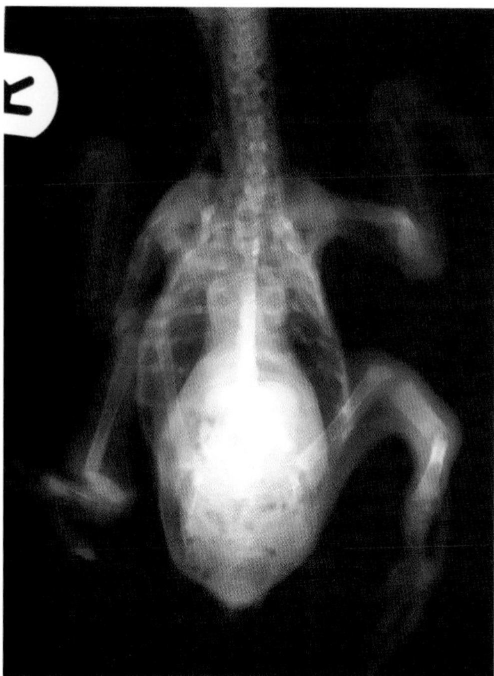

Figure 15.14 Ventrodorsal view of a parrot chick with severe metabolic bone disease due to nutritional secondary hyperparathyroidism. Note the deformed long bones and ribcages, the growth plates and the poor bone quality.

Metabolic bone disease is common in juvenile birds that are fed inappropriate diets, and the bones most commonly affected are the long bones, especially the tibiotarsus, which may bend significantly under the weight of the growing bird (see Figure 15.14).

Other skeletal changes include polyostotic hyperostosis, which is often associated with compulsive egg-laying and/or cystic ovarian disease and persistent hyperoestrogenaemia, leading to a mottled appearance to the long bones, but can also be associated with ovarian and testicular neoplasia (see Figure 15.15); primary or secondary bone neoplasia which often has a 'punched-out' appearance to the bone although proliferative changes to the periosteum may also be seen; and osteomyelitis which can frequently be associated with a mottled appearance associated with erosion of the bone and proliferation of the periosteum and is perhaps most commonly seen in the digits of waterfowl and birds of prey with pododermatitis, often accompanied by joint infections (see Figure 15.16).

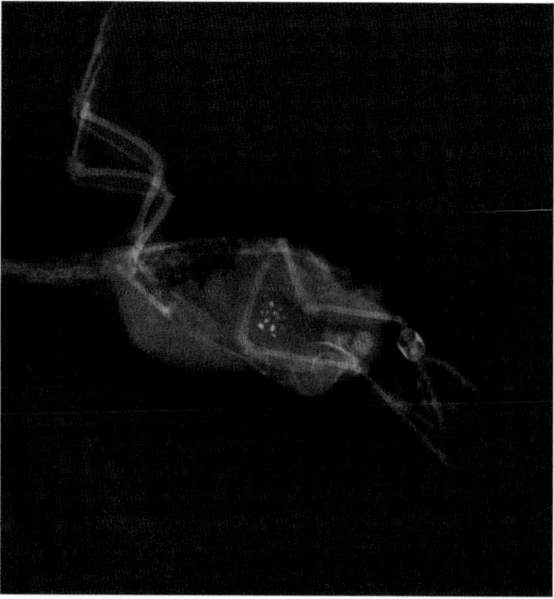

Figure 15.15 Lateral view of a small psittacine bird with polyostotic hyperostosis. Note the increased density of the long pelvic-limb, humerus and coracoid bones. Note also the partially collapsed eggshell in the caudal ventral body cavity with herniation of the caudal body ventral wall. Ventral body-wall herniation is commonly associated with hyperoestrogenism and compulsive egg-laying in small cage birds such as psittacines.

Soft tissue

Enlargement or reduction in size may be noted in any of the internal organs if affected by disease.

On the ventrodorsal view, an enlarged liver often presents in Psittaciformes as a reduction in the 'waist' of the hourglass shape created by the heart and liver shadows due to an increase in the width of the liver area and narrowing of the caudal air sacs (see Figure 15.17). Lines can be drawn on the ventrodorsal radiograph from the shoulder joint to the hip joint and the liver 'shadow' in Psittaciformes should lie medial to these lines. It should be noted however that an enlarged proventriculus can sometimes mimic an enlarged liver and so a contrast study to define what is liver and what is proventriculus may be required (see Figure 15.18).

A reduction in the size of the liver may be seen as a visible gap between the caudal border of the heart and the cranial border of the

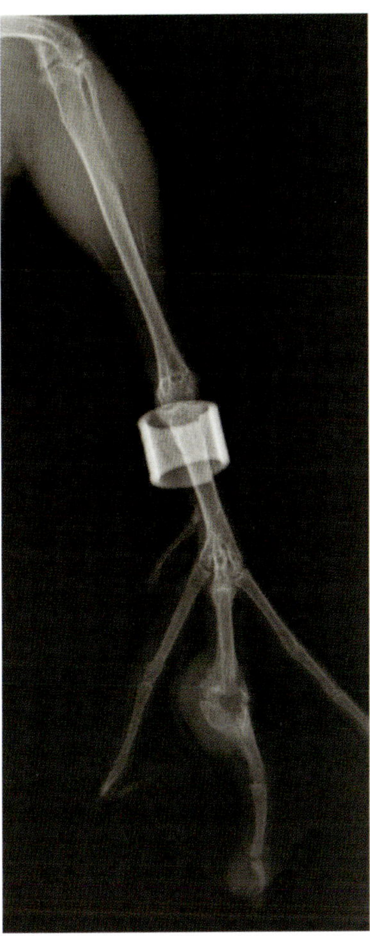

Figure 15.16 Dorsoventral view of a duck's foot showing septic arthritis and osteomyelitis.

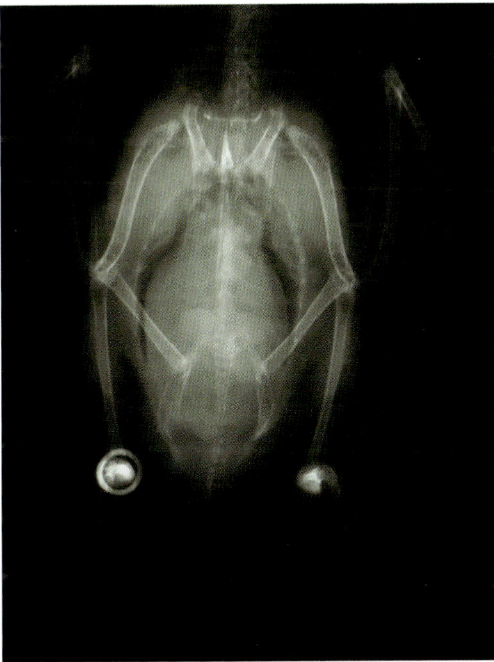

Figure 15.17 Ventrodorsal view of an Amazon parrot with hepatomegaly. Note the reduced caudal air-sac space, the reduction in the 'waist' of the hourglass shape of the major body organs and the increase in width of the liver shadow.

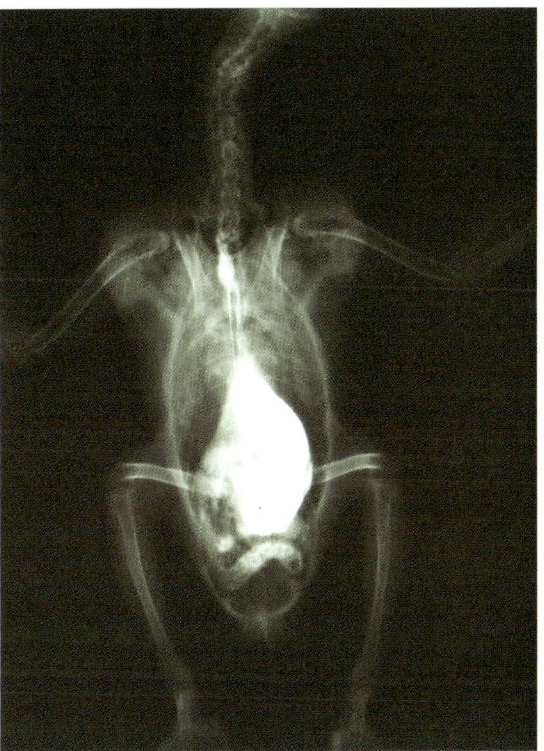

Figure 15.18 Ventrodorsal positive contrast view of a parrot with proventricular dilatation disease showing an enlarged proventriculus and slow gut transit time (4 hours post administration and the contrast media has not yet reached the cloaca).

liver, but note that this may be a normal finding in some larger macaws and cockatoos.

An enlarged proventriculus may be seen in gastric dilatation syndrome, and is shown by a radiodense organ dorsal and caudal to the heart and dorsal to the liver shadows on a lateral radiograph. On a ventrodorsal view, the enlarged proventriculus, which lies on the left-hand side, can be mistaken for an enlarged liver shadow which overlies it unless positive contrast media is used (see Figure 15.18). Proventriculus diameter at the junction of the last thoracic vertebra and the synsacrum can be compared to the maximum dorsoventral height of the keel and for healthy psittacine birds the ratio should be less than 0.48 (Dennison *et al.*, 2008).

Intestinal disease can result in gas production and dilatation, intestinal wall thickening, evidence of foreign bodies and sometimes intussusceptions (see Figure 15.19).

An enlarged spleen, as mentioned previously, may be seen on lateral radiographs, dorsal to the liver shadow, around the mid-femur level, particularly with chlamydiosis/psittacosis in Psittaciformes (see Figure 15.20) but can become enlarged with any infectious disease state, includin parasitic diseases such as malaria (*Plasmodium* spp. infection) in Sphenisciformes (penguins) and Passeriformes.

Enlarged or damaged kidneys may appear more radiodense, or they may project cranially out from the boundaries of the pelvis on a lateral view, or may move dorsocaudally to obliterate a section of the abdominal air sac which normally lies over the dorsal aspect of the caudal kidney area. Care should be taken to avoid confusing cranial enlargement of the kidneys with enlargement of the gonad(s) which sit immediately cranial to them.

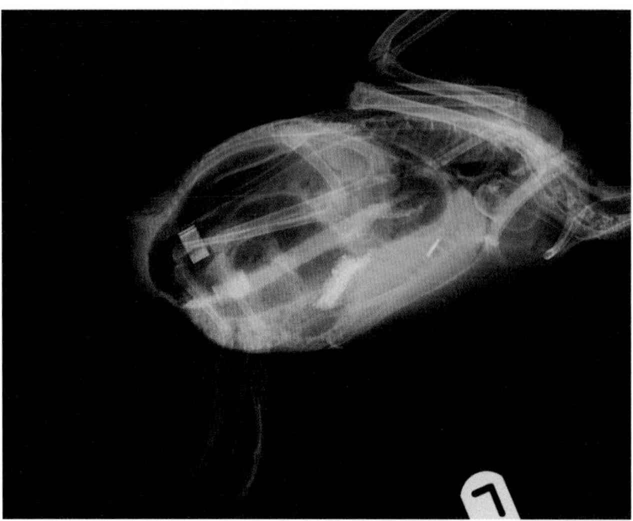

Figure 15.19 Lateral view of a duck with severe parasitic intestinal disease that has resulted in an intussusception. Note this is a male duck as shown by the significant syringeal bulla at the caudal end of the trachea.

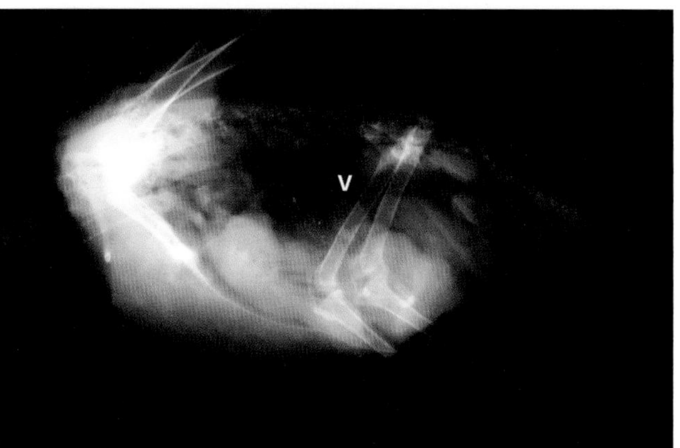

Figure 15.20 Lateral view of a macaw with psittacosis/chlamydiosis showing an enlarged spleen (indicated by the white arrowhead).

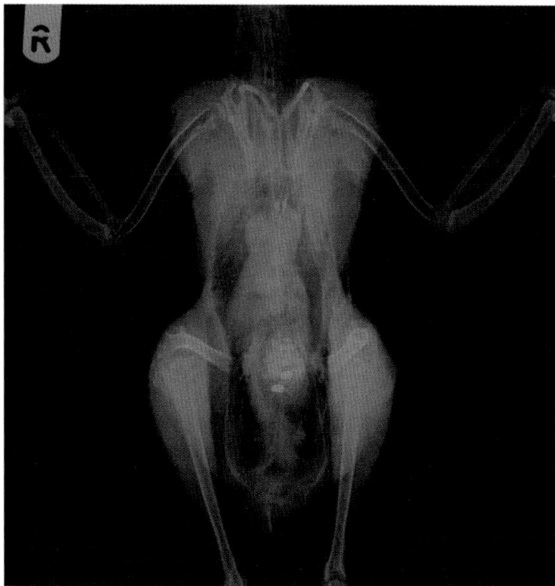

Figure 15.21 Ventrodorsal view of a Galliformes with lead poisoning. Note the radiodense metallic particles present in the ventriculus (gizzard).

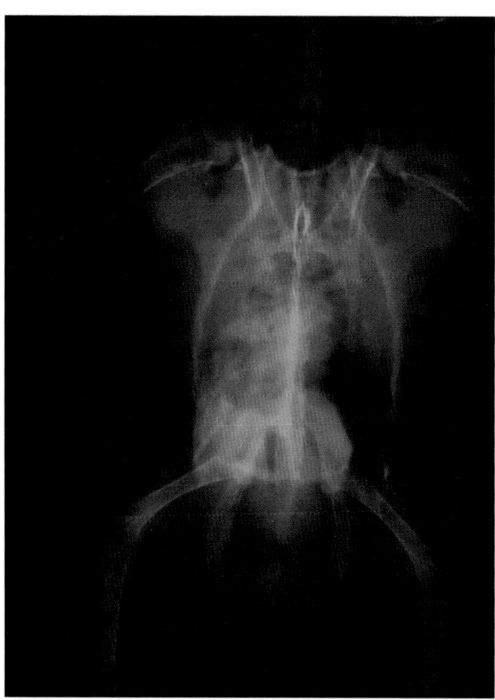

Figure 15.22 Ventrodorsal view of an Amazon parrot with advanced chronic aspergillosis. The bird's right side (our left) is completely obliterated with fungal growth obscuring the air sacs and anatomical structures.

The great vessels exiting the heart may become dilated, or more radiodense, with either atherosclerosis or metastatic mineralisation. The heart itself may also become enlarged with progressive failure in older or diseased birds, with cor pulmonale (due to an increased outflow resistance to the right ventricle because of lung disease) and in younger birds due to dilated cardiomyopathy.

Foreign bodies may also be seen using radiography, particularly metallic elements that may be associated with heavy metal (e.g. lead and zinc) poisoning. They will often lodge in the ventriculus (gizzard) in Psittaciformes and Galliformes (see Figure 15.21).

Infections of the air sacs are common in psittacine birds and raptors. The most frequently seen disease is perhaps aspergillosis, a fungal infection of the lungs and air sacs. This may produce subtle changes initially but may go on to produce significant radiographic changes in advanced chronic disease (see Figure 15.22). These include the production of fungal granulomas causing radiodense structures in the lungs, but also the air sacs. Air sacs affected are often the caudal thoracic and abdominal in Psittaciformes and raptors, but interestingly more typically in the cervical and cranial thoracic air sacs in penguins likely due to their predominantly paleopulmonic lung structure (see Chapter 9). Other infectious agents such as viruses and bacteria can also cause lung and air-sac disease either directly or through systemic spread. Avian tuberculosis (infection with *Mycobacterium avium* subsp. *avium*) typically affects the gastrointestinal tract including the liver but may spread

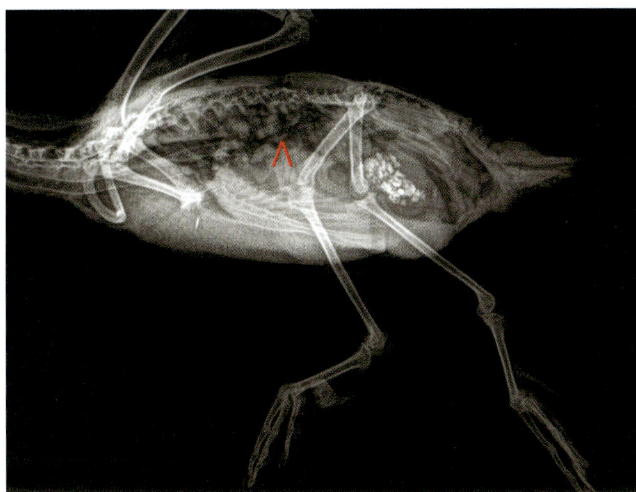

Figure 15.23 Lateral view of a duck with systemic avian tuberculosis. There is a noticeable lesion in the caudal lung field (indicated by the red arrowhead) as well as numerous smaller granulomas. Lesions in this area may penetrate the spinal cord dorsally and result in pelvic limb and caudal body neurological disease.

throughout the body via the bloodstream or by direct extension and occasionally can appear in the lungs (see Figure 15.23)

Ultrasonography

Positioning

The transducer is usually applied to the skin caudal to the keel, ventrally, or in Galliformes and other species where the ribs do not extend as far caudally, such as Columbiformes, access may be gained from the lateral body wall just in front of the leg. Therefore, restraint (preferably chemical) in lateral or dorsal recumbency, with the head elevated to allow the organs to fall towards the transducer, is preferable. It may be possible to image raptors in a conscious state on their perches if they are hooded.

Normal ultrasound findings

For most imaging of birds above 150–200 g, it is preferable to use a 7.5-MHz sector probe. A 10-MHz probe or a stand-off is generally required for such a small species as a budgerigar or canary. Adequate amounts of coupling gel should be applied and allowed to soak into the skin before imaging. It may be necessary to pluck a few feathers as well, although careful wetting and parting of the feathers, particularly immediately caudal to the sternum on the ventrum, will allow access to the skin without this. All these procedures result in potential chilling of the bird and this should be accounted for by using a heated examination room and warmed fluids for the patient.

The main problem with ultrasound examination of birds is the presence of the air sacs, which of course completely block the passage of ultrasound waves. It is possible to use organs as 'windows' to view other organs, and this is usually the case with the liver which is easily accessible from the caudal sternum position and may be used to image the heart for example. Where ascitic/coelomic fluid is present of course this modality becomes much more useful.

Liver: The liver is easily imaged from a ventral approach immediately caudal to the sternum. As with mammals, the normal liver is homogeneous in density (see Figure 15.24). Blood vessels may be seen readily within the parenchyma as hypoechoic areas. Many of the commonly seen species in veterinary practice do not possess a gall bladder, for example the domestic pigeons, many parrots and ostriches. Many Anseriformes such as ducks and Galliformes such as the domestic chicken, quail and turkey do possess a gall bladder.

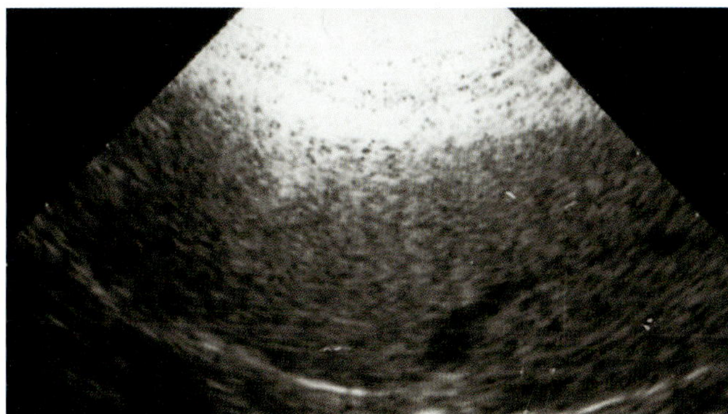

Figure 15.24 Liver structure should be homogeneous. Note the blood vessel creating a hypoechoic line arcing across the lower right of the structure.

Heart: The heart can be seen as a four-chambered structure, although there is a disproportionate difference between the size of the larger left ventricle and the smaller right ventricle (see Figure 15.25). It is generally difficult to see all four chambers in one section as the right and left atria are in a slightly different plane from the ventricles and, as mentioned, the liver is generally used as a 'window' to access it. The left ventricle also has a thinner wall than the right ventricle. The right ventricle ends before reaching the cardiac apex.

The valves of the heart may also be distinguished. The right atrioventricular (AV) valve is normally thickened, muscular and singular. The left AV valves are similar to those seen in the cat and dog but species variation exists and left AV valves can be bicuspid or tricuspid

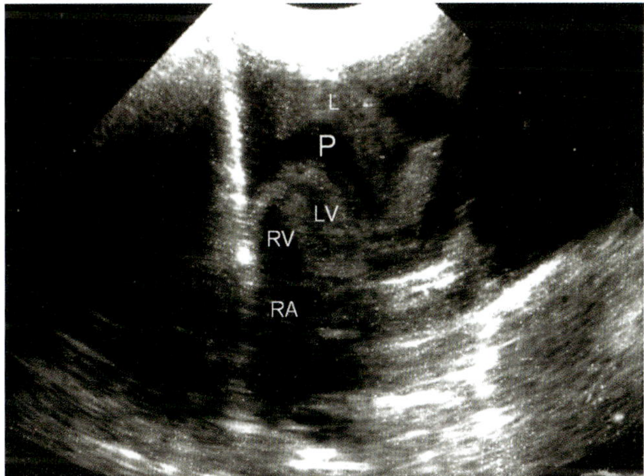

Figure 15.25 Ultrasound image of a parrot heart using the liver as an acoustic 'window'. The liver is at the top of the image (L) with the apex of the heart below. A pericardial effusion (P) is seen in this case, which is an abnormal finding and can be associated with primary heart disease, hypoproteinaemia and anaemia amongst other conditions. LV, left ventricle; RV, right ventricle; RA, right atrium.

according to the species. The aortic valves are also easily seen and are generally paired.

Normal values for heart echocardiographic parameters have been published for African grey and Amazon parrots by Pees *et al.* (2004). Two approaches are typically used (Cornelia and Krautwald-Junghanns 2022).

1. *Parasternal approach*: may be more appropriate for birds such as Columbiformes and Galliformes where the heart can be accessed from a lateral approach above the sternum but caudal to the last rib; provides a cross-sectional view of the heart.
2. *Caudal sternal approach*: often the only available route for species such as Psittaciformes using the liver as an acoustic window; accessed via midline, ventral, caudal to the sternum.

Other organs: It is not normally possible to easily image many of the healthy organs of birds such as Psittaciformes due to the presence of the air sacs combined with a small ventral abdominal scanning window. The kidneys can be particularly challenging unless ascites is present. In birds such as chickens and pigeons, greater coelomic access is possible. Shelled eggs in the oviduct appear obviously hyperechoic, but laminated eggs (i.e. those without a shell yet formed around the yolk and albumen) may also be seen in the oviduct. The yolk tends to be more hyperechoic and the albumen hypoechoic in structure.

Abnormal ultrasound findings

Liver: Enlargement of the liver is difficult to assess using ultrasound as the full extent of the organ cannot be determined in one view. However, the protrusion of the liver beyond the caudal sternum/xiphoid is usually taken as an indication of hepatomegaly.

Where the liver is markedly enlarged, it may be possible to see dilated vessels within the parenchyma and increased echogenicity of their walls. Hepatic lipidosis (fatty liver degeneration) is seen as increased echogenicity and liver size. Hepatic tumours, whether primary or secondary, may of course be identified with ultrasound techniques as areas of increased and decreased echogenicity, although these may be difficult to separate from granulomas and areas of hepatic necrosis unless a discrete capsule to the neoplasm is seen. Hepatic enlargement and necrosis seen as large hypoechoic areas is a common finding in liver diseases such as haemochromatosis (iron storage disease).

Heart: The presence of a pericardial effusion, as with mammals, is considered abnormal in birds (see Figure 15.25). Overall cardiac enlargement, as associated with cardiomyopathies, is also easily diagnosed. Valvular defects have been reported in birds and ultrasound may be used to diagnose these (Rosenthal and Stamoulis, 1993).

Kidneys: Renal tumours, such as those commonly seen in budgerigars, may be diagnosed, as they often enlarge rapidly from the cranial pole of a kidney and may be cystic in nature.

Reproductive system: Coelomic deposition of eggs (so-called 'internal laying') may occur with some cage birds and may result in egg yolk peritonitis. Such eggs may be seen as either hypoechoic or multilaminate structures.

Other organs: Where ascitic/coelomic fluid is present, most of the organs may be imaged easily (see Figure 15.26). In cases of cystic ovarian disease, the classical hypoechoic 'bunches of grapes' may be seen as the ovary becomes sufficiently enlarged to push ventrally. Egg yolk peritonitis will present with a marked coelomic effusion which has a turbid appearance, and so has areas of increased echogenicity whereas a true ascitic effusion tends to be hypoechoic in nature.

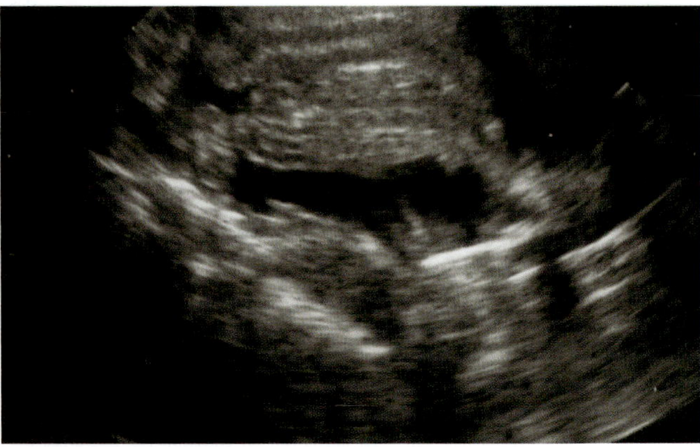

Figure 15.26 Ultrasound image of a toucan with iron storage disease and secondary ascites. Note the layered appearance of the intestines and the anechoic ascitic fluid surrounding them.

Dilatation of the proventriculus may also be imaged, due to its distended size, and a thinning of its wall may further enhance a diagnosis. Splenomegaly, particularly in cases of chlamydiosis in Psittaciformes and malaria in penguins and Passeriformes, may also be diagnosed by ultrasound, as the spleen pushes ventrally towards the body wall caudal to the proventriculus. The spleen in most Psittaciformes is rounded and will have increased echogenicity in comparison to the liver but is normally homogeneous in character. Splenic tumours are rare but may also present as with mammals with hypoechoic areas within the parenchyma.

Magnetic resonance imaging and computed tomography

Both these modalities have been used to good effect in avian patients. CT scanning of the skeleton is commonly performed, particularly the head to examine fractures of jawbones such as the quadrate bone which is easily damaged when birds fly into windows and is far easier than trying to make the diagnosis using traditional radiography. CT scans are also commonly used to identify atherosclerosis, with or without angiography using radiopaque intravenous media (see Figure 15.27). They are also used frequently to identify respiratory tract lesions (aspergillomas in air sacs for example) but may also be used to highlight renal disease, again often with the use of intravenous contrast media, generally an iodine-based product at 2 mL/kg, to produce an excretory urogram.

Magnetic resonance imaging (MRI) of the heart and liver is useful as these are sometimes difficult to visualise on radiographs and ultrasound examinations owing to their encasement within the ribcage and sternum. MRI may also be used to examine other soft tissues such as the brain, kidneys and gonads. Its largest drawback is the much longer periods of time that an MRI scan takes to run as compared with CT, therefore requiring longer periods of anaesthesia for the patient.

Endoscopy

Rigid endoscopes are extremely useful for enabling visualisation and guided sampling of internal lesions. They can be used to look

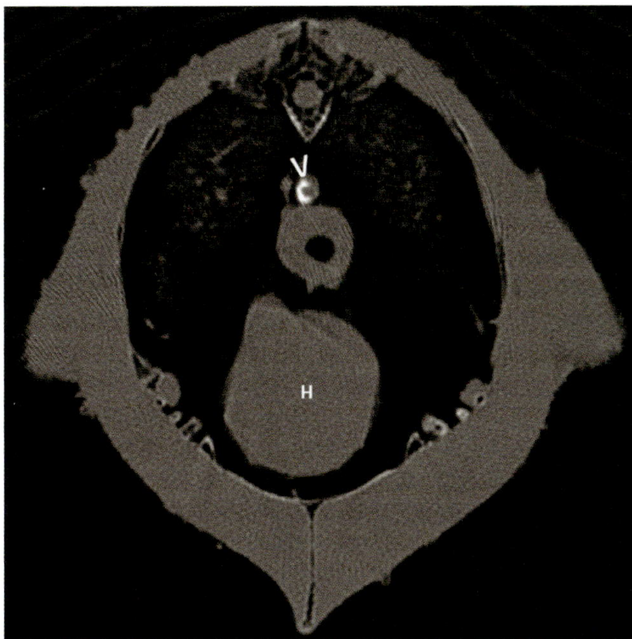

Figure 15.27 Cross-section CT image of an African grey parrot with atherosclerosis of the aorta (indicated by white V; the heart is indicated by H). Either side and dorsal to the aorta are the lungs with the thoracic vertebrae immediately dorsal. Ventral to the aorta and dorsal to the heart is the oesophagus. *Source:* Courtesy of Tobias Schwarz, University of Edinburgh.

down the trachea for syringeal aspergillomas and tracheal parasites such as *Capillaria* spp. and *Syngamus trachea*; into the crop and on into the proventriculus for upper gastrointestinal tract examination; and into the cloaca to look for papillomas, retained eggs, etc.

In addition, the presence of air sacs and a rigid body wall in birds makes them an ideal candidate for laparoscopic endoscopy as the insufflation gas that is used in mammals is not required.

Access to coelom

The point of access is the lateral body wall. The boundaries of the entrance point are usually taken as the cranial edge of the iliotibial muscles (with the bird in lateral recumbency and the legs pulled caudally) and the caudal edge of the pectoral muscles. This site is between the last two ribs for a psittacine bird (may be just caudal to the last rib in a passerine or raptor) (see Figure 15.28). The skin is incised with scissors and the body wall muscles are bluntly dissected using a pair of mosquito haemostats.

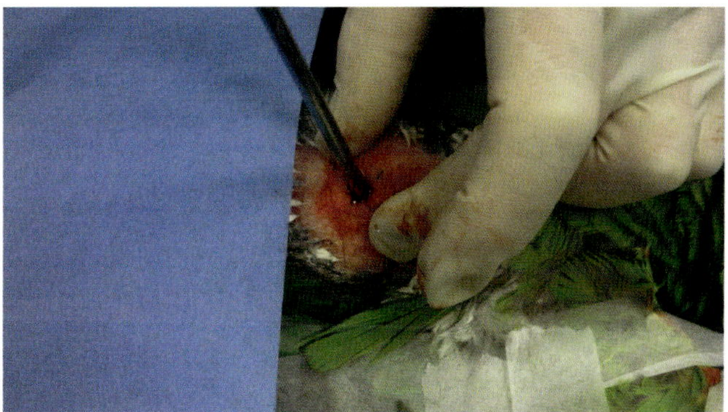

Figure 15.28 Site and positioning of the avian patient for standard rigid endoscopic examination of the coelomic cavity.

The left flank is used when wishing to examine the gonads for sexing, as well as being useful for examining the spleen, gizzard, pancreas, left kidney and left lung. The right flank is preferable for examining the right testis, right kidney and right lung. Either side may be used to view the dorsal surface of the liver.

For views of the ventral surface of the liver, the bird should be in dorsal recumbency and the access point is immediately caudal to the sternum and midline.

References

Cornelia, K. and Krautwald-Junghanns, M.E. (2022) Heart disease in pet birds: diagnostic options. *Veterinary Clinics of North America: Exotic Animal Practice*, **25**, 409–433. doi: 10.1016/j.cvex.2022.01.004.

Dennison, S.E., Paul-Murphy, J.R. and Adams, W.M. (2008) Radiographic determination of proventricular diameter in psittacine birds. *Journal of the American Veterinary Medical Association*, **232**(5), 709–714. doi: 10.2460/javma.232.5.709.

Hein, R.F., Kiefer, I. and Pees, M. (2022) A spectral computed tomography contrast study: demonstration of the avian cardiovascular anatomy and function. *Veterinary Clinics of North America: Exotic Animal Practice*, **25**(2), 435–451.

McMillan, M.C. (1994) Imaging techniques. In: *Avian Medicine: Principles and Applications* (eds B.W. Ritchie, G.J. Harrison & L.R. Harrison), pp. 246–326. Wingers, Fort Worth, FL.

Pees, M., Straub, J. and Krautwald-Junghens, M.E. (2004) Echocardiographic examinations of 60 African grey parrots and 30 other psittacine birds. *Veterinary Record*, **155**, 73–76.

Rosenthal, K. and Stamoulis, M. (1993) Diagnosis of congestive heart failure in an Indian hill mynah (*Gracula religiosa*). *Journal of the Association of Avian Veterinarians*, **7**(1), 27–30.

Straub, J., Pees, M. and Krautwald-Junghanns, M.E. (2002) Measurement of the cardiac silhouette in psittacines. *Journal of the American Veterinary Medical Association*, **221**, 76–79.

Chapter 16 Avian Emergency and Critical Care Medicine

Initial clinical assessment of the avian patient

Physical restraint of a bird may not be advisable where the avian patient is in respiratory distress. Severe respiratory distress is obvious, with respiratory stertor, wheezes and whistles, but subtle changes such as an increase in respiratory rate, tail bobbing and nasal discharge/blocked nares may all be associated with a serious underlying respiratory pathology. Birds have no diaphragm and therefore rely on the outward movement of the ribcage and downward movement of the keel to allow inspiration. Any restriction of this (coupled with an increase in oxygen demand when physically restrained and stressed) will lead to hypoxia, possible cardiac ischaemia and arrest.

Therefore it is preferable to make an assessment of the bird in its cage first, using dimmed/blue/red lighting, which can reduce visual stimulation. If there is any evidence of respiratory difficulty, then it is advisable to place the bird's cage/carry box in an oxygen-enriched atmosphere, ideally with increased humidity via nebulisation with 0.9% saline.

An initial visual assessment should look at the following points.

1. Feather condition: is there evidence of chewed feathers, fret lines, discolouration, feather loss, etc.?
2. Are the feathers fluffed up?
3. Are the eyes closed?
4. Are the corneas bright?
5. Is there respiratory noise?
6. Is there tail bobbing when breathing indicating dyspnoea/hyperpnoea?
7. Are the nares clear or is there a serous or purulent discharge?
8. Is there any faecal clumping to the feathers around the vent?
9. What is the recent faecal output like?
10. Are the urates green/mustard yellow (which may indicate liver disease/biliverdinuria)?
11. Is there any blood in the faeces (may indicate haematuria such as is seen in heavy metal poisoning)?
12. Is there undigested seed in the faeces (may indicate proventricular dilatation disease or pancreatitis)?
13. What is the stance of the bird like (upright on the perch, on the floor, leg weakness, respiratory distress, etc.)?
14. Is there evidence of vomitus/regurgita on the feathers around the head?

All of these assessments can be made relatively quickly and often without actually handling the patient.

Detailed examination of the avian patient

Once it is assumed safe to handle the patient, a more detailed examination may be made. It may in some cases be safer if the examination is carried out under isoflurane/sevoflurane anaesthesia with intubation as oxygenation should be good, intermittent positive pressure ventilation is possible and, once anaesthetised, stress levels and heart rates in the patient are likely to be lower.

See Table 16.1 for some normal biological parameters of selected birds.

Examination

A detailed examination should include the following.

1. An intraoral examination should be carried out, using a mouth gag to encourage the bird to open its beak. This should allow close examination of the tongue, the internal nostril or choanal slit (the communication between the nasal passages and the mouth), and the palate. The glottis may also be visualised. Abnormalities such as a discharge from the choanal slit, loss of papillae on the palate, an abnormal or foul odour and evidence of white or yellow plaques on the mucosa should all be noted and, if possible, sampled with a sterile swab dampened with sterile water.
2. A detailed examination of the nares and the eyes should be undertaken. This will allow an assessment of any upper respiratory tract disease. Clinical signs of this include abnormal-shaped nare(s); loss of the rostral concha(e) (operculum); sinking of the globe of the eye; swelling below the globe of the eye (the region of the infraorbital sinus); discharge from the eye itself; swelling of the conjunctiva; and corneal blemishes.
3. A detailed examination of the feathers themselves is important, particularly with regard to the newly emerged so-called 'blood' or 'pin' feathers. These may be plucked from the body area and the sheath carefully slit to reveal the pulp, which may then be made into a smear and stained. This can give evidence for skin/feather pulp infections. Examination of the shaft and vane of the feather may also reveal evidence of lice and mites.
4. A detailed auscultation of the lungs and air sacs should be performed. The lungs are best auscultated from the dorsum between the wings as they are closely attached to the ventral aspect of the notarium/thoracic vertebrae. The air sacs are dispersed throughout the body. The most easily auscultated, and thankfully those with often the most pathology in cage birds and raptors, are the

Veterinary Nursing of Exotic Pets and Wildlife, Third Edition. Simon J. Girling.

Table 16.1 Biological parameters for selected bird species.

Species	Order	Heart rate at rest (beats per minute)	Respiration rate at rest (breaths per minute)	Average weight
Canary	Passeriformes (perching birds)	275	60–80	25–30 g
Zebra finches	Passeriformes (perching birds)	300	90–110	15–20 g
African grey parrot	Psittaciformes (parrot)	150	15–45	400–500 g
Blue-fronted Amazon	Psittaciformes (parrot)	150	15–45	400–550 g
Blue and gold macaw	Psittaciformes (parrot)	100	20–25	650–850 g
Budgerigar	Psittaciformes (parrot)	250	60–75	25–45 g
Cockatiel	Psittaciformes (parrot)	200	40–50	50–60 g
Ringed-neck parakeet	Psittaciformes (parrot)	175	30–45	80–100 g
Barn owl	Strigiformes (owl)	150	15–40	400–500 g
Tawny owl	Strigiformes (owl)	150	15–40	400–550 g
Golden eagle	Falconiformes (bird of prey)	90	10–20	3–6 kg
Harris hawk	Falconiformes (bird of prey)	100	20–40	0.75–1.5 kg
Peregrine falcon	Falconiformes (bird of prey)	125	30–45	0.65–1 kg

NB: The body temperature of all birds is higher than that of mammals, and all are broadly similar at around 41–42°C.

abdominal and caudal thoracic air sacs that may be auscultated on the lateral aspect of the body caudal to the keel bone. The heart may be auscultated from the lateral body wall just underneath the wings or cranioventrally over the sternum.

5. A detailed examination of the wings may be made. When anaesthetised, an idea of wing integrity and the elasticity of the propatagium (wing web) may be made by placing the bird on its sternum and extending both wings laterally to an equal distance and then letting them go. They should both recoil equally. Any asymmetry should be noted and may indicate joint or propatagial injury.
6. A detailed examination of the vent and caudal abdomen should also be made. The caudal abdomen, unprotected by the keel bone, should be naturally concave in Psittaciformes. Any convexity may indicate a space-occupying mass in the coelomic cavity of the bird, such as hepatomegaly, or the presence of ascites. In smaller birds (<300 g) slightly wetting the feathers over the ventrum in this region will allow the clinician to see through the thin skin of the body wall, and if hepatomegaly is present, the dark black-brown shadow of the liver will be seen. Normally, the liver does not extend caudal to the keel bone.
7. An accurate assessment of the bird's weight and muscle condition of the pectoral area should be carried out. Muscle condition can be scored using a scale from 0 to 5, with 0 representing no significant pectoral muscle, 3 being ideal coverage but still with a keel bone midline being palpable, and 5 being obese where instead of being able to feel the keel bone midline, a groove exists due to the fat deposits over the pectoral area either side.

Triage

Any bird presented unconscious, fitting, or with evidence of head trauma or respiratory distress should be attended to immediately. Birds, such as parrots, that are off colour and dull should be moved into a quiet, warm (29–32°C), dimly lit area with supplemental oxygen if there is any evidence of tachypnoea/hyperpnoea and should be examined as soon as possible.

Cardiopulmonary resuscitation in birds

The ABC may be followed for birds as for mammals, although there is now some feeling that the correct order should be CAB as the circulation contains enough oxygen to maintain life, providing it can keep moving around the body even with temporary loss of breathing.

A for airway and B for breathing

During anaesthesia with isoflurane or sevoflurane, cardiac arrest is usually preceded by respiratory arrest. The prognosis, providing the bird is intubated and respiratory arrest is spotted before cardiac arrest, is good. The anaesthetic should be stopped immediately and mechanical ventilation initiated. If intubation is not possible, a tight-fitting face mask may be used, but it may be preferable to consider placing an air-sac tube (see below). Doxapram has historically been used to stimulate respiration but concerns have been raised that it may worsen central nervous system (CNS) damage if the bird is already hypoxic and so it is not now regularly used in emergency care.

Where the trachea may be blocked, as with a foreign body or an aspergilloma, it may be necessary to place an air-sac tube. The tube is inserted through the body wall and so directly into an air sac. As the bird can extract oxygen from the air on both inspiration and expiration, it does not matter which way the air enters the respiratory tract. A typical air-sac tube is placed as follows.

1. Place the bird in the right lateral recumbency position. This may be done with the bird anaesthetised, but in an emergency in the conscious bird.
2. Elevate the uppermost wing (left). Another operator pulls the uppermost leg caudally.

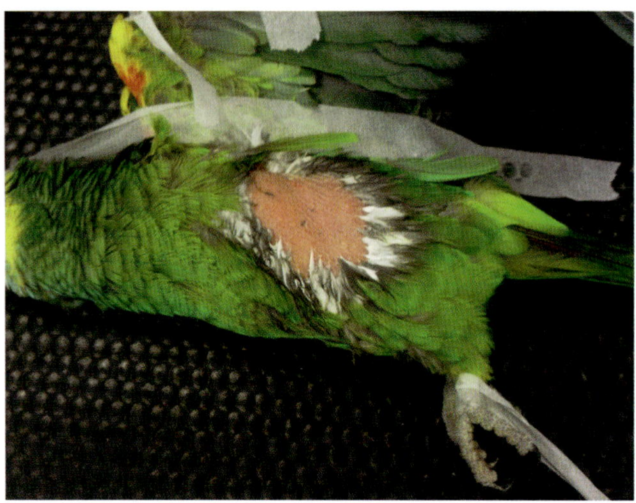

Figure 16.1 Area prepared for insertion of an avian air-sac tube typically just caudal to the last rib.

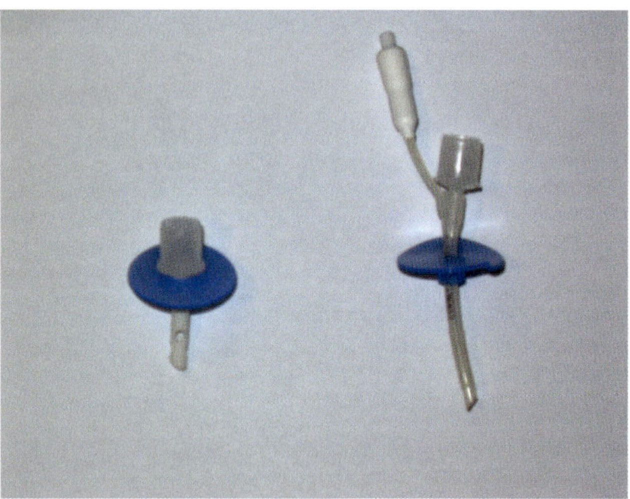

Figure 16.2 Commercially available air-sac tubes (Cook Veterinary Products®).

3. Make a small skin incision just caudal to the last rib, and just ventral to the pelvis at its conjunction with the spine (see Figure 16.1).
4. Pass either a specifically designed air-sac tube (see Figure 16.2) through the body wall or a short length of 2–3.5 gauge endotracheal (ET) tubing. The cuff on the ET tube or air-sac tube may be inflated and the tube sutured to the body wall to prevent removal.
5. The outlet of the anaesthetic circuit may then be attached to the free end of the tube to administer oxygen and, if needed, anaesthetic. An air-sac tube may be left in place for 3–4 days whilst the bird's condition is treated if required.

Respiration rates of 10–12 breaths per minute are typically recommended; if a ventilator is being used, pressures of around 15 cmH_2O will avoid trauma to air sacs (Costello, 2004; Hall, 2023).

C for cardiovascular support

Bradycardia often precedes cardiac arrest and is commonly due to heart blocks developing (similar to those in small mammals). If this is detected quickly, administration of atropine 0.01–0.02 mg/kg intramuscularly or intravenously or glycopyrrolate 0.01 mg/kg intramuscularly/intravenously may be enough to reverse this.

If cardiac arrest has occurred, then the prognosis in birds is poor. One study suggested that a return to spontaneous circulation only occurred in 7% of patients after cardiac arrest and cardiopulmonary resuscitation (CPR), with only 2% surviving (Crawford *et al.*, 2020). As the heart is protected behind the keel/sternum and ribs, external massage is often less effective than in mammals. In addition, there is no diaphragm and so clinicians cannot use the thoracic pump mechanism to increase overall negative thoracic pressure. Adrenaline 0.01–0.02 mg/kg may be administered, preferably intratracheally, with atropine 0.02–0.04 mg/kg. Application of regular compressions on the caudal sternum can be attempted to start cardiac massage. The patient is best placed in dorsal recumbency to allow better compression of the heart with the sternum but be aware that positive pressure ventilation is more difficult in this position owing to the pressure of the viscera on the lungs and air sacs. In one study in the domestic chicken, caudal keel compression with the bird in dorsal recumbency increased arterial blood pressure by up to 28% which was significantly greater than that achieved with lateral chest compressions (Eisenbarth *et al.*, 2022).

D for drugs

See Table 16.2 for tabulated information on emergency drugs in birds. If cardiac arrest occurs, then intubation and intratracheal administration of adrenaline (0.05 mL of 1 : 1000 concentration for a budgerigar and up to 0.5 mL for an African grey parrot) followed by compression of the cranial chest wall between finger and thumb five times in a row, followed by five breaths via an ET tube, and then five compressions of the chest wall may allow revival. As mentioned above, in the larger birds, placing the bird in dorsal recumbency and pressing on the caudal sternum to compress the heart may be more effective. Intubation should be attempted wherever possible. However, if it is not possible, then a face mask with 100% oxygen is used and the resuscitator places the bird in lateral recumbency and grasps the uppermost wing at the carpal joint and rhythmically pumps the wing up and down. This has the effect of raising and depressing the chest wall, thus simulating inspiration and expiration.

In the case of birds such as African grey parrots or in laying hens/birds on poor-quality diets where a possible calcium deficiency may be a cause for collapse of the patient, the use of calcium gluconate is advised. Doses of 50–100 mg/kg intramuscularly have been quoted. Diazepam 0.2–0.5 mg/kg may be needed to control seizures initially in some of these cases. Midazolam has been used intranasally at 2 mg/kg in a variety of birds to cause sedation and may be used to control seizuring.

Where heavy metal poisoning (mainly lead or zinc) is suspected, the chelating agent sodium calcium edetate should be used at 20–50 mg/kg intramuscularly twice daily. Fluid therapy should always be used as heavy metals, and possibly the drug itself, may be nephrotoxic. Alternatively, D-penicillamine 50–55 mg/kg orally twice daily can be used.

Table 16.2 Commonly used emergency and recovery medications for birds.

Drug	Dosage	Notes
Adrenaline (1 : 1000, i.e. 1 mg/mL)	0.01 mg/kg IV/IO 0.02–0.04 mg/kg IT	If cardiac arrest or ECG suggests fine ventricular fibrillation (VF), must use adrenaline to convert to coarse VF before cardiac massage is likely to work
Amoxicillin/clavulanate	125 mg/kg b.i.d.	Useful where anaerobes and *Pasteurella* spp. may be present (e.g. cat bites)
Amphotericin B	1.5 mg/kg IV	Aspergillosis: always use aggressive fluid therapy as drug is nephrotoxic
Atropine	0.02 mg/kg IV/IO	Used where heart block is detected (profound bradycardia)
	0.2–0.5 mg/kg IV/IM	Higher dosage used to reverse cholinesterase inhibitor toxicosis, e.g. organophosphate poisoning
Calcium EDTA (sodium calcium edetate)	20–50 mg/kg IM b.i.d.	Chelating agent for lead or zinc poisoning. Always use aggressive fluid therapy to avoid renal damage
Calcium gluconate	50–100 mg/kg IM	Hypocalcaemic fits, particularly African grey parrots
Dextrose (50%)	125–250 mg/kg IV slow bolus diluted 1 : 1 with 0.9% saline	Hypoglycaemia
Diazepam	0.2–0.5 mg/kg IM/IV	Muscle necrosis if given IM
Dopamine	5–10 μg/kg per minute IV	May be used to support blood pressure where significant hypotension exists (used experimentally in Hispaniolan Amazon parrots to reverse isoflurane-induced hypotension (Schnellbacher *et al*., 2012))
Doxycycline	75–100 mg/kg IM every 5–7 days for 42 days	Treatment for psittacosis/chlamydiosis in parrots. Human IV drug formulations typically used (doxycycline hyclate). Causes muscle necrosis
Enrofloxacin	10 mg/kg b.i.d.	Useful against Gram-negative bacteria but not against anaerobes. Has some effect against *Chlamydia psittaci*. Can cause muscle necrosis
Furosemide	0.1–2 mg/kg	Diuretic. Lories (type of nectar-eating parrot) are very sensitive
Itraconazole	5–10 mg/kg b.i.d.	Aspergillosis: use at lower dose range in African grey parrots
Midazolam	0.2–0.5 mg/kg IM/IV 2 mg/kg intranasally	Less likely to cause muscle necrosis than diazepam. Can be used intranasally
Meloxicam	0.2–0.5 mg/kg IM/PO s.i.d to b.i.d.	Beware use if already has renal damage Twice-daily dosing at 0.5 mg/kg for 14 days has been used in African grey parrots without organ damage or haematological/biochemical changes (Montesinos *et al*., 2015). Species variation exists, e.g. brown pelicans (*Pelecanus occidentalis*) dosed at 0.2 mg/kg s.i.d. developed signs of renal damage after 2–3 days as the half-life appears to be 36.3 hours leading to a gradual toxicity issue if dosed once a day (Horgan *et al*., 2020)
Penicillamine	50–55 mg/kg orally every 12–24 hours	Used as an alternative heavy metal chelation agent to calcium EDTA. May cause vomiting
Prostaglandin E_2 gel	Apply 0.1 mL per 100 g bird	Apply direct to oviduct sphincter inside vent to relax sphincter, increase uterine tone and aid egg passage

IM, intramuscularly; IO, intraosseously; IV, intravenously; IT, intratracheally; s.i.d., once daily; b.i.d., twice daily.
Source: Lichtenberger and Lennox (2016) and Guzman *et al*. (2023).

Where egg binding has occurred, it is vital to keep the patient warm, quiet and well hydrated. Use of prostaglandin E_2 gel applied directly to the oviduct sphincter inside the cloaca is often used to help relax the sphincter and encourage contraction of the uterine muscle. In some circumstances, collapsing the egg inside the bird either by puncturing it through the cloaca with a needle or via a midline ventral abdomen insertion of a needle attached to a syringe may be necessary to relieve pressure from the abdomen, which can cause ischaemic necrosis of the vital organs due to the relatively large size of bird eggs. See Chapter 14 for more information.

Although not strictly emergency drugs, if bacterial sepsis is suspected then combinations of a fluoroquinolone (e.g. enrofloxacin 10 mg/kg twice daily or marbofloxacin 10 mg/kg once daily) and a potentiated penicillin (e.g. amoxicillin/clavulanate 125 mg/kg twice daily) are commonly used as these will cover most of the bacterial pathogens seen in avian medicine. If aspergillosis is suspected, then nebulisation of drugs such as amphotericin B and F10® (Health and Hygiene Pty Ltd.) may be of some help, as is an intravenous bolus of amphotericin B 1.5 mg/kg or oral itraconazole 5–10 mg/kg twice daily or oral terbinafine 10–15 mg/kg twice daily.

E for ECG

ECG traces may be taken from birds, although it is preferable to do so with the patient anaesthetised. It is advisable to use adhesive ECG pads rather than alligator forceps as bird skin is very fragile and damages easily. The bird is placed in dorsal recumbency and the pads attached to the skin of the thighs and the skin of the propatagium (the bit of skin between the shoulder and carpus of the wing on the wings' leading edge). If pads are not available, hypodermic needles can be inserted through the skin of the wings and thighs and alligator clamps can then be attached to these.

In most avian species, the lead II trace appears as a mammalian one, except the QRS complex appears inverted. This is not the case, but rather occurs because the S wave is the dominant deflection and the Q wave hardly records at all. For this reason, bird QRS waves are often referred to as 'rS' waves. P and T waves are as for mammals (see Figure 16.3). Occasionally in some species (pigeons, some parrots), there is a small depression wave known as a Ta wave immediately after the P wave and this is normal (it represents atrial repolarisation) (see Figure 16.4). In addition, the P-on-T phenomenon (where the P wave is superimposed onto the following T wave) is a normal finding in some African grey and Amazon parrots.

Values for ECGs in birds have been published but vary between species and exceed the scope of this text. Many birds have very fast heart rates but some of the more important arrhythmias are due to heart blocks which result in bradycardia, a common abnormality before cardiac arrest in anaesthetised birds.

Monitoring of CPR responses

Assessment of the success of CPR by using end-tidal CO_2 levels as with mammals can be performed (Lichtenberger, 2007). A steady increase in end-tidal CO_2 during CPR should occur and if it has not exceeded 10 mmHg after resuscitation has been ongoing for 15–20 minutes, the prognosis is poor.

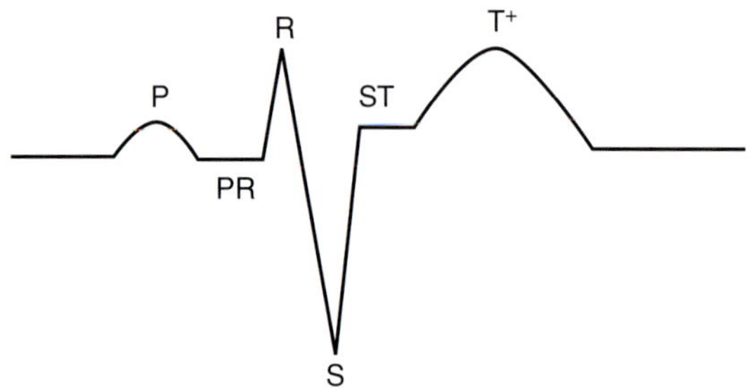

Figure 16.3 Normal lead II annotated ECG trace for a bird.

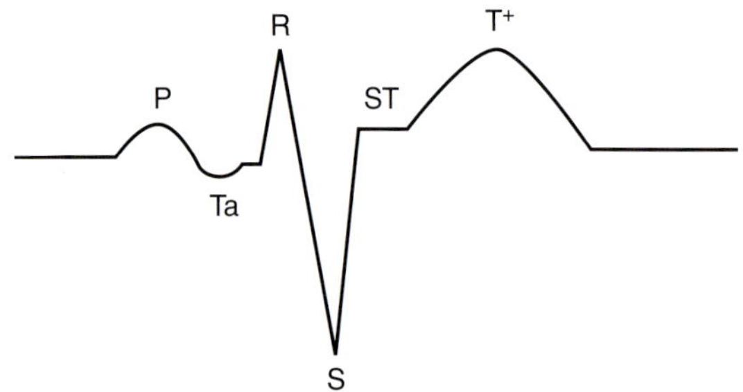

Figure 16.4 Normal lead II annotated trace for pigeons and some psittacine birds showing the Ta wave associated with atrial repolarisation.

Although arterial blood is commonly used for blood gas analysis during anaesthesia, venous blood may be preferable for assessment of blood gases and pH as this more closely represents the status of the body organs than arterial blood does.

Mucous membrane colour should be assessed where possible – the lining of the cloaca or the mouth are the two best sites in birds. Cloacal temperature may also give an indication of peripheral perfusion and should be 40–42°C.

Blood pressure may be monitored as described below under monitoring of hypovolaemia.

Monitoring and treatment of hypotension and hypovolaemia (shock)

Three distinct phases of shock are commonly observed: early/compensatory, early decompensatory and decompensatory.

In early/compensatory shock, the patient has an elevated heart rate and often elevated or normal blood pressure. In these patients, volume replacement fluid therapy is most likely to be effective. Early decompensatory shock in birds has been estimated when 25–30% of fluid loss occurs.

Systolic blood pressure monitoring can be performed by placing a cuff on the distal humerus or femur and the Doppler probe on the medial surface of the proximal ulna (proximal ulnar artery) or tibiotarsus (medial metatarsal artery). Cuff widths should be 40% of the circumference of the humerus or distal femur, which means that the available commercial cuffs are really too large for small avian patients. Systolic blood pressure monitoring using the indirect method correlates better with directly measured blood pressure in birds than is the case in mammals (Lichtenberger and Ko, 2007). Whatever method was used to manually restrain the bird, indirect blood pressure measurements obtained by placing the cuff around the limb proximal to the applied Doppler held over the basilic or cranial tibial artery found that there was considerable variation even when the blood pressure measurement was retaken immediately, throwing into doubt the accuracy of avian indirect blood pressure measurements (Johnston *et al.*, 2011). Central venous pressure monitoring in birds has not been quantified and is technically challenging to measure.

Systolic blood pressure in birds should be at least 90 mmHg, otherwise the bird is hypotensive and likely hypovolaemic. Conversely, anything above 200 mmHg indicates hypertension and maybe hypervolaemia and these patients should not have fluid therapy intravenously or intraosseously.

Slow bolus administration of fluids should be attempted intravenously or intraosseously where systolic blood pressure is below 90 mmHg until correction of blood pressure. Colloids such as hetastarch have been administered at 5 mL/kg – usually one or two boluses are required but they can cause renal damage and have been associated with an increased rate of haemorrhage and so many now question their regular use. Isotonic crystalloids can be administered at a rate of 10 mL/kg and in larger species of bird (>7 kg) at a lower rate of 5 mL/kg but the effects on blood pressure can be short-lived (as little as 30–45 minutes). Bowles *et al.* (2007) and Lichtenberger (2007) advocate the administration of 7.2–7.5% hypertonic saline at 3 mL/kg intravenously/intraosseously as a slow bolus over 10 minutes in cases with acute hypovolaemia. Hetastarch was then administered to maintain the osmotic effects at 3 mL/kg intravenously/intraosseously over 5–10 minutes. Then boluses of 10 mL/kg isotonic crystalloids followed by hetastarch at 3–5 mL/kg until the blood pressure rose above 90 mmHg. Once blood pressure has reached 90 mmHg the rehydration stage of fluid therapy takes over with crystalloids. If the patient is hypoproteinaemic, then hetastarch may be administered as a continuous rate infusion at 0.8 mL/kg per hour during rehydration to maintain the oncotic potential – but be aware of the caveats around the use of colloids in patients with renal disease and internal haemorrhage as both can be worsened.

Dopamine drips have been used successfully at a rate of 5–10 μg/kg per minute to raise blood pressure experimentally in isoflurane-associated hypotensive Hispaniolan parrots (*Amazona ventralis*) and was preferable to dobutamine (Schnellbacher *et al.*, 2012).

Please refer to Chapter 14 for maintenance and moderate rehydration fluid requirements as well as blood transfusion administration in birds.

Pulse assessment

Manually assessing a pulse can be difficult in birds owing to their rapid heart rates and thin-walled vessels which can be easily occluded, but with practice it is possible. Doppler ultrasound probes can also be attached to the following blood vessels to assess pulse:

1. Basilic vein (runs over the ventral aspect of the humerus)
2. Medial metatarsal vein (runs over the medial aspect of the lower unfeathered leg [tarsometatarsus] and may be clearly seen in waterfowl).

Refill times of the basilic or medial metatarsal vessels should be immediate – significant dehydration (>7%) may be associated with refill times of 1–2 seconds. Capillary refill times should be less than 2 seconds as with mammals. They may be assessed on mucous membranes around the mouth and face or vent.

Pulse oximetry

Pulse oximeter probes may be attached to distal legs over the medial metatarsal area, the toes or interdigital web in waterfowl, the propatagium or over the basilic (brachial) vein on the ventral aspect of the elbow in smaller species. However, it should be noted that avian haemoglobin is different in structure from mammalian and therefore the accuracy of pulse oximeter readings is questionable. It is still a useful modality for assessing *changes* in the SpO_2, rather than actual values.

Cardiac and respiratory auscultation

The lungs are best auscultated from the dorsum between the wings as they are closely attached to the ventral aspect of the notarium/thoracic vertebrae. The air sacs are dispersed throughout the body. The most easily auscultated, and often those with the most pathology in cage birds and raptors, are the abdominal and caudal thoracic air sacs, which may be auscultated on the lateral aspect of the body caudal to the keel bone. The heart may be auscultated from the lateral body wall just underneath the wings or cranioventrally over the sternum.

Neurological assessment

Fitting or collapsed birds may be affected by heavy metal poisoning (particularly lead, but also zinc); hypocalcaemia (particularly in a hen bird that is egg-laying and on an unsupplemented diet or in a young African grey parrot as the latter species has a particular hypocalcaemia syndrome); hypoglycaemia (particularly common in birds of prey that are underweight and being flown regularly); or a CNS infection whether it be due to parasites (usually protozoa) or bacteria.

Assess whether the bird can perch using both legs. If held in the hand, see if the bird can grasp a finger/towel with both feet. Unilateral leg paresis through to full paralysis is common, particularly in small psittacine birds such as the budgerigar where it is often associated with a renal or occasionally gonadal tumour. This is due to the mass pressing against the nerves supplying the pelvic limb that pass through the kidneys before entering the leg. Pelvic limb and overall weakness may be seen in toxicities such as heavy metal (lead or zinc) poisoning or organic toxins (gliotoxins) such as those associated with aspergillosis infection of the airways.

Birds of prey that are suffering from lead poisoning, having consumed lead shot in the prey that they have been fed, will often sit on the floor, rocked back onto their 'hocks' (the intertarsal joint) with drooped wings and a sleepy appearance.

Assess whether the bird is holding both wings normally. One wing drooping is most likely to be associated with a muscular/skeletal injury. Both wings drooping is more likely to be a toxicity such as lead or permethrin/organophosphate poisoning.

Birds will not commonly demonstrate eye nystagmus as their eyes are relatively large in comparison to the skull. Instead, birds with CNS disease affecting the vestibular system of the brain will often demonstrate a whole-head nystagmus. In addition, head tilts (torticollis) are common with peripheral and central vestibular disease.

Pupillary reflexes do not work well in birds as they have a significant amount of skeletal muscle in their irises which is under conscious control. The eyes being large and the bone separating them from each other in midline often very thin, any light shone into one eye frequently passes through the bony septum and into the opposite eye as well, meaning the consensual reflex is less useful in birds than mammals.

Blood biochemistry

There are so many species of birds that any meaningfully accurate table would be too large to include here. Instead, Table 16.3 gives broad ranges of common biochemical parameters for cage birds routinely seen in practice. It should be noted that, as with reptiles, uric acid is the only useful indicator of renal function, although usually less than one-quarter of the kidneys needs to be left functioning before uric acid levels become elevated (although a recent meal, particularly in carnivores, will temporarily elevate uric acid levels). Urea and creatinine levels do not provide useful information on renal function in birds and reptiles.

Haematology

As with biochemistry, values vary between species. Some indication of packed cell volume (PCV) across avian species has been given in Chapters 9 and 14. Leucocyte (white cell) counts are in the range of $10–18 \times 10^9$/L. In parrots, three main conditions will typically push the white cell count over 30×10^9/L:

1. Psittacosis/ornithosis (infection with *Chlamydia psittaci*)

Table 16.3 Average plasma biochemistry values for cage birds.

Parameter	Value	Notes
Total protein (g/L)	30–50	
Albumin (g/L)	16–32	
Aspartate aminotransferase, AST (IU/L)	100–350	Not liver specific, also found in muscle so may be elevated with liver or muscle damage and catabolic processes
Creatine kinase, CK (IU/L)	50–300	Only found in muscle so may be elevated with muscle damage and catabolic processes
Lactate dehydrogenase, LDH (IU/L)	150–450	Not liver specific, also found in muscle including cardiac muscle so may be elevated with liver or muscle damage (including heart) and catabolic processes
Calcium (total) (mmol/L)	2–3.25	May be elevated in hen birds around egg production. Total calcium levels may appear within normal range while bird is still showing signs of hypocalcaemia (especially African grey parrots) as ionised calcium is the biologically active fraction (African grey parrot ionised calcium results around 0.96–1.22 mmol/L)
Phosphorus (mmol/L)	1–1.85	Should be less than total calcium. If greater than total calcium may be associated with dietary imbalances (excess seed without calcium/vitamin D_3 supplementation) and renal failure
Glucose (mmol/L)	10–20	Note: Budgerigars may be seen with glucagon-associated diabetes mellitus; birds of prey may be seen with hypoglycaemia associated with exercise when malnourished
Uric acid (µmol/L)	150–350	Gout (precipitation of uric acid) occurs when levels exceed 1500 µmol/L. May be transiently elevated in birds, particularly carnivores, immediately after a meal so to assess for renal function ensure bird is suitably starved

2. Egg yolk coelomitis (equivalent to peritonitis but where the yolk ruptures internally instead of being shed into the oviduct)
3. Mycobacteriosis (uncommon in parrots; more common in waterfowl).

Occasionally, infections such as aspergillosis (a fungal infection usually of the airways) may stimulate a similar response, although more commonly the patient has a low white cell count when severely affected.

The avian equivalent of the neutrophil is the heterophil, so named because of its part basophilic, part eosinophilic staining with Romanowsky stains. It has a bilobed to trilobed nucleus and brick-red cigar-shaped granules in its cytoplasm. Evidence on a blood smear of degranulation of these and rupture of the cells (toxicity) is a strong indicator of active and severe infection. The presence of monocytes in significant numbers is commonly associated with conditions such as aspergillosis, mycobacteriosis and granulomatous disease.

Erythrocytes and platelets in birds are nucleated. The erythrocytes are rugby ball shaped with a similar-shaped nucleus. The platelets are oval and smaller. Other cells are similar to those seen in mammals.

Urinalysis

This is less useful than for mammals owing to the faecal contamination that occurs with avian urine. However, it is important to look at the urates (white portion of the dropping) to see if there is any blood, or if the urates have turned mustard yellow or lime green. If the latter has occurred, this is evidence of biliverdinuria, which in birds is an indicator of liver inflammation/damage (common with psittacosis in parrots and lead poisoning in birds of prey). Biliverdin is the main excretory product of the liver from the breakdown of erythrocytes as opposed to bilirubin in mammals.

Assessment of urine where possible should produce negative results for ketones, glucose and blood. Protein is likely to be identified owing to the combination of faeces, urates and urine in the cloaca.

Volumes of water/true urine should be small in a healthy bird's dropping. If they are very watery, as opposed to diarrhoea, then this may indicate polyuria.

Blood in the urates is often associated with heavy metal, particularly lead, poisoning but can also be associated with nephritis due to infectious causes.

Nebulisation

This can be a good method for delivering medications to the respiratory system and also moisture to aid rehydration, particularly in small species. For further information, see Chapter 14.

Supportive therapy

Ongoing medication

Details of antibiotics useful in birds are given in Table 16.2. Chelation therapy for heavy metal poisoning is also listed. Prokinetics are not often necessary.

Ongoing nutritional supplementation with oral calcium/vitamin D_3 replacers is important in cases of hypocalcaemia in African grey parrots.

Other mineral and vitamin supplements are often required if the diet is poor or restricted to seeds in the case of parrots (as well as trying to introduce fruit and vegetables), particularly vitamin A.

Critical care nutrition including calculation of energy requirements

Calculation of basal metabolic rate (BMR) energy requirements (sometimes referred to as the resting energy requirement or RER; see Chapter 12) in kilocalories per day can be made using the formula:

$$\text{BMR} = k \times \left[\text{weight}(\text{kg})\right]^{0.75}$$

where k the constant is 78 for most non-Passeriformes (pigeons, parrots, etc.) and 129 for Passeriformes. There is a suggestion that temperate species (non-tropical) parrots from Australia and New Zealand have a BMR 21% higher than that of tropical species (Latney, 2023). Remember that maintenance energy requirement (MER) is generally 1.5–2 times the BMR and, if disease is present, then this further amplifies the required calories (sepsis and burns for example may increase MER by two to three times).

Assisted feeding techniques and foods

The majority of cage birds are granivorous/herbivorous/frugivorous. Members of the parrot family should not be fed meat or dairy products as these can result in renal, hepatic and cardiovascular diseases. Many hospitalised cage birds can feed themselves; however, emergency nutrition may be necessary and these patients might require crop tubing. This process preferably involves the use of a purpose-designed, steel, blunt-ended crop tube that can be attached to a syringe containing the food formula. The beak is opened and a gag inserted while the tube is advanced from the bird's left side, dorsally over the base of the tongue and glottis and down to the base of the neck slightly to the right of midline. Several commercially available cage-bird critical care formulas are available in the UK. See the following section on crop tubing for maximum values that may be tubed at one time.

Raptors are by nature carnivores and should preferably be fed whole prey such as rodents or day-old chicks. However, in the practice environment, this may not be possible and therefore crop tubing/gavaging may be necessary. Many commercial companies produce carnivore critical care support formulas (e.g. Lafeber). In an emergency where access to these is not possible, canine/feline critical care formulas can be used, but for anything more than a few days it is better to use formulas designed specifically for avian patients. Care should be taken initially to ensure that the patient is correctly hydrated before loading large amounts of protein into it. It may be better in a severely weakened bird to start off with simple sugar/amino acid products providing calories and fluids before moving on to high-protein/high-fat diets.

Crop tubing/gavaging

Once rehydrated, crop tubing/gavaging with critical care support formulas may be carried out (see Figures 16.5 and 16.6). An idea of maximum volumes that may be safely crop tubed into an avian patient at any one time are given in Table 16.4.

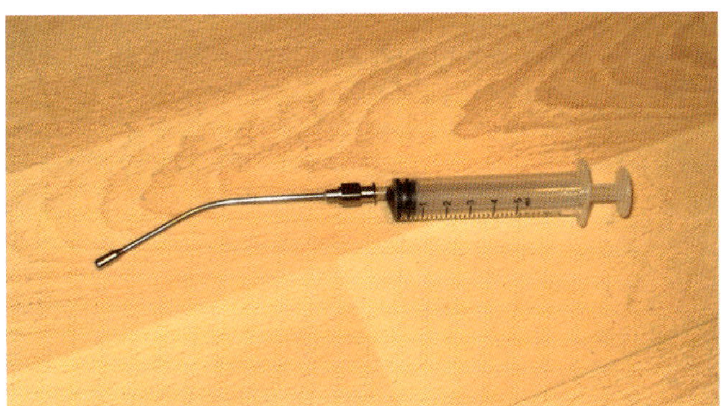

Figure 16.5 A curved, stainless steel crop tube attached to a disposable syringe.

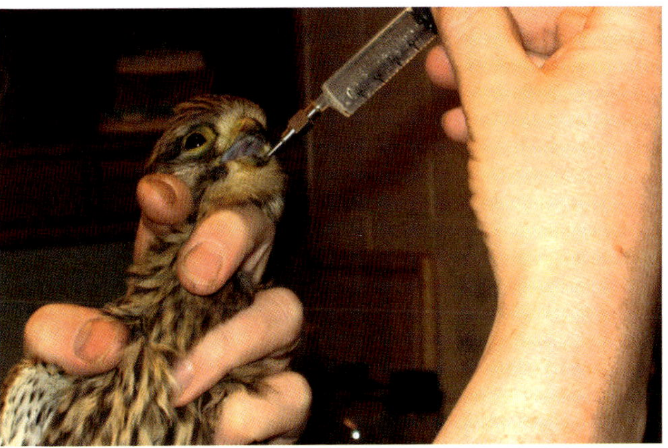

Figure 16.6 Crop tubing a kestrel with support formula.

Table 16.4 Maximum volumes that may be safely administered via crop tube.

Species	Maximum volume (mL)
Budgerigar	0.5–1
Cockatiel	2.5–5
Conures	5–7
Cockatoos	10
African grey	8–10
Macaws	10–15

Nursing of wounds

Avian wounds generally gape as their skin is not very elastic. However, the skin is often very thin and has a low surface bacterial burden, so traumatic wounds if relatively clean may be cleaned briefly with lactated Ringer's solution or isotonic saline (0.9%) as these are the least toxic to the fibroblasts repairing the wound. If gross contamination with microbes is possible (e.g. cat bite wounds) then dilute povidone-iodine or chlorhexidine may be used but care should be taken to make sure they are appropriately diluted to minimise damage to fibroblasts (0.05% for chlorhexidine and 0.1% for povidone-iodine). Pressure can be used to dislodge particulate foreign bodies by using a 30–35 mL syringe with an 18 gauge needle attached to generate around 4.8–5.5 Pa (7–8 pounds per square inch) pressure; more than this will damage fibroblasts.

An Elizabethan collar should be applied to the bird, making sure it is reversed to point caudally as parrots cannot move around their cage or eat with the collar projecting cranially (see Figure 16.7). Alternatively, neck braces may be used to temporarily stop wound trauma located on the body.

For deeper wounds associated with bites etc., particularly if they occur over the legs distally, debridement of the wound under anaesthetic is essential to prevent infections of the avascular tendons or, worse, osteomyelitis. Where skin deficits occur and the wound has exudation (e.g. burns or chronic self-mutilation wounds) they may be dressed with products containing hydrocolloids (e.g. Granuflex®, Convatec UK Ltd.) or hydrogels under non-adhesive dressings. Where a healthy granulation bed exists and there is no skin coverage

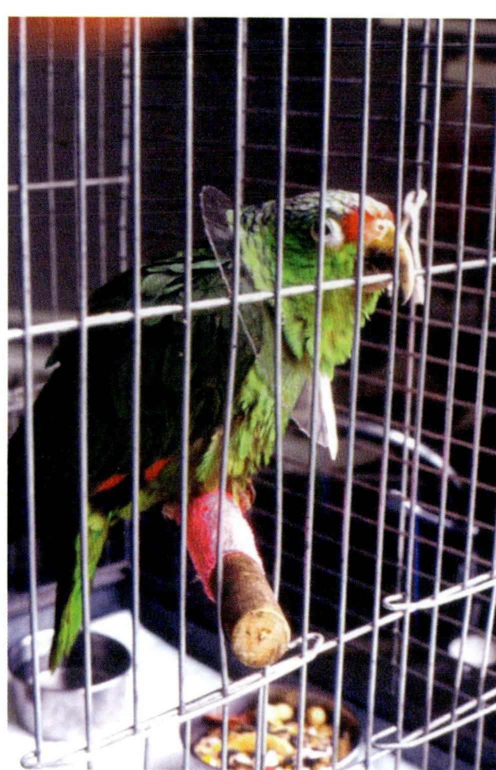

Figure 16.7 When applying an Elizabethan collar to birds, make sure it is positioned to face backwards otherwise the bird cannot eat or limb around its cage.

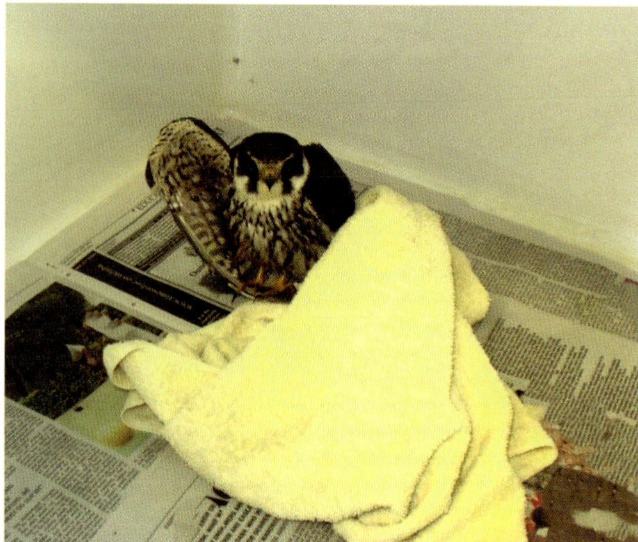

Figure 16.8 Fractures of the wing require stabilisation before surgical fixation can be considered.

possible, wounds have been covered using novel products based on sterilised porcine submucosa or bovine collagen that may be sutured over the deficit so preventing desiccation and protecting the granulation beds (Mickelson *et al.*, 2016). Where bleeding occurs, products containing alginate can be used (e.g. Kaltostat®, Convatec UK Ltd.). Where gross contamination or granulation beds in distal limbs are present, manuka honey dressings have been used with success in birds (Mickelson *et al.*, 2016). Secondary and tertiary bandage material may be applied over the top to protect the wound further, but the primary dressings in some cases may be sutured to the skin edges to facilitate retention.

Various gels (usually simple hydrocolloid), creams and ointments have been used on wounds in birds but care should be taken with the use of any that contain corticosteroids as these can lead to immunosuppression in birds as they are particularly susceptible.

Negative pressure wound therapy, which creates negative pressures of −80 to −120 mmHg to pull exudates out of the wound and into a reservoir bag thus increasing blood supply to the wound, has been used in birds (Knapp-Hoch and de Matos, 2014). It is particularly useful where there are chronic non-healing wounds or grossly infected wounds, but should not be used where the wound has exposed blood vessels, nerves, tendons or ligaments as excessive bleeding and tissue damage will occur. It should also not be used where neoplastic disease is present. Not all bird species or individuals are amenable to its use and good analgesia and often sedation are required as clearly the patient needs to be attached to a suction device and psittacines for example often chew tubing and dressings.

For fracture stabilisation, a figure-of-eight bandage using a non-adherent material may be used on wing fractures for a short period (<48 hours) to contract the wing and bind it to the lateral body wall. Any longer immobilisation leads to fibrosis of the joints and will result in severe impairment in wing function. A figure-of-eight bandage starts on the ventral aspect between the radius/ulna and the humerus. The bandage is then brought over to cover the elbow joint and distal humerus. It then passes dorsally over the wing up to the end of the digits, then moves ventrally to reach the starting point. After a second layer is applied the bandage moves forward along the ventral surface towards the distal aspect of the radius and ulna, then loops around the dorsal aspect of the carpometacarpus and finally loops back to the starting point to create the figure-of-eight. The process is repeated a few times and may be topped off with a cohesive flexible bandage. Care should be taken not to damage the propatagium as excessive pressure on this area can result in necrosis. A simpler technique is to just wrap the wing flat to the body wall in a folded position and pass the bandage around the body of the bird, but this can result in restriction on breathing and so the tension under which the bandage is applied should be carefully assessed (see Figure 16.8).

Leg fractures in small cage birds such as canaries may be stabilised using the so-called 'Altman' splint. This is simply two pieces of heavy zinc tape applied laterally and medially to the fractured leg, sandwiching the leg between them. These can be left on or replaced as the bird chews them off for the duration of the healing process.

Finger splints (e.g. aluminium-backed foam splints) or tongue depressors may be used in larger birds for temporary stabilisation of long bone fractures but, as with wing fractures, these are designed to be temporary and will require a surgical fixation if accurate healing is required.

Placement of tubes

Feeding tubes are generally not used in birds owing to the fragile nature of their skin, the presence of air sacs throughout the body and their ability to commonly interfere with the tubing. Air-sac tubes are mentioned above.

References

Bowles, H., Lichtenberger, M. and Lennox, A. (2007) Emergency and critical care of pet birds. *Veterinary Clinics of North America: Exotic Animal Practice*, **10**(2), 345–394.

Costello, M.F. (2004) Principles of cardiopulmonary cerebral resuscitation in special species. *Seminars in Avian and Exotic Pet Medicine*, **13**(3), 132–141.

Crawford, A., Abelson, A., Gladden, J. and Rozanski, E. (2020) Retrospective evaluation of cardiopulmonary arrest and resuscitation in hospitalized birds: 41 cases (2006–2019). *Journal of Veterinary Emergency and Critical Care*, **32**, 491–499.

Eisenbarth, J., Cummings, C.O., Rozanski, E., Karlin, E. and Rush, J. (2022) Evaluation of cardiac compression techniques for cardiopulmonary resuscitation in laying hens (*Gallus gallus*). *Abstracts of the International Veterinary Emergency and Critical Care Symposium*, 7–11 September, San Antonio, Texas, p. 53

Guzman, D.S.-M., Beaufrere, H., Welle, K.R. *et al.* (2023) Birds. In: *Exotic Animal Formulary* (eds J.W. Carpenter & C.A. Harms), 6th edn, pp. 222–443. Elsevier, St Louis, MO.

Hall, N.H. (2023) Cerebro-cardiopulmonary resuscitation and post-arrest care in exotic animal critical care. *Veterinary Clinics of North America: Exotic Animal Practice*, **26**, 737–750.

Horgan, M.D., Knych, H.K., Siksay, S.E. and Duerr, R.S. (2020) Pharmacokinetics of a single dose of oral meloxicam in rehabilitated wild brown pelicans (*Pelecanus occidentalis*). *Journal of Avian Medicine and Surgery*, **34**(4), 329–337. doi: 10.1647/1082-6742-34.4.329.

Johnston, M.S., Davidowski, L.A., Rao, S. and Hill, A.E. (2011) Precision of repeated, Doppler-derived indirect blood pressure measurements in conscious psittacine birds. *Journal of Avian Medicine and Surgery*, **25**(2), 83–90.

Knapp-Hoch, H. and de Matos, R. (2014) Clinical technique: negative pressure wound therapy – general principles and use in avian species. *Journal of Exotic Pet Medicine*, **23**(1), 56–66.

Latney, L. (2023) Nutritive support for critical exotic patients. *Veterinary Clinics of North America: Exotic Animal Practice*, **26**, 711–735.

Lichtenberger, M. (2007) Shock and CPCR in small mammals and birds. *Veterinary Clinics of North America: Exotic Animal Practice*, **10**(2), 275–291.

Lichtenberger, M. and Ko, J. (2007) Critical care monitoring. *Veterinary Clinics of North America: Exotic Animal Practice*, **10**(2), 317–344.

Lichtenberger, M. and Lennox, A. (2016) Critical care. In: *Current Therapy in Avian Medicine and Surgery* (ed. B. Speer), pp. 582–588. Elsevier, St Loui, MO.

Mickelson, M.A., Mans, C. and Colopy, S.A. (2016) Principles of wound management and wound healing in exotic pets. *Veterinary Clinics of North America: Exotic Animal Practice*, **19**(1), 33–53.

Montesinos, A., Ardiaca, M., Juan-Salles, C. and Tesouro, M.A. (2015) Effects of meloxicam on hematologic and plasma biochemical analyte values and results of histological examination of kidney biopsy specimens of African grey parrots (*Psittacus erithacus*). *Journal of Avian Medicine and Surgery*, **29**, 1–8.

Schnellbacher, R.W., da Cunha, A.F., Beaufrere, H. *et al.* (2012) Effects of dopamine and dobutamine on isoflurane-induced hypotension in Hispaniolan Amazon parrots (*Amazona ventralis*). *American Journal of Veterinary Research*, **73**(7), 952–958.

Part III Reptiles and Amphibians

Chapter 17 Basic Reptile and Amphibian Anatomy and Physiology

Classification

Reptiles are classified into many different family groups, according to a number of physical, anatomical and evolutionary factors. It is useful to know to which group a reptile belongs, as this gives an indication of the other reptiles to which it is related. This is of some help when faced with a species that you have not seen before.

Table 17.1 contains some of the more commonly encountered family groups of reptiles seen in general and reptile-orientated practices. Classification historically was based on anatomical details but increasingly genetic relatedness has also been used and has led to differing opinions as to the grouping of many species. This has led to some significant changes in classification.

SNAKES

Like the bird, the snake has no diaphragm, so no separate thorax and abdomen. Instead it has a coelomic, or common, body cavity. Figure 17.1 is a schematic drawing of the layout of a typical snake's coelomic cavity.

Musculoskeletal system

All true snakes have no obvious external limbs and have fused transparent eyelids (the so-called 'spectacle'). These are some of the things that distinguish them from species that may look like snakes such as the slow worm (*Anguis fragilis*), which is actually a lizard without obvious limbs and mobile eyelids. However, there is some external evidence of the previous presence of limbs in one or two of the evolutionary older species of snake such as the Boidae family (pythons and boas). These can possess vestigial pelvic remnants, with claw-like spurs either side of the vent being all that is left of the hindlimbs.

The snake skull possesses a small calvarium containing the brain and a large nasal cavity.

The anatomy of the snake's head has a number of adaptations that allow it to swallow large prey. In all snakes, the two halves of the mandible are loosely held together rostrally and the symphysis can separate to increase their gape. In addition, the snake has no temporomandibular joint. Instead, it possesses a quadrate bone that articulates between a hemi-mandible and the skull and allows the hemi-mandibles to be moved rostrally and laterally in a manoeuvre that looks like the jaw is dislocating itself but helps to move the prey caudally into the oropharynx. The maxilla also hinges only loosely with the rostral aspect of the cranium via a kinetic hinge, so allowing the 'nose' of the snake to be raised in relation to the calvarium, increasing the oral aperture.

The skull articulates with the atlas vertebra via a simple joint containing only one occipital condyle, rather than the mammalian two. The coccygeal vertebrae (those caudal to the vent) are the only vertebrae with no ribs attached. Instead, they have paired, ventral, haemal processes between which the coccygeal artery and vein are located. This vein can be used for venepuncture for both sampling and intravenous injections. The recommended site for venepuncture is one-third the distance from the vent to the tail tip on the ventral aspect.

The ventral scales, known as scutes or gastropeges, overlie the muscular casing of the snake's torso. This muscle is segmental and supplied by intervertebral nerves. It is by alternately contracting and relaxing these segmental muscles that the snake can propel itself across the ground, the caudal edge of each ventral scute providing friction.

Nervous system

The brain is smooth and lacks gyri but has both a forebrain and hindbrain. The central nervous system of snakes is similar to that of lizards but only has 11 cranial nerves rather than the mammalian and lizard 12 (they are missing cranial nerve XI, the accessory). However, some suggest that they do have 12 cranial nerves if the nervus terminalis (cranial nerve 0) is included; this is involved in olfaction and exists in other vertebrates and supplies the nasal mucosa. The spinal cord extends to the tip of the tail unlike mammals and there is no subarachnoid space so that myelography cannot be performed. Extensive nerve supply to infrared receptors in the skin of snakes is common in boas, pythons and vipers. More information on these cutaneous adaptations can be found in the section on special cutaneous adaptations in snakes.

Respiratory system

Upper respiratory system

The nostrils are paired and open into the roof of the mouth. Snakes do not have a hard palate similar to chelonia and lizards. When the mouth is closed, the internal nostrils are positioned directly above the entrance to the trachea. This is guarded by the glottis. An epiglottis may be present in vestigial form and in some species it appears to play a role in vocalisation (such as hissing for example in pine snakes). The glottis and proximal trachea has a fusion of cartilage here forming a glottal tube. This tube is rigid enough to withstand the pressures placed upon it when the snake is swallowing whole prey and still maintain a patent airway. At rest the proximal glottal opening is held closed, only opening when the snake breathes. The trachea in snakes is supported by C-shaped cartilages similar to those of mammals such as the domestic dog.

Veterinary Nursing of Exotic Pets and Wildlife, Third Edition. Simon J. Girling.

Table 17.1 Basic classification of reptiles.

Clade	Description
Archosauria	Contains all shelled reptiles (Chelonia), e.g. order Testudines which itself contains most turtles and tortoises such as the true 'tortoises' (within which is the family Testudinidae, e.g. *Testudo* spp. that covers most Mediterranean tortoises); crocodilians containing the families Alligatoridae (alligators and caimans), Crocodilidae (crocodiles) and Gavialidae (the gharial); and now birds as well (Crawford *et al.*, 2015)
Lepidosauria	This clade contains: Order Rhyncocephalia, which contains the single species the tuatara (*Sphenodon punctatus*) Order Squamata, which contains the following: Suborder Serpentes: the snake families such as the Elapidae (e.g. king cobra), Colubridae (e.g. garter snakes and corn snakes), Pythonidae (e.g. Burmese pythons) and Boidae (e.g. boa constrictors) Suborder Lacertilia: lizard families such as the Iguanidae (e.g. green iguana), Agamidae (e.g. bearded dragon and Chinese water dragon), Chamaeleonidae (e.g. veiled chameleon), Gekkonidae (e.g. tokay gecko), Eublepharidae (e.g. leopard gecko), Varanidae (e.g. savannah monitor lizard), Scincidae (e.g. blue-tongued skink), and Amphisbaenidae (the worm-lizards) amongst others NB: considerable debate about lizard classification still exists and some divide lacertids into the clade Iguania (that contains the families Iguanidae, Agamidae and Chamaeleonidae) that is further divided into a group with acrodont dentition known as the Acrodonta (Agamidae and Chamaeleonidae) and those with pleurodont dentition known as the Pleurodonta (Iguandidae). All other remaining non-Iguania lacertids being placed in the clade Scleroglossa

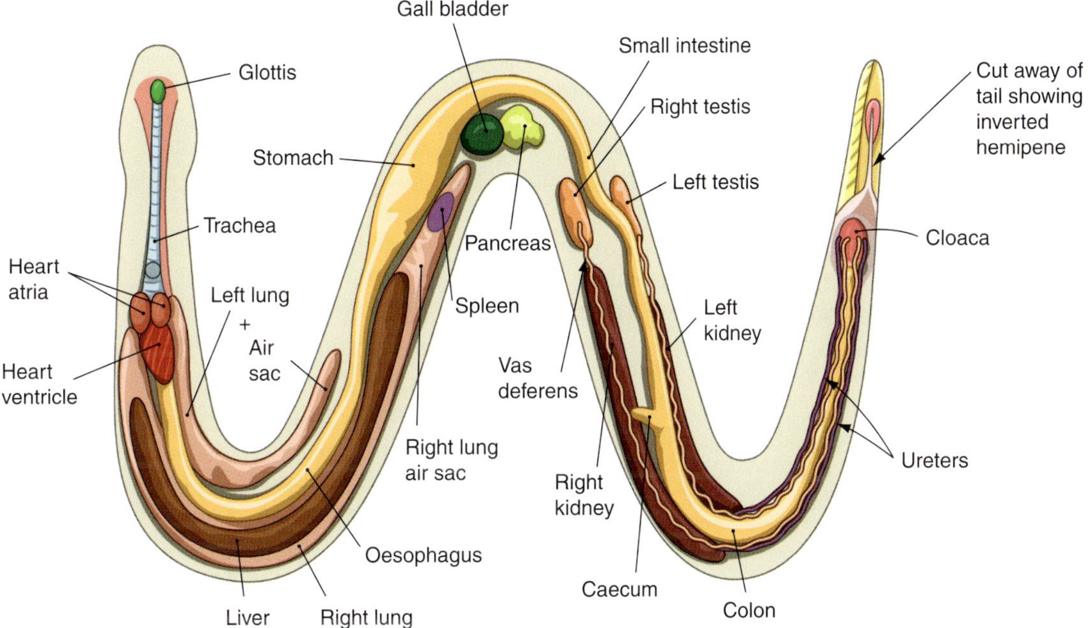

Figure 17.1 Schematic diagram of a male snake from the ventral aspect.

Lower respiratory system

In many colubrid species, such as rat snakes and kingsnakes and some Viperidae, the right lung is the major lung, the left having regressed to a vestigial structure. The vestigial left lung is often replaced by a vascularised air sac and so can still take part in gaseous exchange. In the evolutionary older species such as the Boidae there are two lungs. The right lung often starts near the heart and extends the majority of the length of the snake's body to the level of the right kidney, with the cranial part of the lung being vascular and where the majority of gaseous exchange occurs and the caudal part of the lung being more of an air sac. The vascular lung has structures referred to as faveoli that form a honeycomb pattern and increase surface area for gaseous exchange. Some species of aquatic snakes may have even greater lengths of air sac, stretching caudally the full length of the coelomic cavity and used for buoyancy.

The trachea bifurcates at the level of the heart, and in some species vascular lung tissue may be found in the distal trachea (a so-called 'tracheal lung'). As there is no diaphragm, inspiration is driven by the contraction of intercostal muscles resulting in the outward and cranial movement of the ribs causing negative pressure inside the coelomic cavity. Expiration occurs with inward movement of the ribs and body wall and is aided by elastic tissue present within the lung structure, which allows the lungs to recoil. A tracheal lung is often present as an outpouching of the lining of the trachea. This is thought to aid respiration when the main lungs are being compressed during the swallowing of large prey items.

Respiratory physiology

Peripheral oxygen receptors in reptiles seem to respond to a reduction in oxygen content (i.e. hypoxaemia) or to the rate of delivery of oxygen to the receptor, which includes blood flow, rather than to systemic hypoxia (i.e. a reduction in PO_2) (Taylor *et al.*, 2010). This has implications for recovery from gaseous anaesthesia where the volatile anaesthetic is being delivered in 100% oxygen (see Chapter 19 for further details). As reptiles are ectothermic, an increase in environmental temperature also acts as a stimulus for respiration by increasing the metabolic rate and therefore cellular oxygen demand. Elevated arterial carbon dioxide is also a strong stimulus for increased ventilation but intrapulmonary chemoreceptors may also be suppressed by very high levels of carbon dioxide and result in a reduction in ventilation (Milsom, 1995).

Digestive system

Oral cavity

The tongue sits in a basal sheath at the rostral end of the oral cavity just in front of the glottis and can be pushed out through the lips even when the mouth is closed through the labial notch. The tongue is bifid (split into a forked end) and is used to catch odours on its moist surface that are then guided towards the vomeronasal organ (also known as Jacobson's organ) situated in the roof of the mouth. The vomeronasal organ is connected to the olfactory region of the brain and is a primitive but effective pheromone and scent detector. The oral cavity contains salivary glands that are stimulated to release saliva during mastication. The mouth is normally free of excess saliva at other times.

The maxilla typically has four rows of teeth, two on either side. The mandible has two rows of teeth. The teeth vary somewhat between the genera. Non-venomous species such as the colubrid family (containing the kingsnakes and rat snakes) and the boid family have simple, caudally curved, peg-like teeth. Some of the venomous species have specialist adaptations. Rattlesnakes, for example, have hinged, rostrally situated maxillary fangs which swing forward as they strike and are connected to venom glands situated below the eyes. Other venomous species such as the boomslang (*Dispholidus typus*) may have caudally located fixed maxillary fang teeth. All teeth are replaced as they are lost, including fang teeth in venomous species. It is worth mentioning that private owners of venomous species of snake, such as pit vipers and rattlesnakes, must be licensed and registered in the UK through their local authority government under the Dangerous Wild Animals Act 1976 and need to renew this licence annually.

The oropharynx passes on into the oesophagus, which is an extremely distensible muscular tube travelling ventral to the lungs and entering the stomach halfway through the middle third of the snake's body.

Stomach, associated organs and intestine

The stomach is a tubular organ, populated with compound glands secreting both hydrochloric acid and pepsinogen (mammals having two separate cells) and separate mucus-secreting glands. There is no well-defined cardiac sphincter. The majority of the digestive process occurs in the stomach but is continued by the small intestine. The only substance from rodent prey that cannot be digested is the hair, known as the 'felt' and some of the larger bones which are passed out in the stool.

The stomach empties into the duodenum. The transitions of the duodenum to jejunum and then jejunum to ileum are poorly defined. The spleen, pancreas and gall bladder are found at the point where the pylorus empties into the small intestine. Some snakes have a fused splenopancreas. The gall bladder is found at the most caudal point of the liver, which is an elongated structure extending from the mid-point of the lungs to the caudal stomach.

The small intestine empties into the large intestine, which is distinguished from it by its thinner wall and larger diameter. In the Boidae there may be a caecum at this junction.

The large intestine empties into the coprodeum portion of the cloaca, which, as with birds, is the common emptying chamber for the digestive, urinary and reproductive systems.

Urinary system

There are paired elongated kidneys, situated in the distal half of the caudal third of the snake's body, attached to the dorsal body wall. The right kidney is cranial to the left and both have a single ureter each that travels across their ventral surface to empty into the urodeum of the cloaca, caudal to the proctodeum. There is no urinary bladder in snakes. The caudal portions of the kidneys in male snakes are the 'sexual segments', enlarging during the breeding season as they produce seminal fluid.

Renal physiology

As with the majority of reptiles, terrestrial snakes are uricotelic, that is, like birds, their primary nitrogenous waste product is not urea but uric acid. This compound is relatively insoluble so allowing conservation of water. This is particularly important for reptiles, as they have no loops of Henle in their kidneys; therefore, they cannot create hypertonic urine as mammals can. To further conserve water, urine in the urodeum portion of the cloaca can be refluxed back into the terminal portion of the gut where more water reabsorption can occur. If the reptile becomes dehydrated, or renal blockage or infection occurs, then excretion of uric acid is reduced and can lead to hyperuricaemia followed by visceral gout as seen in birds.

Cardiovascular system

Heart and thyroid

The heart lies in the caudal half of the proximal third of the snake's body, and is mobile, to allow the passage of large food items through the oesophagus above it. However, the position of the heart can vary according to the species and is generally found more caudally in aquatic and terrestrial snakes and more cranially in arboreal species of snake (Schilliger and Girling, 2019). Immediately cranial to the heart is the thyroid gland, often encased in fat.

The heart is generally considered as three-chambered, with two atria and a common ventricle situated within the pericardial sac, but despite this it can separate oxygenated and deoxygenated blood in the ventricle. This is most acutely observed in the pythons, where separation of deoxygenated and oxygenated blood within the ventricle is considerable due to a prominent muscular intracardiac ridge (the horizontal septum) (Hynes and Girling, 2019), although why this has developed in pythons and not in other 'sit and wait' predatory snakes is not fully understood (Jensen *et al.*, 2010). Due to the pressure difference between the systemic and pulmonary sides of the heart in pythons, any heart disease has the ability to increase blood pressure in the delicate vascular structure of the lungs and so dyspnoea, respiratory airway fluid build-up and cyanosis are commonly reported (Jenson and Wang, 2009; Schilliger *et al*., 2010).

The ventricle in all non-crocodilian reptiles is itself divided into three chambers: the cavum pulmonale, functionally similar to the mammalian/avian right ventricle and exiting to the pulmonary artery; the cavum arteriosum, functionally similar to the mammalian/avian left ventricle and exiting to the aortae; and the cavum venosum, which has no direct comparison in mammals and birds but receives blood from the right atrium, although during intracardiac shunting may also receive blood from the cavum arteriosum (i.e. the left side of the ventricle). The cava venosum and arteriosum are dorsally located and partially divided by the vertical/interventricular septum (which attaches to the ventrally located horizontal septum) and so they are sometimes referred to collectively as the cavum dorsale. The cavum pulmonale is ventrally located and so sometimes referred to as the cavum ventrale. The right atrium is significantly larger than the left particularly in snakes.

There are two cranial venae cavae and one caudal vena cava entering via the sinus venosus which creates a further smaller chamber to the heart, a narrow tube leading to the right atrium, from which it is separated by the sinoatrial valve. The sinus venosus in all reptiles is thought to be the dominant cardiac pacemaker as it contains spontaneous contractile myocardial tissues. It often has a septum (division) within it in snakes and lizards (squamates).

Interestingly, snakes have been shown to increase the size of their hearts after feeding. Burmese pythons (*Python bivittatus*), in particular, can increase the heart size by up to 40% after eating, associated with an increased oxygen demand that requires increased cardiac mass to adequately supply oxygenated blood to body tissues (Anderson *et al*., 2005; Slay *et al*., 2014).

Blood vessels

Snakes have paired aortae exiting one from each of the two sides of the single ventricle of the heart (the ventricular chamber known as the cavum venosum to be precise) and bicuspid instead of tricuspid (as seen in mammals and birds) valves typically exist.

The left aortic arch produces a series of arteries supplying abdominal organs: the coeliac, cranial mesenteric and left gastric arteries. The left aortic arch then fuses caudal to these arteries with the right aortic arch into a single abdominal aorta caudally in the main body of the snake.

The pulmonary artery that leads to the lung(s) arises from the cavum pulmonale portion of the ventricle and has significant amounts of smooth muscle that can constrict when a snake swallows food to allow blood to be shunted away from the lungs and back around the body via intracardiac right-to-left shunting from the 'right ventricle' (cavum pulmonale) back through the cavum venosum into the 'left ventricle' (cavum arteriosum) and so to the aortae.

As with birds, snakes have a renal portal system. The blood supply from the caudal portion of the snake in the coccygeal vessels splits into two and can enter the renal circulation or may bypass it via a series of valves. This is important when administering drugs that are nephrotoxic, or which may be excreted by the kidneys, as it means they might be concentrated there. These should therefore be administered in the cranial part of the snake.

There is also a hepatic portal system from the intestine to the liver. A ventral abdominal vein lies in the midline, just beneath the ventral abdominal musculature, and must be avoided when performing surgery.

Two external jugular veins run just medial to the ventral cervical ribs and may be reached to place catheters for intravenous fluid administration via a surgical cut-down procedure. The ventral tail vein has already been mentioned and is useful for venepuncture for blood collection.

Lymphatic system

There are no specific separate lymph nodes as seen in mammals, a situation similar to birds. Instead, as with birds, there are discrete accumulations of lymph tissue within most of the major organs, particularly the liver and intestines. There is also a spleen, as mentioned above, which has loosely arranged red and white pulp, and a thymus (cranial to the heart along with the thyroid), the source of T lymphocytes as in mammals and birds. Significant amounts of lymphatic tissue deposits are found throughout the digestive system (gut-associated lymphatic tissue or GALT) and particularly in the oesophagus (often referred to as the oesophageal tonsils).

Lymphatic vessels are found throughout the body. A lymphatic sinus, for example, runs the length of the snake just ventrolateral to the epaxial musculature immediately below the skin surface on either side of the body. This may be used for small volumes of fluid administration. In the walls of many of the lymphatic vessels there are muscular swellings known as 'lymph hearts' which aid in the return of the straw-coloured lymphatic fluid to the true heart.

Reproductive system

Male

The paired testes lie within the coelom and are generally oval in shape. They are situated cranial to each kidney, and caudal to the pancreatic tissue, with the right testis slightly cranial to the left. In those species that have a distinct breeding season, the testes enlarge during the season, often reaching two to three times their quiescent state. Close to the testes lie the adrenal glands. Each testis has a solitary vas deferens leading down to the urodeum portion of the cloaca, where seminal fluids from the reproductive sexual segment of the kidneys are added.

In the tail base, the male snake has paired intromission sexual organs, known as hemipenes. At rest they are like two inverted sacs either side of the midline and lie ventral to two other small invaginations in the tail which form the anal glands. When a hemipene's lining becomes engorged with blood it everts, forming a finger-like protrusion beside the vent. As with the domestic cat, the hemipenes are often covered in spines and barbs, and they each have a dorsal groove into which the sperm drops from the cloaca, and so is guided into the female's cloaca during a successful mating. The hemipenes therefore do not play any part in urination.

Female

The female has paired ovaries, cranial to the respective kidneys, with the right ovary cranial to the left. There are two coiled oviducts starting with the fimbriae opposite each ovary and moving through the tubular portion of the infundibulum and on into the magnum. From here the tract merges into the isthmus and then the shell gland or uterus before opening into the muscular vagina. This organ ensures

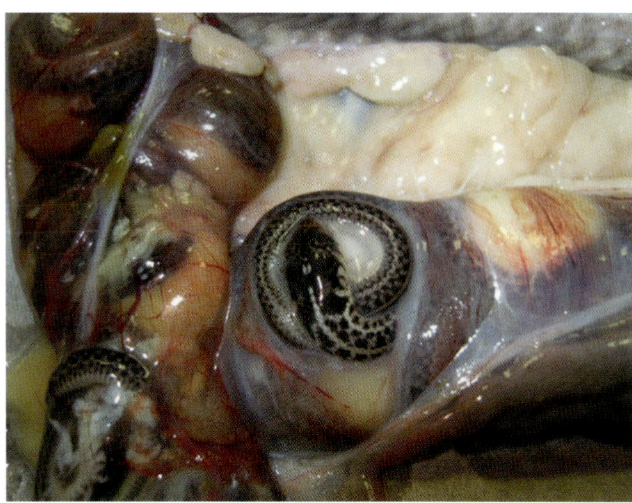

Figure 17.2 Female garter snake (*Thamnophis sirtalis*) post mortem. The oviduct has been incised to show the fetuses. Note the lack of a shell and the presence of a yolk for each fetus.

that the eggs are laid only when the timing is correct. The vagina empties into the urodeum section of the cloaca. The vascular supply to each oviduct involves multiple vessels orientated perpendicular to the oviduct, travelling in the dorsally located oviductal mesentery.

Most seasonally breeding female snakes are stimulated to reproduce in the spring, when the weather warms and the day length increases. However, tropical boids (such as the boa constrictor and Burmese python) start breeding when the temperature drops slightly during the cooler portion of the year.

Some species of snake are oviparous (i.e. they lay eggs), others are viviparous (i.e. they are so-called 'live bearers', that is they give birth to precocious unshelled juveniles although the internal development of the fetus occurs in a rudimentary egg-like sac). Examples of viviparous species are the garter snake (*Thamnophis sirtalis*) and the boid family, which produce a vestigial egg-like structure that has no shell only membranes surrounding the developing snake and the yolk inside the oviduct (see Figure 17.2). The fetus develops inside this structure, staying in the oviduct until gestation is complete. Oviparous species lay eggs in nests and this is the commonest form of reproduction in reptiles. Most will leave the eggs unguarded and untended but many species of python will incubate eggs by contracting and relaxing skeletal muscles, so creating warmth.

Incubation, sex determination and identification

It is recommended to use an incubator for successful egg incubation. The basic components of a reptile egg incubator are as follows: ideally a Perspex® or toughened glass tank with a lid containing aeration holes that can be covered to regulate humidity and temperature; nesting substrate placed into small open containers within the tank; and the eggs placed in slight depressions within the substrate – a useful substrate is vermiculite, although alternative substrates include damp sand, sphagnum moss or even peat.

When the eggs are retrieved from the nest site, particular care should be taken to not rotate the egg in the incubator as this can cause significant fetal mortality. The tank requires a source of humidity and heat production. There are two methods for providing these.

Table 17.2 Typical incubation times and temperatures for some commonly kept snakes.

Species	Egg incubation time (days)	Incubation temperature (°C)
Boa constrictor (*Boa constrictor*)	120–240	28–34
Burmese python (*Python bivitattus*)	58–63	28–32
Corn snake (*Pantherophis guttatus*)	55–70	28–30
Garter snake (*Thamnophis sirtalis*)	90–110	22–30

The containers containing the eggs and substrate may be placed onto a wire mesh which divides the tank into a top and a bottom compartment. The bottom compartment may then be three-quarters filled with filtered water, and a thermostatically controlled water heater placed into it. This technique will provide heat and moisture, and is good for the higher moisture-requiring species (e.g. garter snakes) that need an average 80% humidity.

An alternative set-up is to attach a thermostatically controlled radiant heat mat to the outside of the tank. The tank is then completely filled with the substrate, which is kept moist by regular misting with a plant sprayer, and by placing shallow containers of filtered and previously boiled water in amongst the eggs. This provides a drier atmosphere, more suitable for desert-dwelling species. Care should be taken not to allow the humidity to drop below 50%, as reptile eggs are porous and excessively dry conditions will dehydrate the fetus inside and lead to high levels of mortality. Equally, excessive levels of humidity will lead to an increased risk of fungal infection of the shell and contents and again higher mortality rates. It is therefore important to have both a thermometer and a humidity gauge within the incubator, and both should be monitored regularly.

Snakes are completely chromosomally dependent for sex determination, similar to mammals. This is in contrast with the chelonians, crocodilians and some lizards, in which the sex is determined by the temperature at which the egg was incubated. Some examples of incubation periods and temperatures are given in Table 17.2.

Sex identification is best made by a technique known as probing. A fine, sterile, blunt-ended probe is inserted through the vent and advanced just to one side of the midline in a caudal direction. If the snake is a male, then the probe will pass into one of the inverted hemipenes to a depth of 8–16 subcaudal scales (see Figures 17.3 and 17.4). In the female, there are anal glands in this region, and so the probe may still be inserted, but only to a depth of two to six subcaudal scales. In some species, such as the boid family, the males possess a paracloacal spur. This is the remnant of the pelvic limb and may be found on either side of body, ventrally, at the level of the cloaca. In very young snakes it may be possible carefully to evert the hemipenes manually, a technique known as 'popping'.

Skin

The outer epidermal layer in snakes is thrown into a series of folds forming scales, which cover the whole surface of the snake. There are different sizes of scale over the body, with smaller, less raised ones covering the head and larger, more raised scales over the main portion of the body. Some species have scales with ridges on their surface to add greater grip; other species have smooth scales. In sea snakes

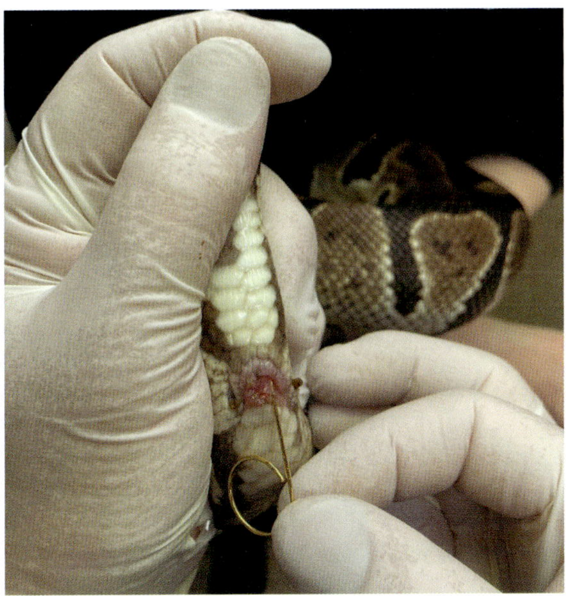

Figure 17.3 Insertion of a sterile metal probe into the inverted hemipene of a live male snake. Care should be taken to ensure good hygiene measures are observed and not to traumatise the delicate tissues.

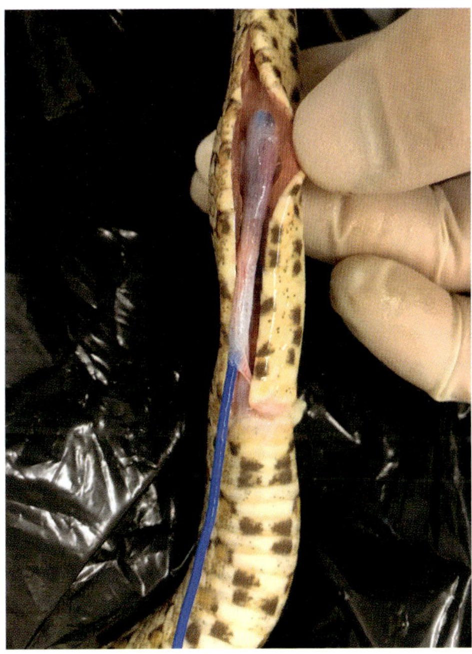

Figure 17.4 Insertion of a probe into the hemipene of a male snake at post-mortem demonstrating the depth the probe will typically allow insertion.

for example, the skin is very loose fitting, and apparently has few elastic fibres. Other snakes have elastic skin which relatively quickly returns to its normal shape. The reptile skin has little or no skin glands. Its outer layer, or stratum corneum, is heavily keratinised and composed of three layers of dead cells filled with keratin. These cells become progressively more flattened as they approach the surface. On the ventral surface of the snake there is a single row of scales which span the width of the snake and are known as the ventral scutes or gastropeges. The caudal edge of each overlaps the cranial edge of the following scale. In most non-venomous species of snake the ventral scutes are paired caudal to the cloaca, but in many venomous species they are single.

Ecdysis

In snakes, ecdysis is the regular shedding of the entire skin including the fused clear eyelids (so-called 'spectacles'). Other reptiles also shed their skin, but Chelonia and Crocodilia may shed individual scutes, and lizards shed in patches. The stimulus can be dependent on time of year, health status and age of the snake and the process is partly controlled by the thyroid gland.

The first phase of ecdysis is the formation of the new layer of skin deep to the old one. Once it is complete, the snake secretes a proteinaceous lymph fluid between the new layer of skin and the old one. Because of this fluid, the snake will become dull in colour, and often exhibits blueing of the eyes (see Figure 17.5). The fluid forces the outer layer of old skin to separate from the new, and often contains enzymes to help in this process by breaking down the connections between cells (desmosomes/hemidesmosomes). Once separation has been achieved the fluid is reabsorbed, and this coincides with the snake's colouration and eyes appearing to return to normal. A few days later the snake will shed the old skin. It starts the process by rubbing the corners of its mouth on some abrasive surface. The shedding proceeds with the head skin first and the snake then rolls the old skin back until the tail is the last to emerge.

In a healthy snake, all of the skin should come away at once. If the skin does not shed cleanly, or at all, the condition is known as dysecdysis. There can be many reasons for this: disease, malnutrition (which causes a reduction in new cell growth and enzyme production), dehydration (which causes too little fluid to be produced between the new and old skin layers), scars on the skin surface (which tie down old and new skin layers) or lack of an abrasive surface upon which to remove the skin. Regular bathing and soft but abrasive damp surfaces may be needed to aid shedding, and any underlying disease should be attended to.

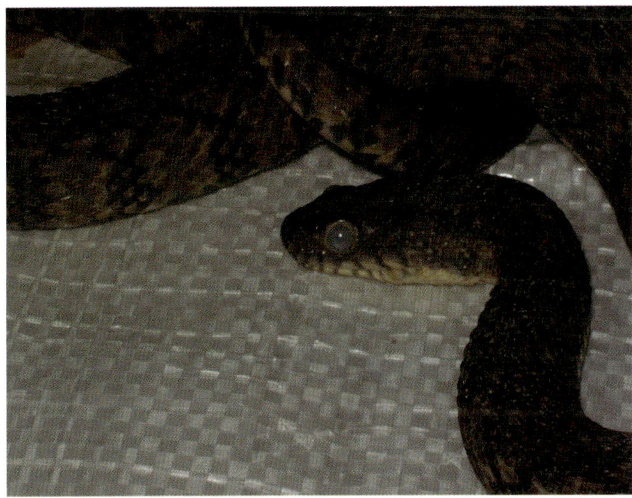

Figure 17.5 Ecdysis in a snake. Note the blueing of the eyes due to the presence of proteinaceous fluid between the old 'spectacle' and the new one beneath.

Special cutaneous adaptations in snakes

There are several special structures associated with the skin of snakes. These include the lateral spurs of the Boidae, which have been mentioned earlier; the male possesses larger spurs than the female.

Snakes do not have mobile eyelids. Instead, the eyelids have become fused together and transparent, forming the so-called 'spectacle'.

Many snakes also have special sense organs on the head. The evolutionary older snake families such as the Boidae have labial pits, a series of depressions running along the rostrolateral margin of the upper or lower lip. These function as rudimentary heat sensors. In evolutionary newer species, such as the pit vipers, the heat-sensing organs are composed of bilateral forward-facing pits midway between the nares and the eyes. These can actually focus on their prey in a 'binocular' fashion. They are supplied by branches of the trigeminal nerves and, in the case of pit vipers, may be sensitive enough to detect changes of heat as small as 0.002°C.

Pigment cells (chromatophores) in snakes, as with other reptiles, are found in the dermis deep to the epidermis.

Snakes do not possess an external eardrum or middle ear. They can, however, hear airborne sounds and can of course detect ground tremors through other sensors in the skin and jaws.

LIZARDS

Musculoskeletal system

Lizards have a musculoskeletal system more familiar to those used to dealing with mammalians. They possess, in the majority, four limbs, an axial skeleton and much of the anatomical layout of small mammals. There are some exceptions, one being the slow worm, a native of mainland Britain and northern Europe which resembles a snake, having no obvious external limbs. It is actually, however, a highly evolved lizard with rudimentary limbs and is related to other limbless lizards such as the glass lizards (*Ophisaurus* spp.) which are sometimes confusingly called glass snakes. They all have mobile eyelids and ears, another difference from snake species.

The lizard skull is more rigid than its snake counterpart, having less mobile jaws and lacking the kinesis at the junction of maxilla and calvarium.

The skull articulates with the atlantal cervical vertebra via a single occipital condyle. The thoracic vertebrae and lumbar vertebrae generally have paired ribs on either side. The coccygeal vertebrae possess ventral haemal arches, between which it is possible to access the ventral tail vein for venepuncture.

In many lizards, the tail possesses one or more fracture planes which allow the tail to break off during escape from a predator, a process known as autotomy. These fracture planes occur in the mid to caudal portions of the tail, but generally not proximally, where vital structures such as the male reproductive organs and fat pads are stored; there also appears to be a difference between some species as to whether it occurs intravertebrally (through a vertebra) or intervertebrally (between vertebrae) (Gordeev *et al.*, 2020). Only certain species exhibit this tail autotomy. This includes most of the Iguanidae (e.g. green iguana), many of the Gekkonidae (e.g. day geckos) and Eublepharidae (e.g. leopard gecko), but does not include the Agamidae (e.g. bearded dragons), Varanidae (e.g. monitor lizards) and true chameleons. When the tail is regrown in these species, the

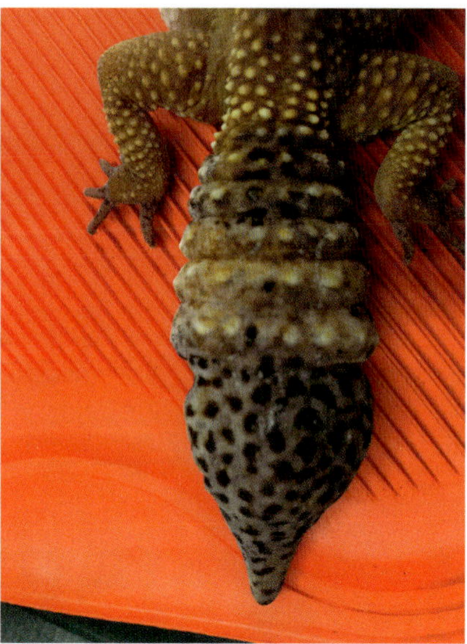

Figure 17.6 Regrowth of the tail is possible in many species of lizard such as this leopard gecko (*Eublepharis macularius*), but the tail nearly always differs from the original and the vertebrae lost are replaced by a rod of cartilage.

coccygeal vertebrae are not regrown, and instead a cartilaginous rod of tissue forms the rigid structure. In addition, the rows of scales over the new tail surface are often haphazardly arranged and do not match the size and shape of the rest of the tail (see Figure 17.6). Some species do not regrow their tails, although they can shed them and some species may lose the ability to regrow their tails with age or if the fracture occurs very close to the tail base.

Nervous system

The brain consists of a forebrain and hindbrain. The cerebrum tends to lack gyri/folds but the cerebrum and cerebellum are generally larger than those of other lower vertebrates such as fish or amphibians (see Figure 17.7). Overall, though, the brain tends not to exceed 1% of body weight. As with snakes, the spinal cord extends to the very end of the tail tip. There is no subarachnoid space which means that myelography cannot be performed. Lizards have a full 12 cranial nerves (13 if the nervus terminalis or cranial nerve 0 is included; see section on the nervous system in snakes).

Respiratory system (see Figure 17.8)

Upper respiratory system

Lizards have paired nostrils situated rostrally on the maxilla. The nostrils enter into the rostral part of the oral cavity, there being no proper hard palate in iguanids and agamids and many geckos. However, in some species of lizard such as tegus, a hard palate is present and therefore the nasal passages communicate more caudally with the oral cavity (see Figure 17.9).

To the side, or just inside each nostril, particularly in iguanids and varanids, there is often situated a salt-secreting gland. These are responsible for excreting excess potassium or sodium as their chlorides so helping to maintain electrolyte balance and conserve water (Hazard, 2004). Potassium levels may become elevated in herbivorous species through their naturally occurring diet; this is why species such as the green iguana (*Iguana iguana*) have these

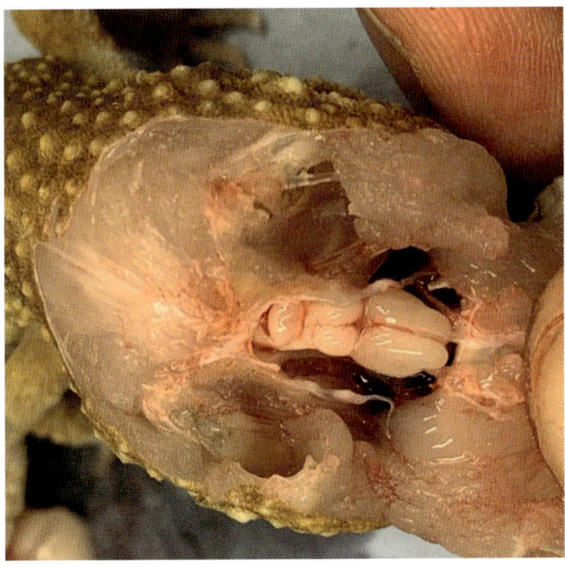

Figure 17.7 Post-mortem view of the dorsal surface of the brain of a leopard gecko showing the relatively small size in relation to body size and lack of gyri.

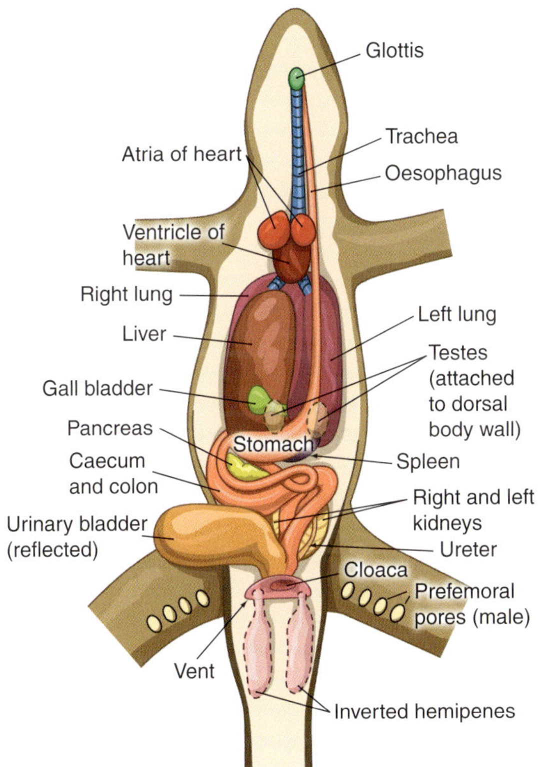

Figure 17.8 Diagram of male green iguana (ventral aspect).

glands, and indeed may excrete potassium as urate salts as for example the blue-chinned, rough-scaled lizard (*Sceloporus cyanogenys*), acting as a route other than the kidneys to rid the body of uric acid (Davis *et al.*, 1976). Conversely, marine iguanas (*Amblyrhynchus cristatus*) live in a sodium chloride-rich environment and excrete predominantly sodium chloride through these glands as a result. The potassium and sodium chloride may be seen as a white crystalline deposit around the nostrils, which is often sneezed out by the lizard.

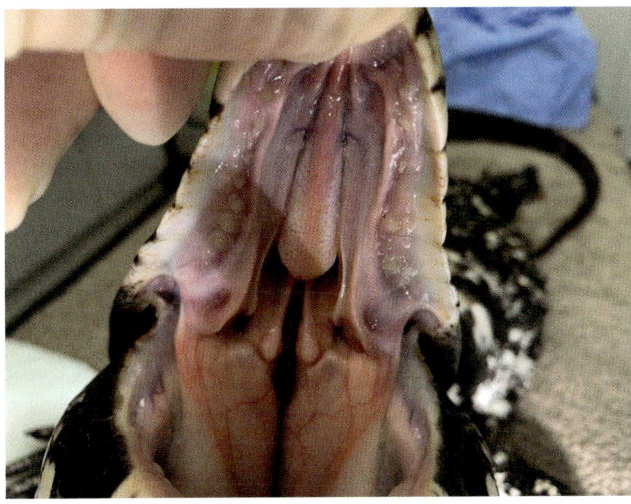

Figure 17.9 View of the nasal and oral cavity in a tegu demonstrating the presence of a hard palate. Note also the short crowned but strong teeth that are more dagger-like rostrally and flatter and more grinding caudally.

The entrance to the trachea is guarded by a rudimentary larynx which often lacks an epiglottis and vocal folds. Some species, such as the Gekkonidae, do possess vocal folds and are capable of producing a variety of sounds. In most species, the trachea is supported by incomplete cartilaginous C-shaped rings similar to those of the cat and dog.

Lower respiratory system

The trachea bifurcates into two main bronchi in the cranial coelomic cavity to supply two lungs, although some chameleons have a tracheal lung lobe cranioventral to the pectoral girdle as well. The lizard lung may be a simple one-chambered sac covered with uniform trabeculae supporting the faveolar parenchyma where gaseous exchange occurs. This is also known as a unicameral lung and is seen in lizards such as the tegu (*Tupinambis* spp.). Other lizards may have a few chambers, also known as a paucicameral lung such as the chameleons, or multiple chambers (multicameral) such as the monitor lizards (*Varanus* spp.) (Perry and Duncker, 1978). The lungs of the savannah monitor lizard (*Varanus exanthematicus*) have been examined using computed tomography (CT) to determine that they have a functional structure with similarities to birds, such as unidirectional flow of air through certain parts. It appears that air moves predominantly caudally through the prominent intrapulmonary bronchus (not present in unicameral and paucicameral lungs) and predominantly cranially through secondary bronchi (Cieri and Farmer, 2020). The Iguanidae have also been shown to have some unidirectional airflow similar to that of the Varanidae. Other families that have not been shown to have unidirectional airflow include the Gekkonidae and Chamaeleonidae. Lizards will often overinflate their lungs in an attempt to make themselves look bigger when threatened. Chameleons in particular have finger-like projections from the edges of the lung fields that are effectively air sacs that facilitate this.

There is no true diaphragm in any lizard species, so there is no clear distinction between the thorax and abdomen, rather there is a common body cavity, known as the coelom, as in snakes and birds. However, the varanids (e.g. savannah monitor lizard) do have a complicated post-pulmonary septum structure that divides the lungs from the pericardium/heart and the digestive tract.

Respiratory physiology

Respiration, as for snakes, is thought to be stimulated by falling partial pressures of oxygen in the bloodstream as well as increasing levels of carbon dioxide, although increased levels of carbon dioxide in the lungs may suppress intrapulmonary receptors. Carotid chemoreceptors have been identified in varanid lizards, innervated by the vagus and possibly glossopharyngeal nerves (Taylor *et al.*, 1999). Increased environmental temperatures also increase respiration due to their ectothermic nature. The act of inspiration is due to the mechanical contraction of the intercostal muscles causing an upwards and outwards movement of the ribcage. Expiration occurs through the reverse process and is aided by the elastic tissues and smooth muscles that are present within the lung structures themselves as well as sometimes caudal body wall muscle contractions.

Digestive system

Oral cavity

The majority of lizards have a large, fleshy tongue which is often highly mobile. In some species such as the chameleons, the tongue has become specialised. It lies coiled in the lower jaw and can be projected out at a flying insect or other potential prey item. The green iguana has a more traditional fleshy tongue, which has a much darker red tip. This is not to be confused with pathological changes. Bearded dragons tend to have a paler body to the tongue with a more yellow coloured tip (see Figure 17.10). The tip of the tongue in many lizards may also be seen to have two small fork-like projections. These are used to push scent into the two entrances of the vomeronasal organ which is present in the rostral maxilla. In varanids and tegus the tongue is more deeply forked, similar to snakes.

There are four rows of teeth, one to each jaw. These are peg-like in shape and are continually replaced in lizards such as the Iguanidae and Varanidae. These species are often referred to as pleurodont in

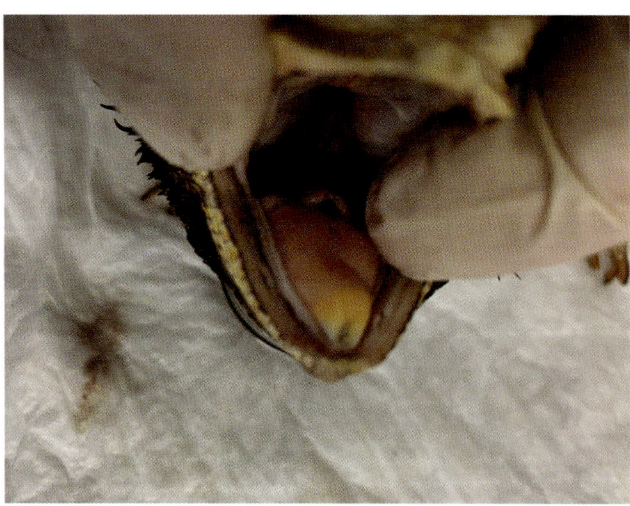

Figure 17.10 Intraoral view of a bearded dragon (*Pogona vitticeps*). Note the pale pink fleshy base to the tongue and the yellow rostral tip that has two small fork-like projections similar to snakes. Also note the glottis at the caudal base of the tongue and the trachea beyond.

dentition as the teeth are not only shed and replaced but also attach to the inner/lingual side of the mandible. In species of the Agamidae and Chamaeleonidae, the teeth are not replaced (except the most rostral teeth in some Agamidae) and the teeth are located on the actual biting edge of the jaws rather than the lingual side. This form of dentition is referred to as acrodont.

There are no fang teeth in lizards, but the beaded lizard (*Heloderma horridum*) and the Gila monster (*Heloderma suspectum*) have grooved mandibular teeth which allow the venom from sublingual venom glands to ooze through these grooves into the prey when they bite/chew them. In the UK, these two species are some of the few lizards currently classified as dangerous wild animals under the Dangerous Wild Animals Act 1976 (as amended), therefore requiring a licence to keep them in private ownership.

Stomach, associated organs and intestine

The stomach is a simple sac-like structure in most species. The glands that line the walls of the stomach secrete both hydrochloric acid and pepsinogen. There are also separate mucus-secreting glands for lubrication.

The small intestine is better developed in more carnivorous species such as the monitor lizards and the insectivorous water dragons. In herbivorous species it is relatively short, with the majority being the duodenum. The division between jejunum and ileum is often not clear. In a few, mainly herbivorous, species, at the junction between the small and large intestines lies the caecum. The liver is roughly bilobed in structure and is situated ventral to the stomach and lungs. There is usually a gall bladder, with the primary bile pigment being biliverdin, as with birds, rather than the bilirubin of mammals.

The large intestine is more highly developed in herbivorous species than in carnivorous or omnivorous species. Examples include the green iguana and the chuckwalla. These have a large intestine which is often sacculated and divided into many chambers by leaf-like membranes. The green iguana has five chambers to the proximal colon created by these membranes which help to slow the transit time down to around three and a half days assuming the iguana is kept within its preferred optimum temperature zone (see Chapter 18) (Troyer, 1984; King, 1996). These membranes increase the surface area so that microbes, upon which these species depend for digestion of vegetation, may colonise it.

The large intestine then empties into the coprodeum portion of the cloaca. The cloaca itself is then continued, as with birds and snakes, by two segments, the urodeum which receives the urogenital openings, and the proctodeum, which is the last chamber before waste exits the cloaca through the vent.

Urinary system

The kidneys are paired and often bean-shaped organs. Their position is variable depending on the species. In some, such as the green iguana and leopard gecko, they are both situated in the pelvis, attached to the dorsal body wall (see Figure 17.8). Other species, such as chameleons and varanids, have longer kidney structures that extend cranially into the coelomic cavity. As with snakes, the males of some species have a specially developed caudal portion of the kidneys known as the 'sexual segment', which enlarges during the breeding season and contributes to the production of seminal fluid. The kidneys empty into the ureters (one per kidney) which empty into the urodeum portion of the cloaca.

Most lizards have a urinary bladder although some like the tegus and varanids do not. The urinary bladder, where present, is not like the sterile bladder of mammals, as it is not connected directly to the ureters. Instead, it is joined to the cloaca, and so urine has to enter the cloaca (urodeum) before entering the bladder. There is some evidence that the bladder is able to absorb some fluid from its contents, or it may function as a fluid storage chamber, flushing its contents back into the caudal large intestine for further fluid absorption.

Renal physiology

The renal physiology is similar to that already described for snakes. The main differences lie in the variable presence of the urinary bladder, which may have some water reabsorption capabilities.

Cardiovascular system

Heart

The lizard heart is generally contained within the pectoral girdle. However, in varanids, tegus and the *Heloderma* it is more caudally located in the coelomic cavity. The heart structure is very similar to the snake model, with paired atria and a single common ventricle, which nevertheless functions as two separate chambers keeping deoxygenated and oxygenated blood apart. A sinus venosus also exists that empties into the right atrium and likely acts as the cardiac pacemaker.

The majority of the deoxygenated blood is channelled to the pulmonary arteries and the oxygenated blood enters the paired aortas; however, lizards, like other reptiles, can perform intracardiac shunting moving blood from the right side to the left and so bypassing the lungs. This may occur due to anoxia and/or increased vagal tone.

Varanids (e.g. savannah monitor lizard) have a different heart structure from many other lizards, being similar in function to pythons. Their heart keeps deoxygenated and oxygenated blood separated to a greater extent within the common ventricle than other squamates due to the presence of a prominent muscular intracardiac ridge (the horizontal septum) that acts to physically divide a significant part of the ventricle into right and left and create a pressure difference between the pulmonary and systemic circulation (Schilliger and Girling, 2019). They do, however, unlike pythons, have a more complex meshwork of trabecular tissue within the heart that interacts with the atrioventricular valve anatomy of the ventricle (Hynes and Girling, 2019). Because of the pressure difference between the systemic and pulmonary sides of the heart in varanids, any heart disease has the ability to increase blood pressure in the delicate vascular structure of the lungs and so dyspnoea, respiratory airway fluid build-up and cyanosis are commonly reported.

Blood vessels

The two aortae fuse caudodorsally, after giving off paired carotid trunks, to form the abdominal aorta. Lizards also possess a hepatoportal venous supply and a renal portal system; hence, as with birds and snakes, intravenous injection into the caudal half of the lizard of medications which are excreted through the renal tubules could result in their failure to reach the rest of the lizard's body. It could also increase the toxicity of substances known to be renally toxic if given by this route.

Lizards, like snakes, also possess a large ventral abdominal vein, which returns blood from the tail area and passes just beneath the body wall, ventrally and in the midline. This must be avoided when performing abdominal surgery. This vessel can be used, carefully, for venepuncture for blood sampling in lizards, although the preferred vessel is the ventral tail vein. For intravenous use, in the larger species the cephalic vein may be accessed on the cranial aspect of the antebrachium, via a cut-down procedure.

Lymphatic system

The lymphatic system is similar to that of snakes, with no discrete lymph nodes but with significant lymphoid deposition within organs such as the liver and digestive tract (gut-associated lymphatic tissue). Lizards possess a spleen (close to the left side of the stomach) and a cervically located thymus (the latter a source of T lymphocytes).

Reproductive system

Male

The paired testes are situated cranial to the respective kidneys in those species which have abdominally positioned kidneys (see Figure 17.8). In those where the kidneys are more pelvic in position (iguanids, geckonids, agamids), the testes are located just caudal to the end of the lungs and liver, in the middle part of the coelomic cavity. They are supplied by several arteries each and drained by several veins. Both are very tightly adhered to their vascular supply, the left testicle being separated from the left renal vein (into which the left testicular veins drain) by the left adrenal gland. The right testicle is tightly attached to its right renal vein, which separates it from the right adrenal gland. This positioning, so close to such vital structures, makes castrating aggressive male lizards such as the green iguana a difficult operation. In those species that exhibit a breeding season, the testes enlarge during the breeding season and regress out of it. Each testis drains into a vas deferens which has a tightly coiled course over the ventral surface of the respective kidney before emptying into the urodeum portion of the cloaca. Some species, such as the Chamaeleonidae, have a pronounced epididymis extending caudally from each testicle.

The male lizard has paired phalluses, as with the snake, known as hemipenes. These lie in the base of the tail structure, either side of midline, and function as with the snake family. At rest they are inverted sacs in the tail base. During copulation, one will engorge with blood and evert itself, creating a groove along its dorsal surface. Into this groove sperm and spermatic fluid will drop from the cloaca, and the hemipene will guide this into the female lizard's cloaca. They play no part in urination and so if lost will not affect the function of the urinary tract.

Female

The female lizard has much the same anatomy as that described for the snake.

Egg-producing physiology

Reproductive physiology in the female lizard is broadly similar to that of the avian patient. Some species, such as some of the Chamaeleonidae, are (ovo)-viviparous. That is, they produce live young instead of laying eggs, although the eggs are produced internally. Some species are viviparous, in which a form of placenta or thin-walled egg structure allows the fetus to develop and live young are produced. Many other species are oviparous – they lay eggs externally that then hatch.

One or two species are parthenogenic – the females produce entire females with no need for a male lizard. Some species of *Lacerta* ('true' lizards) and *Hemidactylus* (geckos) are capable of this.

Reptile eggs are generally soft-shelled and more leathery than those of their avian cousins. Sexual maturity varies according to the species, green iguanas, for example, reaching it at 2–3 years.

Incubation, sex determination and identification

Incubation first principles are described in the section on incubation, sex determination and identification for snakes. Sex determination is largely dependent on chromosomes. However, geckos as a family are temperature dependent, with 99% of eggs incubated between 26.7 and 29.4°C being female, whereas if the temperature is greater than 32.2°C, 90% of the offspring would be male. In leopard geckos, temperatures at or below 29°C will produce predominantly females, intermediate temperatures of 30–32°C produce mostly males and temperatures above 34°C will again produce mostly females (although the latter temperatures are not recommended as they are close to the lethal limit for incubation). It is interesting to note that leopard geckos incubated at cooler temperatures are also more darkly pigmented than those incubated at higher temperatures. Incubation periods in lizards vary from 45–70 days in smaller lizards to 90–130 days for iguanas and larger lizards but is clearly heavily dependent on the temperature ranges the reptile egg is incubated at, with longer hatching times associated with cooler temperatures (see Table 17.3 for more information).

Sex may be identified by hemipenal probing as for snakes. This is often the only method available for some species such as the beaded lizard, some monitors and the Gila monster, although some monitors may show signs of ossification of the hemipenes that can be detected on radiography when they are sexually mature. However, in most other species there are external physical differences. These include the prominent prefemoral pores of males that are seen on the caudoventral aspect of the thigh of iguanids and agamids (see Figures 17.11 and 17.12). Some male lizards have a series of pre-anal pores just cranial to the vent. Males have wider tail bases than the females to house the large hemipenes (see Figure 17.13). Some males have greater ornamentation (see section Special cutaneous adaptations in lizards).

Table 17.3 Typical incubation times and temperatures for some commonly kept lizards.

Species	Egg incubation time (days)	Incubation temperature (°C)
Green iguana (*Iguana iguana*)	60–90	25–30
Inland bearded dragon (*Pogona vitticeps*)	65–90	28–32
Leopard gecko (*Eublepharis macularius*)	55–60	25–32

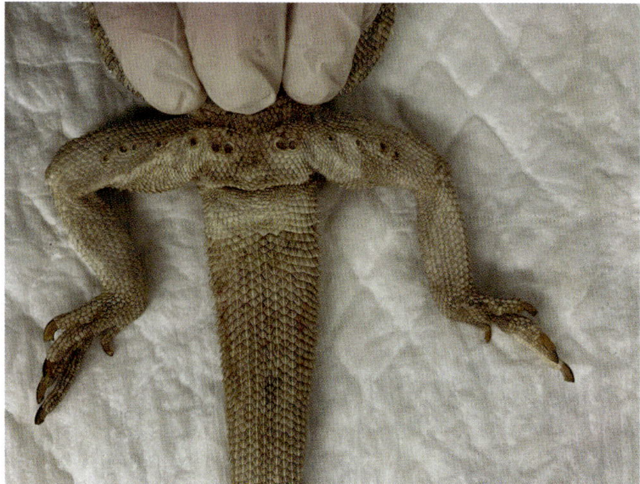

Figure 17.11 Ventral aspect of the pelvic area in a male bearded dragon showing large prefemoral pores.

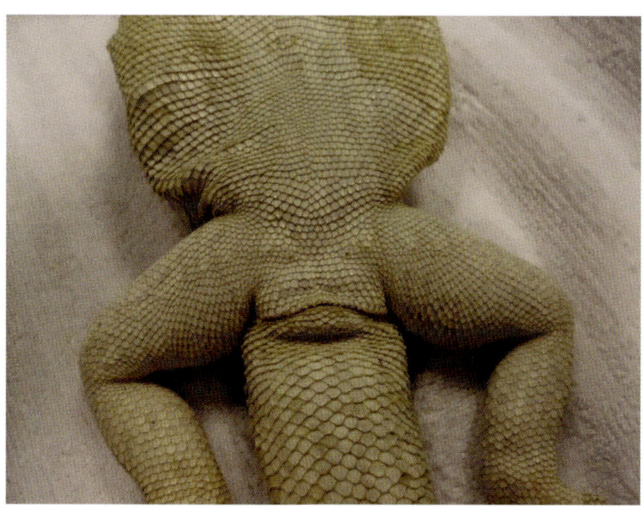

Figure 17.12 Ventral aspect of the pelvic area in a female bearded dragon showing small prefemoral pores.

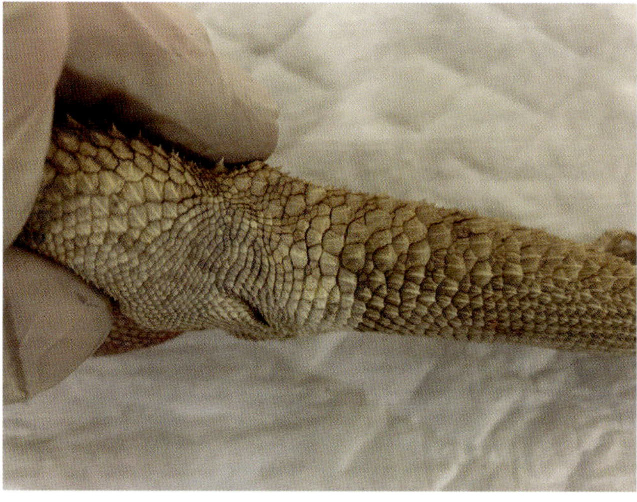

Figure 17.13 Lateral aspect of the tail base and vent in a male bearded dragon showing the ventral bulge associated with the hemipenes.

Skin

Lizard skin is much the same as that of snakes. The scales in most cases are much smaller than the snake equivalent.

Special cutaneous adaptations in lizards

There are some specialised skin glands and structures in lizards. The males of certain species, such as the green iguana, have larger secretory glands or pores than their female counterparts. The green iguana's are on the ventrocaudal aspect of the femoral area. Some geckos have precloacal pores in a chevron pattern.

Many lizards have large numbers of chromatophores in the dermis. These are connected to neural networks, allowing them to alter the colour they produce according to external stimuli and mood. This ability is seen in the chameleons and, to a lesser extent, in green iguanas and many other species.

Unlike snakes, lizards have a tympanum, located ventrocaudal to the eye, and a middle ear.

Many males will have large amounts of ornamentation on their body surface for display purposes. Examples include the male green iguana, which often has large coloured scales on the head and a bluish sheen to the head and neck colouring. Others, such as male anoles (*Anolis* spp.), have extendable chin flaps which are often brightly coloured and can be 'flashed' in display. Some males, such as plumed basilisks (*Basiliscus plumifrons*), have larger nuchal crests than the female. Some males such as Jackson's chameleon (*Trioceros jacksonii*), have triceratops-like horns to the head in males.

Many lizards, such as the green iguana have a parietal eye. This is a special adaptation on the very top of the skull midway between the eyes. It is connected directly, via neural pathways, to the pineal gland in the brain and it is responsible for informing the lizard about light intensity and daytime lengths. These in turn influence feeding and reproductive behaviour. In the tuatara (*Sphenodon punctatus*), found in New Zealand, a primeval lizard in its own class of the reptile family, this parietal eye actually has a vestigial lens within it.

CHELONIA (TORTOISES, TURTLES AND TERRAPINS)

Musculoskeletal system

Chelonia have a rigid upper and lower jaw structure similar to that of the lizard family, but unlike lizards they have no teeth. Instead, the maxillae and mandibles are edged with tough keratin to form a horny beak, similar to that seen in birds. The skull articulates with the atlantal cervical vertebra via a single occipital condyle, similar to birds and other reptiles. There are two strong muscles attached to the back of the chelonian skull, connecting it to the point of fusion of the cervical vertebrae with the shell. These are responsible for the retraction of the head in Cryptodira, those species which can pull their heads back into the shell. There are some turtles (the side-necked or Pleurodira turtles) which, as their name suggests, fold their head sideways into the shell, rather than fully retracting it in a craniocaudal manner. The thoracic vertebrae are fused with the dorsal shell, becoming flattened and elongated. The same is true of the lumbar and sacral vertebrae. The coccygeal vertebrae emerge distally to form the mobile tail.

Chelonia are distinguished from other reptiles by the presence of their shell. This structure is composed of fused living dermal bone covered by keratinised epidermis. It therefore can feel sensations and pain and so should never be used to tether tortoises to ropes or chains. The shell is composed of an upper section known as the carapace (see Figure 17.14), and a lower, flatter, ventral section known as the plastron (see Figure 17.15). These two sections of the shell are connected either side between the forelimbs and hindlimbs by the pillars of the shell. The carapace is a fusion of dermal bone, ribs, thoracic and lumbar vertebrae. The scutes (the individual segments of the shell epidermis)

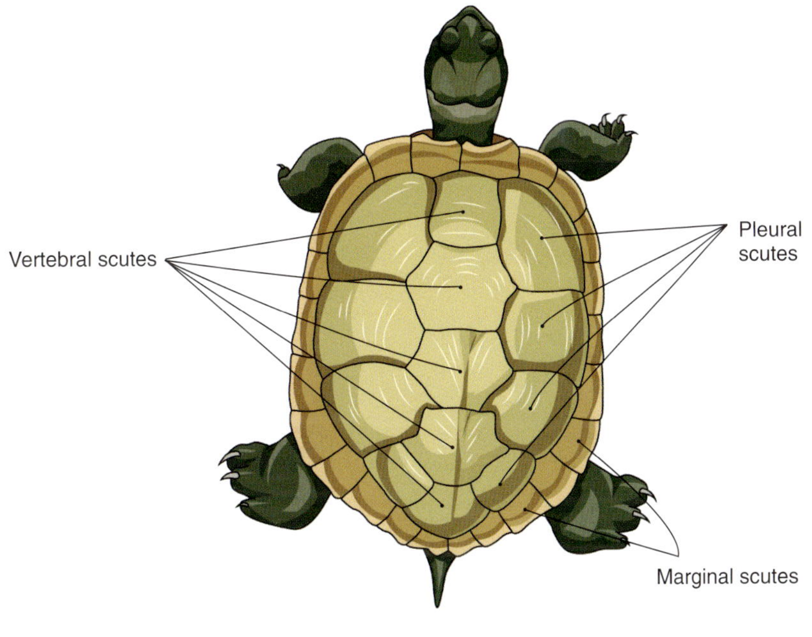

Figure 17.14 Dorsal view of carapace.

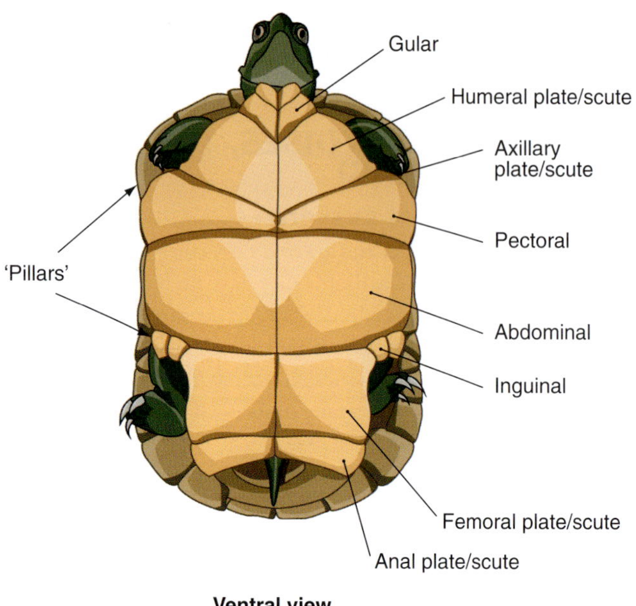

Figure 17.15 Ventral view of plastron.

are given specific names. They do not directly overlie the bone sections of the shell, but there is some overlap. Some tortoises, such as the box turtle (*Terrapene carolina*), possess a hinge to the plastron allowing them to close themselves into their shells even further. Some of the Mediterranean species of tortoise such as the spur-thighed tortoise (*Testudo graeca*) can have caudal plastral hinges. This can be particularly useful in females, when they can increase the caudal exit space of the shell for egg-laying. Others may have a hinge to the caudal carapace, such as the eponymous hingeback tortoises (*Kinixys* spp.).

Another unusual feature of Chelonia is that the scapulae are to be found on the inside of the shell (i.e. inside the ribcage) due to the shell structure. This is unique in the animal world. In addition, the elbow joint is effectively rotated through nearly 180° to cause the twisted forelimb so characteristic of tortoises.

The forelimbs and hindlimbs are supplied with extensive muscles making them extremely strong for their size. The Horsfield's tortoise (*Testudo horsfieldii*) differs from most Mediterranean *Testudo* species in that it is generally smaller than most but has four toed/clawed forelimbs whereas the rest have five.

Nervous system

The brain of Chelonia is similar to that of squamates. They have 12 cranial nerves (13 if the nervus terminalis or cranial nerve 0 is counted; see snakes). The spinal cord extends to the tip of the tail but also is encased within the dorsal carapace as the vertebrae merge with the carapacial shell. This means any midline carapacial damage may involve the spinal cord. There is no subarachnoid space.

Respiratory system (see Figure 17.16)

Upper respiratory system

Chelonia have paired nostrils leading to the rostral portion of the oral cavity. As with other reptiles (excepting the crocodilians) there is no hard palate. The entrance to the trachea is guarded by the glottis, which, as with lizards and snakes, is closed at rest. It opens into the trachea, which has complete cartilaginous rings, and in many chelonia such as the *Testudo* spp. bifurcates into two bronchi relatively far cranially, often in the neck area, allowing the chelonian to breathe easily even when the neck is withdrawn deep into the shell.

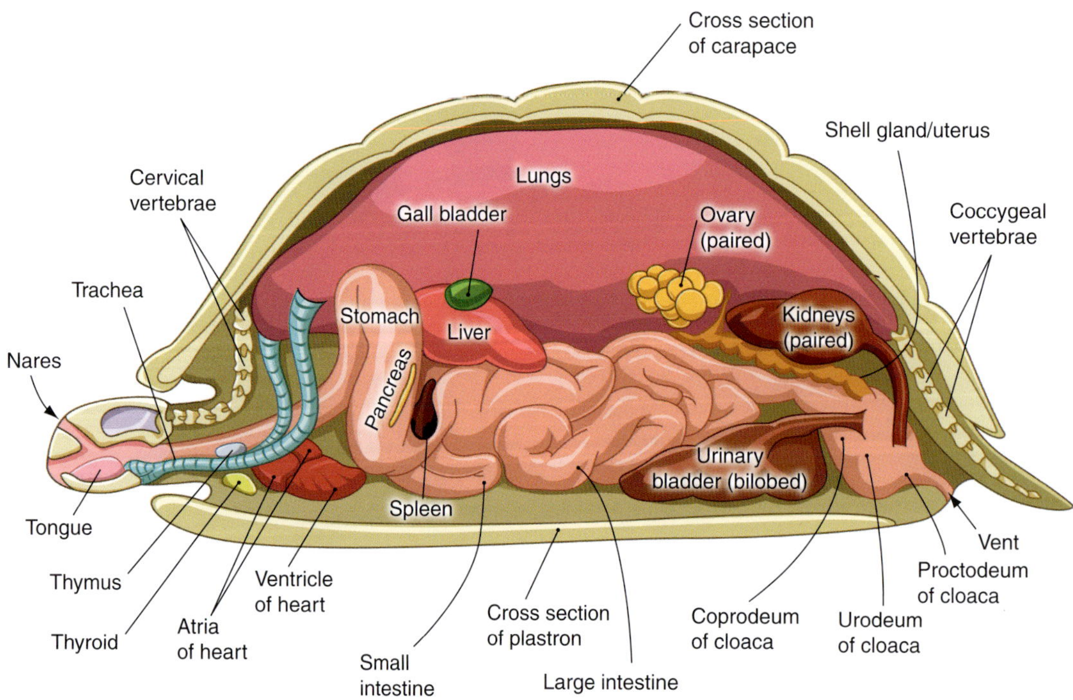

Figure 17.16 Section through the midline of a female tortoise.

Lower respiratory system

The two bronchi each supply a lung and extend the length of each lung with exits along their length. The lungs are situated in the dorsal aspect of the coelomic cavity against the inside of the carapace, and above the liver and digestive system. Between the lungs and the rest of the body organs, there is a connective tissue membrane but no true diaphragm. The lungs are sponge-like in structure and contain smooth-muscle and elastic fibres, forming essentially a non-collapsible structure that connects to the periosteum on the inside of the carapace and the connective tissue sheet separating the lungs from the rest of the coelomic cavity. The lungs themselves are described as faviform in nature and divided into five to six compartments from cranial to caudal. In some aquatic species the lungs have air sacs that act to increase buoyancy.

Respiration is aided by movement of the forelimbs and neck, which act to pump the air into and out of the confined lungs. In addition, there are muscles attached to the membrane that separates the lungs from the rest of the viscera, which during breathing contract and relax. Many chelonians can survive without breathing for several hours if necessary, relying on intracardiac shunting of blood to bypass the lungs if required. It is interesting to note that many chelonians such as red-eared terrapins (*Trachemys scripta elegans*) have been shown to have chemoreceptors that respond to a drop in oxygen located in the aortic arch and chemoreceptors responsible for detecting an increased arterial carbon dioxide level, both of which drive respiration. However, reptiles such as Chelonia also have intrapulmonary chemoreceptors whose discharge frequency has been shown to be inversely proportional to the carbon dioxide present in the lungs, showing that carbon dioxide may have an inhibitory effect if high (Milsom, 1995). Wasser and Jackson (1988) in studies with turtles placed in 100% nitrogen (anoxic) and 95% nitrogen with 5% carbon dioxide (anoxic/hypercapnic) environments identified an anoxic hyperventilation which they believed depended on peripheral hypoxic chemoreceptor control rather than on arterial pH and central chemoreceptor control. A decline in minute ventilation occurred during prolonged anoxic breathing which the same authors believed occurred from a metabolic arrest response and/or a depression in central nervous function.

Digestive system

Oral cavity

The tongue is relatively tightly attached to the inside of the mandible but is fleshy in structure with the glottis at its base. Salivary glands secrete mucus only when eating to lubricate food. The pharynx is wide and passes into a distensible, smooth muscle-covered oesophagus. Many of the aquatic turtles have caudally curved spines present in the caudal pharynx and oesophagus, which are thought to aid in swallowing slippery prey such as fish.

Stomach, associated organs and intestine

The stomach sits on the left side ventrally in the mid-coelomic cavity. It has a strong cardiac sphincter, making vomiting in the healthy chelonian rare. The stomach leads to the duodenum along which lies the pancreas. Following the duodenum is a short but highly coiled jejunum and small ileum. At the junction of the small and large intestine lies the caecum, which is often a rounded bag-like object. The large intestine itself has a large diameter and, for herbivorous chelonians such as tortoises, is the principal site of fermentation. It then narrows to form the rectum. Next come the coprodeum and the urodeum, then the proctodeum of the cloaca, and finally the vent.

The liver is a bilobed structure situated transversely across the mid-section of the coelomic cavity, dorsal to the digestive system, and ventral to the lungs. There is a gall bladder to the right of the midline.

Urinary system

The paired kidneys are situated caudally within the shell, tightly adhered to the ventral surface of the inside of the carapace and caudal to the acetabula of the pelvis. There is a difference in the marine species where the kidneys are situated cranial to the acetabula. Two ureters empty into a urogenital sinus, a common chamber for the opening of the urinary and reproductive systems, which also connects with the urinary bladder that is present in all chelonians. The urinary bladder is a large, bilobed, thin-walled structure which has some ability to reabsorb water. The urogenital sinus empties into the urodeum portion of the cloaca.

Cardiovascular system

Heart

As with lizards and snakes, the chelonian heart is a three-chambered organ situated within the pericardial sac. The two cranial venae cavae and one caudal vena cava merge to form the sinus venosus, which enters the right atrium on the more dorsal aspect.

Blood vessels

Paired aortae give rise to the carotid arteries that supply the head and neck. They then curve dorsally to fuse into the abdominal aorta. Just before fusing, the left aortic arch gives rise to arteries supplying the digestive tract, and the right aortic arch produces the brachiocephalic trunk that supplies the head and forelimbs. The abdominal aorta then courses down the ventral aspect of the vertebrae, supplying the shell and dorsal structures via intercostal arteries. The shell itself has a blood supply arising from cranially placed subclavian and caudally placed iliac arteries which anastomose widely.

The venous return of blood follows a similar pattern to that of lizards and snakes. Another bypass system exists whereby blood from the caudal vessels may cross from one side of the body to the other via transverse pelvic veins. From these, the blood may enter the paired abdominal veins which run along the floor of the coelomic cavity. It is these latter vessels which must be carefully negotiated when performing abdominal surgery/plastral surgery in chelonians.

Lymphatic system

The lymphatic system is similar to other reptiles. The spleen is situated close to the caecum, attached to the left side of the stomach.

Reproductive system

Male

The testes are internal and often yellow cream-coloured oval organs cranial to the kidneys. As with the liver, there may also be some dark pigmentation to the testes. The testes empty into the associated epididymal organs that overlie their surface. The sperm then enter

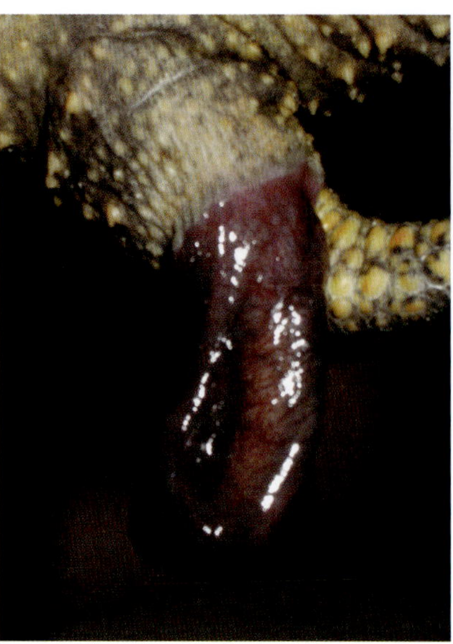

Figure 17.17 Phallus of an alligator snapping turtle (*Macrochelys temminckii*).

the vas deferens, which courses over the ventral surface of the kidneys and enters the urogenital sinus adjacent to the urodeum portion of the cloaca.

The phallus is a large fleshy organ and, unlike in snakes and lizards, there is only one of them. It lies on the ventral aspect of the cloaca at rest. When engorged, the free caudal end of the phallus is projected through the vent and curves cranially. In so doing, a dorsal shallow seminal groove is formed to guide sperm into the female's vent (see Figure 17.17).

Female

Paired ovaries are suspended from the mid-dorsal aspect of the coelomic cavity. They shed their ova into the infundibulum portion of each one of two oviducts. The oviducts have a similar structure to those in snakes and lizards, including the presence of a magnum and a uterus. This finally connects to the smooth muscle-lined vagina which is responsible for keeping the oviduct closed to the outside world until egg-laying occurs. The oviducts empty into the urogenital sinus and then into the urodeum portion of the cloaca.

Reproductive physiology

Folliculogenesis is stimulated by the time of year. In those chelonians such as the Mediterranean species of tortoise, hibernation is an important factor. This period is necessary for the preprogramming of the thyroid gland and the reproductive cycle. Two bouts of egg production can occur per year. On average, 10–30 eggs are laid each year depending on the species. Most Mediterranean tortoise species do not become sexually mature until they are 7–10 years of age.

The female tortoise will start to form fertile eggs after a successful mating. These are carried in her reproductive system for a period of time varying anywhere from 4 weeks to 3–4 years which means that it is possible for Mediterranean species to carry eggs through hibernation. The female can also store the sperm from a successful mating for long periods of time, eventually allowing fertilisation to occur many months to years after exposure to the male, a factor which makes paternal identification sometimes rather difficult.

Incubation, sex determination and identification

Incubation first principles are described in the section on incubation, sex determination and identification for snakes. As with many reptiles, tortoise sex determination depends on the temperature at which the eggs were incubated. Hermann's tortoises (*Testudo hermanni*) will produce males if the eggs are kept at or below 29.5°C and females if kept at or above 32°C. It seems that this fact can be applied to a large number of other tortoise species, with males being predominantly produced at the lower temperatures, and females at the higher ones. It is generally advised for these species that the temperature range is kept at 29–32°C, so that a mixture of sexes is achieved.

Male Chelonia have longer tails, the vent being found on the tail caudal to the edge of the carapace, in order to house the single phallus. Males of many Mediterranean species of tortoise and turtles possess a dished plastron, and a narrower angle to the caudal plastron in front of the cloaca than the egg-bearing female. Some female Mediterranean species have a hinge to the caudal part of the plastron to allow easier egg-laying. The male of the box turtle (*Terrapene carolina*) has red-coloured irises whereas the female has yellow/brown ones. The female leopard tortoise (*Stigmochelys pardalis*) and Indian starred tortoise (*Geochelone elegans*) have longer hindlimb claws for digging than the males. The male red-eared terrapin (*Trachemys scripta elegans*), has longer forelimb claws than the females. Some males, such as Hermann's tortoise (*Testudo hermanni*), have a large, hooked scale at the tip of their long tails (see Figure 17.18). In some species there is a size difference between the sexes, for example the female of the Indian starred tortoise and the red-eared terrapin is larger than the male when full grown, but the reverse is true of the red-footed tortoise (*Chelonoidis carbonaria*).

See Table 17.4 for details of typical incubation periods and temperatures of commonly kept chelonians.

Skin

The skin covering the head, neck, limbs and tail of the chelonian is similar in structure to that of snakes and lizards. Many species of tortoise have enlarged scales over their forelimbs, and some have horny spurs on their hindlimbs. The skin is particularly tightly adhered to the underlying bony structures over the distal limbs and the head.

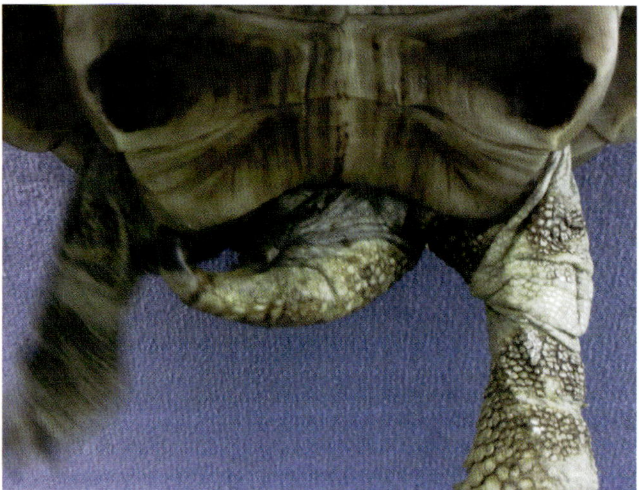

Figure 17.18 The male Hermann's tortoise (*Testudo hermanni*) has a long tail with a curved scale to the tip.

Table 17.4 Typical incubation times and temperatures for some commonly kept chelonians.

Species	Egg incubation time (days)	Incubation temperature (°C)
Hermann's tortoise (*Testudo hermanni*)	85–100	30–33
Horsfield's tortoise (*Testudo horsfieldii*)	60–75	28–32
Leopard tortoise (*Stigmochelys pardalis*)	140–155	28–32
Spur-thighed tortoise (*Testudo graeca*)	56–70	29–32

Tortoises and most other Chelonia have visible auditory membranes covering the entrance to the middle ear. These lie caudoventral to the eyes at the rear of the skull.

The shell is formed from the fusion of islands of bone produced within the chelonian's dermal layer the skin, rather than from the limbs or ribs. The overlying epidermis is highly keratinised and pigmented and contains more beta-keratin, which is tougher than the alpha-keratin found in greater amounts over the limbs, head and neck. The lines joining individual scutes on the shell are not directly above the corresponding suture lines in the bony part of the shell. There is some considerable overlap which reinforces the structure.

CROCODYLIA (CROCODILES, ALLIGATORS, CAIMANS AND GHARIALS)

Musculoskeletal system

The body plan for the Crocodilia is not dissimilar to that of the lizards. The basic structure is a quadruped reptile, with an elongated tail, but instead of the short- to medium-length head, the crocodilians have elongated jaws. This is particularly accentuated in the long thin jaws of the fish-eating gharial family.

The articulation point of the upper and lower jaws is located at the rear of the skull, giving more room for teeth and allowing a larger gape. The jaws are powered by strong temporal and pterygoid muscles, allowing immense crushing forces to be applied. Interestingly, though, the muscles responsible for opening the jaws are relatively weak; hence once closed and taped shut, a crocodilian cannot easily open its mouth again.

The spinal column tends to have between 55 and 67 vertebrae depending on the species. Of these 8–9 are cervical vertebrae, 15–16 thoracolumbar vertebrae, 2 sacral vertebrae and the majority (30–40) caudal (coccygeal) vertebrae.

There are eight pairs of true ribs arising from the thoracic vertebrae, with additional dermal bones embedded in the ventral body wall known as gastralia or floating ribs. There are also thickened transverse processes of the sacral vertebrae which float freely alongside the respective vertebral bodies and have also been called ribs. The coccygeal vertebrae have ventral spinous processes known as haemal arches protecting the ventral tail blood vessels.

The femur is proportionally longer than that of the lizards, leading to a raised appearance to the crocodilian hindquarters. The four limbs have five toes and the hindlimbs have four. Both forelimbs and hindlimbs have claws on the medial three digits. The hindlimbs often have webs between the digits.

Nervous system

The crocodilian brain is small in relation to body size (around 0.004%) but they have good cognitive capabilities and the ability to learn. They have 12 cranial nerves (13 if the nervus terminalis or cranial nerve 0 is included; see snakes), with the fifth (trigeminal or cranial nerve V) is particularly prominent in relation to other reptiles as it innervates the integumentary sense organs. The spinal cord extends to nearly the end of the tail.

Respiratory system

Upper respiratory system

The nares of the Crocodilia are frequently protected by lateral skin flaps which can be contracted medially to close them when submerged. The nasal passages have excellent neural endings in the ethmoid/olfactory chamber area, allowing an acute sense of smell. The crocodiles have a true hard palate that separates the oral and nasal passages. The internal nostrils open caudally; therefore, the glottis guarding the trachea is also situated caudally.

The entrance to the larynx is guarded by the glottis but also by a gular and basihyal fold which originate in, respectively, the floor and roof of the oropharynx and can close access to the glottis from the mouth when a crocodilian is submerged. This allows them to drag prey underwater at the same time as preventing any water from entering the caudal aspect of the pharynx. Providing its nostrils are above water, the crocodilian can still draw air in through the nasal passages.

The trachea is composed of complete cartilage rings, similar to chelonians and birds.

Lower respiratory system

The trachea bifurcates within the 'chest' into two primary bronchi, each supplying a well-formed lung structure. The lungs are basic in design, and do not contain well-defined lobules, as do their mammalian counterparts, although they are very well vascularised and multisaccular. More importantly, they can function as a gas reserve, allowing them to remain submerged for up to 1–2 hours before anaerobic respiration takes over. The lungs are also different from those of other reptiles in that there is a crude muscular diaphragmatic structure separating the dorsally situated lung fields from the ventrally situated heart and digestive system and connects the caudal lungs to the liver and the liver to the pelvic girdle. The diaphragm and the intercostal muscles are important for respiration in crocodilians.

Respiratory physiology

It is interesting that increasing inspired carbon dioxide levels increase the respiration rates and depth in crocodilians, whereas hypercarbia typically depresses ventilation in snakes and lizards (Milsom, 1995). Airflow through the lungs is believed to be unidirectional.

Digestive system

Oral cavity

The teeth are continually replaced throughout life as they are lost and are held in simple alveolar sockets. They are hollow and rootless. One of the distinguishing features between crocodiles and alligators is that the fourth mandibular tooth on either side is visible along its entire length in the crocodiles. In the alligator subfamily the tooth tip is hidden in a maxillary pocket.

The crocodilian tongue is large and fleshy, but immobile and contains lymphatic tissues, mucous glands, taste receptors and salt-secreting glands. Caudally, the floor of the mouth forms a transverse fold, as does the palate above. This shuts the oropharynx off completely from the glottis, internal nostrils and nasopharynx. There is more lymphoid tissue caudal to the internal nostrils in a fold of tissue either side around the area where the Eustachian tubes enter the nasopharynx and this area is commonly sampled at post-mortem for signs of infectious disease.

Stomach, associated organs and intestines

The crocodilian stomach is large and has a well-developed cardiac sphincter. It is divided into two areas, known as the body and the pars pylorus. The body area is heavily populated by mucous-secreting glands and surrounded by a thick band of smooth muscle. It is in this area that stones swallowed by the crocodilian may be found, and therefore this area seems to be responsible for grinding and massaging food into smaller pieces, similar to the action of the avian ventriculus. The pars pylorus then empties into the small intestine through a well-developed pyloric sphincter. The stomach has acid- and pepsinogen-secreting glands and produces a highly acidic pH, and shunting of deoxygenated blood through the left aortic arch and so to the coeliac artery helps this by increasing the supply of hydrogen ions. Because of the very high hydrochloric acid production in the stomach, chloride ions are sequestered from sodium chloride in the plasma, leaving sodium ions in the plasma that react with carbonic acid to create sodium bicarbonate. This produces a significant metabolic alkalosis, which is normal in crocodilians after a large meal.

The duodenum has the descending limb of the pancreas between its loops. The small intestine meets the large intestine at the ileocaecal sphincter. The large intestine empties into the coprodeum portion of the cloaca, which opens into the urodeum, then the proctodeum before ending at the vent to the outside world.

The liver is divided into a right and left lobe with the right being larger and associated with a triangular fat pad. There is a gall bladder draining both lobes and, interestingly, crocodilians produce bilirubin, like mammals, rather than biliverdin as their main bile pigment.

Urinary system

There are paired kidneys located in the caudal abdomen, and extending into the pelvis. The aquatic crocodile kidney excretes waste protein nitrogen as ammonia rather than as the more usual terrestrial reptile uric acid, although the latter can also be produced, particularly when the animal is dehydrated. Osmoregulation, the maintenance of the electrolyte and water balance within the body, is not solely performed by the kidneys, as with many other reptiles. Instead, there are salt-secreting glands in the mouth (usually on the tongue) which aid excretion of excess sodium as sodium chloride. There are no truly marine crocodilians, although the saltwater crocodile and the American crocodile will spend time in brackish water and will venture out to sea.

The oral salt-secreting glands of the alligator subfamily are not as highly developed as those of crocodiles, reflecting their more fresh-water habitat. The kidneys empty through the ureters which travel into the urodeum portion of the cloaca. There is no urinary bladder.

Cardiovascular system

Heart

The crocodilian heart is different from that of other reptiles in that it has four main chambers, similar to the mammalian model. There is also a reduced sinus venosus leading into the right atrium. The left ventricle ejects blood into the right aorta while the right ventricle ejects blood into the left aorta and pulmonary artery.

Despite the crocodilian heart being four-chambered, there is a small 'hole in the heart' between the base of the two aortic arches, immediately after the ventricles, known as the foramen of Panizza, which allows some mixing of oxygenated and deoxygenated blood. The rate of mixing is dependent on the pressures within the left and right ventricles. While the animal is breathing normal air, deoxygenated blood goes from the right ventricle to the lungs and oxygenated blood goes from the left ventricle to the body. It does this despite the fact that the left ventricle has higher pressure than the right as the foramen of Panizza and the dorsal artery (see below) allow the blood pressure in the two aortae to become equalised. This means that the bicuspid valve at the base of the left aorta (which confusingly exits the right ventricle) closes, stopping blood being forced from the left side of the heart to the right. More important for the crocodilian is what happens when it is submerged and not breathing. The increased pulmonary resistance so produced, combined with cog-like valves at the base of the pulmonary artery, increases the pressure in the right ventricle over the left aorta. This forces blood from the right ventricle into the left aorta predominantly, although through the foramen of Panizza blood also enters the right aorta as well. The left ventricular blood, still returning from the lungs and so still relatively well oxygenated, is diverted through the brachiocephalic trunk to the head and heart muscle which need more oxygen to keep functioning. This allows the crocodilian to function in conditions of reduced oxygen and anaerobic metabolism for up to 6 hours.

The heart sits in a pericardial sac which commonly has free fluid within it.

Blood vessels

There are paired aortae from the right and left ventricles which are connected at two points: one is the foramen of Panizza immediately after the ventricles and the other is the mid-coelomic cavity dorsal to the lungs by a dorsal artery. The right aortic arch gives rise to the brachiocephalic trunk and arteries to the head and neck before becoming the dorsal aorta after the dorsal artery connecting it with the left aorta. The left aortic arch becomes the coeliac artery supplying the gastrointestinal system after the dorsal artery connection with the right aorta.

The venous system has many parallels with the lizard's. There is a hepatoportal system supplying the liver directly from the intestines and a renal portal system wherein the blood returning from the hindlimbs and tail enters a venous circle around the kidneys.

There is a large venous sinus caudal to the occiput of the skull on either side of the midline which may be used for venepuncture. Alternatively, the ventral tail vein may be used for blood sampling purposes, although in larger individuals accessing the ventral coccygeal vessels from the lateral aspect may be necessary due to the thickness of the tail and presence of haemal arches protecting the vessels.

Lymphatic system

The lymphatic system parallels the lizard's system. The spleen lies close to the mesenteric root, near the base of the duodenum and is pear-shaped. Significant amounts of GALT is found throughout the gastrointestinal tract but particularly the intestines.

Reproductive system

Male

The testes are long thin organs situated medial to their respective kidneys either side of the caudal vena cava. The vasa deferentia travel to the urodeum portion of the cloaca. The testes enlarge during the reproductive season.

On the ventral aspect of the cloaca lies the phallus. This is a fibrous organ which has little erectile tissue, but once everted forms a dorsal groove into which the semen is deposited. There are two accessory ducts entering this groove which supply seminal fluids from the caudal kidney area.

Female

The paired ovaries are also to be found medial to their respective kidneys. Each ovary is slightly flattened and has a central medullary area which is supplied with nerves and blood vessels. The rest of the reproductive system consists of the fimbria or ostium which catches the ova, and then there is a muscular portion followed by the isthmus and the shell gland or uterus. The paired oviducts open into the urodeum of the cloaca, adjacent to the clitoris.

Reproductive physiology

Follicular activity is triggered by increasing day length in March–May, there being one cycle per year (the exception being the Indian mugger crocodile, *Crocodylus palustris*, which has two cycles/clutches per year). An average clutch of follicles varies from 20 to 80 per cycle. All crocodilians are oviparous.

Sex determination and identification

This varies with species. In the case of alligators and caimans, the lower incubation temperatures (28–to 31°C) produce all females. An intermediate temperature (31–32°C) produces males and females, and a higher temperature (32–34°C) produces all males. In the case of crocodiles, temperatures at the lower end of the range (28–to 31°C) also produce all females. Intermediate temperatures (31–33°C) produce some females but predominantly males. For higher temperatures (33–34°C), predominantly female crocodiles, with some males, are produced.

The best method of sex identification is by manual palpation of the ventral surface of the cloaca for the presence of the phallus. This is an obvious structure if present, although the female crocodilian does have a prominent clitoris which may be confused with a phallus. The crocodilian involved must be in dorsal recumbency and adequately restrained in order to perform this.

Skin

The epidermis and dermis of Crocodilia are composed of thickened scales that are joined together like a patchwork quilt by elastic tissue (see Figure 17.19). Beta-keratin is present to a greater extent within the outer layers of scales, with alpha-keratin, which is more flexible, in between the scales. The skin is tightly attached to underlying bone over the feet and the skull. The skin covering the dorsum has layers of dermal bone present within it (osteoderms), making this area extremely thick and impossible to penetrate for injections. The caimans have areas of bone in the skin covering their ventral surface as well.

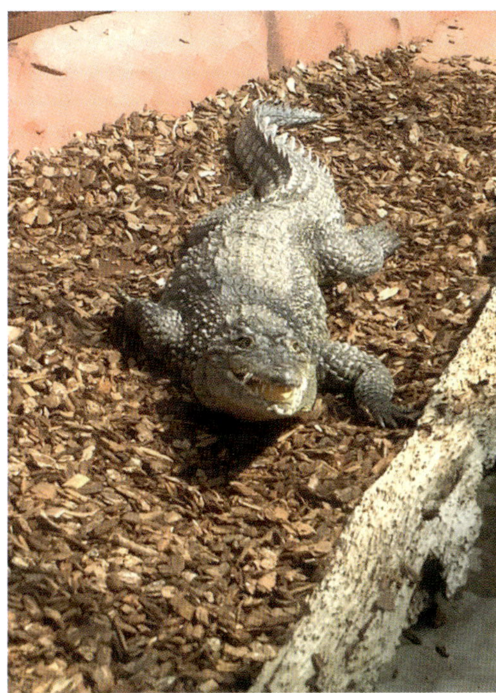

Figure 17.19 The integument of crocodilians is composed of thickened scales and has layers of dermal bone for protection particularly over the dorsum.

Specialised skin areas

Present within the majority of the scales of the Crocodilia are integumentary sense organs. These are believed to be absent from the body (torso) of the alligators but are found on their head region. They have large amounts free nerve endings and their function is to determine underwater pressure sensations which can be used to locate prey while submerged.

Significant paracloacal scent glands exist that each empty through a single duct lateral to the vent and submandibular/gular scent glands exist in the caudal mandibular area.

The tympanic membranes are found either side of the head immediately caudal to the eye. They are covered by a flap of skin most of the time and so may be difficult to see.

OVERVIEW OF REPTILIAN AND AMPHIBIAN HAEMATOLOGY

The cells found in the reptilian bloodstream broadly mirror those seen in mammals. However, there are a few important differences.

- The reptilian (and amphibian) erythrocyte is oval in shape rather than biconcave and has a nucleus even when fully matured.
- The reptile, like the avian patient, has a slightly different version of the mammalian neutrophil, known as the heterophil. The heterophil has a multilobed nucleus, like the neutrophil, and

contains cytoplasmic granules, but these stain a variety of colours with Romanowsky stains, rather than remaining neutral as seen in neutrophils. The heterophil performs similar functions to the neutrophil, being a first line of defence against infection. However, although its numbers may be increased during infections, they may stay the same, in which case the only tell-tale sign of an inflammatory process occurring is vacuolation and degranulation of the cell (the so-called 'toxic' cell). This makes cytological examination as important as cell counts in reptiles.
- An additional cell is the azurophil. It stains a blue-red colour and is a large single-nucleated cell with moderate cytoplasm present. It is found normally in small numbers, particularly in snakes, but if elevated in numbers and sometimes found in low numbers in lizards and chelonians, it suggests an inflammatory/infectious process. It is particularly associated with chronic granuloma formation.
- Eosinophils and basophils are present in most species, basophils being more common in turtles. Basophils generally stain intensely basophilic (blue), and are small spherical cells with a non-lobed nucleus. The eosinophil is a larger spherical cell with eosinophilic cytoplasmic granules and a mildly lobed to elongated nucleus. However, in the green iguana they often stain blue.
- Lymphocytes may vary with the season, showing a decrease in the 'winter'/colder months. Unlike mammals, the B lymphocyte can change into the plasma cell form within the bloodstream during chronic or severe infections of reptiles. Hence, the eccentrically placed nucleus and pale-staining 'clock-face' cytoplasm of the plasma cell may be seen in blood smears of reptiles.
- The thrombocytes (platelets) of reptiles, like avian species, are also nucleated and in addition to performing coagulation will also become phagocytic in the face of severe infection.

Most importantly, when collecting blood samples from reptiles, it is better to do so into heparinised containers for haematology, rather than the potassium ethylenediaminetetraacetic acid (EDTA) tubes used in birds and mammals. This is because the blood cells, particularly erythrocytes, of many species (particularly the Chelonia) will rupture in potassium EDTA. An air-dried smear for staining made at the time of sampling is also useful, as heparin interferes with the Romanowsky stains often making the overall background appear basophilic (blue).

AMPHIBIANS

Classification

Amphibians are classified into many different family groups, according to a number of physical, anatomical and evolutionary factors. It is useful to know to which group an amphibian belongs as this gives an indication of the other amphibians to which it is related. This is of some help when faced with a species that you have not seen before.

Table 17.5 lists some of the more commonly encountered family groups of amphibians seen in general and exotic species orientated practices.

Musculoskeletal system

The body plan of Amphibia in general varies greatly, from the classic lizard shape of the salamanders and newts, to the tail-less quadruped form of the anurans (frogs and toads) and the worm-like caecilians.

Table 17.5 Basic classification of amphibians.

Order	Description
Anura (Salientia)	Includes frogs and toads
Caudata (Urodela)	Includes salamanders and newts
Gymnophiona (Apoda)	Includes caecilians (legless amphibians)

In the case of the anurans and the salamanders, the skeletal structure is very basic but similar to the lizard model described above. The main differences lie in the anurans, which have long femurs, tibias and fibulas, and metatarsals which are developed into the well-muscled hindlimbs, even in the smaller species (see Figure 17.20). There is a basic spinal column of cuboid vertebral bodies joining to the primitive pelvis caudally and the single occipital condyle of the skull cranially.

The skull possesses a mandible and maxilla with, in many cases, simple peg-like and continually replaced teeth. The eye sockets are large in anurans, as is the well-developed eardrum that leads to the middle ear. Sight is better at detecting movement rather than sharp focus, but the sense of hearing is very good, although low-frequency sounds are transmitted through the bones of the forelimbs, and high-frequency ones through the actual eardrum.

The majority of anurans have five digits on the forelimbs and four on the hindlimbs. Many salamanders and newts have four digits on

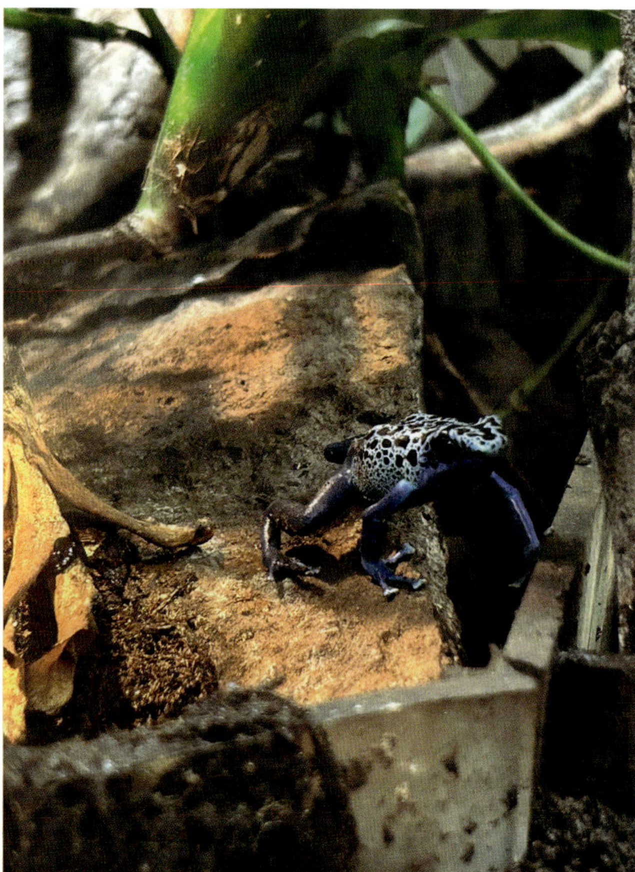

Figure 17.20 A blue poison dart frog (*Dendrobates azureus*).

their forelimbs and four or five digits on their hindlimbs. Many salamanders will show autotomy or tail shedding when roughly handled as with many lizards.

Many amphibians possess vestigial rib structures, and the majority also have a sternum. The pectoral and pelvic girdles are fused to the spine, giving increased rigidity to the body structure.

The caecilians have a much simpler body plan with few if any bones. Their body plan is more worm-like, although they are amphibians rather than insects, but they do possess jaws, a primitive skull and a fibrocartilaginous spinal column. They also have small eyes and nostrils in the head.

Nervous system

The brain has a cerebrum, midbrain and cerebellum. Amphibians have only 10 cranial nerves (11 if the nervus terminalis or cranial nerve 0 is included; see snakes). The amphibian spinal cord extends to the end of the vertebral column. Amphibians are capable of pain sensation for which there is considerable evidence and are considered sentient and protected in the UK by the animal welfare acts.

Respiratory system

As an amphibian metamorphoses from egg to larval or tadpole form it will possess external gills, although these are generally lost as the adult form is reached. In some aquatic amphibians such as the axolotl, external gills are still present in the adult and function as the main gaseous exchange organ even though axolotls have rudimentary lungs.

The majority of amphibians have lungs (although the majority of salamanders do not). These are often no more than a simple, single, vascular-lined, sac-like structure. There are no internal alveolar areas to this lung, although it may be folded to increase its surface area. No diaphragm is present, giving a continuous body cavity or coelom; hence respiration for those amphibians possessing lungs occurs due to intercostal muscle and limb movements pulling the chest wall up and outwards. A few amphibians do not have lungs at all (e.g. many salamanders) and rely totally on cutaneous and orobuccal (i.e. transmucosal) oxygen exchange.

Many amphibians will use the skin surface for gaseous exchange, whether they possess an internal lung structure or not. Indeed, the skin is often solely used for gas exchange during periods of low oxygen requirement, such as during hibernation. For other skin breathers, such as the plethodontid salamanders, other adaptations are necessary, such as increasing the skin surface area by having folds of skin, by having 'hairs' on their surface (e.g. the African hairy frog, *Trichobatrachus robustus*) or by reducing oxygen demands/metabolic rates,.

Digestive system

All adult amphibians and all larval salamanders, newts and caecilians are carnivorous and their digestive systems are adapted to this diet. The majority of adults possess a tongue which can be projected at high speed towards their prey. It is covered in fine sticky cilia, as in many anurans, enabling it to capture flying prey. The salamanders, newts and most anurans have vestigial peg-like teeth. There are frequently cilia within the oral cavity and oesophagus, which aid in the propelling of food into the stomach. Terrestrial amphibians also have mucus-secreting salivary glands to aid in the swallowing of prey.

The stomach is simple in nature, possesses mucus-secreting glands and, in the majority of cases, combined acid- and pepsinogen-secreting glands. The small intestine is short, and little defines its finish and the start of the rectum which empties into the cloaca.

The liver is frequently dark coloured due to melanin pigmentation for protection from ultraviolet light, necessary due to the thin nature of amphibian skin and also associated with melanomacrophages, an important part of the immune system. In anurans the liver is usually bilobed, in caecilians and Caudata often elongated and has a gall bladder.

Urinary system

As with the reptile family, amphibians cannot concentrate urine beyond plasma tonicity. The main excretory product of aquatic amphibians, such as caecilians and aquatic newts and the axolotl, is ammonia. This is actually excreted, as with fish, through the gills if present, and the skin if not, rather than the kidneys.

In terrestrial amphibians, urea is the main waste product of nitrogen metabolism and this is excreted through a primitive paired kidney structure. The cloaca of these species (chiefly the anuran toad family) may also have a pocket forming a primitive bladder. One or two amphibians can produce uric acid. The kidneys empty into ureters which travel to the urodeum portion of the cloaca, before either refluxing into the bladder (if present) or emptying through the vent.

Cardiovascular system

Heart

The circulatory system changes dramatically during the metamorphosis of the amphibian. At the larval stage the circulatory system is more fish-like, with a two-chambered heart possessing only one atrium and one ventricle. When the adult form is achieved, the heart has divided itself into three chambers by producing an intra-atrial septum, and the circulation has also rerouted away from the gill arches of the larva to the adult respiration organ (the skin, lungs or again gill arches). There are some exceptions, such as the axolotl, which still retains external gills.

Blood vessels

As far as the more peripheral vascular system is concerned, the amphibians differ from the reptiles in that the caudal body drainage goes predominantly through the hepatic portal system rather than the renal portal system. This is important for the administration of hepatically metabolised drugs or hepatotoxic drugs in the caudal half of an amphibian. However, the fact that there is still some renal portal blood flow does also mean that potentially nephrotoxic drugs may be more harmful if given in the caudal half of the body.

The ventral midline abdominal vein is commonly used in Caudata and anurans for venepuncture and the ventral tail vein may be used in caecilians and Caudata. In larger anurans the femoral vein can also be used (when the amphibian is anaesthetised) for venepuncture.

Lymphatic system

There is a large lymphatic drainage system, with paired dorsal lymph sacs in anurans lying cranial to the hindlimbs laterodorsally. These help to propel lymph fluid as well as draining it via lymph hearts back to the true heart. They may also play a role in electrolyte balance through the skin overlying them.

Reproductive system

Reproduction in amphibians is generally driven by changes in environmental temperatures or humidity/rainfall.

There are paired internal testes or ovaries depending on the sex. There is some variation in the size of the gonads during the reproductive season and basic hormones resembling the activity of follicle stimulating hormone (FSH) and luteinising hormone (LH) are produced.

In the female, there are paired oviducts that are responsible for producing the jelly-like material that coats the ova. Most amphibians, particularly anurans, fertilise their eggs outside the body, but some species of anurans, salamanders, newts and all the caecilians do have a form of phallus and/or copulate to allow for internal fertilisation. It is also interesting to note that while amphibians are oviparous, some may also produce a form of lipid milk to feed their offspring once they are hatched. An interesting example is the caecilian *Siphonops annulatus* that produces milk from the oviducts that the altricial caecilians drink from the mother's vent (Mailho-Fontana *et al.*, 2024). Many of the poison arrow frogs also nutritionally supplement their tadpoles with skin secretions.

When hatched, the amphibian then metamorphoses through a series of changes, often known as instars, one of which we all know as the 'tadpole' of the anurans which has external gills and a tail and no legs initially. The stimuli for the metamorphosis seem to come from various external sources, such as environmental iodine levels, as well as internal hormonal influences from the thyroid gland.

Interestingly, a number of Caudata will offer parental care of offspring, guarding the eggs and tadpoles from predators.

Sex determination and identification

Many of the amphibians commonly seen are sexually dimorphic, that is the male and female look physically different. In the anurans males are nearly always smaller than the females. In Caudata the males have a swollen tail base (particularly during the breeding season) as well as significant ornamentations such as dorsal crests along the length of the spine, or greater coloration. Many anuran males develop 'nuptial pads' or glandular thickening of the skin over the digits (usually medial) of the forelimbs.

Skin

The terrestrial amphibian has a thin stratum corneum which provides extra cutaneous protection above that seen in aquatic species. It also reduces water loss from the skin. The skin is shed regularly, similarly to a snake, and is frequently then eaten by the amphibian. The skin contains many glands which secrete oils and mucus to further protect against water loss, but amphibians always require access to damp conditions or free water to survive.

The skin of amphibians is not only an important osmoregulatory organ, it can also be used for gaseous exchange. Indeed, in many Caudata the skin is the only organ through which gaseous exchange and so oxygenation of body tissues occurs. Osmoregulation through the skin is important and many anurans have a so-called 'drink-patch' on the pre-pelvic ventrum area where the skin is more permeable to allow water uptake through osmosis. It follows therefore that any damage to the skin of an amphibian may have very serious consequences for water, electrolyte and blood gas regulation.

The Caudata (salamanders and newts) have no subcutaneous space as the dermis is closely connected to the underlying tissues, which has implications for injectable medications.

The caecilians are thought to be the only amphibians that like reptiles have scales. These are located in the deeper skin or dermis.

Many of the toad family have poison glands located in their parotid glands which are used as a form of protection. A similar ploy is used in the poison arrow tree frogs which secrete neurotoxins (batrachotoxin) onto the surface of their skin along the back and behind the ears in particular. However, captive-bred poison arrow frogs are not considered a hazard as the toxins they secrete in the wild are not manufactured by the frog, but are found in the insects (beetles) that they eat and which are absorbed from the gut and then secreted through the skin.

Some anurans, such as the midwife toad *Xenopus laevis*, have claws, but most have very fragile skin which, as mentioned above, may have capabilities for gas exchange as well as water and electrolyte exchange.

Some male amphibians can be identified by skin colour or ornamentation. The male great crested newt has a larger crest than the female, for example, and many male frogs and toads have a swelling in the 'thumb' area of the hand that contains scent glands. Male caecilians often have a phallus in the cloaca.

References

Anderson, J.B., Rourke, B.C., Caiozzo, V.J. *et al.* (2005) Postprandial cardiac hypertrophy in pythons. *Nature*, **434**, 37–38.

Cieri, R.L. and Farmer, C.G. (2020) Computational fluid dynamics reveals a unique net unidirectional pattern of pulmonary airflow in the Savannah monitor lizard (*Varanus exanthematicus*). *The Anatomical Record*, **303**, 1768–1791.

Crawford, N.G., Parham, J.F., Sellas, A.B. *et al.* (2015) A phylogenomic analysis of turtles. *Molecular Phylogenetics and Evolution.*, **83**, 250–257. doi: 10.1016/j.ympev.2014.10.021.

Davis, L.E., Schmidt-Nelson, B. and Stolte, H. (1976) Anatomy and ultrastructure of the excretory system of the lizard *Sceloporus cyanogenys*. *Journal of Morphology*, **149**, 279–326.

Gordeev, D.A., Ananjeva, N.B. and Korost, D.V. (2020) Autotomy and regeneration in Squamate reptiles (Squamata, Reptilia): defensive behavior strategies and morphological characteristics (using computer microtomography methods). *Biology Bulletin*, **47**(4), 389–398.

Hazard, L.C. (2004) Sodium and potassium secretion by Iguana salt glands: acclimation or adaptation? In: *Iguanas: Biology and Conservation* (ed. A. Alberts), pp. 84–95. University of California Press.

Hynes, B. and Girling, S. (2019) Cardiovascular and haemopoietic systems. In: *BSAVA Manual of Reptiles* (eds S.J. Girling & P. Raiti), 3rd edn, pp. 323–341. BSAVA Quedgeley, Glos.

Jensen, B., Nyengaard, J.R., Pedersen, M. and Wang, T. (2010) Anatomy of the python heart. *Anatomical Science International*, **85**(4), 194–203.

Jenson, B. and Wang, T. (2009) Hemodynamic consequences of cardiac malformations in two juvenile ball pythons (*Python regius*). *Journal of Zoo and Wildlife Medicine*, **40**, 752–756.

King, F. (1996) Lizards. In: *Reptile and Herbivory*, pp. 29–42. Chapman and Hall, London.

Mailho-Fontana, P.L., Antoniazzi, M.M., Coelho, G.R. *et al.* (2024) Milk provisioning in ovoparous caecilian amphibians. *Science*, **383**(6687), 1092–1095.

Milsom, W.K. (1995) Regulation of respiration in lower vertebrates: role of CO_2/pH chemoreceptors. *Advances in Comparative Environmental Physiology*, **21**, 63–104.

Perry, S.F. and Duncker, H.-R. (1978) Lung architecture, volume and static mechanics in five species of lizards. *Respiration Physiology*, **34**, 61–81.

Schilliger, L. and Girling, S. (2019) Cardiology. In: *Mader's Reptile and Amphibian Medicine and Surgery* (eds S.J. Divers & S.J. Stahl), 3rd edn, pp. 669–698. Elsevier, St Louis, Missouri.

Schilliger, L., Trehiou-Sechi, E., Petit, A.M.P. *et al.* (2010) Double valvular-insufficiency in a Burmese python (*Python molurus bivittatus* Linnaeus, 1758) suffering from concomitant bacterial pneumonia. *Journal of Zoo and Wildlife Medicine*, **41**(4), 742–744.

Slay, C., Enok, S., Hicks, J. and Wang, T. (2014) Reduction of blood oxygen levels enhances postprandial cardiac hypertrophy in Burmese python (*Python bivittatus*). *Journal of Experimental Biology*, **217**(10), 1784–1789.

Taylor, E.W., Jordan, D. and Coote, J.H. (1999) Central control of the cardio-vascular and respiratory systems and their interactions in vertebrates. *Physiological Reviews*, **79**, 855–916.

Taylor, E.W., Leite, C.A.C., McKenzie, D.J. and Wang, T. (2010) Control of respiration in fish, amphibians and reptiles. *Brazilian Journal of Medical and Biological Research*, **43**(5), 409–521.

Troyer, K. (1984) Structure and function of the digestive tract of a herbivorous lizard *Iguana iguana*. *Physiological Zoology*, **57**(1), 1–8.

Wasser, J.S. and Jackson, D.C. (1988) Acid–base balance and the control of respiration during anoxic and anoxic-hypercapnic gas breathing in turtles. *Respiration Physiology*, **71**(2), 213–226. doi: 10.1016/0034-5687(88)90017-5.

Chapter 18 Reptile and Amphibian Housing, Husbandry and Rearing

There are many good books available on the husbandry of reptiles and amphibians. This chapter therefore provides only an overview of the main points in housing and caring for reptiles and amphibians. It is essential when treating a reptile or amphibian patient for the first time that a thorough history is taken. This is particularly important as many problems can arise through improper care and inappropriate environmental conditions.

Vivarium requirements

Dimensions and construction

Vivarium designs vary, as does their construction material. The main aim though is to ensure that they are durable, easily cleaned for hygiene reasons, have enough complexity to stimulate the reptile or amphibian, provide appropriate heat, light and humidity, and offer enough space for the animals to demonstrate normal behaviour. Strict cage dimensions are therefore difficult to quantify, as each situation should be judged on its own merits. However, some general principles apply. Size of the vivarium/terrarium will depend on the species, number of individuals housed and sexual maturity. It is important that the vivarium is large enough to allow a temperature gradient to be created.

For species that are more arboreal (tree climbing) in nature, for example the green iguana and many snakes such as the boa constrictor and Burmese python, the emphasis in cage design should be more on vertical height rather than horizontal space. For terrestrial reptiles such as tortoises, however, the provision of too much vertical space is pointless. Barnard (1996) and Animal Welfare Committee (2023) have provided some minimum dimensions detailed in Table 18.1.

Construction materials of the vivaria commonly used include Perspex®, reinforced glass, sealed wood and fibreglass (see Figure 18.1). Wood should be avoided unless it is sealed to prevent moisture damage and rotting, as well as being difficult to cleanse and disinfect. Glass and clear Perspex are useful when showing off a collection, but care should be taken as many reptiles cannot see the vivarium sides, and so may continually rub their snouts along the inside of the vivarium, causing abrasions which can become infected. Often the provision of a visual barrier on the inside or outside of the glass at reptile level allows them to appreciate that a solid barrier exists and prevents this problem. However, it should also be noted that this problem may be an indication of physiological stress for the reptile due to lack of space, overcrowding or aggression from vivaria-mates, all of which should be considered in attempting to prevent or treat the issue (Warwick *et al.*, 2013). Some species are very flighty and easily disturbed, such as the Thai water dragon (*Physignathus cocincinus*) and may injure their snouts on the inside wall of the vivarium, allowing infection to gain hold (see Figure 18.2). Visual barriers are therefore important for these species to prevent them being startled by someone walking past the vivarium.

Heating

Reptiles are ectothermic by nature, that is they rely on the environment to provide sufficient heat to warm them to their preferred body temperature (PBT). Their PBT is the body temperature at which their organs and biochemical processes function optimally. To maintain their PBT, the reptile must be provided with a preferred optimum temperature zone within which it may position itself. This necessitates the provision of some form of artificial heating within the vivarium to create a temperature gradient within which the reptile can place itself to either cool down or warm up.

Two main forms of heating are advised. A background, continuous heat source is important to raise the vivarium temperature above the background room temperature. This is often provided in the form of a radiant heat mat, which emits heat continuously and is placed on the outside wall of the vivarium. It then radiates heat through the vivarium wall. Placing it on the outside of the vivarium avoids the possibility of the reptile chewing, urinating or defecating on it, so increasing hygiene and safety. The size of available mats varies, but a rough rule is that one-third to half of the longest side of the vivarium should be covered with the mat. Some form of insulation on the outside of the mat, increasing reflection of heat into the vivarium, is also useful.

In addition, the vivarium requires a focal hot spot, which may be provided in the form of a ceramic infrared heat or combination heat/ultraviolet (UV) bulb. This should be suspended from the ceiling of the vivarium, and should be protected from the reptile to avoid the risk of burns. The bulb should be attached to a thermostat, which will allow maximum and minimum vivarium temperatures to be set. A form of heated, plastic moulded rock has been used to provide a basking point for reptiles. These should be avoided, as should the thermostat break within such a device it can overheat and the animal will injure itself; this is because, being ectotherms, reptiles do not respond to thermal pain in the same way as mammals and birds and will therefore not move away. This can be a particular problem for larger reptiles, as work by De Vosjoli (1999) and Warwick *et al.* (2013) has clearly shown that the size of the heat source versus the size of the reptile is important. Basically, if the focal heat source is producing a hot spot smaller than the body of the reptile, there is an increased likelihood of thermal damage as the reptile would place itself closer to the heat source.

Veterinary Nursing of Exotic Pets and Wildlife, Third Edition. Simon J. Girling.

Table 18.1 Some minimum vivarium sizes suggested for reptiles.

Type of reptile	Minimum vivarium sizes
Semi-aquatic chelonians	Height should be enough to prevent escape Floor dimensions should be a minimum of five times the reptile's length by three times the reptile's length Water depth should be a minimum of half the length of the reptile
Terrestrial chelonians	Floor dimensions should be minimum of five times the reptile's length by five times the reptile's length
Arboreal lizards	Height should be two to three times the reptile's length Floor dimensions should be minimum of twice the reptile's length by three times the reptile's length
Burrowing lizards	Height should be a minimum of half of the reptile's length above substrate and 30 cm depth of substrate Floor dimensions should be a minimum of three times the reptile's length by twice the reptile's length
Terrestrial lizards	Height should be sufficient to prevent escape Floor dimensions should be a minimum of twice the reptile's length by three times the reptile's length
Arboreal snakes	Height should be a minimum of the reptile's length* Floor dimensions should be a minimum of the reptile's length by two-thirds the reptile's length
Burrowing snakes	Height should be a minimum of half of the reptile's length above the substrate and 30 cm depth of substrate Floor dimensions should be a minimum of three times the reptile's length by twice the reptile's length
Terrestrial snakes	Height should be a minimum of one-third of the reptile's length Floor dimensions should be a minimum of the reptile's length by two-thirds of the reptile's length

* Height requirement for arboreal snakes is the author's opinion and is greater than that proposed by either of the source references.
Source: Data from Barnard (1996) and AWC (2023).

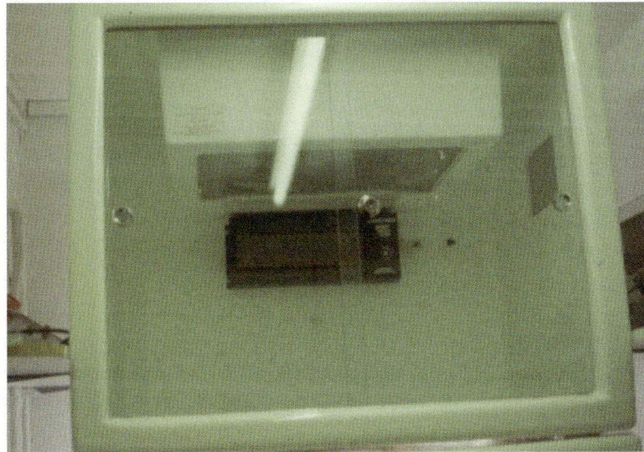

Figure 18.1 Vivarium made of moulded fibreglass.

The importance of a focal heat source is that it provides a temperature gradient, allowing the reptile to bask underneath the heat source or to escape to a cooler end of the vivarium when overheated. The reptile can then maintain its PBT by positioning itself at different points in the vivarium during the course of the day.

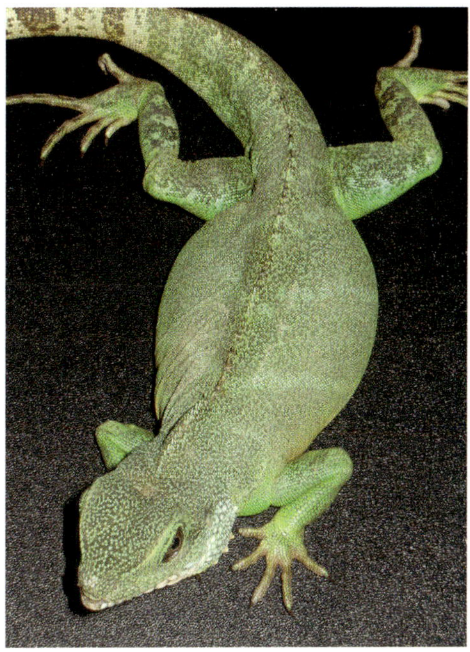

Figure 18.2 Thai water dragons (*Physignathus cocincinus*) are easily startled, requiring visual barriers in their vivaria in order to prevent this. When startled they may run into the side of the vivaria damaging their upper jaw in particular as seen here.

Table 18.2 Preferred optimum temperature zones and relative humidity for selected species of reptile.

Species	Temperature range (°C)	Relative humidity (%)
African spurred tortoise (*Centrochelys sulcata*)	25–35	40–75
Bearded dragon (*Pogona vitticeps*)	25–35	30–40
Boa constrictor (*Boa constrictor*)	28–30	50–80
Burmese python (*Python bivittatus*)	25–30	50–80
Californian kingsnake (*Lampropeltis californiae*)	25–30	30–70
Chinese water dragon (*Physignathus cocincinus*)	24–30	80–90
Corn snake (*Pantherophis guttatus*)	23–30	30–70
Garter snake (*Thamnophis sirtalis*)	21–28	50–80
Green iguana (*Iguana iguana*)	25–35	75–100
Leopard gecko (*Eublepharis macularius*)	25–34	30–40
Leopard tortoise (*Stigmochelys pardalis*)	25–35	40–75
Mediterranean tortoises (*Testudo* spp.)	20–28	30–50
Red-footed tortoise (*Chelonoidis carbonarius*)	21–27	50–60
Royal python (*Python regius*)	25–30	50–80
Veiled chameleon (*Chamaeleo calyptratus*)	21–38	75–80

The temperatures required for different species of reptile will naturally differ. A list of some species and their temperature requirements is given in Table 18.2.

Humidity

Humidity is also important. Many species of reptile come from dry desert regions, but equally many originate in tropical rainforests. Therefore, their tolerance of water moisture in their environment will vary. A water dragon, basilisk or garter snake, all used to living near or in water, will require a 75–100% humidity level. This may be difficult to maintain in a heated environment; the hotter the air, the more water droplets the air can hold, and so the relative humidity drops. Thus, spraying the enclosures frequently, using a hand-held plant mister with previously boiled, and then cooled, water is useful. Alternatively, automatic misting devices or the provision of water baths or damp substrate within the vivarium can be used to increase humidity. Care should be taken over hygiene levels, though, as an excessively damp and soiled substrate can lead to environmental fungal and bacterial build-up that results in skin infections such as blister disease, a common problem in garter snakes. In the case of reptiles from more arid climates, a relative humidity between 25 and 50% is often adequate (see Table 18.2). This is around the normal level of the average centrally heated home. However, at certain times even these species require increased levels of humidity. One such example is during the shedding cycle when the old skin layer is sloughed. At this time an increase in humidity is essential to prevent the old skin drying out before it has a chance to peel off and so resulting in constrictions around extremities such as the digits. This is a common problem in leopard geckos amongst others and many adults have lost the ends of their toes through avascular necrosis. To prevent this, it is useful to provide a hide that has an increased humidity level in addition to a normal hide (i.e. creating a 'dry' or normal hide and a 'wet' hide to provide choice). This can be achieved by placing a shallow dish of water with some cotton wool in it within the wet hide.

Ultraviolet lighting

Lighting is particularly important for the growing juveniles of many species but is also important for the health of adult reptiles. In the wild, many reptiles live in parts of the world where the intensity of the sun's UV rays is high. However, even in species that are crepuscular in nature, some UV light may still be important.

Ultraviolet rays stimulate a number of functions in the reptile, often encouraging mating at certain times of year, and may act as a general appetite stimulus as many reptiles can see in UV-A, which has a wavelength from around 350 nm. The UV-B waveband of the spectrum is important in all species in encouraging the production of pre-vitamin D_3 from precursors (7-dehydrocholesterol) in the reptile's skin. Provitamin D_3 (cholecalciferol) is converted first by the liver to 25-hydroxycholecalciferol and then by the kidneys to 1,25-dihydroxycholecalciferol, which is the active form of vitamin D_3 (calcitriol) and is intimately involved in the metabolism of calcium and bone growth in the reptiles as with other vertebrates. A lack of UV-B light can therefore be responsible for the presence of metabolic bone disease in several species, for example the green iguana and Mediterranean *Testudo* spp. tortoises (see Chapter 21).

UV-B lighting should be provided on the inside of any vivaria or at least not passed through standard glass or Perspex as these will filter out the UV-B rays. It is important to note that the type of UV-B lighting should be tailored to the species. Some species prefer to bask in full sunlight and so a 'sunbeam' method of lighting should be provided using a high UV-B mercury vapour or metal halide light ideally in combination with an incandescent lamp to produce the equivalent of a sunbeam in the basking zone. This should be big enough to allow the whole reptile inside the basking zone. This is most suitable for reptiles noted for basking, such as fence lizards (*Sceloporus* spp.), bearded dragons (*Pogona* spp.) and frilled lizards (*Chlamydosaurus kingii*). Others do not bask and prefer more dappled shade, provided by an incandescent lamp at one end of the vivarium controlled by a dimming thermostat. This creates a suitable temperature gradient and a focal UV-B source, which then creates a UV gradient in the vivarium as well as a high point underneath the heat lamp. Shelter is then provided using vegetation and plenty of hides so that the reptile is not continuously exposed to UV light. This is most suitable for reptiles such as rat snakes (e.g. *Elaphe* spp.), anoles (*Anolis* spp.) and water/garter snakes (*Thamnophis* spp.). Indeed Ferguson *et al.* (2010) describe four groups of reptiles that can be categorised into a series of UV-B zones (Table 18.3). Commercial hand-held UV meters are available, but the Ferguson zones focus on those which limit their analysis to the longer UV-B wavelengths, from 290 to 400 nm (Baines *et al.*, 2016). This is further complicated as some that require more intense UV light provision associate this with sun-basking and so heat emission in a focal area whereas the

Table 18.3 'Ferguson' zones describing four groups of reptiles according to their likely UV light exposure in their wild habitat (summarised from Ferguson *et al.*, 2010).

Zone and type of environment	Typical species of reptile	Zone range UV index	Zone maximum UV index
1. Shade-dweller or crepuscular reptile. Likes a thermoneutral zone and does not bask	Burmese python (*Python molurus bivittatus*) Corn snake (*Pantherophis guttatus*) Leopard gecko (*Eublepharis macularius*)	0–0.7	0.6–1.4
2. Occasional sun-basking reptile which requires a temperature gradient	Boa constrictor (*Boa constrictor*) Chinese water dragon (*Physignathus cocincinus*) Red-footed tortoise (*Chelonoidis carbonarius*)	0.7–1.0	1.1–3.0
3. Open or partial sun-basking reptile which requires a temperature gradient	Bearded dragon (*Pogona vitticeps*) Leopard tortoise (*Stigmochelys pardalis*) (see Figure 18.3) Red-eared terrapin (*Trachemys scripta elegans*) Spur-thighed tortoise (*Testudo graeca*)	1.0–2.6	2.9–7.4
4. Full sun (midday) basking reptile which requires a temperature gradient	Bell's dab lizard (*Uromastyx acanthinura*) Chuckwallas (*Sauromalus* spp.)	2.6–3.5	4.5–9.5

Note that the UV index is unitless and focuses, in the publication by Ferguson *et al.* (2010), on the longer UV-B wavelengths, i.e. 290–400 nm (Baines *et al.*, 2016), that coincide with maximum vitamin D_3 conversion.

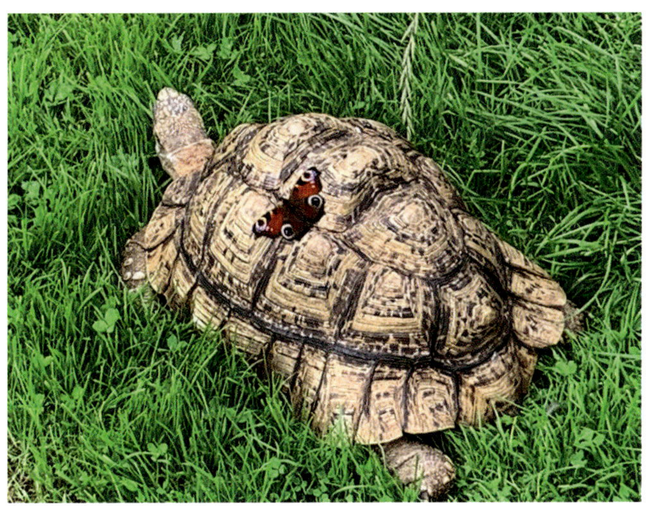

Figure 18.3 Species such as this leopard tortoise (*Stigmochelys pardalis*) have been categorised as a zone 3 UV-B requiring reptile.

lower intensity UV-requiring reptiles need a more widespread UV provision, although clearly at a lower level and not associated with a heat source specifically.

If excessive levels of UV-B light are given to a species of reptile (e.g. a UV index of 3 is given to a leopard gecko) then serious consequences such as serious skin burns, eye damage and increased risk of neoplasia are likely.

More information can be found in Baines and Brames (2010), Ferguson *et al.* (2010) and Baines *et al.* (2016).

Ventilation

It is important that air quality is preserved within the vivarium. This may be simply achieved in smaller vivaria with vent holes in the top of the structure. However, in larger vivaria or more densely stocked vivaria, maintaining air quality may require an extraction system with inlet vents to allow a through-flow of air. In this latter situation it should be noted that temperature and relative humidity levels may be more difficult to maintain. The downsides of not providing adequate ventilation are the build-up of irritant gases such as ammonia, associated with bacterial breakdown of excretory proteins and the likelihood that this will increase the risk of respiratory disease in the housed reptiles.

Vivarium 'furniture' and environmental enrichment

Many reptiles are relatively poorly adapted to captivity, being wild animals in a confined space, and so it is important to ensure that their environment adequately caters for their needs both physically and mentally.

As previously mentioned, many arboreal species enjoy exploring vertical space. They should therefore be provided with branches and ramps up which they may climb. It is often useful to provide an elevated basking spot which they can lie out on near to the focal heat source.

In the case of terrestrial species, the provision of some form of floor furniture is important. Tortoises are best kept singly, except when breeding of course, or in the case of small hatchlings which prefer to be in groups. In these cases, the provision of visual barricades which they can hide behind and so escape from one another is useful.

All reptiles should be provided with a hide. This is important particularly for many snakes, which will often refuse to eat their prey in the open, but rather prefer to take it back into the hide area away from view. The size of these areas should be a minimum of 2–2.5 times the size of the reptile being housed but not so excessively large that the reptile does not feel 'secure'. The number of hides should ideally be a minimum of the number of reptiles housed in the vivarium, plus one. Dry and wet hides, with low and high humidities respectively, are also advisable to reduce the incidence of dysecdysis.

As previously mentioned, provision of visual barriers to reduce stress and injury is essential for some species such as water dragons.

Substrate

The substrate of the vivarium, or floor covering, is important. The substrate used should be non-toxic to the reptiles housed and easily cleaned. In many cases the provision of newspaper or unbleached household paper is perfectly sufficient, although possibly not so aesthetically pleasing as more naturalistic substrates. Care should be taken with smaller reptiles with newspaper, as the ink from the newsprint may prove irritant.

Other substrates used commonly include bark chippings, calcite sand and peat substitute. Bark chippings are a good choice for deep litter situations, particularly when providing enough substrate for a pregnant female to dig a nest in which to lay eggs. However, the chips should not be of cedar as the resins from this can be irritant. It is also more difficult to monitor the cleanliness of bark chippings as faeces and urine may fall into the substrate and so avoid detection.

Sand is useful for desert species such as leopard geckos, collared lizards and sand boas, but care should be taken with any reptile on this substrate. If the diet contains mineral deficiencies, the reptile is fed directly on the sand, or if there is intestinal parasitism present, many species will consume the sand and may suffer intestinal blockages.

Peat substitutes can be useful for species requiring damper conditions such as water dragons and red-footed tortoises, but care again should be taken with the hygiene of this substrate, as waste materials may build up unnoticed.

Certain types of substrate are best avoided. Peat is not advised as a substrate for ecological reasons and coral for the same reason, as well as the tendency for reptiles to eat the substrate and suffer gut impactions. Corn cobs should also be avoided as these are often inadvertently eaten, swell and cause intestinal blockages.

Aquatic species and amphibians

Some reptile species, such as the terrapins and turtles, require large areas of free water; some, such as frogs and toads, a small area but damp environmental conditions (see Figure 18.4).

In the case of freshwater species, tap water may be used, but it should be dechlorinated. This may be done by standing chlorinated tapwater in an open container for 24 hours prior to use or by using any commercial dechlorinating tablets, available from commercial aquarist suppliers. In addition, the water should be allowed to come up to vivarium temperature before being introduced to avoid cold shocking the reptile or amphibian.

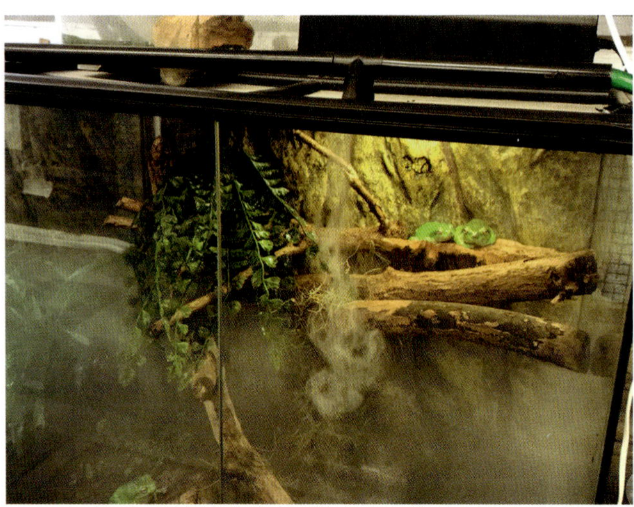

Figure 18.4 Example of suitable housing for tree frogs with a misting system to maintain humidity.

Where large areas of water are provided, it is important to keep them clean. It is advisable for terrapins and soft-shelled turtles that their habitat provides an area in which they can immerse themselves completely in water, and an area into which they can pull themselves out to bask and dry themselves off, preferably with a focal heat source above it. It is often advisable to remove them from the water and place them in a separate, dry or water-containing feeding tank. This is because they are extremely messy eaters and will quickly contaminate their water with food. The food acts as a nutritional resource for bacteria, resulting in a bacterial population explosion, and this can increase the risk of shell infections and septicaemia. An alternative would be a powerful water filtration device placed in the vivarium to cope with the large volumes of organic debris produced. Even if a feeding tank is provided, regular water changes or filtration is required, as they will of course still urinate and defecate in their water (see Figure 18.5).

Many anurans will appreciate a small amount of free water, but the rest of their vivarium should be well supplied with moisture-retaining substrate such as mosses or peat substitute mulches. These retain moisture and increase the humidity of the vivarium, ensuring protection of the sensitive amphibian's skin. Other amphibians, such as newts and salamanders, require more access to free fresh water and precautions similar to those mentioned for freshwater turtles and terrapins should be taken. In addition, for all these species, the construction of the vivarium should ensure that it is watertight.

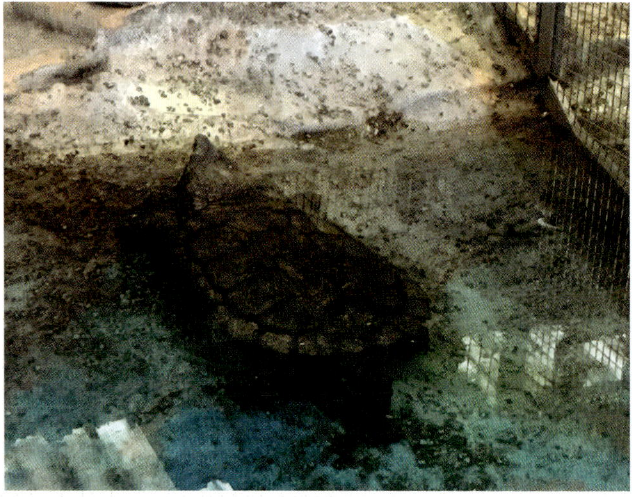

Figure 18.5 In order to maintain water quality for semi-aquatic species that feed in water, such as this alligator snapping turtle (*Macrochelys temminckii*), a good-quality filtration unit with regular water changes is required.

Solitary housed versus group housed reptiles and amphibians

Some species of reptile and amphibian are aggressive and so should be housed singly. For example, kingsnakes eat other snakes and so should be kept on their own. Even herbivorous species such as *Testudo* spp. tortoises and green iguanas can show aggression between the sexes particularly when breeding, with males often harassing and injuring females. It is also known that housing some females, particularly lizards such as the green iguana, leopard gecko and bearded dragon, may increase the chances of developing preovulatory stasis as the sight and scent of a male is thought to be required for ovulation to occur (see Figure 18.6). Some species, however, seem to thrive in group situations such as many of the *Anolis* spp. of lizard and many anurans such as tree and dart frogs.

Quarantine

There are an increasing number of viral diseases being discovered in reptiles as well as other known pathogens that can have long incubation periods and may be difficult to detect ante-mortem. For this reason, it is important to consider quarantining any new reptile before adding it to a collection. Periods of quarantine suggested have varied from 6 weeks to 9–12 months. Veterinary health tests should be carried out where possible during this period. The new reptile should be housed preferably not only in a separate vivarium but in a separate room to avoid sharing the same airspace as some of the pathogens are aerosol transmitted. Separate utensils should be used, and the new arrivals should be cleaned out and fed last to avoid cross-contamination. Disinfection is important for avoiding potential spread of disease. Typical disinfectants suitable for reptiles include quaternary

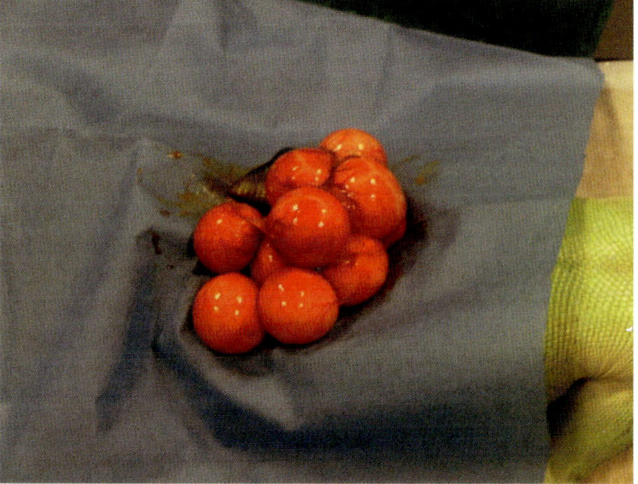

Figure 18.6 Preovulatory stasis, as seen here, may be more commonly seen in solitary housed females such as this green iguana (*Iguana iguana*).

ammonium compound-based products such as Ark-Klens® (Vetark Professional Ltd.) and F10® (Health and Hygiene Pty Ltd.).

Hospitalised reptiles

The guidelines given above for UV light, humidity and temperature should be applied for any hospitalised reptile. However, some important differences may be made with regards to substrate which in most cases can be of newspaper (avoid coloured print which may be irritant) or unbleached paper towelling to ensure good hygiene and facilitate faecal collection. Space provision may also be compromised for short periods of hospitalisation, but for periods of more than 2–3 days, every effort to keep the reptile in the minimum dimensions detailed should be made.

It is vitally important that the vivarium is cleansed thoroughly between patients to avoid disease spread. The use of povidone iodine-based cleansing agents such as Tamodine-E (Vetark Professional Ltd.) or quaternary ammonium compounds such as F10® (Health and Hygiene Pty Ltd.) should be considered.

Some have suggested having separate facilities for carnivores (such as snakes) and herbivores (such as many tortoises) as the latter may carry organisms that are not necessarily always harmful to them (protozoa such as *Entamoeba* spp.) but which can be lethal to carnivores.

References

Animal Welfare Committee (2023) AWC opinion on the space requirements for snakes in vivaria within pet selling establishments. DEFRA, UK Government. https://www.gov.uk/government/publications/awc-opinion-on-the-space-requirements-for-snakes-in-vivaria-within-pet-selling-establishments (accessed 30 March 2024).

Baines, F. and Brames, H. (2010) Preventive reptile medicine and reptile lighting. *Proceedings of the 1st International Conference on Reptile and Amphibian Medicine*, Munich, 4–6 March, pp. 3–13.

Baines, F., Chattell, J., Dale, J. *et al.* (2016) How much UV-B does my reptile need? The UV-tool, a guide to the selection of UV lighting for reptiles and amphibians in captivity. *Journal of Zoo and Aquarium Research*, **4**(1), 42–63.

Barnard, S.M. (1996) *Reptile Keepers Handbook*. Krieger Publishing, Malabar, FL.

De Vosjoli, P. (1999) Designing environments for captive amphibians and reptiles. *Veterinary Clinics of North America: Exotic Animal Practice*, **2**, 43–68.

Ferguson, G.W., Brinker, A.M., Gehrmann, W.H. *et al.* (2010) Voluntary exposure of some western-hemisphere snake and lizard species to ultraviolet-B radiation in the field: how much ultraviolet-B should a lizard or snake receive in captivity? *Zoo Biology*, **29**(3), 317–334.

Warwick, C., Arena, P., Lindley, S. *et al.* (2013) Assessing reptile welfare using behavioural criteria. *InPractice*, **35**, 123–131. doi: 10.1136/inp.f1197.

Chapter 19 Reptile and Amphibian Handling and Chemical Restraint

Handling the reptilian patient

Is there a need to restrain the reptilian patient?

Reptiles are less easily stressed than their avian cousins, and so restraint may be performed without as much risk in the case of the debilitated animal. However, it is still worthwhile considering factors that may make restraint dangerous to animal and nurse alike.

- Is the patient in respiratory distress where excessive manual manipulation can be dangerous?
- Is the species a fragile one? Day geckos (*Phelsuma* spp.) are extremely delicate and prone to shedding their tails (autotomy) when handled. Similarly, some species such as green iguanas are prone to conditions such as metabolic bone disease where spontaneous fractures occur if roughly handled.
- Is the species an aggressive one? Some are naturally so, for example snapping turtles (*Macrochelys* spp.), tokay geckos (*Gekko gecko*) and rock pythons (*Python sebae*)
- Does the reptile patient require medication or physical examination? If yes, is restraint essential?

It should be noted that many species of reptile have *Salmonella* spp. present normally in their gut without the bacterium causing clinical disease in the reptile. Personal hygiene is therefore very important when handling these patients to prevent zoonotic diseases.

Techniques and equipment involved in restraining reptile patients

Lizards

Their main dangers to the handler are their claws and teeth and, in some species such as iguanas, their tails, which can lash out in a whiplike fashion. A few are venomous, such as the *Heloderma* and varanids such as the Komodo dragon.

Geckos, other than tokay geckos (*Gekko gecko*), are generally docile as are lizards such as bearded dragons (*Pogona* spp.). Others, such as green iguanas (*Iguana iguana*), may be aggressive, particularly sexually mature males. They may also be more aggressive towards female owners and handlers as they are able to detect pheromones secreted during the menstrual cycle.

They are best restrained by grasping around the shoulders (the pectoral girdle) with one hand, from the dorsal aspect, so controlling one forelimb with forefinger and thumb and the other between middle and fourth finger. The other hand is used to grasp the pelvic girdle from the dorsal aspect, controlling one limb with thumb and forefinger, the other again between middle and fourth finger (see Figure 19.1). The handler may then hold the lizard in a vertical manner, with head uppermost, placing the tail underneath his or her arm. It is then possible to present the head and feet of the lizard away from the handler to avoid injury. The handler should allow some flexibility as the lizard may struggle and overly rigid restraint could damage the spine.

More aggressive iguanas may need to be pinned down first. The use of a thick towel to control the tail and claws is useful. Gauntlets may be necessary for particularly aggressive large lizards or for those which may have a venomous bite. It is important to ensure that you do not use too much force when restraining the lizard, as those with skeletal problems, such as metabolic bone disease, may be seriously injured. In addition, lizards do not have a diaphragm and so overzealous restraint will lead to increasing pressure on the lungs.

Day geckos (*Phelsuma* spp.) and other fragile species are best examined in a clear plastic container. Other geckos have easily damaged skin, so latex-free gloves and soft cloths should be used for examination. When handling small lizards, they may be cupped in the hand and their heads controlled by holding between the index finger and thumb to prevent biting.

It is important that lizards (and some snakes) are never restrained by their tails. Many will shed their tails at this time, but not all of them will regrow. Green iguanas, for example, will only regrow their tails as juveniles (less than 2.5–3 years of age). Once they are older than this, they will be left tail-less. However, there are plenty of lizards that do not undergo autotomy, such as many agamids and chameleons.

Vasovagal reflex

The vasovagal reflex can be used to place members of the lizard family into a trance-like state. The eyelids are closed and gentle digital pressure is applied to both eyeballs. This stimulates the autonomic parasympathetic nervous system, resulting in a reduction in heart rate, blood pressure and respiration rate. Providing there are no loud noises or environmental stimulation, after 1–2 minutes the lizard may be placed on its side, front, back, etc. allowing radiography to be performed without using physical or chemical restraint. A loud noise or physical stimulation will immediately cause the lizard to revert to its normal wakeful state.

Snakes

Snakes are all characterised by their elongated form and absence of limbs. The danger areas for the handler are their teeth and in the case of the most venomous species, which are more likely to strike a handler (such as the viper family), their fang teeth. However, rear-fanged species also exist, such as the boomslang (*Dispholidus typus*), which generally only envenomates when handled or provoked. In the case of non-venomous species such as the constrictor and python family,

Veterinary Nursing of Exotic Pets and Wildlife, Third Edition. Simon J. Girling.

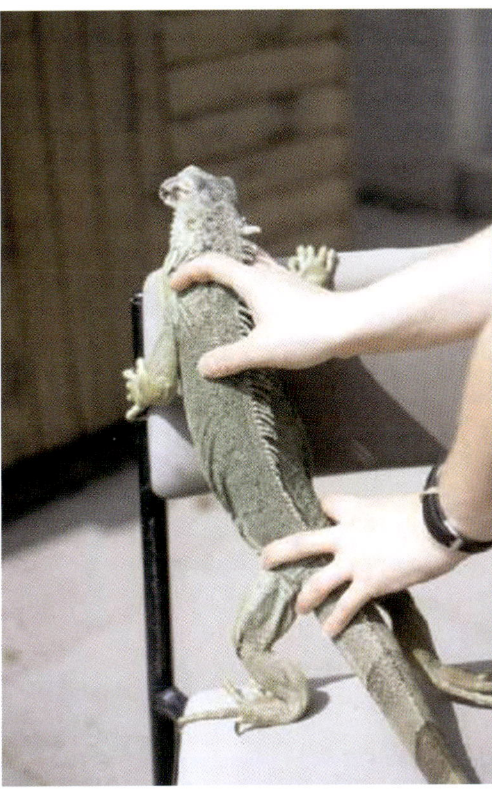

Figure 19.1 The iguana should be approached from above grasping over the pectoral and pelvic areas dorsally and may then be firmly but gently controlled. Tucking the tail underneath the arm prevents eye injuries.

their ability to asphyxiate their prey by winding themselves around the victim's chest and neck is also a significant concern to the handler.

With this in mind, the following restraint techniques may be employed. Non-venomous snakes can be restrained by controlling the head initially. This is done by placing the thumb over the occiput and curling the fingers under the chin. Reptiles, like birds, have only one occipital condyle, so it is important to stabilise the occipito-atlantal joint (see Figure 19.2). It is also important to support the rest of the

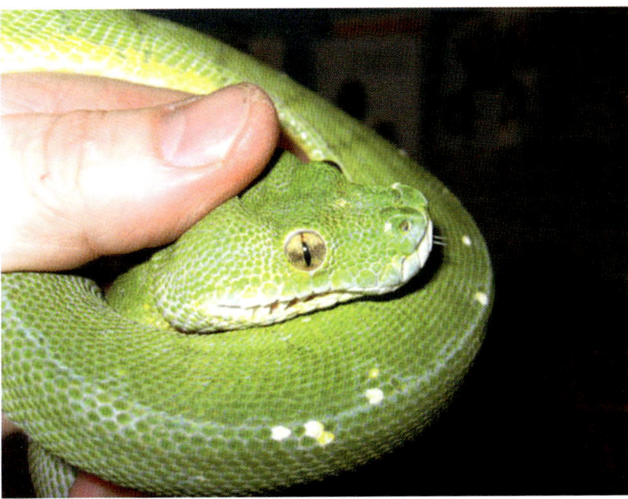

Figure 19.2 Support of the atlanto-occipital joint is important to prevent injury to the snake and the snake biting the handler.

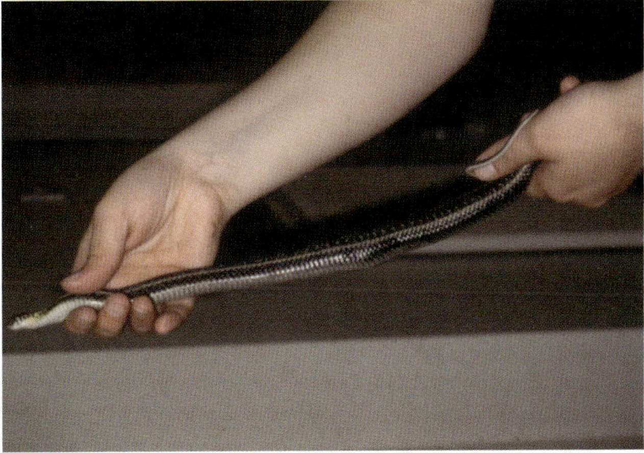

Figure 19.3 Smaller species of snake such as this garter snake can be held by one handler but when allowing the snake to stretch out, both hands should be used to avoid placing undue stress on the cervical area and atlanto-occipital joint.

snake's body so that not all of the weight of the snake is suspended from the head. Allow the smaller species to coil around the handler's arm, so the snake is supporting itself or hold them with a two-handed hold for examination (see Figure 19.3).

In the larger species (longer than 3 m) it is necessary to support the body length at regular intervals. This often requires several handlers. Indeed, it is vital to adopt a safe operating practice with the larger, constricting species of snake. A 'buddy system' should be operated whereby any snake longer than 1.5–2 m in length should only be handled by two or more people (see Figure 19.4). This ensures that if the snake was to enwrap one handler, the other could disentangle him or her by unwinding from the tail end first. Above all, it is important not to grip the snake too hard as this will cause bruising and the release of myoglobin from muscle cells. This can damage the glomerular filtration membrane in the kidneys.

Venomous snakes or very aggressive species may be restrained initially using snake hooks. These are 45–60 cm steel rods with a blunt shepherd's hook on the end. They are used to loop under the body of a snake to move it at arm's length into a container. The hook may also be used to trap the head flat against the floor before grasping it with the hand. Once the head is controlled safely the snake is rendered harmless. Exceptions include the spitting cobra family where handlers should wear plastic goggles or a plastic face visor as the snake can spit poison into the prey or assailant's eyes and mucous membranes causing blindness and paralysis.

Chelonia

The majority of chelonians are harmless, although surprisingly strong. For Mediterranean species (*Testudo* spp.), when being restrained the tortoise may be held with both hands, one on either side of the main part of the shell behind the front legs (see Figure 19.5). To keep the tortoise still for examination, it may be placed onto a cylinder or stack of tins, raising its legs clear of the table as it balances on the centre of the underside of the shell (plastron).

For aggressive species (e.g. snapping turtle and the alligator snapping turtle), it is essential that you hold the shell on both sides

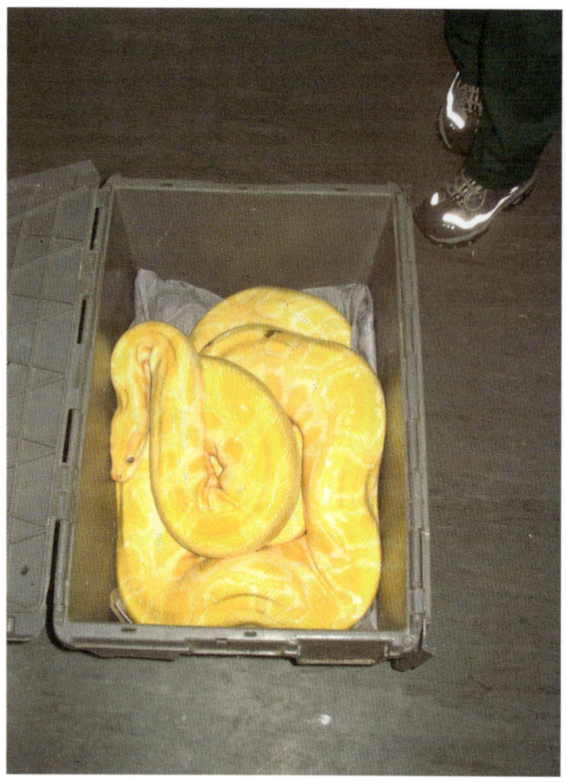

Figure 19.4 Larger species of snake over 1.5–2 m in length such as this Burmese python require two or more people to handle for both the handler's and snake's safety.

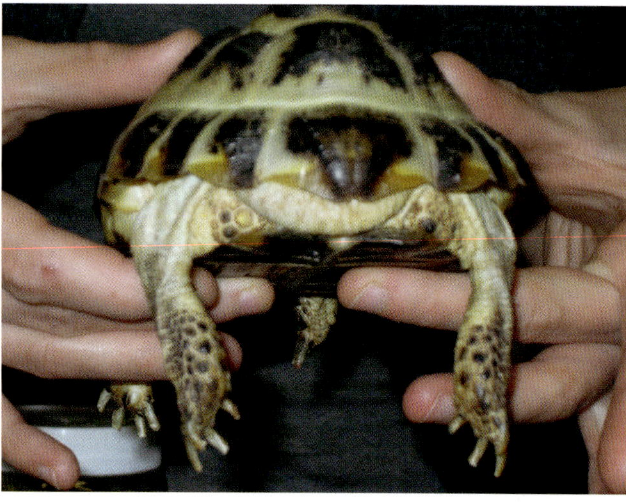

Figure 19.5 Even in small examples of herbivorous chelonia it is wise to hold them with both hands between the forelimbs and hindlimbs as they are surprisingly strong and can seriously injure themselves if dropped.

behind and above the rear legs to avoid being bitten. Chemical restraint is necessary in order to examine the head region in these species. Large species such as the Aldabran tortoise (*Aldabrachelys gigantea*) may also require chemical restraint to safely examine or blood sample.

For the soft-shelled and aquatic species, soft cloths and latex-free gloves should be used to prevent damaging the shell.

Crocodilia

The Crocodilia include freshwater and saltwater crocodiles, alligators, fish-eating gharials, and caimans. Their dangers to the handler lie in their impressively arrayed jaws and often their sheer size – an adult bull Nile crocodile (*Crocodylus niloticus*) may weigh many hundreds of kilograms. Saltwater crocodiles have a bite force of around 16 460 N, equivalent to a jaw crushing pressure of 25 510 kN/m^2 (3700 lb/in^2).

Small specimens may be restrained by grasping the base of the tail in one hand while the other is placed behind the head. For slightly bigger specimens, a rope halter or noose may be tied around the snout so securing it closed. All of the major muscles in the crocodilian jaws are involved in closing not opening them, hence relatively fine rope or tape can be used to keep the mouth closed. The rest of the animal is restrained by pinning it to the ground.

Always approach crocodilians from head on, as their binocular vision is poor (although the alligator family does have some). Care should be taken when close to the crocodilian for head and tail movements are both directed at the assailant at the same time.

Much larger crocodiles require teams of people, with nets and snout snares in order to quickly clamp the jaws closed and to restrain the dangerous thrashing tail. Chemical immobilisation via dart guns should always be seriously considered.

Principles of chemical restraint

Chemical restraint is necessary for many procedures in reptile medicine, ranging from minor procedures such as extracting the head of a leopard tortoise or box turtle from its shell to enabling a jugular blood sample to be taken or to carrying out coeliotomy procedures because of egg binding. Before any anaesthetic or sedative is administered, an assessment of the reptile patient's health should be made. Considerations include the following.

- Is sedation or anaesthesia necessary for the procedure required?
- Is the reptile suffering from respiratory disease or septicaemia?
- Is the reptile's health likely to be made worse by sedation or anaesthesia?

Before discussing the administration of chemical restraint, it is important to understand the reptilian respiratory system.

Overview of reptilian respiratory anatomy and physiology relevant to anaesthesia

The reptile patient has a glottis similar to the avian patient, which lies at the base of the tongue. This is more rostral in snakes and lizards and more caudal in Chelonia. At rest, the glottis is permanently closed, opening briefly during inspiration and expiration. In crocodiles, the glottis is obscured by the basihyal valve which is a fold of the epiglottis. This fold has to be deflected before they can be intubated (Bennett, 1998).

The trachea varies between species. In Chelonia and Crocodilia, complete cartilaginous rings similar to those of the avian patient are found, with chelonians having a very short trachea that generally bifurcates into the two bronchi in the neck region. Snakes and lizards have incomplete C-rings, with snakes having a very long trachea.

No reptile has a diaphragm, although crocodilians have a pseudodiaphragm which changes position with the movements of the liver and gut so pushing air in and out of the lungs. Most reptiles use intercostal muscles to move the ribcage in and out in a manner similar to birds. The exception to this is members of the Chelonia. These species need to move their limbs, neck and head into and out of the shell in order to bring air into and out of the lungs.

Some species can survive in oxygen-deprived atmospheres for prolonged periods – many chelonian species may survive for 24 hours or more, and even green iguanas may survive for 4–5 hours. This makes induction of anaesthesia via inhalation of a gaseous anaesthetic agent almost impossible in these animals. The stimulus for respiration in reptiles is also driven by lowered PO_2 as well as an elevated PCO_2 and many reptiles when breath-holding show right-to-left shunting of blood in the heart, so bypassing the lungs.

Many snakes have both intrapulmonary chemoreceptors and stretch receptors whereas many chelonians have only stretch receptors; hence when there are high levels of carbon dioxide, snakes can override the volume-related feedback and continue to breathe. Hypercapnia tends to increase the tidal volume by suppressing the stretch receptors. Hypoxia increases breathing frequency by reducing or eliminating the non-breathing periods and these effects are increased at higher environmental temperatures.

In snakes, the central control of respiration can also override the stretch receptors allowing them to control breathing even when constricting prey or swallowing large prey which may impinge on the lungs.

The presence of a renal portal system, where the blood from the caudal half of a reptile's body may pass through the kidneys before returning to the heart, has implications for drugs which are excreted by the kidneys (e.g. ketamine) as they may be removed from the body before they have had a chance to take effect. Similarly if the drug is nephrotoxic, then higher concentrations of the drug may end up in the kidneys if injected in the caudal body. A hepatoportal system also exists in many reptiles where again blood from the caudal half of the body may pass through the liver parenchyma before being circulated around the rest of the body. Drugs that are metabolised by the liver (e.g. alfaxalone and many of the opiates) may be removed before having a systemic effect.

Pre-anaesthetic preparation

Weight measurement

This is important for accuracy as some species of reptile may be very small. Scales accurate to 1 g are therefore advised for smaller reptiles to ensure correct dosage.

Blood testing

It may be advisable to test biochemical and haematological parameters before administering chemical immobilising drugs. Blood samples can be taken from:

- Jugular veins in Chelonia
- Dorsal tail vein in Chelonia
- Ventral tail vein in snakes, Crocodilia and lizards
- Palatine vein or cardiac puncture in snakes (although they frequently need to be sedated or anaesthetised to collect blood from these routes).

Fasting

Fasting is necessary in snakes to prevent regurgitation and pressure on the lungs or heart. It is advisable to ensure that no prey has been offered in the 2 days prior to anaesthesia in small snakes and more than a week in large species such as pythons or boas.

Other reptiles require less fasting, for example chelonians rarely if ever regurgitate and so require little fasting. However, it is important not to feed live prey to insectivores such as leopard geckos 24 hours prior to an anaesthetic as the prey may still be alive when the reptile is anaesthetised.

Pre-anaesthetic medications

Premedications are used to provide cardiopulmonary and central nervous system stabilisation, a smooth anaesthetic induction, muscle relaxation, analgesia and a degree of sedation.

Antimuscarinic medications

Atropine 0.01–0.04 mg/kg intramuscularly (IM) or glycopyrrolate 0.01 mg/kg IM may be used to reduce oral secretion and to reduce bradycardia; however, these are not usually of concern in reptiles. Indeed, antimuscarinics may increase the thickness of mucus secretions, leading to more rapid blocking of the airways. In addition, in herbivores it can result in prolonged periods of ileus. In one study, atropine at a high dosage (1 mg/kg) decreased the minimum alveolar concentration (MAC) requirements for isoflurane in red-footed tortoises by apparently preventing the right-to-left intracardiac shunting so maintaining blood flow to the lungs (Greunz *et al.*, 2018).

Tranquillisers

Acepromazine (0.05–0.5 mg/kg IM) may be given 1 hour before anaesthetic induction to reduce the levels of anaesthetic required, as can diazepam (0.22–0.62 mg/kg IM in alligators) and midazolam (2 mg/kg IM in turtles) (Bennett, 1998).

Alpha-2 adrenoceptor stimulants

Xylazine at 1 mg/kg can be used 30 minutes prior to ketamine in crocodilians to reduce the dose of ketamine needed. Medetomidine, used at doses of 100–150 μg/kg, markedly reduces the dose of ketamine required in chelonians, and has the advantage of being reversible with atipamezole at 500–750 μg/kg. They both create a drop in blood pressure and cardiac output and so should be used with caution in debilitated reptiles.

Opioids

Butorphanol (0.4–1.5 mg/kg IM) can be administered 20–30 minutes before anaesthesia. This drug may be combined at 0.4 mg/kg with midazolam at 2 mg/kg. More recently there is some question over whether butorphanol is an effective analgesic and while it can cause sedation at higher dosages and by some thought to aid anaesthesia induction, there may be species variations as in green iguanas it did not have an anaesthetic-sparing effect when used at 1 mg/kg prior to isoflurane (Mosely *et al.*, 2003).

Fluids

Fluid therapy is very important, and correction of fluid deficits should be attempted prior to surgery. Maintenance levels in reptile patients have been quoted as 25–30 mL/kg per day (see Chapter 22 for more information on fluid therapy in reptiles).

Induction of anaesthesia

It should be noted that reptiles should never be immobilised by chilling or cooling them down. This does not provide analgesia and has serious welfare implications.

Injectable agents

Table 19.1 describes the advantages and disadvantages of injectable anaesthetic agents.

Dissociative anaesthetics

Ketamine: Recommended levels range from 22 to 44 mg/kg IM for sedation to 55–88 mg/kg IM for surgical anaesthesia. Lower levels are needed if combined with a premedicant such as midazolam or medetomidine (Bennett, 1996). Doses in excess of 110 mg/kg will produce profound bradycardia and the death of the reptile.

Effects are seen in 10–30 minutes but may take anything up to 4 days to wear off, particularly at low environmental temperatures. Its main use is therefore at the lower dose range, to allow sedation, facilitate intubation and allow maintenance of gaseous anaesthesia in species such as chelonians that hold their breath during gaseous induction. Doses of 5–10 mg/kg have been used in chelonians to allow extraction of the head from the shell.

It is, however, frequently painful on administration. Also, because ketamine is actively excreted by the kidneys (via the proximal tubules), it is recommended that it is administered in the cranial half of the body. This is because blood from the caudal half of the body travels to the kidneys before returning to the heart and the anaesthetic may thus be excreted before it has a chance to work. In addition, its use in reptiles with renal disease will result in prolonged recovery periods.

Ketamine (5 mg/kg) may be combined with 100 μg/kg (0.1 mg/kg) medetomidine to facilitate intubation of small reptiles (<2 kg) or at 7.5 mg/kg ketamine plus 75 μg/kg (0.075 mg/kg) medetomidine for reptiles over 2 kg. It has also been used at 5–10 mg/kg combined with medetomidine 100–150 μg/kg (0.1–0.15 mg/kg) in adult alligators (Heaton-Jones *et al.*, 2002) and at 15 mg/kg combined with medetomidine at 300 μg/kg (0.3 mg/kg) in juvenile Nile crocodiles (Monticelli *et al.*, 2019) to facilitate induction of anaesthesia.

Other injectable anaesthetics

Alfaxalone: This can be used to aid induction, allowing intubation within 3–5 minutes when administered intravenously (IV). It may be administered intramuscularly but induction takes longer via this route (25–40 minutes). Doses of 6–15 mg/kg have been advised but it appears in many reptiles not to be capable of inducing full anaesthesia but rather permitting intubation and causing immobilisation (Sheelings *et al.*, 2010). Doses of 30 mg/kg intramuscularly in green iguanas induced surgical anaesthesia within 4–5 minutes and lasted around 40 minutes (Bertelsen and Sauer, 2011). In royal (ball) pythons (*Python regius*) the hepatoportal system has been blamed for the reduced efficacy of alfaxalone when injected in the caudal half of the body (James *et al.*, 2018; Yaw *et al.*, 2018).

Propofol: Propofol produces rapid induction and recovery. Its advantages include a short elimination half-life and minimal organ metabolism, making it relatively safe to use in debilitated reptiles which often have some liver damage.

Its disadvantage is that it requires intravenous access, although use of the intraosseous (IO) route is useful in green iguanas at a dose of 10 mg/kg (Bennett *et al.*, 1998). Propofol also produces a transient period of apnoea and some cardiac depression. In this situation, intubation and positive pressure ventilation are necessary.

Doses of 10–15 mg/kg in chelonians given via the dorsal coccygeal (tail) vein have successfully induced anaesthesia in under 1 minute. This allows intubation and maintenance on a gaseous anaesthetic if required. Alternatively, propofol can be used alone providing a period of anaesthesia of 20–30 minutes. For giant species of Chelonia, lower doses of 1–2 mg/kg IV/IO have been used and doses of 5–10 mg/kg have been used intravenously via the coccygeal tail vein in green iguanas to allow intubation (Bertelsen, 2014).

Table 19.1 Advantages and disadvantages of injectable anaesthetics.

Advantages	Disadvantages
Ease of administration	Recovery often dependent on organ metabolism
Prevention of breath-holding on induction	Difficult to reverse rapidly
Reduced costs	Often prolonged recovery times
Easy to administer	Muscle necrosis at site of injection
Lower risk to anaesthetist versus gaseous anaesthesia	

Depolarising muscle relaxants

Succinylcholine: This is a neuromuscular blocking agent and produces immobilisation without providing analgesia. Therefore, it should only be used to aid the administration of another form of anaesthetic or for transportation, and not as a sole source of anaesthesia. Recovery is dependent on liver metabolism and its use in animals with possible liver disease should be avoided.

It can be used in giant Chelonia at doses of 0.5–1 mg/kg IM and will allow intubation and conversion to gaseous anaesthesia. Crocodilians can be immobilised with 3–5 mg/kg IM, with immobilisation occurring within 4 minutes and recovery in 7–9 hours. Respiration usually continues without assistance at these doses but it is important to have assisted ventilation facilities to hand as paralysis of the muscles of respiration occurs and results in significant hypoxia.

Reversal of succinylcholine is not possible and the patient must be ventilated until the drug has been excreted.

Gallamine: This has been used in crocodiles (0.3–2 mg/kg) to achieve immobility in 15–30 minutes with a recovery time of 1.5–3 hours. In alligators it should not be used above 1 mg/kg and there is some question in general over its safety in American alligators or false gharials (Lloyd, 2003). Its advantage over succinylcholine is that it is reversible with neostigmine (0.25 mg/kg).

Gaseous agents

The gaseous anaesthetics used for induction are discussed in the next section on maintenance of anaesthesia; however, Table 19.2 lists their advantages and disadvantages.

Table 19.2 Advantages and disadvantages of gaseous anaesthetic.

Advantages	Disadvantages
Ease of administration via face mask	Breath-holding (Chelonia particularly)
Absence of pain associated with some injectable drugs	Environmental pollution
Minimal tissue trauma	Health risk to anaesthetist
Rapid induction where breath-holding is not an issue	Risk with dangerous reptiles during handling

Maintenance of anaesthesia

Injectable agents

Dissociative anaesthetics

Ketamine: Ketamine may be used on its own for anaesthesia at doses of 55–88 mg/kg IM. It is worthwhile noting though that as the dosages get higher the recovery time also increases, and in some cases it can be as long as several days. Also, doses above 110 mg/kg will cause respiratory arrest and bradycardia with often fatalities.

Ketamine may be combined with other injectable agents to provide surgical anaesthesia. Examples of these combinations include the following.

- Midazolam 2 mg/kg IM with ketamine 40 mg/kg in turtles (Bennett, 1996)
- Xylazine 1 mg/kg IM, given 30 minutes prior to ketamine 20 mg/kg in large crocodiles (Lawton, 1992)
- Medetomidine 100 µg/kg (0.1 mg/kg) IM with ketamine 50 mg/kg in kingsnakes (Malley, 1997)
- Medetomidine 100–300 µg/kg (0.1–0.3 mg/kg) IM with ketamine 10 mg/kg in most species (Sladky *et al.*, 2023).

Other injectable anaesthetics

Alfaxalone: This can be used for induction and also for short periods of anaesthesia (average 25 minutes) at 9 mg/kg IV/IO. Topping up of the anaesthetic allows maintenance of light anaesthesia for longer procedures but caution should be observed as it may not produce enough anaesthesia to allow invasive procedures in all species. Kischinovsky and Bertelsen (2011) showed that 30 mg/kg was required in green iguanas to achieve surgical anaesthesia, but many became apnoeic. Recovery times are often 1–4 hours.

Local anaesthesia: Drugs such as bupivacaine at 1 mg/kg and lidocaine at 2–4 mg/kg can be used for regional/local anaesthesia. They may also be used intrathecally, particularly in the tail region when trying to replace cloacal organ prolapses in reptiles. Injections are often carried out near to the tail base between sacral and coccygeal or coccygeal and coccygeal vertebrae. More advanced surgery has been carried out combining intrathecal lidocaine (2 mg/kg) with morphine (0.1 mg/kg) in desert tortoises (*Gopherus agassizii*) undergoing gonadectomy as this combination produced adequate analgesia in the caudal half of the chelonian (Proenca *et al.*, 2014a,b).

Propofol: Propofol may be used to give 20–30 minutes of anaesthesia after administration, allowing minor procedures such as wound repair, intraosseous or intravenous catheter placement, or oesophagostomy tube placement to be carried out.

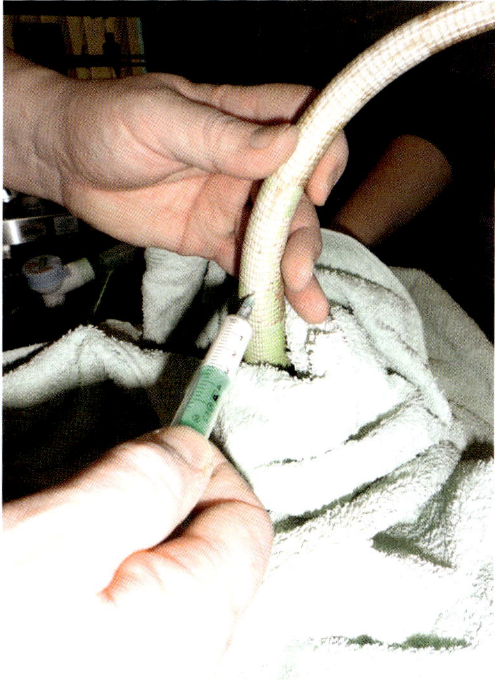

Figure 19.6 Intravenous administration of propofol via the ventral tail vein to induce anaesthesia in a green iguana.

It may be topped up at 1 mg/kg per minute IV/IO, but apnoea is extremely common and intubation and ventilation with 100% oxygen is required (see Figure 19.6).

Gaseous agents

Isoflurane

Isoflurane is a commonly used gaseous maintenance anaesthetic (see also Table 19.2). Isoflurane is minimally metabolised in the body (0.3%) and has a very low blood–gas partition coefficient (1.4 compared with 2.3 for halothane in human trials). This means that it has a very low solubility in blood, so as soon as administration is stopped the reptile starts to recover, exiting the anaesthetic from the lungs. In addition, it has low fat solubility and so is not stored. Isoflurane still has excellent muscle relaxing properties and is a good analgesic during anaesthesia, although no effects post recovery. Apnoea precedes cardiac arrest, unlike the case with halothane anaesthesia. MACs have been derived for a few species (although some argue that MAC should stand for minimum anaesthetic concentration in reptiles as they do not have alveoli) and are around 2–2.1% for green iguanas and 1.5% in monitors (*Varanus dumerilii*) (Mosely *et al.*, 2003; Bertelsen *et al.*, 2005a; Barter *et al.*, 2006).

It can be used to induce anaesthesia in those species not exhibiting breath-holding at levels of 4–5%, by induction chamber. It is also possible to adapt the cases of 20- and 60-mL syringes to form long, thin face masks to induce snakes. Isoflurane can then be used to maintain anaesthesia, preferably via endotracheal (ET) tube, at levels from 2 to 3% depending on the procedure.

Sevoflurane

As with isoflurane, this drug may be safely used. It is highly insoluble in the bloodstream, though, and so ventilation rates may need to be increased above the usual 4–6 breaths per minute to maintain anaesthesia, although intracardiac shunting can also complicate the issue and make induction with this anaesthetic gas alone difficult in some species. MACs for sevoflurane published for reptiles include 3.4% in green iguanas and 2.5% in Dumeril's monitor lizards (Bertelsen *et al.*, 2005b; Barter *et al.*, 2006).

Induction and maintenance levels of sevoflurane are higher than for isoflurane, being typically 6–8% and 3–4%, respectively.

Nitrous oxide

Nitrous oxide can be used in conjunction with isoflurane, reducing the percentage of gaseous anaesthetic required for induction and maintenance of anaesthesia. Its other advantages include good muscle relaxation and excellent analgesic properties, making it useful in orthopaedic procedures.

Disadvantages of nitrous oxide include its tendency to accumulate in hollow organs. This may prove a problem for herbivorous reptiles as they often have capacious hindguts and nitrous oxide can accumulate there and in species with air sacs. Nitrous oxide also requires some organ metabolism for full excretion and so may be a problem in a seriously diseased patient. It also prolongs anaesthetic recovery times by up to 50%.

Aspects of gaseous anaesthesia maintenance for reptiles

Inhalant gaseous anaesthesia is becoming the main method of anaesthetising reptiles for prolonged procedures. The reptile patient should preferably be intubated to allow the inhalant anaesthetic to be delivered in a controlled manner.

Intubation

Intubation is straightforward in reptiles as they do not have an epiglottis and the glottis, which acts as the entrance to the trachea, is relatively cranial in the majority of species. It is useful to note that the glottis is kept closed at rest, so the operator must wait for inspiration to occur to allow intubation. Reptiles produce little or no saliva when at rest or not eating, so blockage of the tube is uncommon unless there is underlying respiratory disease.

In snakes, the glottis sits rostrally on the floor of the mouth just caudal to the tongue sheath and is easily visible when the mouth is opened (see Figure 19.7). Intubation may be performed in the conscious patient if necessary, as reptiles do not have a cough reflex. The mouth is opened with a wooden or plastic tongue depressor and the ET tube inserted during inspiration. In the main, however. it is preferable to administer an induction agent before intubation is attempted.

In Chelonia, the glottis sits slightly more caudally at the base of the tongue. The trachea is very short and the ET tube should only be inserted a few centimetres, otherwise there is a risk that only one or the other of the bronchi will be intubated, leading to only one lung receiving the anaesthetic. An induction agent such as ketamine or propofol is advised for chelonians prior to intubation due to their ability to breath-hold and difficulty in extracting the head from the

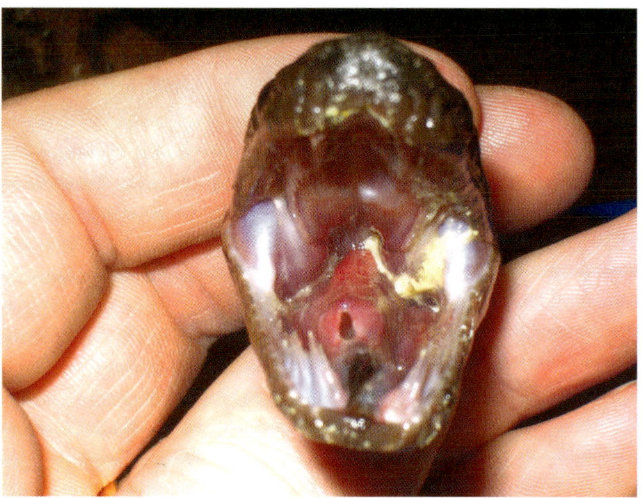

Figure 19.7 Intraoral view showing the rostral position of the glottal opening and tube in a boa.

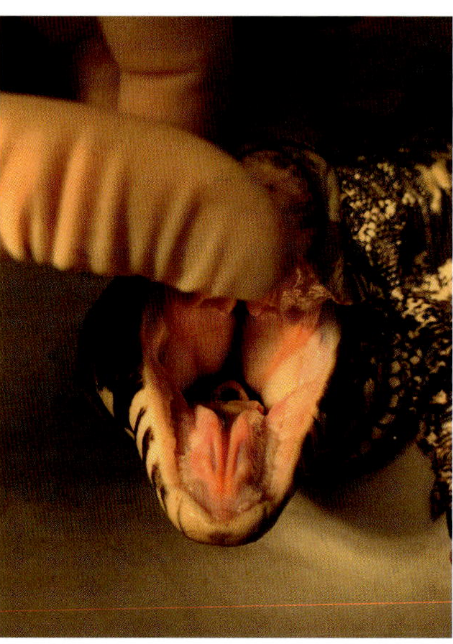

Figure 19.8 Intraoral view of a tegu showing the glottis at the base of the tongue.

shell. Chelonia have complete O-rings of cartilage to the trachea and so the cuff on the ET tube should not be inflated to avoid postoperative stricture formation, as can occur in birds.

Lizards vary depending on the species, most having just a glottis guarding the entrance to the trachea (see Figure 19.8). Some species possess vocal folds, notably some species of gecko (Porter, 1972). Some may be intubated consciously, but most are better induced with an injectable preparation or by face mask using gas. Some species may be too small for intubation. The larger species may also require a mouth gag to avoid biting down on the tube (see Figure 19.9).

Crocodilia have a basihyal fold (Bennett, 1998) that acts as an epiglottis and needs to be depressed prior to intubation. Because they are potentially dangerous, these species require some form of injectable chemical sedation or induction agent to have taken full effect prior to an attempt to intubate. Crocodilia have complete

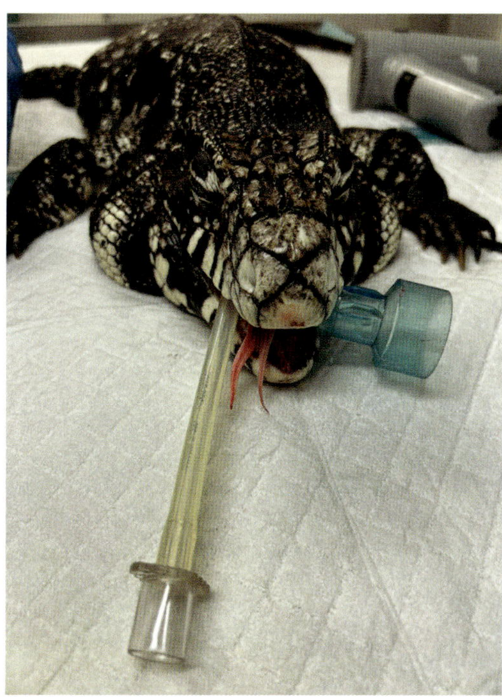

Figure 19.9 A mouth gag may be needed in larger species such as this black and white tegu (*Salvator merianae*) to prevent them biting down on the tube.

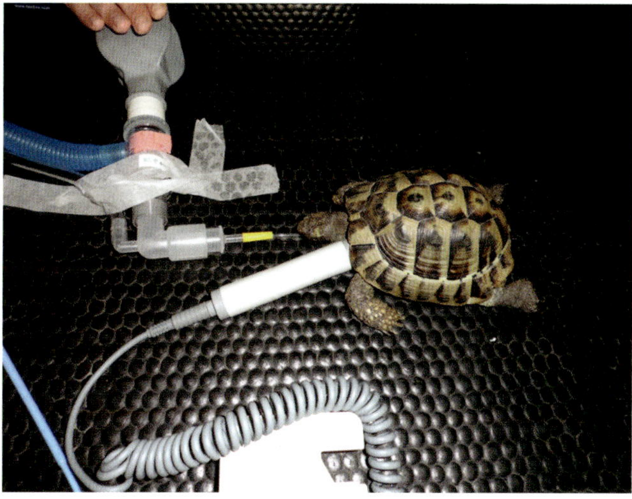

Figure 19.10 Manual bagging of a tortoise. Note Doppler probe to monitor heart sounds at the cervical inlet, and Mapleson C circuit typically used for smaller species.

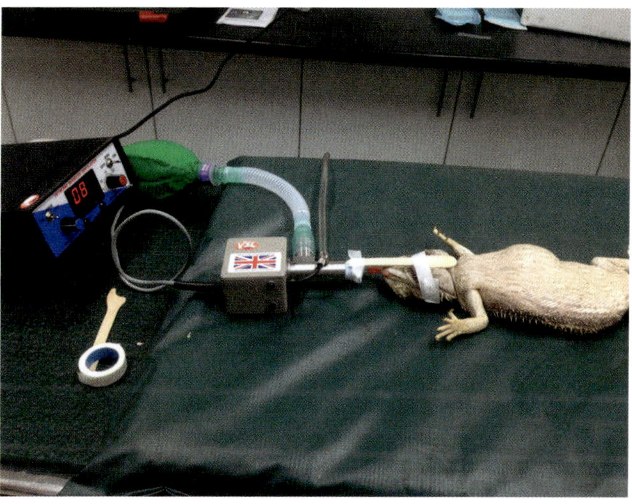

Figure 19.11 Mechanical IPPV using a ventilator in a bearded dragon (*Pogona vitticeps*). Note the use of a wooden tongue depressor taped to the jaw and the endotracheal tube to stabilise the airway connection.

O-rings of cartilage to the trachea and so the cuff on an ET tube should not be inflated or stricture formation can occur postoperatively, similar to birds.

Intermittent positive pressure ventilation

Reptiles generally require positive pressure ventilation during the course of an anaesthetic. The aim of intermittent positive pressure ventilation (IPPV) is to inflate the lungs with an oxygen and anaesthetic mixture sufficient for an adequately oxygenated state to be maintained and for the animal to remain anaesthetised. To this end it is sufficient to ventilate most reptiles two to six times a minute and no more, at a pressure of 10 cmH_2O. As with birds, a ventilator unit makes life much easier, but with experience manual 'bagging' of the patient with enough pressure just to inflate the lungs and no more can be achieved (see Figures 19.10 and 19.11). A rough guide is to inflate the first two-fifths of the reptile's body at each cycle (Malley, 1997).

Anaesthesia even with IPPV can become complicated as there is often right-to-left intracardiac shunting of blood which can be worsened by the presence of intracoelomic masses such as eggs, food or effusions. In addition, the position of the reptile and its lack of a diaphragm may also create a perfusion mismatch as many reptiles require to be placed in dorsal recumbency for coeliotomy, thus allowing the dorsally located lungs to be squashed by the liver and gastrointestinal tract.

Anaesthetic circuits

For species weighing less than 5 kg, a non-rebreathing system with oxygen flow at twice the minute volume is suggested (Bennett, 1998). This approximates to 300–500 mL/kg per minute for most species. Ayres T pieces, modified ('mini') Bain circuits and Mapleson C circuits may all be used.

Note that normal tidal volumes vary in reptiles widely, from 12.5 mL/kg in boas to 45 mL/kg in freshwater turtles. In general, for most pet snakes a tidal volume of 15–30 mL/kg is assumed to be ideal.

Additional supportive therapy

Recumbency

Many chelonians are placed in dorsal recumbency for intracoelomic surgery. Other groups of reptiles may also be placed in this position for similar techniques. The use of foam wedges, or positional polystyrene-filled vacuum bags, is essential for maintaining stability.

Snakes may become extremely flaccid during surgery. In order to provide stability, they may be strapped to a long board or wedged in place with foam wedges or vacuum bags. In any case, it is important to keep the body wall of non-chelonian species free of constraint and to use IPPV if necessary.

Maintenance of body temperature

Maintaining body temperature is important for successful recovery. Body temperature can be monitored using a cloacal probe attached to a digital thermometer. Reptiles should be maintained as near to their preferred body temperature (PBT) as possible, which lies in the range 25–30°C for temperate and 30–35°C for tropical species. This can be achieved by placing the reptile onto a circulating water or air heating pad during anaesthesia. Maintaining warm room temperatures will also clearly help reduce losses. Warmed subcutaneous or intracoelomic fluids can be given during and after surgery.

Hot water bottles or hot water-filled latex gloves may also be used but must be wrapped in towelling to prevent direct contact with the reptile which might result in thermal burns. Care should also be taken when these cool down, as they may then draw heat away from the patient rather than supply it. The use of clear drapes will also help to keep heat in while maintaining visibility as will the utilisation of light sources for surgery, many of which radiate heat.

Fluid therapy

Fluid therapy is covered in more detail in Chapter 22. However, it should be noted that, as with small mammals, postoperative fluid therapy will enhance the recovery rate and improve the patient's return to normal function. Recommended fluid volumes are 20–25 mL/kg every 24 hours across the species (Frye, 1991). They should not exceed 2–3% body weight in chelonians.

Monitoring anaesthesia

Box 19.1 shows the stages of anaesthesia seen in reptiles. It should be noted that in most reptile species when being deepened by gaseous anaesthesia, loss of reflexes tends to occur from cranial to caudal with tail tone being the last to disappear. One publication (Mans *et al.*, 2019) suggested that appropriate anaesthetic depth in lizards for example included:

1. Lack of spontaneous movement in response to a toe or tail pinch
2. Good overall muscle relaxation
3. Absence of the righting reflex
4. Absence of the palpebral reflex
5. Reduced cloacal tone.

It should be noted that despite the above, species variations exist, for example the tongue retraction reflex may still be present in varanids.

Monitoring the heart rate and rhythm can be difficult with a conventional stethoscope due to the rough scales of the reptile interfering with sound transmission and the three-chambered heart of reptiles which reduces the clarity of the heartbeat. Some of this can be overcome by placing a damp towel or gauze swab over the area to be auscultated so deadening the sound of the scales, but in many cases the best solution is to resort to using a Doppler probe which may be placed over the heart outlet at the base of the neck in lizards and Chelonia (see Figure 19.10) and directly over the heart in snakes (see Figure 19.12). Changes in rate and intensity of flow can then be monitored.

Pulse oximetry is not so useful in reptiles due to the differences in haemoglobin structure from mammals, which alters the dissociation curve and so makes accurate determination of values impossible. General trends though may be monitored but even then, due to the complex intracardiac shunting of blood which can occur in reptiles, understanding the significance of trends is still challenging.

Blood gas measurement has been suggested as important particularly in terrestrial species of snakes, which seem to be more sensitive to hypercapnia than hypoxia. Therefore, in the majority of terrestrial

Box 19.1 Stages of anaesthesia in reptiles.

Stage 1

- Limb movements reduced
- Righting reflex present (reptile will flip back onto its feet after being inverted)
- Snake tongue withdrawn after being grasped
- Responds to noxious stimuli
- Muscles are tense
- Writhing movements occur
- Vent stimulation reflex present
- Palpebral reflex present

Stage 2

- Righting reflex ceases
- Tongue withdrawal reflex much reduced
- No response to noxious stimuli
- Muscles start to relax
- Writhing movements cease
- Vent reflex reduced
- Palpebral reflex diminished

Stage 3

- Righting reflex ceased
- No voluntary motion
- Tongue withdrawal reflex totally absent (but may still be present in varanids)
- No response to noxious stimuli
- Muscles totally relaxed
- Snakes: Bauchstreich reflex (where stroking the ventral scales produces reflex contraction of the body wall) much reduced
- Laryngeal reflexes lost in alligators
- Chelonia (and varanids) may still have a corneal reflex
- Vent reflex much reduced: loss of this indicates anaesthesia is too deep

Stage 4

- Extreme depression and death (chelonians lose corneal reflexes just before entering this phase)

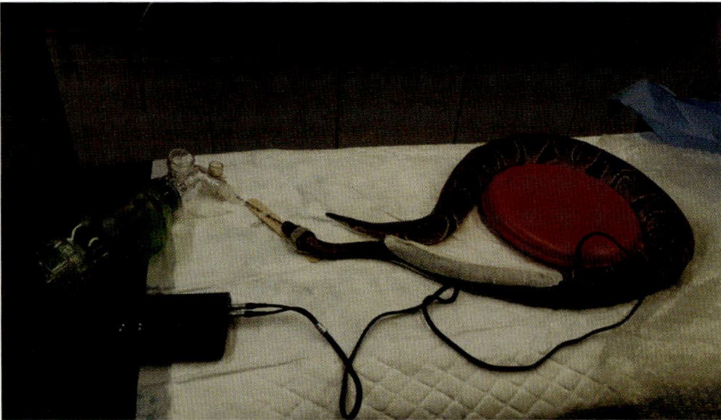

Figure 19.12 Doppler probe monitoring heart sounds in an anaesthetised royal python (*Python regius*). Note also the tape securing the endotracheal tube and the snake's head to prevent dislodgement and the supplemental heat sources.

species of snake, Wang *et al.* (1998) suggest keeping the arterial carbon dioxide levels ($PaCO_2$) between 15 and 35 mmHg. $PaCO_2$ levels are controlled by pulmonary ventilation. If the ventilation is increased, then a decrease in $PaCO_2$ occurs and vice versa. Hypoxia in reptiles tends to stimulate respiratory rate and hypercapnia respiratory depth.

Capnography can be difficult to interpret, again due to intracardiac shunting of blood which means that expired carbon dioxide levels do not always reflect blood levels ($PaCO_2$).

ECG leads may be attached to the patient to give an electrical trace of heart activity. The alligator forceps on the leads may be attached to hypodermic needles which can then be attached to the patient to minimise the crushing effects of the forceps on small fragile patients. Sticky pads are now routinely used in mammals and work well in reptiles to connect the ECG leads to the patient. In snakes, ECG can still be used even in the absence of limbs. The forelimb leads are placed two heart lengths cranial and the hindlimb leads two heart lengths caudal to the heart. In some lizards, such as iguanas, skinks, chameleons and water dragons, the heart is situated very cranially and therefore the forelimb leads are better placed cervically either side of the mid-neck. Heart rate (HR) may be measured and compared with the metabolic scaling formula:

$$HR = 33.4 \times \left[\text{Body weight}(\text{kg})\right]^{-0.25}$$

assuming the reptile is kept in its preferred optimum temperature (i.e. it is at its PBT).

Respiratory flow monitors are not so useful due to the need for IPPV in most reptile species.

Recovery

Reptiles often recover rapidly from isoflurane anaesthesia. However, if other injectable drugs have been used, such as alfaxalone or ketamine, recovery may be prolonged. It is essential at this time to keep the reptile patient calm, stress-free and at its optimum PBT. It is also necessary to keep the patient intubated and on IPPV with oxygen until the reptile is once again breathing for itself. The use of doxapram 5 mg/kg by intramuscular or intravenous injection is useful to help stimulate respiration. The stimulus for reptiles to breathe is thought to be associated with the delivery rate of oxygen, so one theory is that IPPV with 100% oxygen for recovery may actually inhibit respiration. Therefore, recovery using room air, or increasing the intervals between ventilations from one every 10 seconds to one every 20–30 seconds may be helpful in lowering PO_2 and so aid in stimulating spontaneous breathing. However, the return to spontaneous respiration with lowered oxygen supply does not necessarily mean that the recovery from anaesthesia is quicker using this technique, more that hyperoxygenation can inhibit respiration. Odette *et al.* (2015) in bearded dragons demonstrated a marginally, though not clinically significant, faster recovery when using 21% oxygen versus 100% oxygen and Justo *et al.* (2023) found in green sea turtles that while the time to bite was faster with 21% oxygen versus 100% oxygen, the overall recovery times were not meaningfully different.

Recovery will be speeded up if the reptile is kept to its PBT and conversely slowed down if it becomes cold (see Figure 19.12).

Fluid therapy during this period will also help to speed recovery, especially from agents such as ketamine which are cleared through the kidneys. Once recovery is complete, the reptile should be encouraged to eat or, if anorectic, the patient should be hand fed, stomach tubed, etc.

Many snakes will start to show sinuous movements from the tail end first as they recover. Chelonians will start to move hindlimbs and then forelimbs and lizards will start uncoordinated hindlimb movements followed by forelimb movements. It can therefore be generally considered that a reptile has recovered completely when the head and cranial end of the reptile has regained normal function.

Analgesia for reptiles

Pain assessment in reptiles

Reptiles which have been provided with analgesia have been shown to have a quicker return to normality, eating, normal behaviour, etc. than those who do not receive analgesia. However, assessing pain in reptiles is extremely difficult owing to the huge species variations. Mosley (2011) has derived an approach to pain assessment which tries to encompass behaviour (taking into account species variations, stage of ecdysis, hibernation status, socialisation, concurrent illness, and owner assessment of their pet), environmental considerations (enclosure and temperature range), locomotor activity (taking into account posture, gait) and miscellaneous attributes (including appetite, eyelid position, colour changes and abnormal respiratory movements). These are compared with the anticipation of pain levels based on our understanding in mammals and birds.

General but non-specific signs of pain in reptiles include immobility, anorexia, abnormal locomotion and posture, increased aggression and, in those species which can control chromatophore expression in their skin, a dull or dark colouration (e.g. chameleons and bearded dragons). Many snakes with visceral pain will adopt an S-shaped position.

Analgesics used in reptiles

Butorphanol

Despite its wide historic use many newer studies suggest that butorphanol may not be an effective analgesic in reptiles, even at excessive dosages. It has been used at 0.4 mg/kg prior to anaesthesia and believed to aid induction particularly in aquatic chelonians. Actual studies where painful stimuli have been given to reptiles suggest, however, that butorphanol is not an effective analgesic in those reptiles so far tested (red-eared terrapins, cornsnakes, green iguanas, tegus, ball pythons and bearded dragons) (Greenacre *et al.*, 2006; Sladky *et al.*, 2007, 2008; Olesen *et al.*, 2008; Kinney *et al.*, 2011; Fleming and Robertson, 2012; Leal *et al.*, 2016).

Buprenorphine

Buprenorphine 0.01–0.02 mg/kg IM has been recommended but doses of 0.075–0.1 mg/kg were needed in red-eared terrapins in order to maintain therapeutic levels for 24 hours (Kummrow *et al.*, 2008). Some difference was noted in concentrations needed, depending on where the drug was administered, with significantly reduced levels being achieved if injected in the hindlimb versus the forelimb (thought to be hepatic removal); enterohepatic recycling has also been noted. Buprenorphine did not show analgesic properties in a couple of studies in green iguanas and red-eared terrapins, making it largely questionable in reptiles (Greenacre *et al.*, 2006; Mans *et al.*, 2019).

Fentanyl

Fentanyl 0.05 mg/kg subcutaneously (SC) has been used in red-eared terrapins and provided analgesia effective against an interdigital forceps pinch (Kaminishi *et al.*, 2019). Interestingly, in snakes such as ball (royal) pythons, a fentanyl transdermal patch (12.5 μg/hour) seems to work, pharmacokinetically at least (Kharbush *et al.*, 2017). Sladky (2023) suggests that snakes less than 5 kg in body weight are a suitable size for a 12.5 μg/hour patch; for snakes that are 5–10 kg body weight, a 25 μg/hour patch is appropriate. The patch is usually placed dorsally, to one side of midline over the epaxial muscles, close to the heart area.

Hydromorphone

Hydromorphone at around 0.5 mg/kg SC or IM has been used as an analgesic successfully in reptiles (Sladky, 2023). It should be administered into the cranial half of the reptile's body, similar to other medications that are metabolised by the liver, to avoid the analgesic being removed from the body before reaching its effective systemic concentration.

Morphine

Morphine has been shown to be effective at high doses (10 mg/kg) in bearded dragons (Greenacre *et al.*, 2008), but at 1.5–6.5 mg/kg in turtles with a duration of activity which lasted 24 hours (Sladky *et al.*, 2007). At high doses, morphine can act as a significant respiratory depressant in some species (Sladky *et al.*, 2007, 2008, 2009) and that its onset of action can be prolonged (2–8 hours) due to unknown factors.

NSAIDs

All non-steroidal anti-inflammatory drugs (NSAIDs) are potentially nephrotoxic and can have gastrointestinal ulcerative side-effects, and hence fluid therapy and close monitoring should be performed when administered to reptiles.

The two most reported NSAIDs in reptile medicine at the current time are carprofen and meloxicam. Carprofen has been used at 2–4 mg/kg IM once, and then 1–2 mg/kg every 24–72 hours thereafter. Meloxicam has been trialled in a pharmacokinetic study in green iguanas that suggested a dosage of 0.2 mg/kg orally every 24 hours was likely to reach therapeutic levels (Hernandez-Divers *et al.*, 2004). The same study showed that high doses of 5 mg/kg meloxicam administered orally for 12 days in green iguanas produced no clinically apparent abnormalities or histopathological lesions associated with toxicity. Dosages of 0.4 mg/kg IM were effective as an analgesic in bearded dragons (Greenacre *et al.*, 2008).

However, dosages of meloxicam 0.3 mg/kg in ball pythons (*Python regius*) showed no decrease in physiological stress after a surgical procedure, suggesting it did not provide adequate analgesia (Olesen *et al.*, 2008). However, this study did acknowledge that it was difficult to see any increase in physiological stress response in the control animals after surgery.

Other NSAIDs such as ketoprofen have been assessed for toxicity in bearded dragons, with dosages of 2 mg/kg IM showing no adverse physical or biochemical changes and dosages of 20 mg/kg (way in excess of expected therapeutic dosages) showing only damage to the muscles around the injection site (Vigneault *et al.*, 2022). Dosages of ketoprofen 2 mg/kg IM once daily have been used in sea turtles such as loggerheads for three consecutive days with no evidence of harm with regard to blood clotting times and haematological or biochemical parameters (Harms *et al.*, 2021).

Other analgesics

Tramadol: Tramadol works similarly to opioids through the mu-opioid receptors but also inhibits central serotonin and noradrenaline (norepinephrine) reuptake. It has some advantages over morphine in that it produces less respiratory depression and its major metabolite is also an active analgesic so prolonging its activity. Tramadol has been used at 11 mg/kg in bearded dragons (Greenacre *et al.*, 2008) and at 10–25 mg/kg in red-eared terrapins (Cummings *et al.*, 2009) and found to increase the threshold to noxious stimuli; it is thought to work via its weak opioid activity on mu receptors. Duration in the terrapins was between 6 and 96 hours when given orally (10–25 mg/kg) and 12–48 hours when given parenterally (10 mg/kg).

Ketamine: Ketamine appears to be well tolerated in reptiles and has been used as an adjunct to multimodal analgesia, although strong evidence of its efficacy in reptiles is lacking. The alpha-2 drugs such as medetomidine and dexmedetomidine may also be useful in analgesia without sedation but they do seem to produce similar undesirable effects as in mammals, namely bradycardia, hypotension and a reduction in arterial PO_2 levels (Sleeman and Gaynor, 2000; Dennis and Heard, 2002).

Local anaesthesia

Local anaesthetics may be used as ring blocks around amputations to reduce the chances of postoperative self-mutilation. Doses should not exceed 4 mg/kg of lidocaine (known toxic doses in mammals are 10–22 mg/kg) and should be diluted to at least 1 : 10. Bupivacaine should not exceed 5 mg/kg but typically doses of 1 mg/kg are used.

Overview of amphibian anaesthesia and analgesia

Techniques and equipment involved in restraining amphibian patients

Examination of the amphibian patient should be performed at that species' optimum PBT, as with reptile patients. A rough guide is between 21 and 24°C, which is lower than the more usual 22–32°C for reptile housing conditions.

The examination table should be covered with paper towels (unbleached) that have been soaked in dechlorinated water (preferably purified water). More purified water should be on standby to be applied to the amphibian patient to prevent dehydration during the examination.

Initially, it is useful not to restrain the amphibian patient until the extent of any problem is assessed, as many have severe skin lesions that are extremely fragile. Once an initial assessment has been made, the patient may be restrained manually. First, it is advisable to put on a pair of latex-free gloves in order to minimise irritation to the amphibian's skin caused by either the handler's normal acidic skin environment or by the powder in many prepacked latex gloves. The wearing of gloves is also essential in many species of anurans whose skin can produce irritant or even potentially deadly toxins which can be absorbed through unprotected human skin. It may also be necessary to wear goggles when handling some species of toad; the giant toad (*Bufo marinus*) can squirt a toxin from its parotid salivary glands over a distance of several feet.

When handling the amphibian patient, the method of restraint will obviously depend on the animal's body shape. The elongated form of salamanders and newts will require similar restraint to that of a lizard, with one hand grasping the pectoral girdle from the dorsal aspect, index finger and thumb encircling one forelimb, second and third fingers the other, with the opposite hand grasping the pelvic girdle, again from the dorsal aspect in a similar manner. Some salamanders will shed their tails if roughly handled, so care should be taken with these species.

Large anurans can be restrained by cupping one hand around the pectoral girdle immediately behind the front limbs with the other hand positioned beneath the hindlimbs. Care should be taken with some species which have poison glands in their skin, as mentioned above, and in the case of species such as the Argentinian horned frog, care should be taken as they bite. Aquatic urodeles should be examined only in water as removal causes skin damage. Some of the larger urodeles, such as the hellbender species (*Cryptobranchus* spp.) can also inflict unpleasant bite wounds on handlers, so firm restraint is required.

Smaller species and aquatic species may be best examined in small glass jars.

Aspects of chemical restraint in amphibians

There are three main routes of administration of anaesthetic and sedative agents to amphibians: injections, inhalant gaseous anaesthetics and in-water methods. Most amphibians should be fasted for 24–48 hours prior to anaesthesia to reduce stomach and gut loading.

Stomach eversion may occur in anurans during induction of anaesthesia even if they are starved for a period of time. In most cases this may be simply reinserted with moistened cotton-buds with a likely full return to function assuming no physical damage has occurred to the stomach lining or wall.

In-water anaesthetic agents

There are two main anaesthetics: MS-222 and benzocaine. Water should be ideally distilled water at room temperature. If the amphibian's tank water is in good condition, then that may also be an alternative. Chlorinated (e.g. tap) water should always be avoided as chloramines are toxic to amphibians. Partial immersion of amphibians so they can continue to breathe room air is recommended.

MS-222: This is tricaine methanesulphonate, an anaesthetic used commonly in fish restraint. It is a water-soluble white powder. A range of 1–2 g/L water is required to anaesthetise most adult frogs and urodeles, 2 g/L for axolotls but a solution of 3 g/L is required for most adult toads (Wright, 1996). Immersion times are typically around 20 minutes and produce anaesthesia for 15–30 minutes. A reduced level of 0.2–0.5 g/L can be used for tadpole anaesthesia. Sodium bicarbonate (at the same to twice the weight of MS-222) is often added to the water to counteract MS-222's tendency to acidify the solution. The aim is to try to create a near neutral solution (pH 7–7.4) so that it is not irritant and also is better absorbed by the amphibian.

It is best to use distilled water or the amphibian's own water at room temperature to minimise environmental changes, and to place this into a plastic bag or plastic-lined box. This is useful as many amphibians go through an excitation stage during anaesthesia, and the slight give in the plastic bags reduces skin damage. It is also important to ensure any anurans and other non-gilled amphibians can raise their nostrils above the water, otherwise they will drown.

Anaesthesia induction will take 20 minutes or so, with reducing respiration rates. Respiration may even stop, although cardiac function persists. During the induction period, the ventrum of the amphibian will redden and anurans will become excited, making leaping movements.

Initial anaesthesia is manifested by the inability of the amphibian to right itself, and loss of the corneal reflex, but with pain reflexes still intact. A deep plane of anaesthesia is when all of these are abolished and only the heartbeat can be seen as a sign of movement. The level of anaesthesia can be maintained by trickling the anaesthetic solution over the amphibian's body once the amphibian is removed from the solution. Reversal is achieved by trickling fresh, distilled, oxygenated water over the amphibian's skin.

Benzocaine: This can be used to anaesthetise African clawed frogs (*Xenopus laevis*) within 3–4 minutes in a bath of concentration 1 g/L (0.1%) which lasts around 40 minutes (Smith *et al.*, 2018). Solutions of 0.005–0.01% can be used for tadpoles (DiGironimo and Balko, 2021). Benzocaine is more soluble in ethanol than in water and so is often dissolved in a small volume of this before it is added to the water. Recovery occurs some 60 minutes after rinsing the amphibian with benzocaine-free water.

It may be necessary to add a buffer solution to the water to correct acidification as with MS-222.

Other in-water anaesthetics: Clove oil, or to be accurate its active ingredient isoeugenol, can be added to the bath water at 350 μL/L to anaesthetise African clawed frogs for 15–30 minutes (Goulet *et al.*, 2010).

Injectable anaesthetic agents

Alfaxalone: Alfaxalone does not appear to be able to induce full anaesthesia in amphibians and so is rarely used for restraint.

Ketamine: Ketamine may be used, but is less preferable to MS-222. This is because relatively large volumes are required (75–100 mg/kg; Bennett, 1996), and the anaesthetic takes a variable period to take effect, from 10 minutes to 1–2 hours. Injections may be made intramuscularly or intravenously into the midline ventral abdominal vein or subcutaneously. Muscle rigidity is also a problem with ketamine usage and this, combined with its often prolonged effects (sometimes up to 24 hours to recover), means it is uncommonly used on its own. Lower dosages of 20–40 mg/kg have been used as sedation or premedication. Combinations of ketamine (100 mg/kg) with dexmedetomidine (5 mg/kg) and midazolam (40 mg/kg) have been used in poison arrow frogs, producing a loss of the righting reflex (Yaw *et al.*, 2019).

Propofol: Propofol anaesthesia has been attempted in amphibians but results are inconsistent and as vascular access is difficult in the conscious amphibian, it is not commonly used.

Inhalant gaseous anaesthetic agents

Isoflurane: This may be used via induction chamber at a dose of 2.5–3%, or, in the larger species of toads, by applying it via a gel directly onto the amphibian's skin. The latter technique involves mixing 3 mL isoflurane with 1.5 mL water and 3.5 mL of a water-based soluble lubricant and then using 0.025–0.035 mL of this per gram of amphibian (Wright, 2001). Some of the larger species may also be intubated but some amphibians have no trachea, making intubation complicated. Gaseous anaesthesia can be erratic, as alternative respiratory routes are available to amphibians such as cutaneous or buccopharyngeal routes (i.e. the amphibian can breathe through its skin or oral membranes). Some of the more fragile species, such as the smaller urodeles or caecilians may actually suffer severe skin damage during gas chamber induction due to the direct irritant effect of the anaesthetic on the skin.

Analgesia

There is limited research and knowledge into pain and its control in amphibians. Recognising pain in amphibians is also difficult, but studies by Pezalla (1983) showed that the wiping response (where the hindlimb wipes the affected limb) to increasing levels of acetic acid was a specific response to pain. These tests showed that opioids (e.g. morphine, butorphanol and buprenorphine) could raise the pain threshold in amphibians. Indications are that mu and kappa receptors exist in the spinal cord of amphibians.

In addition, other tests showed the analgesic efficacy of alpha-2 agonists such as xylazine (Brenner *et al.*, 1994; Terril-Robb *et al.*, 1996). NSAIDs produced weaker but still significant analgesic effects. Barbiturates, however, did not seem to provide analgesia in a similar study.

Suggested analgesics for frogs include butorphanol (25 mg/kg intracoelomically), buprenorphine (14 mg/kg intracoelomically), flunixin meglumine (25 mg/kg intracoelomically once) and xylazine (10 mg/kg intracoelomically every 12–24 hours) (Terril-Robb *et al.*, 1996; Stevens, 2011). I have also used meloxicam at 0.2–1 mg/kg per os every 24 hours in anurans and newts as postoperative analgesia. Dosages of buprenorphine 50 mg/kg intracoelomically once daily for 3 days in newts after limb amputation appeared effective (Koeller, 2009).

References

Barter, L.S., Hawkins, M.G., Brosnan, R.J. *et al.* (2006) Median effective dose of isoflurane, sevoflurane, and desflurane in green iguanas. *American Journal of Veterinary Research*, **67**(3). doi: 10.2460/ajvr.67.3.392.

Bennett, R.A. (1996) Anaesthesia. In: *Reptile Medicine and Surgery* (ed. R. Mader), pp. 241–247. W.B. Saunders, London.

Bennett, R.A. (1998) Reptile anaesthesia. *Seminars in Avian and Exotic Pet Medicine*, **7**, 30–40.

Bennett, R.A., Schumacher, J., Hedjazi-Haring, K. and Newell, S.M. (1998) Cardiopulmonary and anaesthetic effects of propofol administered intraosseously to green iguanas. *Journal of the American Veterinary Medical Association*, **212**, 93–98.

Bertelsen, M.F. (2014) Squamates (snakes and lizards). In: *Zoo Animal and Wildlife Immobilization and Anesthesia* (eds G. West, D. Heard & N. Caulkett), 2nd edn, pp. 351–363. Wiley-Blackwell, Ames, IA.

Bertelsen, M.F. and Sauer, C.D. (2011) Alfaxalone anaestheisa in the green iguana (*Iguana iguana*). *Veterinary Anaesthesia and Analgesia*, **38**, 461–466.

Bertelsen, M.F., Mosley, C.A.E., Crawshaw, G.J. *et al.* (2005a) Minimum alveolar concentration of isoflurane in mechanically ventilated Dumeril monitors. *Journal of the American Veterinary Medical Association*, **226**, 1098–1101.

Bertelsen, M.F., Mosley, C.A.E., Crawshaw, G.J. *et al.* (2005b) Anesthetic potency of sevoflurane with and without nitrous oxide in mechanically ventilated Dumeril monitors. *Journal of the American Veterinary Medical Association*, **227**(4). doi: 10.2460/javma.2005.227.575.

Brenner, G.M., Klopp, A.J., Deason, L.L. and Stevens, C.W. (1994) Analgesic potency of alpha adrenergic agents after systemic administration in amphibians. *Journal of Pharmacology and Experimental Therapeutics*, **270**, 540–545.

Cummings, B.B., Sladky, K.K. and Johnson, S.M. (2009) Tramadol analgesic and respiratory effects in red-eared slider turtles (*Trachemys scripta*). *Proceedings of the Association of Reptilian and Amphibian Veterinarians*, Milwaukee, Wisconsin, p. 115.

Dennis, P.M. and Heard, D.J. (2002) Cardiopulmonary effects of a medetomidine–ketamine combination administered intravenously in gopher tortoises. *Journal of the American Veterinary Medical Association*, **220**, 1516–1519.

DiGironimo, P.M. and Balko, J.A. (2021) Sedation and anesthesia of amphibians. *Veterinary Clinics of North America: Exotic Animal Practice*, **25**, 31–47.

Fleming, G.J. and Robertson, S.A. (2012) Assessments of thermal antinociceptive effects of butorphanol and human observer effect on quantitative evaluation of analgesia in green iguanas (*Iguana iguana*). *American Journal of Veterinary Research*, **73**, 1507–1511.

Frye, F. (1991) *Biomedical and Surgical Aspects of Captive Reptile Husbandry, Volume 1 and 2*. Krieger Publishing, Malabar, FL.

Goulet, F., Helie, P. and Vachon, P. (2010) Eugenol anesthesia in African clawed frogs (*Xenopus leavis*) of different body weights. *Journal of the American Association for Laboratory Animal Science*, **49**(4), 460–463.

Greenacre, C.B., Tackle, G., Schumacher, J.P. *et al.* (2006) Comparative antinociception of morphine, butorphanol, and buprenorphine versus saline in the green iguana, *Iguana iguana*, using electrostimulation. *Journal of Herpetological Medicine and Surgery*, **16**, 88–92.

Greenacre, C.B., Massi, K., Schumacher, J.P. and Harvey, R.C. (2008) Comparative antinociception of various opioids and nonsteroidal anti-inflammatory medications versus saline in the bearded dragon (*Pogona vitticeps*) using electrostimulation. *Proceedings of the Association of Reptilian and Amphibian Veterinarians*, Los Angeles, California, pp. 87–88.

Greunz, E.M., Williams, C., Ringgaard, S. *et al.* (2018) Elimination of intracardiac shunting provides stable gas anesthesia in tortoises. *Scientific Reports*, **8**(1), 17124. doi: 10.1038/s41598-018-35588-w.

Harms, C.A., Ruterbories, L.K., Stacy, N.I. *et al.* (2021) Safety of multiple-dose intramuscular ketoprofen treatment in loggerhead turtles (*Caretta caretta*). *Journal of Zoo and Wildlife Medicine*, **52**(1), 126–132.

Heaton-Jones, T.G., Ko, J. and Heaton-Jones, D.L. (2002) Evaluation of medetomidine–ketamine anesthesia with atipamezole reversal in American alligators (*Alligator mississippiensis*). *Journal of Zoo and Wildlife Medicine*, **33**, 36–44.

Hernandez-Divers, S.J., McBride, A., Koch, T., et al. (2004) Single dose oral and intravenous pharmacokinetics of meloxicam in the green iguana (*Iguana iguana*). *Proceedings of the Association of Reptilian and Amphibian Veterinarians*, Naples, Florida, p. 106.

James, L.E., Williams, C.J., Bertelsen, M.F. and Wang, T. (2018) Anaesthetic induction with alfaxalone in the ball python (*Python regius*): dose response and effect of injection site. *Veterinary Anaesthesia and Analgesia*, **45**(3), 329–337.

Justo, A.A., Dutra, G.H.P., Carregaro, A.B. and Cortopassi, S.R.G. (2023) The fraction of inspired oxygen does not affect the time to extubation in mechanically ventilated, sevoflurane-anesthetized green sea turtles (*Chelonia mydas*). *American Journal of Veterinary Research*, **84**(5), ajvr.23.01.0008. doi: 10.2460/ajvr.23.01.0008.

Kaminishi, A.P.S., de Freitas, A.C., Avila Jnr, R.H. *et al.* (2019) Antinociceptive and physiological effects of subcutaneous administration of fentanyl in

Trachemys spp. (Testudines: Emydidae). *International Journal of Advanced Engineering Research and Science*, **6**(11), 311–316.

Kharbush, R., Gutwillig, A., Hartzler, K. *et al.* (2017) Antinociceptive and respiratory effects following application of transdermal fentanyl patches and assessment of brain μ-opioid receptor mRNA expression in ball pythons. *American Jounral of Veterinary Research*, **78**(7) https://doi.org/10.2460/ajvr.78.7.785.

Kinney, M., Johnson, S.M. and Sladky, K.K. (2011) Behavioral evaluation of red-eared slider turtles (*Trachemys scripta*) administered either morphine or butorphanol following unilateral gonadectomy. *Journal of Herpetological Medicine and Surgery*, **21**, 54–62.

Kischinovsky, M. and Bertelsen, M.F. (2011) Alfaxalone anaesthesia in green iguanas and red-eared sliders. *Proceedings of the European Association of Zoo and Wildlife Vets*, Lisbon, Lisbon, Portugal, p. 113.

Koeller, C.A. (2009) Comparison of buprenorphine and butorphanol analgesia in the eastern red-spotted newt (*Notophthalmus viridescens*). *Journal of the American Association of Laboratory Animal Science*, **48**, 171–175.

Kummrow, M.S., Tseng, F., Hesse, L. and Court, M. (2008) Pharmacokinetics of buprenorphine after single dose subcutaneous administration in red-eared sliders (*Trachemys scripta elegans*). *Journal of Zoo and Wildlife Medicine*, **39**, 590–595.

Lawton, M.P.C. (1992) Anaesthesia. In: *Manual of Reptiles* (eds P.H. Beynon, M.P.C. Lawton & J.E. Cooper), 1st edn, pp. 170–183. BSAVA, Cheltenham, Gloucestershire.

Leal, W.P., Carregaro, A.B., Bressan, T.F. *et al.* (2016) Antinociceptive efficacy of intramuscular administration of morphine sulfate and butorphanol tartrate in tegus (*Salvator merianae*). *American Journal of Veterinary Research*, **78**, 1019–1024.

Lloyd, M.L. (2003) Crocodilia. In: *Zoo and Wild Animal Medicine* (eds M.E. Fowler & R.E. Miller), 5th edn, pp. 59–70. Elsevier Saunders, Philadelphia, PA.

Malley, D. (1997) Reptile anaesthesia and the practising veterinarian. *InPractice*, **19**, 351–368.

Mans, C., Sladky, K. and Schumacher, J. (2019) General anesthesia. In: *Mader's Reptile and Amphibian Medicine and Surgery* (eds S. Divers & S. Stahl), 3rd edn, pp. 447–464. Elsevier, St. Louis, MO.

Monticelli, P., Ronaldson, H.L., Hutchinson, J.R. *et al.* (2019) Medetomidine–ketamine–sevoflurane anaesthesia in juvenile Nile crocodiles (*Crocodylus niloticus*). *Veterinary Anaesthesia and Analgesia*, **46**, 84–89.

Mosely, C.A.E., Dyson, D. and Smith, D.A. (2003) Minimum alveolar concentration of isoflurane in green iguanas and the effect of butorphanol on minimum alveolar concentration. *Journal of American Veterinary Medical Association*, **222**, 1559–1564.

Mosley, C. (2011) Pain and nociception in reptiles. *Veterinary Clinics of North America: Exotic Animal Practice*, **14**, 45–60.

Odette, O., Churgin, S.M., Sladky, K.K. and Smith, L.J. (2015) Anesthetic induction and recovery parameters in bearded dragons (*Pogona vitticeps*): comparison of isoflurane delivered in 100% oxygen versus 21% oxygen. *Journal of Zoo and Wildlife Medicine*, **46**(3), 534–539. doi: 10.1638/2014-0193.1.

Olesen, M.G., Bertelsen, M.F., Perry, S.F. and Wang, T. (2008) Effects of preoperative administration of butorphanol or meloxicam on physiologic responses to surgery in ball pythons. *Journal of the American Veterinary Medical Association*, **233**, 1883–1888.

Pezalla, P.D. (1983) Morphine-induced analgesia and explosive motor behaviour in an amphibian. *Brain Research*, **273**, 297–305.

Porter, K.R. (1972) *Herpetology*. W.B. Saunders, Philadelphia, PA.

Proenca, L.M., Fowler, S., Kleine, S. *et al.* (2014a) Coelioscopic-assisted sterilization of female Mojave desert tortoises (*Gopherus agassizii*). *Journal of Herpetological Medicine and Surgery*, **24**, 95–100.

Proenca, L.M., Fowler, S., Kleine, S. *et al.* (2014b) Single surgeon coelioscopic orchiectomy of desert tortoises (*Gopherus agassizii*) for population management. *Veterinary Record*, **175**, 404–409.

Sheelings, T.F., Holz, P., Haynes, L., et al. (2010) A preliminary study of the chemical restraint of selected squamate reptiles with alfaxalone. *Proceedings of the Annual Conference of the Association of Reptilian and Amphibian Veterinarians*, South Padre Island, Texas, pp. 114–115.

Sladky, K.K. (2023) Treatment of pain in reptiles. *Veterinary Clinics of North America: Exotic Animal Practice*, **26**, 43–64.

Sladky, K.K., Miletic, V., Paul-Murphy, J. *et al.* (2007) Analgesic efficacy and respiratory effects of butorphanol and morphine in turtles. *Journal of the American Veterinary Medical Association*, **230**, 1356–1362.

Sladky, K.K., Kinney, M.E. and Johnson, S.M. (2008) Analgesic efficacy of butorphanol and morphine in bearded dragons and corn snakes. *Journal of the American Veterinary Medical Association*, **233**, 267–273.

Sladky, K.K., Kinney, M.E. and Johnson, S.M. (2009) Effects of opioid receptor activation on thermal antinociception in red-eared slider turtles (*Trachemys scripta elegans*). *American Journal of Veterinary Research*, **70**, 1072–1078.

Sladky, K.K., Klaphake, E., Di Girolamo, N. and Carpenter, J.W. (2023) Reptiles. In: *Carpenter's Exotic Animal Formulary* (eds J.W. Carpenter & C.A. Harms), 6th edn, pp. 101–221. Elsevier, St Louis, MO.

Sleeman, J.M. and Gaynor, J. (2000) Sedative and cardiopulmonary effects of medetomidine and reversal with atipamezole in desert tortoises (*Gopherus agassizii*). *Journal of Zoo and Wildlife Medicine*, **31**, 28–35.

Smith, B.D., Vail, K.J., Carroll, G.L. *et al.* (2018) Comparison of etomidate, benzocaine and MS-222 anesthesia with and without subsequent flunixin meglumine analgesia in Africa clawed frogs (*Xenopus laevis*). *Journal of American Association for Laboratory Animal Science*, **57**, 202–209.

Stevens, C.W. (2011) Analgesia in amphibians: preclinical studies and clinical applications. *Veterinary Clinics of North America: Exotic Animal Practice*, **14**, 33–44.

Terril-Robb, L., Suckow, M. and Grigdesby, C. (1996) Evaluation of the analgesic effects of butorphanol tartrate, xylazine hydrochloride and flunixin meglumine in leopard frogs (*Rana pipiens*). *Contemporary Topics in Laboratory Animal Science*, **35**, 54–56.

Vigneault, A., Lair, S., Gara-Boivin, C. *et al.* (2022) Evaluation of the safety of multiple intramuscular doses of ketoprofen in bearded dragons (*Pogona vitticeps*). *Journal of Herpetological Medicine and Surgery*, **32**(2), 123–129.

Wang, T., Smits, A.W. and Burggren, W.W. (1998) Pulmonary function in reptiles. In: *Biology of the Reptilia, Volume 19, Morphology G, Visceral Organs* (eds C. Gans & M.H. Gault), pp. 297–374. Society for the Study of Amphibians and Reptiles, Ithaca.

Wright, K.M. (1996) Amphibian husbandry and medicine. In: *Reptile Medicine and Surgery* (ed. D. Mader), pp. 436–458. W.B. Saunders, Philadelphia, PA.

Wright, K.M. (2001) Restraint techniques and euthanasia. In: *Amphibian Medicine and Captive Husbandry* (eds K.M. Wright & B.R. Whitaker), pp. 111–122. Krieger Publishing, Malabar, FL.

Yaw, T.J., Mans, C., Johnson, S.M. *et al.* (2018) Effect of injection site on alfaxalone-induced sedation in ball pythons (*Python regius*). *Journal of Small Animal Practice*, **59**(12), 747–751.

Yaw, T.J., Mans, C., Martinelli, L. and Sladky, K.K. (2019) Comparison of subcutaneous administration of alfaxalone–midazolam–dexmedetomidine with ketamine–midazolam–dexmedetomidine for chemical restraint in juvenile blue poison dart frogs (*Dendrobates tinctorius azureus*). *Journal of Zoo and Wildlife Medicine*, **50**, 868–873.

Chapter 20 Reptile and Amphibian Nutrition

Classification

Reptiles and amphibians may be classified in a number of different ways, one of which is according to their diet. Of the commonly seen species, there are four main categories as defined by the diet.

- Carnivores such as snakes, monitor lizards, snapping turtles and Crocodilia, which will eat whole avian, amphibian or mammalian prey. To do this, snakes have recurved often long teeth, flexible jaws and significant jaw muscles. Some snakes have venom glands and fangs while others, such as the boa and the python species, rely on constricting their prey. The Crocodilia have powerful crushing jaws and simple peg-like teeth.
- Herbivores are generally found in the chelonians and lizard species, from tortoises such as the Greek or spur-thighed tortoise (*Testudo graeca*) to lizards such as the green iguana (*Iguana iguana*).
- Insectivores are predominantly lizards such as leopard geckos (*Eublepharis macularius*), collared lizards (*Crotaphytus collaris*), chameleons and many amphibians such as the poison arrow frogs (*Dendrobates* spp.) and many salamanders (*Ambystoma* spp.)
- Omnivores are from a variety of reptile species such as box turtles (*Terrapene* spp.), terrapins (*Trachemys* spp.), water dragons (*Physignathus* spp.), many skinks (*Tiliqua* spp.) and tegus (*Salvator* spp.). The term may be used to refer to reptiles which change their eating habits during the course of their life. For example, the inland bearded dragon (*Pogona vitticeps*) starts off as a predominant insectivore, but becomes more and more dependent on leafy greens as it gets older.

In all these cases, many individual species have become highly evolved to cope with certain types of food. We also know that many of these creatures in the wild have a changing food supply throughout the year, so what may form a staple diet in the summer does not necessarily apply come the winter.

General nutritional requirements

Water

As mentioned in Chapter 12 (avian nutrition), the most important thing about the water provided is its quality and presentation.

Reptiles may defecate in their water bowls, and turtles and terrapins eat in their water. These habits cause pollution which leads to disease. To prevent this, either the water must have a powerful filter system, or the terrapins/turtles be fed in a separate feeding tank which may be cleaned out after feeding.

Vitamin and mineral supplements administered in the water will allow rapid bacterial growth over 24 hours, so these are generally not recommended or if they are then bowl hygiene must be rigorous.

The amount of water consumed by individual reptiles and amphibians will depend on the diets being offered as well as on the species. On dry insect-based diets, water consumption will generally be higher than for reptiles and amphibians which consume large amounts of fresh vegetables. Even so a leopard gecko may only consume 5 mL of water in a 24-hour period and daily water consumption for reptiles in general is roughly 20–30 mL/kg per day. These figures are derived from water turnover rates in the wild, also known as field water budgets, and can be described by the equation:

$$R = 20.6\,W^{0.84}$$

where R is water turnover or loss (mL/day) and W is body weight (kg) (Minnich, 1982).

Tap water contains chlorine, which may irritate the skin of sensitive aquatic species such as amphibians or soft-shelled turtles. It is advised therefore that tap water be allowed to stand for 24 hours to let the chlorine escape and to allow it to attain room temperature. Alternatively, dechlorinating tablets (often containing sodium sulphite) can be added to the tap water to remove chlorine prior to being offered.

Renal disease as a result of chronic dehydration is common in captive reptile species. Reptiles, like birds, are susceptible to renal disease because the waste product of protein metabolism is predominantly the insoluble uric acid. If the reptile is not kept adequately hydrated, it will reduce the excretion of uric acid through the kidneys. This leads to deposition of uric acid inside the body, a condition known as visceral gout. Once deposited, the uric acid forms a tough mineralised coating to the lining of blood vessels, and organs such as the kidneys and heart, leading to hypertension and multiple organ failure.

Many reptiles, such as green iguanas and water dragons, have high relative humidity in their natural habitats, anywhere from 60 to 100%. If these species are kept in vivaria at their correct temperatures, it can be difficult to maintain the necessary relative humidity as the warmer air is, the more water it can hold. Many reptiles will also not drink from water bowls, instead preferring to lick moisture from leaves or cage furniture (Figure 20.1). Combining these two factors, we can see that chronic dehydration, and therefore renal damage, can occur. Regular misting of the vivaria for these high humidity-requiring species can help and so can the presence of an organic substrate that can hold a reserve of moisture. Sprinkler or drip feed systems are also useful and can be set on a timer to create water droplets in the vivaria.

High humidity is of course not required for desert-dwelling species, such as leopard geckos and pancake tortoises, but even these

Veterinary Nursing of Exotic Pets and Wildlife, Third Edition. Simon J. Girling.

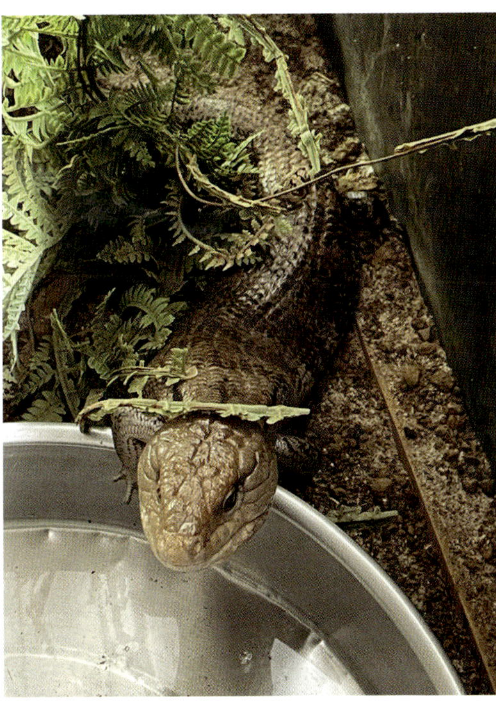

Figure 20.1 Many tropical species of reptiles (unlike this skink) that require higher humidity will not choose to drink from water bowls but prefer to lick water droplets from surfaces within the vivarium.

species benefit from being misted every now and then and a 'wet' hide with a higher humidity as well as a 'dry' hide in their vivarium.

Energy requirements

Every species has a level of daily energy consumption that is needed to satisfy the basic maintenance requirements. This is the energy used purely to maintain current status under minimal activity and is the minimum energy required to support the reptile's or amphibian's life. However, as reptiles are ectotherms, their energy requirements vary with the environmental temperature even when they are inactive, the term 'basal metabolic rate' (BMR) used in mammals and birds being replaced by the term 'standard metabolic rate' (SMR). It therefore follows that SMRs should always be accompanied by the temperature the reptile was kept at when the rate was calculated.

The SMR can be calculated for a reptile very crudely using the following equation:

$$\text{SMR} = k \times \left[\text{weight}(\text{kg})\right]^{0.75}$$

The constant, k, varies with family groups, and has been estimated at 10 for reptiles in general (Sedgwick, 1993). However, there are several publications that have now more accurately derived the SMRs for individual species (Table 20.1).

In the wild, reptiles may choose to place themselves in lower environmental temperature zones to reduce their energy requirements, making calculating their needs in captivity sometimes more complicated. The term 'field maintenance requirement' (FMR) is often used instead of maintenance energy requirement (MER) to reflect this, although MERs are still often quoted. Standard FMR values are often around 1.5 times the SMR, but energy requirements will also vary according to the animal's stage of life. For example, the energy requirements will be more than doubled in active egg-laying females and during disease or growth.

Table 20.1 Species-specific SMR equations and the temperatures they were measured at.

Species	Temperature (°C)	SMR equation (kJ/day)
Boidae snakes (boas)	20	$7.48 \times [\text{weight(kg)}]^{1.09}$
Colubridae snakes (e.g. cornsnakes, kingsnakes, milksnakes, garter snakes)	20	$18.37 \times [\text{weight(kg)}]^{0.98}$
Desert tortoise (*Gopherus agassizii*)	30	$12.5 \times [\text{weight(kg)}]^{0.75}$
Green iguana (*Iguana iguana*)	30	$36.78 \times [\text{weight(kg)}]^{0.734}$
Inland bearded dragon (*Pogona vitticeps*)	37	$52.85 \times [\text{weight(kg)}]^{0.80}$
Varanidae (monitor lizards)	35	$91.6 \times [\text{weight(kg)}]^{0.84}$

Sources: Data from Galvao *et al.* (1965); Brand *et al.* (1991); Thompson and Withers (1992); Barboza (1995); Secor and Phillips (1997); Maxwell *et al.* (2003).

If the foods offered are so low in kilojoules that the reptile or amphibian has to eat more of it than will fit into its digestive system in 24 hours, that animal will rapidly lose condition. For example, vegetables such as lettuce and celery have an energy content of 12.6 kJ/g dry matter (or in real terms 0.75 kJ/g wet food), whereas meat-based foods such as rodent prey have a much higher energy density of 19–21 kJ/g dry matter (or in real terms 6–7.5 kJ/g wet food) (Donoghue, 1998). From this we can see that in 'as fed' terms (i.e. wet food) one would need to feed eight times as much weight of vegetable matter to give the same energy in animal prey. This volume may well exceed the gut capacity of the reptile or amphibian.

Conversely, many pet reptiles and amphibians will continue eating until their digestive tracts are full, and if all they are offered is high-energy-density food then they will rapidly achieve their MER, exceed it and become obese. Nagy (1982), for example, showed that the daily FMR requirements for a 100-g lizard (8.9 kJ/day) was only 5.5% that of a 100-g rodent (162 kJ/day).

Weighing and body condition scoring

Considering the information above, it is therefore helpful to regularly weigh reptiles to assess whether they are gaining weight. Weight gain may clearly be appropriate in young growing reptiles or those recovering from illness associated with previous weight loss, but is unlikely to be appropriate in a mature adult healthy reptile.

Weight to carapace lengths have been derived for some *Testudo* spp. (*T. graeca* and *T. hermannii*) of tortoises and the following formula (Jackson, 1980) has been derived:

$$W = 0.191 \times L^3$$

where W is body weight in grams and L is the carapace length in centimetres.

In green iguanas (*Iguana iguana*), their body weight could be related directly to the snout-to-vent length (SVL) by the following formula (Donoghue *et al.*, 1998):

$$W = (61 \times \text{SVL}) - 859$$

where *W* is body weight in grams and SVL is in centimetres.

Body condition scoring may also be very helpful in some species. Many body condition scoring scales have been derived but a simple one, from 0 (emaciated) to 5 (morbidly obese), can be applied with the aim of targeting 2.5–3 as a healthy score. For example, in species such as leopard geckos, which store fat in their tails, the fat reserves of the reptile may easily be seen and a crude score derived: from 0, no fat at all and the spinous processes of the caudal vertebrae clearly visible through to 5, the tail so full of fat that it becomes pear-shaped.

In many snakes, the epaxial area in the last third of the body can be assessed. Again, a scoring system could be applied: from 0, the snake's dorsal spinous processes of the vertebrae are clearly very prominent and where there is no significant epaxial musculature through to 5, where the dorsal spinous processes have disappeared and instead due to subcutaneous fat deposits, the epaxial areas are dorsal to the midline creating an axial gutter or groove.

In many lizards, the pelvic area and base of the tail can be used in a similar fashion to snakes: from 0, the lizard's dorsal spinous processes of the vertebrae are clearly very prominent and where there is no significant epaxial musculature or covering of the pelvic bones though to 5, where the dorsal spinous processes of the tail base have disappeared and instead due to subcutaneous fat deposits, the cross-section of the tail base has become circular and the pelvic bones are not discernible.

Protein and amino acid requirements

Proteins are assembled from groups of amino acids; indeed a protein can contain up to 22 amino acids. In general terms, for humans, and it seems for many reptiles, 10 amino acids are essential and need to be provided in the diet. The others may be manufactured from these 10 in herbivores. The essential amino acids are:

- leucine
- lysine
- methionine
- phenylalanine
- threonine
- tryptophan
- isoleucine
- valine
- arginine
- histidine.

In addition, it is known that for diets low in the amino acids methionine or arginine, an extra supplement of the amino acid glycine is required. Strict mammalian carnivores also need additional amino acids such as taurine. It is not fully understood if strict reptilian carnivores such as snakes and the carnivorous amphibians have a similar requirement, but it is likely.

Proteins are therefore assessed on their ability to provide these essential amino acids, with poor proteins supplying only non-essential ones. This is quantified by the term 'biological value', indicating a high biological value foodstuff containing more of the essential amino acids.

For herbivorous reptiles, levels of 25% protein content as metabolisable energy in the diet have been shown to be adequate (Donoghue, 1998). Most of this protein source in herbivores seems to come from leafy greens, but deficiencies are seen in herbivorous reptiles fed high-cellulose, low-protein foods such as the ubiquitous lettuce, and fruits. Chronic protein deficiencies are often presented as gradual wasting conditions, with increased susceptibility to infections. In one study by Donoghue et al. (1998), increasing dietary protein levels up to 30% dry matter fed increased the rate of growth in the green iguana; however, above 30% dry matter failed to produce further increases.

For omnivorous reptiles, protein levels of 15–40% dry matter have been suggested as adequate (Rendle, 2019). Deficiencies in amino acids in carnivorous reptiles and the amphibians are extremely rare because they eat whole vertebrate/invertebrate prey. This gives them 30–60% protein content as metabolisable energy. Herbivorous species may experience deficiencies in specific amino acids, although these are not well documented.

In general, waste products of protein metabolism in land-based reptiles are converted into the relatively insoluble uric acid. Alligators may produce ammonia as the waste product, as may many amphibians, depending on their state of hydration, but adult frogs may excrete urea. Protein excesses, such as those produced by feeding cat or dog foods to predominantly herbivorous species, can lead to excess production of uric acid, which may result in visceral gout, renal failure and death.

Fats and essential fatty acids

Fats provide high concentrations of energy. They also supply the reptile or amphibian with essential fatty acids (EFAs), which are required for cellular integrity and as the building blocks for internal chemicals such as prostaglandins (which play a part in reproduction and inflammation). Fats also provide a carrier mechanism for the absorption of fat-soluble vitamins such as vitamins A, D, E and K.

The primary EFA for reptiles is linoleic acid, as it is for mammals, with the absolute dietary requirement of this fatty acid being 1% of the diet. If the diet becomes deficient in linoleic acid, a rapid decline in cellular integrity occurs. This is manifested clinically by the skin becoming flaky, inelastic and prone to recurrent infections and also to fluid loss through the skin, which in turn leads to polydipsia (Wallach and Hoff, 1982a,b).

In herbivores, less than 10% of the diet on a dry matter basis is composed of fats, the chief energy sources being carbohydrates and proteins. However, fermentation of fibre in the lower bowel produces short-chain fatty acids that can be used for energy.

For carnivores, fat forms a major part of the energy source in the diet (as much as 40–70% of the calories), with protein chiefly making up the rest. It is assumed that strict carnivores such as snakes cannot manufacture arachidonic acid, similar to the situation in strict mammalian carnivores, and so this must be present in the diet. However, as they eat whole vertebrate prey it is unlikely such a deficiency will occur.

The problem of overconsumption of fats in pet reptiles which are not exercising regularly is well known, and high-fat foods such as dog and cat food fed to herbivores, or extremely fat rodent prey fed to snakes, are prime culprits for this. Obesity can lead to a number of problems, the most frequent of which is fatty degenerative change in the liver (hepatic lipidosis), which can lead to liver failure. This is particularly common in tortoises. Varanids (monitor lizards) are more active than many reptiles and have higher energy and fat requirements but are still prone to obesity in captivity.

Carbohydrates

Carbohydrates are primarily used for rapid energy production. This is particularly important in herbivores which consume plant matter only, and so gain the majority of their energy source from carbohydrates and proteins. Typical values for carbohydrates (including fibre) for herbivorous reptiles are around 55–75% of the diet, with crude fibre being between 15 and 40% depending on the species (Rendle, 2019).

Carnivorous reptiles do not utilise carbohydrates much at all, making blood glucose from proteins (gluconeogenesis) in a similar fashion to carnivorous mammals. Complex carbohydrates (fibre) are important for herbivores.

Omnivorous reptiles may have a carbohydrate range of 20–75% of the diet but there is significant variation within the trophic group. Many require less fibre than the strict herbivores, and more in the way of leafy greens.

Fibre

Dietary fibre is extremely important for herbivorous reptiles. Indeed, the presence of fibre acts both as a bulking agent, encouraging gut motility, and as a source for fermentation by the intestinal microflora, essential for fatty acid and B vitamin production. Snakes and other strict carnivores do not have a dietary fibre requirement, and indeed if provided with fibre it will not be utilised. Ultimately in carnivores, fibre will dilute the energy concentration of the diet, necessitating feeding more frequent and larger meals. Many of the grassland chelonia, for example leopard tortoises (*Stigmochelys pardalis*) and African spurred tortoises (*Geochelone sulcata*), have a particularly high requirement for dietary fibre, typically 50–60% of the dietary intake. Green iguanas in colonies often have moderate numbers of intestinal nematodes of the pinworm family (Oxyuridae) and there is a suggestion that these nematodes also help in the utilisation of fibre by the iguana (Iverson, 1980). Adequate fibre in herbivorous reptiles is therefore important, although excessive levels may lead to reduced growth through reduced energy and protein intake. This has been reported in juvenile green iguanas if neutral detergent fibre levels exceed 24% as dry matter with 29% protein (Baer et al., 1997).

Vitamins

These compounds are grouped together although they are widely differing in nature, but all animals have a requirement for various numbers of these. They are categorised into fat-soluble (vitamins A, D, E and K) and water-soluble (the B vitamin complex and vitamin C).

Fat-soluble vitamins

Vitamin A: In herbivorous reptiles, beta-carotene is the most important plant precursor in terms of how much vitamin A can be produced from it. Carnivorous reptiles and amphibians will gain the preformed vitamin A in their prey food and cannot convert beta-carotene to vitamin A.

Hypovitaminosis A is a frequently seen problem in chelonians, particularly in tortoises and young red-eared terrapins. If a deficiency in vitamin A occurs, then mucous membranes become thickened and oral and respiratory secretions dry up. This is due to blockage of salivary and mucous glands with cellular debris, a condition known as squamous metaplasia. This leads to poor functioning of the ciliary mechanisms that have a role in removing foreign particles from the airways. Swelling of the periorbital membranes and failure of the tear glands to produce tears may also be seen, a condition known as xerophthalmia (Figure 20.2).

Vitamin A's role in immune system function means that a deficiency makes respiratory and digestive tract infections more common. The most frequently seen example of this is the increased susceptibility to pneumonias seen in semi-aquatic carnivorous chelonians and can present as a turtle that adopts a lopsided position when swimming. This is because of lung collapse or congestion which reduces buoyancy on the affected side.

Tortoises may suffer more frequently from upper respiratory tract infections when a deficiency is present. Evidence of sterile pustules and cornified plaques inside the mouth are commonly seen, with overgrowth of the beak due to hyperkeratosis (Figure 20.3).

Vitamin A also has a role in bone growth and structure, the normal function of secretory glands such as the adrenals and also in reproductive function. Finally, renal damage may occur in hypovitaminosis A, with evidence of oedema in the inguinal and axillary regions secondary to failure of the renal tubular filtration system.

Because it is fat soluble, vitamin A can be stored in the body, primarily in the liver. Recommended minimum dietary levels are 200–300 IU/kg for most reptiles (Wallach and Hoff 1982a,b). Abate *et al.* (2003) suggested vitamin A doses of 1000–2000 IU/kg per week in panther chameleons. Carnivores may need higher levels and Allen and Oftedal (1994) suggest dietary levels of 5000–10 000 IU/kg dry matter of food fed.

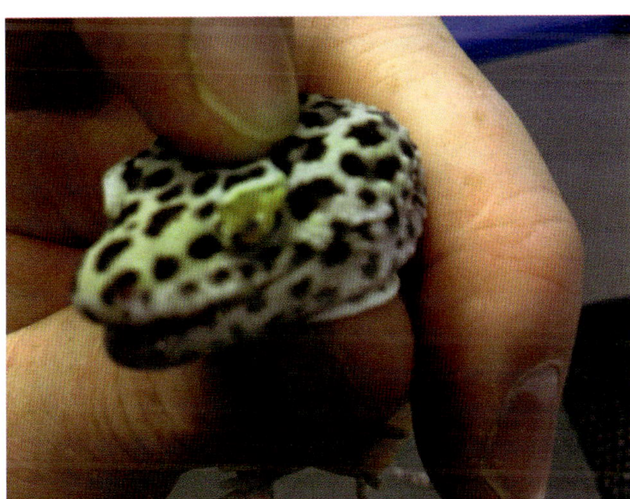

Figure 20.2 Hypovitaminosis A can result in squamous metaplasia of many epithelial structures including the tear glands. The latter can result in 'dry-eye' with conjunctivitis, keratitis and build-up of fibrinous material in the eye aperture as seen here in a leopard gecko (*Eublepharis macularius*).

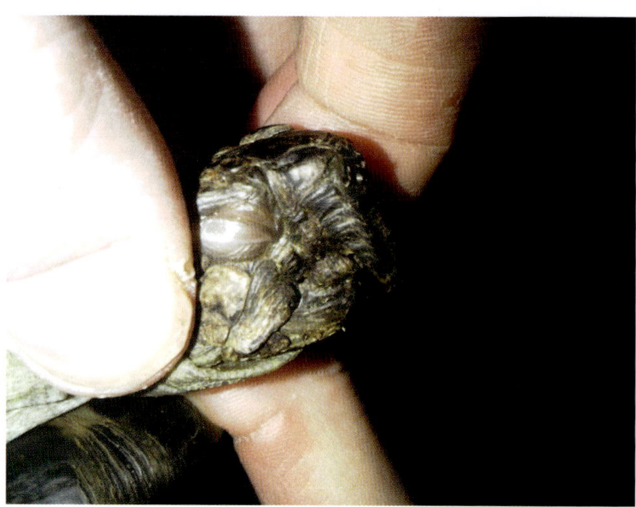

Figure 20.3 Hyperkeratosis of the 'beak' of chelonians can occur due to a number of conditions including hypovitaminosis A, high-protein diets and lack of abrasive surfaces to eat off.

Hypervitaminosis A rarely occurs naturally but may be induced by overdosing with vitamin A injections at 1000 times or more the daily recommended doses. If this occurs, acute toxicity develops, with mucous membrane and skin sloughing and frequently death within 24–48 hours. Vitamin A supplements are therefore often given orally as, due to slower absorption, this reduces the risk of this condition developing.

Vitamin D: Vitamin D_3 is the most active form for calcium homeostasis, and plants are not effective as suppliers of this compound, with leafy greens tending to contain ergocalciferol (also known as vitamin D_2).

Cholecalciferol (vitamin D_3) is manufactured in herbivorous and many omnivorous reptile's skin from a precursor (7-dehydrocholesterol) in a process controlled by ultraviolet (UV)-B light and heat. Carnivorous reptiles tend to get their vitamin D_3 preformed from consumed animal tissues. Cholecalciferol must then be activated, first in the liver (to become 25-hydroxycholecalciferol) and then by the kidneys (to become 1,25-dihydroxycholecalciferol), before it becomes fully functional as a hormone important for calcium metabolism (calcitriol). It works with parathyroid hormone to increase reabsorption of calcium at the expense of phosphorus from the kidneys. It also increases absorption of calcium from the intestines and mobilises calcium from the bone, increasing the blood's calcium levels. UV-B provision is a vital component of vitamin D_3 synthesis in many reptiles and even species viewed as crepuscular, such as the leopard gecko, still benefit from UV-B lighting, albeit at a much lower intensity than basking species such as pancake tortoises.

Hypovitaminosis D_3 causes problems with calcium metabolism and leads to a form of metabolic bone disease. This is exacerbated by low calcium, high phosphorus-containing diets. A typical scenario would be seen in a young growing herbivorous reptile, kept indoors with no UV-B light supplementation and fed on a low-calcium diet (e.g. lettuce, celery, cucumber) for herbivores. The situation can be seen in carnivores fed only skeletal meat or a poor calcium/vitamin D_3-containing diet such as unsupplemented invertebrates such as mealworms and waxworms or day-old chicks or very young rodents.

An animal so affected can appear 'well-muscled', due to poorly mineralised bones which increase their thickness to maintain their strength. There is often flaring of the epiphyseal plates at the ends of the long bones, with concomitant bowing of the limbs due to the lack of skeletal mineralisation. Green iguanas and other herbivorous species such as chelonian *Testudo* spp. are particularly susceptible, with the lizards showing rachitic rosettes due to flaring of the epiphyses in the ribs at the costochondral junction (Frye, 1991). Chelonia develop 'lumpy shell', a deformity of the carapace in particular, where the edges roll upwards creating a 'Cornish pasty' effect, and the muscles which attach the limbs to the inside of the shell pull the carapace downwards creating pits either side cranially and caudally.

However, shell pyramiding in chelonia is often more complicated, with other factors playing a role:

1. High environmental temperatures (particularly focal hotspots of narrow diameter)
2. High dietary protein
3. Low calcium, vitamin D_3 and UV-B
4. Reduced humidity causing the keratin to dry out.

In African spurred tortoises, low relative humidity had some of the most significant effects on pyramiding along with a smaller positive effect associated with high protein levels (Wiesner and Iben, 2002).

Recommended vitamin D_3 levels for adults are 50–100 IU/kg every other day. Allen and Oftedal (1994) recommend dietary levels of 500–1000 IU/kg of dry matter fed for carnivorous reptiles. It should be noted that vitamin D_3 as cholecalciferol is always preferred as an oral supplement over vitamin D_2 (ergocalciferol), as although the latter can be converted into the active calcitriol, it is much less effective.

Hypervitaminosis D_3 occurs due to oversupplementation with D_3 and calcium and leads to calcification of soft tissues, such as the medial wall of the arteries, and the kidneys, creating hypertension and organ failure. This can occur in herbivores such as *Testudo* spp. fed on tinned cat and dog food. A maximum dosage has been suggested of 5000 IU/kg dry matter of food fed (Donoghue, 2006).

Vitamin E: Hypovitaminosis E may occur due to a reduction in fat metabolism or absorption, such as can occur in small intestinal, pancreatic or biliary diseases, or due to a lack of dietary green plant material for herbivores. A relative deficiency will occur in species eating large amounts of polyunsaturated fats (e.g. marine fish such as tuna and mackerel). These use up the body's vitamin E reserves. A condition called steatitis, wherein body fat starts to necrose, has been seen in gharials (a fish-eating crocodilian) (Frye, 1991) and terrapins.

Recommended levels are approximately 1 IU/kg dry matter food fed (20–80 mg/kg). Note that ratios of vitamins A, D and E in human supplements typically follow a pattern of 100 : 10 : 1 as interactions between the three can alter their efficacy and toxicity.

Hypervitaminosis E is extremely rare

Vitamin K: Because of its production by gut bacteria, it is very difficult to get a true deficiency, although absorption will be reduced when fat digestion or absorption is reduced, as in biliary or pancreatic disease. The consumption of warfarin- and coumarin-derived compounds (as found in sweet clovers) can increase the demand for clotting factors, and this may also be seen in snakes consuming prey which has consumed rodenticides. Disease so caused is characterised by increased internal and external haemorrhage, but vitamin K also has some function in calcium/phosphorus metabolism in bone so this may also be affected. Frye (1991) has recorded disease in crocodiles exhibiting gingival bleeding without petechiation. Recommended minimum levels for reptiles are 1 ppm (Wallach and Hoff 1982a,b).

Water-soluble vitamins

Vitamin B_1 (thiamine): Deficiencies can occur in two ways. The most common is when presented with a significant source of thiaminases, enzymes which destroy thiamine, in the diet. Examples of such foods include raw saltwater fish, which may be fed to some snakes, crocodilians and turtles, for example garter snakes, red-eared terrapins and gharials. Thiaminases are increased in fish that has been frozen for a period of time and then defrosted. The second way is associated with the thiamine antagonists that can be found in foods such as blackberries, beetroot, coffee, chocolate and tea and may be occasionally seen in herbivores fed such foods. When a relative deficiency occurs, neurological signs such as opisthotonus, weakness and head tremors may be seen. In garter and water snakes, a classical inability to right itself occurs, with the snake continually flipping onto its back. In addition, fungal infections are reported as more likely after a B_1 deficiency. The recommended minimum level for reptiles is 20–35 mg/kg food offered. In addition, if sea fish such as smelt, which are particularly high in thiaminases, are to be fed, cooking the fish for 5 minutes at 80°C deactivates the thiaminase. In a reptile with thiamine deficiency, doses of 50–100 mg/kg body weight should be given. To avoid the problem altogether it is often advised that garter and water snakes are fed on rodent prey rather than sea fish. They may be encouraged to eat this by wiping the rodent prey with the fish to which it is accustomed to cover the scent. Care should be taken to avoid excessive amounts of fully furred rodent prey for such species as this can lead to constipation.

Biotin: Deficiencies do occur, commonly in Gila monsters, beaded lizards and monitor lizards, all of which enjoy raw eggs in the wild. In the wild the majority of eggs are fertile and contain little avidin (an anti-biotin vitamin). However, unfertilised hen's eggs are high in avidin so a relative biotin deficiency may occur. Deficiencies produce muscular weakness, occasionally with skin lesions. It is therefore recommended that minimal levels of raw eggs are fed to such reptiles.

Folic acid: A deficiency of folic acid is rare but can lead to severely impaired cellular division. This can lead to the failure of maturation of female reptile's reproductive tracts, macrocytic anaemia due to failure of red blood cell maturation, and immune system cellular dysfunction. A relative deficiency of folic acid may occur in some individuals fed a very high protein diet, as folic acid is needed to produce uric acid, the waste product of protein metabolism in the majority of reptiles. In addition, there are inhibitors of folic acid in some foods, such as cabbage and other brassicas, oranges, beans and peas. The use of trimethoprim sulfonamide drugs also reduces gut bacterial folic acid production.

Vitamin B_{12}: Vitamin B_{12} is generally produced by intestinal bacteria and so deficiencies are uncommon but may occur after prolonged antibiotic medication. Deficiency produces slow growth, muscular dystrophy in the legs, poor hatching rates, high mortality rates and hatching deformities in young reptiles and amphibians.

Choline: Choline may be synthesised in the body, but not in sufficient quantities for the growing reptile. Because of interactions, the need for choline is dependent on levels of folic acid and vitamin B_{12}. Excess protein, as with folic acid, therefore increases choline requirements, as does a diet high in fats. Deficiency causes retarded growth, disrupted fat metabolism and fatty liver damage.

Vitamin C: There is no direct dietary need for this vitamin in reptiles and amphibians as vitamin C may be produced from glucose in the outermost portions of the kidneys. However, during disease processes, particularly those which affect liver function, it may be beneficial to the recovery process to provide a dietary source of vitamin C. It is required for the formation of elastic fibres and connective tissues and is an excellent antioxidant similar to vitamin E. Deficiency leads to scurvy, in which there is poor wound healing, increased bleeding due to capillary wall fragility and bone alterations. Deficiency has been postulated as the cause of skin splitting in snakes fed rodent prey that had been starved for 24–48 hours before being fed (Frye, 1991). This allowed the emptying of their gastrointestinal tract, and hence reduced levels of vitamin C from the plant material therein. It has also been suggested that increasing vitamin C levels by supplementation at 10–20 mg/kg intramuscularly or orally (Frye, 1991) may be useful in the treatment of chronic infections, such as 'mouth rot' in snakes.

Minerals

As with mammals, there are two main groups of minerals: macrominerals (i.e. those present in large amounts in the body, such as calcium and phosphorus) and microminerals, or trace elements (e.g. manganese, iron and cobalt), which are all necessary for normal bodily function.

Macrominerals

Calcium: Calcium has a wide range of bodily functions, the two most obvious being its role in the formation of the skeleton and mineralisation of bone matrix, and its requirement for muscular contractions. The active form of calcium in the body is the ionic double charged molecule Ca^{2+}. Low levels of this form, even though the overall body reserves of calcium are normal, leads to hyperexcitability, fitting and death, conditions commonly seen for example in gravid female egg-bound green iguanas.

The ratio of calcium to phosphorus in the diet is important: as one increases, the levels of the other decreases and vice versa. Calcium levels in the blood are controlled by the hormones calcitonin and parathyroid hormone and the accessory hormone vitamin D_3. A dietary ratio of 2 : 1 calcium to phosphorus is desirable in growing reptiles and 1.5 : 1 for adults. In high egg-laying periods in oviparous species, to keep pace with the output of calcium into the shells, a dietary ratio of 10 : 1 may be needed.

Calcium deficiency causes nutritional osteodystrophy, or metabolic bone disease, and is often accompanied by a deficiency in vitamin D_3. However, normal levels of vitamin D_3 in the presence of low dietary calcium ironically may exacerbate this disease once it is present as they encourage further calcium resorption. Dietary calcium deficiency may be seen in lizards such as green iguanas and herbivorous chelonians fed on diets high in mineral-poor fruit, lettuce, celery, etc. Diets with excessive levels of oxalates, compounds which bind calcium and prevent it being absorbed, such as spinach and beetroot or rhubarb leaves, can also lead to a deficiency. Ideally for herbivorous reptiles the feeding of leafy greens with a good calcium content is advised (e.g. chard, dandelion leaves, watercress, spring greens, kale, nasturtium leaves), although supplementation of leaves with a dusting powder containing calcium, vitamin D_3 and other minerals and vitamins can also be performed.

Calcium deficiency may also be seen in insectivorous species, such as geckos, and bearded dragons, fed on insects without supplementation. Insects commonly fed in captivity (crickets, waxworms, mealworms, etc.) have little or no calcium, their tough outer coat being made of a protein known as chitin. Consequently, to provide adequate calcium the insect should be fed a calcium supplement (often with other minerals and vitamins) prior to the insect itself being fed to the reptile. This is mixed in with the insect's food and fed for the 24–48 hours before feeding the reptile, so that the insect's gut is preloaded with calcium. An alternative is to use a dusting powder containing calcium on the insects immediately prior to feeding, but this has a habit of falling off the insect and so is less effective.

Extensive resorption of calcium occurs from the bones during dietary deficiencies, leaving only fibrous tissue. This is considerably weaker and so the 'bones' thicken their diameter to maintain their strength. Even so, the bones are weakened, and bowing of long bones and spontaneous fractures can occur in lizards, the collapse of spinal vertebrae and deformities can occur in most reptiles, and deformed lumpy shells can occur in chelonians.

Excessive calcium in the diet (>1–2% as dry matter) reduces the use of proteins, fats, phosphorus, manganese, zinc, iron and iodine, and can lead to soft tissue mineralisation if in conjunction with adequate or excessive vitamin D_3 levels. Newly hatched and therefore growing red-eared terrapins have been shown to have a requirement for 2% calcium on a dry matter basis with 0.5% being insufficient even though all diets had 1.2% phosphorus and, as mentioned, ideally any diet should have a 2 : 1 calcium to phosphorus ratio for growing animals (Kass *et al.*, 1982).

Phosphorus: Phosphorus is widespread in plant and animal tissues, but in the former it may be bound up in unavailable form as phytates. Levels of phosphorus are controlled in the body as for calcium, the two being in equal and opposite equilibrium with each other. Therefore, if dietary phosphorus levels exceed calcium levels appreciably, the parathyroid glands become stimulated to produce more parathyroid hormone and nutritional secondary hyperparathyroidism occurs. This leads to progressive bone demineralisation and renal damage due to high circulating levels of parathyroid hormone. High dietary phosphorus also reduces the amount of calcium which can be absorbed from the gut, as it complexes with the calcium present there, particularly as phytates. This can be a problem in reptiles fed pure meat with no calcium or bone supplement, and in herbivores which are predominantly fruit and lettuce consumers, as these are high-phosphorus, low-calcium foods. Green vegetables or supplementation with calcium powders may therefore be necessary. In addition, low-calcium/high-phosphorus levels frequently allow bladder stones to form in those species (such as chelonians, green iguanas) that have a urinary bladder.

Magnesium: Most magnesium is absorbed from the small intestine and is affected by large amounts of calcium in the diet which reduce magnesium absorption. Deficiencies rarely occur, but muscular weakness can be the result.

Potassium: As with mammals, potassium is the major intracellular positive ion. Rarely is there a dietary deficiency, but severe stress can cause hypokalaemia through increased kidney excretion because of elevated plasma proteins. This can lead to cardiac dysrhythmias, muscle spasticity and neurological dysfunction.

Sodium: Sodium is the main extracellular positive ion and regulates the body's acid–base balance and osmotic potential. In conjunction with potassium, it is responsible for nerve signals and impulses. Rarely does a true dietary deficiency occur, but hyponatraemia may occur due to chronic diarrhoea or renal disease. Many reptiles have salt glands found outside the kidneys, responsible solely for the excretion of excess sodium whilst conserving water. For example, the marine iguana's salt glands are present inside the nostrils, and white crystalline deposits of salt may be seen here and are frequently sneezed out. It may be necessary to supplement the diet of marine species with sodium chloride if kept in freshwater situations, or if fed freshwater plants or fish.

Chlorine: This is the major extracellular negative ion and is responsible for maintaining acid–base balance in conjunction with sodium and potassium. Deficiencies are rare.

Microminerals (trace elements)

These elements include zinc, copper, iron, manganese, cobalt and sulphur, all of which have an important part to play in cellular function. However, so far, no actual deficiencies specifically related to these elements have been reported in reptiles or amphibians. The exception is iodine.

Iodine: Iodine's sole function is in thyroid hormone synthesis, which affects metabolic rate. Deficiency causes goitre and fluid retention (myxoedema). It has knock-on effects on growth, causing stunting and neurological problems and in amphibians may prevent metamorphosis from intermediate tadpole stages to the adult form. In reptiles it is most often encountered in giant terrestrial tortoises, which will exhibit goitre swelling of the neck. It can also occur due to overfeeding with iodine-binding plants, such as cabbage, cauliflower, broccoli, kale and Brussel sprouts (brassicas). Excess iodine added to the water may cause species such as the amphibian axolotl (a neotenic salamander, i.e. its 'adult' form has the external gills more typical of a tadpole or intermediate life stage) to shed its external gills. Levels of 0.3 mg/kg body weight have been quoted (Donoghue and Langenburg, 1996).

Specific nutritional problems in reptiles

Below are some common presentations of nutritional problems in reptiles.

Post-hibernation (brumation) anorexia

Post-hibernation anorexia, or often now referred to as post-brumation anorexia (PBA), is seen most commonly in the Mediterranean *Testudo* species of tortoise (Hermann's, Greek or spur-thighed, marginated and Horsfield's), which brumate during the colder months of the year. The commonest presentation is that of an inappetant tortoise after coming out of brumation/hibernation, often with signs of systemic or respiratory tract infections (e.g. 'runny nose syndrome') and often with a low body weight in relation to length (a low Jackson's ratio). In addition, the blood glucose levels are frequently below 3.2 mmol/L, which appears to be the minimum level required for appetite stimulation, with high levels of urea and often leukopenia (Lawrence, 1987). More severe cases often have evidence of renal disease with elevated uric acid and potassium levels. Many have become ketoacidotic with the production of ketones such as beta-hydroxybutyrate.

Dehydration is apparent in these cases, and treatment requires aggressive fluid therapy and nutritional support, using glucose-containing fluids and liquid food stomach tubing, as well as warming the tortoise to its preferred body temperature.

Causes of this condition could involve any one of the following:

- Disease during or prior to hibernation
- Poor nutrition leading to poor fat reserves prior to hibernation
- Owner failure to observe recovery from brumation/hibernation for several days, so no food or sufficient heat offered at the critical time, or
- A period of cold weather immediately after recovery.

It is the rising plane of blood glucose after hibernation that acts as the stimulus for appetite in these chelonians, and failure of this rise, due to malnutrition or failure to eat whilst the levels are still high, may lead to a subsequent unresponsive anorexia.

To prevent PBA, therefore, it is important to treat any disease prior to hibernation, and if severely affected or underweight, the tortoise should not be brumated/hibernated, but kept indoors at its optimum temperature range and fed throughout the winter. The tortoise should also be checked regularly during brumation/hibernation, around once or twice a week, to ensure that if it does come out early, it has food and water and sufficient heat available immediately. Bathing the tortoise immediately after waking in warm water, cleaning the nose, eyes and mouth especially can also stimulate appetite, and no tortoise having recovered from brumation/hibernation should be allowed to re-hibernate that same winter. If not voluntarily eating and/or evidence of dehydration is seen, then correction of fluid deficits with intravenous or intraosseous fluid therapy and nutritional support via stomach tubing/oesophagostomy feeding with a commercially available reptile critical care herbivore support formula should be initiated.

Visceral and articular gout

Gout is a condition caused by the unique way that many reptiles deal with the waste products of protein metabolism. Most reptiles are uricotelic – the main excretory product of protein metabolism is uric acid. This compound is relatively insoluble in water, which has its advantages as reptiles are therefore able to reduce the water lost in excreting it. Unfortunately, if the reptile becomes significantly dehydrated (either acutely or chronically) or consumes diets with excessive levels of protein (particularly those containing high levels of purines) or suffers functional kidney damage, then uric acid levels build up in the bloodstream. If allowed to do so, they will eventually exceed the precipitation point and form crystals inside the body.

Diet is important, as purines, which are found mainly in animal protein, are converted readily to uric acid on degradation in the body. Therefore, if herbivorous species, such as green iguanas, which are not used to large volumes of purines, are fed a diet rich in animal protein, such as cat or dog food, they will produce excessive amounts of uric acid and develop gout.

There are two presentations of gout commonly seen: visceral and articular. Articular gout can more easily be diagnosed ante-mortem, as it often causes gross swelling and inflammation in the joints where the uric acid crystals form. Visceral gout is more difficult to diagnose ante-mortem early on, because it occurs where uric acid crystals are deposited in the soft tissues of the body, primary sites of visceral gout deposition being the kidneys, pericardial sac, lungs, spleen and liver. Once deposited, it is almost impossible to move the crystals medically and permanent damage is often done.

Obesity

Obesity is a common problem in many reptiles and amphibians kept in captivity. Many species are overfed because of owner ignorance of natural feeding amounts and intervals and also of food types commonly eaten in the wild. Examples include feeding dog food to *Testudo* spp. of tortoises and green iguanas, both of which are almost totally herbivorous in the wild but both of which will eat meat if offered it. The resulting problems are, as mentioned above, with excess protein causing gout, excess calcium and vitamin D_3 causing soft tissue mineralisation, and excess animal fat causing fatty liver syndrome (hepatic lipidosis) wherein the liver cells are filled with fat deposits impeding their function (Figure 20.4). Bearded dragons change their dietary preferences as they age in the wild, moving from predominantly insect orientated to

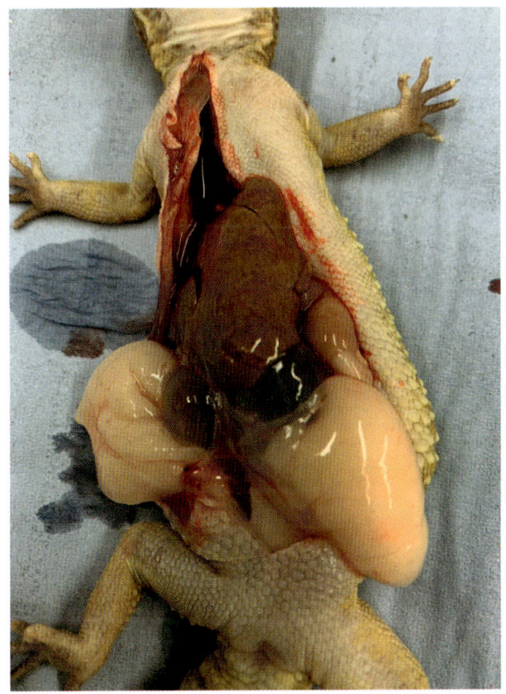

Figure 20.4 Post-mortem of a leopard gecko (*Eublepharis macularius*) with hepatic lipodosis. Note the prominent coelomic fat pads and the tan/pale-coloured liver.

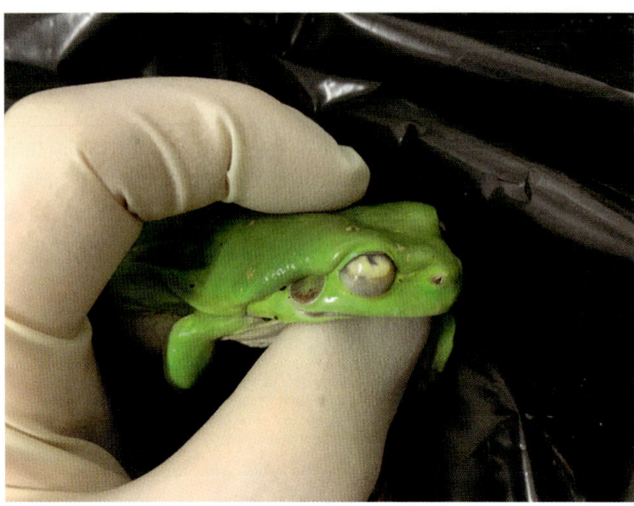

Figure 20.5 Corneal lipidosis is seen in many amphibians and reptiles where higher than required levels of cholesterol-containing fats and calories are consumed.

Table 20.2 Feeding frequencies and food types for various reptile species.

Species	Feeding frequencies and food types
Herbivores (e.g. iguanas, tortoises)	Daily grazing of food advised
Small insectivores (e.g. leopard geckos, collared lizards)	Fed two to three times weekly on live insect prey, supplemented with mineral/vitamins
Small carnivores (e.g. garter snakes, corn snakes)	Fed once to twice weekly on rat pups, fuzzies (furred baby mice) or pinkies (nude baby mice) up to adult mice according to size. Try not to feed anything more than 50% the maximum width of the snake
Medium carnivores (e.g. kingsnakes, rat snakes)	Fed once weekly to once every 2 weeks, adult mice or small rats according to size. Try not to feed anything more than 50% the maximum width of the snake
Large carnivores (e.g. boa constrictors, Burmese pythons)	Fed once weekly or fortnightly (the larger the snake, the less often) on adult rats or small rabbits. Try not to feed anything more than 50% the maximum width of the snake Large adult pythons (such as Burmese) may require feeding only once every 5–6 weeks Large boas (such as boa constrictors) may require feeding once every 4–5 weeks

predominantly leafy greens as adults. However, they will readily accept invertebrates as adults and can easily become obese. Snakes also suffer from these conditions when fed overly fatty laboratory rodents, or simply fed too often. A reptile has on average one-seventh the energy requirements, gram per gram, of a placental mammal. Amphibians and reptiles may develop corneal lipidosis when fed higher than required calories due to the amount of fats containing cholesterols (Figure 20.5). A rough idea of feeding frequencies is given in Table 20.2.

The aim should be a reptile which does not appear emaciated, but lean.

Hypoglycaemia in crocodilians

It has been reported that crocodiles kept in high-density conditions, or are otherwise stressed, are prone to hypoglycaemic fits (Scott, 1992). It is interesting to note that blood sugar levels of crocodiles vary throughout the year, being lowest in the winter and highest in the summer. A rising blood sugar level appears to be the stimulus to eat, as seems to be seen with Mediterranean tortoises after hibernation.

Environmental temperature and its effects on nutrition

Because reptiles and amphibians are ectothermic and rely on their surroundings to maintain their body temperature, environmental temperature is important in all aspects of husbandry.

There is an optimum preferred temperature zone that will allow them to maintain their preferred body temperature at which their enzymes and metabolic pathways function at optimum levels, so environmental temperature will influence the rate of digestion of the food offered. It may take 2–3 days for a rat consumed by a large boa constrictor to pass through its digestive system if kept within its preferred temperature zone of 25–30°C, but if kept 5–10°C cooler this will often slow down to 5–7 days, and if kept much lower than this, digestion may not occur before the prey item becomes rancid inside the snake. Similarly, if kept at too high a temperature, the reptile may not be stimulated to eat at all and dehydration and heat stress may set in.

A general guide to feeding reptiles

Fresh food should always be fed to reptiles. It should also be remembered that at the increased temperatures of most vivaria, the food offered will spoil very quickly and will need to be replaced frequently.

Snakes

It is important to note that it is technically illegal to feed live vertebrate prey to another animal in some countries. It is recommended therefore to maintain animal welfare that all rodent prey fed to snakes and lizards should be humanely killed prior to feeding. In addition, live prey may damage the reptile if the latter is not hungry and does not kill the prey quickly.

To encourage anorectic snakes to eat, a number of tricks may be employed.

- Warm the defrosted vertebrate prey briefly before offering or feeding fresh recently killed vertebrate prey.
- Break the prey item open to release the scent of blood.
- Tease the snake by moving the dead prey item around the cage with forceps, to mimic live prey movements.
- Try a variety of pelage colours of prey – some snakes will only take dark-furred rodents.
- To get a snake (e.g. garter or water snake) used to eating rodent prey after only eating fish or amphibians (hog-nosed snakes), wipe the rodent to be offered with the previously taken food item to transfer scent.
- Ensure that there are plenty of areas to hide; some boids and pythons like to consume their prey in a box or hide.
- Leave the prey in overnight because some species prefer to hunt at night.
- Choose the next smallest size of rodent, so if adult mice were previously offered try fuzzies; if juvenile rats, try adult mice, etc.

Note that the term 'pinkies' refers to nude neonatal rat and mice pups, 'fuzzies' refers to week-old rat and mice pups with a thin covering of fur, and 'furries' refers to juvenile rat and mice pups between 1 and 3 weeks of age which have a soft but longer covering of fur. Even mildly dehydrated snakes can become constipated if fed heavily furred rodents as the fur is indigestible.

Refeeding syndrome

If anorexia in a snake or other reptile has persisted for some time, it is essential to rehydrate the patient before attempting to feed. Indeed, initial feeding after this should be started off at very low levels and gradually built up over several weeks. This is because excess calories and proteins once absorbed from the gut will then result in a rapid uptake of glucose from the bloodstream into the tissue cells, which also takes potassium and phosphorus with it. After a prolonged period of anorexia, whole-body levels of potassium and phosphorus can be reduced and therefore this can lead to a life-threatening hypokalaemia and hypophosphataemia in the bloodstream that in turn can result in serious cardiac arrhythmias and potential failure. The monitoring of blood phosphorus and potassium is therefore to be recommended when treating chronically anorectic reptiles, whether carnivores or herbivores.

Herbivores

Commercial pelleted diets are a useful adjunct to the diet of herbivorous reptiles and many commercial companies now produce iguanid and chelonian diets that are well supplemented with minerals and vitamins and also contain moderate levels of fibre for gut motility enhancement. If using a commercial pelleted food for herbivorous reptiles such as iguanas or land-based tortoises, then be sure to soak the pellets thoroughly before feeding, otherwise they can swell up inside the reptile causing colic and bloat.

The feeding of certain foods to strict herbivores should be controlled or prevented. Animal proteins (because they cause increased uric acid production) and certain fruit and vegetables can be problematic to strict herbivores. We have already discussed the problems of excessive volumes of largely water-containing vegetables such as lettuce, cucumber and celery, the goitrogenic properties of cabbage, kale, broccoli and cauliflower, and the anti-calcium effect of oxalate-containing plants such as spinach, beetroot and rhubarb leaves. In addition, fruits such as banana can cause a sugar ferment in herbivorous reptiles causing colic, as well as adhering to the mouthparts and encouraging local infection and dental disease. Avocados have an extremely high fat content and should not be fed to herbivorous reptiles due to potential secondary fatty degeneration of the liver.

Sample diet for green iguanas

If pelleted soaked commercial food is to be fed, then it should not exceed 25% of daily food intake. Alternatively, a typical fresh diet would be as follows (Rendle 2019):

1. 32% winter squash, red pepper, sweet potato, parsnip (provides calories, low oxalates and good vitamins A and C but the squash may need to be steamed or microwaved to soften before feeding)
2. 24% green beans and peas providing protein and fibre
3. 16% alfalfa (lucerne) hay providing good protein, fibre and calcium
4. 15% leafy greens such as dandelions, watercress, spring greens, cabbage, kale, nasturtium leaves as well as dandelion, nasturtium and rose flowers providing fibre and water
5. 4% fruit such as raspberry, blueberry, fig, melon, etc. providing enrichment/palatability, antioxidants (and in the case of figs calcium) but watch for diarrhoea and oral infections due to sugars and bacterial fermentation. Some recommend feeding a lower level (1–2%) of fruit to avoid this.

This combination should be thoroughly mixed so as to prevent selective feeding, and to it should be added a supplement of calcium in the form of calcium lactate or gluconate. In addition, the use of a vitamin D_3/calcium supplement once or twice a week, particularly for growing iguanas and egg-laying females, is advised as well as access to suitable UV-B lighting/basking areas.

Sample diet for *Testudo* spp. tortoises

The majority of the diet is to be composed of vegetable matter of a leafy nature such as dandelions, kale, watercress, land cress, flat-leaved parsley, chicory and bok-choy. To this may be added pea leaves/pods, beans, hay or dried grass, fresh grass (not cut), alfalfa, grated carrot, grated pumpkin and sweet peppers. Interestingly in the wild, *Testudo graeca* has a leaf diet of 30% plantains (*Plantago* spp.), 26% daisies (Compositae) and 10% bedstraw plants (Rubiaceae). *Testudo hermannii* and *T. horsfieldii* have a wild-type diet of 25% Rubiaceae, 22% Leguminosae (pea flower family), 10% Compositae and 8% Ranunculaceae (buttercup family) (Rendle, 2019). Flowers such as dandelion, nasturtium and rose petals may also be well accepted.

To this may be added very small volumes of fruit (1% maximum) such as apples, pears, melon, papaya, passion fruit, strawberries and plums.

Other species of Chelonia

For more tropical species of Chelonia, such as the red- and yellow-footed tortoises (*Chelonoidis carbonarius* and *Chelonoidis denticulatus*), the amount of fruit and flowers may be doubled over that offered for *Testudo* spp.

For grassland species of Chelonia, such as leopard tortoises (*Stigmochelys pardalis*), African spurred tortoises (*Geochelone sulcata*) and Indian starred tortoises (*Geochelone elegans*), a good provision of fresh uncut grass or good-quality hay and alfalfa is advised and fruit generally excluded.

For more omnivorous species of Chelonia, such as box turtles (e.g. *Terrapene carolina*), up to 50% of the above vegetable diet may be replaced with adult maintenance dry dog foods (soaked), mealworms, crickets, earthworms and even baby mice (pinkies). Juveniles of this species tend to be more carnivorous than the adults.

In all of these diets it is recommended that daily supplementation with calcium lactate or gluconate be included, with a vitamin D_3 supplement added once or twice weekly depending on whether the tortoise is a juvenile (higher requirement) or an adult (lower requirement). Suitable UV-B provision is also required (see Chapter 18).

References

Abate, A.L., Coke, R., Ferguson, G. and Reavill, D. (2003) Roundtable: chameleons and vitamin A. *Journal of Herpetological Medicine and Surgery*, **13**(2), 23–31.

Allen, M.E. and Oftedal, O.T. (1994) The nutrition of carnivorous reptiles. In: *Captive Management and Conservation of Amphibians and Reptiles* (eds J.B. Murphy, K. Adler & J.T. Collins), pp. 71–83. Society for the Study of Amphibians and Reptiles, Ithaca NY.

Baer, D.J., Oftedal, O.T. and Rumpler, W.V. (1997) Dietary fibre influences nutrient utilization, growth and dry matter intake of green iguanas (*Iguana iguana*). *Journal of Nutrition*, **127**, 1501–1507.

Barboza, P.S. (1995) Digesta passage and functional anatomy of the digestive tract in the desert tortoise (*Xerobates agassizii*). *Journal of Comparative Physiology B*, **165**, 193–202.

Brand, M.D., Couture, P., Else, P.L. *et al.* (1991) Evolution of energy metabolism. *Biochemical Journal*, **275**, 81–86.

Donoghue, S. (1998) Nutrition of pet amphibians and reptiles. *Seminars in Avian and Exotic Pet Medicine*, **7**, 3.

Donoghue, S. (2006) Nutrition. In: *Reptile Medicine and Surgery* (ed. D. Mader), 2nd edn, pp. 287–288. Elsevier Saunders, St Louis, Missouri.

Donoghue, S. and Langenburg, J. (1996) Nutrition. In: *Reptile Medicine and Surgery* (ed. D. Mader), pp. 148–174. W.B. Saunders, Philadelphia, PA.

Donoghue, S., Vidal, J. and Kronfeld, D. (1998) Growth and morphometrics of green iguanas (*Iguana iguana*) fed four levels of dietary protein. *Journal of Nutrition*, **128**(12), S2587–S2589.

Frye, F. (1991) *Biomedical and Surgical Aspects of Captive Reptile Husbandry*, Volume 1 and 2. Krieger Publishing, Malabar, FL.

Galvao, P.E., Tarasantchi, J. and Guertzenstein, P. (1965) Heat production of tropical snakes in relation to body weight and body surface. *American Journal of Physiology*, **209**, 501–506.

Iverson, J.B. (1980) Colic modifications in Iguanine lizards. *Journal of Morphology*, **163**, 79–93.

Jackson, O.F. (1980) Weight and measurement data on tortoises (*Testudo graeca* and *Testudo hermanni*) and their relationship to health. *Journal of Small Animal Practice*, **21**(7), 409–416.

Kass, R.E., Ullrey, D.E. and Trapp, A.L. (1982) A study of calcium requirements of the red-eared slider turtle (*Pseudemys scripta elegans*). *Journal of Zoo Animal Medicine*, **13**, 62.

Lawrence, K. (1987) Post hibernational anorexia in captive Mediterranean tortoises (*Testudo graeca* and *T. hermanii*). *Veterinary Record*, **120**, 87.

Maxwell, L., Jacobson, E.R. and McNab, B.K. (2003) Intraspecific allometry of metabolic rate in green iguanas (*Iguana iguana*). *Comparative Biochemistry and Physiology A*, **136**(2), 310–310.

Minnich, J.E. (1982) The use of water. In: *Biology of the Reptilia, Volume 12* (eds C. Gans & F.H. Pough), pp. 323–395. Academic Press, London and New York.

Nagy, K.A. (1982) Energy requirements of free-living iguanid lizards. In: *Iguanas of the World* (eds G.M. Burghardt & A.S. Rand), pp. 49–59. Noyes Publications, Park Ridge, New Jersey.

Rendle, M. (2019) Nutrition. In: *BSAVA Manual of Reptiles* (eds S.J. Girling & P. Raiti), 3rd edn, pp. 49–69. BSAVA, Quedgeley, Glos.

Scott, P.W. (1992) Nutritional diseases. In: *Manual of Reptiles* (eds P.H. Beynon, M.P.C. Lawton & J.E. Cooper), pp. 138–152. BSAVA, Cheltenham, UK.

Secor, S.M. and Phillips, J.A. (1997) Specific dynamic action of a large carnivorous lizard, *Varanus albigularis*. *Comparative Biochemistry and Physiology A*, **117**, 515–522.

Sedgwick, C.J. (1993) Allometric scaling and emergency care: the importance of body size. In: *Zoo and Wild Animal Medicine* (ed. M.E. Fowler), 3rd edn, pp. 34–37. W. B, Saunders, Philadelphia, PA.

Thompson, G.G. and Withers, P.C. (1992) Effects of body mass and temperature on standard metabolic rates for two Australian Varanid lizards (*Varanus gouldii and V. panoptes*). *Copeia*, **1992**(2), 343–350.

Wallach, J.D. and Hoff, G.L. (1982a) Nutritional diseases of mammals. In: *Non-infectious Diseases of Wildlife* (eds G.L. Hoff & J.W. Davis), pp. 133–135. Iowa State University Press, Ames IA, 143–144.

Wallach, J.D. and Hoff, G.L. (1982b) Metabolic and nutritional diseases of reptiles. In: *Non-infectious Diseases of Wildlife* (eds G.L. Hoff & J.W. Davis), pp. 155–168. Iowa State University Press, Ames, IA.

Wiesner, C.S. and Iben, C. (2002) Influence of environmental humidity and dietary protein on pyramidal growth of carapaces in African spurred tortoises (*Geochelone sulcata*). *Journal of Animal Physiology and Animal Nutrition*, **87**, 66–74.

Chapter 21 Common Reptile and Amphibian Diseases

Skin disease

Ecdysis

The process of ecdysis involves the formation of a new skin beneath the old one. Once this is complete, a series of proteolytic enzymes and lymphatic fluid is secreted between the new skin layer and the overlying old one. This fluid lifts and separates the two layers, and makes the snake appear dull and lacklustre with the eyes noticeably bluing (see Figure 21.1). This lasts for 5–7 days on average in the snake. Once complete, the fluid is reabsorbed, and the snake appears to return to its normal hue. After a further 5–7 days the skin is shed, in the case of the snake in one whole go from the head end first. It is initiated in snakes by rubbing the face on an abrasive surface to loosen the first piece of skin. The regularity at which the process of ecdysis occurs depends on a number of factors:

1. Age of the reptile (younger animals shed more frequently as they are growing faster)
2. Nutritional status (high-protein and high-calorie diets increase the frequency of ecdysis)
3. Seasonal influences such as day length, humidity and temperature may all have an effect depending on the species involved.

When the separation fails to occur, whether in part or totally, the condition is known as dysecdysis.

Dysecdysis

Dysecdysis is when ecdysis fails. It can occur in any reptile but is most commonly observed in snakes and lizards (see Figure 21.2).

The causes of dysecdysis are many and varied and include any condition which can cause dehydration, so reducing lymphatic fluid available to separate the skin layers. If the reptile is malnourished, dysecdysis may occur due to a lack of proteolytic enzymes. Alternatively, old scars, a lack of an abrasive surface in the vivarium upon which to start the process or severe ectoparasitism may also cause dysecdysis.

Scale rot

Scale rot is a colloquial term for a range of conditions affecting the reptile skin which result in severe infections.

Septicaemic cutaneous ulcerative disease

Septicaemic cutaneous ulcerative disease (SCUD) is seen most often in semi-aquatic chelonians. *Citrobacter freundii* has been implicated which, once it has gained access to the bloodstream, produces ulcers in the skin and loosening of scales with debilitation and, in some cases, organ failure and death. Other bacteria such as *Pseudomonas* and *Aeromonas* spp. are also involved (see Figures 21.3 and 21.4).

Blister disease

This is a form of scale rot seen in semi-aquatic species such as garter or water snakes. It can, however, occur in any species exposed to a persistently damp substrate. The outer layer of skin develops blisters of a clear fluid which become secondarily infected with environmental bacteria such as *Aeromonas* spp., *Serratia* spp. or *Pseudomonas* spp. These can progress to septicaemia. Occasionally these conditions may involve a fungus such as *Aspergillus* spp.

Abscesses

Reptile abscesses, sometime referred to as fibriscesses (Huchzermeyer and Cooper, 2001), form in the presence of certain bacterial infections. Instead of liquid pus, reptiles and birds form solid, caseous, dried pus surrounded by a thick shell of fibrous tissue. This is due to the lack of lysozymes and the secretion of huge amounts of fibrinogen which converts to fibrin in the abscess producing a caseous or solid abscess (see Figure 21.5). These may form anywhere, but a common site in chelonians is the middle ear (often associated with squamous metaplasia due to hypovitaminosis A), causing a bulging of the eardrum. The bacterial pathogens involved are frequently Gram-negative species, although the presence of fungi has been well recorded.

Erythema, petechiae and ecchymoses

These three conditions may all be present at the same time or may appear individually.

Erythema is the reddening of skin tissues due to vascular congestion beneath. It can be seen in reptiles as a pink hue to the areas between scutes in the case of chelonians and crocodilians, or the more generalised reddening of the skin seen in snakes and thin-skinned reptiles such as leopard geckos (see Figure 21.6). Erythema is often suggestive of septicaemia.

Petechiae are pinpoint subepithelial haemorrhages. They can be seen in the mouth and cloaca. In the mouth they are often associated with oral infection such as 'mouth rot'. They may be seen over the body suggesting septicaemia. Other conditions producing petechiae include clotting deficiencies, for example consumption of rodent prey which has itself consumed a warfarin-type poison.

Ecchymoses are larger areas of haemorrhage and may be caused by severe local infection, disseminated intravascular coagulation or conditions mentioned above.

Veterinary Nursing of Exotic Pets and Wildlife, Third Edition. Simon J. Girling.

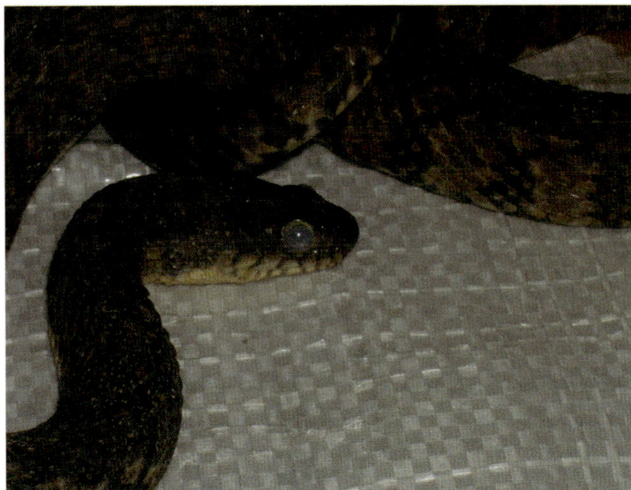

Figure 21.1 During the process of ecdysis in snakes, the eyes appear to go cloudy due to secretion of lymphatic fluid between the new and old spectacles.

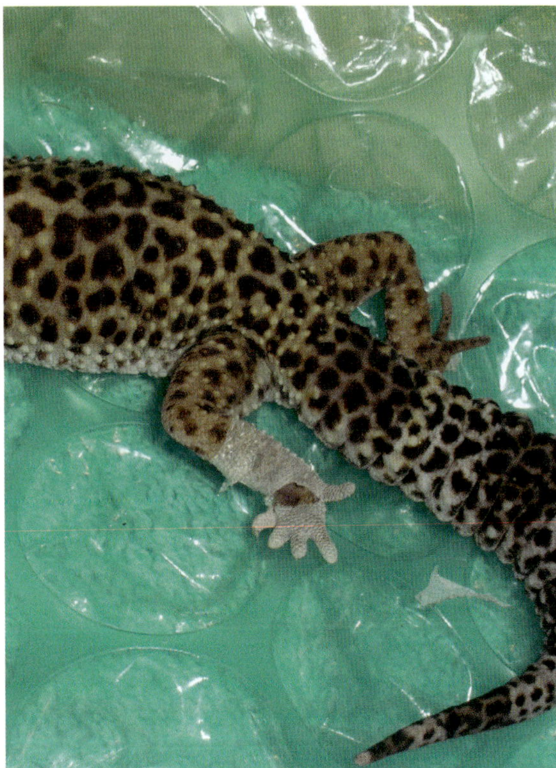

Figure 21.2 Dysecdysis in a leopard gecko (*Eublepharis macularius*). Note the retained skin over the distal left hindlimb and the fact that previous loss of the distal digits have occurred, most likely from a similar dysecdysis resulting in ischaemic necrosis.

Overgrown beaks and claws

Overgrown beaks are common in chelonians and are often due to a lack of abrasive foodstuffs or abrasive surfaces from which to eat them.

However, it should be noted that some species have perfectly normal apparently 'long' claws. An example is the male red-eared terrapin, which uses its claws as a mating display aid to attract a female.

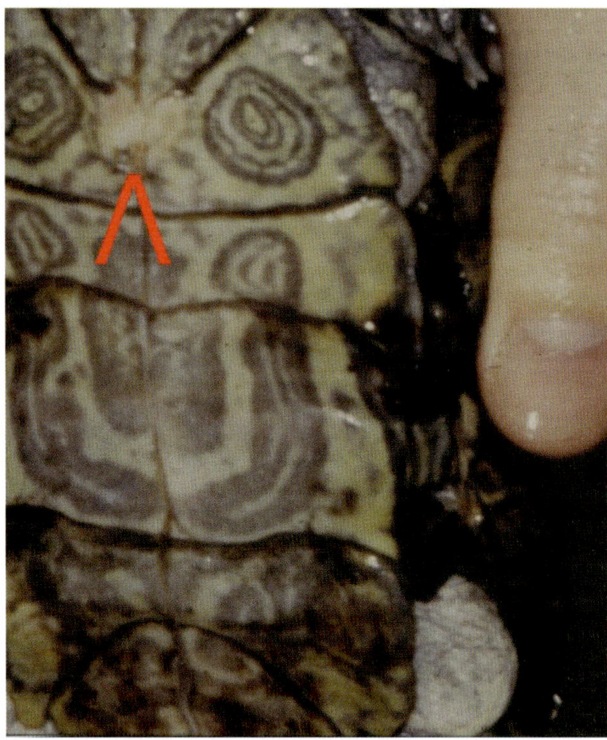

Figure 21.3 SCUD in a red-eared terrapin (*Trachemys scripta elegans*). Note the red arrowhead pointing to the ulceration in the keratin overlying the bony shell.

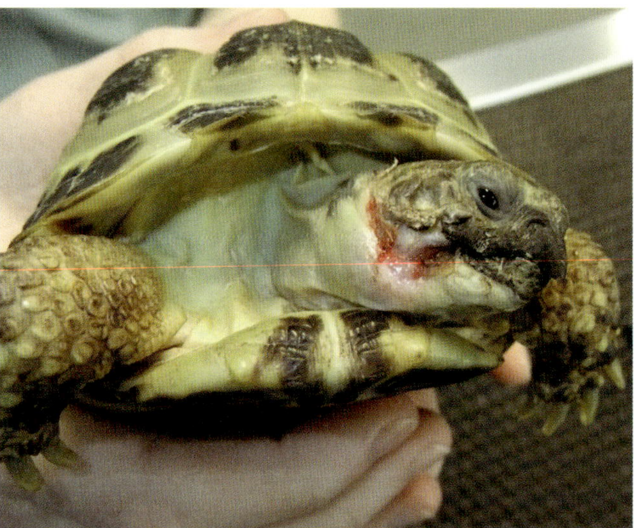

Figure 21.4 Skin infection with *Pseudomonas aeruginosa* causing ulceration and erythema in a Horsfield's tortoise (*Testudo horsfieldii*).

Pigment changes

An example of a physiologically normal colour change is seen in the Chamaeleonidae which will often darken in colour as they become stressed. Green iguanas often become yellow-brown in colour as they become stressed or unwell, bearded dragons often become dark coloured and many of these species will exhibit darkening at the site of an injection. Areas of previous trauma may become whitened.

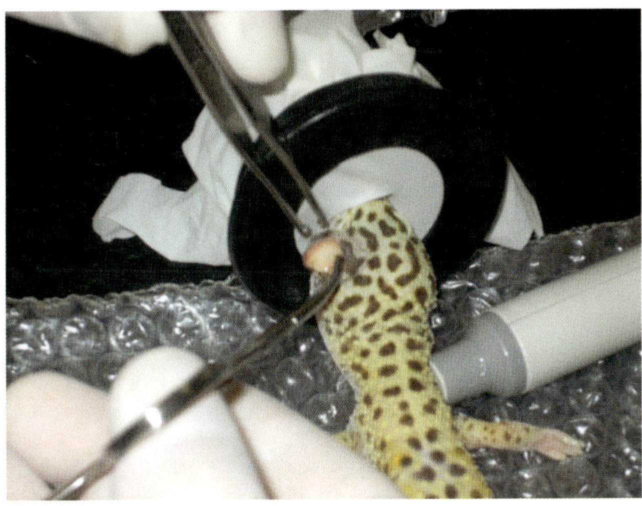

Figure 21.5 Caseous abscess in a leopard gecko (*Eublepharis macularius*) associated with hypovitaminosis A.

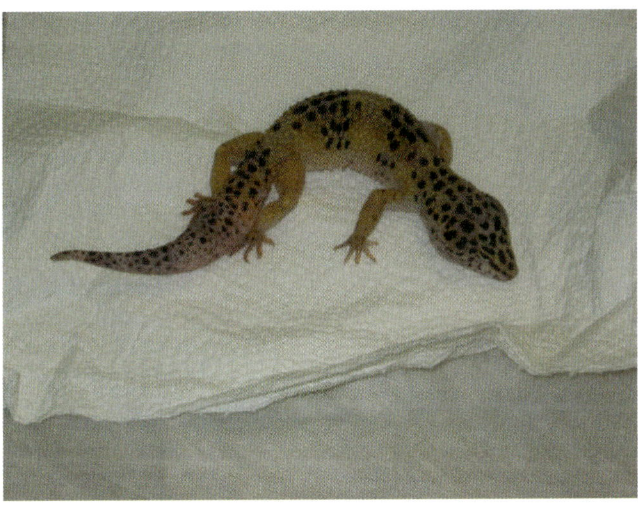

Figure 21.6 Generalised erythema associated with bacterial septicaemia in a leopard gecko (*Eublepharis macularius*).

Ectoparasitic

Mites

The snake mite *Ophionyssus natricis* appears as red to dark-coloured pin-head mites hiding under the overlapping edges of scales, although they are also commonly found around the commissures of the mouth. They may be seen in water dishes in which the reptile has been bathing. They can cause severe irritation, pruritus and self-trauma, as well as causing anaemia and dysecdysis. In addition, they can transmit *Aeromonas* spp. bacteria, which may cause septicaemia, and viruses such as inclusion body disease (IBD). Other mites include the cloacal mites (*Cloacarus* spp.) of aquatic turtles and *Hirstiella* spp. of mites in lizards (although the snake mite can also be found on reptiles other than snakes). In addition, there is of course the non-parasitic harvest mite *Neotrombicula autumnalis*, which may be brought in on straw and hay bedding material. The adult itself is not an irritant but the six-legged larval stage is and may cause the reptile to traumatise itself.

Ticks

In the UK, *Ixodes ricinus* (the sheep or deer tick) and *Ixodes hexagonus* (the hedgehog tick) are seen in outdoor tortoises. These are often found around the neck inlet and in front of the hind legs. They may cause local damage and can transmit pathogens. These include bacteria (*Staphylococcus aureus*, the cause of tick pyaemia and *Borrelia burgdorferi*, the cause of Lyme disease) as well as haemoparasites and viruses. Some of the soft-bodied ticks (*Amblyomma marmoreum* and *A. sparsum*) have been implicated in the transmission of *Cowdria ruminantium* the cause of heartwater disease in mammals. These ticks are more commonly seen in the UK on wild-caught imported reptiles as they are non-native. In the USA, *Aponemma*, *Hyalomma* and *Ornithodoros turicata* have all been seen as well as other species of *Ixodes*.

Blowfly myiasis

Myiasis is a problem for any reptile kept in unsanitary conditions or those with diarrhoea. Primary blowfly strike is seen associated with the larvae (maggots) of blowflies such as green (*Lucilia* spp.), black (*Phormia* spp.) and blue (*Calliphora* spp.) bottles. The larvae can develop from egg to the L2 stage that causes the tissue damage in as little as 2 hours in hot weather. These larvae then burrow away from the light, eating into the body of the tortoise causing severe trauma, infections, shock and ultimately death.

Leeches

Leeches tend not to be a significant problem in the UK, but can affect semi-aquatic species all over the world. The family Annelidae are the most dangerous, and can cause large wounds which continue to bleed after the leech has detached. These may then become secondarily infected. They can also transmit haemoparasites, bacteria and viruses.

Traumatic and spontaneous damage

Traumatic damage can be due to attacks by predators or other reptiles, for example males fighting over a female. In some species, for example green iguanas, the male mounting the female during mating bites the shoulder area vigorously, often causing open wounds. Dog attacks are common in tortoises. The feeding of live vertebrate and invertebrate prey to reptiles may occasionally result in the reptile being attacked and damaged by the prey. Unprotected heat sources frequently cause severe burns.

In some chelonians, scutes may be seen to lift off, often weeping clear fluid beneath them. This is frequently associated with underlying renal disease or septicaemia.

Iatrogenic causes of skin damage are also seen in some reptiles such as chelonians. This can occur after over-administration of vitamin A, which can cause sloughing of the epidermal layer on the head, neck and limbs, exposing the underlying dermis.

Tumours

Fibrosarcomas and squamous cell carcinomas may be seen in lizards and snakes. Melanomas are also seen in pigmented species such as the bearded dragon (*Pogona vitticeps*). Viral-induced fibropapillomas are frequently seen in green turtles (*Chelonia mydas*), where herpesviruses have been implicated. Another herpesvirus is a common cause of 'grey-patch disease' in this species, where circumscribed papular grey lesions appear over the whole body. In addition, papillomas have been regularly reported in Lacertidae (sand, wall and emerald lizards), occurring over the dorsum of the individual lizard.

Bacteria associated with skin problems

Gram-negative bacteria can cause skin abscesses, septicaemia and areas of skin sloughing and commonly seen organisms include *Aeromonas hydrophila*, *Edwardsiella*, *Klebsiella*, *Salmonella*, *Serratia* and *Pseudomonas* spp. Others such as *Mycobacterium* spp. may be seen associated with the appearance of classical tuberculous lesions. The mycobacteria found are more commonly environmental ones, for example *Mycobacterium marinum* (Girling and Fraser, 2007) and *Mycobacterium chelonae* rather than the human or cattle TB organisms.

Dermatophilus congolensis has been associated with skin disease in a number of lizards and snakes and *D. cheloniae* has been isolated from captive chelonians (Masters *et al.*, 1995). Tamukai *et al.* (2016) reported an outbreak of a related organism, *Austwickia chelonae*, in 100 bearded dragons associated with a ranavirus infection, with around half showing skin lesions and 15 dying. Dermatophilosis is technically zoonotic (Burd *et al.*, 2007).

Dermabacter spp. related bacteria have been associated with a proliferative cheilitis syndrome in agamid lizards (Koplos *et al.*, 2000). This has also been seen to cause proliferative lesions around the cloaca and over the legs (Pasmans *et al.*, 2010) and is now thought to be due to the Gram-positive bacterium *Devriesea agamarum*. Gram-negative bacterial infections of the hind feet of savannah monitor lizards seems to be another common condition and is associated with an overly abrasive and damp substrate leading to foot abrasion and secondary infection (Stahl, 2003).

Fungal

The incidence of fungal infections in reptiles has been quoted as ranging between 0.4% (Austwick and Keymer, 1981) and 4% (Jacobson, 1980). These include *Aspergillus* spp. (Austwick and Keymer, 1981; Tappe *et al.*, 1984; Girling, 2002a,b,c; Girling and Fraser, 2009); *Mucor* spp. (Lappin and Dunstan, 1992; Heatley *et al.*, 2001); *Paecilomyces* spp. (Heard *et al.*, 1986; Schumacher, 2003; Diaz-Figueroa *et al.*, 2008); *Candida albicans* (Austwick and Keymer, 1981; Migaki *et al.*, 1984); *Fusarium* spp. and *Chrysosporium* spp. (Austwick and Keymer 1981; Schumacher, 2003); *Sporothrix schenckii*, *Pestalotia pezizoides* and *Geotrichum candidum* (Cheatwood *et al.*, 2003); *Beauveria bassiana* (Gonzalez Cabo *et al.*, 1995); *Penicillium griseofulvum* (Oros *et al.*, 1996); *Alternaria* spp. (Rossi and Rossi, 2000); *Cryptococcus* spp. (Hough, 1998); *Scolecobasidium humicola* (Weitzman *et al.*, 1985) and the primary fungal pathogen the *Chrysosporium* anamorph of *Nannizziopsis vriesii* (CANV) in bearded dragons, brown tree snakes and chameleons (Pare *et al.*, 1997; Nichols *et al.*, 1999; Bowman *et al.*, 2007; Abarca *et al.*, 2009). (see Figure 21.7). CANV has now been reclassified into several species of fungus through molecular analysis which suggests three lineages (genus): *Nannizziopsis*, *Paranannizziopsis* and *Ophiodiomyces* spp. Of these, *N. guarroi* has been associated with yellow fungal skin disease in bearded dragons and iguanas and *Ophidiomyces ophidiicola* has been associated with white nose fungal disease in snakes both in captivity and the wild (Sigler *et al.*, 2013; Cabanes *et al.*, 2014).

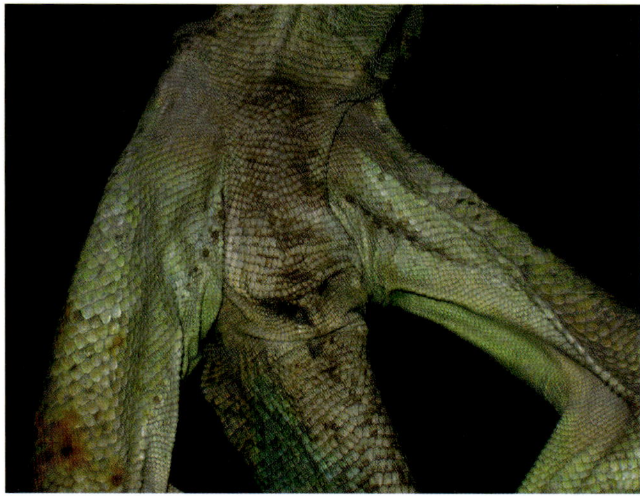

Figure 21.7 *Nannizziopsis guarroi* fungal infection in a green iguana (*Iguana iguana*) is frequently fatal and can produce yellow skin lesions. This individual eventually went into renal failure.

Many of these fungal infections appear to enter the reptilian body via the skin (Austwick and Keymer, 1981). With increasing use of antibiotic therapy in pet reptiles, climate change and the discovery of new fungal species associated with disease, the incidence of fungal disease appears to be on the increase (Fraser and Girling, 2004, 2019).

Emydomyces testavorans is an emerging keratinophilic fungal organism that has been linked to ulcerative skin and shell disease in a range of semi-aquatic chelonians but has not so far been confirmed as a primary pathogen (Woodburn *et al.*, 2021).

Viral

There are more and more cases of novel viral diseases being diagnosed in reptiles each day. Herpesviruses causing grey patch disease have been found in turtles, papillomaviruses in lizards, and poxviruses in caimans (a member of the family Crocodilia). West Nile virus infection (a flavivirus) is transmitted by haematophagous invertebrates and has caused lymphohistiocytic skin lesions in wild American alligators (*Alligator mississipiensis*). Interestingly, arenaviruses such as IBD may not directly cause skin lesions but as they often affect the central nervous system (CNS) can result in dysecdysis in snakes.

Hereditary

Many species exhibit scale and skin abnormalities. These vary from cleft palates to failure of scales to develop at all. In addition, many colour variations have been specifically bred for.

Hyperthyroidism

This has been diagnosed in green iguanas and corn snakes, although it is rare. It is associated with an increased turnover of skin and so an increase in ecdysis. It may also be associated with loss of dorsal spines in iguanas, tachycardia, increased aggression, polyphagia and weight loss overall (Hernandez-Divers *et al.*, 2001). Normal thyroid hormone reference ranges are difficult to find, but 0.21–6.78 nmol/L have been reported for *Calotes* and *Sceloporus* lizards.

Hypothyroidism

This has been reported in giant Chelonia (Frye, 1991). It may also be due to the presence of goitrogens in the diet such as brassicas. Myxoedema and heart failure are the most commonly seen clinical signs.

Thermal burns

Reptiles can sense pain but do not appear to respond to thermal pain in the same way that birds and mammals do; that is, they often do not remove themselves from the heat source even when it is resulting in severe burns. Unprotected heat lamps which allow reptiles close contact are dangerous, as are so-called 'hot-rocks' when the thermostat breaks. Full skin thickness burns and even death of the reptile may occur as a result. (see Figure 21.8).

Hypervitaminosis A

This can occur if parenteral vitamin A is given in doses exceeding 10 000 IU/kg. Initially it presents as dry skin but may progress to whole skin sloughing.

Hypovitaminosis A

This is mainly seen in aquatic chelonians and chameleons. The presenting signs include ocular oedema, xerophthalmia, middle ear abscessation, hyperkeratosis, lethargy and anorexia. It is preferable that vitamin A supplements should be given orally to minimise toxicity. Doses of 200 IU per 30 g body weight have been quoted, administered twice, 7 days apart (Harkewicz, 2001).

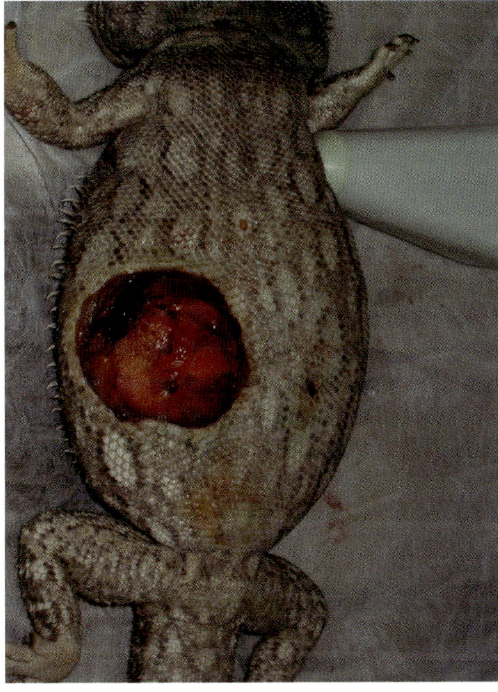

Figure 21.8 Full skin thickness burns can be seen where heaters are incorporated into synthetic 'rocks' to provide a basking area and the thermostat is faulty/inappropriately set. This bearded dragon (*Pogona vitticeps*) had preovulatory stasis and climbed onto the heated device and remained there for several days resulting in the full skin and body wall thickness thermal burn.

Hypovitaminosis E

This has been reported in caimans and other reptiles which eat marine fish. The presence of free radicals in oily frozen marine fish can result in a relative vitamin E deficiency which can lead to steatites, skin sloughing, and necrosis of fat and secondary infections.

Biotin deficiency

This may be seen in reptiles which consume large amounts of eggs, such as some snakes and monitor lizards. Unfertilised eggs contain avidin, an anti-vitamin to biotin which may lead to a relative deficiency. The main signs are neurological, but fracturing and splitting of keratin structures such as scales and claws and beaks along with abnormal sloughing may be seen. Removal of eggs from the diet results in a cure in most cases.

Hypocalcaemia/hypovitaminosis D

This can result in shell deformities in chelonians and is often associated with poor calcium-containing diets and a lack of ultraviolet (UV)-B provision. See the section on musculoskeletal diseases for further information. In addition, calcinosis cutis and circumscripta have been reported in reptiles with multifocal crusting and thickened skin which can then ulcerate. These two conditions are often related to calcium imbalances, more often hypercalcaemia, but also to areas of skin damage.

Digestive disease

Oral (mouth rot)

'Mouth rot' is the colloquial term for stomatitis, commonly seen in many reptiles particularly in snakes and chelonians.

The causes are many and varied. It can be caused by secondary infections with Gram-negative bacteria. The initial cause of the damage can be rubbing of the snout on vivarium glass, particularly in snakes. The use of opaque tape stuck to the outside of the glass helps the snake to 'see it', preventing this injury. Stomatitis may also be due to the overzealous force-feeding of anorectic reptiles or to other disease or stresses leading to reduced immune system function. Uric acid crystals deposited around the base of the teeth, due to visceral gout and renal failure, can allow infections to occur. Herpesvirus and ranavirus infections in terrestrial tortoises are also a cause, with oral ulceration and diphtherisis (see Figure 21.9). *Mycoplasma* spp. infections may also be associated with stomatitis in tortoises. *Devriesea agamarum*, a bacterium, has been reported in agamid lizards as a cause of proliferative cheilitis, pericloacal disease and dermatitis. Adenoviruses have been implicated in snakes and lizards and IBD in snakes.

Diagnosis is made on impression smears and bacterial swab and culture of samples. A polymerase chain reaction (PCR) for diagnosing many of the reptilian viral diseases is now commercially available, and reptile cell lines are available in some laboratories to attempt virus isolation where PCR is not accessible. Alternatively, electron microscopy of samples may aid the diagnosis.

Periodontal disease

This is particularly common in Agamidae and Chamaeleonidae which possess acrodont teeth. These teeth are not replaced when lost during the course of the lizard's life. This is as opposed to pleurodont teeth

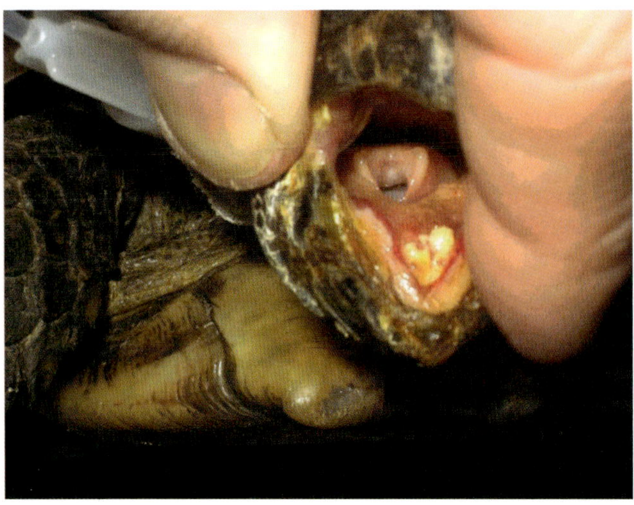

Figure 21.9 Oral ulceration in a spur-thighed tortoise (*Testudo graeca*) associated with herpesvirus and secondary *Pseudomonas* spp. infection.

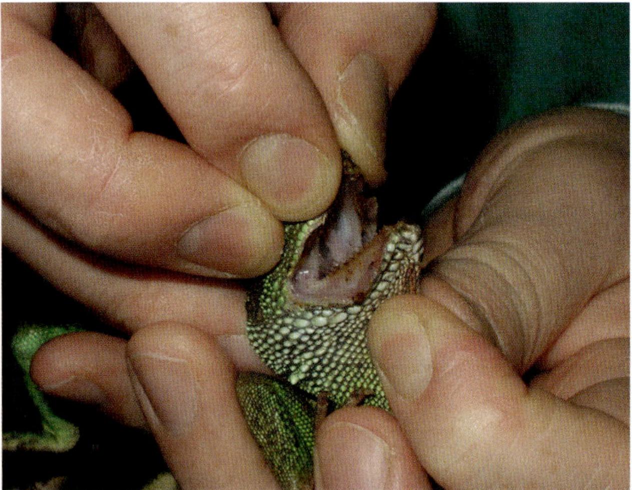

Figure 21.10 Periodontal disease is common in species fed inappropriate diets particularly if they have acrodont dentition and so do not replace their teeth regularly.

(present in Iguanidae amongst other species) where the teeth are continually replaced. If inappropriate food is provided, such as soft fruit, which adheres readily to the teeth and rots, periodontal disease will develop (see Figure 21.10). As the species with acrodont teeth cannot shed and replace the teeth, infection, often with osteomyelitis, ensues.

Vomiting and regurgitation

In snakes, regurgitation may simply occur due to rough handling, particularly soon after the snake has eaten. Snakes will also regurgitate if fed or force-fed and then kept at suboptimal environmental temperatures. Lizards and chelonians rarely vomit.

Parasitic causes of vomiting and regurgitation

In snakes, one of the most important stomach diseases is cryptosporidiosis due to a single-celled parasite, *Cryptosporidium serpentis*, which invades the outer membrane of cells lining the stomach. With time, it causes a thickening of the stomach, narrowing the lumen and so reducing its elasticity and digestive powers and causing vomiting. In lizards, cryptosporidiosis mainly affects the intestines, making vomiting less likely. Cryptosporidiosis was implicated in an outbreak of vomiting in juvenile Hermann's tortoises (McArthur *et al.*, 2004). It is therefore currently thought that there are lizard-, snake- and chelonian-specific forms of *Cryptosporidium* spp.

Diagnosis is made on clinical signs and demonstrating oocysts shed in the faeces or recovered from a stomach wash, or biopsy of the stomach wall. In snakes, the course of the disease can vary from 4 days in severe cases to 2 years in chronic ones. Externally, the snake often shows signs of a mid-body swelling, due to the thickening of the stomach wall associated with the host's immune system response to the parasite. The parasite is passed directly from one snake's faeces or regurgitated fluids to another. The condition is difficult to treat, the organism is hardy in the environment and infection frequently results in the death of the snake.

Other forms of parasitism may cause vomiting or regurgitation in snakes, for example *Kalicephalus* spp. (the snake hookworm), which may cause extensive ulceration of the digestive system; ascarids; and in the python family the tapeworm *Bothridium* spp. have all been reported.

Bacterial and fungal causes of vomiting and regurgitation

Bacterial and fungal infections, granulomas and abscesses may also cause damage to the stomach and its outflow or result in pressure on it, and so lead to regurgitation or vomiting.

Viral causes of vomiting and regurgitation

IBD, an arenavirus, has been associated with chronic regurgitation in boids although there are usually other clinical signs such as respiratory disease and neurological disease.

Tumours

Stomach tumours, for example gastric adenomas and adenocarcinomas, have been reported and may cause swelling. Bearded dragons are commonly affected by a form of stomach cancer known as a gastric neuroendocrine carcinoma which frequently causes anorexia, vomiting, hyperglycaemia and anaemia (Ritter *et al.*, 2009).

Intestinal disease

Parasitic causes of intestinal disease

Snakes: Species involved include the strongylid hookworm *Kalicephalus* spp., threadworms such as *Strongyloides* spp., and tapeworms such as *Bothridium* spp. in pythons and *Ophiotaenia* spp. in garter and water snakes. Ascarids do occur in the wild but generally in snakes they require an intermediate rodent or amphibian host and so tend to be uncommon in captive snakes.

Entamoebiasis caused by the single-celled parasite *Entamoeba invadens* can cause diarrhoea in snakes. Its life cycle is direct, with infection spread directly from one reptile to another. After incubating in the lining of the small intestine, each infective cyst produces eight uninucleate amoebae which invade cells lining the large intestine of the same snake. The amoebae may also penetrate into the bloodstream and so end up in the liver, causing necrotising hepatitis. Diagnosis is by finding the small amoebae or cysts in the faeces (×400 magnification is required).

Other single-celled parasites of snakes include the flagellate family (e.g. *Trichomonas* spp.). Clinical signs again include large bowel distension with fluid and gas, diarrhoea and increased thirst.

Chelonians: The ascarid family, for example *Angusticaecum* spp. (10–20 cm in length), is most significant as it can result in intestinal blockage, weight loss and anaemia. It has a direct life cycle and so can be perpetuated relatively easily in captivity. It can be detected by finding thick-walled ovoid eggs in the faeces that can survive for months to years in the soil (see Figure 21.11). Oxyurid pinworms may be asymptomatic, but some may be large enough to debilitate a tortoise, particularly prior and subsequent to hibernation. Roundworms are passed directly from chelonian to chelonian in the faeces in the infectious egg form and may be diagnosed by the detection of these eggs in a faecal smear.

The most important group of intestinal parasites of Chelonia is the flagellate family. These include *Trichomonas* and *Hexamita* spp. The clinical signs produced are rapid in onset and include anorexia, occasionally diarrhoea and frequently the passage of undigested food in the faeces. There is often polydipsia, due partly to the inability of the damaged intestines to absorb water and partly, in the case of *Hexamita parva*, to kidney damage, as this organism migrates up the ureters from the cloaca into the kidneys. Diagnosis is made by viewing the very fast-moving organisms microscopically using ×400 magnification, although a fresh faecal specimen is required. Transmission is faeco-oral. The prognosis may be extremely poor for any chelonian severely parasitised by this organism, due to its ability to cause irreparable damage to the intestinal mucosa.

Another family of motile protozoans afflicting herbivorous Chelonia are ciliates such as *Balantidium coli* and *Nyctotherus* spp. They may be seen normally in the stool of healthy animals, but they may be present in such large numbers as to cause weight loss and intestinal damage and *Balantidium* spp. may affect the liver causing a hepatitis.

Entamoeba invadens has caused large intestinal and hepatic disease in herbivorous and omnivorous chelonians. Juvenile individuals appear more susceptible particularly with reduced food in their digestive tracts. Clinically, anorexia and wasting with diarrhoea are seen.

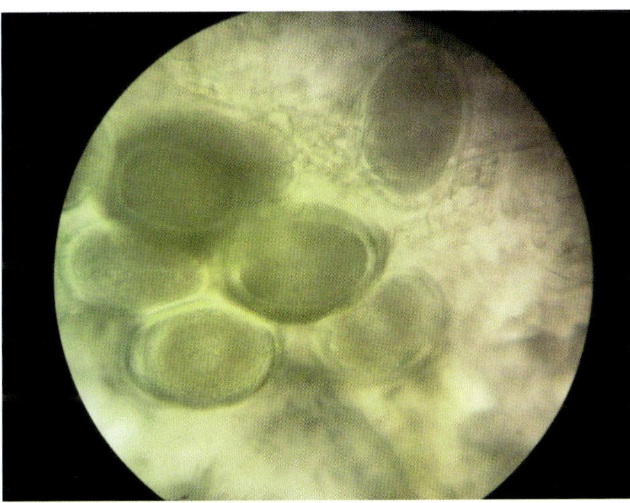

Figure 21.11 Ascarid eggs such as *Angusticaecum* spp. are typically thick-walled and often ovoid in shape.

As mentioned, *Cryptosporidium* spp. can affect the small intestine and stomach of chelonians and has been implicated in pancreatitis as well.

Intranuclear coccidiosis is of growing concern in some chelonians, particularly testudines (known as testudine intranuclear coccidiosis or TINC), affecting the intestines and liver as well as the kidneys and pancreas and can be difficult to diagnose as the organism may be intermittently shed into the faeces and the oocysts are small (6–7 µm) and spherical. PCR tests are now commercially available and increase testing sensitivity. There may be some species variability in susceptibility as in one study Greek spur-thighed tortoises (*Testudo graeca*) and leopard tortoises (*Stigmochelys pardalis*) rapidly died after diarrhoea, coelomic effusion and renal failure but Hermann's (*T. hermanni*), Horsfield's (*T. horsfieldii*) and African spurred (*Centrochelys sulcata*) did not show clinical signs (Hofmannova *et al.*, 2019). Radiated tortoises (*Astrochelys radiata*) also appear to be very susceptible.

Lizards: Oxyurid nematodes (so-called pinworms) are common (e.g. *Ozolaimus* spp. in iguanids and *Tachygonetria* spp. in agamids) and in herbivorous lizards such as the green iguana may even help to digest cellulose/hemicellulose in the gut and so some think are beneficial (Iverson, 1980). However, due to the direct life cycle of these parasites and the, often confined, spaces associated with captivity, environmental levels may become very high resulting in significant burdens, sufficient to produce intestinal damage and debilitation. Diagnosis is by finding the eggs in the faeces (see Figure 21.12). Ascarids do occur but generally in lizards require an intermediate rodent or amphibian host and so tend to be uncommon in captive lizards.

The coccidian family are also important parasites in lizards, particularly geckos and chameleons. Clinical signs include anorexia, weight loss, diarrhoea, dysentery and general debilitation. *Isospora amphiboluri* is a cause of stunting and runting in bearded dragon neonates, often associated with an adenovirus (see Figures 21.12 and 21.13). Diagnosis is by finding the typically isosporean oocysts in the faeces, and disease spread is direct.

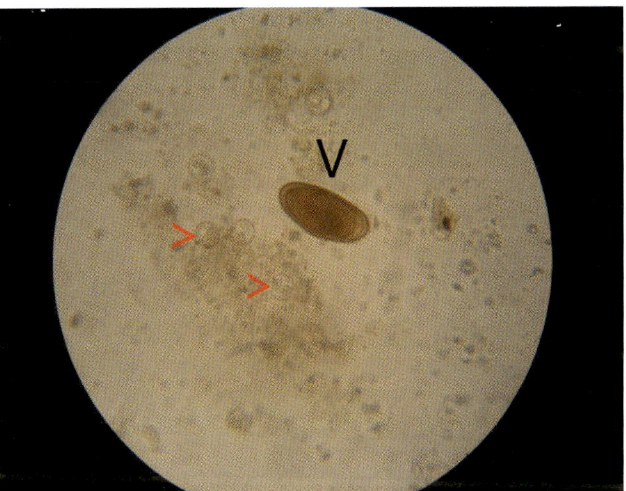

Figure 21.12 Oxyurid nematode infections are common in reptiles such as bearded dragons and may be diagnosed by finding these classical eggs in the faeces (shown by the black arrowhead). The red arrowheads point to *Isospora amphiboluri* coccidial occysts which, in conjunction with atadenoviral infections, can result in stunting and mortalities in bearded dragons.

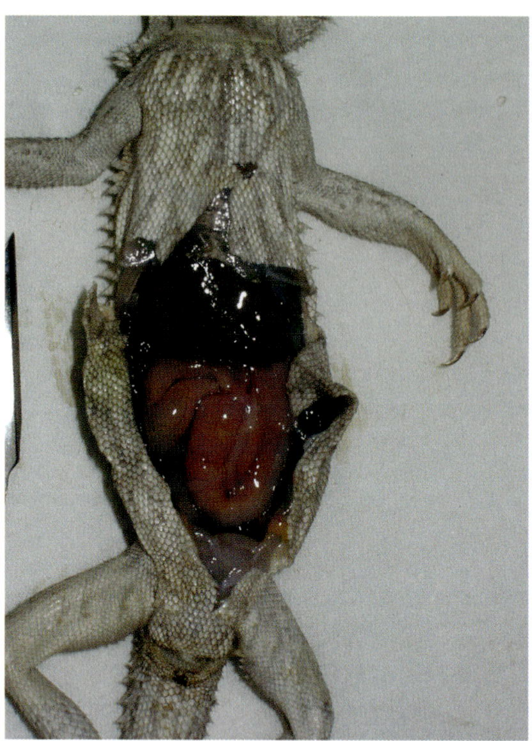

Figure 21.13 Infections with *Isospora amphiboluri* and atadenovirus can lead to mortalities in bearded dragons. Note the intestinal intussusception in the centre of the image.

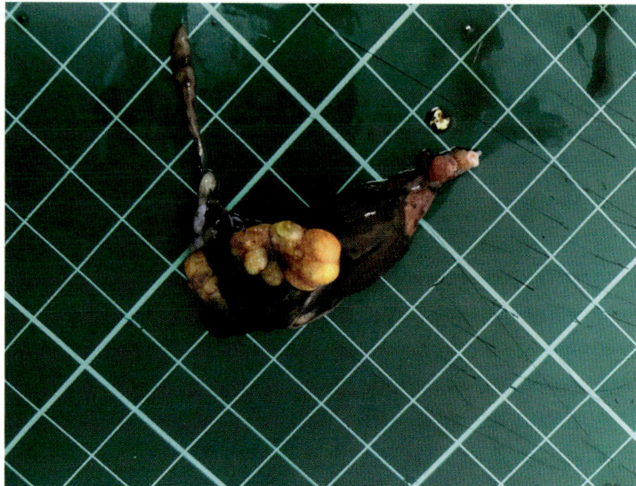

Figure 21.14 Post-mortem view of the liver and gastrointestinal tract of a lizard affected by *Mycobacterium* spp. infection. Note the yellow-white spherical abscesses in the intestines. Mycobacterial disease tends to gain access via the oral route and can result in chronic wasting and mortality as it is often unresponsive to a wide range of antimicrobials.

Intestinal cryptosporidiosis is a problem in geckos and the species is now known as *C. varanii*. Clinical signs include weight loss, diarrhoea and anorexia. It typically affects young hatchlings, most presenting as geckos that basically fail to thrive. The pathology has been described above.

Entamoeba invadens may also be seen in carnivorous lizards, producing colic and progressive weight loss with diarrhoea.

Bacterial causes of intestinal disease

In all species, but particularly snakes and chelonians, members of the zoonotic family Salmonellae are commonly recovered. Current advice is that providing they are not causing clinical disease, no antibiotics should be given. This is to prevent the development of antibiotic resistance, and on a practical basis no one has satisfactorily proven that such treatment can clear a reptile permanently of *Salmonella* spp.

Other bacteria found in the normal digestive system of reptiles can act as opportunistic pathogens, including many members of the *Escherichia coli* family, *Klebsiella* spp., *Pseudomonas* spp., *Campylobacter* spp., *Clostridium* spp. and *Aeromonas* spp. In addition environmental mycobacteria such as *Mycobacterium marinum* and *M. cheloniae* may result in significant digestive tract disease that can be difficult to treat and is often fatal (see Figure 21.14).

Fungal causes of intestinal disease

Published reports of gastrointestinal fungal disease are rare, but fungal overgrowth appears to be a relatively common finding particularly after prolonged antibiotic use. Documented cases of intestinal fungal overgrowth include *Candida albicans*, *Penicillium* spp., *Basidiobolus ranarum* and *Paecilomyces* spp.

Physical causes of intestinal disease

Foreign bodies are not uncommon in chelonians and lizards, which may consume stones, sand, soil or any other substrate present. Crocodilia commonly consume stones that sit in the stomach and may help mechanically break down food. Surgery may be required to remove some foreign bodies where a blockage occurs, although many may be passed with the aid of oral liquid paraffin and fluid therapy.

Other physical obstructions include tumours within the intestines. These are not uncommon, particularly in snakes, and may present as a swelling, or produce clinical signs such as vomiting, diarrhoea, constipation or anorexia.

Lead poisoning

This has been reported in chelonians such as common snapping turtles (*Chelydra serpentina*) and spur-thighed tortoises (*Testudo graeca*). Clinical signs included ileus, anaemia, lethargy and renal failure. Blood tests can confirm exposure and radiography will highlight larger lead particles in the gastrointestinal tract.

Liver disease

Snakes

Entamoeba invadens can cause hepatitis and has already been mentioned above. Other parasitic causes include some forms of the coccidian family which gain access to the liver from the small intestine via the bile ducts.

Herpesviruses, caliciviruses and atadenoviruses have been isolated from damaged snake livers.

Chelonia

The protozoan *Hexamita parva* has been associated with intestinal, renal and hepatic disease in chelonians.

Adenoviruses (siadenovirus and testadenovirus) have been associated with hepatitis in a range of chelonians and may cause mortalities although they may also produce no clinical signs. Herpesviruses have also been associated with hepatitis in semi-aquatic chelonians.

Hepatic lipidosis is common in tortoises fed inappropriate high-fat diets. Fat becomes deposited within the liver cells themselves, enlarging the liver and, more importantly, severely affecting its function. This can lead to jaundice, anorexia and death.

Post-hibernation jaundice is often a temporary finding in tortoises, but it may persist, indicating liver damage due to any one of the above or to hepatitis from bacteria such as *Salmonella* spp. and *Aeromonas hydrophila*. In addition, some forms of herpesviruses and iridoviruses have been isolated from damaged tortoise and other chelonian livers.

The liver may become calcified due to oversupplementation of the diet with calcium and vitamin D_3.

Lizards

A coccidial parasite, *Choleoeimeria* spp., affects the lining of the gall bladder and biliary system of lizards and can result in their proliferation and eventual blockage. This can result in jaundice and liver failure as a result.

Bacterial hepatitis due to *Salmonella* spp., *Aeromonas* spp. or *Pseudomonas* spp. has been recorded. This may or may not be associated with heavy worm burdens, many of which may migrate through or to the liver, often carrying bacteria with them.

Viral hepatitis has been reported due to atadenoviruses in bearded dragons (*Pogona* spp.). It is generally seen in young animals and often associated with coccidiosis resulting in poor-thriving young. Pathology can include hepatitis, nephritis and CNS damage resulting in opisthotonus. Serological tests are available for detection of this disease as is a PCR test. Herpesviruses and ranaviruses have been associated with hepatitis as well as pneumonia in the case of herpesviruses in other iguanids and agamids. Yellow-green urates may be seen in reptiles associated with hepatic dysfunction due to the presence of increased levels of biliverdin.

Hepatic lipidosis, or fatty liver syndrome, has been well documented in lizards, particularly monitors and bearded dragons. This is frequently seen when they are fed inappropriate high-fat diets. In bearded dragons, the feeding of excessive amounts of insects to adults (which are supposed to become more herbivorous once they reach maturity) has also been implicated. In lizards with preovulatory stasis, lipidosis occurs due to the high levels of circulating yolk lipids. Lipidosis can lead to jaundice, anorexia and death. The liver may become calcified due to oversupplementation of the diet with calcium and vitamin D_3.

Pancreatic diseases

Pancreatitis

This may be associated with bacterial infections as well as herpesvirus disease and cryptosporidiosis in chelonians (McArthur *et al.*, 2004). Frye (1999) describes a spontaneous autoimmune pancreatitis and diabetes mellitus in a Western pond turtle.

Diabetes mellitus

This has been reported in chelonians associated with damage to the beta islet cells and a reduction in insulin secretion (McArthur *et al.*, 2004). Reptiles such as herbivorous chelonians are insulin resistant, so insulin therapy is rarely effective. Ketoacidosis and hepatic lipidosis are often also present.

Neoplasia of the digestive tract

Neoplasia of the pancreas has been mentioned. Neoplasia of the stomach and intestines are not uncommon, particularly in snakes. Hepatic neoplasia has been reported most frequently in chelonians. Onset tends to be gradual, and unless the neoplasm involves an intestinal obstruction, may pass unnoticed until advanced.

Respiratory disease

Signs of respiratory disease

Respiratory disease in reptiles is exacerbated by the lack of a cough reflex as reptiles have no true diaphragm. Secretions therefore pool in the dependent parts of the lungs and so make the course of the disease more chronic and difficult to treat. Signs of respiratory disease are given in Table 21.1.

Causes of respiratory disease

Parasitic causes

Entamoeba invadens can cause respiratory disease in snakes. The commoner parasites, though, are nematodes, represented by the following.

- *Kalicephalus* spp.: the early larval stages can migrate through the skin of the snake or be eaten. The larvae then migrate through the body, often through the lungs as the snake develops/moults, before finally ending up as the adult hookworm in the gut.
- Family Ascaridae: in carnivorous reptiles, ascarid infection is frequently acquired via amphibian or rodent prey, which acts as an intermediate/paratenic host. The worm larvae, once consumed, migrate through the liver and lungs of the reptile again before ending up in the digestive tract or encysted in muscle.
- *Rhabdias* spp. (lungworm of snakes): the snake ingests the infective eggs from the faeces of other snakes, or the infective larvae may penetrate the skin of the snake as with *Kalicephalus* spp. The larvae then migrate to the lungs, where they all develop into adult female worms. Eggs are therefore produced by parthenogenesis (female giving birth to female).
- *Entomelas/Neoentomelas* spp. (lungworm of lizards): the life cycle is similar to that of the lungworm of snakes.

Other less common parasitic causes of respiratory disease in reptiles include the following.

- Flukes (e.g. *Dasymetra* spp.), which live in the oral cavity and respiratory tract of snakes. These parasites are rarely pathogenic. Diagnosis is made by finding the fluke eggs in the snake's faeces.

Table 21.1 Signs of respiratory disease in reptiles.

Common signs of respiratory disease in reptiles	Less frequently seen signs associated with respiratory disease in reptiles
Mouth breathing (particularly snakes)	Hypopyon (pus in the anterior chamber of the eye, particularly Chelonia)
Excess mucus at nares and mouth	Abscess beneath the eye spectacle (snakes)
Increased respiratory noise	
Lethargy	
Anorexia	

- Pentastomes, also known as 'tongue worms', are the adult stage of an arachnid organism related to spiders and ticks, rather than a true worm. It uses the lungs of snakes, crocodiles or lizards as the final host, shedding eggs which are coughed up and swallowed and passed in the faeces. These then are ingested by an intermediate host such as rodents, or even humans, making this a significant zoonotic disease. The larvae encyst in the intermediate host. If this is then consumed by the reptile, the larvae are reactivated and migrate to the lungs where they can grow to several centimetres in length, causing severe damage. They are generally only found in wild-caught specimens, due to the lack of native prey to transmit the parasite in captivity.
- Intranuclear coccidiosis, although typically associated with the gastrointestinal tract, has been reported in the lungs of chelonians by biopsy. A PCR test has been developed (Garner *et al.*, 2006).

Bacterial causes

Examples of the bacteria seen in pneumonias include *Acinetobacter* spp., *Actinobacillus* spp., *Aeromonas* spp., *Bacteroides* spp., *Corynebacterium* spp., *Klebsiella* spp., *Pasteurella* spp., *Pseudomonas* spp., *Salmonella* spp. and *Serratia marcescens*.

Mycoplasmas are regularly recovered from chelonians with herpesvirus infections, particularly *Mycoplasma agassizii*. One study suggested an incidence of 15.8% in UK tortoises (Soares *et al.*, 2004). This may result in oedema and swelling of the neck and tissues between neck and forelimbs in chelonians. A *Mycoplasma. agassizii*-like mycoplasma has also been identified as a cause of a proliferative interstitial pneumonia and tracheitis in Burmese pythons (Penner *et al.*, 1997). PCRs and culture have been used to diagnose mycoplasmal infections.

Chlamydia spp. infections have also been reported particularly in snakes resulting in pneumonia, and occasionally environmental mycobacteria such as *Mycobacterium marinum* may cause systemic disease with lung involvement (Girling and Fraser, 2007).

Bacterial sampling

There are two main techniques involved in sampling bacteria or parasites that cause pneumonias.

- Lung wash: a sterile catheter is passed into the trachea of the reptile and may be done in the conscious animal due to lack of the cough reflex. Fractious animals may require sedation. Through this catheter, sterile saline may be infused, at doses equal to 0.5–1 mL per 100 g body weight, and immediately aspirated. This sample can then be cultured to identify the pathogen. Sample collection may be enhanced by holding the reptile upside down whilst aspirating.
- Direct sampling: this involves taking a swab directly from the site of the problem. This may be done via laparotomy or endoscopy. In the case of Chelonia, the reptile may be anaesthetised, the shell overlying the pneumonic lesion aseptically prepared and a small hole drilled through to enable the bacteriological swab to be passed.

Fungal causes

Fungal infections of the respiratory tract are more commonly seen in chelonians than in other species of reptile. The infections are often due to saprophytic opportunistic environmental fungi and so are often secondary to bacterial infections or traumatic injuries. Fungi associated with disease include *Aspergillus*, *Paecilomyces*, *Candida*, *Sporotrichum*, *Cladosporium* and *Penicillium* spp.

Viral causes

Herpesviruses: This has been recorded in tortoises, particularly *Testudo* spp., and is associated with upper respiratory tract infections. Clinical signs include lethargy, rhinitis, conjunctivitis, stomatitis and anorexia. Diphtheritic plaques may form inside the oral cavity and oesophagus. One serological study reported that 42.5% of spur-thighed tortoises and 18.5% of Hermann's tortoises were positive (Frost and Schmidt, 1997). *Testudo graeca* appears more resilient and *T. hermanni* and *T. horsfieldii* appear more susceptible (Marschang and Chitty, 2019). Routes of transmission are not fully understood but studies have shown success via oral, aerosol and intramuscular routes. Any infected tortoise should be considered as infected for life and so can spread herpesvirus particles even after resolution of clinical signs.

Diagnosis is by serology or PCR. A serum neutralisation test was the first to be developed, but a more effective and sensitive ELISA now exists. A PCR real-time assay also exists and is the most useful in an acute outbreak as serological conversion can take 6–8 weeks post infection to occur. Histopathology may also demonstrate classical eosinophilic intranuclear inclusion bodies.

Inclusion body virus: This was thought to be a retrovirus but has been reclassified as an arenavirus. It causes digestive and CNS system diseases and has been associated with pneumonia in snakes, primarily pythons and boas. There is no treatment. It is thought to be spread by direct contact or aerosol and by the snake mite *Ophionyssus natricis*, although there is some suggestion that it can pass through the egg (vertical transmission). Diagnosis, using biopsies of lung, liver, spleen or kidney tissue, is made by PCR or by demonstrating eosinophilic intracytoplasmic viral inclusions. Occasionally it may be possible to see the viral inclusions in pneumocytes dislodged during a lung wash, particularly in boids in my experience.

Iridovirus: Iridoviral respiratory infections, particularly ranavirus infections, are most commonly reported in chelonians and can produce a severe, extensive, necrotising ulcerative tracheitis, pneumonia, pharyngitis and oesophagitis producing so-called 'red neck' disease. It seems that amphibians are the reservoir host as the ranavirus isolated in cases of upper respiratory tract disease in chelonians is of amphibian origin. PCR and neutralisation tests are available (Westhouse *et al.*, 1996).

Paramyxovirus: The virus family *Paramyxoviridae* contains the genus *Ferlavirus* which is highly infectious, being shed in respiratory secretions. It causes a haemorrhagic pneumonia and viraemia that affects other organs as well. Diagnosis is generally made by PCR, serology or histopathology. Seroconversion does take 6–8 weeks to occur post infection, so false-negative results early in the course of the disease are possible. Disease including pneumonia has been reported most commonly in viperid, boid and elapid snakes but it has also been reported in lizards and tortoises.

Reoviruses: Reovirus infections have been reported in lizards causing respiratory and neurological disease

Hypovitaminosis A

This has been reported in aquatic and semi-aquatic carnivorous chelonians. Typical lesions of squamous metaplasia, periocular oedema and xerophthalmia, and secondary bacterial infections of the gastrointestinal and respiratory tract are seen.

Trauma and respiratory tract disease in reptiles

Trauma to the carapace of chelonians is a frequent cause of non-infectious lung disease. It is often associated with dog attacks, car accidents or lawnmower injuries.

Cardiovascular disease

Congenital defects

These have been reported in a number of species and include atrial septal defects and valve dysplasias.

Cardiomyopathy

Dilated cardiomyopathy has been reported, particularly in snakes (Barten, 1980; Wagner, 1989). Some causes appear to be similar to those described for birds and mammals but are not fully understood. Both visceral gout and vitamin E deficiencies can lead to myocardial damage and potential development of cardiomyopathies.

Infectious disease

Many pathogens which cause systemic illness and septicaemia are responsible for cardiac damage. Damage can be due to bacterial endocarditis causing microthrombi to seed off into the rest of the body. Many of the Gram-negative bacteria seen in reptiles, such as *Aeromonas* spp., *Salmonella* spp. and *Pseudomonas* spp., are associated with heart disease. In aquatic chelonians, species of bacteria commonly seen in fish and other aquatic species, such as *Flavobacterium* and *Vibrio* spp., have been linked to myocarditis and septic endocarditis (Jacobson *et al.*, 1989a). *Mycobacterium* spp. have also been associated with granulomatous myocarditis in a frilled lizard (Murray, 1996). Chlamydial myocarditis has been reported in puff adders (Jacobson *et al.*, 1989b) and mycoplasmal myocarditis due to *Mycoplasma alligatoris* has been reported in American alligators as well as other pathology including mortalities, pneumonia and septic arthritis (Brown *et al.*, 2001). Viruses such as IBD may affect many body organ systems including the heart and may result in cardiac failure.

Pneumonia often accompanies endocarditis and septicaemic situations in reptiles (Pees *et al.*, 2010).

Diagnosis requires ultrasonography and radiology to determine heart size and internal structure. Pericardial effusions associated with cardiac failure are commonly seen (see Figure 21.15). Electrocardiograms may also be helpful. Final proof of the organism involved depends on blood culture.

Haemoparasites

Filarids

The adults often live subcutaneously and release microfilariae, microscopic young, which may be transmitted from reptile to reptile by mosquitoes and ticks. These parasites may cause thrombi to develop in any of the major blood vessels, causing ischaemic necrosis or cardiac damage.

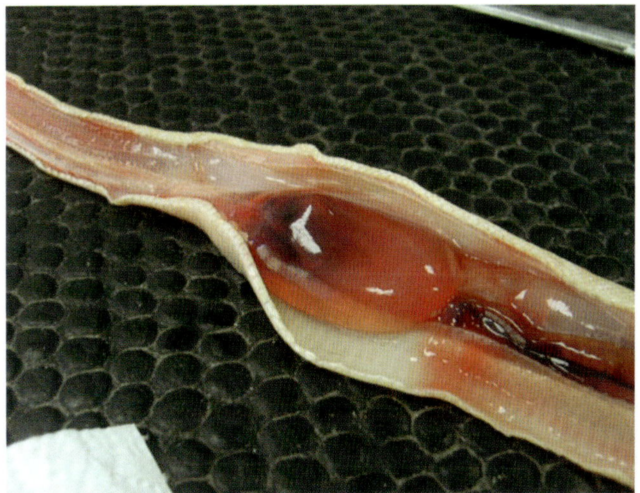

Figure 21.15 Post-mortem view of the heart within its pericardium of a snake that died of inclusion body disease (IBD). Note the significant pericardial effusion.

Trematodes

Trematodes (flukes) have been identified in marine chelonians. The adult fluke is not normally the problem, but the eggs laid into the bloodstream cause thrombi to form and so can block capillary beds in vital organs.

Protozoa

A wide range of haemoprotozoans have been identified in wild and captive reptiles. Many cause no obvious clinical disease; however, *Plasmodium* spp. have been shown to cause haemolytic anaemia and mortality in chelonians. They are transmitted by mosquitoes predominantly and schizonts, gametocytes and trophozoites may be found in the peripheral blood. The gametocyte is the most obvious stage, as it is refractile with pigment granules in the cytoplasm of white and red blood cells and thrombocytes.

Haemogregarina spp. are widespread and found typically in freshwater turtles, *Testudo* spp. tortoises and some snakes and lizards and are commonly transmitted by leeches and sometimes dipteran flies. They are rarely pathogenic, with perhaps the exception being the American alligator infected with *H. crocodilinorum*.

Haemoproteus spp., another protozoan, can be found as gametocytes in the cytoplasm of erythrocytes and have refractile pigment granules. There is no known effective treatment for this condition but it rarely causes clinical disease.

Hepatozoon spp. is seen in terrestrial snakes and is transmitted by the snake mite *Ophionyssus natricis*. It rarely causes clinical disease but erythrocyte inclusions are commonly seen.

Karyolysus spp. is transmitted through the faeces of mites such as the lizard mite *Hirstiella trombidiiformis* and the protozoan may infect numerous organs such as the liver, spleen and lung as well as getting into the bloodstream. It tends to be seen in Old World lizards and tree snakes.

Trypanosomes, *Schellackia* spp. and piroplasms (e.g. *Sauroplasma*) have all been reported in reptiles and are nearly always asymptomatic. Treatment is rarely needed.

Nutritional disease

Hypoiodinism in chelonians has been associated with cardiac disease and goitre. The feeding of mineral-poor foods such as cucumber and lettuce or goitrogenic foods such as brassicas (e.g. cabbage, Brussel sprouts) may lead to this.

Oversupplementation with vitamin D_3 and calcium may lead to calcification of the tunica media of the major arteries, causing a decrease in their elasticity and so increased blood pressure. This may lead to heart failure or aneurysm formation. It is also the case that renal failure can lead to monosodium urate and calcium crystal deposition in blood vessels as well.

Dietary deficiencies in vitamin E and/or selenium can lead to a condition known as white muscle disease and can cause a dilated cardiomyopathy to develop. It may occur due to a dietary deficiency, or to overfeeding with high-fat foods, such as snakes fed overweight rodents or fish (e.g. tuna and mackerel) which are high in polyunsaturates and increase the demand for vitamin E.

Atherosclerosis

This has been reported in green iguanas (Schuchman and Taylor, 1970) and bearded dragons (Schilliger *et al.*, 2010b) and may be a precursor to mineralisation of major arteries.

Neoplastic disease

Leukaemias have been regularly reported in many reptiles, particularly in snakes. They are often tissue-bound lymphomas, that is they are typically seen in body organs such as the liver, spleen and thymus rather than the bloodstream. However, some may become leukaemic overspill cases with the presence of neoplastic cells in the circulation. Up to 30.8% of cancers in reptiles have been associated with the haemopoietic system (Catao-Dias and Nichols, 1999). There is some suggestion that, as with birds, some lymphomas are virus associated.

In addition, other tumours have been reported including fibrosarcomas, mast cell tumours and chondrosarcomas in snakes (Schumacher *et al.*, 1998; Schmidt and Reavill, 2010). Fibrosarcomas seem to have a predilection for the right atrium. Haemangiomas, whilst benign, can rupture and result in fatal blood loss (Girling, 2019).

Urinary tract disease

Renal disease and gout

Aetiology

Damage to kidney function in the average terrestrial reptile can lead to increasing blood levels of uric acid, the main excretory product of protein metabolism. Uric acid is poorly water soluble, and so rapidly reaches its precipitation point in the bloodstream so that crystals form and come out of solution. This may occur in internal organs (visceral gout; see Figure 21.16) and also the joints (articular gout).

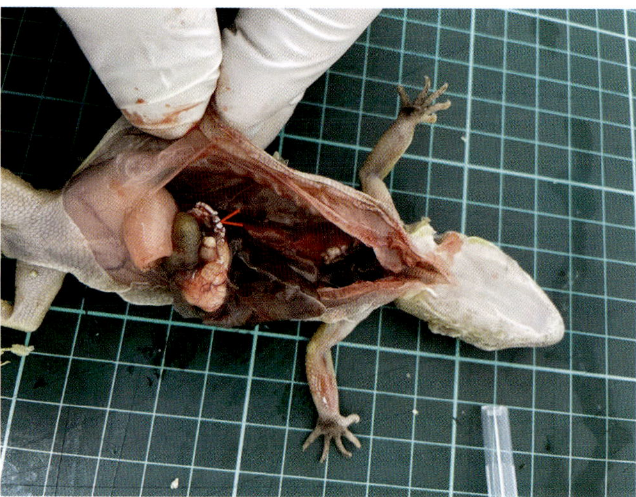

Figure 21.16 Visceral gout is the deposition of uric acid crystals on body organs (identified by the red arrowhead) due to excessively high blood levels of uric acid, usually associated with renal failure, as seen here in this post-mortem of a leopard gecko.

Factors contributing to renal failure include the following.

1. Diets high in protein, fed to herbivores, automatically lead to excessive production of uric acid, the main waste product of protein metabolism.
2. Diets with excessive levels of vitamin D_3 and calcium lead to calcification of soft tissue structures, such as the tunica media of the arterial walls, and the kidneys themselves. It should be noted that high deposition of monosodium urate and calcium crystals can occur in vessels associated with chronic renal failure.
3. Diets low in vitamin A result in squamous metaplasia of the proximal tubules of the kidneys.
4. Iatrogenic causes: certain nephrotoxic drugs such as the aminoglycoside antibiotic family (e.g. gentamicin, amikacin, sulfonamides), and the diuretic furosemide.
5. Toxic heavy metals such as lead.
6. If sufficient muscle bruising occurs, such as too firm a grasp of the patient when handling, then myoglobin is released. This causes damage to the kidney filtration membrane.
7. Glomerulonephritis occurred in approximately 27% of kidneys examined in one survey (Zwart, 2006). This can be associated with a number of infectious organisms including:
   a. Flagellates such as *Hexamita* spp., *Trichomonas* spp. and *Giardia* spp. have been reported in chelonians, snakes and lizards. *Hexamita* spp. are particularly damaging to the kidneys of chelonians.
   b. *Entamoeba invadens* has also been reported in snakes where it often becomes systemic and so can cause extensive areas of renal necrosis.
   c. Kidney flukes (trematodes) have been found in kingsnakes, and members of the Boidae. They may block renal tubules, and in high enough quantities, cause kidney failure.
   d. Coccidial parasites (e.g. *Klossiella boae*) in boids parasitise the collecting ducts and ureters. Intranuclear stages of coccidia have also been found in chelonians causing tubular necrosis.
   e. Myxosporidia of the genus *Myxidium* have been reported in the kidneys of chelonians but little is known about their pathogenicity.
   f. Microsporidia have also been reported in bearded dragons associated with infection of renal epithelial cells.
   g. Almost any bacterium found in the digestive system or environment of the reptile has the potential to cause renal disease if that reptile is stressed or debilitated in any way

(e.g. *Salmonella* spp., *Aeromonas* spp., *Pseudomonas* spp. and *E. coli*). In some chelonians, the bacteria responsible for septicaemic cutaneous syndrome, *Citrobacter freundii*, is also implicated. Mycobacteria have also been associated with renal disease in chelonians.

h. IBD of snakes has been associated with inclusions and damage to the kidneys with glomerulonephritis. Herpesvirus has been seen in chelonians causing the same.
i. Any systemic mycosis or local extension from a fungal pneumonia may lead to infection of the kidneys. *Penicillium griseofulvin*, *Geotrichum nigra* and *Colletotrichum acutatum* have all been reported associated with renal disease in chelonians.

Diagnosis of renal disease

Clinical signs can include lethargy, polydipsia, polyuria, collapse, visceral and articular gout, obstipation due to renomegaly pressing on the cloaca/rectum and dystocia (remember that the kidneys are in the pelvis in lizards and chelonians) and fluid retention with oedema.

Haematological parameters may alter with a leukocytosis in acute infectious renal disease. Chronic renal failure may have a non-regenerative anaemia. Uric acid measurement will allow an assessment of the severity of renal damage, with visceral gout starting when levels in the blood rise above 1500 μmol/L. Remember, though, that uric acid measurement is not a sensitive indicator of early renal disease, as less than 25% of the renal mass has to be left functioning before uric acid levels will rise significantly. Also, any reptile, particularly a carnivore that has eaten a meal recently, will have elevated uric acid levels. A starved sample (and remember that may mean 1–2 weeks in larger snakes) is required to ascertain a baseline blood uric acid level. In aquatic Chelonia, urea is a consistent fraction of nitrogen and therefore may be of use. In terrestrial species, urea is not a useful indicator of renal disease.

Calcium and phosphorus levels have been used as early indicators of renal disease in reptiles. The product of calcium and phosphorus (both measured in mmol/L) should be less than 9. If it exceeds this, and particularly if it exceeds 12, then metastatic mineralisation occurs and phosphate binders should be used. Gamma-glutamyltransferase is found in the brush border of the renal tubule and so is released when damaged. At this stage there is not enough evidence to determine what is significant.

Potassium levels may significantly elevate in chelonians with renal disease.

Urinalysis is less useful in reptiles than birds as there is usually post-renal modification of the urine in either the urinary bladder (where present) or the rectum, as urine is refluxed and more water (and solutes) is absorbed. No urine sample will be sterile either. However, assessment for protein casts, haematuria and, of course, parasites is useful.

Radiography demonstrating renomegaly can aid diagnosis. In lizards the kidneys should be within the pelvis. In renomegaly the cranial pole often projects into the caudal coelomic cavity and can be seen. Radiopaque dye may be injected intravenously to perform a urogram (800–1000 mg/kg of aqueous iodine). Finally, loss of bone density may occur with secondary hyperparathyroidism, although there has to be a significant drop in bone density for conventional radiographs to detect it.

Ultrasound examination of kidney structure can also be helpful for indicating overall increases in echogenicity and size. It is particularly useful in chelonians where radiography is not useful in detecting changes in size. The probe is placed in front of the hindlimb and angled caudally onto the inside of the carapace to examine the kidneys.

Endoscopy and biopsy, as with birds, is perhaps the definitive technique for determining the cause and severity of renal disease in reptiles. Even then, they have their limitations; in lizards, the kidneys are generally in the pelvis and may be difficult to visualise due to the presence of the fat pads, and in chelonians their position on the dorsum of the internal carapace means a rigid endoscope may find access difficult. Ultrasound-guided needle biopsy may also be attempted.

Bladder stones

These are common in reptiles, but obviously some reptiles do not have a urinary bladder. Chelonia and lizards such as the green iguana are the most commonly seen species. The stones are generally uric acid based and may form around a nidus of bacteria, a refluxed egg in females or a parasite. They may reach significant sizes, resulting in cystitis and cause considerable pain and discomfort.

Reproductive tract disease

Egg-binding or post-ovulatory stasis

Dystocia is common in many species of reptile. It is often associated with hypocalcaemia/hypovitaminosis D_3 in herbivorous chelonians and lizards. Other causes include malformed eggs, fractured pelvic bones, cystic calculi, lack of nesting material or malnutrition of the female.

Dystocias can be difficult to diagnose in snakes, as they tend to be relatively quiet creatures. This difficulty is exacerbated in those species (e.g. garter snakes) which are viviparous (giving birth to 'live' young rather than eggs) in that any abdominal swelling is much less pronounced. Any previous history of passing eggs, and then the presence of a persistent caudally located mass, is of course highly suggestive. In addition, any evidence of a prolapse of the cloaca or distal reproductive tract can indicate dystocia.

In lizards, the patient may be obviously distended with eggs, and become progressively more moribund and lethargic. Many snakes can survive prolonged periods of dystocia, but lizards are not so resilient and dystocia may prove fatal within days.

Chelonia may show signs of discomfort and straining or they may show no signs at all. Radiographs are often the only way to tell if a chelonian is gravid.

Preovulatory stasis

A condition recorded in both lizards and chelonians, and to a lesser extent in snakes, is preovulatory stasis. This is when the ovaries produce follicles that enlarge but do not shed into the reproductive tract. This results in ovaries containing anywhere up to 30 or 40 yolks, displacing all other coelomic organs (see Figure 21.17). Over time the affected reptile becomes anorectic and lethargic and often succumbs to secondary diseases (e.g. egg yolk coelomitis) and malnourishment. The cause of the condition is not fully understood but is thought to be associated with a long-term absence of a male or a brief exposure to a

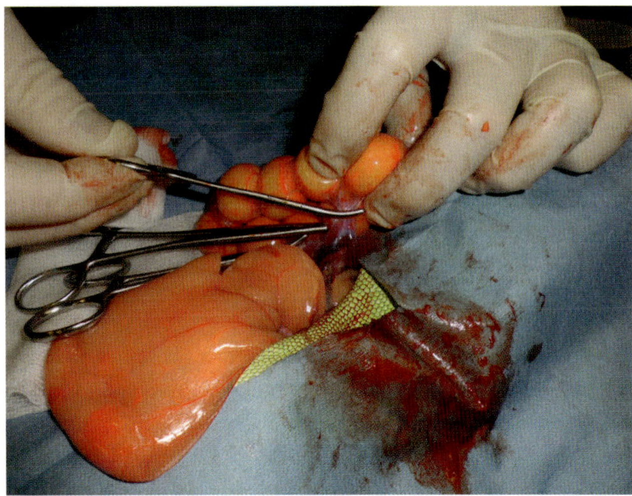

Figure 21.17 Preovulatory stasis is common and a potentially life-threatening condition in species such as the green iguana (*Iguana iguana*), particularly when they are kept as solitary individuals. Note one of the two coelomic fat pads to the left of the image and the numerous spherical 'yolks' on the clamped ovarian pedicel.

male after prior isolation. Radiographs show spherical rather than oval densities in the abdomen without the characteristic thin-walled part-calcified shell. Ultrasound can be useful to help diagnose the condition where moderately echo-dense spherical structures may be seen in the region of the ovaries.

Yolk coelomitis

This is often associated with preovulatory stasis when a follicle ruptures, leaking the irritant yolk into the coelomic cavity. This can in turn become secondarily infected and result in a septic coelomitis. Ultrasonography and radiography may help in identifying the cause. Clinical signs include lethargy, anorexia, coelomic distension and diarrhoea. There may be evidence of hyperproteinaemia, an increase in beta-globulins, leukocytosis, hypercalcaemia and azotaemia.

Hemipenal and phallus prolapse

This is often seen in weakened cachectic reptiles, or those with gastrointestinal, urinary or cloacal disease that results in persistent straining. In addition, many reptiles prolapse their phallus due to sexual frustration or to infection or to the formation of dried secretions (so-called hemipenal plug) within the hemipene which are irritants.

Oviduct prolapse

This may be seen in female reptiles, as a result of conditions described for phallus prolapse in males, and as a consequence of dystocia/egg binding or salpingitis. Severe prolapses, which have been present for some time, may necessitate emergency surgery and replacement of the prolapse via a coeliotomy, with the possibility of a salpingectomy at the same time.

Musculoskeletal disease

Metabolic bone disease

Aetiology

Metabolic bone disease (MBD) is common in young growing lizards and chelonians on a calcium-deficient diet, often in conjunction with deficiency of vitamin D_3/ UV-B. This results in nutritional secondary hyperparathyroidism (NSHP), the main form of MBD seen in reptiles. Another cause is renal secondary hyperparathyroidism due to renal failure producing hyperphosphataemia.

The clinical signs of MBD due to NSHP in lizards include a reptile that is weak and lethargic, and unable to support its body off the ground. The limbs appear swollen due to fibrous thickening (fibrous osteodystrophy) of the bones. Pathological fractures are common. Bowing of the lower jaw is also common in lizards due to tongue muscle contraction of softened bone. Hyperaesthesia may also be seen due to the hypocalcaemia, manifested as twitching digits when standing at rest and this may extend to the gastrointestinal tract, with ileus and cloacal prolapses made more likely.

In chelonians, the disease is seen as a softening and pyramiding of the shell (although other factors also contribute to this condition such as low humidity and excessive dietary proteins). The plastron and carapace are weakened due to hypomineralisation, which allows the internal skeletal muscles to deform their structure. This is particularly obvious over the internal attachments of the forelimbs and hindlimbs, where depressions in the shell may subsequently be seen. In some chelonians for example, the softened shell allows the corners of the carapace to roll upwards.

The source of cholecalciferol (vitamin D_3) for snakes and carnivorous lizards and chelonians is entirely from their food. For most insectivorous or herbivorous lizards and some chelonians, UV-B (280–315 nm wavelength) is necessary to activate the production of cholecalciferol (see Chapter 20).

Diagnosis of MBD

A history of poor diet and lack of UV-B provision is typical with NSHP-induced MBD. Plasma/serum ionised calcium levels are a more accurate indicator of the bioavailable calcium than total calcium levels. Values of 1.47 mmol/L have been calculated as the mean ionised calcium in green iguanas (Dennis *et al.*, 2001). Hypocalcaemia, hyperphosphataemia and a calcium to phosphorus ratio of less than 1 : 1 are often associated with MBD. Studies have also looked at blood calcitriol levels in reptiles (the active form of vitamin D_3) but there is often a lack of published normal values for individual species. Values for 25-hydroxyvitamin D_3 of 51–393 nmol/L have been determined for green iguanas (Nevarez *et al.*, 2002).

Radiography has been used as a primary, though not very sensitive, tool for diagnosing MBD. Poor bone mineralisation, widening of the bone diameter and deformity in the long axis of bones with general bone fractures and kyphotic/scoliotic spines may be seen.

Prevention of MBD

Klaphake (2010) has described UV light provision for reptiles to prevent MBD as follows.

1. Desert diurnal lizards/chelonians: high UV-B levels (10% or full unfiltered sun for 12 hours).
2. Diurnal arboreal lizards or semi-aquatic basking chelonians: moderate UV-B (5%, 12 hours).
3. Diurnal terrestrial lizards or chelonians from forests: low UV-B (5%, 6 hours).
4. Nocturnal lizards: low levels UV-B (2%, 6 hours).
5. Snakes: dietary calcium and vitamin D_3 is sufficient.

Calcium supplementation should be provided for young growing lizards and chelonians, and preferably in its more readily absorbable forms (i.e. calcium gluconate or calcium glubionate). For insectivores, gut loading their invertebrate prey is preferred as this guarantees the reptile will get the nutritional supplement. Commercially available insects need supplementation as most have inverted calcium to phosphorus ratios. Dietary deficiencies of calcium in herbivores can also occur where large amounts of leaves containing oxalates (e.g. spinach and beetroot tops) that bind calcium in the gut and prevent absorption are present. Fruit should be kept to a minimum in the vast majority of herbivorous species as it contains little or no calcium as well as causing bacterial fermentation and dental disease. Studies into shell pyramiding in Chelonia (*Geochelone sulcata*) showed that pyramiding was more likely to occur in individuals kept under dry environmental conditions than those in more humid ones, with small variations occurring due to higher levels of dietary protein. This study showed no significant impact on pyramiding of the dietary calcium to phosphorus ratio just to add further confusion to the MBD debate (Wiesner and Iben, 2003).

Fractures

These may be pathological, as is seen in cases of MBD, or they may be truly traumatic in origin. Repair of these fractures depends on their cause (see Chapter 22).

Joint swelling

This can be due to tumours, sepsis and articular gout. Systemic or local mycobacteriosis due to *M. marinum* has also been reported (Girling and Fraser, 2007).

Autotomy (tail shedding)

Autotomy, or spontaneous shedding of the tail sometimes with subsequent regrowth, is seen in some lizard species, for example many geckos and iguanas. These lizards have 'fracture planes' in their tails which will allow a clean break, with minimal bleeding, to occur should a predator attack or overzealous restraint is used. The tail will subsequently often (although not always) regrow, but when it does the coccygeal vertebrae are replaced with a rod of cartilage, and the scale pattern is frequently much more haphazard (see Figure 21.18).

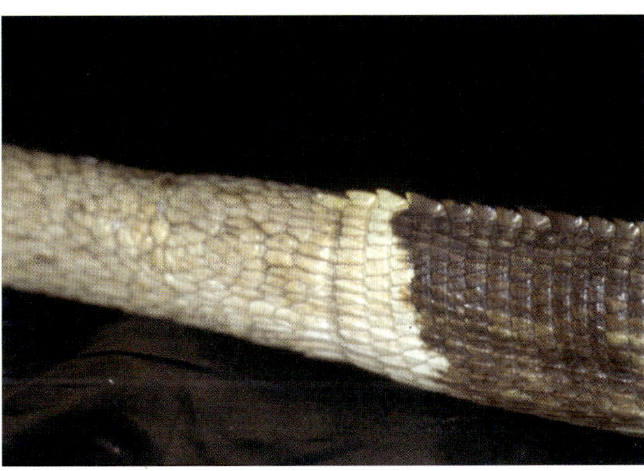

Figure 21.18 Autotomy followed by regrowth of the tail in a green iguana (*Iguana iguana*). Note the haphazard arrangement of scales distal to the break and the lack of dorsal spines.

When treating such lizards where the tail has broken off, it is important to avoid suturing the skin of the lizard over the stump of the tail left, as this may well prevent regrowth. Instead, the area should be treated as an open wound with topical antiseptics such as dilute povidone-iodine. In iguanids, once the individual matures, autotomy often ceases. This can occur over the age of 2.5–3 years in the green iguana for example.

If the tail wound is very proximal, such as through the area where the inverted hemipenes are situated in the male species, or in species of lizard where autotomy does not occur (such as many species of agamid lizards), routine closure of the skin over the stump under a general anaesthetic is required.

Neurological disease

Parasitic causes of neurological disease

Acanthamoebic meningoencephalitis is a condition seen primarily in snakes due to *Entamoeba invadens*. Fits and opisthotonic seizures are seen. Treatment is generally unsuccessful.

Toxoplasma and *Encephalitozoon* infections have also been reported as a cause of meningoencephalitis in reptiles.

Bacterial causes of neurological disease

Bacterial abscesses/granulomas of the spinal cord or the brain may result in neurological disease. These are usually as a result of septicaemia which is common in reptiles. Most are Gram-negative in nature, but mycoplasma and chlamydophilal organisms have also been reported as have mycobacterial infections.

Middle ear infections in aquatic chelonians are common and may result in peripheral vestibular disease. There is often an underlying vitamin A deficiency problem.

Fungal causes of neurological disease

Migration of fungal disease from other body organs such as the lungs can involve the spinal column or disseminate into the CNS and cause neurological disease.

Viral causes of neurological disease

Paramyxovirus

These have been reported in many species of snake, with the *Ferlavirus* genus being most significant. The virus causes haemorrhagic pneumonias but will also cause neurological signs such as the loss of righting reflexes. There is no current treatment.

Inclusion body disease

This has been seen in a range of snake species including boas and pythons, elapids and colubrids. It is thought to be an arenavirus. In pythons, the disease is severe with infectious stomatitis, pneumonia and neurological signs such as loss of the righting reflex, disorientation and blindness often followed rapidly by death. In boas, the disease is fatal in young individuals. In older patients, the disease produces more chronic neurological signs with chronic anorexia, vomiting and pneumonias. Neurological signs are milder, with a loss of ability to chew and swallow prey, and a loss of the striking reflex. Diagnosis is currently based on biopsy of affected organs, principally the liver, kidney, spleen and oesophageal tonsils, which will show classical eosinophilic intracytoplasmic inclusion bodies. Early in the course of the disease there may be a leukocytosis (white blood cells >30×10^9/L).

There is no treatment for this disease.

Other viruses

Chelonian herpesviruses have been associated with neurological disease. Adenoviruses have been associated with opisthotonus and death in chameleons (Jacobson and Gardiner, 1990).

Nutritional causes of neurological disease

Hypocalcaemic collapse

This is commonly seen in gravid lizards, such as green iguanas, when the blood calcium levels drop too low. The female becomes flaccidly paralysed and unresponsive. Fine muscle tremors will often be seen prior to the final paralysis stage.

Hypovitaminosis B_1

It is seen in primarily fish-eating reptiles such as garter snakes. The thiaminases present in previously frozen and then defrosted fish break down the vitamin B_1 present in the food leading to a functional deficit. The presenting signs include opisthotonus and lack of a righting reflex.

Biotin deficiency

This is seen in species fed mainly on unfertilised hen's eggs that contain large amounts of the anti-biotin vitamin, avidin. This produces a relative deficiency in biotin which leads to muscle tremor and general weakness. Monitor lizards are commonly affected.

Hypoglycaemia

This is a condition seen in crocodiles. It is unknown why it occurs, but muscle tremor and weakness are seen.

Environmental causes of neurological disease

This can occur due to freezing injuries. These are seen in chelonians overwintering outside in the UK. Frost damage causes blindness, vestibular disease and death. There is no treatment.

Toxic causes of neurological disease

Pyrethrin/organophosphate poisoning

These are most likely to be associated with home-administered antimite treatments. Overdose will result in opisthotonus, head tilts, fits and death. Management with atropine in cases of organophosphate poisoning may be successful but is rarely so in pyrethrin cases. Supportive therapy in mildly affected animals may be sufficient to allow recovery.

Lead toxicosis

This has been reported in chelonians with access to lead piping or lead paints commonly used in older houses on internal woodwork. It usually results in gut stasis and liver/kidney problems, but may present as neurological disease in reptiles.

Diseases of amphibians

Bacterial diseases

Redleg

Redleg is caused by the bacterium *Aeromonas hydrophila*. It produces ulcerating red wounds, which give it its name. The bacterium also causes a septicaemic syndrome with the amphibian becoming bloated and developing renal and hepatic failure. Skin lesions may occur late on in the course of the disease. Poor environmental conditions are often blamed for increasing bacterial burden and reducing amphibian immune system responses.

Mycobacteria

Mycobacterial infections due to environmental species such as *Mycobacterium marinum*, *M. chelonea*, *M. ulcerans*, *M. liflandii*, *M. ranae* and *M. xenopi* can cause classical tuberculous lesions mainly on the limbs or internal organs (see Figure 21.19). The affected amphibian loses weight rapidly, becoming emaciated, but often maintains a good appetite in the earlier stages unlike other bacterial diseases. There is no effective treatment.

Flavobacteria

These Gram-negative, yellow pigment-producing bacteria are widely present in aquatic environments and are a known cause of oedema disease in adult amphibians, producing a syndrome that resembles some viral conditions and dermatosepticaemia and so is a differential diagnosis with *Aeromonas hydrophila* infection. Diagnosis is based on detection of the bacteria either after culture or using PCR technology.

Chlamydiosis

The bacteria *Chlamydia* spp. have been associated with disease in large anurans including the European common frog. Clinical signs include petechiation, sloughing of the skin and abdominal swelling. Diagnosis is based on clinical signs, use of generic PCR tests on swabs of affected areas for chlamydial organisms and histopathology.

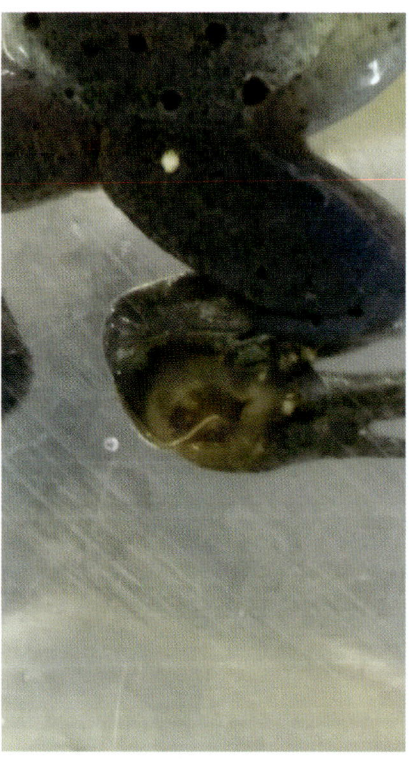

Figure 21.19 Environmental mycobacterial disease can gain access through skin wounds and create significant tuberculous lesions in amphibians as seen here.

Fungal diseases

Chytridiomycosis

This is the single most important fungal disease affecting amphibians in the world today and has resulted in a massive decline in amphibian numbers. The organisms involved *Batrachochytrium dendrobatidis* in anurans and Caudata and *B. salamandrivorans* in Caudata. The fungus has motile zoospores that will swim towards an amphibian and once attached, in the case of *B. dendrobatidis*, feeds off the keratin of the skin. This means that adult amphibians are more likely to be affected as the tadpoles only have keratin in their mouthparts. *Batrachochytrium salamandrivorans* produces a rapid decline in the newt/salamander, with numerous ulcerated skin lesions and often death within a week of infection. *Batrachochytrium dendrobatidis* produces skin ulceration, and invades deeper tissues that results in dehydration, secondary bacterial infections and death in adult amphibians over a more protracted course. Diagnosis is by clinical signs and PCR of swabs associated with infected tissues, particularly the toes of anurans and the drink patch on the ventrum.

Saprolegniasis

This is a common environmental fungal disease seen in all aquatic species. It occurs classically as strands of white, cotton wool-like material adhering to the skin surface. The condition is worsened in warmer waters.

Phycomycosis

This is due to common moulds such as *Mucor* spp. These are often darkly pigmented and so the condition can be referred to as chromomycosis. Infections can become systemic (which is uncommon with saprolegniasis). These moulds will often affect amphibian eggs.

Viral diseases

Herpesvirus

A herpesvirus (ranid herpesvirus 1) in the North American leopard frog induces a form of renal adenocarcinoma, known as Lucke's renal tumour. The tumour grows during the warmer months, with the virus being shed in the spring to infect other frogs. Renal failure occurs with chronic weight loss and death. There is no treatment for this condition.

Tadpole oedema virus

Again, this is thought to be due to an iridovirus in the genus *Ranavirus*. As its name suggests it produces oedema in affected tadpoles and internal haemorrhage. There is no treatment.

Spindly leg syndrome

This has been associated with a ranavirus in the family *Iridoviridae* but other causes of this condition have also been suggested, such as poor diet, particularly vitamin B deficiencies. As its name suggests, it affects mainly young growing anurans by causing a failure in the development of the forelimbs. Once developed there is no treatment. A scoring system from 0 (no limbs affected) through to 5 (hindlimbs very stunted and forelimbs do not develop) has been devised (Claunch and Augustine, 2015).

Parasitic diseases

Nematodes

The commonest nematode seen in anurans is the lungworm *Rhabdias* spp. In large numbers, this parasite may cause pneumonia. The parasite has a direct life cycle and can penetrate the skin of the amphibian to infect it.

Other nematodes such as *Strongyloides* spp. may parasitise the gut and coelomic cavity, with large burdens resulting in poor growth and intestinal blockages.

Protozoa

Entamoeba ranarum: Can cause damage to the large intestine of anurans, as well as the liver. This may lead to weight loss, diarrhoea with blood, anorexia and dehydration. It can also cause nephritis with ascites and oedema of the limbs. The trophozoites are 16–18 μm in diameter and are shed in the faeces.

Oodinium pillularis: A motile protozoan that affects many aquatic animals including amphibians. It damages the skin, and in tadpole stages damages the gills leading to anoxia. It is able to swim through the water from amphibian to amphibian and can therefore spread rapidly.

Trematodes

Trematodes such as *Ribeiroia ondatrae* have been linked with the production of extra limbs in anurans. Adult trematodes can be found in many places including the lung, gastrointestinal tract, skin, kidney and urinary bladder. They may block the intestines if present in large enough numbers and result in a wasting condition.

Mesomycetal diseases

These are organisms that cross the fungal–animal divide and so have characteristics of both. They include organisms such as *Amphibiocystidium*, *Amphibiothecum* and *Ichthyophonus* spp. All produce spores that are usually motile and cause nodular skin lesions in amphibians. Most self-resolve but *Ichthyophonus* spp. can cause muscle damage in anurans and Caudata.

Toxicity

Amphibians are highly susceptible to toxicities associated with environmental agents such as chlorine (e.g. mains tap water) and ammonia. Many commonly used veterinary antiseptics and disinfectants can be toxic to amphibians, including most of the chlorine-, chlorhexidine- and quaternary ammonium-containing compounds. Tap water should always be dechlorinated by allowing it to stand for 24 hours or more after pouring or adding dechlorinating agents such as sodium thiosulphate. Alternatively, spring water should be used when providing water for amphibians.

Heavy metal toxicosis is also possible as amphibians are susceptible to the toxic effects of lead, zinc, chromium and copper, amongst others. All of these can cause renal, liver and bone marrow damage.

Metabolic bone disease

Metabolic bone disease due to NSHP is common, particularly in frogs and toads (anurans). Earlier in the course of the condition, tetany can be seen after leaping/exercise in anurans and swimming can become incoordinated. Skeletal changes include softening of the lower jaw which bulges laterally, weakness and paralysis of the limbs, with spontaneous fractures and kyphosis and scoliosis of the spine. Limb paralysis and bloating can also be associated with hypocalcaemia in amphibians. Some recommend access to cuttlebone for tadpoles in all species in order to provide sufficient calcium in the diet (Whitaker and Wright, 2019).

Hypovitaminosis A

Hypovitaminosis A is a potential risk to captive amphibians as they are unable to manufacture it from precursors (pre-carotenoids) and so must obtain preformed vitamin A through their diet. Clinical signs can include squamous metaplasia of epithelial and glandular structures including the mucous secretions of the tongue, which may inhibit the ability of anurans for example to catch their prey (Pessier *et al.*, 2002). Squamous metaplasia can occur in the kidneys and may result in hydrocoelom, the retention of fluid in the coelomic cavity. There is also a suspicion that due to skin cell changes, increased susceptibility to skin infections, particularly chytrid, may also occur.

Stomach impaction

This can be seen in some of the larger anurans that may take small rodent prey. Should these amphibians be overfed (and they will often eat if presented with a food item that is moving even if already full), then the enlarged stomach will press on the lungs above resulting in decreased respiration. The food in the stomach is also more likely to become rancid if in excess as the digestive enzymes cannot cope with such an overload. This can lead to a bacterial population explosion and subsequent septicaemia.

References

Abarca, M.L., Martorell, J., Castella, G. *et al.* (2009) Dermatomycosis in a pet inland bearded dragon (*Pogona vitticeps*) caused by a *Chrysosporium* species related to *Nannizziopsis vriesii*. *Veterinary Dermatology*, **20**(4), 295–299.

Austwick, P. and Keymer, I. (1981) Fungi and actinomycetes. In: *Diseases of the Reptilia* (eds J.E. Cooper & O.F. Jackson), pp. 93–231. Academic Press, San Diego, CA.

Barten, S. (1980) Cardiomyopathy in a kingsnake (*Lampropeltis calligaster rhombomaculata*). *Veterinary Medicine Small Animal Clinician*, **75**, 125–129.

Bowman, M.R., Pare, J.A., Sigler, L. *et al.* (2007) Deep fungal dermatitis in three inland bearded dragons (*Pogona vitticeps*) caused by the *Chrysosporium* anamorph of *Nannizziopsis vriesii*. *Medical Mycology*, **45**(4), 371–376.

Brown, D.R., Nogueira, M.F., Schoeb, T.R. *et al.* (2001) Pathology of experimental mycoplasmosis in American alligators. *Journal of Wildlife Diseases*, **37**(4), 671–679. doi: 10.7589/0090-3558-37.4.671.

Burd, E.M., Juzych, L.A., Rudrik, J.T. and Habib, F. (2007) Pustular dermatitis caused by *Dermatophilus congolensis*. *Journal of Clinical Microbiology*, **45**, 1655–1658.

Cabanes, F.J., Sutton, D.A. and Guarro, J. (2014) *Chrysosporium*-related fungi and reptiles: a fatal attraction. *PLoS Pathogens*, **10**, e1004367.

Catão-Dias, J.L. and Nichols, D.K. (1999) Neoplasia in snakes at the National Zoological Park, Washington, DC (1978–1997). *Journal of Comparative Pathology*, **120**, 89–95.

Cheatwood, J.L., Jacobson, E.R., May, P.G. *et al.* (2003) An outbreak of fungal dermatitis and stomatitis in free-ranging population of pigmy rattlesnakes (*Sistrurus miliarius barbouri*) in Florida. *Journal of Wildlife Diseases*, **39**(2), 329–337.

Claunch, N. and Augustine, L. (2015) Morphological description of spindly leg syndrome in golden mantilla (*Mantella aurantiaca*). *Journal of Herpetological Medicine and Surgery*, **25**, 72–77.

Dennis, P.M., Bennett, R.A., Harr, K.E. and Lock, B.A. (2001) Plasma concentration of ionized calcium in healthy iguanas. *Journal of the American Veterinary Medical Association*, **219**(3), 326–328.

Diaz-Figueroa, O., Mitchell, M.A., Ramirez, S. *et al.* (2008) *Paecilomyces lilacinus* pneumonia in a free-ranging Gopher tortoise, *Gopherus polyphemus*. *Journal of Herpetological Medicine and Surgery*, **18**(2), 52–60.

Fraser, M.A. and Girling, S.J. (2004) Dermatology. In: *BSAVA Manual of Reptiles* (eds S.J. Girling & P. Raiti), 2nd edn, pp. 184–198. BSAVA, Quedgeley, UK.

Frost, J.W. and Schmidt, A. (1997) Serological evidence for susceptibility of various species of tortoises to infections by herpesvirus. *38th Intemationalen Symposiums uber Erkrankungen der Zoo und Wildtiere*, 7–11 May 1997, Zurich, pp. 25–28.

Frye, F. (1991) *Biomedical and Surgical Aspects of Captive Reptile Husbandry*, Volume 1 and 2. Krieger Publishing, Malabar, FL.

Frye, F.L. (1999) Spontaneous autoimmune pancreatitis and diabetes mellitus in a Western pond turtle *Clemmys m. marmorata*. *Proceedings of the Association of Reptilian and Amphibian Veterinarians, Columbus, Ohio*, pp. 103–106.

Girling, S.J. (2002a) Plasma protein electrophoresis: variations in health and disease in the family Psittaciformes. Dissertation as part-fulfilment for the RCVS Diploma in Zoological Medicine, RCVS Library.

Girling, S.J. (2002b) A fungal granuloma in a corn snake (*Elaphe guttata guttata*) due to *Aspergillus fumigatus* associated with a previously treated abscess. *Bulletin of the British Veterinary Zoological Society*, **2**(1), 27–35.

Girling, S.J. (2002c) Mammalian imaging and anatomy. In: *Manual of Exotic Pets* (eds A. Meredith & S. Redrobe), 4th edn, pp. 1–12. BSAVA, Quedgeley, UK.

Girling, S.J. (2019) Vascular, hematopoietic and immune systems. In: *Mader's Reptile and Amphibian Medicine and Surgery* (eds S.J. Divers & S.J. Stahl), 3rd edn, pp. 917–921. Elsevier, Philadelphia.

Girling, S.J. and Fraser, M.A. (2007) Systemic mycobacteriosis in an inland bearded dragon (*Pogona vitticeps*). *Veterinary Record*, **160**, 526–528.

Girling, S.J. and Fraser, M.A. (2009) Treatment of *Aspergillus* species infection in reptiles with itraconazole at metabolically scaled dosages. *Veterinary Record*, **165**(2), 52–54.

Gonzalez Cabo, J.F., Espejo Serrano, J. and Barcena Asensio, M.C. (1995) Mycotic pulmonary disease by *Beauveria bassiana* in a captive tortoise. *Mycoses*, **38**(3–4), 167–169.

Harkewicz, K.A. (2001) Dermatology of reptiles: a clinical approach to diagnosis and treatment. *Veterinary Clinics of North America: Exotic Animal Practice*, **4**, 441–461.

Heard, D.J., Cantor, G.H., Jacobson, E.R. *et al.* (1986) Hyalophomycosis caused by *Paecilomyces lilacinus* in an Aldabran tortoise. *Journal of the American Veterinary Medical Association*, **189**, 1143–1145.

Heatley, J.J., Mitchell, M.A., Williams, J. *et al.* (2001) Fungal periodontal osteomyelitis in a chameleon *Furcifer pardalis*. *Journal of Herpetological Medicine and Surgery*, **11**(4), 7–12.

Hernandez-Divers, S.J., Knott, C.D. and MacDonald, J. (2001) Diagnosis and surgical treatment of thyroid adenoma-induced hyperthyroidism in a green iguana (*Iguana iguana*). *Journal of Zoo and Wildlife Medicine*, **32**, 465–475.

Hough, I. (1998) Cryptococcosis in an eastern water skink. *Australian Veterinary Journal*, **76**(7), 471–472.

Fraser, M.A. and Girling, S.J. (2019) Dermatology. In: *BSAVA Manual of Reptiles* (eds S.J. Girling & P. Raiti), 3rd edn, pp. 257–272. BSAVA, Quedgeley, UK.

Garner, M.M., Gardiner, C.H., Wellehan, J.F.X. *et al.* (2006) Intranuclear coccidiosis in tortoises: nine cases. *Veterinary Pathology*, **43**, 311–320.

Hofmannova, L., Kvicerova, J., Bizkova, K. and Modry, D. (2019) Intranuclear coccidiosis in tortoises: discovery of its causative agent and transmission. *European Journal of Protistology*, **67**, 71–76.

Huchzermeyer, F.W. and Cooper, J.E. (2001) Fibriscess, not abscess, resulting from localised inflammatory response to infection in reptiles and birds. *Veterinary Record*, **147**, 515–516.

Iverson, J.B. (1980) Colic modifications in Iguanine lizards. *Journal of Morphology*, **163**, 79–93.

Jacobson, E.R. (1980) Mycotic diseases of reptiles. In: *The Comparative Pathology of Zoo Animals* (eds R.J. Montali & G. Migaki), pp. 283–290. Smithsonian Institution Press, Washington, DC.

Jacobson, E.R., Gardiner, C.H., Barten, S.L. *et al.* (1989a) *Flavobacterium meningosepticum* infection of a Barbour's Map Turtle (*Graptemys barbouri*). *Journal of Zoo and Wildlife Medicine*, **20**(4), 474–477.

Jacobson, E.R., Gaskin, J. and Mansell, J. (1989b) Chlamydial infection in puff adders (*Bitis arietens*). *Journal of Zoo and Wildlife Medicine*, **20**(3), 364–369.

Jacobson, E.R. and Gardiner, C.H. (1990) Adeno-like virus in oesophageal and tracheal mucosa of a Jackson's chameleon (*Chameleo jacksonii*). *Veterinary Pathology*, **27**, 210–212.

Klaphake, E. (2010) A fresh look at metabolic bone diseases in reptiles and amphibians. *Veterinary Clinics of North America: Exotic Animal Practice*, **13**, 375–392.

Koplos, P., Garner, M., Besser, T. *et al.* (2000) Cheilitis in lizards of the genus *Uromastyx* associated with filamentous gram positive bacterium. *Proceedings of the 7th Annual Association of Reptile and Amphibian Veterinarian Conference*, 73–75.

Lappin, P.B. and Dunstan, R.W. (1992) Difficult dermatologic diagnosis. *Journal of the American Veterinary Medical Association*, **200**, 785–786.

Marschang, R. and Chitty, J. (2019) Infectious diseases. In: *BSAVA Manual of Reptiles* (eds S.J. Girling & P. Raiti), 3rd edn, pp. 423–442. BSAVA, Quedgeley, UK.

Masters, A.M., Ellis, T.M., Carson, J.M. *et al.* (1995) *Dermatophilus cheloniae* sp. nov. isolated from chelonids in Australia. *International Journal of Systemic Bacteriology*, **45**, 50–56.

McArthur, S., McLellan, L. and Brown, S. (2004) Gastrointestinal disease. In: *Manual of Reptiles* (eds S.J. Girling & P. Raiti), 2nd edn, pp. 210–229. BSAVA, Quedgeley, UK.

Migaki, G., Jacobson, E.R. and Casey, H.W. (1984) Fungal diseases in reptiles. In: *Diseases of Amphibians and Reptiles* (eds G.L. Hoff & E.R. Jacobson), pp. 183–204. Plenum Press, New York.

Murray, M.J. (1996) Cardiology and circulation. In: *Reptile Medicine and Surgery* (ed. D. Mader), 1st edn, pp. 95–103. WB Saunders, Phialdelphia.

Nevarez, J.G., Mitchell, M.A., Le Blanc, C., *et al.* (2002) Determination of plasma biochemistries, ionized calcium, vitamin D_3, and hematocrit values in captive green iguanas (*Iguana iguana*) from El Salvador. *Proceedings of the Annual Conference of the Association of Reptilian and Amphibian Veterinarians*, pp. 87–91.

Nichols, D.K., Weyant, R.S., Lamirande, E.W. *et al.* (1999) Fatal mycotic dermatitis in captive brown tree snakes (*Boiga irregularis*). *Journal of Zoo and Wildlife Medicine*, **30**(1), 111–118.

Oros, J., Ramirez, A.S., Poveda, J.B. *et al.* (1996) Systemic mycosis caused by *Penicillium griseofulvum* in a Seychelles giant tortoise (*Megachelys gigantean*). *Veterinary Record*, **139**(12), 295–296.

Pare, J.A., Sigler, L., Hunter, D.B. *et al.* (1997) Cutaneous mycoses in chameleons caused by the *Chyrsosporium* anamorph of *Nannizziopsis vriesii (Apinis)* Currah. *Journal of Zoo and Wildlife Medicine*, **28**(4), 443–453.

Pasmans, K., Hellebuyck, T., Haesebrouck, F. and Martel, A. (2010) Dermatitis and septicaemia caused by *Devriesea agamarum*: an overview including recent developments in disease management. *Proceedings of the 1st International Conference on Reptile and Amphibian Medicine, Munich, Germany*, pp. 105–106.

Pees, M., Schroff, S., Kiefer, I. and Krautwald-Junghanns, M.E. (2010) Ultrasonographic examination of the heart and the great vessels in boid snakes and demonstration of a case of valvular insufficiency in a Burmese python (*Python molurus bivittatus*). *Proceedings of the 1st International Conference on Reptile and Amphibian Medicine, Munich*, pp. 211–212.

Penner, J.D., Jacobson, E.R. and Brown, D.R. (1997) A novel *Mycoplasma* sp. associated with proliferative tracheitis and pneumonia in a Burmese python (*Python molurus bivittatus*). *Journal of Comparative Pathology*, **117**, 283–288.

Pessier, A.P., Roberts, D.R., Linn, M., Garner, M.M., Raymond, J.T., Dierenfield, E.S. and Graffham, W. (2002) Short tongue syndrome, lingual squamous metaplasia and suspected hypovitaminosis A in captive Wyoming toads (*Bufo baxteri*). *Proceedings of the 9th Annual Conference of the Association of Reptilian and Amphibian Veterinarians*, pp. 151–153.

Ritter, J.M., Garber, M.M., Chilton, J.A. *et al.* (2009) Gastric neuroendocrine carcinomas in bearded dragons (*Pogona vitticeps*). *Veterinary Pathology*, **46**(6), 1109–1116. doi: 10.1354/vp.09-VP-0019-K-FL.

Rossi, J. and Rossi, R. (2000) Fungal dermatitis in a large collection of Brazos water snakes, *Nerodia harteri harteri* housed in an outdoor enclosure, and a possible association with slugs. In: *Proceedings of the Association of Reptilian and Amphibian Veterinarians* (eds M.M. Willette & L.C. Boyer), pp. 81–83.*Reno, Nevada*

Schilliger, L., Lemberger, K., Bourgeois, A. and Charpentier, M. (2010b) First case of atherosclerosis associated with pericardial effusion in a bearded dragon (*Pogona vitticeps* AHL 1926). *Proceedings of the Annual Conference of the Association of Reptilian and Amphibian Veterinarians*, 70–74.

Schuchman, S.M. and Taylor, D.O. (1970) Arteriosclerosis in an iguana (*Iguana iguana*). *Journal of the American Veterinary Medical Association*, **157**, 614–616.

Schumacher, J. (2003) Fungal diseases of reptiles. *Veterinary Clinics of North America: Exotic Animal Practice*, **6**(2), 327–355.

Schumacher, J.R., Bennett, A., Fox, L.E. *et al.* (1998) Mast cell tumor in an eastern kingsnake (*Lampropeltis getulus getulus*). *Journal of Veterinary Diagnostic Investigation*, **10**, 101–104.

Sigler, L., Hambleton, S. and Pare, J.A. (2013) Molecular characterization of reptile pathogens currently known as members of *Chrysosporium* anamorph of *Nannizziopsis vriesii* complex and relationship with some human-associated isolates. *Journal of Clinical Microbiology*, **51**, 3338–3357.

Soares, J.F., Chalker, V.J., Erles, K. *et al.* (2004) Prevalence of *Mycoplasma agassizii* and chelonian herpesvirus in captive tortoise (*Testudo* spp.) in the United Kingdom. *Journal of Zoo and Wildlife Medicine*, **35**(1), 25–33.

Stahl, S.J. (2003) Pet lizard conditions and syndromes. *Seminars in Avian and Exotic Pet Medicine*, **12**(3), 162–182.

Tamukai, K., Tokiwa, T., Kobayashi, H. and Une, Y. (2016) Ranavirus in an outbreak of dermatophilosis in inland bearded dragons (*Pogona vitticeps*). *Veterinary Dermatology*, **27**, 99–105.

Tappe, J.P., Chandler, F.W., Lui, S.K. and Dolensk, E.P. (1984) Aspergillosis in two San Esteban chuckwallas. *Journal of the American Veterinary Medical Association*, **185**(11), 1425–1428.

Weitzman, I., Rosenthal, S.A. and Shupack, J.L. (1985) A comparison between *Dactylaria gallopava* and *Scolecobasidium humicola*: first report of an infection in a tortoise caused by *S. humicola*. *Sabouraudia*, **23**(4), 287–293.

Westhouse, R.A., Jacobson, E.R., Harris, R.K. *et al.* (1996) Respiratory and pharyngoesophageal iridovirus infection in a gopher tortoise (*Gopherus polyphemus*). *Journal of Wildlife Diseases*, **32**, 682–686.

Whitaker, B.R. and Wright, K.M. (2019) Amphibian medicine. In: *Mader's Reptile and Amphibian Medicine and Surgery* (eds S.J. Divers & S.J. Stahl), 3rd edn, pp. 992–1013. Elsevier, Philadelphia.

Wiesner, C.S. and Iben, C. (2003) Influence of environmental humidity and dietary protein on pyramidal growth of carapaces in African spurred tortoises (*Geochelone sulcata*). *Journal of Animal Physiology and Animal Nutrition*, **87**, 66–74.

Woodburn, D.B., Kinsel, M.J., Poll, C.P. *et al.* (2021) Shell lesions associated with *Emydomyces testavorans* infection in freshwater aquatic turtles. *Veterinary Pathology*, **58**(3). doi: 10.1177/0300985820985217.

Schmidt, R.E. and Reavill, D.R. (2010) Metastatic chondrosarcoma in a corn snake (*Elaphe guttata*). *Proceedings of the 1st International Conference on Reptile Amphibian Medicine, Munich, Germany*, p. 147.

Wagner, J. (1989) Clinical challenge case number one. *Journal of Zoo and Wildlife Medicine*, **20**, 238–239.

Zwart, P. (2006) Renal pathology in reptiles. *Veterinary Clinics of North America: Exotic Animal Practice*, **9**, 129–159.

Chapter 22 An Overview of Reptile and Amphibian Therapeutics

FLUID THERAPY

Maintenance requirements

Every reptile or amphibian has a fluid maintenance requirement. These losses, as for cats and dogs, occur in several ways, for example urine output, insensible losses through respiration, panting (i.e. gular fluttering) and salivation.

In most reptiles, very little water is lost through the skin – reptiles have little to no true sweat glands. Amphibians, however, will lose fluid readily across their semipermeable skin membranes, and so need to remain close to a water source for nearly all of their lives.

Some reptiles will lose water through gular fluttering, for example members of the Crocodilia as well as many desert-dwelling lizards.

Reptiles are well adapted to conserve water. Most species are uricotelic, excreting uric acid instead of urea as the main waste product of metabolised protein. Uric acid requires very little water to be excreted with it, unlike urea in mammals, as it is actively excreted via the proximal tubules of the nephron and so maintenance fluid requirements are lower for reptiles than mammals. However, not all reptiles produce predominantly uric acid; many aquatic and semi-aquatic species excrete ammonia and urea. In the case of totally aquatic amphibian species such as caecilians, ammonia is also excreted, whereas the more terrestrial amphibian species such as toads excrete urea and one or two may produce uric acid.

Maintenance requirements, although lower than an equivalent-sized mammal, can vary widely. A desert-dwelling uricotelic species may be able to cope with some water deprivation, while an ammonotelic (ammonia-excreting) species, such as an aquatic turtle or amphibian, is used to large, regular fluid intakes and outputs and therefore has a higher maintenance requirement.

However, if a uricotelic reptile is deprived of water for prolonged periods of time, reduced renal blood flow leads to reduced uric acid excretion. This leads to a build-up of uric acid in the bloodstream. Once uric acid levels exceed 1200–1500 µmol/L precipitation of uric acid crystals occurs inside the body, a condition known as 'visceral gout'. Once uric acid crystals are deposited in and around vital organs, such as the kidneys and heart, they cannot be removed and permanent damage has been done.

The volume of water consumed daily varies from species to species as do the sources of water. Many herbivorous reptiles such as *Testudo* spp. tortoises obtain the majority of their daily fluid requirement from their diet, which is generally composed of leafy greens. However, other herbivorous species, such as the green iguana, while consuming plenty of leafy greens are used to living in tropical rainforest conditions where the relative humidity is 100%. Place this reptile into an arid vivarium and it will, with time, lose fluid through its skin and mucous membranes if it is not also provided with daily misting of its tank. This is compounded by the fact that many reptiles will not readily drink from water bowls, only taking water from droplets on surfaces in the wild, for example many chameleons as well as the green iguana.

To add to this, in ectothermic species, it is important to take into account the environmental temperature requirements of that species. If the reptile is not kept within its preferred optimum temperature zone (POTZ), then it cannot achieve its preferred body temperature (PBT) and its internal physiological processes will not operate at their optimal rates, leading to inefficient water usage and consumption.

The effect of disease on fluid requirements

Fluid loss may be rapid, due to water loss alone, for example with acute diarrhoea, thermal burns or vomiting. In this case, the remaining extracellular fluid (ECF) becomes reduced, but is still of the same composition (isotonic). Alternatively, fluid loss may be due to long-term anorexia, producing a reduction in electrolytes and creating a hypotonic ECF. Finally, water deprivation or oral trauma that prevents drinking will lead to increases in the tonicity of the ECF, and create a hypertonic dehydration.

With any disease, the need for fluids increases, even if no obvious fluid loss has occurred. This is due to a number of reasons. It may involve renal changes, such as increases in the glomerular filtration rate or reduction in water reabsorption by the collecting ducts so causing increased urine output. Or there may be reduced absorption of water from the small or large intestine.

Respiratory disease is common in reptiles, with increased respiratory secretions being the result. Fluid loss via this route can be appreciable.

Another less obvious route is fluid and electrolyte loss through skin disease. Reptiles often suffer serious burns from unprotected basking lamps and faulty heaters. Not only will there be serious fluid and electrolyte loss via full-thickness skin burns but these reptiles will succumb to secondary skin infections from environmental bacteria such as *Pseudomonas* spp. These produce lesions that resemble chemical or thermal burns, and leave large areas of weeping exudative skin for further fluid loss.

Finally, we have to consider the need for fluid therapy during other forms of medical therapy, such as antibiotic treatment. Many bacterial infections in reptiles are caused by Gram-negative bacteria and therefore the aminoglycoside family of antibiotics (gentamicin, tobramycin, amikacin, etc.) has been widely used for treatment. This

Veterinary Nursing of Exotic Pets and Wildlife, Third Edition. Simon J. Girling.

family of antibiotics has several serious side-effects, of which the most serious is renal damage. This can be heightened if there is reduced renal perfusion because of dehydration. The renal damage so caused can be severe enough to kill even a healthy reptile.

Anaesthesia fluid requirements

Causes of fluid loss during anaesthesia include the possibility of intra-surgical haemorrhage. This will call for vascular support with an aqueous isotonic electrolyte solution or, in more serious blood losses (>10% blood volume), colloidal fluids or even blood transfusions.

Even if surgery is relatively bloodless, there are inevitable losses via the respiratory route. This is due to the drying nature of the gases used in anaesthesia. As many of these species are small in size, they have a large lung surface area in relation to volume and hence a greater loss of fluid per unit time/per breath than larger animals. To exacerbate the situation, many patients are not able to drink immediately after surgery, and so the period without water or food intake may stretch to several hours. Finally, some forms of surgery will lead to inappetance for a period, for example oral surgery.

Electrolyte replacement

Other diseases, such as diarrhoea, will cause fluid loss and metabolic acidosis due to the prolonged loss of bicarbonate. This is often due to parasitism, such as amoebiasis, in snakes. There may also be chronic losses of potassium, in cases of chronic diarrhoea, due to the reduced absorption of this electrolyte by the large intestine.

Snakes will vomit after a meal if stressed, and may suffer from diseases of the stomach such as cryptosporidiosis, causing loss of fluid and hydrogen ions, and a resultant potential metabolic alkalosis. Other reptiles such as tortoises will rarely vomit, so the likelihood of fluid loss via this route is less common.

Fluids used in reptilian practice

For many years the osmolarity/tonicity of reptile plasma was assumed to be lower than that of mammals. Osmolarity is measured in milliosmoles per litre (mOsm/L). There is now considerable evidence that many of the commonly seen species of reptiles, such as bearded dragons, green iguanas and corn snakes, have similar plasma osmolarity to mammals such as dogs and cats (generally between 290 and 330 mOsm/L), although there are wide variations within reptiles as a whole (Fitzsimons and Kaufman, 1977; Dallwig *et al.*, 2010; Guzman *et al.*, 2011). In addition, reptiles are more tolerant of variations in osmolarity than mammals and so fluids that are isotonic in mammals (typically 0.9%) are considered safe to use in reptiles.

It is important that whatever fluid is administered is warmed to the reptile or amphibian's PBT (approximately 30–35°C) before being given.

Lactated Ringer's/Hartmann's

As with cats and dogs, lactated Ringer's solution is useful as a general purpose rehydration and maintenance fluid. It is particularly useful for reptiles and amphibians suffering from metabolic acidosis, such as those described above with chronic gastrointestinal problems, but can also be used for fluid therapy after routine surgical procedures. Care should be taken in the use of lactated fluids where moderate to severe liver damage is present as they require the liver to metabolise the lactate into bicarbonate for the fluids to be considered alkalinising.

Saline and saline combinations

Saline 0.9% is an acidic solution with a pH of around 5 and is considered isotonic in most reptiles and can be considered a replacement crystalloid fluid, useful where hyperkalaemia and alkalosis is present.

Saline/glucose combinations are useful for reptiles and amphibians suffering from simple water loss or where hypernatraemia is present as although many are isotonic at the point of administration, metabolism of the glucose into water renders most hypotonic fairly quickly. They may be useful where simple water loss has occurred as many reptiles have been through periods of anorexia prior to treatment, and therefore may well also be borderline hypoglycaemic. Hypotonic fluids should not be used intravenously as a rapid bolus administration as they can lead to cerebral oedema and they are not effective at expanding the intravascular volume where it is reduced.

Hypertonic saline

Hypertoninc saline (7.2–7.5%) may be used in reptiles with acute hypovolaemia. It works by rapidly drawing fluid from the cellular and pericellular space into the circulation to support central venous pressure. See Chapter 24 on reptile emergency and critical care medicine for further details of its use. It must be administered intravenously or intraosseously and with care as reptiles in general have a lower blood pressure than mammals or birds.

Protein amino acid/B vitamin supplements

Protein and vitamin B supplements used in mammals are sometimes useful for nutritional support. Products such as Duphalyte® (Zoetis UK Ltd.) may be used at the rate of 1 mL/kg per day. They are used to replace nutrients in cases where the patient is malnourished or has been suffering from protein-losing enteropathy, such as may occur with heavy parasitism, or a protein-losing nephropathy, as in renal failure. It is also a useful supplement for patients with hepatic disease or severe exudative skin diseases, such as heater burns, in which blood proteins will be reduced.

Colloidal fluids

Colloidal fluids can include natural colloids such as blood and plasma but also include synthetic colloids and have been used in reptilian practice when intravenous/intraosseous administration has been possible. This does limit their usefulness, as some reptiles are just too small to gain full vascular access. They are used when a serious loss of blood occurs, in order to support central blood pressure. This may be a temporary measure while a blood donor is selected or, if none is available, the only means of attempting to support such a patient. Hydroxyethyl starch which has a larger colloid particle size than many colloids and so stays in the circulation for up to 24 hours has been used but concerns have been raised in mammals over adverse effects such as kidney damage and increased clotting times.

Blood transfusions are indicated when the packed cell volume (PCV) has dropped below 0.05–0.1 L/L, and they may be given via intravenous or intraosseous routes. Cross-matching of blood groups does not appear to be necessary for one-off transfusions, but the same species should be used each time; that is, green iguana to green iguana, boa constrictor to boa constrictor. Up to 2% body weight as blood may be taken from healthy species (Klingenberg, 1996), preferably into a pre-heparinised or citrate/phosphate/dextrose/adenine (CPDA) anticoagulant-coated syringe before immediately transfusing into the recipient. Ratios of CPDA to blood should ideally be 1:9. Ratios of heparin to blood should ideally be 5–10 IU of heparin per millilitre of blood. Doses of 10–15 mL/kg every 24 hours at an administration rate of 5–10 mL/kg per hour have been suggested (Schumacher, 2000). A blood giving set with micro-clot filter should be used to administer to the recipient.

Oral fluids and electrolytes

Oral fluid administration may also be used in reptile and amphibian practice for those patients experiencing mild dehydration, and for home administration. Many products are available for cats and dogs, and may be used for reptiles. The inclusion of a probiotic/prebiotic with the electrolytes may aid recovery, particularly in herbivores, by normalising gut flora and digestion. Alternatively, in herbivores transfaunation – the oral administration of faeces from a healthy reptile of the same species – can help repopulate the digestive tract with bacteria and protozoa that can assist in digestion.

Calculation of fluid requirements

Fluid requirements may be calculated as for cats and dogs. It is worth noting that a lot of the fluid intake is normally consumed in food, for example in the form of fresh vegetation for herbivorous species. This is difficult to take into consideration, and therefore it is safer to assume that the debilitated and hospitalised reptile will not be eating enough for this to matter in the calculation.

Frye (1991) recommends that levels of 20–25 mL/kg per day be used for hydration purposes in both reptiles and amphibians, and current literature suggests that maintenance rates across several species vary from 10 to 50 mL/kg per day.

The factor that limits the volume of fluids that can be administered is that, although intravenous and intraosseous routes may also be used, many fluids are given intracoelomically to the debilitated reptile, particularly in species such as snakes. Reptiles and amphibians do not possess true diaphragms and therefore the thorax and abdomen are interconnected in a common coelomic cavity. When fluids are placed in this cavity, it is equivalent to giving intraperitoneal fluids to a mammal, but as there is no diaphragm to protect them, these fluids can cause a greater pressure to build up on the lungs. Excessive fluids may severely compromise respiration and oxygenation, particularly where pre-existing respiratory or cardiovascular disease is present.

One can assume that 1% dehydration equates with a need to supply 10 mL/kg fluid replacement in addition to the maintenance requirements. It is also possible to make some qualitative assessment of the level of dehydration from the elasticity of the skin. Although reptile skin is not as elastic as mammalian, it should be freely mobile and recoil, albeit slowly, after tenting particularly over the epaxial muscles in snakes, the thigh of lizards and antebrachium of chelonians. Other factors to assess are the brightness of the corneas in species with mobile eyelids. In those without mobile eyelids (e.g. snakes), the collapse of the spectacle (the clear fused eyelids) is suggestive of dehydration. Other assessments of thirst and urate output can be made over 24 hours.

It is possible to estimate the degree of dehydration of a reptile patient as follows:

- 3% dehydrated – increased thirst, slight lethargy, decreased urates
- 7% dehydrated – increased thirst, anorexia, dullness, tenting of the skin with slow return to normal, dull corneas, loss of turgor of spectacles in snakes
- 10% dehydrated – dull to comatose, skin remains tented after pinching, desiccating mucous membranes, sunken eyeballs, no urate/urine output.

Table 22.1 Examples of normal packed cell volumes (PCV) and total blood proteins in selected species of reptiles.

Species	PCV (L/L)	Total protein (g/L)
Green iguana (*Iguana iguana*)	0.25–0.38	28–69
Tortoise (*Testudo* spp.)	0.19–0.4	32–50
Rat snake (*Elaphe* spp.)	0.2–0.3	30–60
Boa constrictor (*Boa constrictor constrictor*)	0.2–0.32	46–60

The alternative is to compare PCVs and total protein levels to assess dehydration (Table 22.1), again with 1% increase in PCV suggesting 10 mL/kg fluid replacements are needed (this assumes no anaemia in the patient).

It is important not to exceed 25–30 mL/kg per day as a maximum for the reasons mentioned above, whatever the level of dehydration of the patient. Therefore, rehydration of severely debilitated reptiles may take days to weeks. As with avian patients, therefore, making good the fluid deficit may need to be split over several days. Excessive fluids given intravenously or intraosseously may also overload the circulation and cause pulmonary oedema as the reptile's blood pressure tends to be lower than that of mammals or birds. For example, mean chelonian blood pressures are typically 15–30 mmHg although some of the varanids are closer to mammals at around 60–80 mmHg. Excessive fluids can result in cardiac and renal overperfusion and solute wash-out, with potassium in particular being excreted with the increased diuresis causing a hypokalaemic crisis to develop. This may manifest itself initially as an anorectic reptile, but will progress to cardiac arrhythmias, coma and death.

Equipment for fluid administration

Catheters

Butterfly catheters are useful for the small and fragile vessels typically encountered as they have a short length of tubing attached to the needle into which blood readily flows once correctly inserted. If the syringe or drip set is connected to this piece of flexible tubing, rather than directly to the catheter, there is also less chance of the catheter becoming dislodged if the reptile moves.

To make effective use of a butterfly catheter, it is advisable to flush it with heparinised saline prior to use to prevent clotting. Catheters of 25–27 gauge are recommended. They may also be used to give intracoelomic fluids to reptiles, as the conscious patient may continue to move (particularly common in snakes) without dislodging the needle.

For larger patients, such as adult iguanas, monitor lizards and Crocodilia, 21–25 gauge over-the-needle Teflon®-coated catheters can be used.

Hypodermic or spinal needles

Hypodermic needles are useful for the administration of intraosseous, intracoelomic or subcutaneous fluids.

Intraosseous fluids may be the only method of central venous support in very small patients or patients in which vascular collapse is occurring. The distal femur, proximal tibia or distal humerus may be used. Spinal needles are useful as they have a central stylet to prevent clogging the lumen of the needle with bone fragments after insertion. Spinal needles of 23–25 gauge are usually sufficient for most commonly seen reptiles.

Straightforward hypodermic needles may also be used for the same purpose, although the risks of blockage are higher. Hypodermic needles may also be used, of course, for the administration of intracoelomic and subcutaneous fluids. Generally, 23–25 gauge hypodermic needles are sufficient for the task.

Pharyngostomy or oesophageal tubes

Pharyngostomy tubes are often used in reptiles in order to provide nutritional support in as stress-free manner as possible. They are also useful as a route for some fluid administration, as only liquid formulas will pass through these narrow (3.5–6.5 French) tubes. The exception is Chelonia and larger species such as adult green iguanas, in which Foley catheters may be inserted as oesophageal tubes (see below). It should be noted though that in severely dehydrated individuals there is a real possibility that gut pathology may exist, so this route may need to be supplemented by others. This route therefore has limited use in facilitating fluid replacement, and is used mainly for nutritional support and rehydrating and replenishing the gut microflora.

Syringe drivers and pumps

For continuous fluid administration, as is often required for intravenous and intraosseous fluid administration, syringe drivers are advisable. Their advantage is that small volumes, such as a fraction of a millilitre, may be administered accurately per hour. In some of the smaller species dealt with, an error of 1–2 mL over an hour could be equivalent to overperfusion of 50–100%. In addition, it is almost impossible to keep gravity-fed drip sets running at these low rates without blockage every few minutes. Larger species may be administered fluids via spring-loaded pumps that rely on a specific diameter of drip tubing attached to the pump to determine the fluid rate. The latter pumps are inherently less accurate and so should be avoided or used with caution in smaller species.

Intravenous drip tubing

Particular fine drip tubing is available for attachment to syringes and syringe-driver units. It is useful if these are luer locking as this enhances safety and prevents disconnection when the patient moves. As mentioned above, if using spring-loaded infusion pumps, these rely on the diameter of the tubing to ensure the delivery rate.

Routes of fluid administration in reptiles

As with cats and dogs, the same medical principles broadly apply with five main routes of administration available as follows:

- Oral
- Subcutaneous
- Intracoelomic
- Intravenous
- Intraosseous.

However, many reptiles can also absorb fluids via the cloaca and distal rectum and so bathing reptiles in warmed water can encourage fluid uptake, which is helpful in cases of mildly dehydrated individuals

Table 22.2 lists the advantages and disadvantages of each of the five main routes.

Table 22.2 Advantages and disadvantages of various fluid therapies for reptiles and amphibians.

Route of fluid administration	Advantages	Disadvantages
Oral	Minimal stress with experienced handler Physiological route for fluid intake Less risk of tissue trauma Home therapy possible Rapid administration	Stressful with inexperienced handler No use in cases of digestive tract disease May damage stomach if the stomach tube is inserted too roughly Rehydration rates are slow Risk of aspiration pneumonia Limited volumes may be administered at any one time
Subcutaneous	Large volumes may be given at one time Rapid administration possible, minimising stress Uptake may be better than oral in cases of digestive tract disease Minimal risk of internal organ damage during administration	May be uncomfortable for the patient Risk of muscle and subcutaneous tissue trauma Rates of rehydration poor if severely dehydrated and peripheral vessels are collapsed Only isotonic or hypotonic fluids may be administered Darkening of the skin at the injection site particularly in lizards such as iguanas and chameleons
Intracoelomic	Large volumes may be administered at one time increasing dosing intervals Uptake is faster than subcutaneous Minimally painful route of administration	Large volumes may cause pressure on the lungs (no diaphragm) Rehydration rates may still be slow in severe cases of dehydration Only isotonic or hypotonic fluids may be administered Increased risk of organ damage
Intravenous	Rapid rehydration in even severely dehydrated patients is possible Colloidal and hypertonic fluids and blood transfusions possible Use of intravenous catheters and syringe drivers makes for accurate delivery	Size of reptile may prevent venous access Species of reptile (e.g. snakes) may make venous access difficult without minor surgery Veins are more fragile than mammalian vessels Increased skill levels and equipment required
Intraosseous	Rapid rehydration possible even with collapsed peripheral vasculature Colloidal and hypertonic fluids and blood transfusions possible Use of intraosseous catheters and syringe drivers make for accurate delivery Useful in smaller species or species where venous access is difficult	Not useful in the presence of infection (osteomyelitis) or metabolic bone disease Sedation, local or general anaesthesia is required for catheter insertion Tolerance may be poor in some species

Oral

Snakes

The oral route is not useful for seriously debilitated animals, but is for those with pharyngostomy feeding tubes in place, or if the owner or handler is experienced in stomach tubing. Mild cases of dehydration, where owners wish to home treat their pet, are ideal. A stomach tube is passed by restraining the snake's head gently but firmly, and then inserting a plastic or wooden tongue depressor to open the mouth. A lubricated feeding tube is then passed through the labial notch (the area at the most rostral aspect of the mouth without teeth) and to a depth of one-third of the snake's length (the approximate location of the stomach).

Lizards

Gavage (stomach) tubes or avian straight crop tubes or straightforward feeding tubes can be used to administer fluids directly into the oesophagus or stomach. The reptile needs to be firmly restrained to keep the head and oesophagus in a straight line. The mouth is opened with a plastic or wooden tongue depressor and the tube inserted to a depth of one-third to half the torso length of the reptile. This method is often stressful for the reptile. The alternative is to syringe fluids into the mouth, but this risks inhalation in a debilitated reptile. A pharyngostomy tube may be placed for nutritional support, and so may be used for fluid therapy.

Chelonians

An oesophagostomy tube may be implanted as described below, and levels of 10 mL/kg at any one time can be administered. Alternatively, a stomach tube may be inserted each time it is needed. The feeding tube is first measured from the tip of the extended nose to the line where the pectoral and abdominal ventral scutes connect (the approximate location of the stomach). It can then be lubricated and passed after extending the head and gently prising the mouth open with a wooden or plastic speculum (see Figure 22.1).

Placement of oesophagostomy tubes: Oesophagostomy tubes may be placed in any species of reptile, but are particularly useful in Chelonia which can retract their head deep inside the shell, making repeated stomach tubing difficult and stressful for handler and chelonian alike.

The steps for placement are as follows.

1. Sedation with local anaesthesia or general anaesthesia is required and good analgesia post implantation.
2. Surgically prepare the site with 0.25–0.5% povidone-iodine, being particularly scrupulous as reptile skin is notoriously dirty. In chelonians, the implantation site is the ventral aspect of the lateral neck, 3–4 cm caudal to the angle of the jaw. In snakes and lizards it is the ventrolateral aspect of the throat region, 5–10 cm caudal to the angle of the jaw in the case of most medium-sized snakes and lizards such as iguanas.
3. A pair of curved haemostats is placed in through the mouth and pushed laterally and ventrally, tenting the skin above them.
4. A sharp incision is made with a scalpel blade, over the point of the haemostats, through the skin and the underlying muscle and mucosa.
5. The tubing, preferably as large a diameter as will comfortably fit down the oesophagus and as flexible as possible (Foley catheters are useful in tortoises), is grasped with the haemostats as they protrude out through the incision, and then pulled into the pharynx and pushed down into the oesophagus. NB: The tube should be measured prior to implantation so the depth of insertion is known. It is measured in tortoises from the site of the tube incision to the mid-portion of the plastron, halfway through the abdominal scutes. A further length from the skin surface should then be allowed, in order to attach the end of the feeding tube to the dorsal aspect of the carapace.
6. Once in place, two pieces of zinc oxide tape may be attached to the tube close to the skin surface. Through this, sutures may be placed, attaching this to the skin itself. Alternatively, a finger-snare suture can be performed. The tube may then be attached to the midline

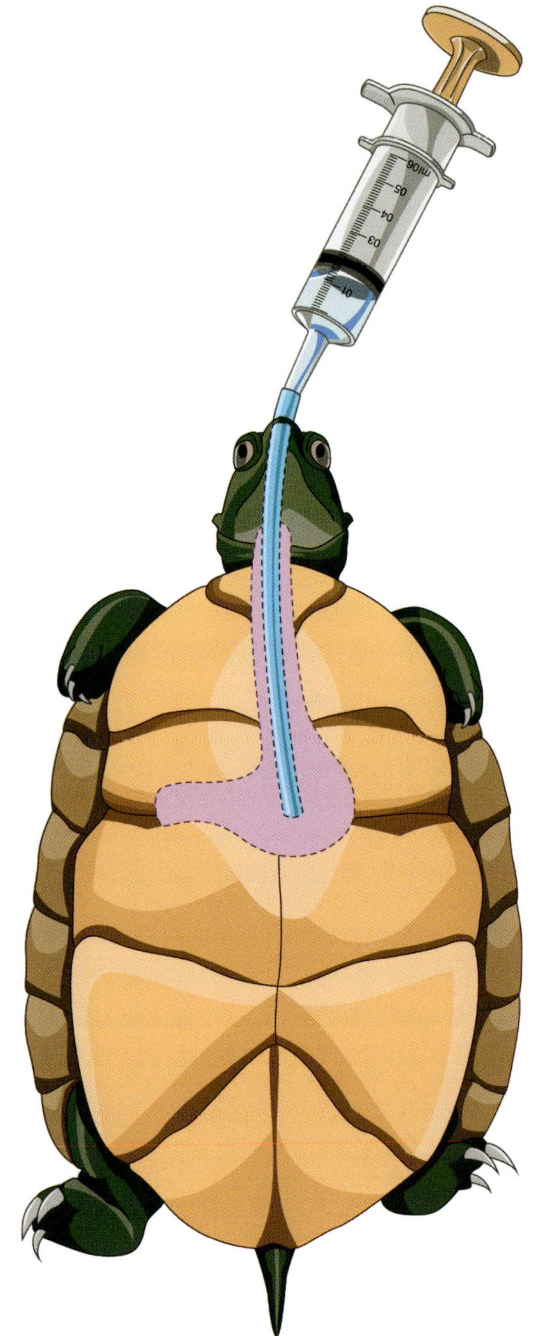

Figure 22.1 Placement and depth of insertion of a stomach tube in a chelonian.

(a)

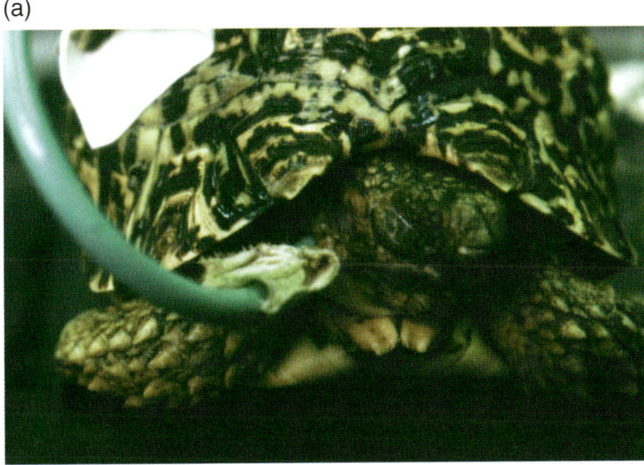

(b)

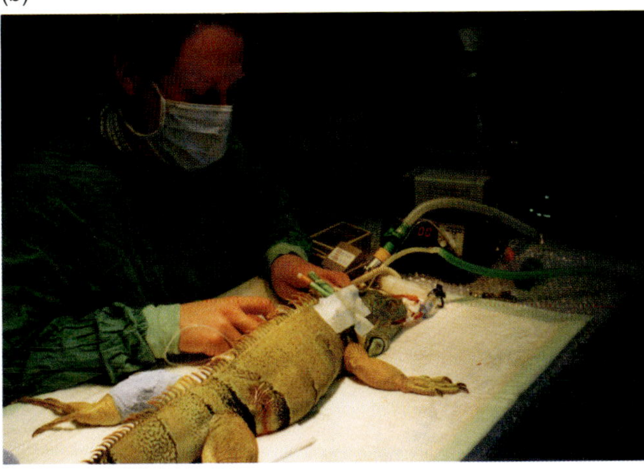

Figure 22.2 (a) An oesophagostomy tube in place in an anorectic leopard tortoise (*Stigmochelys pardalis*). (b) An oesophagostomy tube in place in an anorectic green iguana (*Iguana iguana*).

cranial carapace in tortoises, or taped to the side of the neck for snakes and reptiles, and a bung inserted (see Figure 22.2a,b). Care of the tube is as for nasogastric tubes in cats and dogs: plain water should be flushed through the tube prior to administering food to ensure correct placement. This should also be done after feeding to flush food debris out of the tube.

Subcutaneous

Snakes

The lateral aspect of the dorsum of the snake, in the caudal third of its body, is the ideal site for subcutaneous fluid administration. This is a good technique for routine postoperative administration of fluids to patients undergoing minor surgical procedures such as skin mass removals. If positioned correctly, there is a lymphatic sinus running lateral to the epaxial muscles on either side, just subcutaneously, which can be used for moderately large volumes. It may, however, still be necessary to use several sites.

Lizards

The lateral thoracic ribcage area is easily used for smaller volumes of fluids at any one site. There is a risk of the reptile developing a darkened, pigmented area over the injection site, particularly, though not exclusively, in chameleons.

Chelonians

The subcutaneous route is easily used for postoperative fluids and mild dehydration in this species. Fluids may be given in the area just cranial to the hindlimbs, or in the skin folds just lateral to the neck. Relatively large volumes may be given via this route.

Intracoelomic

Snakes

The intracoelomic route is useful for more seriously dehydrated reptiles, as there is a greater vasculature at this site for absorption. The needle or butterfly catheter is inserted two rows of lateral scales dorsal to the ventral scutes in the caudal third of the snake, but cranial to the vent. The needle is inserted so that it just penetrates the body wall, the plunger of the syringe is pulled back to ensure no organ/viscus puncture has occurred and the fluids administered. If correctly inserted, there will be no resistance to the injection.

Lizards

Because of the positioning necessary for administration, the intracoelomic route may be a stressful method of fluid administration. As for small mammals, the lizard should be placed in dorsal recumbency with its head downwards to encourage the gut contents to fall cranially and away from the injection site. The needle, preferably 25 gauge or smaller, is advanced slowly to just pop through the abdominal wall in the lower right or left ventral quadrant. The syringe plunger should be pulled back to ensure that the fat pads or organs have not been penetrated, and the fluids can be administered without any resistance.

Chelonians

The intracoelomic route can be used in tortoises up to a maximum of 20–25 mL/kg per day only; otherwise, due to the confines of the rigid shell, the fluids will place too much pressure on the lung fields. The area cranial to the hindlimbs is used (i.e. the same site as for subcutaneous delivery), but the chief difference is depth. The concern with this route is that the bladder lies in this area and if full may be punctured. Tilting the chelonian on its side to allow the bladder to fall away from the injection site can assist. The other route is the cranial access site. This is located lateral to the neck and medial to the front limb and is more epicoelomic than truly intracoelomic and so has a limited space. The needle is kept close and parallel to the plastron and a 2-cm needle may be inserted to the level of the hub.

Intravenous

Snakes

There are no major vessels for intravenous use in snakes that are easily accessible. If an intravenous route is to be used, one of the following is required.

Ventral tail vein: This is more of a plexus of veins, and may be accessed from the ventrum. The needle is inserted midline, one-third of the tail length from the vent, and advanced until it touches the coccygeal vertebrae at a 90° angle. The needle is then retracted slightly whilst

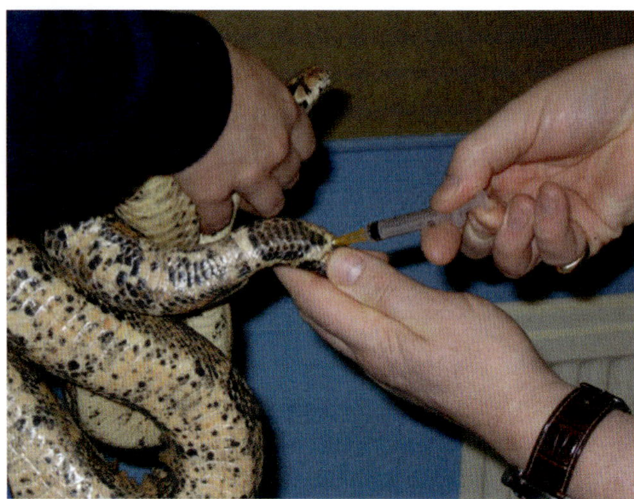

Figure 22.3 Slow bolus intravenous fluid administration may be performed in snakes and lizards via the ventral tail vein.

drawing back on the syringe until blood flows into the hub. Fluids may then be given slowly (see Figure 22.3).

Palatine vein: This is present on the roof of the mouth, as its name suggests, and is paired. Cannulation may be performed with a 25–27 gauge butterfly catheter although the snake has to be sedated or anaesthetised to gain access.

Jugular vein: This can only be accessed in an anaesthetised or sedated snake. A full-thickness skin cut-down procedure is performed 5–7.5 cm caudal to the angle of the jaw, two rows of scales dorsal to the ventral scutes. The jugular vein can then be seen medial to the ribs. An over-the-needle catheter is best for this, and should then be sutured in place.

Intracardiac: This site can be used in emergencies. The heart may be catheterised under sedation or anaesthesia only. On turning the snake onto its back, the heart may be seen to beat against the ventral scales, approximately one-quarter of its length from the snout. A 25–27 gauge over-the-needle catheter may be inserted between the scales, ventrally, in a caudocranial manner at 30° to the body wall into the single ventricle. A bolus may be administered, or it may be taped, glued or sutured in place for 24–48 hours.

Lizards

The intravenous route can be difficult in small lizards, and frequently requires sedation or anaesthesia. Several veins may be tried.

Cephalic vein: This is approached in the anaesthetised lizard by performing a cut-down procedure on the cranial aspect of the middle of the antebrachium, perpendicular to the long axis of the radius and ulna. The vessel may then be catheterised using an over-the-needle catheter, which is then sutured in place. This technique is really only useful for lizards over 0.25 kg in weight.

Jugular vein: This vessel may be accessed via a cut-down technique in the anaesthetised or sedated lizard. An incision is made in a craniocaudal direction 2.5 cm caudal to the angle of the jaw. An over-the-needle catheter may then be sutured in place.

Ventral tail vein: This is more of a plexus of veins. It is accessed from the ventral aspect of the tail and can be performed in the conscious lizard. It is frequently only suitable for one-off bolus injections, and special care should be taken with species that exhibit autotomy (spontaneous tail shedding). The needle is inserted at 90° to the angle of the tail and advanced until it touches the coccygeal vertebrae. It is then withdrawn slightly while drawing back on the syringe. When blood flows into the syringe, the infusion may begin.

Chelonians

There are two main intravenous routes: the dorsal tail vein and the jugular veins.

Jugular veins: These may be accessed for catheter placement in the sedated or anaesthetised tortoise. The neck is extended and the head tilted away from the operator to push the neck towards him or her. The jugular vein runs from the dorsal aspect of the eardrum along the more dorsal aspect of the neck (see Figure 22.4). An over-the-needle catheter may be placed directly or, in thicker-skinned animals, a cut-down technique employed.

Dorsal tail vein: This is more of a plexus of veins. Therefore, it is often not possible to give large volumes of fluids, and certainly not possible to place a catheter. Access is midline, on the dorsal aspect of the tail. The needle is inserted at a 90° angle until it hits the coccygeal vertebrae. The needle is then pulled back, drawing back on the syringe at the same time, until blood flows into the hub.

Intraosseous

Snakes

The intraosseous route is not possible in the snake.

Lizards

The intraosseous is a good route for smaller species of lizards, where venous access is restricted or difficult. There are a few access points to choose from. Hypodermic or spinal needles of 23–25 gauge may be used.

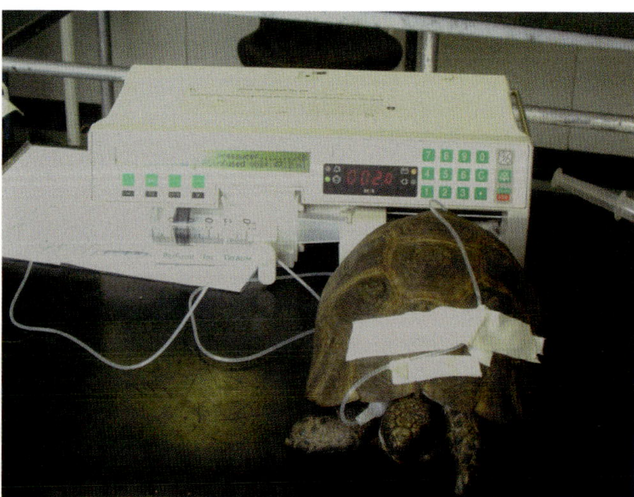

Figure 22.4 Placement of a jugular catheter in a chelonian. Note the taping of the drip tubing to the dorsal carapace midline and the attachment to the syringe driver.

Proximal femur: This may be accessed from the fossa created between the greater trochanter and the hip joint. This route may be difficult due to the 90° angle the femur often forms with the pelvis and so is restricted to species such as chameleons.

Distal femur: This is relatively easy to access from above the stifle joint. It does restrict the movement of the stifle, but it is easier to bandage the catheter into this site and access to the medullary cavity of the femur is certainly easier via this route. Sedation or anaesthesia is required. See below for the placement technique.

Proximal tibia: This again is possible in the larger species. Anaesthesia and sedation is needed, and the spinal needle or hypodermic needle may be screwed into the tibial crest region in a proximodistal manner.

Placement of distal femoral intraosseous catheters in lizards (see Figure 22.5): The technique for placement of a distal femoral intraosseous catheter in a lizard is explained in detail below.

1. Sedation or anaesthesia (local or general) is needed, and in all cases it is advised that good analgesia is administered.
2. Surgically scrub the area overlying the craniolateral aspect of the stifle joint using dilute povidone-iodine. It is important that placement of the catheter or needle is performed as aseptically as possible.
3. Take a 20–23 gauge spinal or hypodermic needle and insert it through the ridge just proximal to the stifle joint, screwing it into the bone in the direction of the long axis of the femur proximally.
4. Flush the needle with heparinised saline (the advantage of a spinal needle is that it has a central stylet which helps prevent it from becoming plugged with bone fragments).
5. Tape the needle securely in place and apply an antibiotic cream around the site. It may be worthwhile radiographing the area to ensure correct intramedullary placement of the needle.
6. Once the needle or catheter has been correctly placed, attach the intravenous tubing and bandage it securely in place by wrapping bandage material around the leg of the patient.
7. It may be necessary to immobilise the limb by bandaging it to a splint to prevent dislodgement of the catheter, which should now be attached to a syringe driver.

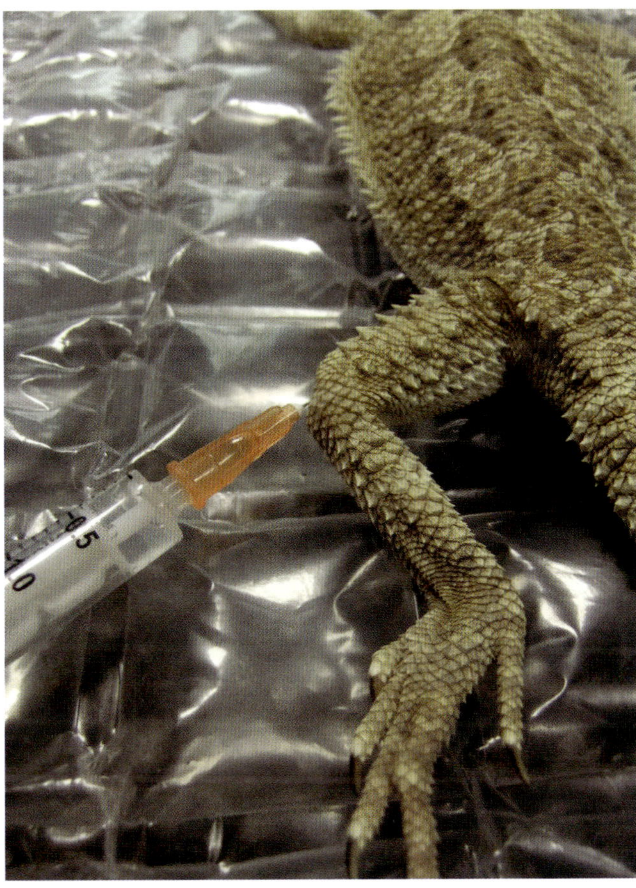

Figure 22.5 Distal femoral intraosseous fluid administration in an inland bearded dragon (*Pogona vitticeps*).

Chelonians

Two main intraosseous sites can be used.

Plastrocarapacial junction/pillar: This is the pillar of shell which connects the plastron to the carapace. It is approached from the caudal aspect, just cranial to one of the hindlimbs. The spinal or hypodermic needle (21–23 gauge) is screwed into the shell attempting to keep the angle of insertion parallel with the outer wall of the shell, so entering the shell bone marrow cavity. In larger, older species, the shell may be too tough to allow penetration.

Proximal tibia: This may be approached as for lizards. The area is thoroughly scrubbed with 0.25–0.5% povidone-iodine and the hypodermic or spinal needle is screwed into the tibial crest in the direction of the long axis of the tibia distally.

The distal femur has also been used but is difficult to maintain when the chelonian withdraws its hindlimb into the shell.

Routes of fluid administration in amphibians

Cutaneous

The cutaneous route is unique to amphibians and makes use of their semipermeable skin. It can be used only with mildly dehydrated amphibians, and should only involve the use of dechlorinated plain water. It should be warmed to the amphibian's PBT and be well oxygenated before immersing the patient. Absorption will occur across the skin membranes.

Oral

This route can be used for hypotonic fluid therapy via a small feeding tube inserted orally. The danger is that trauma can easily occur during restraint and opening of the amphibian's mouth during this procedure. In addition, the process is moderately stressful.

Intracoelomic

This is accessed in the right or left lower ventral quadrant of the 'abdomen'. The amphibian should be placed in dorsal recumbency and with its head down to allow coelom contents to fall away from the injection site.

Intravenous

In the larger anurans and some salamanders, the ventral abdominal vein may be used for bolus fluids or blood transfusions. The vessel lies midline, just below the skin surface and runs from just cranial to the pubis of the pelvis to close to the xiphoid of the sternum. A 25–27 gauge insulin needle may be used to gain access, although the vessel is very fragile and care should be taken not to rupture it.

TREATMENT OF REPTILIAN DISEASES

As this text is aimed at the veterinary nurse or technician, it is not intended to provide exhaustive lists of treatments or drug dosages, but rather to give an idea of the treatments possible and the techniques useful to aid recovery. For drug dosages, the reader is referred to one of the many excellent texts listed in the references at the end of this chapter.

Metabolic scaling of drug dosages

Many drugs have not been evaluated in reptiles and amphibians; however, drug doses may (with care) be extrapolated from known doses in other species. However, to do this, the differences in basal metabolic rate/standard metabolic rate (BMR/SMR) or metabolism should be taken into consideration (see Chapter 20). Reptiles have a much lower metabolic rate than mammals, and this is reflected by the fact that they excrete drugs at slower rates. The environmental temperature at which the reptile or amphibian is kept will also, due to their ectothermic nature, greatly affect its metabolic rate and hence excretion of any drug administered. Therefore, dosages and dose rates can often be much lower in reptiles than in mammals.

A formula has been derived to 'metabolically scale' the dosage of a drug in a tested species, such as a dog, to an untried one, such as a snake, and has been used to derive dosages of medications not commonly used in reptiles (Girling and Fraser, 2009). This is derived from the formula used to calculate the BMR/SMR:

$$\text{BMR/SMR} = k \times (W)^{0.75}$$

where k is a constant dependent on the order of animal being considered (very broadly k is 70 for placental mammals, 78 for non-passerine birds and 10 for reptiles) and W is the weight in kilograms.

From this, it is possible to calculate an animal's specific minimum energy cost (SMEC) as:

$$\text{SMEC} = k \times \left(W^{0.75}/W\right) = k \times \left(W^{-0.25}\right)$$

This then allows you to calculate an SMEC *dose* for any drug by dividing its known dose rate in mg/kg in a species (say a human) by that species' SMEC. For example, if the dose rate of ceftazidime in a human is 20 mg/kg, and that human's SMEC is 24.2, then the SMEC dose is 0.8. Therefore, by simply balancing equations, if you then know the weight of your reptile (say a 2-kg iguana), you can calculate its SMEC as:

$$\text{Iguana SMEC} = k \times (10) \times \left(2^{-0.25}\right) = 8.4$$

And therefore, the dose rate of drug required by multiplying the iguana's SMEC by the SMEC dose as:

$$8.4 \times 0.8 = 6.72 \text{ mg/kg}$$

The next stage is to calculate the dose frequency. Again, by extrapolation from a known dose frequency in humans for the drug of three times per 24 hours, the SMEC *frequency* may be calculated as:

$$\begin{aligned}\text{SMEC frequency} &= \text{treatment frequency / SMEC}\\ &= 3/24.2 = 0.1\end{aligned}$$

Therefore, to calculate the treatment frequency for the iguana you simply multiply the iguana's SMEC by the SMEC frequency for the drug:

$$\begin{aligned}\text{Dose frequency iguana} &= 8.4 \times 0.1\\ &= 0.84 \text{ times in 24 hours}\end{aligned}$$

which is equivalent to one dose (of 6.72 mg/kg) every 28.6 hours.

The technique is crude, but does allow some attempt to derive a dose more suited to the lower metabolic rate of reptiles in comparison with mammals, when extrapolating drug doses and where robust pharmacological studies are not available.

Reptile dermatological disease therapy

Table 22.3 highlights some of the treatments and therapies commonly used for the management of reptilian dermatological diseases.

Table 22.3 Treatment of skin diseases.

Diagnosis	Treatment
Abscesses and bacterial infections	Surgical therapy for most abscesses due to their fibrous nature (see Figure 22.6). Require debridement and topical antiseptic with systemic antibiosis based on culture and sensitivity. Many are Gram-negative infections and therefore fluoroquinolones (e.g. enrofloxacin and marbofloxacin) and third-generation cephalosporins (e.g. ceftazidime) are useful. Aminoglycoside drugs such as amikacin have also been used but caution should be observed as amikacin is potentially nephrotoxic and good hydration is essential. Other aminoglycoside drugs such as gentamicin are highly nephrotoxic and so should not be used systemically in reptiles. Metronidazole may be required where anaerobic bacterial infections are present (commonly associated with liquid pus rather than the normal inspissated abscesses seen in reptiles). Treatment may be prolonged, particularly where bone involvement occurs (see Figure 22.7) *Devriesea agamarum* requires debridement and application of topical doxycycline mixed with a gel such as Orabase. Alternative treatment with ceftiofur at 5 mg/kg q24 hours has been effective as fluoroquinolones such as enrofloxacin are considered ineffective (Pasmans *et al.*, 2010)
Dysecdysis	1. Rehydrate patient 2. Treat underlying cause, e.g. septicaemia causing peripheral arterial disease (the blockage of small arteries by antibody–antigen complexes and infection, so damaging the blood supply to organs and areas of the skin) (see Figure 22.7) 3. Lukewarm water shallow bathing; allow access to abrasive surfaces for snakes (e.g. wet towels) 4. Retained spectacles in snakes may be removed carefully with viscous tear drops and moistened cotton buds

Table 22.3 (continued)

Diagnosis	Treatment
Ectoparasites	
Blowfly miasis	Manual removal, often under sedation, antibiosis and treatment of initiating cause. Management of shock with fluid therapy and good analgesia also vital
Leeches	Manual removal after applying lidocaine to leech
Mites	Ivermectin 0.2 mg/kg injection on two or three occasions at 10–14 day intervals (***Do not use ivermectin in chelonians, crocodilians, skinks or indigo snakes as it has the potential to be lethal***) Can spray environmental mixture of 0.5 mL ivermectin + 1 L water with 1–2 mL propylene glycol to aid mixing to remove remaining mites Fipronil has also been used topically, sprayed onto a cloth and wiped over the reptile but caution should be used particularly in newly sloughed snakes and young animals as fipronil has proved toxic to some Predatory mites such as *Cheyletus eruditus* (taurrus) mites have been used to kill snake mites successfully
Ticks	Manual removal, ivermectin or fipronil on a cloth (however please see warning note regarding both drugs on mites). Treat for secondary bacterial infection
Erythema, ecchymoses and petechiae	Find the cause of the condition which has led to septicaemia If anticoagulant poisoning is suspected, use injections of vitamin K 0.25–0.5 mg/kg
Fungal skin infections	Superficial infections may respond to enilconazole washes Most are deeper and require systemic medication with itraconazole at metabolically scaled doses (Girling and Fraser, 2009) Voriconazole and sometimes itraconazole have been shown to be effective against *Nannizziopsis* spp. in bearded dragons and voriconazole has been shown to be effective against *Ophidiomyces ophiodiicola* in rattlesnakes (Martel *et al.*, 2009; Van Waeyenberghe *et al.*, 2010; McBride *et al.*, 2015)
Hyperthyroidism	Case of the green iguana: a thyroid adenoma was surgically removed (Hernandez-Divers *et al.*, 2001) Case of the corn snake: methimazole was used at 1–1.25 mg/kg q24 hours for 30 days (Frye, 1991)
Scale rot	1. Isolate bacteria/fungi involved and obtain sensitivity 2. Blisters treated topically with dilute povidone-iodine, silver sulfadiazine/enilconazole washes 3. Parenteral antibiosis 4. Prevention geared to reducing substrate moisture and increasing hygiene
Thermal burns	Management of large skin deficits using skin grafts or porcine xerograft patches or suturing granulation pads, e.g. Granuflex® (Convatec) over the wounds once infection has been contained. Antibiotics suitable for Gram-negative infections should be used systemically and topically (e.g. silver sulfadiazine). Repair of large skin deficits may take up to 6 months
Viral skin infections	Some herpesvirus infections may be treated with aciclovir topically or orally once daily at 80 mg/kg (Stein, 1996) Some have suggested three times daily treatment to be more effective (McArthur *et al.*, 2004)

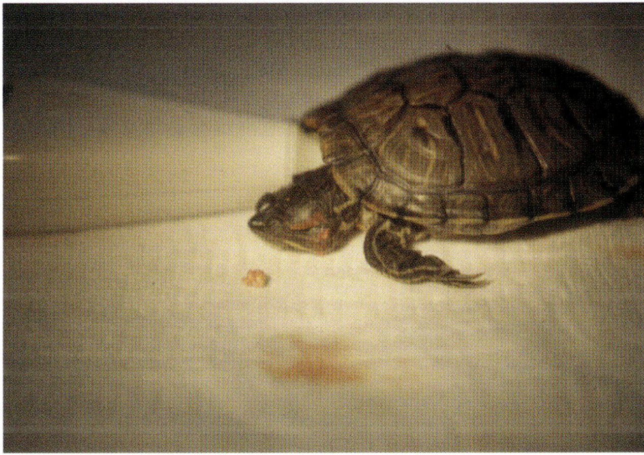

Figure 22.6 Abscesses are generally solid and fibrous in nature and so require surgical debridement such as the aural abscess in a red-eared terrapin (*Trachemys scripta elegans*). In the case of aural abscessation in chelonians such as terrapins, an underlying vitamin A deficiency may also be an issue so the diet should be reviewed as well.

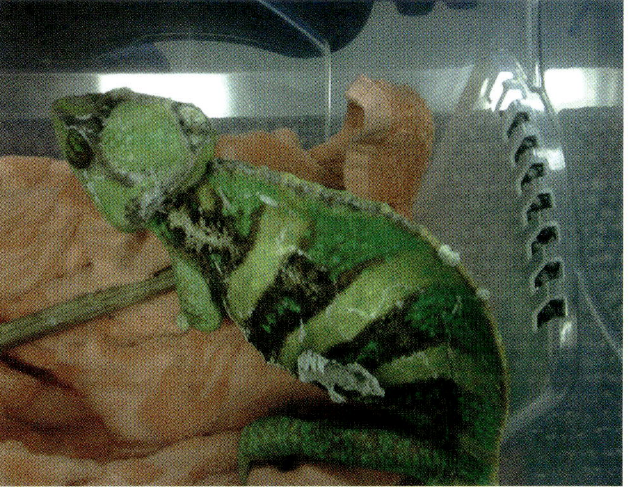

Figure 22.7 Dysecdysis and skin infections can be part of a wider septicaemic syndrome that can involve body organs and bone as seen here in this chameleon. Note the grey colouration of the casque and other bony projections of the skull as well as the dorsal spine associated with osteomyelitis. Note the large attached area of dead skin on the left flank associated with an underlying full skin thickness ulcer caused by peripheral arterial disease. Prolonged antimicrobial therapy (weeks to months) may be required.

Reptile digestive tract disease therapy

Table 22.4 highlights some of the treatments and therapies commonly used for the management of reptilian digestive tract diseases.

Reptile respiratory and cardiovascular disease therapy

Table 22.5 highlights some of the treatments and therapies commonly used for the management of reptilian respiratory and cardiovascular diseases.

Reptile urinary tract disease therapy

Table 22.6 highlights some of the treatments and therapies commonly used for the management of reptilian urinary tract diseases.

Treatment of renal disease

Fluid therapy is an essential part of this (see above and Chapter 24). In severely dehydrated reptiles, an initial fluid rate of 5 mL/kg per hour may be attempted for the first 1–3 hours. Beware of reptiles with hyperkalaemia that potassium-containing fluids are avoided.

If anuria is present, then diuretics such as furosemide (2–5 mg/kg intravenously or intramuscularly once every 24 hours) or mannitol (20% as 2 mL/kg intravenously once every 24 hours) can be given as a last resort.

Allopurinol can be given to reduce blood uric acid levels (10–20 mg/kg orally once every 24 hours).

Bladder lavage, involving the cloacal insertion of a Foley catheter into the urinary bladder (where present) and lavage of its contents, offers possibilities for the stabilisation of the hyperuricaemic and hyperkalaemic patient (Dantzler and Schmidt-Nielson, 1966).

Table 22.4 Treatment of digestive system diseases.

Diagnosis	Treatment
Oral diseases	
Mouth rot	Antibiosis based on culture and sensitivity Necrotic tissue debrided under sedation/anaesthesia Topical compounds containing silver sulfadiazine and framycetin are useful Intralesion injections of antibiotic and vitamin C advised (Frye, 1991) Chelonian herpesvirus: use topical iodine washes and aciclovir ointment/systemic aciclovir 80 mg/kg once to three times daily
Periodontal disease	Ultrasonic scaling of debris and calculus is advised. The use of antibiotics effective against Gram-negative bacteria is advised. The diet should also be corrected
Stomach diseases	
Cryptosporidiosis	Paromomycin is the only drug so far that has been shown to be successful. It has been used successfully in bearded dragons at 100 mg/kg orally once daily for 7 days, then 100 mg/kg orally twice weekly for 6 weeks, then 360 mg/kg orally every 48 hours for the final 10 days of an experimental study (Grosset *et al.*, 2011). It has been used in Gila monsters at 300–360 mg/kg orally every 48 hours for 2 weeks (Pare, 1997) and 360 mg/kg orally twice weekly for 6 weeks in king cobras (Rivas *et al.*, 2018). Metronidazole has been used at high dosages (100–220 mg/kg); however, this can be toxic in all species and particularly in indigo snakes (*Drymarchon* spp.) and kingsnakes (*Lampropeltis* spp.) Increasing the environmental temperature to greater than 27°C, whilst ensuring prevention of dehydration and provision of easily digestible liquid foods has increased the success rates by reducing environmental survival of the organism and speeding up the life cycle. Hospital enclosures should be disinfected between cases. Few disinfectants can be guaranteed, only ammonia (5%) and formol-saline (10%) were considered effective at low temperatures by Cranfield and Graczyk (1996). Most effective method of disrupting the parasite life cycle includes steam cleaning, freezing and desiccation
Granulomas (bacterial/fungal)	Surgical excision for large granulomas, culture and sensitivity testing and antimicrobials for small granulomas
Nematodes	Ivermectin 0.2 mg/kg once; repeat after 2 weeks (***Do not use ivermectin in chelonians, crocodilians, skinks or indigo snakes as it has the potential to be lethal***) Fenbendazole 25–100 mg/kg once and repeat after 2 weeks Oxfendazole has been used at 66 mg/kg orally once and repeated after 2 weeks
Neoplasia	Surgical excision
Intestinal diseases	
Coccidiosis	Ponazuril 15–40 mg/kg orally once daily for 21 days was effective in bearded dragons (Walden, 2009) Sulfadimidine 50 mg/kg orally once daily for 3 days. Clazuril 2–3 mg/kg q48 hours on three occasions has also been used Toltrazuril diluted to poultry concentrations for drinking water and dosed for 2 days has also been used (many preparations must be diluted prior to use as they are intensely caustic so follow data sheets)
Constipation	Rehydration therapy Correction of diet and husbandry (e.g. avoiding highly furred rodents when feeding garter snakes and ensuring the relative humidity is kept high for species such as green tree pythons and green iguanas) Cisapride 0.5–4 mg/kg orally once daily (Wangen, 2013)
Cryptosporidiosis	See section Stomach diseases above

Table 22.4 (continued)

Diagnosis	Treatment
Entamoebiasis	Metronidazole has been used orally at varying dosages, typically around 50 mg/kg every 2 days but this can be toxic in indigo snakes and kingsnakes where it should be avoided or the dosage reduced to around 25 mg/kg once daily and iodoquinol (which works against the cyst protozoal stage) combined
Flagellates	Flagellates may be treated using metronidazole as a single dose of 40–100 mg/kg orally (Frye, 1991); however, beware toxicity in indigo snakes and kingsnakes
Nematodes	See section Stomach diseases above. (***Do not use ivermectin in chelonians, crocodilians, skinks or indigo snakes as it has the potential to be lethal***)
Liver diseases	
Entamoebiasis	See section Intestinal diseases above
Hepatic lipidosis	Hepatic lipidosis may be treated with supportive fluid and nutritional therapy. In addition, use of anabolic steroids (nandrolone) at doses of 0.5–1 mg/kg IM every 7 days and the use of milk thistle (*Silybum marianum*) 4–15 mg/kg orally every 8–12 hours and L-carnitine 100 mg/kg orally once daily may be helpful (Carpenter *et al.*, 2019; Divers, 2019). In chelonians levothyroxine 0.02 mg/kg orally every 2 days may be helpful (Norton *et al.*, 1989), as well as ensuring during this period the diet comprises a high-fibre vegetarian one. It may be necessary to prevent hibernation in chelonians that perform this naturally if the problem occurs in the autumn, and the placement of a pharyngostomy tube for ease of food administration is advisable

Table 22.5 Treatment of respiratory and cardiovascular system diseases.

Diagnosis	Treatment
Respiratory disease	
Bacterial respiratory disease	Based on culture and sensitivity results. Lung washes may be used to collect samples and to flush out infection. Gram-negative bacterial infections predominate, therefore fluoroquinolones, aminoglycosides and third-generation cephalosporins may be useful Mycoplasmal diseases in chelonians have been successfully treated with clarithromycin
Fungal respiratory disease	Itraconazole or voriconazole preferred as ketoconazole is often ineffective against *Aspergillus* spp. and many other fungal pathogens which are commonly found
Nematodes	Ivermectin may be used at 0.2 mg/kg (***Do not use ivermectin in chelonians, crocodilians, skinks or indigo snakes as it has the potential to be lethal***) Alternatively, fenbendazole and oxfendazole may be used (see intestinal disease treatment, Table 22.4)
Pentastomes	Manual removal. Levamisole has been used at 5 mg/kg
Cardiovascular disease	
Heart failure	With little information regarding suitable therapeutics, the following provides a guide only: 1. Maintain at lowest extent of POTZ 2. Enrich local environment with oxygen 3. Minimise stress with minimal handling 4. Withhold food (for the short term) 5. Short-term diuresis when signs of congestive failure are present: frusemide 2–5 mg/kg IV or IM two to three times daily (may also use hydrochlorothiazide 1 mg/kg every 24–72 hours) 6. Broad-spectrum antimicrobial 7. Parasiticides (if suspect haemoparasites/microfilaria, or blood-sucking ectoparasites/endoparasites) 8. Fluids: 15–30 mL/kg per day 9. Digoxin has been used at empirical cat and dog dosages for a case of diagnosed dilated cardiomyopathy in a python, but extreme care should be taken with all of these drugs as no proper studies have been performed to ascertain safe dosages
Filariasis	Nematode filariasis treatment attempted with ivermectin 0.2 mg/kg intramuscularly (see notes above regarding potential toxicity in chelonians, crocodilians, skinks and indigo snakes). Alternatives include raising the environmental temperature to 35–37°C for 24–48 hours causing death of the adult worms Watch for signs of heat stress and dehydration at these temperatures
Goitre	Iodine supplement at 2–4 mg/kg orally once weekly particularly giant chelonians (Stein, 1996)
Leukaemia	Vincristine (0.025 mg/kg IV once weekly) and prednisolone (0.5–1 mg/kg once daily). Resistance can occur with this regimen and more success has been achieved by adding in cyclophosphamide (10 mg/kg) and chlorambucil (0.1–0.2 mg/kg orally once daily) (Willette *et al.*, 2001). Doxorubicin has been used at 1 mg/kg IV once weekly for two treatments, then once every 2 weeks for two treatments and then once every 3 weeks for two treatments (Rosenthal, 1994)
Other haemoparasites	Chloroquine 125 mg/kg orally every 48 hours on three occasions for haemoparasites, e.g. *Plasmodium* spp. (Girling, 2019) Quinacrine 20–100 mg/kg orally every 48 hours for 2 weeks for haemogregarines in snakes (Raiti, 2002)

Table 22.6 Treatment for urinary tract diseases.

Diagnosis	Treatment
Renal disease	See text
Urinary bladder stones	Treatment by surgical removal, or if small enough by endoscope via the cloaca. Antibiotic therapy often required due to concurrent cystitis

Bearing in mind the function of the lower urinary tract, it should be possible to remove excess potassium and uric acid, and to administer fluids (and possibly even medications such as allopurinol) by this route.

Hypocalcaemia is a common finding with renal failure and can cause seizures and tetany. Therapy with calcium gluconate (100 mg/kg every 6 hours) along with aluminium hydroxide (15–45 mg/kg orally once every 24 hours to reduce phosphate absorption) is advised.

In chronic renal failure, anabolic steroids and vitamin B injections may also be given to enhance appetite and stop catabolism and reverse anaemia.

Reptile reproductive tract disease therapy

Table 22.7 highlights some of the treatments and therapies commonly used for the management of reptilian reproductive tract diseases.

Treatment of dystocia (post-ovulatory stasis)

Medical treatment revolves around the administration of oxytocin 5–30 IU/kg intramuscularly or intracoelomically (Stein, 1996). Oxytocin tends to work best in chelonians, less well in lizards and worst in snakes in my opinion. Prior to oxytocin administration (preferably 1 hour), calcium gluconate 100 mg/kg, particularly in lizards and chelonians where hypocalcaemia can be a common problem, is administered. In addition, the use of sterile lubricants injected into the reproductive tract via the cloaca may be helpful. The provision of nesting material such as damp sand or bark chippings for the female to dig into is also useful and may be all that is needed in uncomplicated cases, particularly in chelonians.

Table 22.7 Treatment for reproductive system diseases.

Diagnosis	Treatment
Dystocia (post-ovulatory stasis)	See text
Egg yolk coelomitis	Similar to the condition in birds; however, reptiles will often be more tolerant of advanced disease Surgical option is ovariectomy to prevent recurrence; also allows debridement and flushing of the coelomic cavity. Covering antibiotics with fluid therapy and assist feeding also required
Hemipenal/phallus prolapse	If hemipene/phallus is non-reducible then amputation is advised
Oviductal prolapses	Severe prolapses that have been present for some time may necessitate emergency surgery, and replacement of the prolapse via a coeliotomy ± salpingectomy at the same time
Preovulatory stasis	Surgical ovariectomy

Atenolol 7 mg/kg orally with calcium gluconate has also been used in chelonians followed by 1–3 IU/kg of oxytocin intramuscularly the following morning. This protocol is continued daily, assuming eggs are produced, until all eggs are laid.

As with birds, the application of prostaglandin E gel to the oviduct sphincter per cloaca may help dilation if this is the cause of dystocia.

Surgical methods include, where possible, percutaneous aspiration of the egg contents by bringing the egg to the abdominal wall, surgically scrubbing the skin surface and passing a 21 gauge needle through the body wall into the egg. The needle should be attached to a syringe which should be used to aspirate the yolk and albumen contents. Once collapsed, the eggshells will often be passed of their own accord.

Other methods include salpingotomy. In the case of snakes, this means making very long incisions to ensure removal of all the eggs. In the case of chelonians, this means entering into the shell via the plastron by creating a trapdoor through the shell.

Reptile musculoskeletal system disease therapy

Table 22.8 highlights some of the treatments and therapies commonly used for the management of reptilian musculoskeletal system diseases.

Treatment of metabolic bone disease

This is by correction of the dietary deficiency of calcium and by ensuring that susceptible species are provided with ultraviolet (UV) artificial lighting on the inside of the vivarium. Injectable calcium should not be used for routine cases of metabolic bone disease (MBD)

Table 22.8 Treatment of musculoskeletal diseases.

Diagnosis	Treatment
Fractures	In cases of metabolic bone disease, it is better to correct diet and splint fractures than repair surgically
Lizards	For one forelimb fracture, bandage limb to body wall (see Figure 22.8). For bilateral humeral fractures, use a coaptation splint. For one hindlimb fracture, bandage limb to tail base. For digital fractures, ball bandage as for avian patients
Chelonians	Possible to bandage limb into shell. This is useful in cases of metabolic bone disease. Spinal fractures should be splinted as neural control may be regained. All species may require external coaptation or internal surgical fixation to mend fractures
Metabolic bone disease	See text
Tail loss	Young individuals that exhibit autotomy (e.g. iguanids and geckos), treat the stump as an open wound and dress with topical silver sulfadiazine cream or iodine antiseptic (dilute). For agamids or species not showing autotomy and older iguanids which lose this ability, suture the stump surgically under general anaesthesia

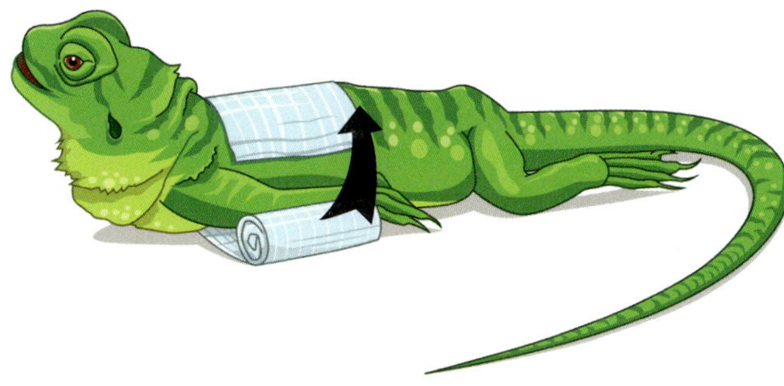

Figure 22.8 Bandaging a forelimb to the body wall as a conservative method of treating a humeral fracture in a lizard.

as it is both painful and if given intravenously may cause fatal arrhythmias. Injectable calcium should only be used if there is evidence of hypocalcaemic tetany or collapse. Treatment should focus on dietary correction of calcium imbalance in combination with vitamin D_3 provision (including UV-B light and dietary cholecalciferol administration).

Salmon calcitonin has been used once blood calcium levels have been corrected to encourage deposition of calcium in the bones. Doses of 50 IU per green iguana once weekly for 2 weeks have been quoted (Mader, 2006). A typical protocol for a green iguana with MBD is to administer 400 IU/kg vitamin D_3 intramuscularly plus 23 mg/kg calcium glubionate orally twice daily plus supportive therapy. The first week after, repeat the vitamin D_3 injection, and assuming normalised blood calcium, give the first salmon calcitonin injection and continue with the oral calcium. The second week, just the calcitonin injection is repeated plus the oral calcium (Mader, 2006).

Unfortunately, some of the shell deformities seen in chelonians are not correctable. Fractures are best repaired by splinting and dietary corrections.

Internal fixation with advanced MBD is generally not advised due to the fragility of the bones.

Prevention of metabolic bone disease

Klaphake (2010) has described UV-B light provision for reptiles to prevent MBD as follows.

1. Desert diurnal lizards/chelonians: high UV-B levels (10% or full unfiltered sun for 12 hours).
2. Diurnal arboreal lizards or semi-aquatic basking chelonians: moderate UV-B (5%, 12 hours).
3. Diurnal terrestrial lizards or chelonians from forests: low UV-B (5%, 6 hours).
4. Nocturnal lizards: low UV-B (2%, 6 hours).
5. Snakes: dietary calcium and vitamin D_3 is sufficient.

Ferguson *et al.* (2010) further summarised UV light intensity requirements for reptiles in a series of four zones ranging from requirements for shade dwellers/crepuscular through to midday basking species (see Chapter 18 for further details).

Calcium supplementation should be provided for young growing lizards and chelonians in particular and the calcium to phosphorus ratio is assumed to be 2 : 1. For insectivores, gut loading their invertebrate prey rather than dusting it is preferred as this guarantees the reptile will receive the nutritional supplement; dusting powders have frequently dropped off the insect before it is consumed. Commercially available insects need supplementation as most have inverted calcium to phosphorus ratios (i.e. they have greater phosphorus levels than calcium). Dietary deficiencies of calcium can occur in herbivores when they are fed large amounts of leaves containing oxalates (e.g. spinach and beetroot leaves), which bind calcium in the gut and prevent absorption. The feeding of fruit for many species should be kept in check as most commercially available fruit contains little or no calcium and is high in sugars that can lead to gastrointestinal and dental disease.

Reptile neurological system disease therapy

Table 22.9 highlights some of the treatments and therapies commonly used for the management of reptilian neurological system diseases.

Treatment of amphibian diseases

Table 22.10 highlights some of the treatments and therapies commonly used for the management of amphibian diseases.

Table 22.9 Treatment of nervous system diseases.

Diagnosis	Treatment
Hypocalcaemic tetany	Over short term use calcium gluconate 100 mg/kg IM. Over long term, administer dietary calcium, vitamin D_3 and appropriate UV-B light supplementation for the species
Hypoglycaemia	Oral administration of 3 g/kg glucose solution Use of dextrose 50% (diluted 1 : 1 with 0.9% saline) administered at 0.25 ml/kg (125 mg/kg) IV
Hypovitaminosis B_1	Over short term, thiamine injections 25 mg/kg once daily. Over the longer term change to a non-thiaminase-containing diet, or supplement the diet with thiamine at 35 mg/kg of food given
Hypovitaminosis B_7 (biotin)	Biotin deficiency: over short term, give a vitamin B complex containing biotin by injection. Over long term, supplement the diet with vitamin B complex powder and stop feeding unfertilised hen's eggs, the most likely cause in omnivorous or specialist feeding reptiles
Lead poisoning	Sodium calcium edetate 10–40 mg/kg every 12 hours with fluid therapy
Meningoencephalitis	There are many causes: entamoebiasis (see section on treatment of intestinal diseases); viral causes (e.g. inclusion body disease) are not treatable; bacterial causes may be treated early on with antimicrobials

Table 22.10 Treatment of diseases of amphibia.

Diagnosis	Treatment
Chlamydiosis	Treatment with oxytetracycline as a 100 mg/L bath for 1 hour daily or doxycycline 50 mg/kg orally once daily
Chytrid (*Batrachochytrium dendrobatidis, B. salamandrivorans*)	Itraconazole 0.01% baths in 0.6% saline, for 5 minutes, daily for 11 days have proved effective (Forzan *et al.*, 2008; Hardy *et al.*, 2015) Spraying with voriconazole at 125 mg/L once daily for 7 days has also been shown to be effective (Martel *et al.*, 2011) Raising environmental temperatures to 25°C for 10 days has been shown to be effective against *B. salamandrivorans* (Blooi *et al.*, 2015)
Hypovitaminosis A	Gut-load invertebrate prey with multivitamin-containing preformed vitamin A (not just beta-carotenes)
Metabolic bone disease	Dietary supplementation with calcium and vitamin D_3. Flaked fish foods also contain these two nutrients. Whitaker and Wright (2019) recommend access to cuttlebone for tadpoles to ensure sufficient calcium access
Mycobacteriosis	Not treatable. Infected inidviduals should be isolated from others. Good biosecurity essential but difficult to eradicate in the environment requiring quaternary ammonium and iodophor-style disinfectants
Phycomycosis	Dilute topical malachite green or itraconazole baths (see Chytrid) NB: treatment frequently not successful as becomes systemic
Parasitic nematodes	Fenbendazole 50 mg/kg orally once, oxfendazole 25 mg/kg orally once or ivermectin 0.2–0.4 mg/kg orally once. All may require repeat treatment in cases of heavy infestations, usually at 14-day intervals
Protozoal diseases	*Entamoeba ranarum* in anurans treated with metronidazole 100 mg/kg orally once; however, metronidazole may be toxic at this higher dosage and so many recommend reducing the dosage to 50 mg/kg orally once every 14 days *Oodinium pilularis*: mild salt solutions of 0.4–0.6% for 2–3 days or a 0.15% formalin dip every 48 hours are useful
Redleg (*Aeromononas hydrophila*)	Enrofloxacin 5 mg/kg orally daily. Tetracyclines (e.g. oxytetracycline) 50 mg/kg orally twice daily
Saprolegnia	Dilute topical malachite green or itraconazole baths (see Chytrid)

References

Blooi, M., Martel, A., Haesebrouck, F. *et al.* (2015) Treatment of urodelans based on temperature dependent infection dynamics of *Batrachochytrium salamandrivorans. Scientific Reports*, **5** [Article number 8037].

Carpenter, J.W., Klaphake, E., Gibbons, P.M. and Sladky, K.K. (2019) Reptile formulary. In: *Mader's Reptile and Amphibian Medicine and Surgery* (eds S.J. Divers & S.J. Stahl), 3rd edn, pp. 1191–1211. Elsevier, St. Louis, MO.

Cranfield, M.R. and Graczyk, T.K. (1996) Cryptosporidiosis. In: *Reptile Medicine and Surgery* (ed. D.R. Mader), pp. 359–363. WB Saunders, Philadelphia, PA.

Dallwig, R.K., Mitchell, M.A. and Acierno, M.J. (2010) Determination of plasma osmolality and agreement between measured and calculated values in healthy adult bearded dragons (*Pogona vitticeps*). *Journal of Herpetological Medicine and Surgery*, **20**, 69–73.

Dantzler, W.H. and Schmidt-Nielson, B. (1966) Excretion in the fresh-water turtle (*Pseudemys scripta*) and desert tortoise (*Gopherus agassizii*). *American Journal of Physiology*, **210**, 198–210.

Divers, S.J. (2019) Hepatology. In: *Mader's Reptile and Amphibian Medicine and Surgery* (eds S.J. Divers & S.J. Stahl), 3rd edn, pp. 649–668. Elsevier, St. Louis, Missouri.

Ferguson, G.W., Brinker, A.M., Gehrmann, W.H. *et al.* (2010) Voluntary exposure of some western-hemisphere snake and lizard species to ultraviolet-B radiation in the field: how much ultraviolet-B should a lizard or snake receive in captivity? *Zoo Biology*, **29**(3), 317–334.

Fitzsimons, J. and Kaufman, S. (1977) Cellular and extracellular dehydration, and angiotensin as stimuli to drinking in the common iguana *Iguana iguana*. *Journal of Physiology*, **265**, 443.

Forzan, M.J., Gunn, H. and Scott, P. (2008) Chytridiomycosis in an aquarium collection of frogs: diagnosis, treatment, and control. *Journal of Zoo and Wildlife Medicine*, **39**(3), 406–411.

Frye, F. (1991) *Biomedical and Surgical Aspects of Captive Reptile Husbandry*, vol. 1 and 2. Krieger Publishing, Malabar, FL.

Girling, S.J. (2019) Vascular, hematopoietic and immune systems. In: *Mader's Reptile and Amphibian Medicine and Surgery* (eds S.J. Divers & S.J. Stahl), 3rd edn, pp. 917–921. Elsevier, Philadelphia.

Girling, S.J. and Fraser, M.A. (2009) Treatment of *Aspergillus* species infection in reptiles with itraconazole at metabolically scaled dosages. *Veterinary Record*, **165**(2), 52–54.

Grosset, C., Villeneuve, A., Brieger, A. and Lair, S. (2011) Cryptosporidiosis in juvenile bearded dragons (*Pogona vitticeps*): effects of treatment with paromomycin. *Journal of Herpetological Medicine and Surgery*, **21**(1), 10–15.

Guzman, D.S.-M., Mitchell, M.A. and Acierno, M. (2011) Determination of plasma osmolality and agreement between measured and calculated values in captive male corn snakes (*Pantherophis [Elaphe] guttatus guttatus*). *Journal of Herpetological Medicine and Surgery*, **21**, 16–19.

Hardy, B.M., Pope, K.L., Piovia-Scott, J. *et al.* (2015) Itraconazole treatment reduces *Batrachochytrium dendrobatidis* prevalence and increases overwinter field survival in juvenile Cascades frogs. *Diseases of Aquatic Organisms*, **122**, 243–250.

Hernandez-Divers, S.J., Knott, C.D. and MacDonald, J. (2001) Diagnosis and surgical treatment of thyroid adenoma-induced hyperthyroidism in a green iguana (*Iguana iguana*). *Journal of Zoo and Wildlife Medicine*, **32**, 465–475.

Klaphake, E. (2010) A fresh look at metabolic bone diseases in reptiles and amphibians. *Veterinary Clinics of North America: Exotic Animal Practice*, **13**, 375–392.

Klingenberg, R.J. (1996) Therapeutics. In: *Reptile Medicine and Surgery* (ed. D.R. Mader), 1st edn, pp. 299–321. WB Saunders, Philadelphia, PA.

Mader, D. (2006) Metabolic bone disorders. In: *Reptile Medicine and Surgery* (ed. D. Mader), 2nd edn, pp. 841–851. Saunders, Elsevier, Philadelphia, PA.

Martel, A., Hellebuyck, T. and Van Waeyenberghe, L. (2009) Treatment of infections with *Nannizziopsis vriesii*, an emergent reptilian dermatophyte. *Proceedings of the Annual Conference of the Association of Reptilian and Amphibian Veterinarians*, pp. 69–70.

Martel, A., Van Rooij, P., Vercauteren, C. *et al.* (2011) Developing a safe antifungal treatment protocol to eliminate *Batrachochytrium dendrobatidis* from amphibians. *Medical Mycology*, **49**(2), 143–149.

McArthur, S., McLellan, L. and Brown, S. (2004) Gastrointestinal disease. In: *Manual of Reptiles* (eds S.J. Girling & P. Raiti), 2nd edn, pp. 210–229. BSAVA, Quedgeley, UK.

McBride, M.P., Wojick, K.B., Georoff, T.A. *et al.* (2015) *Ophidiomyces ophiodiicola* dermatitis in eight free ranging timber rattlesnakes (*Crotalus horridus*) from Massachusetts. *Journal of Zoo and Wildlife Medicine*, **46**, 86–94.

Norton, T.M., Jacobson, E.R. and Caligiuri, R. (1989) Medical management of a Galapagos tortoise (*Geochelone elephantopus*) with hypothyroidism. *Journal of Zoo and Wildlife Medicine*, **20**, 212–216.

Pare, J. (1997) Treatment of cryptosporidiosis in Gila monsters (*Heloderma suspectum*) with paromomycin. *Proceedings of the Association of Reptilian and Amphibian Veterinarians, Houston, Texas*, pp. 23–24.

Pasmans, K., Hellebuyck, T., Haesebrouck, F. and Martel, A. (2010) Dermatitis and septicaemia caused by *Devriesea agamarum*: an overview including recent developments in disease management. *Proceedings of the 1st International Conference on Reptile and Amphibian Medicine, Munich, Germany*, pp. 105–106.

Raiti, P. (2002) Snakes. In: *Manual of Exotic Pets* (eds A. Meredith & S. Redrobe), 4th edn, pp. 241–256. BSAVA, Quedgeley, UK.

Rivas, A.E., Boyer, D.M., Torregrosa, A. *et al.* (2018) Treatment of *Cryptosporidium serpentes* infection in a king cobra (*Ophiophagus hannah*) with paromomycin. *Journal of Zoo and Wildlife Medicine*, **49**(4), 1061–1063.

Rosenthal, K. (1994) Chemotherapeutic treatment of a sarcoma in a corn snake. *Proceedings of the American Association of Zoo Veterinarians/Association of Reptilian and Amphibian Veterinarians*, p. 46.

Schumacher, J. (2000) Fluid therapy in reptiles. In: *Kirks Current Veterinary Therapy XIII* (ed. J. Bonagura), pp. 1170–1173. WB Saunders, Philadelphia.

Stein, G. (1996) Reptile and amphibian formulary. In: *Reptile Medicine and Surgery* (ed. D.R. Mader), pp. 465–472. WB Saunders, Philadelphia, PA.

Van Waeyenberghe, L., Baert, K., Pasmans, F. *et al.* (2010) Voriconazole, a safe alternative for treating infections caused by the *Chrysosporium* anamorph of *Nannizziopsis vriesii* in bearded dragons (*Pogona vitticeps*). *Medical Mycology*, **48**, 880–885.

Walden M.R. (2009) Characterizing the epidemiology of *Isopora amphiboluri* in captive bearded dragons (*Pogona vitticeps*). Thesis, Louisiana State University. http://digitalcommons.lsu.edu/gradschool_dissertations/1402 (accessed 20 April 2024).

Wangen, K. (2013) Cisapride. *Journal of Exotic Pet Medicine*, **22**, 301–304.

Whitaker, B.R. and Wright, K.M. (2019) Amphibian medicine. In: *Mader's Reptile and Amphibian Medicine and Surgery* (eds S.J. Divers & S.J. Stahl), 3rd edn, pp. 992–1013. Elsevier, Philadelphia.

Willette, M.M., Garner, M.M. and Drew, M. (2001) Chemotherapeutic treatment of lymphoma in a king cobra (*Ophiophagus hannah*). *Proceedings of the American Association of Zoo Veterinarians/Association of Reptilian and Amphibian Veterinarians*, pp. 20–24.

Chapter 23 Reptile and Amphibian Diagnostic Imaging

RADIOGRAPHY

The rationale behind diagnostic imaging of reptiles and avian patients is much the same as that behind any species commonly seen in general practice. The main aims are to ensure the rapid detection of internal foreign bodies, the presence of growths, whether tumours, granulomas or abscesses, as well as the enlargement/reduction of internal organs due to diseases. In addition, the detection of gravidity and the confirmation of fractures are common reasons for radiographing a patient.

There are many considerations which need to be made prior to attempting to radiograph a reptile or amphibian patient.

- Is the patient an aggressive or even venomous species and will therefore require anaesthesia or chemical sedation to safely radiograph?
- Is the patient in respiratory distress, and therefore the stress of manual restraint or chemical restraint may be too high to allow safe radiography?
- What is the area that is to be viewed? In the case of reptiles in particular, the absence of a diaphragm makes viewing the lung fields (which are situated generally in the dorsal coelom) almost impossible on normal lateral views, and horizontal X-ray beam radiography with a standing patient is required in lizards and chelonians (see Figures 23.1 and 23.2). Snakes, due to the presence of fascia which holds the coelomic organs in place and their elongated body form, can be radiographed in a conventional vertical beam for both lateral and dorsoventral views but horizontal beam radiography can be particularly helpful when looking for fluid lines associated with effusions.
- What is the size of the patient to be radiographed?

Physical restraint

Many of the more docile reptiles will remain motionless for long enough to take radiographs without the need for chemical restraint. The use of Perspex or even cardboard boxes to constrain the reptile, particularly if they are some of the smaller lizards such as anoles and day geckos, is very useful, although minor reduction in the quality of the radiographs will occur.

Chelonians may be easily positioned for horizontal beam radiography in the conscious state by balancing the mid-part of the plastron on a block or small pile of upturned feeding bowls so as to lift all four feet off the ground, preventing them from walking off.

Snakes may be constrained manually or encouraged to crawl into a Perspex or plastic tube, such as can be made from syringe cases taped together. This has two advantages. One is that the snake is adequately restrained to allow the handler to leave the snake whilst the radiograph is being taken. The second is that it ensures the snake is stretched out and avoids the confusion of interpretation which occurs in the coiled individual.

Lizards such as the green iguana (*Iguana iguana*) may present more difficulty to restrain physically. However, many will quieten down when placed into a dimmed environment. Alternatively, the use of a heavy towel to restrain the iguana initially, long enough to allow the handler to gently close the eyelids and apply firm but careful pressure to the eyeballs through the eyelids, can be employed. This pressure may be maintained manually, or replaced by a ball of cotton wool over each eyelid and the whole wrapped in an elasticated bandage to maintain the pressure. This procedure makes use of the vasovagal reflex, whereby pressure on the eyeballs stimulates the vagus nerve and consequently leads to a reduction in respiration rate and heart rate, so creating a semi-sedated condition. This is sufficient to allow the iguana to be placed in lateral recumbency for limb radiographs, etc., without the need for chemical restraint. However, as soon as a loud noise or other form of stimulation occurs, the effect is abolished and the iguana becomes alert again.

Chemical restraint

This may be necessary for aggressive individuals, very large species or venomous ones. There are many combinations of sedatives and anaesthetic regimens available to practitioners, and it is impossible to describe them all here but more information is given in Chapter 19. However, commonly used chemical restraint drugs include alfaxalone, ketamine (often with an alpha-2 drug such as medetomidine or dexmedetomidine) and propofol to induce, and isoflurane or sevoflurane to maintain, anaesthesia.

Positioning

As with small mammals, the need is to obtain a three-dimensional view of the area under investigation. To obtain this, the traditional two views, at right angles to each other, are required.

However, although a dorsoventral view is performed as for a small mammal patient, a lateral view is often better performed in the standing patient using horizontal beam radiography, as mentioned above. This means images are more representative of normal organ positions and is also extremely useful in cases of coelomic fluid effusion where fluid lines become readily apparent.

In Chelonia, an additional third view is recommended. This is the craniocaudal view, again utilising the horizontal beam X-ray. This view allows comparison of the right and left lung fields, which are situated in the dorsal aspect of the shell, and is useful for diagnosing one-sided lesions such as single granulomas or focal pneumonias.

Veterinary Nursing of Exotic Pets and Wildlife, Third Edition. Simon J. Girling.

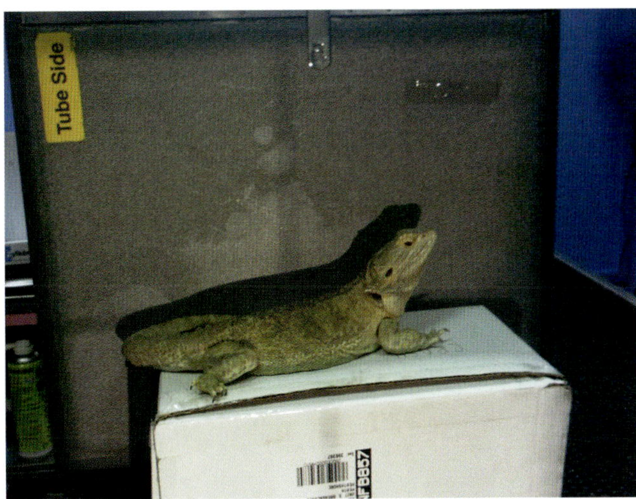

Figure 23.1 Horizontal beam radiography is necessary in lizards and chelonians in particular to obtain anatomically correct views of the coelomic cavity due to the absence of a true diaphragm.

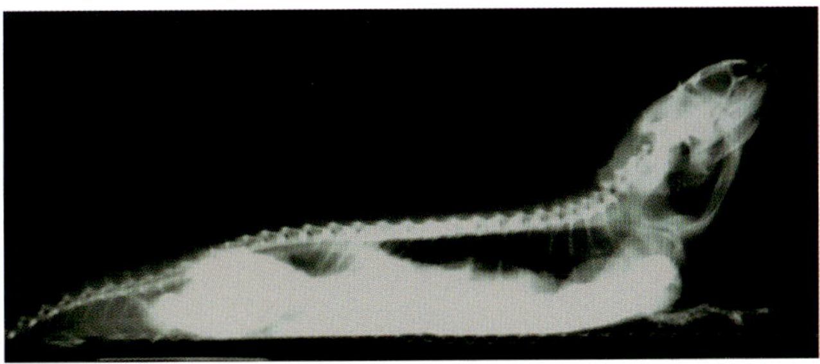

Figure 23.2 Radiographic image of the bearded dragon shown in Figure 23.1 using horizontal beam radiography. This view is useful for assessing skull, spine, lung fields and some coelomic organs.

In snakes, it is advised that the snake be extended in form before radiography is performed, as the traditional coiled-up view of a snake makes for poor interpretation of internal organs and the position of lesions.

Positive contrast techniques

Barium

The use of barium sulphate is useful for positive contrast radiography of the gastrointestinal tract in all reptiles. However, it should not be used where surgery of the gastrointestinal tract is contemplated as, should the barium leak into the coelomic cavity, it is highly irritant. In this scenario, iodine-based contrast media should be considered.

Chelonia

The use of 5–7 mL of a 25–30% solution of barium, administered by stomach tube, is useful for most *Testudo* tortoise species. Stomach emptying time may take up to a day, and the gut transit time from mouth to cloaca may take nearly a month. Barium studies are especially useful in chelonians due to the lack of detail encountered on plain radiographs.

Lizards

As for Chelonia. Transit times are faster, particularly in insectivorous species such as geckos, and may take 24–36 hours if kept at optimal temperatures. Useful for highlighting foreign intestinal bodies in iguanas which are notorious for consuming things they should not.

In one study in bearded dragons the median stomach emptying time with barium contrast was 10 hours (range 4–24 hours) and median time to reach the colon was 31 hours (range 12–72 hours) (Grosset *et al.*, 2014). In another study in green iguanas, stomach emptying times were faster with a median of 8 hours and median time to reach the colon 15 hours (although emptying was nearer 66 hours due to the complicated multipartitioned nature of the colon in this herbivorous species) (Smith *et al.*, 2001).

Snakes

As for Chelonia, with doses of barium of 5 mL/kg, although transit times are much faster with gastric emptying occurring in 2–3 hours and full transit time taking 4–7 days. Air may be injected into the stomach immediately after barium to create a positive contrast technique, which is useful when examining thickening of the stomach wall as is found with some tumours, cryptosporidiosis and abscesses.

Iodine-based contrast

Useful where minimal irritation is required, such as when gut/intestinal surgery may be planned shortly after using positive contrast techniques. If using in the gastrointestinal tract, it is recommended to use the higher concentration (300 mg/mL) solutions to get better resolution. Transit times are generally shorter as the product is more liquid than barium but there are fewer published studies to define the exact timing of transit.

Chelonia

Gastrointestinal transit times are faster, with stomach emptying occurring in 1.5–4 hours and full gut transit time taking 3–8 hours at 21°C. Note that a positive contrast urocystogram may be seen some 8–10 hours after oral administration as the aqueous iodine is absorbed and excreted through the kidneys.

Lizards

Gastrointestinal transit times vary between species although there is less information on iodine than barium. Typically the stomach of a bearded dragon should empty within 2–4 hours and the column of iodine should have reached the caecum and colon by 8–10 hours in my experience (see Figure 23.3 and 23.4)

Intravenous techniques have been used to determine blood flow through the kidneys and may be used to assess the cardiovascular system. Doses of 0.5–1 mL/kg intravenously have been used.

Snakes

As for Chelonia, although gut transit times are even faster, with stomach emptying occurring within 30–45 minutes (see Figures 23.5 and 23.6).

Iodine-based contrast has been used to highlight the hemipenes of snakes to allow identification of the sex of the snake. However, poor filling of the hemipene sulcus resulted in an accuracy rate of 81.4% in one study (Gnudi *et al.*, 2009).

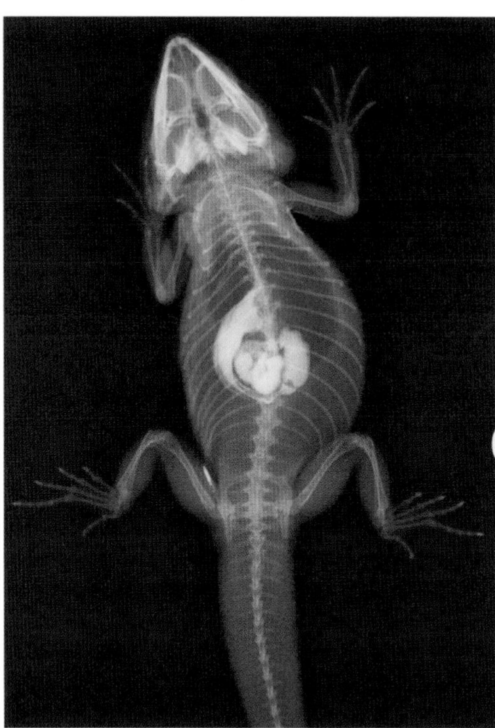

Figure 23.3 Dorsoventral view of a bearded dragon undergoing an iodine-based gastrointestinal positive contrast study. The outline organ to the left making a 'C' shape is the stomach that empties through the pylorus where the column narrows before entering the duodenal 'bulb' to the right of midline. The column continues to the small intestine before entering the caecum and start of the colon in midline.

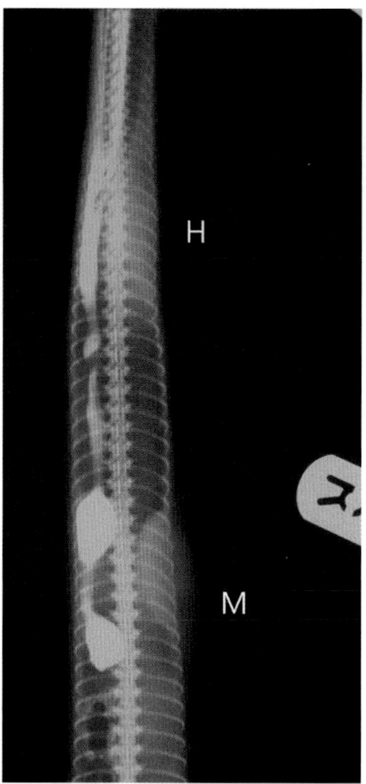

Figure 23.5 Dorsoventral view of a corn snake undergoing gastrointestinal iodine positive contrast radiography to determine the extent of a coelomic mass. Note the heart (H) and the mass (M) and the fact that the column of iodine deviates around the mass.

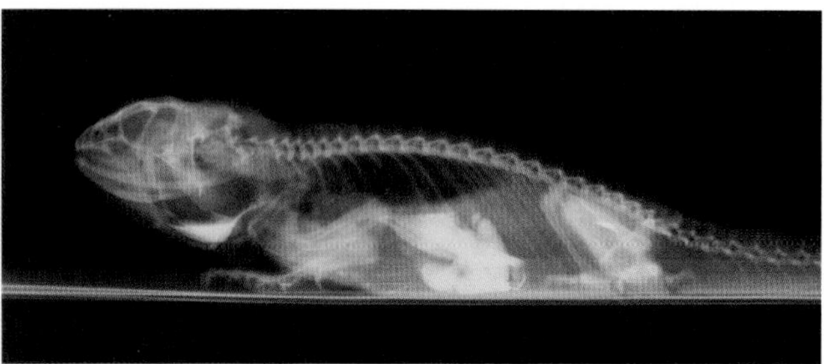

Figure 23.4 Right lateral horizontal beam view of the bearded dragon in Figure 23.3 showing the iodine contrast in the stomach, duodenum and start of the colon. Note also some residual contrast in the oropharynx.

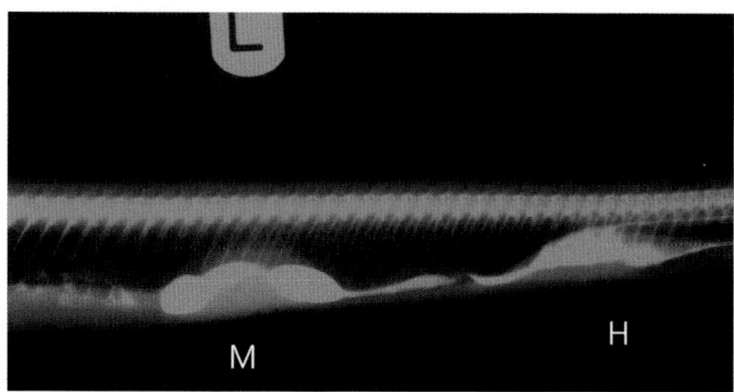

Figure 23.6 Left lateral view of the corn snake in Figure 23.5. Note the heart (H) and the mass (M) and again the fact that the column of iodine in the oesophagus deviates around the coelomic mass.

Normal and abnormal radiographic findings

Chelonia

It is difficult to view many of the chelonian internal organs due to the density of their shell. However, the heart and liver may be seen on lateral views using horizontal beam radiography, and the liver shadow may be enhanced by the use of positive contrast studies and lies in a dumb-bell shape across midline in the caudal part of the cranial half of the chelonian.

Metabolic bone disease (MBD) will generally cause deformities of the carapace and lucencies in the pelvis and pectoral girdle. Oversupplementation with vitamin D_3 and calcium or renal failure leading to hypercalcaemia may result in renal and cardiovascular mineralisation. Bladder stones and gravidity are most easily seen in dorsoventral radiographs. Limb fractures are most easily viewed in dorsoventral images. Articular gout may present as joint swelling with osteolysis and proliferative densities both within and around the joint(s) affected.

Lung fields are best assessed on the lateral horizontal beam radiograph (see Figure 23.7) and the craniocaudal horizontal beam radiograph which combined can help pinpoint lesions such as granulomas and neoplasms. Fluid lines associated with coelomic fluid linked to cardiovascular disease and egg yolk coelomitis may be seen most easily in lateral horizontal beam radiographs.

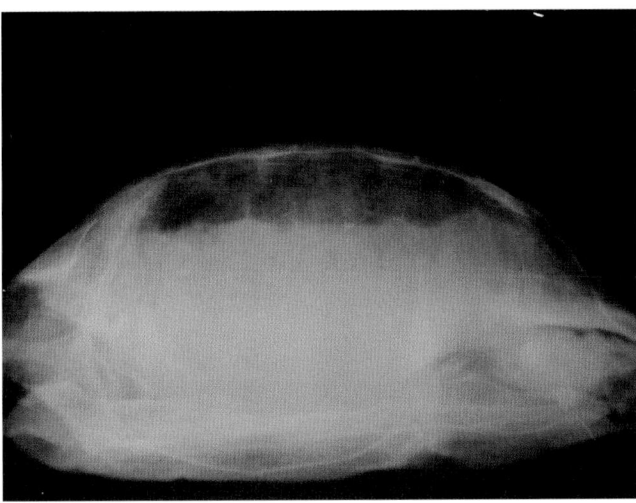

Figure 23.7 Right lateral horizontal beam radiograph of a tortoise with a diffuse pneumonia demonstrated by the increased radiodensity of the dorsally located lung fields.

Gravidity is easily diagnosed in chelonians as the eggshell is radiodense, similar to bird eggs, and the most useful view is the dorsoventral (see Figures 23.8–23.10).

Radiography may, of course, also be used to assess whether intraosseous catheters are correctly sited.

Lizards

Internal organs of most lizards are best viewed on the lateral horizontal beam radiographs. These allow good visualisation of the dorsal lung fields and the liver shadow (see Figures 23.2 and 23.4).

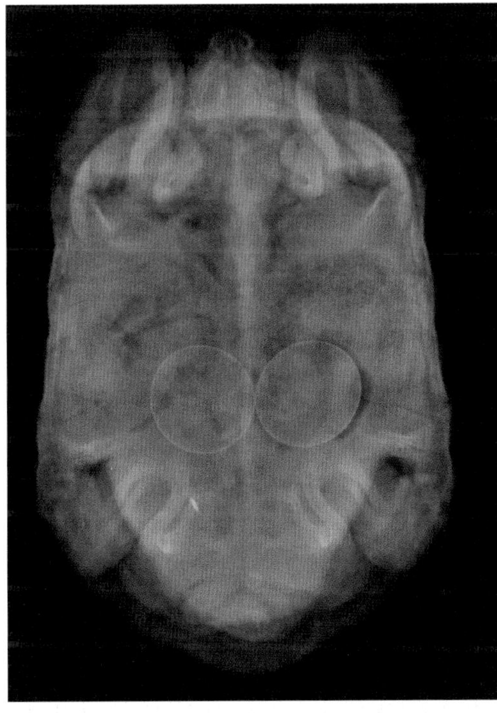

Figure 23.8 Dorsoventral view of a female chelonian showing the outlines of two normal eggs. It is difficult to identify coelomic organs on this view using plain radiography, although some assistance is given by the presence of gas and ingesta in the stomach to the left side and the intestinal mass predominantly to the right.

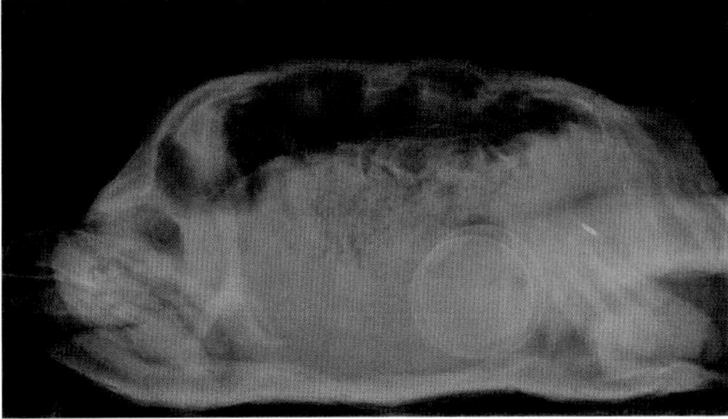

Figure 23.9 Horizontal beam lateral view of the tortoise in Figure 23.8. Note the dorsally situated lungs and their radiolucency in comparison to Figure 23.7. Note also the internal support of the carapace created by the pectoral girdle and pelvis which both have a vertical orientation. Immediately dorsal to the eggs is the intestinal mass with ingesta and gas. Cranial to the eggs is the stomach and liver. The heart is difficult to see as it is immediately caudal to the neck contained within the pectoral girdle.

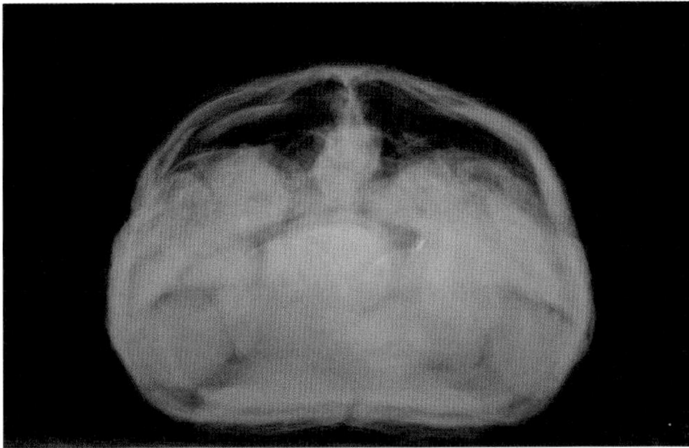

Figure 23.10 Craniocaudal horizontal beam view of the tortoise in Figures 23.8 and 23.9. Note the fact that in this view it is possible to compare right and left lung fields for lesions, although it is less helpful when assessing coelomic cavity organs.

The dorsoventral view, due to the absence of a diaphragm, results in superimposition of the lung fields over the liver and digestive tract, making interpretation difficult without contrast media (see Figure 23.3).

The caudal coelom is occupied by the gut, which may be extensive in herbivorous species such as the green iguana and may contain gas. In insectivorous and more omnivorous species such as geckos and monitors, the gut may be smaller. Large fat bodies fill the ventral and caudal abdomen in many lizards and may make outlining the gut more difficult in obese individuals.

Kidneys cannot be viewed easily in healthy iguanids, geckos and agamids as they are situated in the pelvis, and if visualised projecting cranially from the pelvis tends to suggest renomegaly associated with inflammatory or neoplastic disease. In varanids and chameleons the kidneys are normally located cranial to the pelvis and so may be seen especially on lateral horizontal beam views.

The heart in lizards may be placed so far cranially that it is hidden within the sternal plate (e.g. green iguanas and bearded dragons) and so is not visible on either horizontal beam radiographs or dorsoventral views. In other species (e.g. monitor lizards) the heart is more caudally placed and so better seen. The stomach of many lizards such as the green iguana is actually quite far caudal. Loss of coelomic detail can be associated with coelomitis such as will occur due to a perforated bowel.

Gravidity is usually obvious on radiography although eggshells in lizards are less radiodense than in chelonians. Preovulatory stasis is more difficult to identify due to the less radiodense nature of the egg yolks. A negative contrast technique injecting room air or medical gas into the coelomic cavity can sometimes help with identification of preovulatory stasis.

Some members of the order Geckonidae (*Uroplatus* and *Phelsuma* spp.) store calcium in specialised structures called endolymphatic sacs. These organs, which lie in the cervical area, are readily visible radiographically and are a normal feature for the species (see Figure 23.11). Other species have moderate amounts of mineralisation of the skin (osteoderms) and increased keratin, so that radiography can be less helpful in assessing coelomic organs (see Figures 23.12 and 23.13).

MBD can be confirmed by radiography by comparing soft-tissue density with bone density, with dorsoventral radiographs being the most useful (see Figure 23.14). Long bone deformities are common in this condition, as are swellings and flaring of the epiphyseal plates in cases of rickets due to vitamin D_3 deficiencies (most commonly seen on the costochondral junctions of green iguanas). The exoskeleton often has a moth-eaten appearance with MBD causing the ribs to appear more prominent. In lizards, demineralisation is followed by fibrous tissue proliferation around the shafts of the long bones. Folding fractures are common, particularly in chronic cases of MBD. Fractures in adult reptiles are most commonly due to trauma.

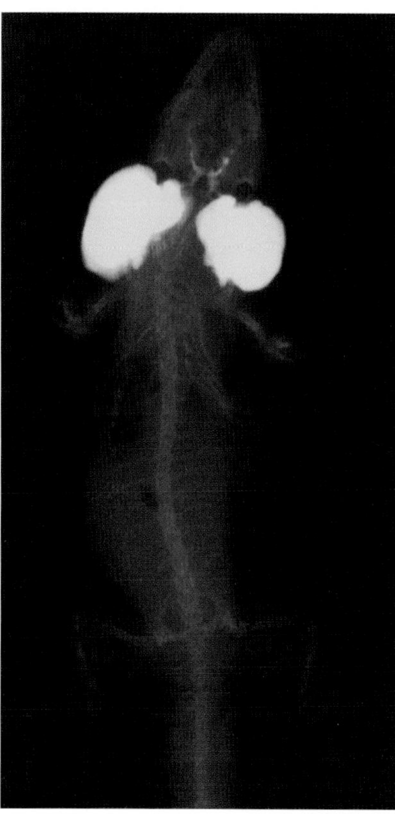

Figure 23.11 Dorsoventral view of a Standing's day gecko (*Phelsuma standingi*) demonstrating the calcium storage glands in the neck. This is a normal radiographic finding in this species.

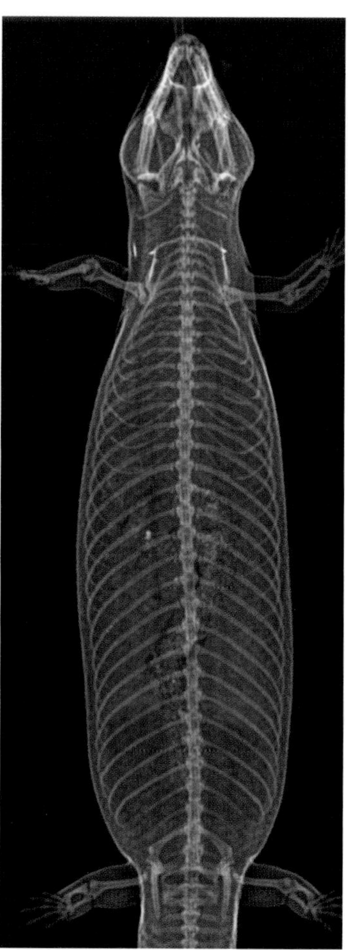

Figure 23.12 Dorsoventral view of a skink showing the presence of widespread increased skin/scale radiodensity which is normal for this species but can obscure some of the detail of coelomic organs.

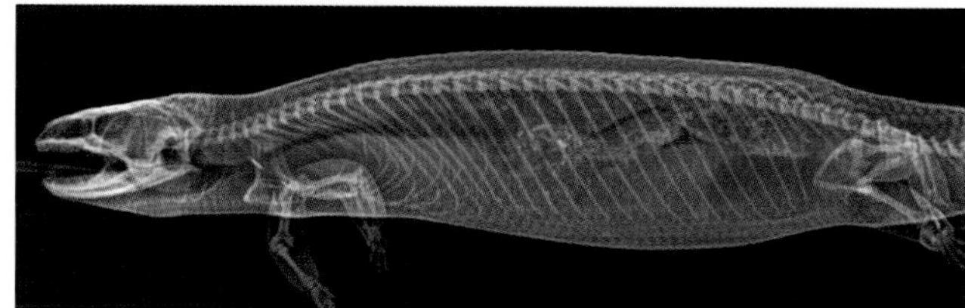

Figure 23.13 Lateral view of the skink in Figure 23.12. The stomach and intestines can be identified due to the presence of ingesta, some of which is radiodense. Below this is the liver but otherwise relatively little detail can be determined due to the overlying very obvious scale structure.

Infectious diseases of bones (osteomyelitis) are characterised by lysis and soft-tissue swelling. With septic arthritis, there is often destruction of the epiphyses of the bones which form the joint. Neoplasia of the bone is less commonly seen but where it does occur seems to be most typically seen in the skull (see Figure 23.15).

In species where autotomy occurs with regrowth of the tail, the vertebral bodies are replaced distally by cartilage, which as a consequence is not as radiodense as the rest of the spinal column (see Figure 23.16).

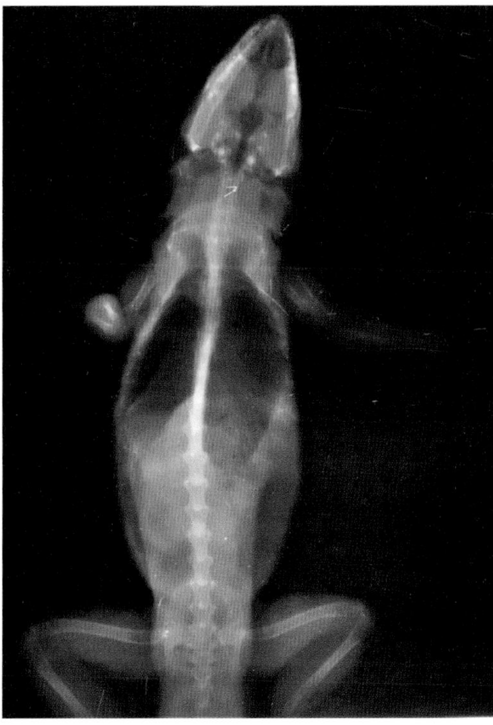

Figure 23.14 Dorsoventral view of a lizard with metabolic bone disease. Note the poorly mineralised bones particularly in the more distal limbs and the presence of a fracture in the right humerus.

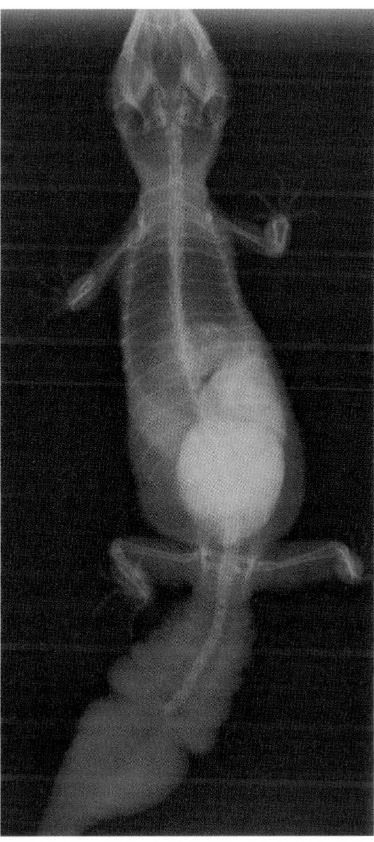

Figure 23.15 Dorsoventral view of a leopard gecko (*Eublepharis macularius*) showing evidence of previous distal tail loss and regrowth as shown by the lack of mineralised vertebrae in the distal tail. This individual also has an appreciable amount of radiodense material (likely substrate) in its distal intestinal tract.

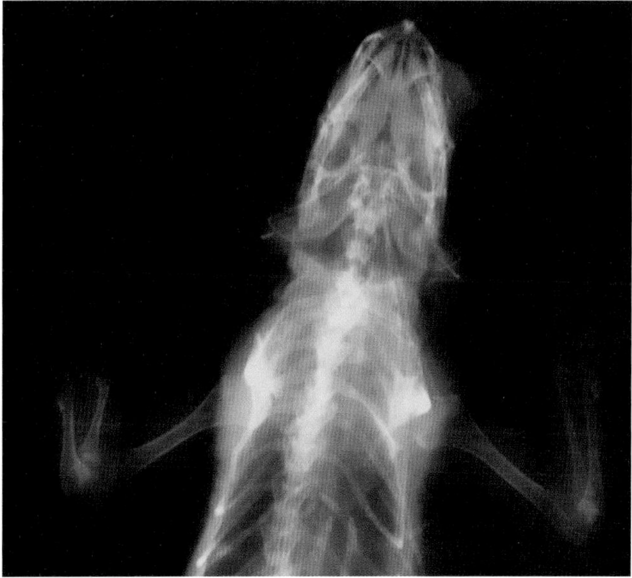

Figure 23.16 Dorsoventral view of a green iguana (*Iguana iguana*) with an osteosarcoma of the right maxilla. Note the proliferative lesion with some ectopic mineralisation.

Dorsoventral views allow the confirmation of pre- and post-ovulatory stasis, two common reproductive diseases of lizards, particularly the green iguana. Preovulatory stasis is shown by up to 70 spherical soft-tissue densities in the cranial mid-coelom, and post-ovulatory stasis is shown by more ovoidal soft-tissue densities with very thin calcium cortices as reptile shells are poorly mineralised in comparison to their avian counterparts. This radiographic view also allows visualisation of bladder stones in species possessing a urinary bladder, such as the green iguana.

Some monitor lizards (*Varanus indicus*, *V. prasinus*, *V. gouldii*) can be sexed radiographically because there is calcification of the hemibacula of the hemipenises although the mineralisation can be inconsistent (Shea and Reddacliff, 1986).

Snakes

The most useful view for snakes is the lateral radiograph, as in the dorsoventral view the body organs are largely obscured by the ribs and spinal column. However, both views are recommended to obtain a three-dimensional image.

Radiographic changes to the spinal column are commonly seen with osteomyelitis and can be both proliferative and osteolytic and result in considerable spinal deformity with time (see Figure 23.17).

In the lateral beam radiograph, the lung fields are clearly seen occupying the caudal half of the first third of the snake, with the heart

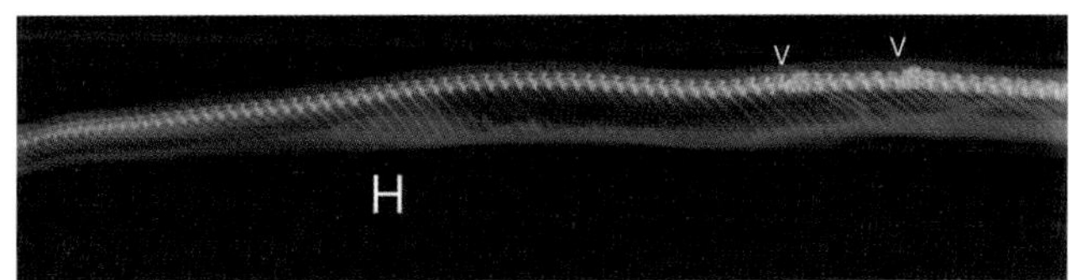

Figure 23.17 Right lateral view of a rat snake with evidence of spinal osteomyelitis. Note the heart (H) and the osteomyelitis lesions (white arrowheads).

PART III: REPTILES AND AMPHIBIANS

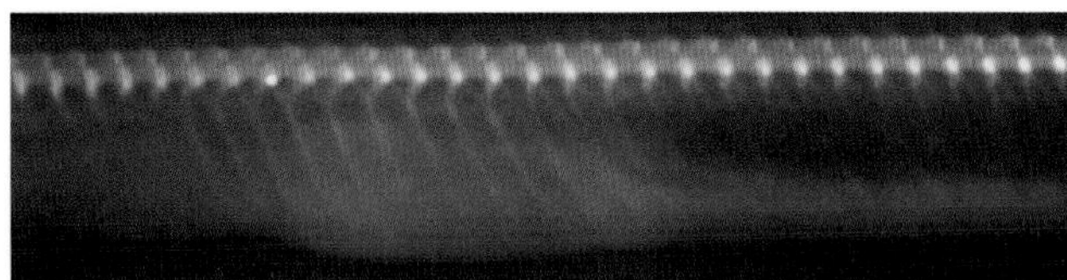

Figure 23.18 Right lateral radiograph of a corn snake with cardiac enlargement due to a cardiomyopathy. The heart is the radiodense object in the centre of the image with the radiolucent lung field starting immediately caudal to it and the thin radiolucent line of the trachea running over the dorsum of the heart.

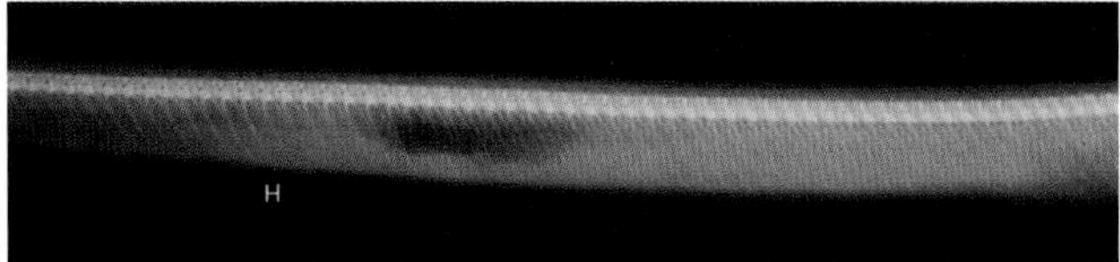

Figure 23.19 Right lateral view of a kingsnake with pneumonia. The heart is denoted by the letter H. Note the radiolucent cranial lung field immediately caudal to the heart, but this rapidly becomes radiopaque due to the presence of inflammatory exudates within the airways, whereas the lung field should extend to nearly the right-hand edge of the image in a healthy snake (see Figure 23.17).

shadow clearly outlined. Cardiac enlargement associated with cardiomyopathies may be seen visually due to the deviation of the ventral body wall, but radiography can be helpful in confirming that the heart is the organ affected (see Figure 23.18).

Pneumonia and fluid lines are occasionally seen where lateral beam radiography is used (see Figure 23.19). Caudal to the heart shadow lies the liver shadow and stomach followed by the gall bladder and small intestine. Blockages of the bowel may be seen on plain radiographs if food material is held back, but determining their severity often requires positive contrast techniques as described above.

In the cranial half of the caudal third of the snake lie the kidneys and reproductive organs along the dorsal surface of the coelom. Radiolucent areas may represent follicular activity, and regular ovoidal soft-tissue densities along the caudal third of the snake may indicate gravidity. For live-bearers, such as garter snakes and boa constrictors, it is possible to see the skeletons of the fetuses in this region in the later stages of gravidity, and in oviparous species such as pythons and corn snakes it may be possible to see eggs shortly before being laid although as with lizards the eggshells are less radiodense than in chelonians. The large intestine and rectum occupy the ventral surface.

AMPHIBIANS

Radiography is increasingly being used in amphibians, particularly to diagnose MBD (nutritional secondary hyperparathyroidism) and trauma. Many will allow radiography without chemical restraint, but as they are delicate and readily desiccate, the time taken to image them should be minimised.

Plain radiography is best performed via two views as for other animals and horizontal beam radiography is again helpful for assessing the correct anatomical position of coelomic organs due to the absence of a diaphragm. Dorsoventral views are often best for assessing skeletal structures but as there is no separate thoracic and abdominal cavity, the lungs (where present) overlie the other

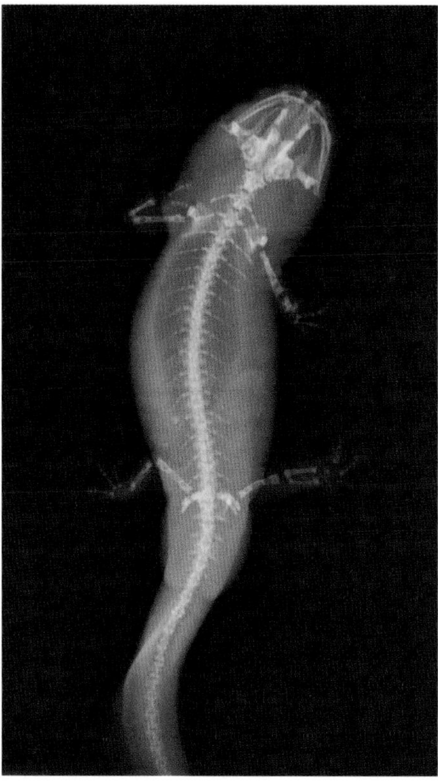

Figure 23.20 Dorsoventral view of an axolotl. Note the very simple skeletal structure, the presence of ribs along the vertebral column and the poorly defined outline of the paired lungs in the cranial coelomic cavity overlying the heart and liver.

coelomic organs and so make their differentiation and assessment difficult (see Figures 23.20 and 23.21). Lateral horizontal beam views, as mentioned, allow a better appreciation of the lung fields (see Figure 23.22).

There is limited information on gut transit times for positive contrast studies but iodine contrast should be avoided in amphibians such as the axolotl and in pre-metamorphic stages of other species as this can cause shedding of the external gills.

ULTRASONOGRAPHY

Physical restraint

This is the preferred method for ultrasound examination as it allows observation of gut movements, which may not be possible in a sedated or anaesthetised reptile.

Equipment

The use of a hard worktop area with a section cut out to allow the ultrasound probe to be applied to the dependent side of the patient is preferred for larger individuals.

As far as the ultrasound equipment is concerned, the preferred size of probe is a 7.5 MHz transducer, as most reptile patients are relatively small. Indeed, it may still be necessary to use a stand-off (an acoustic coupling device) in patients under 50 g in weight and the narrower snakes. A stand-off may be cheaply made from a latex glove finger filled with coupling gel, or more expensive purpose-built ones may be bought. In patients over 1.5 kg, it may be

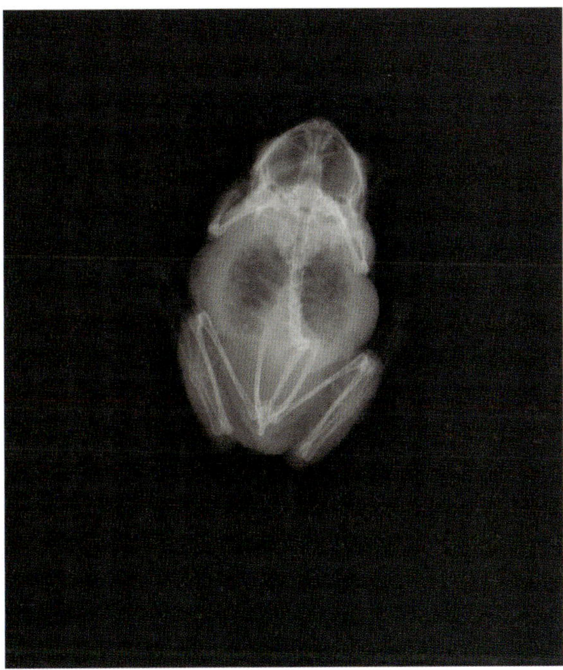

Figure 23.21 Dorsoventral view of a tree frog. Note the elongated hindlimbs typical of anurans. Note also that this individual has a deviation of the lumbrosacral area of the spine.

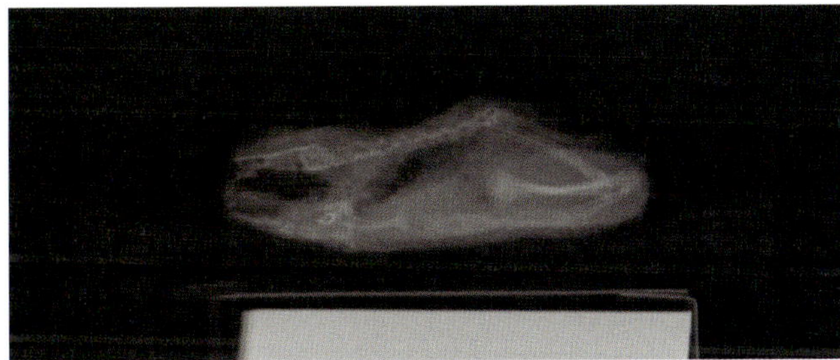

Figure 23.22 Lateral horizontal beam view of the tree frog in Figure 23.21. Note the ability to see the lung fields clearly separated from the other coelomic organs in this view.

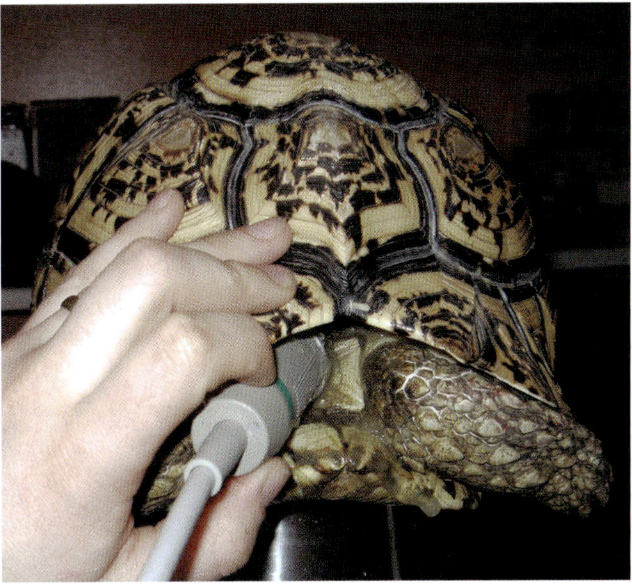

Figure 23.23 Approach to imaging the heart in chelonians using the thoracic inlet to one side of the neck. *Source:* Reproduced with permission from the BSAVA Manual of Reptiles 3rd edition figure 19.14a © BSAVA.

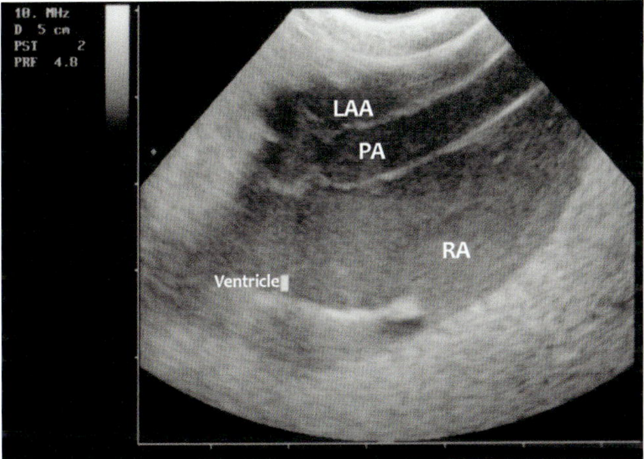

Figure 23.24 Two-dimensional echocardiogram, sagittal view from the right side of the neck in a leopard tortoise (*Stigmochelys pardalis*). LAA, left aortic arch; MPA, main pulmonary artery; RA, right atrium; V, ventricle. *Source:* Reproduced with permission from the BSAVA Manual of Reptiles 3rd edition figure 19.14b © BSAVA.

necessary to use a 5 MHz transducer to see deeper structures such as internal organs more than 10 cm away from the probe head, for example the liver.

Normal and abnormal ultrasound findings

Chelonia

Thoracic inlet

The thoracic inlet allows the heart to be visualised (see Figures 23.23 and 23.24). As with other reptiles (except the Crocodilia), there are two atria and only one ventricle. This may be seen midline on the floor of the plastron, and just cranial to this area is the oval thyroid gland. Enlargement is seen in the thyroid in cases of goitre, due to overfeeding of brassicas for example. The atrioventricular valves appear hyperechoic. It may be possible to examine some of the liver behind the heart structure, allowing the assessment of focal lesions such as abscesses, as well as general increased density as will occur in mineralisation, gout and hepatic lipidosis. The anechoic gall bladder is easily visible in the right lobe.

Inguinal inlet

The inguinal inlets will allow the urinary bladder to be examined, which can be an extensive bilobed structure. Bladder stones are not uncommon.

The kidneys appear homogeneous in outline with a very narrow hypoechoic medulla. They are attached to the dorsal aspect of the caudal shell. Again, gout, abscesses and enlargement may be visualised by changes in density and outline.

The female reproductive tract can be visualised easily when gravid. There are two ovaries, suspended from the underside of the carapace, caudal to the lung field and cranial to the kidneys. Preovulatory stasis will present as the 'cluster of grapes' effect with more than 10–15 follicles in each ovary but these are relatively hyperechoic. From each ovary, a uterine body extends down to the cloaca, and it is here that shelled eggs and post-ovulatory stasis or gravidity may be determined. Shelled eggs are readily apparent, with the lightly mineralised shell, surrounding the hypoechoic albumen, around the denser hyperechoic yolk.

Lizards

The heart again is a three-chambered organ, and may be found anywhere from the thoracic inlet in the case of the green iguana and bearded dragon, to the mid-section of the body in the case of many monitor lizards.

The liver sits on the ventral body wall just caudal to the ribcage, and is a bilobed structure with the gall bladder and caudal vena cava appearing as hypoechoic structures in the right lobe. Abscesses, gross enlargement and tumours as well as gout may be visualised.

The kidneys may be located in the pelvic region in species such as the green iguana, or on the caudal coelomic wall dorsally in species such as bearded dragons and chameleons. As the kidneys enlarge due to inflammation or growths, they will protrude out from the pelvis region and be easier to examine. Gout crystals and mineralisation indicative of advancing renal failure appear as scintillating hyperechoic areas. The urinary bladder in those species that have one, such as the green iguana, is found immediately cranial to the pelvis ventrally. A cloacal bladder is more typically seen in species such as bearded dragons and monitor lizards and appears as an enlargement of the urodeum portion of the cloaca rather than a separate bladder structure. Bladder stones may be present and will appear as hyperechoic structures blocking ultrasound wave transmission.

The bilateral fat pads extend cranially from the pelvis. In cachectic animals they are reduced in size and may even be absent. Adipose tissue is hyperechoic compared to other coelomic organs and is divided into lobes by hyperechoic septae. In obese animals the fat bodies extend to the liver and heart and can significantly interfere with imaging of the coelomic cavity.

The female reproductive tract may be easily visualised. There are two ovaries, suspended from the dorsal body wall caudal to the ribcage, follicles appearing as echogenic densities that increase in density as they mature. Eggs have a hyperechoic rim. In viviparous lizards (e.g. blue-tongue skinks, *Teliqua scincoides*), fetuses are identified by their hyperechoic signals surrounded by anechoic fluid and membranes. In the later stages of gestation, the skeletons and beating hearts become visible. Pre- and post-ovulatory stasis may be determined as described for chelonians.

In sexually monomorphic lizards such as Gila monsters (*Heloderma suspectum*) and prehensile-tailed skinks (*Corucia zebrata*), the hemipenises can be identified in the ventral tail base. They appear as elongated heterogeneous structures compared to the surrounding homogeneous muscle tissue.

Snakes

The heart is situated in the caudal section of the first third of the snake. Under sedation and in relaxed snakes the heart apex beat may be seen moving the ventral scutes. Again, the heart is a three-chambered structure (see Figure 23.25).

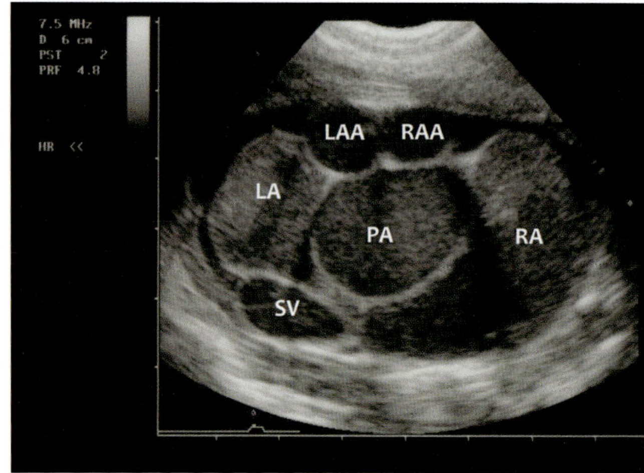

Figure 23.25 Two-dimensional echocardiogram, short axis view demonstrating the normal echocardiographic anatomy of a Burmese python. LA, left atrium; LAA, left aortic arch; PA, pulmonary artery; RA, right atrium; RAA, right aortic arch; SV, sinus venosus. *Source:* Reproduced with permission from the BSAVA Manual of Reptiles 3rd edition (2019) Figure 19.20 © BSAVA.

The liver is a short distance caudal to the heart and is an elongated structure of homogeneous echogenicity. Abscesses, tumours and gout crystals may all disturb this homogeneity. The gall bladder is a separate, hypoechoic, spherical organ situated immediately caudal to the liver, adjacent to the splenopancreas and is usually surrounded by more hyperechoic fat in healthy snakes.

The kidneys are elongated flattened structures extending into the proximal half of the caudal third of the snake and are hyperechoic when compared with the liver but hypoechoic to the fat bodies also present close by.

The female reproductive system is again suspended from the dorsal body wall, with the paired ovaries located cranial to the kidneys and caudal to the stomach. Preovulatory stasis is uncommon, but ultrasonography is useful for determining gravidity as the thin-shelled eggs are easily visualised in oviparous species. Hyperechoic reflections may be seen in viviparous species such as the garter snake and boa constrictor due to reflections from the skeleton of the fetus.

The hemipenises may be seen as hyperechoic areas caudal to the vent and either side of midline. The female has no similar structure, and this method may be used to sex snakes.

MRI AND CT SCANNING

Computed tomography (CT) in chelonians is useful due to its ability to penetrate the bony shell without distortion, allowing examination of the internal organs. Normal chelonian lungs appear as radiolucent air-filled cavities with CT images, separated by septae consisting of pulmonary vasculature and smooth muscle. Soft tissues do not emit high-contrast signals; however, preovulatory follicles and dystrophic calcification may be easily defined on CT images (see Figure 23.26). Positive contrast intravenous iodine studies are commonly used in mammalian CT imaging and can be used in reptiles as well to highlight specific organs and neoplasms/inflammatory processes.

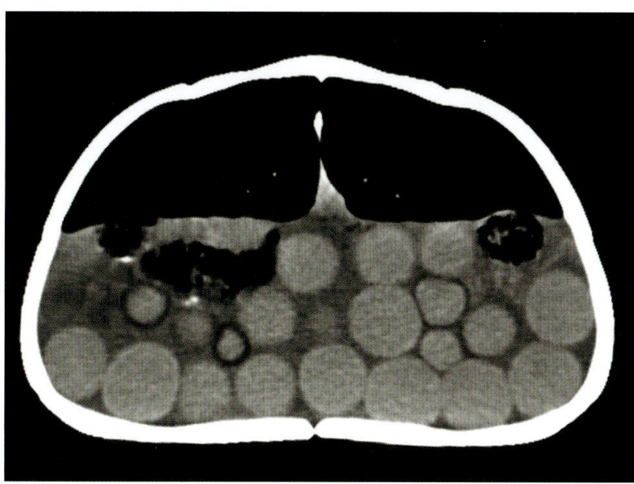

Figure 23.26 CT image of a female tortoise with preovulatory stasis. The tortoise shell is identified as the outer white structure, the lungs are dorsally located and radiolucent (black) and the follicles are the numerous round grey structures. Non-oval shapes, dark rims and layering content are abnormal features in follicles. *Source:* Courtesy of Tobias Schwarz, University of Edinburgh.

Magnetic resonance imaging (MRI) is useful as in other species for determination of soft-tissue growths within organs and may be applied to reptiles in a similar manner. It is particularly helpful in differentiating tumours within organs and haemorrhages (as iron found in all haemoglobins is highly magnetic). However, reptiles with steel implants for fracture repair are not candidates for MRI due to the intense magnetic fields generated.

Both techniques require that the reptile is completely immobilised, and therefore chemical restraint is necessary.

RIGID ENDOSCOPY

This is a useful technique in lizards and particularly chelonians. Similar equipment to that used in avian patients is used; however, due to the absence of air sacs, it is more difficult to perform laparoscopic procedures in reptiles. For this, the use of a positive pressure system to pump either carbon dioxide or room air into the coelomic cavity and so separate the internal organs to aid visualisation is helpful. It is particularly useful in chelonians where the shell may interfere with other imaging modalities such as radiography; however, larger specimens may require purpose-built human bariatric endoscopes to reach some of the deeper body organs. Snakes, due to their elongated nature and multiple internal connective tissue compartments, are not so suited to this modality but if the rough location of a lesion is known can still allow minimal invasive biopsies to be carried out which may aid a diagnosis.

Rigid endoscopy can of course be used to examine body orifices such as the cloaca, pharynx, proximal trachea and nares.

References

Girling, S.J. and Raiti, P. (2004) Appendix 2 a formulary of drugs for use in reptiles. In: *BSAVA Manual of Reptiles* (eds S.J. Girling & P. Raiti), 2nd edn, pp. 352–356. BSAVA, Quedgeley, UK.

Gnudi, G., Volta, A., Di Ianni, F. *et al.* (2009) Use of ultrasonography and contrast radiography for snake gender determination. *Radiology and Ultrasound*, **50**(3), 309–311.

Grosset, C., Daniaux, L., Guzman, D.S.-M. *et al.* (2014) Radiographic anatomy and barium sulfate contrast transit time of the gastrointestinal tract of bearded dragons (*Pogona vitticeps*). *Veterinary Radiology and Ultrasound*, **55**(3), 241–250.

Shea, G.M. and Reddacliff, G.L. (1986) Ossifications in the hemipenes of varanids. *Journal of Herpetology*, **20**(4), 566–568.

Smith, D., Dobson, H. and Spence, E. (2001) Gastrointestinal studies in the green iguana: technique and reference values. *Veterinary Radiology and Ultrasound*, **42**(6), 515–520.

Chapter 24 Reptile and Amphibian Emergency and Critical Care Medicine

Initial assessment of the collapsed reptile

An initial assessment of the reptile patient should be made before it is removed from its carry cage/box. This should focus on the following points.

1. Is it potentially hazardous/dangerous to the handler? For example, male green iguanas, snapping turtles, aggressive snakes and unlikely but possibly venomous snakes and lizards.
2. Is it mouth breathing and therefore in possible respiratory distress?
3. Is it a fragile species? For example, many geckos will shed their tails very easily, as will many iguanas, so do not rush handling.
4. Is it suffering from metabolic bone disease making it a risk to handle? Deformed limbs, shell, spine, etc. and inability to support its own weight in a lizard or chelonian may suggest this condition is present.
5. How large is the animal? Many larger species of tortoise are surprisingly heavy and strong, and snakes longer than 1.5–2 m require more than one handler to avoid damaging the patient and putting the handlers at risk.

While examining the patient from a distance to ascertain if it is safe to handle, it is a good idea to question the owner about the husbandry of the reptile at home.

1. What do they feed it?
2. Do they feed vitamin/mineral supplements?
3. Is there an ultraviolet (UV) lamp and if so what type and where is it situated (may not be necessary for most snakes but is necessary for lizards and chelonians)?
4. What temperature range do they keep the vivarium at and is the UV provision associated with a hot/basking spot dependent on the species?
5. What hides/cage furniture is present in the tank?
6. What humidity do they keep the vivarium at?
7. Do they have any other reptiles/pets and have any new reptiles been recently added?
8. If a snake, when did it last shed its skin, and was it a complete shed?
9. When did the reptile last eat and defecate?
10. Has the owner used any new disinfectants/medications/therapies on the reptile and its vivarium recently?

Detailed examination of the collapsed reptile

Manual restraint

This is covered in the section on anaesthesia and analgesia.

Detailed examination

1. An intraoral examination using a mouth gag or a pen/pencil to encourage the reptile to open its mouth (be careful with chelonians, as they have powerful jaws, and aggressive snakes and of course avoid in venomous species and Crocodilia until safely sedated/anaesthetised). This should allow a close examination of the tongue, the roof of the mouth/nasal passages (there is no hard palate in reptiles other than Crocodilia). The glottis may also be visualised at the base of the tongue. Abnormalities such as a discharge from the nasal passages, petechiae or haemorrhages in the mouth, an abnormal or foul odour, and evidence of white or yellow plaques on the mucosa should all be noted and if possible sampled with a swab dampened with sterile water. Note that many lizards normally have a two-coloured tongue, for example the green iguana has a bright red tongue tip and a pale pink body to the fleshy tongue.
2. A detailed examination of the nares and the eyes. This will allow an assessment of any upper respiratory tract disease. Clinical signs of this include abnormal shaped nare(s), sinking of the globe of the eye, swelling below the globe of the eye, discharge from the eye itself, swelling of the conjunctiva, corneal blemishes and, in the case of snakes, evidence of a retained spectacle or swelling of the spectacle suggesting a build-up of tears underneath as can occur with blocked nasolacrimal ducts.
3. A detailed examination of the skin/shell. This may allow you to see areas of retained slough (snakes should shed in one complete go, lizards in small patches and chelonians only in small patches from the limbs and head/neck/tail). It will also allow any petechiae or ecchymoses to be observed, which may indicate septicaemia. Abscesses appear generally as firm, inspissated, subcutaneous masses, although anaerobic bacteria can produce liquid pus.
4. A detailed auscultation of the lungs and air sacs. The lungs are best auscultated from the dorsum in chelonians and lizards. To improve sound conductivity, a damp towel/cloth may be placed over the

Veterinary Nursing of Exotic Pets and Wildlife, Third Edition. Simon J. Girling.

reptile and the diaphragm of the stethoscope applied to this. Snakes are difficult to auscultate owing to their long thin lungs.

5. The heart is possible to auscultate in snakes but more difficult to auscultate in lizards and chelonians using a stethoscope. The same technique may be used as when auscultating the lungs with a damp cloth to improve sound transmission but it is often preferable to use a Doppler probe to assess blood flow throughout the heart to determine heart rate. Note that heart rate and heart sounds for reptiles are significantly different from those in mammals owing to the three-chambered heart (one ventricle and two atria) and its different construction. In addition, being ectothermic in nature, environmental temperatures will significantly alter heart rates.
6. A detailed examination of the limbs may be made. Palpate the long bones as metabolic bone disease is common, producing fibrous dystrophy where the poorly ossified bone swells due to cartilage deposition and making the limb look fat and muscular. Palpation reveals, however, that it is solid cartilage and not muscle. Shells of chelonians may be deformed and soft to touch. Mandibles of lizards may be bowed and malleable with this condition as well.
7. A detailed examination of the vent and caudal coelom should also be made. Many lizards such as iguanas have kidneys tucked into the pelvic area, and so these should not be palpable in front of the iliac wings in a normal animal. Snakes may be palpated by running a finger along the ventrum to feel for masses or obstructions. Chelonians are obviously difficult to palpate, although gentle ballottement of eggs or masses by placing a finger cranial to a hindlimb and rolling the animal onto its side and away again is possible. If doing this do ensure that someone else holds the end of the limb to prevent the chelonian trapping your fingers.

Triage

Any reptile presented unconscious, fitting, with evidence of head trauma or respiratory distress should be attended to immediately. Reptiles which are off colour and dull should be moved into a quiet, warm (32–38°C) vivarium with supplemental oxygen if there is any evidence of tachypnoea/hyperpnoea and should be examined as soon as possible.

Emergency ABC protocol

A for airway and B for breathing

It should be noted that an important impetus for respiration in the reptile is a lowered PaO_2 as well as the environmental temperature and hypercapnia. This means that if 100% oxygen is administered to a cold reptile, it will in effect often reduce its respiratory rate and depth even if it becomes hypercapnic. Reptiles should therefore be warmed to their preferred body temperature and intermittent positive pressure ventilation (IPPV) may be required to ensure adequate oxygenation of tissues and expulsion of carbon dioxide from the body. However, there is considerable species variation and one study in conscious green iguanas showed that 100% oxygen supplied by face mask increased the PaO_2 but did not alter the respiratory rate (Hernandez *et al.*, 2011).

Intubation of reptiles is straightforward and should be attempted where there is any doubt over whether the reptile is breathing or not (see Figure 24.1). The glottis is situated at the base of the tongue and is easily visualised, particularly in snakes. The glottis is held closed at rest, only opening for inspiration so an introducer may need to be used to allow intubation. If IPPV is used it should aim to allow an approximate 25–30% increase in body diameter, measured in snakes at the level of the end of the first third of the body and in lizards at the level of the elbows. This approximates to around 10 cmH_2O pressure on a mechanical ventilator. A breathing rate of 4–6 breaths per minute is preferred for critical care. Doxapram does work in reptiles but it has the same potential negative effects as it does in higher vertebrates, namely that it increases the oxygen demand of the breathing centre in the brainstem and if this area is already anoxic may hasten the death of neurons controlling respiration. So whilst it is helpful in stimulating respiration, care around its use should be taken.

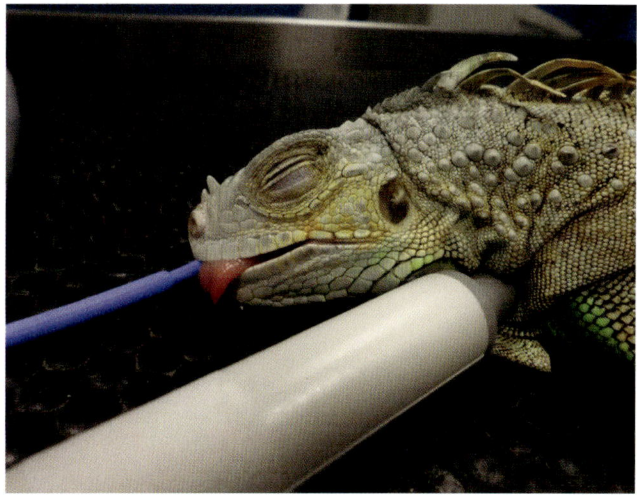

Figure 24.1 Intubation to secure an airway is important in any reptile where there is doubt over respiration. Note the Doppler probe placed over the thoracic inlet to detect cardiac output.

C for cardiovascular

The prognosis for respiratory arrest without cardiac arrest in reptiles is good. With IPPV and 100% oxygen, reversal of any anaesthesia where possible (e.g. use of atipamezole where medetomidine/dexmedetomidine has been used; use of naloxone where morphine or fentanyl has been used) and judicious administration of doxapram, recovery is likely.

However, cardiac arrest in reptiles carries a worse prognosis than for mammals. This is partly due to the robustness of the heart in most reptiles, meaning that should arrest occur, there is usually significant myocardial hypoxaemic damage or in those suffering from hypoproteinaemia from long-term malnutrition often a significant pericardial effusion (see Figure 24.2). Most reptiles become bradycardic immediately before arrest, and if this is recognised, rapid administration of atropine 0.02 mg/kg can be effective. Adrenaline (epinephrine) may be given if cardiac arrest has occurred prior to cardiac massage. It can be given intravenously, intraosseously or intratracheally in most reptiles and in snakes may be given by intracardiac injection. Because of the protected nature of the heart within the shell (chelonians) and often pectoral girdle (many lizards), intracardiac administration is less easy in non-snake reptiles.

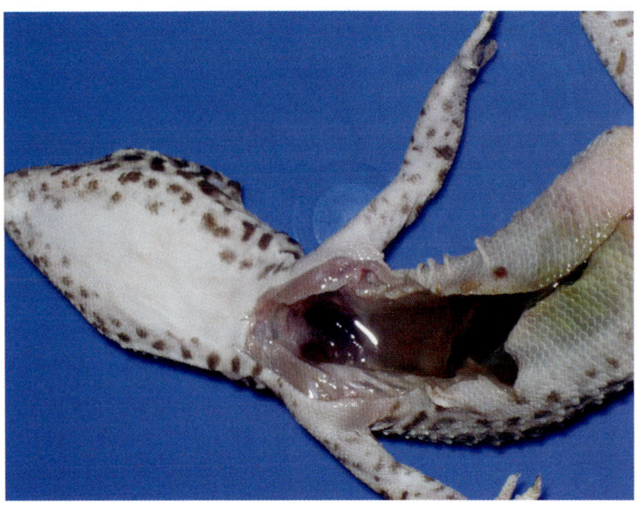

Figure 24.2 Underlying cardiac disease may be severe, including those affected by long-term malnutrition leading to hypoproteinaemia which can then lead to significant pericardial effusions making reversal of cardiac arrest difficult.

D for drugs

See Table 24.1 for a list of commonly used 'emergency' drugs in reptiles. Whilst not typically considered as emergency drugs, antimicrobials are often included as most sick reptiles are borderline or fully septicaemic. They tend to be attacked by their own gut bacteria, which are generally Gram-negative in nature and often comprise *Salmonella* and *Pseudomonas* spp. bacteria. Therefore, a bacteriocidal antibiotic with good action against Gram-negative bacteria should be used. These include the fluoroquinolones and third-generation cephalosporins. However, other injuries may be sustained, such as dog attacks, and so anaerobic bacteria may also be implanted into wounds (see Figure 24.3).

Garter and water snakes, which are fed saltwater fish that has been previously frozen, may suffer from a relative deficiency of vitamin B_1 (thiamine), which can lead to a neurological condition manifesting as an inability to right itself and continual star gazing. Injections of vitamin B_1 25–35 mg/kg may be effective if administered quickly, and sedation with midazolam/diazepam or anaesthesia may be necessary to prevent seizuring.

Table 24.1 Commonly used emergency and recovery medications for reptiles.

Drug	Dosage	Notes
Adrenaline	0.5–1 mg/kg IV/IC/IT/IO	Used where no cardiac output detected or where fine ventricular fibrillation is detected by ECG to convert to coarse ventricular fibrillation to improve success of cardiac massage. Can be used intratracheally after intubation and IPPV with 100% oxygen
Allopurinol	10–50 mg/kg PO every 24 hours	Reduces uric acid production to aid management of gout
Atropine	0.01–0.5 mg/kg IM/IV/IT/ICo/IO	Counteracts early heart block and increases heart rate (Hernandez *et al.*, 2011 used 0.2 mg/kg). Used for organophosphate poisoning and to reduce excessive respiratory secretions. Wide ranges published with higher doses being used in emergency situations and via non-vascular routes
Calcium EDTA	10–40 mg/kg IM every 12 hours	Heavy metal (e.g. lead) poisoning. Ensure well hydrated
Calcium gluconate	100 mg/kg IM/SC/ICo	Hypocalcaemic tetany especially in female egg-bound green iguanas
Ceftazidime	20–40 mg/kg SC/IM/IV every 72 hours	Broad-spectrum bacteriocidal third-generation cephalosporin; particularly effective against Gram-negative bacteria
Diazepam	0.2–0.5 mg/kg IM/IV	Anticonvulsant. Muscle necrosis if given IM
Doxapram	5–10 mg/kg PO/IM/IV	Respiratory stimulant. Intubate and use IPPV
Enrofloxacin	5–10 mg/kg every 24 hours	Useful against Gram-negative bacteria but not against anaerobes. Can cause muscle necrosis at injection site. May cause painful reaction response particularly in chelonians after injection
Furosemide	1–5 mg/kg PO/IM/IV	Diuretic often used in cardiovascular disease
Hydrochlorothiazide	1 mg/kg PO/IM every 24–72 hours	Diuretic
Midazolam	0.5–2 mg/kg IM/IV	Anticonvulsant. Less likely to cause muscle necrosis than diazepam
Meloxicam	0.1–0.5 mg/kg IM/PO once every 24 hours	Analgesic anti-inflammatory. Beware use if already has renal damage
Naloxone	0.04–2 mg/kg SC/IM	Reversal of respiratory depression associated with previous administration of potent opiates such as morphine or fentanyl
Oxytocin	Chelonians 10 IU/kg IM Lizards 5–20 IU/kg IM Snakes 20–40 IU/kg IM	Uterine muscle stimulant to encourage egg-laying where a non-obstructive dystocia has been diagnosed. May be repeated on maximum of four occasions. Important to ensure calcium blood levels are within normal bounds or to administer calcium gluconate first. In chelonia the use of atenolol 7 mg/kg PO with calcium gluconate 100 mg/kg IM followed by oxytocin 1–3 IU IM 6–12 hours later may be helpful in conjunction with adequate hydration and provision of a nest site
Silver sulfadiazine	Topical product on burns/wounds	Effective against many Gram-negative bacteria and some fungi
Vitamin B_1	25–35 mg/kg IM/PO/SC	Thiamine deficiency (fish-eating snakes)

PO, per os; SC, subcutaneously; IM, intramuscularly; IV, intravenously; IC, intracardiac; IT, intratracheally; IO, intraosseously; ICo, intracoelomically.

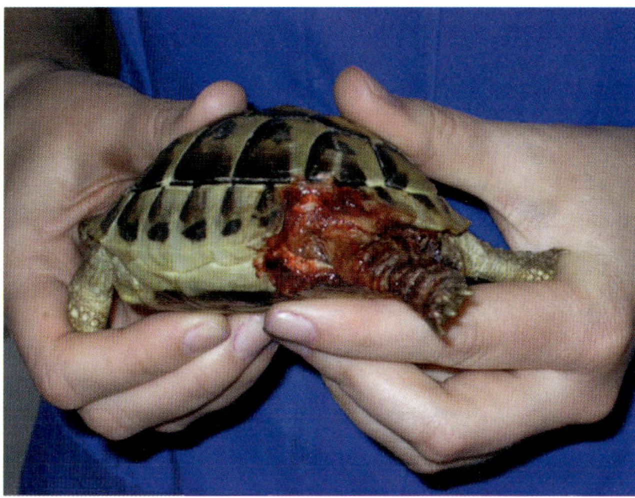

Figure 24.3 Dog-attack wounds in terrestrial chelonians are common and may result in serious trauma and infections.

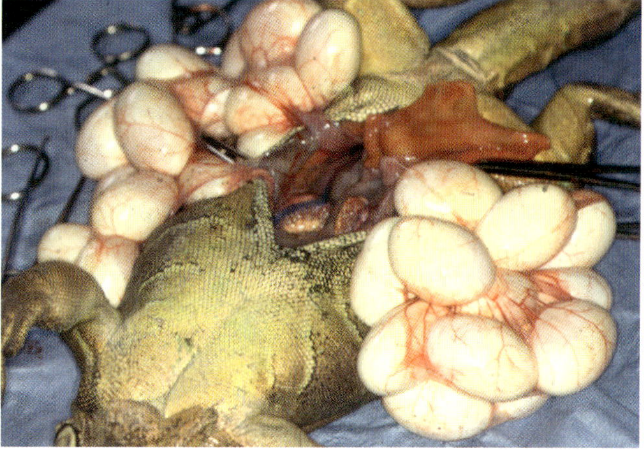

Figure 24.5 Post-ovulatory stasis can become an emergency as it is often associated with hypocalcaemia that may result in collapse and neurological disease including seizuring.

Cardiovascular and respiratory diseases are relatively common, and pneumonia or lung oedema may result. Use of diuretics such as furosemide and hydrochlorothiazide may be helpful in the short term and many will require antimicrobial therapy (see Figure 24.4). Oxygen therapy can be used, but care should be taken as the impetus for breathing in reptiles is a lowered PaO_2 rather than an elevated $PaCO_2$ as in mammals, therefore providing 100% oxygen for even short periods of time can stop breathing altogether. As reptiles do not have a cough reflex (no diaphragm) and are relatively easy to intubate, conscious intubation of collapsed reptiles can be performed and IPPV administered for a short period.

If cardiac arrest occurs, intubation and administration of adrenaline should be attempted. Reptiles can cope with a degree of hypoxia beyond that tolerated by mammals. IPPV after intubation is essential, although chest massage in the case of lizards and moving limbs into and out of the shell in chelonians may also be successful in aiding the pumping of air into and out of the lungs. Snakes offer the option of easier intracardiac administration of adrenaline and the heart can also be more easily massaged. However, snakes often present with pericardial effusions and significant myocardial damage prior to cardiac arrest and so carry a poor prognosis. Tapping the pericardial effusion to reduce the compression on the heart would also be helpful and requires ultrasound-guided fine needle aspiration.

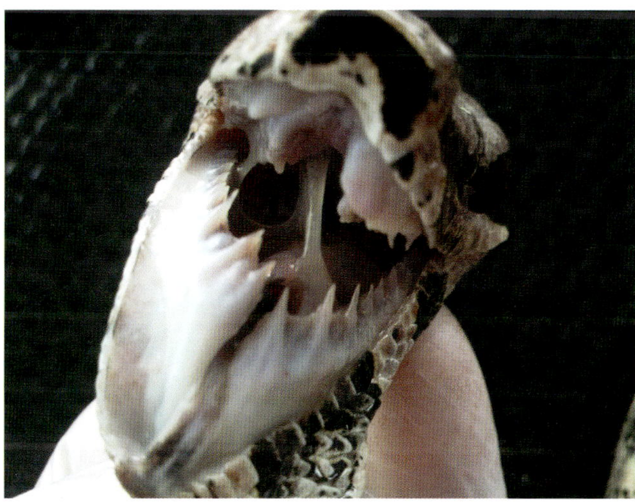

Figure 24.4 Severe respiratory infections may go unnoticed until the final stages of disease and so significant build-up of respiratory fluids may completely block the airways and can be seen in the oral cavity flowing from the glottis as in this snake.

Many nutritional and husbandry diseases are common in reptiles, including metabolic bone disease and hypocalcaemic tetany in egg-bound mature lizards such as the green iguana (see Figure 24.5). Calcium gluconate 100 mg/kg may be administered in an emergency. Some of these lizards may seizure, and diazepam or midazolam may be administered (see Table 24.1). Salpingitis may result in adherence of the eggs to the reproductive tract lining, which can then precipitate significant prolapses that can become an emergency (see Figure 24.6).

E for ECG

ECG deflections are generally small and rates, of course, slow. The rate is dependent on the external temperature at which the reptile is kept.

In snakes, lizards and chelonians, it is preferable to use sticky pads as used in human and domestic veterinary medicine to connect the

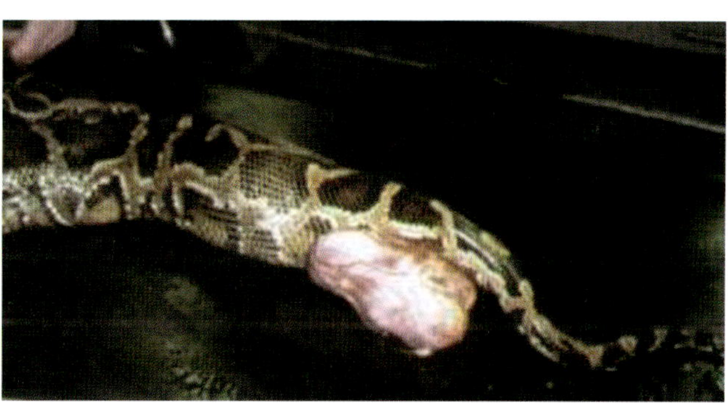

Figure 24.6 Reproductive tract infections can result in post-ovulatory stasis due to the eggs becoming fused to the reproductive tract lining and this can result in significant prolapses of the oviduct as in this python.

electrodes to the skin surface rather than alligator clips which are traumatic.

- Snakes: a base-apex reading is taken with electrodes placed two heart lengths cranial and caudal to the heart on the lateral aspect.
- Lizards such as iguanids and agamids where the heart is in the pectoral girdle: cranial leads are placed on the skin of the axilla, forelimb or neck, caudal leads on the crural or popliteal fold.
- Lizards such as monitors where the heart is at the caudal end of the sternum: cranial leads are placed on the forelimbs in the humeral region and caudal leads on the thighs.
- Chelonians: cranial leads are placed on the cervical or axillary skin folds and caudal leads on the skin fold caudal to the hindlimb.

Reptile ECGs demonstrate a P wave, QRS complex and T wave pattern familiar to cardiologists. An additional SV waveform preceding the P wave that represents depolarisation of the sinus venosus has been described but is rarely seen.

Normal ECG findings include pleomorphism of the P wave, which may be single, peaked or biphasic. The QRS complex is often represented as a single R wave. Long repolarisation phases (longer QT and ST intervals) are present.

Allometric scaling may be used for the prediction of heart rate (HR) assuming the reptile is maintained at its optimal body temperature as follows (Sedgwick, 1991):

$$HR = 33.4 \times (\text{weight } [\text{kg}])^{-0.25}$$

Monitoring and vital sign assessment

Puls-e assessment

This is best performed using a Doppler ultrasound probe. It should be attached to the skin with a generous amount of coupling gel. The main site of attachment is around the outflow of the heart. This is located immediately caudal to the neck inlet in chelonians; around the mid-point of the first third of a snake, ventrally (measured from the snout); or just in front of the point of the shoulder in most lizards (monitor lizards, the caudal end of the sternum).

Cardiac and respiratory auscultation

It is difficult to auscultate reptiles owing to their scaly skin. To aid the passage of sound, wrapping the reptile in a damp cloth first and applying the diaphragm of the stethoscope to the outside of the towel can improve sound transference. Alternatively, a Doppler probe applied over the heart (base of the neck in most lizards and chelonians and 20–30% of the snout–vent length in snakes) can provide an assessment of blood flow that can give an indication of the intensity of flow and turbulence.

The lungs of snakes are particularly challenging to auscultate due to their long extended nature. Chelonian lungs are situated in the dorsal aspect of the carapace, and lizard lungs are encased in the ribcage.

It is not possible to auscultate the heart in the same way as a bird's or mammal's heart due to the slow rate at which it beats and the fact that the heart is three-chambered (there is only one ventricle). Therefore, Doppler probes should be used to gain an idea of cardiac output, strength and any variations in flow.

Neurological assessment

This can be very difficult in reptiles, particularly if they are not within their preferred optimum temperature zone as they will be sluggish and lethargic if too cold. All critically ill reptiles should be gradually warmed to their preferred body temperature to assess them fully and to support their normal physiological functions.

One of the commonest neurological problems is loss of the righting reflex in snakes, so that they continually flip onto their backs. This may be associated with the following conditions.

1. Vitamin B_1 deficiency (garter/water snakes who are fed defrosted frozen fish as this contains large amounts of thiaminases).
2. Permethrin/organophosphate toxicity (overzealous owners treating their snakes for mites).
3. Meningoencephalitis (usually associated with *Acanthamoeba invadens* or Gram-negative bacteria).
4. Inclusion body disease (a retrovirus, particularly prevalent in pythons and boas).

Blindness and head tilts may be seen in tortoises associated with frost damage.

Hypocalcaemic tremors are common in female iguanas on low-calcium diets or where no UV light has been provided.

Panniculus reflexes can be tested as for cats and dogs in snakes and lizards, although of course with less success in chelonians.

Pulse oximetry

This is not so useful in reptiles as reptile haemoglobin is significantly different to that of a mammalian. However, trends of readings are of some help as with birds. The clips/probes may be applied to the vent, tongue (if anaesthetised) or, in thin-skinned smaller reptiles, the extremities.

Blood biochemistry

It should be noted that, as with birds, uric acid is the only useful indicator of renal function, although usually less than one-quarter of the kidneys need to be functioning before uric acid levels become elevated. Urea and creatinine levels do not provide information on renal function in reptiles.

As with birds, no one parameter is specific for liver damage, although aspartate aminotransferase (AST) is more useful than alanine aminotransferase (ALT).

A very rough guide to average plasma biochemistry values is provided in Table 24.2.

Haematology

All blood samples in reptiles should be collected in heparin as potassium EDTA lyses the red cells of many reptiles.

As with biochemistry, values vary between species. Some indication of packed cell volume (PCV) across reptile species has been given in Chapter 17. In general, white cell counts are in the range of $2–8 \times 10^9$/L. During an infection, there is often no change in the overall white cell count and therefore creating a blood smear is a vitally important diagnostic technique.

The reptile equivalent of the neutrophil, as in birds, is the heterophil.

Erythrocytes and platelets in reptiles are nucleated. The erythrocytes are rugby ball-shaped with a similar-shaped nucleus. The platelets are

Table 24.2 Broad range plasma biochemistry values for reptiles.

Parameter	Value	Notes
Total protein (g/L)	44–65	
Albumin (g/L)	13–30	
AST (IU/L)	20–80	Liver leakage enzyme, but not liver specific as it is also found in muscle
Creatine kinase (IU/L)	400–600	Only found in muscle so can be used to determine if elevations in AST are associated with liver damage
Lactate dehydrogenase (IU/L)	200–350	Not liver specific, also found in muscle including cardiac muscle
Calcium (total) (mmol/L)	2–3	May be elevated in female reptiles around egg production
Calcium (ionised) (mmol/L)	1–1.6	Biologically active form of calcium and so preferred over total calcium measurement
Phosphorus (mmol/L)	1–1.85	Calcium to phosphorus ratios can be calculated to help assess renal disease as phosphorus levels will generally increase the worse the renal damage. In the green iguana, for example, the ratio of calcium to phosphorus should be in excess of 0.77
Glucose (mmol/L)	3–12.5	Levels tend to be lower than birds or mammals. Normal low glucose levels may be seen in species undergoing hibernation
Uric acid (μmol/L)	150–350	Gout (precipitation of uric acid) occurs when levels exceed 1500 μmol/L. May be transiently elevated in reptiles immediately after a meal, particularly carnivores such as snakes and this may last for several days in larger species consuming larger prey items that take longer to digest

oval and smaller. Other cells are similar to those seen in mammals except occasionally a circulating plasma cell (type of lymphocyte which produces antibodies) may be seen, particularly in the face of a chronic infection. Also, in snakes, large numbers of so-called 'azurophils' (darkly basophilic staining monocytic cells) may indicate chronic infection.

Urinalysis

This is less useful than for mammals owing to the faecal contamination which occurs with reptile urine. However, it is important to look at the urates (white portion of the dropping) to see if there is any blood, or if the urates have turned mustard yellow or lime green. If the latter has occurred, this is evidence of biliverdinuria, which in reptiles as in birds is an indicator of liver inflammation/damage. Biliverdin is the main excretory product of the liver as opposed to bilirubin in mammals.

Volumes of water/true urine should be small in a healthy reptile's droppings. If they are very watery, as opposed to diarrhoea, then this may indicate polyuria. Specific gravity of reptile urine is around 1.005–1.010.

Monitoring and treatment of acute hypovolaemia

Monitoring of central venous and arterial pressure in reptiles is technically difficult. Non-invasive blood pressure monitoring is also poorly understood in reptiles, and some evidence suggests discrepancies between invasive and non-invasive methods. Part of the problem is that reptiles are ectothermic, and this means the environmental temperature has significant effects on systemic blood pressure.

A study in green iguanas has indicated that mean systolic blood pressure is 43 mmHg and mean diastolic blood pressure is 29 mmHg (Mosley *et al.*, 2004). Another study in green iguanas ($N = 6$) has suggested that mean arterial blood pressure is around 51 ± 2 mmHg (Hernandez *et al.*, 2011). In snakes there appears to be a relationship between the size of the snake and its blood pressure: the larger the snake, the higher the blood pressure (Mosley, 2005). Drugs such as ketamine are likely to increase blood pressure and one study in grey rat snakes has demonstrated a doubling, raising the mean arterial pressure from 46.6 ± 15.8 mmHg to 83.8 ± 16.2 mmHg (Schumacher *et al.*, 1997).

Non-invasive methods can be applied as follows: in chelonians and lizards, a cuff may be placed at the most proximal point on the forelimb and the Doppler probe applied above the carpus on the ventral aspect to cover the brachial artery. The cuff is inflated as with mammals to occlude blood flow and then deflated until flow occurs which is the maximum systolic pressure. In snakes the cuff is applied just caudal to the cloaca, and the probe is applied to the ventral tail artery distal to this. Various studies have suggested that indirect systolic pressure varies from 30 to 63 mmHg (Martinez-Jimenez and Hernandez-Divers, 2007).

Reptiles can survive significant haemorrhage because of the rapid shift of interstitial fluids into the circulation. However, this does not remove the need to replace fluid or blood losses to stabilise blood pressure. The amounts required can be assessed using blood pressure and heart rate. Expected heart rates can be calculated as described in the section on ECGs above. However, it is important that reptiles are maintained at their preferred body temperature to accurately assess this due to their ectothermic nature. Bolus administration of fluids should be attempted intravenously or intraosseously until correction of blood pressure. Crystalloids are administered at a rate of 10 mL/kg and colloids at 5 mL/kg – usually one or two boluses are required. In larger species, 5 mL/kg of 7.5% hypertonic saline may be used once or twice to increase systolic blood pressure.

Calculation of fluid requirements for reptiles

Please see Chapter 22 for fluid therapy and blood transfusions in reptiles.

Supportive therapy

Ongoing medication

Some antibiotics effective against Gram-negative bacteria include the third-generation cephalosporins, third-generation penicillins, aminoglycosides and fluoroquinolones. It is important to note that many reptiles will need to be on antibiotics for considerable periods of time (months rather than weeks) due to their often advanced state of infection – once finally seen – and their slower metabolism.

Ongoing fluid therapy is also very important whether it be regular warm water baths in mildly dehydrated individuals, or intravenous/intraosseous fluids in the severely dehydrated ones as kidney failure is common.

Analgesia is also vitally important where there are serious injuries.

Critical care nutrition including calculation of energy requirements

Calculation of energy requirements can be made using the formula:

$$\text{SMR} = k \times \left(\text{weight}\left[\text{kg}\right]\right)^{0.75}$$

where SMR is standard metabolic rate and k the constant has been crudely assumed to be 10 for reptiles; however, see Table 20.1 in Chapter 20 for some more species-specific equations for SMR.

Remember that field maintenance requirement (FMR), equivalent to maintenance energy requirement (MER) for mammals and birds, is generally 1.5–2 times the SMR and if disease is present then this further amplifies the required calories (sepsis and burns for example may increase FMR by two to three times again). See Chapter 20 for more information on energy requirements for reptiles.

Nebulisation

Achieving therapeutic levels of any antibiotic in infected reptile lungs is difficult. The blood–air barrier is thicker in reptiles than in mammals, plus reptiles have a poorly developed or absent cough reflex. Add to this, the fact that caseous, impenetrable, purulent discharges are common and that many of the most effective antibiotics such as aminoglycosides are potentially toxic if given in effective doses systemically, it can be seen that a topical respiratory method such as nebulisation of a drug is attractive. Although the possibility exists that a significant proportion of the drug could be absorbed across an inflamed respiratory epithelium, signs of, for example, aminoglycoside-related nephrotoxicity are not seen following aerosolised administration of these drugs. Other drugs suitable for nebulisation include antiseptic disinfectants (F10, Health and Hygiene Ltd.), soluble steroids in inflammatory conditions, bronchodilators and agents aimed at reducing the viscosity of respiratory secretions.

Assisted feeding techniques and foods

For information on oesophagostomy tube placement, see Chapter 22. For initial emergency nutrition, as with birds, the use of commercial reptile-designed critical care products are useful and should be appropriate to the species trophic group (herbivore, omnivore, carnivore).

Anorexia in snakes may be associated with an emergency critical care situation but can also be associated with changes in husbandry and routine and in some species such as ball pythons (*Python regius*) can commonly be linked to over-handling. To encourage non-emergency but anorectic snakes to eat, a number of tricks may be employed including the following.

1. Warm the prey before offering by heating it in a pot of hot water.
2. Break the prey item open to release the scent of blood.
3. Tease the snake by moving the dead prey item around the cage with forceps, to mimic live prey.
4. Try a variety of colours of prey; some snakes will only take dark furred rodents.
5. To get a snake used to eating rodent prey after only eating fish (e.g. garter and water snakes) or amphibians (hog-nosed snakes), wipe the rodent to be offered with the previously taken food item to transfer scent.
6. Ensure that there are plenty of areas to hide; some boids and pythons like to consume their prey in a box/ hide.
7. Leave the prey in overnight, as some species prefer to hunt at night.
8. Feed the next smallest size of rodent, so if adult mice were previously offered, try fuzzies; if juvenile rats, try adult mice, etc.

The term 'pinkies' refers to nude neonatal rat and mice pups, 'fuzzies' refers to week-old rat and mice pups with a thin covering of fur, and 'furries' refers to juvenile rat and mice pups of 1–3 weeks of age which have a soft but longer covering of fur.

If the reptile will not eat, then most species of snakes and chelonians may be stomach tubed relatively easily if they do not want to feed of their own accord.

In snakes, a dog urinary catheter is used and inserted to approximately the caudal end of the first third of the snake (roughly where the stomach lies). The volume given depends on the size of the snake, with a 100-g garter snake receiving a maximum of 4–5 mL and a 30-kg Burmese python up to 100–200 mL.

Tortoises can be stomach tubed by measuring from the extended tip of the head to the caudal edge of the large abdominal scutes on the plastron. Most tortoises of 2–3 kg may be stomach tubed with 10–15 mL of feed at one time (see Figure 24.7).

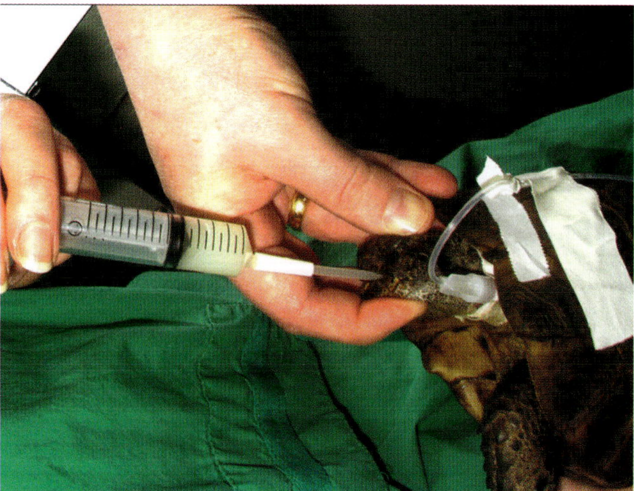

Figure 24.7 Nutritional support is essential for recovery of the debilitated reptile and may include initially the administration of liquid formulas via stomach tubing.

Lizards may be gavaged liquid feed as for mammals, or again tubed. It is important to use a mouth gag when tubing reptiles to prevent the tube being bitten in half.

In all cases, feeding a reptile by stomach tube should be the final intervention before putting it back into its vivarium, otherwise the reptile will become distressed and regurgitate its feed.

Refeeding syndrome

It is very important to ensure that in snakes in particular, the patient is rehydrated before feeding high-protein meals. This is because of the refeeding syndrome, which can be defined briefly as follows: if anorexia in a snake or other reptile has persisted for some time, it is essential to rehydrate the patient before attempting to feed. Initial feeding after this should be started off at very low levels: 50% of the requirement for the current weight of the reptile. Otherwise, excess calories and proteins cause a rapid uptake of glucose from the bloodstream into the cells, and this takes potassium and phosphorus with it. This can lead to a life-threatening hypokalaemia/hypophosphataemia. The monitoring of blood phosphorus and potassium levels is therefore to be recommended when treating chronically anorectic reptiles whether carnivorous or herbivorous.

Nursing of wounds

Open wounds are generally of two main types in reptiles: thermal burns and infections. It is important therefore to ensure correct antibiotic coverage for these wounds. As most reptile infections are due to Gram-negative bacteria, it makes sense to use fluoroquinolones and third-generation cephalosporins.

Povidone-iodine diluted to 0.05% with water may be used to clean infected wounds. Topical medications such as silver sulfadiazine creams have good efficacy against Gram-negative bacteria as does the use of topical eye drops containing gentamicin, ofloxacin or chloramphenicol. Where an infected wound is present, daily changing of any dressings is advised.

Dressings which may be sutured to the skin around large wound deficits include Granuflex®, Melolin® and Veterinary BioSISt®. The former should be used where the infection is under control and is excellent for encouraging granulation tissue to form. In many cases this primary dressing is all that is required, particularly when sutured to the patient as reptiles rarely remove dressings, the problem being, especially in snakes, that dressings are difficult to attach in the first place unless sutured.

Aqueous gels may be used to cover the surface of wounds and promote further healing.

References

Hernandez, S.M., Schumacher, J., Lewis, S.J. *et al.* (2011) Selected cardiopulmonary values and baroreceptor reflex in conscious green iguanas (*Iguana iguana*). *American Journal of Veterinary Research*, **72**(11), 1519–1526.

Martinez-Jimenez, D. and Hernandez-Divers, S.J. (2007) Emergency care of reptiles. *Veterinary Clinics of North America: Exotic Animal Practice*, **10**(2), 557–586.

Mosley, C. (2005) Anaesthesia and analgesia in reptiles. *Seminars in Avian and Exotic Pet Medicine*, **14**, 243–262.

Mosley, C., Dyson, D. and Smith, D. (2004) The cardiovascular dose-responsive effects of isoflurane alone and combined with butorphanol in the green iguana (*Iguana iguana*). *Veterinary Anaesthesia and Analgesia*, **31**, 64–72.

Schumacher, J., Lillywhite, H.B. and Norman, W.M. (1997) Effects of ketamine HCl on cardiopulmonary function in snakes. *Copeia*, **2**, 395–400.

Sedgwick, C.J. (1991) Allometrically scaling the database for vital sign assessment used in general anesthesia of zoological species. *Proceedings of the American Association of Zoo Veterinarians*, pp. 360–369.

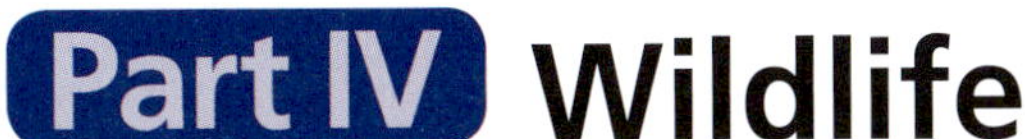

Wildlife

Chapter 25 Common Mammalian Wildlife Species Biology, Anatomy and Physiology

Classification

Wildlife species considered here will largely focus on northern European species, most of which but not all are found in the UK. Because of the shortage of space and to avoid duplication with some of the previous chapters on rodents, birds, reptiles and amphibians, the focus in this chapter will be on specific mammal species.

Mammalian species considered here fall into the following broad classification groups.

1. Artiodactyls (even-toed ungulates), including:
   a. Bovidae such as European bison, mouflon
   b. Cervidae such as muntjac, roe, red, sika, fallow and Chinese water deer
   c. Suidae such as wild boar
2. Carnivora, including:
   a. Canidae such as foxes, jackals and wolves
   b. Felidae such as wildcats and lynx
   c. Mustelidae such as badgers, weasels, stoats, martens and otters
   d. Phocidae such as harbour/common and grey seals
3. Chiroptera, including bats such as pipistrelle, Daubenton's, horseshoe
4. Eulipotyphla (previously known as Insectivora), including:
   a. European hedgehog
   b. European mole
   c. Shrews
5. Lagomorpha, including rabbits and hares
6. Rodentia, including:
   a. Castorimorpha that contains beavers
   b. Myomorpha that contains
      i. Cricetidae such as voles and hamsters
      ii. Muridae such as rats and mice
   c. Sciuromorpha such as red and grey squirrels

Wild avian species commonly seen in the UK in wildlife rehabilitation centres and veterinary practices include many of the following.

1. Accipitriformes: including hawks, eagles, kites and Old World vultures
2. Anseriformes: including swans, geese and ducks
3. Charadriiformes: including gulls, waders and auks
4. Columbiformes: including pigeons and doves
5. Falconiformes: including falcon species
6. Galliformes: including pheasants, partridges, quail and grouse
7. Passeriformes: include, but are not restricted to:
   a. Alaudidae: Larks such as the skylark
   b. Corvidae: Crows, rooks, magpies and jays
   c. Fringillidae: Finches such as chaffinches and greenfinches
   d. Hirudinidae: Martins and swallows
   e. Paridae: Tits such as blue tits and great tits
   f. Passeridae: Old World sparrows
   g. Sturnidae: Starlings
   h. Troglodytidae: Wrens
   i. Turdidae: Thrushes
8. Pelecaniformes: including herons such as the grey heron
9. Strigiformes: all owl species (such as barn, great grey, tawny, snowy, eagle owls, etc.)

Wild reptile and amphibian species commonly seen in the UK in wildlife rehabilitation centres and veterinary practices include many of the following.

1. Anura: including the frog and toad families
2. Caudata: including the salamanders and newts
3. Squamata: including
   a. Lacertilia: the lizards such as the slow worm, common (viviparous) and sand (green) lizards
   b. Serpentes: the snakes such as the European adder, smooth and grass snakes
4. Testudines (Chelonia): including shelled reptiles such as red-eared terrapins which are considered an invasive species in the UK and European Union and are commonly found in the wild, particularly in the southern UK.

ARTIODACTYLS

We will not consider the Bovidae here as wild members of this family are rare in the UK and most of Europe and even more rarely presented to wildlife veterinary practices for treatment. Suidae will also not be considered here as they are non-native to the UK and as such any release of injured suids is prohibited.

Cervidae (deer)

Distribution

Chinese water deer (Hydropotes inermis): This species prefers dense woodland, often close to water courses. It is native to China and Korea but is now found in the UK (predominantly in the southern counties of England), Ireland, the USA and parts of western Europe. It is unusual among cervids in that the male does not have antlers but rather prominent tusks, particularly in the maxilla, which project ventrally well below the jawline and are used in fighting, inflicting serious lacerations on other deer, potential predators and, if not careful, human handlers.

Fallow deer (Dama dama): This species prefers deciduous woodland but may be seen in open countryside with areas of broken forest. It is found all over Europe in lowland situations. It has also been

Veterinary Nursing of Exotic Pets and Wildlife, Third Edition. Simon J. Girling.

introduced into New Zealand, the USA, North Africa, the Caribbean and South America.

Red deer (Cervus elaphus): The largest deer species in the UK and despite Landseer's painting *The Monarch of the Glen* and the popular image of this species as a Scottish Highland deer, red deer generally prefer open woodland and broken lowland countryside. They are found extensively throughout Europe, northern and western Africa, Asia Minor and parts of Asia. They have also been introduced into New Zealand, the USA, Canada and parts of South America.

Reeve's muntjac deer (Muntiacus reevesi): This species prefers dense deciduous or coniferous woodland. In the UK it is found mainly in the south where it has been introduced but individuals have been seen as far north as Northumberland. It has also been introduced to Ireland and northern Europe. Its native habitat is southwestern China and Taiwan. It is related to the common or Indian muntjac (*Muntiacus muntjak*) and a further 10 species of the genus *Muntiacus*.

Roe deer (Capreolus capreolus): This common UK species prefers open deciduous or coniferous woodland, but is found in open moorland situations as well. It is found all over Europe and western Asia.

Sika deer (Cervus nippon): This species was introduced to the UK and prefers the fringes of dense deciduous or coniferous woodlands. It is found throughout UK, Europe and eastern USA. It was originally native to Japan and the Far East.

Anatomy and biology

Musculoskeletal system

Cervids considered here vary in size from the largest, the red deer, an adult male of which may reach just over 1.5 m at the shoulder and weigh 200–240 kg to the Chinese water deer which may measure only 0.46–0.6 m at the shoulder and weigh 9–12 kg. In terms of size and weight, the descending order is red deer (120–240 kg), fallow deer (60–100 kg), sika deer (25–90 kg), roe deer (18–28 kg), Reeve's muntjac deer (9–18 kg) and Chinese water deer.

Cervids are digitigrade, that is they all walk on the tips of the digits.

The head is elongated and narrow, but in the male the frontal sinuses and their bony walls which cover the crown and caudal part of the muzzle may be extensive, giving strength to the skull when sparring and as a resonance chamber. The red, fallow and sika deer male will develop extensive neck muscles to support the head and often significant antler production during the rut.

Digestive system

The permanent dentition in each half of the mouth in red deer, sika deer, Chinese water deer and Reeve's muntjac deer is as follows (where I is incisor, C canine, Pm premolar and M molar, and the numbers represent in order: right side maxilla/right side mandible):

I0 / 3C1 / 1Pm3 / 3M3 / 3

The permanent dentition of fallow deer and roe deer is as follows:

I0 / 3C0 / 1Pm3 / 3M3 / 3

Many deer often do not have visible canines in the mouth, as these can be hidden below the gum margin, particularly in females. In male Chinese water deer, though, the maxillary canine is highly developed to form a tusk which may be seen projecting below the lower jawline, and is used when fighting other males. The male Reeve's muntjac deer also has a long maxillary canine which may just protrude below the upper lip margin and is again razor sharp and is a hazard when handling either species (see Figure 25.1). The premolars and molars form an arcade of teeth, all closely packed together, as is seen in other herbivores such as the domestic horse, cow and rabbit. For this reason, the premolars and molars are often referred to collectively as the 'cheek teeth'.

The rostral opening of the mouth is relatively small, making visualisation of the oral cavity and intubation difficult.

The deer has a ruminant digestive system and so has four stomachs, the first of which is the reticulum, followed by the rumen, the omasum and the abomasum. Of these four stomachs, only the last, the abomasum, functions as a true acidic glandular stomach. The other three act as fermenting chambers where the plant material consumed is broken down by microorganisms which colonise this area. The smallest of the four stomachs is the reticulum into which the oesophagus empties. The food then moves into the rumen, which is the largest of the four chambers and situated on the left side of the cranial abdomen, although it reaches caudally to around the point of the ilium of the pelvis (see Figure 25.2). Here the majority of microbial fermentation occurs. The rumen contracts and churns the food, mixing it. Part-chewed food can then be regurgitated up the oesophagus into the oral cavity and rechewed as a 'cud' to help break it down further. The food particles when sufficiently small are passed from the rumen into the omasum, which is filled with fine leaf-like folds. Further bacterial breakdown of fibre occurs here and then the food particles move on into the glandular acidic environment of the abomasum. From here the rest of the digestive system is similar to many other mammals, with a moderately long small intestine, starting with the duodenum moving into the jejunum and then ileum, followed by the large intestine.

The liver is a flattened structure lying between the rumen/abomasum and diaphragm on the right-hand side and possesses a gall bladder. A spleen exists as a strap-like organ along the greater curvature/left-hand side of the abomasum.

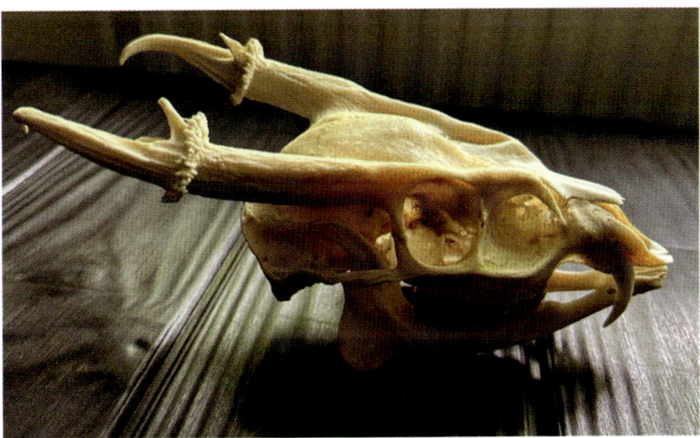

Figure 25.1 Skull of a male muntjac deer. Note the significant maxillary canines and small (but sharp) antlers.

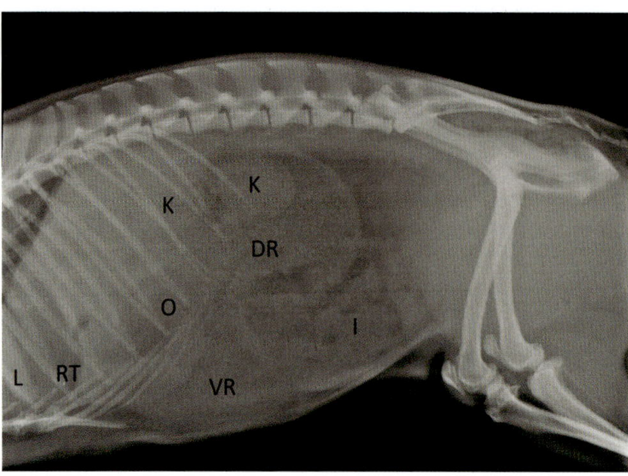

Figure 25.2 Right lateral radiograph of a deer showing the significant extent of the forestomachs. Note that the abomasum is not clearly visible in this image as it lies behind the omasum and ventral rumen. K, kidneys; DR, dorsal rumen; VR, ventral rumen; O, omasum; RT, reticulum; L, liver; I, intestines.

Skin and associated structures

Antlers: Antlers are one of the most significant features of cervids. Many of the species here (red, fallow, roe, sika for example) will develop antlers only in the male, just before the rut (breeding season). The Chinese water deer does not possess antlers in either sex. The female Reeve's muntjac deer does possess a couple of bony protrusions in the area where the male would develop antlers. These are accentuated by tufts of fur. Antler size varies according to age of the stag, and species. Red deer can have some of the most impressive antlers which may be almost a metre long on each side with 10–15 tines (the side spurs of the antlers) per antler being commonly seen. In sika and roe deer the antlers may be much shorter, only 0.15–0.31 m with two to three tines.

In species such as reindeer, or caribou (*Rangifer* spp.) both males and females can develop antlers although generally at different times of the year (if Rudolf existed then 'he' would have been a 'she' as female reindeer have antlers at Christmas but males have shed them by November/mid-December typically).

The antlers of most northern temperate cervids are produced in midsummer, as a development of the skin itself. This is different to the situation in cattle and sheep and other Bovidae, where the horns are extensions of the bone of the skull and therefore a permanent year-round feature that grows with age. Antlers do contain bone but it is produced by the skin growth bud, and therefore antlers may be shed without damaging the skull. It also means that when the antlers are initially produced, they are covered with skin (known as the 'velvet') and therefore blood vessels, nerves and other structures that one would expect to find in the skin (see Figure 25.3). If the antlers are damaged while they are 'in velvet' then they will bleed copiously. Once bone growth underneath the velvet is fully developed, the velvet dies off, as the blood supply retracts to the base of the antler.

The velvet is then shed, a process known as 'cleaning the velvet', leaving just the bare 'bone' of the antler. This occurs just before the rut, typically in the autumn in northern species, allowing the male to use the antlers as an offensive/defensive weapon without any risk of haemorrhage. The antlers are then carried through the winter and into the following spring (with the exception mentioned above in male reindeer), when they are shed, known as 'casting the antlers'. In red deer the age of the male deer has historically been classified according to antler development, as the antlers become more and more impressive with successive years, developing increasing branching and points or 'tines' (see Figure 25.4). This has given rise to some interesting English terminology for ageing deer (particularly red deer). One of many versions for naming deer according to antler development is as follows (Bell, 1839).

1. A deer in its first year is known as a 'calf' and the male has no antlers.
2. A second-year antlered male is known as a 'brocket' and has no antler branching (sometimes also referred to as a 'pricket').
3. A third-year antlered male is known as a 'spayard'.
4. A fourth-year antlered male is known as a 'staggard'.
5. A fifth-year antlered male is known as a 'stag'.
6. A sixth-year antlered male is known as a 'hart'.
7. A seventh-year or older male is known as a 'great hart'.

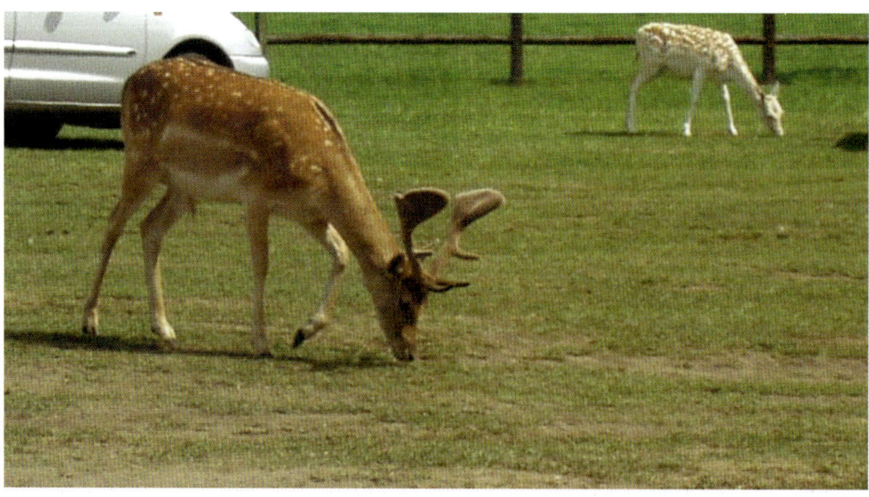

Figure 25.3 Fallow deer stag in 'velvet'. The covering of the growing antler is plentifully supplied with blood vessels and nerves, meaning trauma to this can result in copious bleeding (and can also be painful).

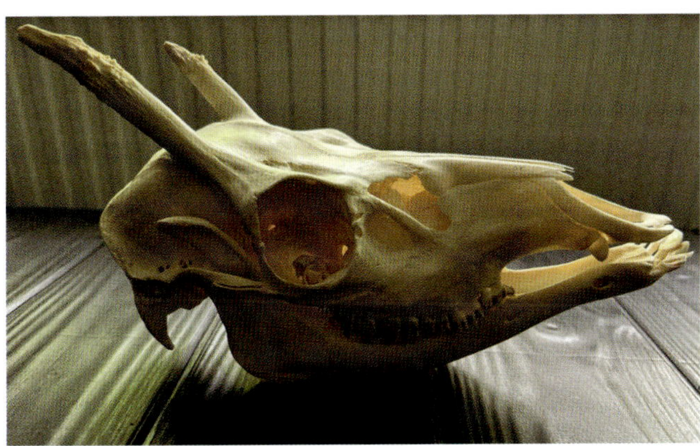

Figure 25.4 Skull of a red deer male showing reduced maxillary canines, cheek teeth and, in this case, unbranching antlers which in a live deer with full antler growth for that year is associated with a second-year male.

In addition, a number of terms have been applied to the number of points or 'tines' seen on the antlers, with the afore-mentioned *Monarch of the Glen* painting by Landseer referring to a red deer male with 16 points or 'tines' per antler.

A mane of fur is often produced just prior to the rut that lasts throughout the winter in some stags, particularly red deer, roe deer and sika males. Fallow deer have the most distinctive coat possessing the characteristic white spots, although there are many variations, with some fallow deer herds in parks being all white in colour.

Skin glands: Many deer have obvious preorbital or lacrimal glands just cranial to the medial canthus of the eye that may ooze secretions particularly during the breeding season. Several deer possess interdigital glands which will sent mark a trackway and some (particularly reindeer) make a clicking noise associated with tendon movement when walking that allow deer to follow in single-file in poor visibility. In addition, there are hock glands and ventral tail glands all used for marking territories and identifying individuals.

Chinese water deer have a pair of inguinal glands, muntjac deer have a 'V'-shaped row of glands across the brow, and sika deer have prominent white metatarsal glands that are located in the region of the hock joint.

Senses

Sight in cervids is a fairly well-adapted sense, although fine detail of vision is perhaps not so good. Colour vision does exist but it is relatively poor. Deer in general respond more to movement, although their laterally situated eyes give a good near-360° field of view, but very little if any binocular vision.

Hearing is an acute sense in deer. They are quick to detect changes in sound and their highly mobile ears can pinpoint a sound source rapidly. Muntjac are often referred to as the 'barking deer' as they will readily vocalise and so communicate with each other but many deer can vocalise.

Smell is well adapted in cervids and they are able to detect the scent of a predator many hundreds of metres away down-wind. Stags also exhibit a condition known as flehmen when excited by a female during the breeding season. This is where pheromones given off by a hind are solubilised into saliva by the male and enter the vomeronasal organ, which sits in the rostral hard palate and is connected directly to the sensory portion of the brain responsible for detecting and interpreting smell. The male curls the upper lip, extends the head and neck and froths saliva at the mouth, drawing more pheromones into this area. A stag may also do this during the rut when displaying against another stag.

Touch is a well-developed sense in cervids as with other mammals and they possess vibrissae. Physical contact between hind and calf reinforces bonding.

Reproductive biology, sexual cycle, reproduction and neonatology

Male cervids are generally referred to as stags, females as hinds and unweaned cervids as fawns.

All hinds have two mammary glands. They have a bicornuate uterus similar to other ruminants and the placenta is referred to as cotyledonary. This means the uterus produces many mushroom-like projections (known as caruncles) from its surface that interlock with cupped projections on the placenta (known as cotyledons). This allows maternal blood flow to come into close contact with placental blood flow.

Stags have scrotally located testes that sit caudally in the inguinal region close to the body. In the seasonally breeding species, these enlarge often significantly during the breeding season.

Chinese water deer

Females pair with one male during the rut that lasts from November to December in Europe. The gestation period is 180–210 days, and the young are therefore born May to July, with one to two offspring born. The fawn is weaned after 2 months, and becomes sexually mature from 6 months of age, although females will not breed until the following season.

The male Chinese water deer has no antlers but will use his impressive tusks. The male is a solitary creature for most of the year, pairing up with a female in winter and sometimes remaining with her throughout the winter and into the spring.

Fallow deer

The fallow deer oestrus cycle is 22–24 days in length, and she is seasonally polyoestrus and a spontaneous ovulator, with the breeding season running from September to late October/early November. Oestrus lasts for around 15 hours and if successfully mated the hind's gestation period is an average of 229 days, with the hind producing one fawn or occasionally two. Hinds become sexually mature at 15–18 months of age, assuming they are healthy. Hinds group together in small numbers of up to five, led by a dominant hind.

The stag becomes sexually mature at around 12 months of age. Antlers start to grow in late June to July, with the velvet being removed in late August and September. The antlers are typically shed in April of the following year. The stags form bachelor groups of up to five individuals during the non-breeding season from February to September. Once into the breeding season, stags start to compete for female harems, and may mark out a territory. A group of these standing grounds where the males will challenge other stags for hinds is known as a 'lek'. Once mating has occurred, stags generally leave the hinds and stop defending a territory.

Red deer

The red deer hind is seasonally polyoestrus and a spontaneous ovulator, with the cycle lasting 18 days on average with true oestrus lasting 12–24 hours. The breeding season for the red deer hind runs from October to February the following year in the northern hemisphere. Gestation length is as for the fallow deer, with generally one fawn born, although occasionally two may be produced. Weaning can be performed at 4–6 months of age. Red deer hinds become sexually mature at 28–40 months of age on average. Hinds form hierarchical groups outside the breeding season with a dominant hind in overall charge

The red deer stag will defend a harem and territory during September to November. Antler development is as for the fallow deer. Stags become sexually mature at 12–18 months of age but are only large enough to manage a harem of hinds when they reach 4–6 years of age. Stags will form bachelor groups that are strongly hierarchical. These will break up during the rut when dominant stags will defend a harem of hinds and their local territory.

Reeve's muntjac deer

Unlike the fallow and red deer hind, the Reeve's muntjac hind is not seasonally polyoestrus; instead in Europe she may mate all year round but is a spontaneous ovulator. The reproductive cycle lasts for 14–21 days with truc oestrus lasting 2 days. Gestation length is around 210 days. Generally, one fawn per gestation is produced. The muntjac hind becomes sexually mature at around 6–12 months of age. The hinds are solitary, as are the stags, but they may pair with one stag for periods of time.

The muntjac stag develops small antlers that appear in July to August with the velvet being cleaned in September to October. They are then shed in May to June.

Roe deer

The roe deer hind is unusual in that she is seasonally monoestrus, having just one heat a year, usually in late July to early August. The gestation period is 273–294 days, but this includes a period of 150 days of delayed implantation, which occurs at the early blastocyst stage of development and makes them somewhat unique among artiodactyls. This means that the young are born from May to June. Twin calves are common. The young are weaned at around 12 weeks of age and stay with the mother until the following breeding season when they reach sexual maturity at around 14 months of age.

The roe deer stag is also unusual in that he defends a territory all year round, the hind defending a separate and often overlapping territory, usually with one or two other hinds and their young.

Sika deer

Sika hinds are seasonally polyoestrus, with the breeding season running from September to October. The oestrus cycle lasts for 21 days, with true heat lasting 12–24 hours. Gestation length is roughly 220 days, with parturition occurring in May and June of the following year, with on average one fawn born. The young are usually weaned at 4–6 months of age with sexual maturity being reached at around 2 years of age. Females group together during the year in small herds of six to eight females led by a senior matriarchal hind.

The sika stag develops a thick dark fur mane during the rut, similar to the red deer stag. The rut starts in October, with stags gathering a harem at this time. During the rest of the year, the sika deer stags form small groups separate from the female groups. Antler development starts in June/July, with the antlers being cleaned in August and September just prior to the rut. The antlers are then shed/cast the following March to April.

Sex identification

The stags of all breeds have scrotally located testes that sit caudally in the inguinal to perineal region that enlarge markedly during the breeding season. In addition, as mentioned above only the males of the current wild UK species have antlers at any time during the year with the exception of the Chinese water deer in which neither sex has antlers but the male has long maxillary canines or tusks. Reindeer or caribou are cervids where both sexes carry antlers but often at slightly different times of year as previously mentioned. Stags are generally 50% larger than the hinds once sexually mature.

Neonatology

The young are referred to as fawns and are born precocial, that is their eyes and ears are open and they can walk and run from soon after birth. When suckling, the milk consumed bypasses the poorly developed rumen via a reticular groove, similar to that in domestic cattle, which is formed due to the suckling action. The groove formation can be difficult to stimulate when stomach tubing fawns during hand rearing, leading to the milk entering the developing rumen where, due to its neutral pH, it is more likely to ferment and result in bacterial overgrowth. Encouraging a sucking reflex prior to stomach tubing is therefore important as this action stimulates closure of the groove. Some have also used copper sulphate (10% solution, 5 mL given orally) which stimulates closure of the groove for a few minutes so allowing any subsequently administered oral liquid to enter the abomasum and bypass the rumen.

CARNIVORA

Canidae: red fox (*Vulpes vulpes*)

For Canidae the red fox will be examined in closer detail as a commonly seen wild representative canid in the UK.

Distribution

Red foxes are one of the most successful wild canids and are found throughout Europe, Asia, North America and North Africa, and have been introduced to Australia; they are often considered a pest species in many of these countries due to their strong predatory habits on domestic poultry. They prefer open countryside, with access to woodland and hedgerows for cover. A fox's den is often made out of previous rabbit warrens or constructed in the wall of a bank or ditch. The urban red fox is a successful scavenger of human food waste, often raiding bins and refuse centres.

Red foxes are crepuscular in nature in the countryside, less so in urban settings. In the daytime they will rest but when active at night they can cover distances up to 8 km. The male red fox is referred to as a dog and the female as a vixen.

Anatomy and biology

Musculoskeletal system

The musculoskeletal system is similar to that of the domestic dog although they generally only have four digits to each hindlimb. The claws do not retract similar to domestic canids.

The skull is elongated (dolicocephalic) in nature. The sagittal crest is prominent particularly in the male and provides strong attachment for the temporal muscles providing the strength of the bite. The male is generally 20–25% larger than the female and weighs around 8–10 kg, with a body length of 0.55–0.8 m with an additional tail length of 0.3–0.5 m.

Digestive system

The adult dental formula of the red fox is as follows:

I3/3C1/1Pm4/4M2/3

The rectal temperature of the red fox is 37.6–38°C (100–102°F).

The stomach is simple and glandular in form. The spleen lies along the greater curvature of the left side of the stomach. The duodenum and jejunum are significant in length with a short ileum. A small caecum exists at the ileocaecal junction. The large intestine is moderately short.

The liver structure is similar to that of the domestic dog. A gall bladder opens into the small intestine along with the pancreatic duct.

Foxes have a prominent set of anal glands that are larger in the male than the female and are used for territory marking.

Skin and associated structures

The pelage of the red fox is, as its name suggests, mainly red-brown coat to the dorsal body surface, with a white to cream chin, bib and ventrum, and white tail tip. There may be some black on the ear tips and muzzle and darker fur during the winter, when a longer and denser coat develops. Red foxes typically moult twice a year, once in the spring and once in the autumn and this is also seen in other northern species of northern hemisphere foxes such as the Arctic fox (*Vulpes lagopus*).

There is a tail gland as is seen in dogs on the dorsal aspect of the tail head and this can become alopecic with age.

Senses

Eyesight is acute with good binocular colour vision, and a well-developed tapetum lucidum behind the retina that increases light transfer to the photoreceptors. The tapetum often appears green in colour in the red fox. Dimmed lighting when holding the species in captivity can therefore help in reducing stress.

Hearing is also acute in foxes and so noise levels should be minimised if holding them in captivity for rehabilitation. They can hear higher frequency sounds than humans similar to other canids. They have large mobile ears that may be used to detect and pinpoint prey.

Sense of smell is well developed in foxes and they avoid new scents. However clearly this can become habituated or lessened in its intensity as many foxes live in close daily contact with humans without any apparent fear.

Significant vibrissae along the snout tip are available for touch receptors that are used for social interaction and potentially detecting prey at close quarters.

Reproductive biology, sexual cycle and reproduction

The reproductive cycle of the red fox vixen is monoestrus in that only one heat generally occurs each year. The breeding season in Europe is generally from January to March; the further north the latitude, the later the season. The oestrus cycle lasts for about 3 weeks, and the true heat lasts for around 3 days when mating can occur.

The gestation period of the red fox averages 52–53 days, with the majority of young being born in March and April. The placentation is similar to the cat and dog being zonary in nature.

The vixen possesses four pairs of mammary glands on average.

Both the vixen and the dog play a part in rearing the young. The dog tends to confine himself to feeding the vixen for the first few weeks after whelping. The red fox is generally monogamous in that one or two vixens will permanently attach themselves to one dog and remain throughout the year in his territory.

The dog red fox testes lie in a well-developed caudally located scrotum. A prostate is present in the dog which is the only accessory sex gland in the fox.

Sex identification

The dog has scrotally located testes in the caudal inguinal area, and a ventrally located prepuce, and is 20–25% larger than the female with a prominent sagittal crest to the skull. The vixen has a perineally located vulva that enlarges noticeably during oestrus and is smaller than the dog fox.

Neonatology

The young fox is known as a cub. Cubs are altricial in nature. They are born blind, deaf with the ears sealed to the top of the head but do have a sparse covering of downy white fur when born.

The eyes open at around 2 weeks of age, and the ears are fully open at 3–4 weeks shown by their erect posture. The milk/deciduous teeth erupt at 3–4 weeks and are fully erupted by 7–8 weeks of age. They are then gradually replaced by the permanent dentition which is fully in by 4–5 months of age. The cubs are weaned by 7–10 weeks of age, and become sexually mature at around 1 year of age.

Mustelidae: Badgers

Distribution

The European badger (*Meles meles*) is found throughout Europe and parts of western Asia. The North American badger (*Taxidea taxus*) is anatomically similar to the European badger and is found throughout the western and central USA, southern and central Canada and northern Mexico. The honey badger or ratel (*Mellivora capensis*) is renowned for its fearsome nature and is native to the middle and far eastern Asia and in body form is more similar to weasels than the rest of the badger family although it has a powerful frame, being around 0.2–0.25 m high and 0.7 m long and weighing up to 16 kg.

The European badger is mainly nocturnal in activity, only coming above ground at dusk and during the night when it forages for food. The badger's main den area is referred to as a 'sett' which is a large network of tunnels and underground dens dug into a sandy bank, often within a wood or forest edge. Badgers are however common in urban areas and so may make use of disused buildings and cellars.

Anatomy and biology

For clarity, the following description of anatomy and biology focuses on the European badger.

Musculoskeletal system

The badger skeleton is similar to that of the dog or ferret. The main differences are the shorter limbs and heavier bone structure.

There are five digits to each limb, the hindlimbs having a 'dew claw' for digit 1. Each digit has long claws that are not retractable and are significantly longer in the forefeet than the hind and used for digging and searching for food. A small web lies between each digit, and the stance is digitigrade.

The overall length of the European badger is 0.6–1 m (smaller for the female), and they can reach a height of 0.3 m at the shoulder in the case of the full-grown male. Their weight averages 10 kg in midsummer, increasing to 15–20 kg in the autumn prior to the winter. In the early spring after an average winter body weight may have dropped to 9 kg. So, there is some considerable weight changes during the course of the year.

The skull is broad and has an interparietal/midsagittal ridge across the top in midline to which the powerful temporal muscles attach meaning that the zygomatic arch is significantly bowed laterally to allow the bulk of the muscle to pass medial to it. This gives the badger's jaws an extremely powerful bite. The attachment of the mandible to the skull is such that dislocation of the jaw is virtually impossible in the adult badger without fracturing the mandible. The size of the calvarium and so brain is large, and the eyes point more forward than lateral. The width of the skull is greater in the male badger. The nasal bones are long and allow the attachment of long cartilages for the mobile nose.

Digestive and urinary system

The teeth of the badger are generally domestic dog-like in shape, but the molars and last few premolars are more flattened to provide crushing grinding surfaces that aid in chewing plant material, as the badger omnivorous in nature.

The dentition of the adult European badger is:

I3/3C1/1Pm4/4M1/2

Occasionally though there are only three premolars in the hemimandible and commonly there are only three premolars in the hemimaxilla as Pm1 is frequently absent (see Figure 25.5). Milk/deciduous teeth are present and start to erupt from 4 weeks of age and are often totally replaced by permanent dentition by 16 weeks of age.

The rest of the digestive system is similar to that seen in the domestic dog.

The rectal body temperature is on average 37°C (98.6°F) (Neal and Cheeseman, 1996).

The kidneys and associated structures are sites for fat deposition in the badger during the late summer and autumn in preparation for the winter months.

Skin and associated structures

The skin is thick and generally loosely attached to the underlying structures which offers some protection during intra- and interspecific fighting and also needs to be considered when repairing any wounds.

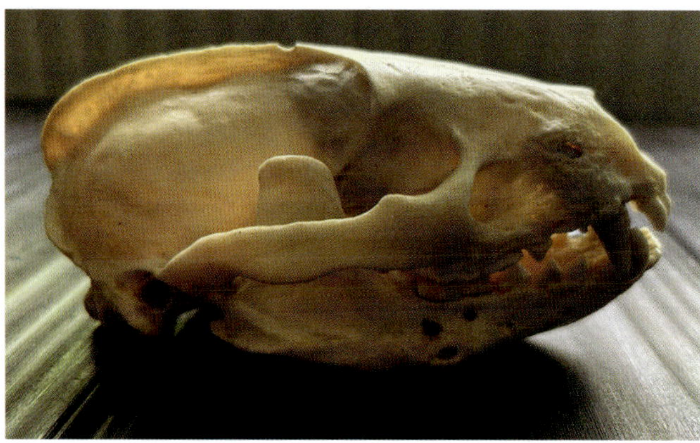

Figure 25.5 Skull of a European badger (*Meles meles*). Many badgers have a reduced number of premolars as a normal feature as shown here. Note also the damage to the skull around the root of the maxillary right canine (104) which has a fractured tip. The skull damage here is likely due to a tooth root abscess which is common.

The fur coat is also extremely thick, each follicle having more than one hair growing from it. A main primary or guard hair arises from each follicle, providing a rainproof outer coat, and a cluster of secondary or undercoat hairs also grows providing insulation. In the winter the coat is particularly thickly clustered with guard hairs which appear slightly grey towards their ends due to a band of pigment near the tip of the hair. Badgers moult twice a year, once in the spring and once in the late summer. The undercoat sheds first.

The hair of the tail lacks any pigment, as do the characteristic white stripes of the face.

Scent glands are present at the base of the tail (subcaudal scent gland) opening into a small fold of skin, in addition to the paired anal glands. These two sets of paired glands can release a strongly odoured oily scent used for territory marking. There are also interdigital scent glands which mark out badger trails.

The snout has a broad planum nasale at the end which is highly mobile and used for rooting in the undergrowth for earthworms and other food items.

Senses

Eyesight is not the badger's strongest sense. Their eyes are small but the retina has large numbers of rods allowing good collection of light, although relatively few cones for colour vision, typical of nocturnal species. Badgers possess a tapetum lucidum helping to further enhance night vision. They are sensitive to increased light intensity so it is important to keep their accommodation during any hospitalisation and treatment in dimmed lighting.

Hearing is acute in the badger, having a higher auditory range than humans. The badger will respond rapidly to any unfamiliar sound with a fear response, first trying to run away and then if this is not possible by standing its ground and attacking. Keeping areas where badgers are being treated extremely quiet, and adopting a routine which allows some prediction of events will reduce stress levels.

Smell is likely the badger's most important sense and they can pick up the scent of a human from a distance of over a couple of hundred yards (180 m) assuming downwind (Neal and Cheeseman, 1996).

The muzzle is covered in vibrissae which are used to hone in on small food items, as well as being used for social interaction between parents and offspring.

Reproductive biology, sexual cycle and reproduction

The female European badger is known as the sow and the male is known as the boar or brock with the young referred to as cubs.

The uterus of the sow is bicornuate. The boar possesses externally located testes in a scrotum.

Badgers are induced ovulators. They are unusual in that they may mate at almost any time of the year, but the cubs are only born between mid-January and mid-March due to delayed implantation. Cubs are born underground in the sett. Litter sizes vary but average at three cubs per litter, although as many as five may be seen. Soon after mating the sow may come back into heat, and it is possible for the sow to be remated during the period of delayed implantation. Gestation lasts for 6–7 weeks on average.

Neonatology

The cubs are altricial in nature with a thin covering of fine grey fur. They measure around 120 mm in length and 75 g in weight. They sow makes a nest often of dried grasses or straw and fur from her ventrum. The cub's eyes do not open until 4–5 weeks of age. They rarely venture above ground before 10 weeks of age and are only fully weaned at around 5–6 months of age, although they are eating solids from 10 to 12 weeks.

Sex identification

This is by the larger size and broader head of the boar, and the presence of an abdominally located prepuce/penis and caudoventrally located testes sited in the scrotum just cranial to the anus. The sow has a semicircular vulval slit ventral to the anus.

Mustelidae: *Martes* and *Mustela* species

Distribution

Pine marten (*Martes martes*)

In the UK the pine marten is restricted to areas of Scotland from Perthshire northwards, in England in some areas of the Lake District, Yorkshire and in North Wales. It is also found in Ireland and throughout northern Europe. It prefers coniferous woodland.

Polecat (*Mustela putorius*)

These are found predominantly in northern and western Europe and North Africa. Their habitat preferences are wide, as with stoats and weasels, although they are reputed to prefer living near to a watercourse (similar to mink). They are much more likely to use human habitations as homes than the stoat or weasel although they are still uncommon in the UK due to persecution.

Stoat (*Mustela erminea*)

These are native to most of Europe, northern Asia and North America and are found throughout the UK.

Weasel (*Mustela nivalis*)

These are native throughout Europe, North Africa, and the USA and have been introduced to New Zealand, Australia and some parts of South America. The weasel has few preferences in habitat type, although woodlands are preferred for shelter in the winter.

Anatomy and biology

Musculoskeletal system

The body form of the weasel, stoat, pine marten and polecat is essentially similar to that seen for the domestic ferret. The skeleton is fine boned and short legged in the weasel and stoat, with a more powerful skeletal structure for the larger marten species. They all possess five digits on both fore and hind limbs.

The largest of the group considered here is the pine marten followed by the polecat (see Figure 25.6). The smallest is the weasel which may only be a matter of 10–20 cm in length.

Table 25.1 outlines some biological values of typical *Martes* and *Mustela* species.

Digestive system

The dental formula of the adult pine marten is as follows (although Pm1 is often missing in both mandibles and maxillae):

I3/3C1/1Pm4/4M1/2

The dental formula of the adult polecat is as follows:

I3/3C1/1Pm3/3M1/2

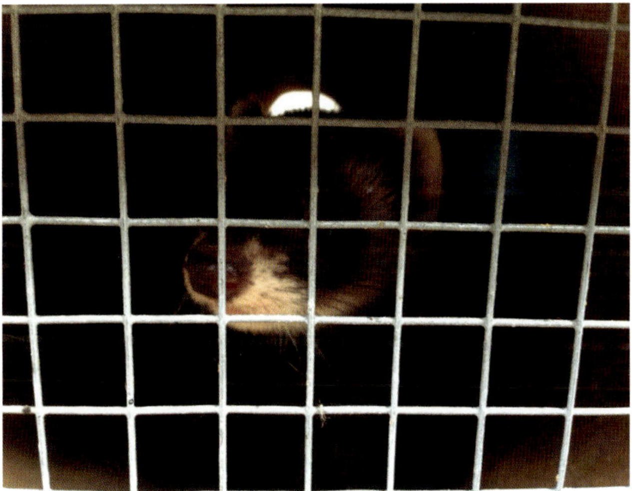

Figure 25.6 The polecat (*Mustela putorius*) is the wild-type of the domestic ferret.

Table 25.1 Biological characteristics of some typical mustelids.

Species	Weight (g) (male/female)	Heart rate (beats per minute)	Rectal temperature (°C)
Pine marten	1500–1800/ 1100–1500	180–300	38.5–39.5
Polecat	800–1700/ 500–900	200–300	39–40
Stoat	200–350/140–250	360–500	38–40
Weasel	150–200/50–90	420–500	39–40

The dental formula of the adult weasel and stoat is as follows (although some reports suggest similar dentition to the polecat (Miles and Grigson, 1990):

I3/3C1/1Pm3/3M1/1

The dentition is that of a carnivore with prominent canines and cheek teeth being of a shearing nature.

The digestive system is a simple one and closely resembles that described for the domestic ferret with a simple glandular stomach, a moderately long small intestine and short large intestine with little or no caecum.

The mustelid family has prominent anal glands which empty into the last portion of the rectum/anus junction, and produce a very strong-smelling secretion. They tend to be more developed in males than females.

Skin and associated structures

The pine marten has a dark brown coat colouration with large numbers of guard hairs. The brisket and throat are a yellow cream colour. During the summer, the coat thins and becomes darker brown. There are the usual two moults per year. There are scent glands on the ventral abdomen which secrete a musk odour and become enlarged during the breeding season and may be involved in courtship behaviour.

The polecat is generally a dark brown to black colour over the majority of the body, with long guard hairs. There are some patches of white fur over the face and brisket. There are two moults per year, one in the spring and one in the autumn.

The stoat also moults twice yearly, the autumn moult often resulting in the production of a white coat known as ermine. This white fur is dependent on the local temperature ranges, the colder the weather, the more likely the coat is to be white. In addition, female stoats are more likely to develop the ermine form than males. The stoat is a larger species than the weasel and has the distinguishing feature of a black tail tip which is retained in the summer red-brown fur coat and the winter white ermine coat. In the summer coat, the ventrum, like the weasel is a cream colour.

The weasel undergoes two moults per year, in the northern hemisphere one in the spring and one in the autumn. The fur colour is a reddish brown over the head and dorsum, with a lighter cream colour to the ventrum.

A variety of small scent glands are present over the face and lips in *Mustela* spp. which may be used to coat burrow entrances and other prominent territory markers when the mustelid rubs its face along these.

Senses

Eyesight is acute in all mustelids as they have excellent binocular colour vision.

Hearing is also acute and as with many species appear to be able to detect sounds well above the upper frequency levels audible to humans. They have mobile ears and can lock onto a sound source and use them to pinpoint prey.

The sense of smell is also well developed and mustelids use a wide variety of odours from anal glands and chin scent glands, as well as abdominal glands in the case of the pine marten, as social and territorial markers.

The sense of touch is one of the lesser senses in comparison to others considered here although they do possess well-developed vibrissae, and undoubtedly use this sense in prey location at close contact.

Reproductive biology, sexual cycle and reproduction

The female small mustelid reproductive system is anatomically essentially similar to that seen in the ferret, being of a bicornuate nature. The reproductive organs of male small mustelids include a single accessory sex gland, the prostate and usually the presence of an os penis.

Pine martens

The pine marten is seasonally polyoestrus and an induced ovulator. The breeding season runs from July to August in the northern hemisphere. The pine marten female performs delayed implantation of 5.5–6.5 months, so that the young are not born until the following March/April. True gestation length following implantation is roughly 30 days. One litter therefore is produced per year. Male and female pine martens become sexually mature over 18 months of age. The female pine marten has on average two pairs of mammary glands.

The male pine marten has its own separate territory from the female, although the two sexes often overlap. There is increased aggression seen between the sexes particularly during the breeding season.

Polecats

The reproductive cycle of the polecat is basically the same as the ferret, to which it is closely related. They are seasonally polyoestrus and induced ovulators. The reproductive season stretches from March/April to June, with the gestation length being on average 42 days. There is usually just one litter per year with on average three to seven kits produced. Sexual maturity in both the male and female is generally reached in the year following their birth. The female polecat has on average five pairs of mammary glands.

The male polecat is territorial, marking out a range often along a river or other water course. Polecats are solitary creatures, only coming together during the breeding season.

Stoats

The stoat's reproductive cycle is similar to the weasel's being seasonally polyoestrus and an induced ovulator. The breeding season stretches from April/May until August. Stoats once mated will often perform delayed implantation with the fertilised ovum only developing as far as an early blastocyst stage before stopping. The early blastocyst is then held at this stage for 9–10 months before implantation the following March. Gestation length is then 28–34 days from this time on average. The female stoat reaches sexual maturity very early on in her life, with the male not reaching it until his first year. On average only one litter per year is produced. Female stoats have five pairs of mammary glands. Only the female stoat rears the young. Female stoats may group together when hunting.

The male stoat is solitary and marks out a territory in much the same way as the male weasel.

Weasels

The reproductive cycle is seasonally polyoestrus with ovulation being induced. The reproductive season runs from February to August, the onset being stimulated by increasing day lengths and warmer temperatures. Sexual maturity is reached at around 3–4 months of age in both sexes. Gestation lasts on average 34–37 days in the weasel, with the average litter size being four to six young. Female weasels may have one to two litters per year. They have four pairs of mammary glands.

The male weasel stakes out a territory as soon as he is sexually active and defends this all year around. The male weasel will attempt to increase his territory size in the spring to encourage females to mate and increase the amount of prey caught. Weasels like most other mustelids are solitary creatures except at mating.

Neonatology

All newborn small mustelids are altricial in nature and so are born blind, deaf and often with a white downy fur coat.

In the pine marten after 5 weeks of age the eyes open, by 7 weeks the deciduous teeth have fully erupted. At 3 months the adult teeth start to appear and by 4–5 months are fully through.

The polecat kit's white fur down is replaced by a darker fur at around the fourth week of life which is about the time that their eyes open. They are weaned at around 5 weeks of age. And are fully independent by 2–3 months.

The stoat kit's white fur is replaced by 3 weeks by a darker fur and by 5 weeks the female kits eyes are open and by 6 weeks the male kits eyes open. The stoat kit is often weaned at 9–10 weeks of age.

The newly born weasel kit is altricial in nature and is blind, hairless and deaf. The eyes open at 3 weeks of age, and the weasel kit is fully weaned at 4–5 weeks of age.

Sex identification

The sexes are generally easily distinguished in the adult animals. The males have a prepuce located on the ventral abdomen and perineally located scrotal sacs containing the testes which enlarge during the breeding season. Females are generally smaller in size and have a perineally located vulva which swells and becomes pinker during the breeding season.

Mustelidae: Otters

Distribution

The European otter (*Lutra lutra*) is found throughout Europe, many parts of Asia and North Africa. It is related to the hairy nosed otter (*Lutra sumatrana*) from Southeast Asia and more distantly to other otter families such as the Asiatic short-clawed otter (*Amblonyx cinerea*) from Southeast Asia, the sea otter (*Enhydra lutris*) from northern and eastern North Pacific coasts and the North American river otter (*Lontra canadensis*). The Eurasian otter was commonly hunted but is now internationally protected and numbers are on the increase throughout its range. They are found close to water sources, although food shortages and severe winters may drive them into contact with humans and away from water. They construct simple rest sites known as holts from small burrows in the river bank or empty tree stumps. More advanced nests are also constructed to create a den to rear young in. These are often lined with leaves and dried grasses.

Anatomy and biology

For clarity the anatomy and physiology of the European river otter (*Lutra lutra*) will be discussed below.

Musculoskeletal system

The European otter body form is similar to that seen in members of the mustelid family. On average the male otter weighs 9–12 kg and is 0.75–1 m in length, the female otter being 7–10 kg and 0.55–0.85 m in length.

The skull of the otter is broad in comparison to many members of the mustelid family, and the eyes, small ears and nostrils are situated more dorsally, all adaptions necessary for a semi-aquatic life.

The limbs are basically the same skeletal formula as many mammals of the mustelid family but are generally shorter and thicker and therefore stronger in character. There are five digits on both fore and hind limbs. The digits are also webbed, aiding their swimming ability.

The tail of the otter is extremely well developed, being long and muscular, and is used as a rudder and aid to propulsion through the water (see Figure 25.7).

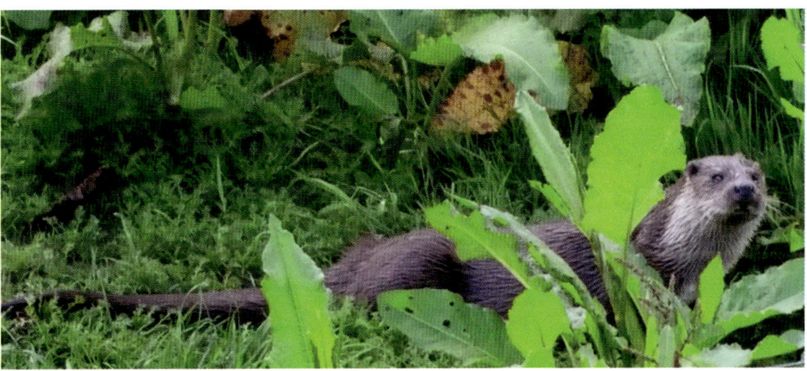

Figure 25.7 The European otter (*Lutra lutra*) has a long body form with a strong and muscular tail.

Digestive and urinary system

The dental formula of the adult European otter is:

I3/3C1/1Pm4/3M1/2

The digestive system is similar to that seen in other mustelids. The stomach is a simple glandular structure, and like many carnivores the small intestine is the larger of the two. The liver, spleen and pancreas are similar to those seen in the pine marten and stoat.

There are two sets of perianal glands at the rear of the otter. The true anal glands empty just at the anal exit, and the proctodeal glands which empty into the rectum.

The kidneys in otters are multilobulated in appearance (reniculate), rather than the smooth surface of the cat or dog kidneys.

Skin and associated structures

The fur of the otter is extremely thick. The dorsal surface of the body is a dark chestnut brown, the ventrum a cream colour. The underfur is densely packed and composed of shorter finer fur. This is overlain with the longer coarser guard hairs.

The interdigital space is covered with skin webs to enhance the swimming ability of the otter. At the end of each digit is a sharp, non-retractable claw.

Senses

Sight is a well-developed sense in the otter, as they have good colour and binocular vision as with many advanced predators.

Hearing is also well developed and acute when hunting prey on land.

The sense of smell is excellent in otters as they can track a scent trail from many miles across land. As with other mustelids they are also very territorial and will scent mark boundaries.

Touch is an important sense in the otter, particularly when hunting underwater in turbid conditions. The vibrissae covering the muzzle are extensive and give fair warning of prey movements through the water.

Reproductive biology, sexual cycle and reproduction

The male otter is referred to as a dog and the female as a bitch. The male otter becomes sexually mature at around 18 months of age. The prepuce is located on the mid ventral abdomen and contains an os penis. The accessory sex gland is the prostate.

The uterus of the female otter is typical of other mustelids in that it is bicornuate. The female otter does not appear to have a set breeding season. Gestation length varies from 61 to 65 days in total.

Female otters have two to three pairs of mammary glands and become sexually mature from around 2 years of age.

Neonatology

The young otter is known as a cub. They are altricial in nature, as they are born blind and deaf, although they are furred. They are able to crawl around the nest at 2–3 weeks of age, and their eyes open at 4 weeks. They are fully weaned at 8–12 weeks, by which time they have learnt to swim – but they have to be taught to swim by their mothers. It is about this time that their permanent dentition appears.

Sex identification

The dog otter is generally larger and has a broader head than the bitch otter. The dog otter also has a prominent ventral mid-abdominally located prepuce and high inguinally located testes.

PINNIPEDIA

Phocidae (true seals)

Distribution

The true seals (Phocidae) or colloquially 'earless' seals will be discussed here and not the 'eared' seals (Otaridae) such as the sealions. The two main species seen in the UK and northern Europe are the common and grey seal.

The common seal (*Phoca vitulina*) is also often known as the harbour seal and is a gregarious species living in small groups close to human inhabited shores, hence their name. They are found all around the North Sea, Irish Sea and North Atlantic Ocean, but particularly around the east coasts of landmasses in these areas. They are also found around the northeastern and northwestern edges of the Pacific ocean.

The grey seal (*Halichoerus grypus*) is more typically seen as a solitary animal off shore, only grouping together during the breeding season. They are often found around the northern coasts of Europe but also in the Baltic seas and around the shores of eastern Canada and USA and southern Iceland.

Anatomy and biology

Musculoskeletal system

The grey seal often exceeds 1.5 m in length (excluding flippers) and weighs 270–320 kg for the male and 140–180 kg for the female, whereas the common seal is generally 1.2–1.5 m excluding flippers which are around 0.2–0.3 m, and weighs 70–170 kg for the male and 50–150 kg for the female.

The skull of the common seal is broad, shorter and more rounded than the grey seal's. The nostrils are dorsally located as expected in a semi-aquatic species and in the common seal also form a 'V' shape, whereas the grey seal's are parallel to each other, due to the elongated muzzle (see Figure 25.8). The ears of both species are far back on the skull and have no external pinnae (hence the term 'earless' seals). The eyes are also dorsally located.

The neck is extremely thick and well muscled. The forelimbs are much shortened and thickened, particularly the humerus. The radius and ulna are in fact longer than the humerus. The carpal bones are reduced in number, the metacarpals and phalanges are elongated to form the flippers, with five digits present and a small claw on the end of each one. The digits of the forelimb, like the hindlimb, are webbed.

The hindlimbs of both seals are rotated to point caudally, with a short and thickened femur. The tibia is slightly longer, but still stout in proportion. The tarsal bones are reduced in number, and the metatarsals and phalanges are arranged in vertical order with the first and fifth digits being the longest, and the middle or third digit the shortest. At the end of each digit there is a small claw and between the digits there is a thick web of skin. The two hind feet have their ventrum (soles) rotated to touch together. The hindlimbs are longer than the tail.

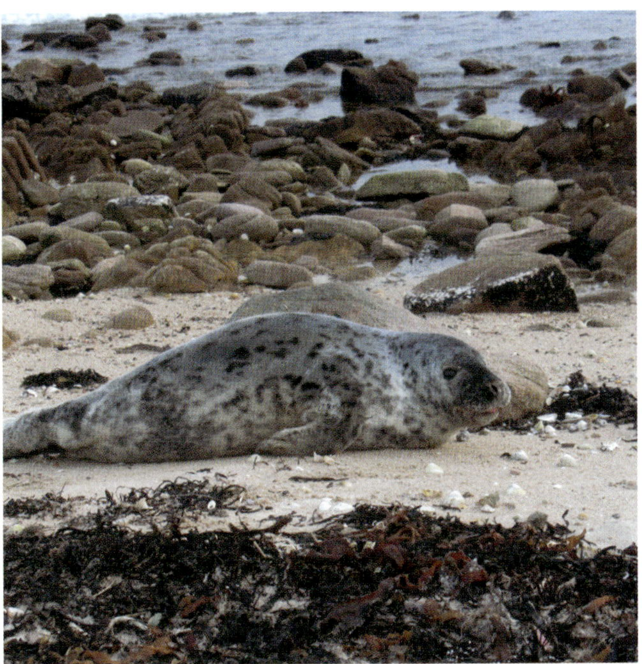

Figure 25.8 Grey seals (*Halichoerus grypus*) have a longer head and their nostrils are more parallel unlike the common seal where they form a 'V' shape.
Source: Courtesy of Kelly Huitson RVN.

Respiratory physiology

Seals have several physiological adaptations to allow diving to significant depths. For example, the condition known as the bends to divers is where nitrogen in the lungs becomes forced into solution in the bloodstream, and so in the tissues as the pressure increases with the depth of the dive. This is fine while continuing to dive, but once surfacing again, the process is reversed and the nitrogen starts to come out of solution. If the ascent is rapid, then the nitrogen is released too quickly, before the blood it was contained in reaches the lungs, and so actual bubbles of nitrogen are formed in the bloodstream, the tissues and joints. This is both painful and potentially fatal. Seals avoid this condition through a couple of measures. One is when diving to great depths, the seal collapses its lungs, so expelling nearly all atmospheric air, and removing the source of much of the nitrogen. This has the downside of also reducing the amount of oxygen in the lungs available for aerobic respiration but seals have a large amount of myoglobin in their muscle and body tissues. This means they can 'store' more oxygen at the site where it is needed when compared to land-based mammals. The heart rate also slows, falling from an average sea surface level of 150 beats per minute in an adult, to 10–20 beats a minute when submerged. This reduces the oxygen requirements of the heart. Finally, blood flow is shunted away from the muscles and towards the brain, and other vital organs such as the kidneys to preferentially support tissues more sensitive to hypoxia. Seals also seem less sensitive to high levels of blood carbon dioxide than most mammals. Rising levels of carbon dioxide act as a respiratory stimulant to all mammals, but this is suppressed in diving seals to reduce the desire to breathe while underwater.

Digestive system

The adult dentition of the grey seal is as follows:

$$I3/3C1/1Pm4/4M1-2/1$$

The common seal is similar although some individuals may only have one maxillary molar each side and only two lower incisors each side. The teeth are mainly peg like, although the molars are more cuspid in nature.

The stomach is of a simple glandular form, and the intestines are of a standard arrangement as seen in carnivores, with a long small intestine split into duodenum, jejunum and ileum with a short large intestine.

The liver, spleen and pancreas are of standard form.

Skin and associated structures

The fur of the common seal is generally thick, short and spotted with light fur on a background of grey-brown. The grey seal has again a thick short coat, with patches of light fur interspersed with larger blotches of grey and brown.

The digits each end in a short but sharp claw.

In both seals, the subcutaneous area is well insulated with extensive fat deposits that insulate the core body temperature against the cold of the sea. This also means that they are more prone to hyperthermia than they are to hypothermia when being treated or anaesthetised.

Senses

Sight is well adapted for underwater vision, although out of the water the seal's sight may be slightly blurred due to the difference in the refraction of light between water and air. They have significantly higher numbers of rods in the retina and a well-developed tapetum lucidum to help vision in low light levels. Interestingly there is no nasolacrimal duct in phocids.

Hearing is an acute sense in seals. They appear to hear well under water as well as above it and seem to suffer no serious reduction in hearing due to a lack of an external pinna.

Smell is probably a very acute sense while on land but is useless when diving as the nostrils are forced closed.

Touch seems to be a very highly tuned sense in seals, as each vibrissa has a well-developed sensory nerve supplying it, suggesting that they may be of some use in sensing prey location and water currents while swimming.

Reproductive biology, sexual cycle and reproduction

The male seal is often referred to as a bull and the female as a cow.

The common seal tends to form almost monogamous pairs. Conversely the grey seal bull tends to mate with a harem of up to 10 females.

The uterus of the grey and common seals is bicornuate in nature. The vulva and anus are found in a common furrow on the ventral caudal aspect of the seal. The grey seal female enters oestrus within 3 weeks of giving birth and is polyoestrus throughout the breeding season which tends to occur in the autumn. The gestation period is long, extending for 11.5 months in total, which is mainly due to a delayed implantation at the early blastocyst stage 1 week into pregnancy. This delayed implantation lasts for around 100 days and the rest of the gestation is thus approximately 240 days in length. On average one pup is produced per year per female. Females become sexually mature from 4 to 5 years of age.

The female common seal also demonstrates delayed implantation and has a similarly long gestation period of 11 months. The common

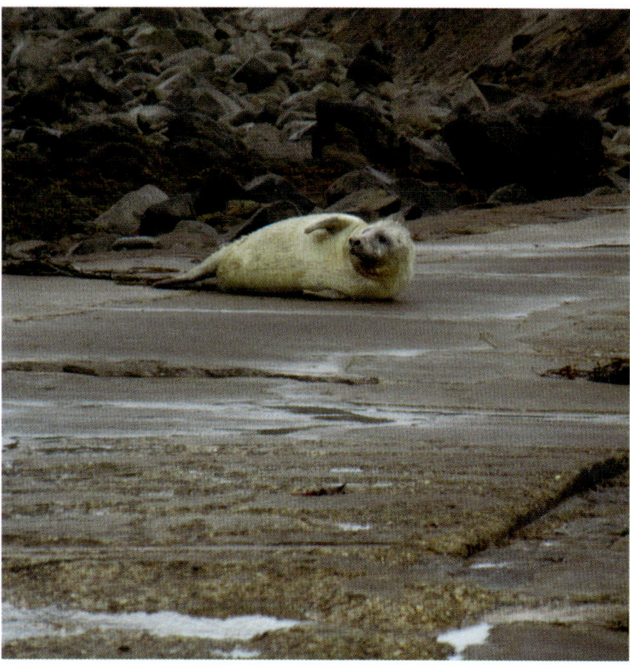

Figure 25.9 Grey seal pups have a white coat and are land-bound for the first few days of life. *Source:* Courtesy of Kelly Huitson RVN.

seal mates in the summer months of June to August and therefore pups around the same time in the early summer.

The two species have one pair of mammary glands.

The male common and grey seals have inguinally located testes and a prominent prepuce cranial to the anus ventrally.

Neonatology

The young phocid seal is referred to as a pup.

The grey seal pup is born with a white coat and is relatively helpless being completely land-bound for the first few days of life (see Figure 25.9). It is weaned at around 16–21 days of age when the coat changes from white to a darker brown-black coat of the adult.

The common seal pup on the other hand is often born without the initial white fur coat, having shed this inside the uterus, and is more precocious being able to swim almost immediately after birth. It is weaned around 3–4 weeks of age. The average seal pup may gain 1.6–1.7 kg per day due to the extremely high fat content (50% or so) of the mother's milk.

Sex identification

The male seal is usually much larger than the female, and generally has more well-developed neck musculature when sexually mature. In addition, the male seal has an obvious prepuce.

CHIROPTERA

Microchiroptera

Distribution

Although somewhat old-fashioned, the term Microchiroptera is still used to refer to those insect-eating bats commonly found in Europe, the Americas, Asia and Africa compared with the Megachiroptera which are often fruit-eating species found in the tropics of Africa, Asia and Australasia. We shall focus on Microchiroptera here.

Examples of Microchiroptera commonly seen in UK and Europe include:

Barbastelle bat (*Barbastella barbastellus*)
Bechstein's bat (*Myotis bechsteinii*)
Brandt's bat (*Myotis brandtii*)
Brown long-eared bat (*Plecotus auritus*)
Daubenton's bat (*Myotis daubentonii*)
Greater horseshoe bat (*Rhinolophus ferrumequinum*)
Leisler's bat (*Nyctalus leisleri*)
Lesser horseshoe bat (*Rhinolophus hipposideros*)
Noctule bat (*Nyctalus noctula*)
Pipistrelle bat (*Pipistrellus pipistrellus*)
Serotine bat (*Eptesicus serotinus*)
Whiskered bat (*Myotis mystacinus*)

Bats in general are found in rural areas with the Daubenton's bat preferring riverside locations, giving its name as the 'water bat' owing to its frequent low dives across the water to drink and catch flying insects.

All of the above species are nocturnal, although many appear at dusk while the sky is still light.

Anatomy and biology

Musculoskeletal system

Bats are the only mammals to have achieved true flight, as opposed to gliding which has been developed by a number of species. Their musculoskeletal system has therefore evolved to become lightweight and to support wing membranes.

The body form is similar to that seen in all mammals, with an appendicular skeleton consisting of a pelvis and four limbs, and an axial skeleton comprising a spinal column of cervical, thoracic, lumbar, sacral and coccygeal vertebrae and a small skull. The skull's zygomatic arch is thinner than most mammals. In addition, the premaxillary bone, which is the most rostral part of the hard palate, is shortened rostrocaudally, and left and right sides are separated from each other leaving a deep notch that also results in the loss of the two central incisors. In horseshoe bats, the second maxillary incisor on either side is also missing.

The spinal column of microchiropteran bats contains seven cervical vertebrae which are generally box-like and mobile. There are a variable number of thoracic, lumbar and sacral vertebrae as many become fused to their neighbours to increase rigidity for flying purposes. Many of the ribs are flattened as is seen in birds. The coccygeal vertebrae vary in number, with the horseshoe family having fewer in number, the short tail often curling dorsally at rest. Other species have longer tails and generally curl the tail ventrally, under the body, at rest.

The humerus articulates with a dorsally located scapula and a strongly curved clavicle on each side. The clavicles articulate with the shoulder joint distally and the sternum proximally. The sternum itself has a midline ventral keel for the attachment of the pectoral muscles in much the same way a bird's skeleton has although it is much smaller than the avian counterpart. The horseshoe bat family has developed the pectoral girdle even further as the last cervical vertebra and the first thoracic vertebra are fused to each other and the first rib. The first rib is then fused to the sternum and the cranial edge of the second rib, thus creating a solid ring of bone to the cranial thoracic cavity.

The humerus communicates distally with the radius and ulna bones at the elbow joint. The radius is the dominant and cranial bone, with the ulna reduced to a thin sliver of bone. The humerus and radius are elongated in the bat family to support the wing membrane. The radius articulates distally with a reduced number of carpal bones (generally reduced to three bones in total) at the carpal joint. The carpal bones articulate distally with the metacarpal bones. The first digit is shortened but is mobile and projects cranially and ventrally from the wing and is supplied with a hooked claw to grasp perches. The second digit supports the leading edge of the distal wing. Digits 3–5 have elongated phalanges and fan out laterally and caudally to support the vane of the wing membrane (see Figure 25.10).

The hindlimb is small in comparison to the forelimbs. The ilium of the pelvis attaches to the sacral vertebrae, and a slender ischium and pubis to each side. The pubic bones are not fused midline, but are joined by a fibrous sheath. The femur articulates with the acetabulum of the pelvis but is rotated outward and backward so that the stifle joint points dorsally. The femur articulates distally with the short tibia and the fibula is much reduced. The tibia articulates distally with the tarsal bones which are again reduced in number. From the tarsal bones a spur of cartilage projects caudomedially to support the wing membrane edge between the hindlimb and the tail. This is known as the calcar or spur. There are five digits, all of relatively short length, and each possessing a claw distally.

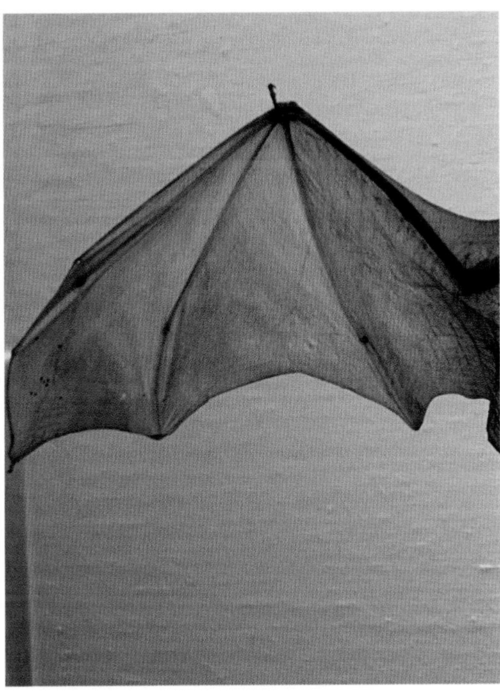

Figure 25.10 The underside of the right wing of a bat. Note the first digit projects cranial to the wing web and is supplied with a hook for roosting. The remaining digits have elongated phalanges to support the wing membrane.

Digestive system

The dental formula of the average adult microchiropteran bat is:

I2/3C1/1Pm2/2M3/3

There is some variation in this formula with horseshoe bats having fewer maxillary incisors due to the much reduced premaxillary bones as discussed, and reduced mandibular incisor numbers.

I1/2C1/1Pm2/3M3/3

The long-eared bat dental formula is slightly different as well having:

I2/3C1/1Pm2/3M3/3

One or two other species, such as the serotine and whiskered bats also differ in having fewer and more premolars, respectively.

The incisors are small, but the canines are prominent in all microchiropterans. The premolars are generally shearing in nature, but the molars are grinding in form, useful for grinding the tough exoskeleton of many insect forms.

The noctule bat has a glandular buccal pad inside the angle of the lip on both sides which may have a role in catching insects due to its sticky and strong-smelling secretions.

Skin and associated structures

The wing membrane is a double layer of skin, with few soft tissue structures except a few blood vessels and nerves between them, stretched over the bones of the forelimb and hindlimb. The wing membrane is an extension of the skin of the body of the bat. Moving from the humeral area, there is a web of skin, known as the antebrachial membrane, from the shoulder to the carpal area cranial to the humerus and radius, mirroring the propatagium found in birds. This area of skin continues caudal to the humerus reaching down to the femur and tibia and moving laterally to form the main portion of the wing which is supported by the outspread digits of the forelimb. The interfemoral membrane lies between the hindlimbs, as its name suggests and is further supported by the tail and the calcar from the tarsal area.

The fur of bats is silky in nature, with guard hairs and dense secondary hairs forming the undercoat. The fur colour in most species is a dark brown, with the underfur being darker and greyer in appearance. The fur on the ventrum of many microchiropterans is often slightly lighter than that on the dorsum. Fur grows all over the body and extends somewhat onto the base of the wings in many cases, such as is seen in the noctule bat where it extends along the ventral aspect of the humerus. In horseshoe bats, the base of the tail is often hairless. The ears are also free of fur and are prominent in species such as the long-eared bat. All microchiropterans have a prominent narrow and long tragus (the flap of skin at the base of the ear partly protecting the external ear canal) except the horseshoe bats in which it is absent.

In many bats (e.g. the noctule bat), there are prominent sebaceous glands forming skin folds around the angles of the lips and nose. They produce an oily secretion that can have a strong rancid smell.

Some bats such as horseshoe bats have developed the skin around the nose into a large skin fold, known as a nose leaf, and the lower part of this which covers the upper lip and nostrils is horseshoe shaped so giving the bats their name. This flap forms a point or lancet dorsally. Its function is not fully understood, but it has some form of sensory function as the branches of the fifth cranial nerve densely innervate this area and may well play a part in echolocation (see below). In addition, there are large numbers of oil and sweat glands over the surface of this nose leaf, as well as an additional sebaceous gland between the nose leaf and the medial canthus of the eye, which may produce so much secretion that the fur is permanently matted.

Immediately beneath the skin in the late summer is an extensive brown fat layer used as an energy source for the winter hibernation. In addition, there are brown fat deposits and extensive lymphatic tissues around the blood vessels of the chest, neck and back, which may well play a role in recovery of hibernation, and maintenance of core body temperature to prevent freezing of body tissues. These areas should be avoided for injections as they are highly innervated and have a good blood supply.

Senses

Eyesight in bats is thought to be poor. This is probably the case in those species which have very small eyes, such as the horseshoe bats, but species such as the noctule bat have large eyes, and these appear to function well, as the bat flies often before sunset, catching prey partly by sight.

Hearing, and particularly echolocation, is the bat's best sense. The technique of echolocation is based on the emission of high-pitched squeaks produced in short pulses of sound, travelling away from the bat, and reflected by any solid surface they meet, such as an insect prey item, or an obstacle. The production of the ultrasonic squeak is performed by the larynx of the bat which is highly modified. In most mammals the larynx is cartilaginous with some fine supporting bones (the hyoid apparatus). In the bat the larynx is entirely composed of bone and is larger in proportion to the body size than in other species with greater musculature. It is not known whether the ultrasonic sounds are emitted through the mouth or the nasal passages, although horseshoe bats have their larynx communicating permanently with the nasal passages, suggesting the nose is the exit route for the sound waves. When the sound wave is reflected, the frequency is lowered slightly due to a loss of energy, and the bat's highly developed ears pick up the echo. The bat can then distinguish between a solid surface and a moving prey item. The ears are highly mobile and can be used to accurately pinpoint the target, much in the same way as many diurnal predators use their binocular vision. Different species of bat have different frequencies and this may be used to track and identify bats on the wing.

Smell is also an acute sense in the bat family. However, the often ornate developments of the nose and the skin surrounding it may be used in the process of echolocation as mentioned above.

Touch plays a part in communication between bats roosting, nursing of young, and in location of prey at close distance. It is also known that even hibernating bats seem able to detect the approach of another animal, possibly by the heat emitted, as they will flex their legs and pull themselves away from the stranger, even though they are to all intents and purposes deeply asleep in a hibernating state.

Reproductive biology, sexual cycle and reproduction

The breeding season in the northern hemisphere is in the late summer and early autumn, when males and females will pair. The female can then store the spermatozoa in the uterus right through the winter before she ovulates and fertilisation occurs in the spring. Alternatively, the female may expel the sperm thus stored and be remated in the spring when another briefer paring will occur.

The gestation period for most bats is around 6 weeks with one young being produced. Young bats are therefore born generally from late May to early July. In the noctule, Leisler's, pipistrelle and serotine bats the young are born into the pouch of the wing between the hindlimbs (the interfemoral membrane). Sexual maturity is reached in the female at around 3 years of age.

The female bat has on average two mammary glands located in the pectoral area, although the mammary tissue extends around to the dorsal aspect of the bat. Horseshoe bats have a pair of false teats which sit near the urogenital tract openings and function as an anchorage for the young bat when roosting.

Neonatology

Young bats are altricial in nature and are born naked clinging to their mother's fur for the first few weeks of life. They have a set of deciduous/milk teeth which are believed to aid this as they are sharp and slender in nature. Their eyes open at around 7–9 days of age and they are fully weaned at around 7 weeks of age.

Sex identification

Female bats have one pair of pectoral-sited mammary glands which are obvious when nursing young. The female horseshoe bat also possesses a pair of false teats just cranial to the anus, used to help the young cling onto the mother. The male bat has internal testes, but the urethral opening is situated further cranially on the ventrum than the urogenital opening in the female.

Hibernation and roosts

European and North American microchiropteran bats will use roosts throughout the summer months to rest during daylight hours. These vary from caves through to trees and buildings.

During the winter more permanent undisturbed sites are often sought which will maintain a relatively constant temperature. Caves, disused mine shafts, tunnels, etc., are then more commonly used. Microchiropteran bats may hibernate from September/October through to April/May in response to a reducing food source, colder weather and decreasing day length. It has been suggested though that one of the main stimuli for hibernation is the laying down of sufficient subcutaneous fat reserves, and so a metabolic stimulus rather than a purely physical external one. The winter roost is often referred to as a hibernaculum, and generally is chosen on its ability to maintain temperatures between 4 and 8°C. Bats may recover rapidly from hibernation in warmer spells and start to hunt for food. Alternatively, if the hibernaculum fails to maintain the correct temperature, they may leave it in search for more suitable accommodation. Some bats such as the pipistrelle, may regularly recover from hibernation throughout the winter, particularly on warmer days.

Physiological changes in bats during hibernation

During hibernation the bat's respiration rate drops from 200 breaths per minute when active, to 25–30 breaths per minute, which may be interspersed with complete pauses in breathing of 3–4 minutes duration. Body temperature may drop from 37.4°C to 9–10°C, and heart rates can drop from 400 to 600 beats per minute to a low of 40–60 beats per minute. The spleen enlarges dramatically as the majority of the erythrocytes are stored here during hibernation. All of this leads to a dramatic reduction in oxygen utilisation – around one-hundredth that of the active non-hibernating bat.

Arousal from hibernation can take some 30–40 minutes or so, during which time the spleen contracts and increases the blood volume and erythrocyte count, and the brown fat reserves mentioned above are stimulated to produce heat to raise the body temperature. This is achieved through branches of the sympathetic autonomic nervous system and via the adrenal glands, and result in an increase in the respiration and heart rates as well.

EULIPOTYPHLA

We will focus on the hedgehog as a common wild species of Eulipotyphyla presented for veterinary care.

European hedgehog

Distribution

The European hedgehog (*Erinaceus europaeus*) is found throughout western and northern Europe. It prefers broken countryside, with access to hedgerows where it can nest in the undergrowth. Other species closely related are the Amur hedgehog (*Erinaceus amurensis*) found across Russia and China, the northern white-breasted hedgehog (*Erinaceus roumanicus*) found in eastern Europe and central Russia and the southern white-breasted hedgehog (*Erinaceus concolor*) found in the Middle East. They are less closely related to the African hedgehogs (*Atelerix* spp. often kept as pets and *Paraechinus* spp.) and Asiatic hedgehogs (*Hemiechinus* and *Mesechinus* spp.).

The European hedgehog is nocturnal in activity, coming out after dark to forage for prey. During the day, the hedgehog will hide up in a nest made of leaves and grasses, often in the bottom of hedges or underneath bramble stems. A more secure den may be made for hibernation purposes, when a small burrow may be dug into a bank or ditch wall, and often places such as compost heaps and bonfire piles.

Anatomy and biology

For clarity the following description of anatomy and biology focuses on the European or western hedgehog (*Erinaceus europaeus*).

Musculoskeletal system

The musculoskeletal system is a standard quadruped mammalian format. Notable features include a long narrow skull with prominent nasal passages and nasal cartilages providing a flexible nose.

The hedgehog has five digits on each forelimb, and five digits on each hindlimb. The stance of the hedgehog is plantigrade.

The forelimbs are slightly out of proportion to the rest of the body being well-developed for digging and searching for invertebrate prey.

All hedgehogs also have a unique anatomical structure, the orbicularis muscle. This is a circular muscle that forms the leading edge of the spiny-covered skin and contracts to roll the hedgehog into a ball and pull the spines over the nose and limbs (see Figure 25.11). The function of this muscle is aided by the contraction of other accessory muscles such as the preorbitalis dorsalis muscle which runs underneath the orbicularis and attaches to the frontal bones of the skull. It helps to pull the spine-covered skin over the face, and is the first defence in a hedgehog that is threatened. The panniculus carnosus is the muscle which lies in concentric rings over the back of the hedgehog, just underneath the skin's surface and is responsible for erecting the bristles when aroused. Finally, the caudo-dorsalis and caudo-abdominalis muscles are responsible for pulling the tail and rear of the hedgehog inside the line of the orbicularis muscle when it contracts.

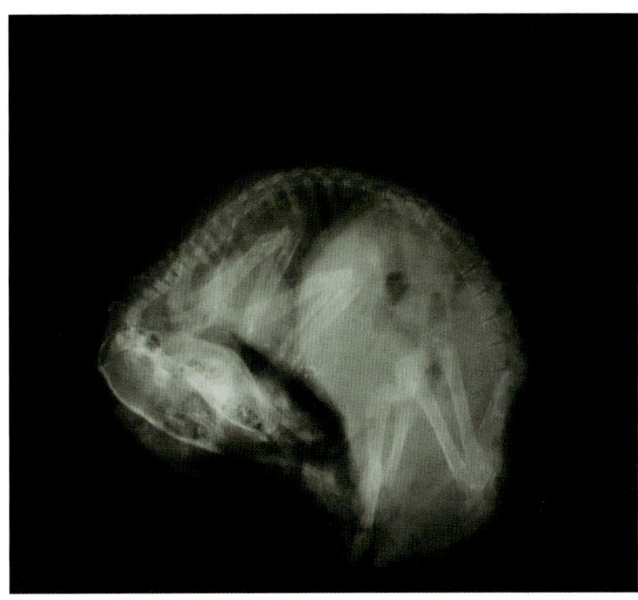

Figure 25.11 Lateral radiograph of a European hedgehog in typical curled up position. Note the increased soft tissue (muscles) around the head and rump that facilitate this posture.

Digestive system

The dental formula of the adult European hedgehog is as follows:

I3/2C1/1Pm3/2M3/3

The upper central incisors are extremely long, project rostrally and have a wide central space. The lower incisors are reduced in numbers and the central incisors also project rostrally. The canines are small, and the premolars and molars are flattened and of a crushing nature to cope with the hard exoskeletons of beetles facilitated by well-developed chewing muscles and zygomatic arches.

Just behind the upper incisors exists the small openings of the vomeronasal organ situated in the hard palate. This is well developed in the hedgehog, pheromones being captured in the saliva on the tongue and pushed into the opening to this sensory organ.

The stomach is of a simple form, and the small intestine is the most extensive part of the digestive system, with a relatively simple large intestine, and no caecum.

The average rectal temperature of the European hedgehog has been reported as 35.4°C (Reeve, 1994).

There is a proctodeal gland present emptying into the last portion of the rectum, and a series of sebaceous glands in the rectal lining. These secrete an obvious strong scent when frightened and coat the faecal stool which may be useful for territorial marking.

Skin and associated structures

The most obvious adaptation of the cutaneous structures are the spines. These form the 'hair' of the head back and flanks of the hedgehog. Each spine grows from a single adapted follicle. The spine grows from a bulb of germinal tissue, and on leaving the skin bends slightly, an adaptation thought to make the spine less likely to break during an impact. The spine itself is hollow, buttressed on the inside of the shaft with a series of divisions. This makes the spines immensely strong and lightweight. In addition, the angle at which the spines point is different in every case, so that they interlock with each other providing enhanced protection. Each spine has its own erector muscle originating from the panniculus carnosus that can erect the spine on contraction.

The first spines, grown in the neonate, are replaced from 2 days of age by pigmented spines, which are still much shorter than the adult ones. By 5–6 weeks of age, the second-generation spines are replaced by adult spines. These are then shed on an individual basis as they are lost.

The rest of the skin structure over the head and dorsum is also unusual. The skin here has no sebaceous or sweat glands, and the epidermis is relatively thin. There are also no hairs in this region, only the spines. Beneath the epidermis in this area is a thick fibrous layer, beneath which lie the blood vessels.

The skin structure over the ventrum, legs, and face is different with the spines being replaced by hairs, and the presence of sweat and sebaceous glands.

Senses

The sense of smell is one of the most highly developed senses in the hedgehog. The nose is mobile and permanently wet. Hedgehogs will often perform an unusual procedure known as 'self anointing'. This tends to occur when the hedgehog is excited or presented with almost any strong-smelling substance. The hedgehog then starts to froth at the mouth and licks the object which has been presented to it, and then spreads the saliva with some of the substance over its flanks. It may well be that this unusual activity has some link to sexual behaviour as it seems to occur predominantly during the breeding months and involves the use of the vomeronasal organ. It is seen in both sexes and even in juveniles which does suggest that there may be other factors not fully understood behind this process.

Eyesight in the hedgehog is moderately poor, and is thought to be principally in monochrome, although some colours can be detected. The eyes are situated slightly pointing forward so there is some binocular vision and are small in size.

Hearing is an acute sense in the hedgehog. Their sound range is mainly in the higher frequency ranges, such as are the noises made by many insect life forms which make the predominant prey of the hedgehog.

Touch plays a large role in food detection. Numerous vibrissae exist around the muzzle and face and allow close contact determination of the position of prey items.

Reproductive biology, sexual cycle and reproduction

The male European hedgehog is often referred to as a boar and the female as a sow.

Female hedgehog

In the female hedgehog the uterus is almost bipartite in structure with two well-developed horns which form the cross-bar of the T shape made by the reproductive tract. There is a single cervical opening, to which each horn communicates with no discernible uterine body. The vagina is split into three different areas. The cranial vagina is thin-walled and relatively wide in diameter, and from the outside looks like the 'body' of the uterus. This then narrows to a mid-vaginal area which is much narrower in diameter and possesses the urethra running in a tract in its ventral muscle wall. In addition, the mid-vagina has two frond-like glands, one on either side opening via a single left and right duct into its lumen. These have been compared with the bulbourethral (Cowper's) glands of the male, and seems to provide mucus secretions. Most caudal is the lower vagina which is 1–2 cm long and has the opening of the urethra on its floor. The lower vagina also possesses the clitoris which is prominent, before opening into the vulva caudally.

The female hedgehog has five pairs of mammary glands.

The female European hedgehog's reproductive cycle is seasonally polyoestrus with the start of the season occurring in April–May and ending in September–October. The hedgehog is a spontaneous ovulator, although the exact length of the oestrus cycle is not truly known. They may however undergo a period of pseudopregnancy after an infertile mating lasting 7–10 days or so. Sexual maturity is reached at around 9 months of age.

If a mating is successful, the gestation length is 35–40 days on average. The placentation is of discoidal and haemochorial in form meaning that in certain areas of the placenta the blood vessels are in direct contact with the maternal blood flow, similar to that seen in many rodents and indeed humans. The average litter size is four to five in the European hedgehog, and the female is reportedly very sensitive to disturbance of the litter which may lead to cannibalisation of the young.

Male hedgehog

The male hedgehog's reproductive system is similar to many rodents. There are two inguinally located testes during the reproductive season. They do not actually come through the inguinal canal but sit in a pouch in the abdominal body wall in the groin area, and they are therefore not detectable from the outside during the non-breeding season. The vas deferens leave the abdominal testes and curve cranially and dorsally before reflecting caudally to join the urethra at the neck of the bladder. At this point the urethra is joined by the ducts of the right and left prostate lobes which sit ventral to the urinary bladder. The next accessory sex gland to join are the prominent seminal vesicles which lie dorsal to the bladder and enter the urethra via a common sheath from the union of the left and right ducts. Outside the caudal aspect of the pelvis the right and left ducts of the two halves of the Cowper's (bulbourethral) glands empty into the urethra. All of these sexual organs change size and enlarge dramatically during the breeding season. As the testes are abdominal they have a fat pad insulating them from the heat of the abdomen and a countercurrent blood supply in the pampiniform plexus of the spermatic cord to allow spermatogenesis to occur.

The urethra reflects ventrally and cranially and runs through the structure of the penis along the ventral body wall. The penis possesses a corpus cavernosum in much the same way as the domestic dog does. This may engorge with blood when mating occurs. The urethra exits through the glans penis which is a green colour in young hedgehogs changing to pink-red in adults. Male hedgehogs play no part in rearing the young.

Neonatology

The young hedgehogs are usually known as piglets and are altricial being born hairless, deaf and blind, and with no obvious spines. However small pimples exist over the dorsum, through which, in a matter of hours after birth, the spines appear. These are replaced gradually by a series of pigmented spines from 2 days of age. The young are born in a nest of dried grasses and leaves, which may be positioned underneath outbuildings, or bramble bushes in hedges or dug into compost heaps and sandy banks. The young are able to raise their spines from around 1 week of age. The eyes and ears open at around the second week of life. At around the 2–3 weeks of age stage, the deciduous teeth erupt, the adult teeth developing over the ensuing months until a total adult formula is seen. The young are weaned at around 5–6 weeks of age.

Sex identification

This is relatively easy in the uncurled hedgehog. Male hedgehogs have a ventral mid abdomen-located prepuce, and inguinally located testes during the breeding season. The female possesses a single urogenital opening situated just cranioventral to the anus.

Hibernation

Hibernation lasts from October/November to April. It is important that a hedgehog's body weight reaches a minimum of 450 g prior to going into hibernation to ensure sufficient fat reserves (Reeve, 1994). The stimulus for entry to hibernation is a combination of factors including a reducing day length, reducing environmental temperatures and a dwindling food resource.

During hibernation, the hedgehog relies on stored energy as fat deposits which are present in two forms, white fat and brown fat. The most important fat reserves for hibernation is brown fat. Prior to hibernation the brown fat reserves accumulate over the thorax, neck and spinal column and can reach up to 3% of the body weight of the hedgehog. The function of this brown fat is to provide heat during the hibernation process to prevent over-chilling and to provide the kick start for recovery from hibernation. The stimulus for the fat breakdown is controlled via the hypothalamus which monitors the body temperature and effected through the sympathetic nervous system.

During hibernation, the hedgehog's metabolism drops to around 1–2% of normal levels, and the heart rate drops from 200–280 beats per minute to around 5 beats per minute. Respiration rates also drop from 25–30 breaths per minute to 10–15 breaths per minute and body temperature drops from 35.4°C to 10–15°C.

The hibernation process in hedgehogs is not a constant situation. The European hedgehog comes out of hibernation every 7–10 days, and may then go straight back into hibernation again, or may move from one nest site to another. If the weather warms sufficiently, it may forage briefly for food, and then return into hibernation once the weather cools again.

LAGOMORPHA

Hares and wild rabbits

Distribution

Eurasian rabbits (*Oryctolagus cuniculus*) are found wild throughout western Europe and western North Africa. They prefer light sandy soils, creating deep burrow systems and a stable community known as a warren. Rabbits may travel over long distances and for shelter may make shallow trenches in the soil to keep out of the wind and worst of the weather; these are known as scrapes. They are related to the cottontail rabbits (*Sylvilagus* spp.) found in the Americas.

The European brown hare (*Lepus europaeus*) is native to Europe and central Asia and the Middle East. It has been introduced into Argentina, eastern USA, eastern Australia and New Zealand. Hares are more solitary than rabbits. They do not dig burrows, but when resting prefer to do so in long grasses and hedges in a shallow scrape known as a 'form'. The female will often build a form or area of flattened grasses under brambles or low shrubs to rear the young.

The blue hare or mountain hare (*Lepus timidus*) is found throughout northern Europe including Scotland and Ireland, Scandinavia, Russia and areas of the Alps in Europe. It is related to the Arctic hare (*Lepus arcticus*) which is found in the north of Canada and Greenland.

Anatomy and biology

Musculoskeletal system

The body form is similar to that seen in the domestic rabbit. Variations include the larger frame of the European brown and the mountain hares. They have longer limbs and narrower skulls. The mountain and Arctic hares are a more sociable species than the brown hare and may form loose colonies of 40–50 individuals in some parts of the world, although in the UK small groups of mountain hares of 4–10 individuals are more common. The brown hare tends to be more solitary.

Digestive system

The digestive system of wild lagomorphs is essentially the same as that already described for the domestic rabbit. Readers are referred to the section on small mammal anatomy for a description of this.

Skin and associated structures

The skin and hair coat of wild lagomorphs is again similar to that seen in domestic rabbits. The hare family often has larger ears, and black tips to these. In addition, the mountain hare when it moults in the autumn, replaces the brown summer coat with a white ermine coat, which is then lost again the following spring. It also undergoes an additional third moult in midsummer.

The rabbit has the same glands as the domestic variety, as has the hare with anal glands either side of the anus, inguinal glands in pouches either side of the genital opening and submandibular glands.

Reproductive biology, sexual cycle and reproduction

The female rabbit is known as a doe and the male as a buck.

The wild rabbit follows much the same reproductive cycle pattern as its domesticated counterpart. The doe has a duplex uterus with two separate cervices as with the domestic rabbit.

The hare family also appears to breed throughout the year, with a reduction in fertility during the winter months from October through to February. The female hare may mate every 7 days through the peak season, which may be interspersed by longer periods of 14 days if a phantom pregnancy occurs. Male hares become much more active and display much more frequently in the early spring months. It is at this time that males can be seen jousting and boxing with females that are not yet in heat and are resisting his advances! The European (brown) hare can also conceive before the last litter has been born (a phenomenon known as superfetation).

All lagomorphs appear to be induced ovulators.

Gestation length in the wild rabbit is 30–33 days, in the hare species it is 50 days on average in the mountain or Arctic hare and 42–43 days in the brown hare.

Neonatology

The young rabbit is known as a kit or kitten, the young hare as a leveret.

Rabbit kittens only suckle once or twice a day, unlike a lot of other mammals. The doe's milk is therefore highly concentrated, which is of importance when hand-rearing rabbits. Young rabbits are weaned at 4–6 weeks of age.

Rabbit kittens are altricial and so born blind, fur-less and deaf. In contrast, leverets are precocial and so are born furred and with their eyes open and able to run from the first day of birth. Young hares are eating solids by 12 days of age, and are weaned by 4 weeks of age.

Sex identification

The female rabbit and hare have a spade-shaped urogenital opening close to the anus. The male has a tubular pointed phallus, and scrotally located testes either side of the anus, although these may be retracted into the abdominal cavity.

RODENTIA

We will focus on the Eurasian beaver and squirrels as they differ significantly from other rodents considered previously in this book. Readers are referred to the small mammal chapters on anatomy for information on other rodents.

Castorimorpha: Eurasian beaver (*Castor fiber*)

Distribution

The Eurasian beaver is now found throughout Europe, including the UK as well as deep into Russia. It is a different species to the North American or Canadian beaver (*Castor canadensis*) having 48 chromosomes as compared to the Canadian beaver's 40. It is semi-aquatic in nature and so always lives close to fresh water. It is famous for creating dams to produce still pools of water that encourage the growth of plants it likes to eat. The Eurasian beaver will also use burrows into river bank walls and will create a lodge, often to the side of a dam. It will fell trees and prefers species such as aspen and alder. It uncommonly travels far from a watercourse. Typically, in the wild they live for 12–14 years and so are a long-lived rodent species.

Anatomy and biology

Musculoskeletal system

The body form is typically that of a rodent but the size is nonetheless impressive with adult male beavers being between 20 and 28 kg in weight with females typically being between 18 and 24 kg.

The length of the body is around 0.8 m and the tail around 0.3 m. Beavers have five digits to both fore and hind feet which makes them unusual among rodents.

Digestive and urinary system

The dental formula of the Eurasian beaver is:

$$I1/1C0/0Pm1/1M3/3$$

Like most herbivorous rodents they therefore have a diastema due to a lack of canines and only two upper and two lower incisors in each jaw. The incisors are continuously erupting but the cheek teeth stop erupting around 2 years of age (see Figure 25.12).

The stomach is simple and sac-like in form but has a significant cardiogastric gland close to the oesophagus (cardia) responsible for producing both digestive enzymes and a significant amount of mucus, thought to protect the lining of the stomach. The digestive system is that of a hindgut fermenting rodent and so has a capacious caecum and large intestine for microbial fermentation and production of volatile fatty acids which are the principal energy source for the beaver. Beavers produce a waste faecal pellet which is dry and fibrous and a caecotroph which is covered in mucus and re-eaten resembling the same process recorded in rabbits and lagomorphs.

At the end of the digestive tract is a cloaca into which the urinary tract and reproductive organs open. Attached to this are two pairs of sacs, the castor sacs and anal glands. Both produce fluids that are used in olfactory communication within the species. Castoreum secretions from beavers have historically been used in the perfume industry and was one of the reasons (along with their pelt and as a food source) they were hunted to extinction in the

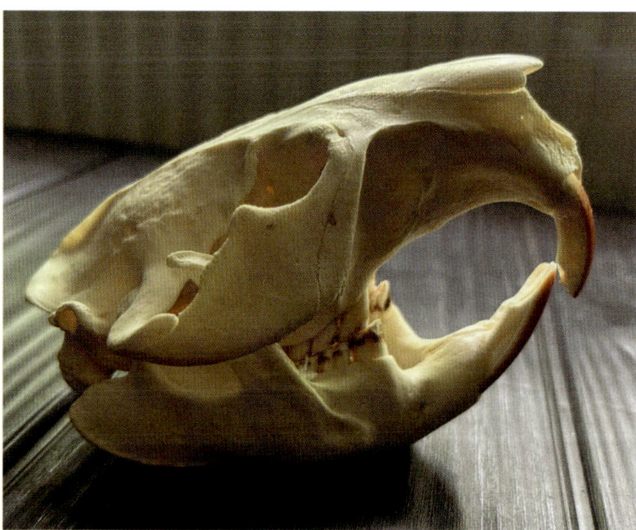

Figure 25.12 Skull of a Eurasian beaver (*Castor fiber*). Note the diastema common with rodents and the pigmented sizeable incisors.

UK. The gland is not a real gland but rather a sac into which urine regularly enters and becomes dehydrated resulting in a build-up of grey material.

The kidneys have short loops of Henle and so produce relatively dilute urine.

Skin and associated structures

The fur or pelage of the Eurasian beaver is dense and highly waterproof as well as insulating against thermal loss. The colour is a red-brown. The guard hairs are around ten times the diameter of the under-fur. The under-fur is not only insulative, it can trap air when the beaver swims and so can aid buoyancy as well as insulation. Density of under-fur hairs is around 12 000–23 000/cm^2 depending on the part of the body assessed (Novak, 1987).

The tail is hair-less and has a scale-like structure to the epidermis. The tail is often assessed to determine the body condition of a beaver as it is a fat deposition site. The second digit of each hindlimb has a double claw which is used for grooming to maintain the waterproofing of the pelage with the medial digit (digit 1) having a mobile claw (see Figure 25.13).

Senses

Beaver's sense of sight is good but not their strongest. The eyes are small and dorsally located as expected in a semi-aquatic species.

Beaver's sense of hearing is very good although their ears are small and dorsally located with valvular flaps in the canal to reduce water ingress.

Beavers have a very good sense of smell and olfaction is an important means of communication between family members and rivals. Their nostrils are situated more dorsally, typical of semi-aquatic species, and they close upon contact with water. The castoreum glands and anal glands are used for chemical communication.

Beaver's sense of touch is good with significant vibrissae around the head and neck used to communicate in the dark interior of a burrow or lodge.

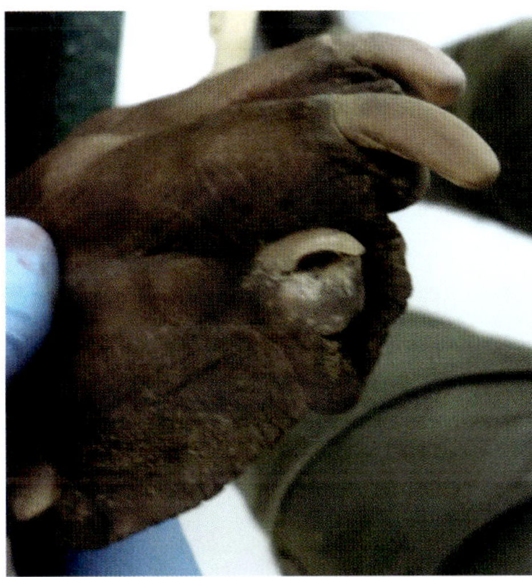

Figure 25.13 Hind foot of a Eurasian beaver demonstrating the double claw on the second digit.

Reproductive biology, sexual cycle, reproduction and neonatology

Beavers typically live in family groups and become sexually mature around 2 years of age. Once an adult male and female are paired they remain together until physically displaced or one or other dies.

Mating occurs in January and gestation lengths are long by rodent standards being 105–107 days.

Beavers produce one to four young in a burrow or dam in late spring/early summer and have only one litter per year. The offspring are referred to as cubs and are altricial in nature although born fully furred and weighing around 0.3–0.5 kg. Their eyes open within a few days of birth and they are eating solids by the first week although they will continue to take their mother's milk for the first 2–3 months.

Male beavers have many secondary sex glands, including prostate, seminal vesicles and bulbourethral (Cowper's) glands. Their testes are intra-abdominally located. There is an os penis in the phallus in adult male beavers. Many male beavers have the remnants of the paramesonephric (Müllerian) ducts that appear to look like a uterus and are referred to as the uterus masculinus.

Sex identification

This can be difficult as unlike many rodents, the Eurasian beaver has a single external orifice leading to a cloaca and the testes in the male are intra-abdominal. Expression of the anal glands of the beaver may be performed and in the case of the female Eurasian beaver the secretion is grey and semi-solid and in the male is an oily yellow/brown colour. Females that are lactating have four obvious pectorally located nipples, and an os penis may be palpable in sexually mature males per cloaca.

Sciuromorpha: squirrels

Distribution

The red squirrel (*Sciurus vulgaris*) is found across Europe and into northern Asia and the Far East. In the UK it is found in Scotland from Perthshire northwards, in central Wales and the lowland forests of East Anglia in the Thetford Hundreds and on the south coast of England. It is also found throughout Ireland and Italy in particular.

The eastern grey squirrel (*Sciurus carolinensis*) is commonly seen throughout Europe including the UK and of course its native eastern North America. It prefers wooded areas, mainly of a deciduous nature, but is a common sight in parks and gardens in towns and cities. The western grey squirrel (*Sciurius griseus*) is found only in western USA.

Both the red and eastern grey squirrels are diurnal species and do not hibernate but may remain within their nest/dray for several days during bad weather.

Anatomy and biology

Musculoskeletal system

The average weight of a male red squirrel is around 240–440 g with a body length (excluding tail) of 22–24 cm, and that of the female is 220–350 g with a body length of 18–22 cm.

The average body weight of the male eastern grey squirrel is 440–650 g with a body length of 25–30 cm, that of the female is 400–720 g with a body length of 28–32 cm.

The skull is narrow and pointed rostrally. The eyes located laterally to give a wider field of view. The jaw has powerful attachments for the large chewing muscles involved in gnawing and grinding hard items of food and wood.

The hind legs are much longer than the fore limbs and are supplied with powerful muscles which allow them to leap easily from branch to branch. They have four digits to each fore limb and five digits to each hind limb.

The coccygeal vertebrae are extensive in number and characteristically carried arched over the back.

Digestive system

The dental formula of the adult squirrel is as follows:

$$I1/1C0/0Pm1-2/1M3/3$$

The incisors are rodent-like in their form, continuously erupting and can inflict a seriously unpleasant bite. A diastema is present (see Figure 25.14). The red squirrel possesses large sebaceous glands inside the commissures of the mouth which are used to territory mark.

The stomach is of a simple glandular form, and the small intestine and large intestine are quite extensive, although not as developed as strict hind-gut fermenters.

Skin and associated structures

The squirrel family has a wide variety of scent glands, some being in the lips, others present in the interdigital skin folds and used to mark territories on branches of trees. Others are found in the perineal and anal areas and are used to mark territories via the stools.

The fur of the grey squirrel frequently is not a real grey, but may have a reddish tinge confusingly, particularly over the head. The tail though is often grey in nature. The ventrum is often white or light grey.

The fur of the red squirrel is more chestnut in colour dorsally, with redder areas over the head and into the tail. The ears are marked with red tufts of fur, and the feet may have tufts as well (see Figure 25.15).

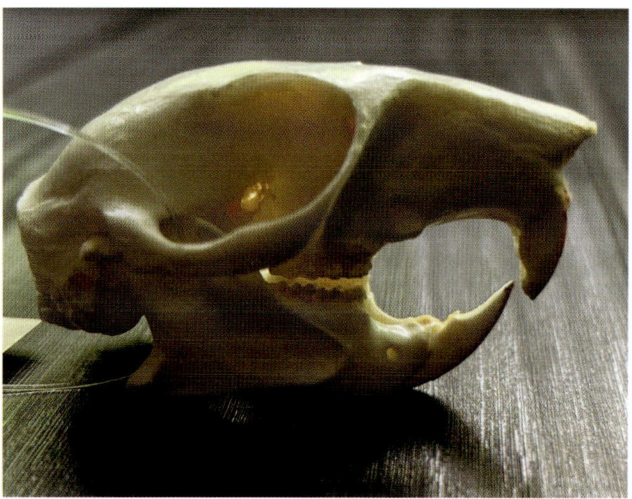

Figure 25.14 Skull of a squirrel showing the diastema and significant pigmented incisors.

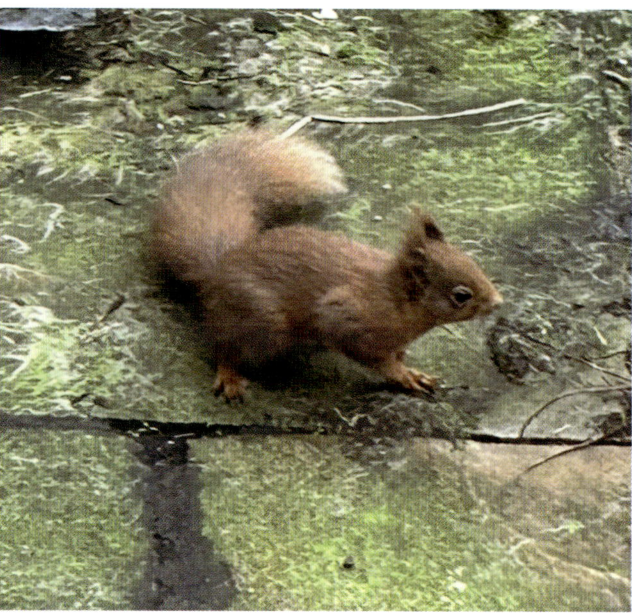

Figure 25.15 Red squirrels have prominent ear tufts and their colouring is chestnut dorsally with redder areas over the head, flanks and the tail which may have a lighter tip.

There are generally two moults in these species per year, one in the spring and one in the autumn.

Senses

Sight is a highly tuned sense in squirrels, they have a near 360° field of vision with some colour appreciation.

Hearing is again acute, with squirrels able to hear higher frequencies of sound than humans.

The sense of smell is also well-developed in squirrels as they territory mark with a variety of body odours which play an important role in the social hierarchy.

Touch is a sensitive sense in squirrels as they possess an extensive array of vibrissae around the nose and lower jaw.

Reproductive biology, sexual cycle and reproduction

The female squirrel is seasonally polyoestrus from January through to August. The uterus is similar to that seen in the rest of the squirrel family having 2 long horns to the uterus. The gestation length is 38 days on average for the red squirrel, and 40 days for the grey, with three to five young produced. It is therefore possible for a female to have more than one litter per year. The females become sexually mature from 12 months of age. It is only the female that rears the young, which are born into a nest of twigs, or a hollow tree stump, lined with dried grasses and mosses, fur and leaves known as a dray. The female tends to stake out a home territory around her dray which she will defend against other females, and after mating, other males. The territory size is larger for the red squirrel than for the grey. The females of both breeds have four pairs of mammary glands.

The male squirrel will hold a territory of his own, and these may overlap with the females. The male squirrel has a prostate, and scrotally located testes during the breeding season, although these are often retracted into the abdomen and shrink in size during the rest of the year.

Neonatology

The young squirrel is often referred to as a kitten or kit. They are born altricial in nature, being blind, deaf and fur-less. By 8–9 days the fur starts to appear in red squirrels, 2 weeks for grey squirrels. At around 4 weeks of age the eyes and ears open in both species. By 8–10 weeks they are fully weaned.

Sex identification

The ano-genital distance is shorter in the female than the male similar to other rodents. Externally otherwise there is little between the sexes, although as the female ages, the nipples become darkly pigmented, and the male possesses scrotal testes during the breeding season.

References

Bell, J. (1839) The game laws. *The New Sporting Magazine*, **17**, 272–276.

Miles, A.E.W. and Grigson, C. (1990) *Colyer's Variations and Diseases of the Teeth of Animals*. Cambridge University Press.

Neal, E. and Cheeseman, C. (1996) *Badgers. Poyser Natural History*. T & D Poyser Ltd, London.

Novak, M. (1987) Beaver. In: *Wild Furbearer Management and Conservation in North America* (eds M. Novak, J.A. Baker, M.E. Obbard & B. Mallock). Queens Printer for Ontario, Toronto.

Reeve, N. (1994) *Hedgehogs. Poyser Natural History*. Academic Press, London.

Chapter 26 Wildlife Species Temporary Captive Husbandry and Nutrition

TEMPORARY HOUSING OF SELECTED WILDLIFE SPECIES

Deer housing during treatment

In the short term, for emergency cases a relatively small area is best to prevent deer from bolting and reaching enough speed to damage themselves against the walls of the enclosure. Ideally this space requirement equates for small deer to around 1.2–1.6 m^2 and for larger deer 1.8 × 2.5 m, i.e. enough space for lying, feeding/watering and a latrine area. It is important that the enclosure is kept in dim lighting and very quiet again to reduce stress. Dimmed lighting may be less effective for roe deer as they are often active at night, but it still has some effect.

The flooring of an enclosure should be solid concrete, which is sloped to allow efficient drainage. This may then be covered with heavy duty rubber matting, such as that used for cows in cowsheds, and then deep littered with straw. The straw can be banked up around the walls to provide some cushioning should the deer become agitated and start crashing around. This may be taken a stage further by using padded walled enclosures, such as those used for horses during recovery from anaesthesia. It is important to ensure that the accommodation is also kept warm, so the use of sheep/lamb heat lamps, which are suspended well above the height of the deer, is advised to heat the environment. It is also vitally important not to group together different species and different sexes when hospitalising deer. Only females and their young should be housed together. Males should always be kept separate. Red lighting can be used to check on deer as they generally do not see well in this spectrum and so allows observation without disturbance.

For longer hospitalisation, larger stabling is required, with purpose-built stable blocks or converted sheds/outbuildings well away from noise and disturbance. If attempting rehabilitation before release, then the animals will require secluded paddocks with field shelters and surrounded by deer fencing (wide wire mesh to a height of 2.5 m under little tension so if a deer runs into it the fence line 'gives').

Red fox housing during treatment

The average dog kennel is sufficient for housing a red fox for short periods of time during treatment. Bedding can be provided using shredded newspaper. Foxes are messy and will tip bowls which ideally should be of a stainless-steel, non-spill design. The environment should be kept slightly dimmed, as foxes are not keen on bright light, and noise levels kept to an absolute minimum.

Longer periods of housing require the construction of a kennel-like shelter and a small enclosed paddock. The latter should have a wall height of about 2 m with a mesh roof or an overhang of wire of 0.3 m depth at the top as foxes are good climbers and can jump nearly 2 m. The fence line should also be buried in the soil to a depth of 0.6 m as they can also dig very well. Ideally the fence should be solid or if of mesh the dimensions should be small enough to prevent foxes biting at the fence and trapping and damaging their canines.

Badger housing during treatment

Badgers are immensely strong and any housing provided must reflect this. They are particularly good at digging and will make short work of any pens that do not have a solid concrete floor and brick walls. Vertical stainless-steel bars may also be used for part of the perimeter of their enclosure as is typical with domestic dog veterinary kennelling.

Housing environments should be quiet and have dimmed lighting to reduce stress levels. The cage dimensions should ensure that the badger has enough space to provide a toilet area, a feeding area and a sleeping area, and that these are kept distinct. This often requires a cage size two and a half to three times the badger's length in two dimensions. Height is not as important for a badger but should allow easy access for the keeper. Sleeping quarters should be deeply bedded in straw/hay, and if longer-term housing is required then they may benefit from being slightly enclosed, such as may be provided by a rabbit hutch-style construction although these often are destroyed and are less favoured due to difficulties in cleaning them between patients.

Small mustelid housing during treatment

In general, for most mustelids the provision of a relatively fine wire mesh cage, of 1-cm mesh or smaller, is advisable. This allows ventilation, but at the same time prevents escape, and is easy to clean between patients. Inside this cage should be provided a hide of some form, so that the mustelid may escape from view. This may be provided as a small wood laminate box, a plastic container, or even a cardboard box (the latter is less suitable as it may disintegrate). In any case it is helpful to have a hide that can fully contain the patient and possesses a lid so that the patient may be boxed in and removed from the wire cage without too much stress and handling. In addition, the use of a wire divider within the wire cage is useful for penning the patient into one half or the other to allow cleaning and feeding to be carried out without the stress of handling and capture every time.

Veterinary Nursing of Exotic Pets and Wildlife, Third Edition. Simon J. Girling.

Cage dimensions for the short-term hospitalisation of mustelids should allow sufficient space for a nest box, which should be just high enough for the mustelid in question to get into, and 20–50% wider and deeper than the length of the patient. There should also be space for a feeding area and a latrine area. The use of straw or hay for bedding is acceptable, although shredded paper is also useful. The floor of the cage may be covered with newspaper, or left clear, and the whole wire cage placed inside a standard dog or cat recovery kennel.

Water and food bowls should be made of a durable and cleanable material such as ceramics or metal (although the latter are often very noisy and may frighten the patient). Sip feeders are not advised for water as wild animals generally will not drink from them.

Factors to consider in the housing of mustelids include the requirement for heat, quiet conditions and dimmed lighting, all of which will reduce stress levels. Heat supplementation is important for any sick or injured wildlife case but is particularly so for the smaller species such as the weasel which has a large body surface area in relation to its mass.

Otter housing during treatment

Short-term accommodation for a hospitalised otter can be made from an existing dog kennel. The main requirements are to ensure complete quietness, dimmed lighting and provision of heat. The floor of the caging should be concrete with a slope and good drainage. The floor may be covered with rubber matting for a better grip. A secluded area can be provided for a nest, made from a rabbit hutch or similar construction, and lined with straw/shredded paper.

For longer-term care, an enclosure with an outside pen is required. This should be surrounded by a fence, buried 0.75 m deep or more into the ground to prevent burrowing, and with a height of 1 m or greater with an inward pointing overhang to prevent climbing. The provision of some form of watercourse, if possible running water, is important for long-term rehabilitation.

The ability of an otter to climb should not be underestimated. They can and will climb chain link fencing of over 2 m in height unless it has a significant inward-directed overhang. They are also pretty good at chewing their way through wooden structures and so do not rely on thin wooden doors or walls to contain adult otters. Otters may also damage their teeth on mesh fencing so solid perimeters are often preferred or mesh small enough to prevent canine entrapment.

Seal housing during treatment

This is the most specialised housing of the species considered here. The most basic of housing for short periods of hospitalisation may be provided with a straightforward large concrete-floored dog kennel but clearly this is not suitable for most adult seals although these are rarely presented for treatment, seal pups being more typical.

It is important not to overheat the accommodation; therefore, unless dealing with a newly born seal, the environmental temperature should be kept between 10 and 15°C, since anything much over 15°C could lead to hyperthermia. Very young pups may need to be warmed in an environment around 18°C but again this should not be exceeded. For this reason, outside stable blocks may be suitable for seal housing. The floor should be concreted and then covered with rubber matting and have good drainage. The accommodation should be quiet and darkened to reduce stress levels.

For long-term housing the provision of a pool for swimming is necessary. This should be shallow (0.6–0.9 m deep) but around 6–9 m long. It is not essential to fill this with salt water, although this is preferable if close to the coast. However, saline may need to be applied to the seal's eyes as they will develop corneal lesions if kept away from salt water for too long, a problem compounded if they are fed freshwater fish, as this can lead to serious leaching of salts from the seal's body.

Bat housing during treatment

Short term it is advisable to provide the bat patient with a small container such as a commercial plastic aquarium box, or rodent carry box. A well-ventilated lid is important. The inside of the container should be lined with a soft towel, which should be draped up the sides of the container to allow the bat to cling to a semi-vertical surface (see Figure 26.1). The entire container should then be placed inside a vivarium or incubator to ensure that the environmental temperature is kept between 22 and 28°C as these species have a very large surface to body ratio and so lose heat rapidly.

If the hospitalisation is to last longer than a few days, then a more permanent enclosure should be considered with heating, a source of increasing the humidity of the environment (microchiropteran bats require humid roosting areas, approaching 80–90%), and a secluded area to roost that allows the bat to grip to the side/roof of an enclosure and is out of view. Butterfly cages/netting may be used to create a fully enclosed cage, as it is soft, thus avoiding traumatic damage to the fine skin, and yet provides an open mesh which is easy to cling to. Alternatively, a large rabbit or guinea pig hutch may be adapted as a roost cage, although care should be taken to ensure that the wood used is not treated with any chemicals. The inside of the hutch is completely covered with fine nylon or wire mesh to provide a surface to which the bat may cling to. It is often helpful to divide the hutch into two sections, one which contains an opening to let light in, and the other completely enclosed. The aperture for lighting the box should also be covered by fine nylon/wire mesh. The fully enclosed smaller section of the hutch should possess a door for easy access and

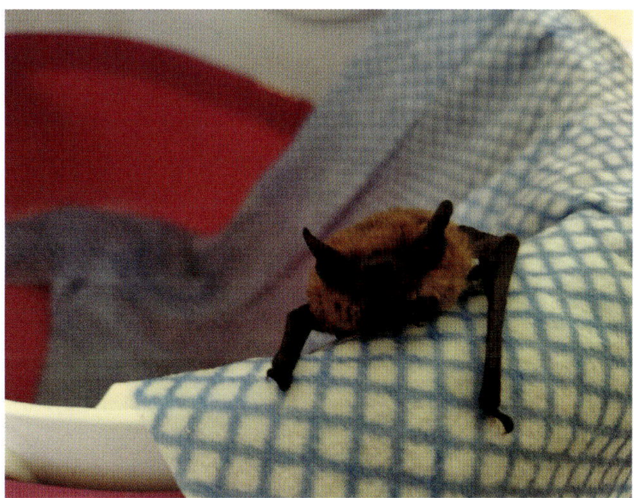

Figure 26.1 Temporary housing for a debilitated pipistrelle bat made from a plastic pet carrier lined with soft towelling. *Source:* Courtesy of Kelly Huitson RVN.

capture of the bats, and air holes to ensure good circulation. The whole of the hutch may be placed into a larger dog or cat kennel with supplemental heat sources such as an infrared heat lamp, to ensure environmental temperatures stay above 20–25°C.

The floor of such an enclosure can be covered with paper towelling to ease daily cleaning of droppings. Food bowls are placed in the larger section of the hutch with the light aperture.

Dimensions obviously depend on the number of bats kept and the species. The larger horseshoe bats may require a hutch which measures some 0.6 m high by 0.6 m deep by 3–4.5 m long. Smaller species though can cope with cage dimensions of 0.3 m high by 0.3 m deep by 1.5 m wide.

Long-term rehabilitation of bats requires specialist outside aviary-style constructions which often require dimensions of 3 m high by 3 m deep by 6 m wide. This should be covered by a mesh of 0.5–1 cm^2 which will allow the bat to cling to it without escaping but will also allow insect life to enter. The roost facilities should comprise a wooden box with a slit opening in its floor to mimic the eaves of a house. The dimensions of the roost box should be roughly 0.3 m wide by 0.3 m deep by 0.15 m high, and is attached to a wall of the cage, towards its top. The use of ultraviolet (UV) light sources to attract insects into the cage has been suggested as helpful.

Hedgehog housing during treatment

Wire enclosures should be avoided as the hedgehog frequently gets its spines and feet caught in the mesh. The provision of a smooth-sided Perspex or plastic vivarium-style cage should be considered; alternatively, for very temporary care a semi-solid plastic pet carrier may be used (see Figure 26.2). Care must be given to ensure that such a cage construction has sufficient ventilation, as poor ventilation can lead to respiratory problems due to the build-up of ammonia gas from the urine and faeces produced. Ventilation holes ideally should be at hedgehog height, avoiding placing any in a direct line with each other across the cage as this will cause a draft.

Heating is important – to prevent hibernation and ensure a good recovery, the environmental temperature should be 18–24°C. This may be provided by using a radiant heat mat, as for reptiles, on the side of one section of the tank providing the housing is in a warm indoor room.

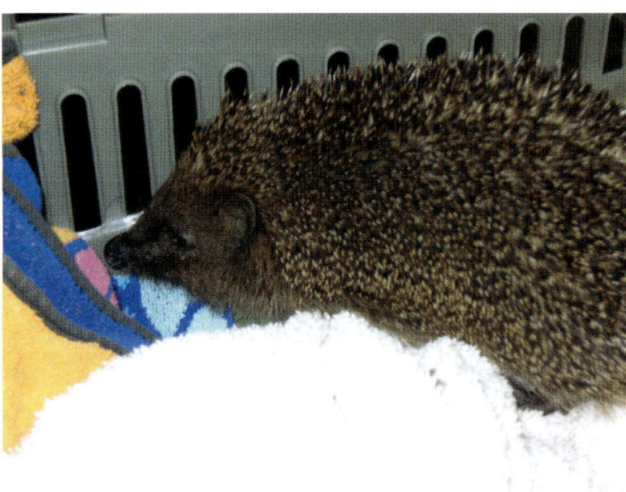

Figure 26.2 Temporary housing for a few days for hedgehogs can be made out of suitably sized semi-solid pet carriers.

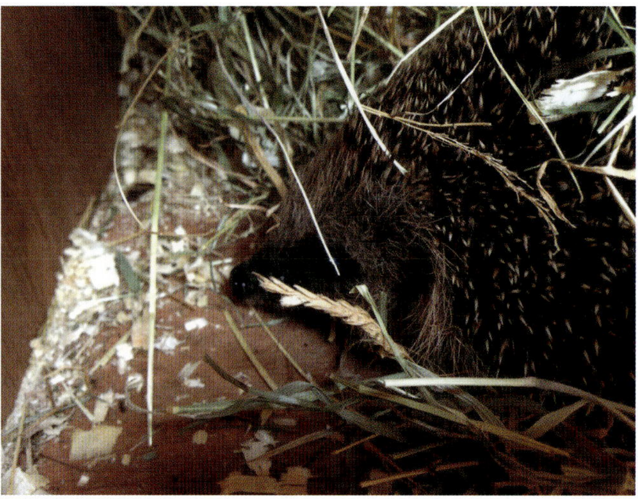

Figure 26.3 Longer-term housing for hedgehogs should provide bedding material such as shredded paper or short-cut hay or straw to avoid entanglement of limbs.

The hedgehog should also be provided with a hide for privacy. This may be constructed from a disused cardboard box, cut with an opening and upturned. The size should be as tall as the hedgehog height wise, and 50% wider and deeper than the length of the hedgehog. Bedding may be provided with shredded paper or short cut hay or straw ideally to minimise the likelihood of becoming entangled (see Figure 26.3).

Lagomorph housing during treatment

Wild rabbits require dimmed lighting and an absence of noise as they are extremely sensitive to disturbance. It is advisable to provide some form of covered shelter within the cage structure so that the rabbit is able to hide from intruders and they feel more secure when in a sheltered darkened confined area.

Hares have similar requirements, although they are often twice the size of rabbits. Hares are generally even more timid than rabbits and do not do well in captivity. They like a sheltered area within the cage, out of the sight of intruders, but they do not enjoy roofed enclosures as rabbits do, which reflects their more open lifestyle where they rest in the open rather than digging burrows.

Squirrel housing during treatment

For short-term hospitalisation (1–2 days) the main needs are to provide an escape-proof container that will keep the squirrel quiet, warm and dark. To this end any large plastic container or box will probably suffice. It should be lined with hay/straw or shredded newspaper for insulation. It may be necessary to provide additional warmth by placing the container in a vivarium or incubator, or for smaller individuals a hot water bottle in a towel. Temperatures should be kept around 18–24°C.

For longer-term hospitalisation, the use of a sturdy wire cage is useful as cardboard and wooden structures may be gnawed through. The cage should be large enough to allow the presence of a nest box/sleeping quarters, a feeding/watering area, and sufficient space to allow the insertion of one or two vertical branches for climbing and gnawing on. The floor may be littered with shavings or paper.

Other rodent housing during treatment

Small rodents are some of the easiest to house during rehabilitation, but they pose an escape risk. Fine mesh or solid plastic or glass tanks are typically used although the latter may cause problems with poor ventilation, leading to an increase in respiratory disease, and therefore ventilation holes should be pre-drilled in any fish tank-style enclosure used. Bedding should be as naturalistic as possible but beware potential ectoparasites and pseudo-ectoparasites such as harvest mites that may be brought in with hay and straw and which may lead to skin irritation (see Figure 26.4).

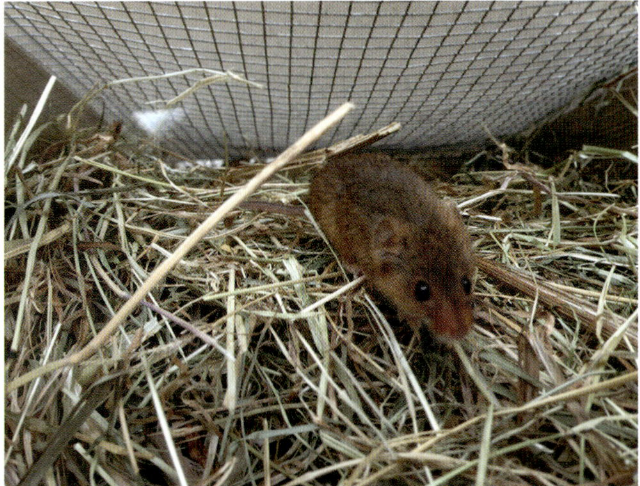

Figure 26.4 Fine mesh is commonly used for smaller rodents to allow good ventilation while preventing escape. Use of naturalistic bedding is ideal but can provide a source of potential parasites.

The Eurasian beaver is now a commonly found rodent in mainland Britain, particularly in Scotland, and is increasingly presented to rehabilitation centres. It is a more complicated species to house safely due to its size and requirements for water. Any holding facility that intends to hold beavers for more than a day should have a water source that the beaver can immerse itself in and this should be taken into consideration before attempting to treat.

Wild bird housing during treatment

Housing should be heated to 20–26°C, dimly lit, and above all quiet. The cage used may be a standard aviary cage for pet species but should be sited away from predators such as cats in the clinic to avoid stress. The size of the cage should be sufficient to allow perching, a feeding and watering area and enough room for the bird to be able to stretch and move its wings in all three dimensions (minimum dimensions can be found in the UK under the Wildlife and Countryside Act 1981 as amended). For short-term purposes (1–2 days) the cage does not need to be much larger than this, as the bird may injure itself on the inside of the cage if frightened. For longer-term rehabilitation, purpose-built aviary flights are required which are large enough to allow short flights within them (see Figure 26.5). These are best constructed with a concrete floor with good drainage, wire mesh sides and wooden or steel post supports. A roosting box should be provided and the flights constructed out of the prevailing wind, and not in direct sun during the hotter part of the year. Waterfowl in rehabilitation will need access to a pond or pool, which brings its own problems when considering how to keep such an area clean. These pools ideally should be netted to prevent access from wild waterfowl which may be attracted to them.

Nestlings are a particular problem. They are best reared in small plastic containers lined with soft towelling or kitchen paper. Attention to supplemental heating is important and the use of incubators designed for domestic bird rearing or reptiles can be helpful (see Figure 26.6).

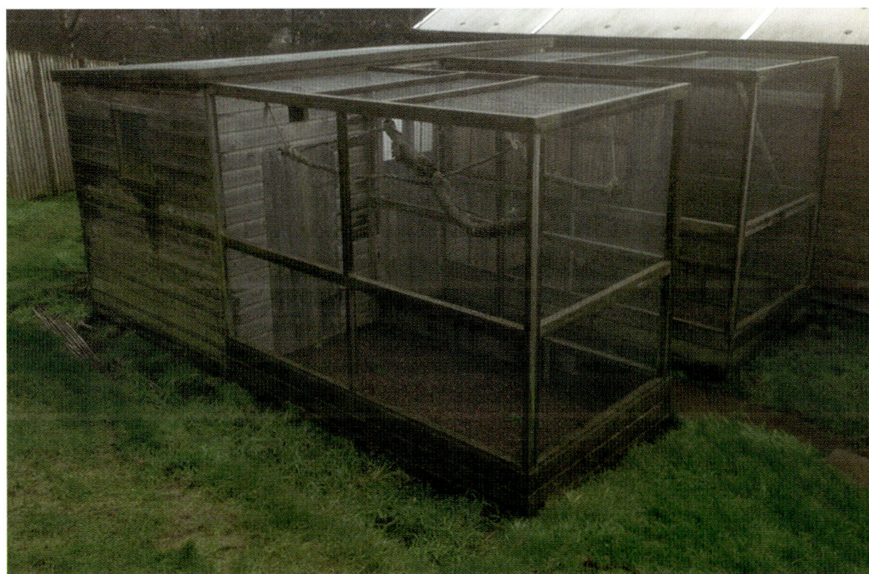

Figure 26.5 For rehabilitation and longer-term housing of wild birds, aviary flights are recommended to assess flying capabilities and progress to therapy.

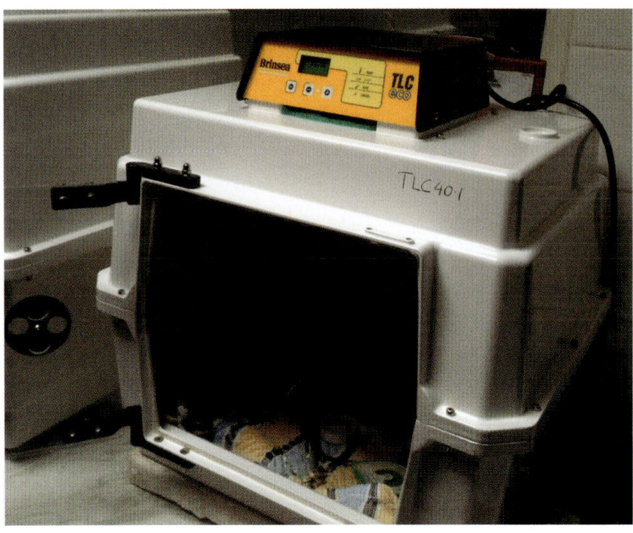

Figure 26.6 For neonates and chilled birds, the use of incubators available for domestic bird and reptiles can be invaluable.

NUTRITION

Classification

Carnivores

These include members of the mustelid, seal and wildcat family predominantly which will eat purely mammalian, avian or fish prey. Their dentition and digestive tracts are reflective of their diet with shearing premolars and molars and prominent canines as well as simple stomachs and short large intestines.

Herbivores

These include a variety of species such as deer, hares, rabbits and many wild rodents such as voles and beavers. They all have flat grinding premolars/molars, some of which are open rooted and grow continuously, and sharp incisors for cropping grass and herbage. They also possess dilated gastrointestinal systems to allow fermentation of plant material by bacteria to allow digestion of the cellulose contained therein, some being foregut fermenters (deer) and others hindgut (herbivorous rodents and lagomorphs).

Omnivores

These include species such as the red fox, which in addition to rodent and avian prey will also consume roots and berries and insects, as will the European badger. European hedgehogs will eat predominantly invertebrates and so are sometimes classified as insectivores but they will also eat fruit; similarly, squirrels will sometimes consume some birds' eggs and small rodents in addition to plants.

General nutritional requirements

Water

This is not so much a nutritional requirement but is of course a necessity. Its real importance lies in the quality of water provided. This should, in the best interests of hygiene, always be presented in a clean and unpolluted form. In addition, the method of provision should be considered as wild animals will not take water readily from sip feeders and so open-topped bowls should be provided.

The amount of water consumed by wild animals will obviously depend on the diets being offered in captivity. Those species offered and consuming dry biscuit or seed-based diets will consume more water than animals eating large amounts of fresh fruit and vegetables.

In the case of marine mammals such as seals, if they are hospitalised for a short period of time, a pool is not provided but more specialist facilities for longer-term rehabilitation may provide pools. If these are fresh water, then the addition of sodium chloride to their diet (often given as a so-called 'fish eater tablet') is required to replace salt lost.

Maintenance energy requirements

Basal metabolic rate (BMR) may be typically calculated from the following formula:

$$\mathrm{BMR} = k \times \left(\text{body weight}\left[\text{kg}\right]\right)^{0.75}$$

where k is a constant that varies from species to species and has been estimated at 70 for placental mammals as a whole. There is a degree of variation within this group though, with the smaller species having higher BMR constants. Lagomorphs have values around 100, hedgehogs nearer 200, and the smaller bats 350–400 when not hibernating. Values of 129 have been calculated for k for passerine wild birds in general.

BMR is the minimal energy requirement, and it is more useful to determine maintenance energy requirement (MER) and this is related crudely to BMR according to the formula:

$$\mathrm{MER} = 1.5 \times \mathrm{BMR}$$

It should be noted however that some forms of movement may increase the MER significantly, for example the flapping flight of birds (23× BMR) compared with gliding flight (3× BMR) (Barboza *et al.*, 2009). Species undergoing torpor/hibernation may of course have a reduction in their energy needs, although this is also highly variable, with brown bears reducing it to 73% of their BMR as they only reduce their core temperature to 35°C whereas Arctic ground squirrels reduce their core body temperature to 5°C and so reduce their energy requirements to 2.4% of their non-torpid BMR (Buck and Barnes, 2000).

Proteins

Proteins are assembled from groups of amino acids and for most mammals and birds 10 amino acids are essential and need to be provided in the diet, allowing the others to be manufactured from these 10, which are leucine, lysine, methionine, phenylalanine, threonine, tryptophan, isoleucine, valine, arginine, and histidine. In addition, it is known that with diets low in methionine or arginine, an extra supplement of glycine is required. Strict carnivores have a requirement for additional amino acids such as taurine.

Deer: Dietary protein varies from the predominantly grazing species such as red deer, fallow deer and Chinese water deer, which consume between 10 and 18% protein primarily from grasses, to species such as roe deer and muntjac deer which need 13–20% protein and obtain some significant proteins from shrubs and tree leaves (Wallach and Hoff, 1982).

Red foxes: Foxes have similar protein requirements to the domestic dog. As with the domestic dog, foxes are capable of utilising plant proteins as well as animal proteins. Levels overall of 22–25% have been recommended, and any commercial brand of tinned canine maintenance diet will suffice for adult foxes (Wallach and Hoff, 1982). Deficiencies may be seen in the wild due to poor availability of protein, which is mainly from rodent, lagomorph, avian and often insect sources. A dull coat and retarded growth rates and fertility will result. Taurine deficiencies can result in increased heart disease. In extreme cases death will ensue.

Wildcats: Their nutrition is basically similar to that of domestic cats with all of their protein coming from animal sources. Being a strict carnivore, they therefore have a need for several additional amino acids, including lysine and taurine, the latter at 500 mg/kg dry matter fed. Minimum levels of protein required are at 20% of the calorific intake, but for growth and reproduction levels of 30% or more are advised (Wallach and Hoff, 1982).

European badgers: This species is omnivorous and as such can utilise plant proteins as well as animal ones. Dietary protein sources and requirements resemble that for foxes.

Wild mustelids: These require a minimum of 25% (Wallach, 1970). Most commercial ferret diets have a range of 35–40% as protein. Any protein fed must be from an animal source as they are strict carnivores and plant proteins result in hyperammonaemia and neurological disease. Taurine and lysine are additional amino acids necessary in their diet. Taurine levels are unknown but assumed to be similar to those of felids (Kirkwood, 1992). Otters obtain most of their proteins from aquatic species, primarily fish and crustaceans. Martens, stoats and weasels get theirs from terrestrial rodents and small birds.

Seals (phocids): Protein levels are estimated around 40–80% of the diet on a dry matter basis and are derived from an animal source, primarily fish and occasionally crustaceans (Gili *et al.*, 2018).

Microchiropterans: Bats in northern Europe are insectivorous. They may be managed on mealworm-based diets which offer 30–35% protein levels and supplemented with other flying insects such as moths, and with mineral vitamin supplements (Constantine, 1993).

European hedgehogs: Most of the protein source of this species is derived from insects. Protein levels vary but 18–25% is recommended (Kirkwood, 1992). They are less able to utilise plant proteins and their main source of non-insect foods is fruit which frequently has extremely poor protein sources. The use again of a canine maintenance dry or tinned diet is recommended in captivity (dry food does have the advantage that it reduces food adhesion to the teeth and reduces periodontal disease which is common in hedgehogs).

Hares: These have similar requirements to those of domestic rabbits and squirrels, with 15% minimum crude protein levels being advised, all of which comes from a grass and herbage source.

Squirrels: Most of their protein sources are from seeds and foliage. Levels of proteins are estimated at a minimum of 15%, with a need for methionine and lysine, deficiencies of which could lead to alopecia and loss of coat colour (Sheldon, 1971).

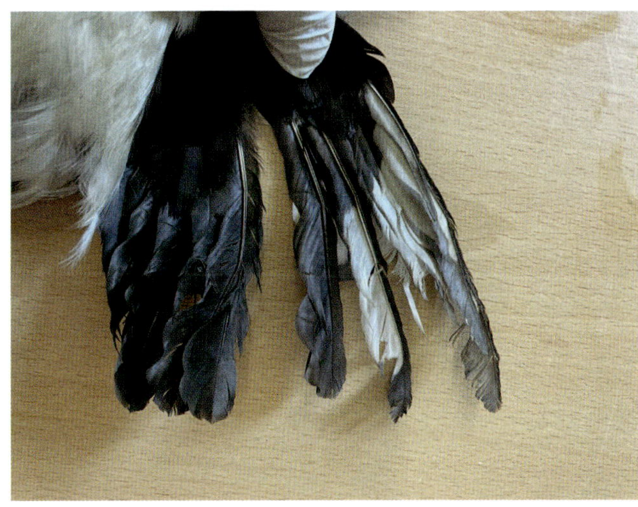

Figure 26.7 Feather abnormalities in wild birds can be due to amino acid deficiencies as seen here in a juvenile magpie.

Wild birds: The variation possible here is huge depending on whether the species is a raptor, passerine or gallinaceous, etc. Many passerines may well be able to cope with a 10–13% protein level from a plant source, but raptors and many seabirds require much higher protein levels from an animal source, needing additional amino acids such as taurine. Deficiencies in amino acids such as methionine, cysteine and lysine can lead to feather abnormalities (see Figure 26.7). See also Chapter 12 for further information on bird nutrient requirements.

Fats and essential fatty acids

Fats provide high concentrations of energy but also supply the animal with essential fatty acids (EFAs) which are required for cellular integrity and as the building blocks for cellular constituents such as prostaglandins which play a part in reproduction and inflammation.

Fats also provide a carrier mechanism for the absorption of fat-soluble vitamins such as vitamins A, D, E and K.

The primary EFA for mammals is linoleic acid as it is for birds, with the absolute minimum dietary requirement of this fatty acid being 1% of the diet. If the diet becomes deficient, a rapid decline in cellular integrity occurs, seen clinically as the skin becoming dry, flaky and prone to recurrent infections. Fluid loss through the skin also increases leading to polydipsia. Other EFAs thought to be important for strict carnivores (mustelids, wildcats, seals and raptors, etc.) include alpha-linolenic acid and arachidonic acid, necessary for some prostaglandin/eicosanoid production.

The problem of overconsumption of fats in wild animals producing obesity is hardly ever seen in the wild.

Deer: Additional dietary fat is not required by wild deer, the vegetable source of fats being sufficient at 2–5% (Wallach and Hoff, 1982). All EFAs can be made by fermentation of vegetable matter consumed by the gut microflora.

Wildcats: Dietary fat requirements are as for domestic cats with a need for an animal source of fat at levels of 20–25% in order to provide arachidonic, linolenic and linoleic acids.

Red foxes: Require similar levels to domestic dogs, which can be 10–15% of the diet (Wallach and Hoff, 1982). Foxes do not seem to have a definite need for arachidonic acid in their diets as true strict carnivores do, but linoleic and alpha-linolenic acids are needed.

European badgers: Require much the same types and levels of fats as foxes and domestic dogs.

Wild mustelids: These have the same high requirements as domestic cats, with a need for animal fats to provide both linoleic acid and arachidonic acid. There is some fluctuation in the fat levels, from 25% or so in the autumn to 20–22% in the winter/early spring, due to the changing fat levels in their rodent prey. Otters consume large volumes of fish oils, which are unsaturated and liquid at much lower temperatures than saturated mammal fats. This may cause a problem if otters are fed large amounts of rodent/mammal-based foods with subsequent constipation.

Seals (phocids): Fat levels of 25% are not uncommon in their diets and are chiefly presented as unsaturated fats in the form of fish oils. Large volumes of saturated fats may therefore cause digestive upsets.

Microchiropterans: Fat levels similar to those described for hedgehogs are advised, mealworms being a useful basis for diets offered in captivity and have a fat content of 10–18%. Other winged insects frequently have lower fat levels. There is no evidence that they can utilise vegetable fats.

European hedgehogs: Again, similar fat levels as those seen for domestic dogs of 10% dry matter are advised. In the wild these are derived from an insect source, but commercial adult maintenance canine diets seem to provide the necessary EFAs.

Hares: Diets do not need to be high in fats. The 2–5% vegetable fats found in forage are sufficient as microbial breakdown of complex carbohydrates occurs in the hindgut producing EFAs.

Squirrels: Diets as for rodents should contain a minimum of 1% fat as linoleic acid. Deficiencies are less likely if seeds/nuts are obtainable as the linoleic acids are present in large amounts in these food sources.

Wild birds: Dietary requirements of a minimum of 1% fat levels as linoleic acid are advised for passerines which is easily provided in seeds. Raptors and other carnivorous birds are likely to require additional fatty acids such as arachidonic and alpha-linolenic acids found in prey items.

Carbohydrates

Carbohydrates, as previously mentioned, are primarily used for rapid energy production. They may be presented in two main forms: in an easily digestible form such as the starch from plants or the glycogen from animals, or as more complex carbohydrates such as fibre/cellulose/hemicellulose fractions found in the structural parts of plants. The biology of species obviously influences the need for these carbohydrates, with strict carnivores unable to cope with large volumes of fibre unlike ruminant and hindgut-fermenting species. Lactose is rarely tolerated by adult animals, and indeed many juveniles, so should be avoided where possible.

Deer: Deer are supremely adapted to coping with large amounts of fibre in their diet. But this is not the same for all species, some being predominantly grazing animals and therefore consuming large amounts of grasses containing high-fibre, low-soluble carbohydrates, while others are more browsing in nature and have a lower-fibre diet.

- Red and sika deer: spend half their time grazing. They frequently require higher levels of food/calories in the October after the rutting season during which males do not eat and lose up to 15% of their body weight. Some root crops such as turnips, carrots, etc., will be taken in addition to hay or cattle/grass pellets.
- Fallow deer: spend more time grazing than browsing in the wild. Their diet is basically similar to that of red deer, but they will also take soft fruits.
- Roe deer: spend most of their time browsing. It seems their chief dietary intake is the leaves of shrubs and brambles, but will also consume acorns and chestnuts and will take root crops readily.
- Chinese water deer: spend most of their time grazing. Their diet is chiefly grass based but some root crops and cattle/grass pellets can be fed.
- Muntjac deer: will graze and browse and will take root crops and grains such as oats, wheat and maize. They tend not to take hay, preferring fresh grass and leaves.

Red foxes: As with domestic dogs, foxes can utilise a source of soluble carbohydrate present in vegetables, as well as the limited sources of glycogen in animal prey. No actual minimum requirement has been calculated, but a maximum of 65% of the diet has been suggested to avoid the displacement of essential fats and proteins from the diet (Wallach and Hoff, 1982). A commercial canine maintenance food is a perfectly acceptable source of carbohydrate. Fibre, although useful to prevent constipation, is not a dietary necessity.

Wildcats: Like domestic cats, wildcats do not need dietary fibre and need limited levels of dietary soluble carbohydrate. Blood glucose is manufactured from deamination of amino acids present in prey muscle protein (gluconeogenesis).

European badgers: The same principles as with foxes apply.

Wild mustelids: These species have very little requirement for carbohydrates other than those present as glycogen in their prey. They exhibit gluconeogenesis, being able to manufacture glucose from amino acids.

Seals (phocids): Carbohydrate sources in seals' prey are small, and their dietary requirements as adults seem small also.

Microchiropterans: Carbohydrate requirements for insectivorous bats would seem to be very small, as the levels found in their prey are similarly so.

European hedgehogs: Hedgehogs will eat some fruits, particularly in the autumn when they are most plentiful, and so fructose and other fruit carbohydrates seem to be tolerated. Levels of these have not been calculated and it has been generally assumed that their carbohydrate, protein and fat requirements are best satisfied by feeding a canine maintenance diet.

Hares: Hares like rabbits are hindgut fermenters and so have a dietary requirement for fibre, needing a minimum of 12–16% for normal dental wear and gut stimulation, as well as providing food for the gut microflora to ferment into fatty acids which the hare can then utilise for glucose production.

Squirrels: Carbohydrate levels similar to those in rodents apply, with a recommended level of 40–50% of the diet as carbohydrate, generally in the form of seeds and soluble sugars in young leaves/shoots.

Wild birds: Carbohydrate levels vary from almost nil in the case of raptors, to an important 40–50% in the case of seed-eating passerines. There is some requirement for fibre in species with fermenting caeca such as the red grouse which eats heather shoots predominantly.

Vitamins

These compounds are grouped together although they are widely differing in nature, but all animals have a requirement for various numbers of these vitamins. They comprise the fat-soluble vitamins (A, D, E and K) and the water-soluble vitamins (B vitamin complex and vitamin C).

Fat-soluble vitamins

Vitamin A

This vitamin comes in a variety of different forms, such as retinol, retinal and retinoic acid. In herbivores and omnivores the most important form, in terms of how much vitamin A can be produced from it, is beta-carotene, whereas in the case of strict carnivores such as mustelids, seals and wildcats, preformed animal vitamin A is needed.

Hypovitaminosis A can occur in species consuming a seed-heavy diet because seeds such as millet and sunflower are notoriously low providers of beta-carotenes. This is unlikely to happen in the wild but may occur in captivity, for example birds kept in rehabilitation for long periods. Deficiencies may also be seen by feeding strict carnivores on plant sources, and in herbivorous grazing species such as deer when the grass pastures have become dry and large amounts of dead/dying vegetation is seen. Vitamin A is required for a number of functions, from maintaining the function of the rods and cones in the retina to epithelial cellular turnover and keratinisation. If a relative deficiency in vitamin A occurs, then night blindness and thickening of mucous membranes can occur. Oral and respiratory secretions dry up due to blockage of salivary and mucous glands with cellular debris. This leads to poor functioning of the ciliary mechanisms in the airways that have a role in removing foreign particles. This, combined with vitamin A's role in immune system function, makes respiratory and digestive tract infections more common. Vitamin A also has a role in bone growth and structure as well as the function of secretory glands such as the adrenals and in reproductive function. Congenital deformities such as diaphragmatic hernias and cleft palates can be seen with deficiencies in carnivores and poor coat quality have also been reported in all species.

Because it is fat soluble, vitamin A can be stored in the body, primarily in the liver. Recommended minimum dietary levels are shown in Table 26.1 (Mitchell, 1967; Wallach and Hoff, 1982).

Hypervitaminosis A rarely occurs naturally but may be induced by overdosing with vitamin A injections at 1000 times or more the daily recommended doses. If this occurs, acute toxicity develops with mucous membrane and skin sloughing. Excessive doses in rats produced teratogenic effects.

Table 26.1 Recommended minimum dietary levels of vitamin A.

Deer	22 000–44 200 IU/kg feed offered (higher values for smaller deer)
Red foxes/badgers	99 IU/kg per day for adults and 198 IU/kg per day for growing canids
Seals (phocids)	25 000 IU/kg feed offered per day
Squirrels/hares	55 000 IU/kg feed offered or 7000 IU/kg body weight of hare
Wild birds	Levels of 8000 IU/kg feed offered per day for a minimum value in passerines

Vitamin D

Further information regarding vitamin D sources for small mammals and birds can be found in Chapters 4 and 12. Suffice to say, strict carnivores such as wildcats and mustelids must have preformed vitamin D_3 in their diet, being unable to manufacture it from plant sources via UV light action on the skin.

Hypovitaminosis D_3, as mentioned elsewhere, causes problems with calcium metabolism, and leads to conditions such as rickets. This is exacerbated by low calcium-containing diets, a typical sufferer being on an all-seed diet in the case of a rodent/squirrel with no UV-B exposure, or a diet composed entirely of skeletal meat and no calcium supplement in the case of a mustelid, wildcat, raptor or other strict carnivore. The animal can appear well muscled, but poorly mineralised bones and flaring of the epiphyseal plates at the ends of the long bones, with concomitant bowing of the limbs especially the tibial bones, can be seen in juveniles in particular. Typical requirements are 5.5–6.6 IU/kg body weight for a small ruminant and 4–5 IU/kg body weight for large ruminants (Wallach, 1970). Recommended maximum levels are 2000 IU/kg dry matter of food fed for most small mammals (Wallach and Hoff, 1982) but in rabbits, because of their efficient absorption of dietary calcium, maximum dietary levels of 1000–1300 IU/kg feed have been recommended (Mateos *et al.*, 2020).

Hypervitaminosis D_3 leads to calcification of soft tissues such as the medial walls of arteries resulting in hypertension, and affects the kidneys eventually causing organ failure. It is also possible to find the same condition in grazing stock consuming plants such as golden oat grass that contain a compound similar to vitamin D_3.

Vitamin E

This compound is found in several active forms in plants, the most active being alpha-tocopherol. It is important for cell wall integrity and mops up free radicals and peroxides produced during the metabolism of molecules such as polyunsaturated fats in the diet. To do this vitamin E is combined with a number of trace elements in enzymes, one of these being selenium in the metalloenzyme glutathione peroxidase. Vitamin E enhances immune system function and has positive effects on reproductive function.

Hypovitaminosis E can cause increased susceptibility to infection due to increased disruption of cells lining the gut and skin and

Table 26.2 Recommended minimum dietary levels of vitamin E.

Deer	55–176 IU/kg of food offered (higher doses for smaller deer)
Seals	50–100 IU/kg fish fed per day
Hares	89 IU/kg of food offered
Squirrels	40 IU/kg of food offered

respiratory system. Deficiency produces a condition known as white muscle disease, especially in deer associated with capture stress or trauma. In mustelids it leads to anasarca, and the formation of necrotic fat deposits under the skin along the ventrum. In canids such as the fox an association with myocardial damage has been shown. In seals, a retarded growth rate, alopecia, cessation of blubber development and muscular dystrophy has been reported. Hypovitaminosis E may occur due to a reduction in fat metabolism or absorption as can occur in small intestinal, pancreatic or biliary diseases, or due to a lack of green plant material, the chief source of the compound in the diet of herbivores. In some species such as otters and seals, the presence of large amounts of unsaturated fats in the diet from rancid fish, or fish such as herring, consume vitamin E at an accelerated rate and can induce relative deficiencies, necessitating higher levels of vitamin E in the diet. Freezing fish for prolonged periods of time increases the degradation of fats and depletes vitamin E.

Hypervitaminosis E is extremely rare.

Recommended minimum dietary levels of vitamin E are shown in Table 26.2 (Wallach and Hoff, 1982).

Vitamin K

There are three main sources of vitamin K precursors: green plants, bacteria and synthetic sources. Because of its production by bacteria, it is very difficult to observe a true deficiency, although absorption will again be reduced when fat digestion/absorption is reduced as in, for example, biliary or pancreatic disease. The consumption of compounds derived from warfarin and coumarin (as found in sweet clovers) can increase the demand for clotting factors, and may be seen in mustelids, wildcats and raptors consuming prey that has been poisoned by these rodenticides, an increasingly common occurrence. Disease caused is associated with increased clotting times and resultant haemorrhage, but vitamin K also has some function in calcium/phosphorus metabolism in the bones and this may also be affected at low levels of poisoning.

Water-soluble vitamins

Vitamin B$_1$ (thiamine)

Thiamine is found widely in plants and animal tissues alike. It is concerned with a number of cellular functions, one of which involves the integrity of the central nervous system (CNS).

Hypovitaminosis B$_1$ is uncommon, but the presence of thiaminases in the diet, particularly where raw saltwater fish is fed (e.g. to some raptors such as sea eagles and ospreys, and of course mammals such as otters and seals), can lead to a deficiency. Ruminant species consuming large amounts of grain produce an acid stomach fermentation that in turn produces thiaminases and so induces a deficiency. Thiamine antagonists are also present in some plant food sources, for example blackberries and beetroot. When a relative deficiency occurs, the neurological signs that result include ataxia, opisthotonus, weakness and head tremors. In mustelids and foxes the condition is known as Chastek paralysis and clinical signs may appear 2–4 weeks after exposure to the thiaminase due to its progressive damage on the myelin sheaths in the CNS.

Table 26.3 Recommended minimum dietary levels of vitamin B$_1$.

Foxes	0.013–0.017 mg/kg body weight per day
Wildcats	5.6 mg/kg dry matter of food fed as a minimum (assumed to be the same as domestic cats)
Mustelids	25.3–26.4 mg/kg fish fed
Rodents	6.6 mg/kg of diet fed minimum
Seals (phocids)	100–500 mg thiamine given per day per seal depending on size. NB: generally given in captivity whether deficient or not as frozen and defrosted fish are a high source of thiaminases
Hares/squirrels	Minimum 6.6 mg/kg dry matter of diet offered

Recommended minimum dietary levels are shown in Table 26.3 (Wallach and Hoff, 1982; National Research Council (NRC), 2006).

Vitamin B$_2$ (riboflavin)

This is present in many plants, where it is bound up in flavin complexes and in animal tissues. Little is present in seeds and so primarily seed-eating birds/rodents can become deficient. Supplementation can be achieved via commercial powder supplements or simple brewer's yeast.

Hypovitaminosis B$_2$ produces growth retardation, scaly dermatitis, muscular weakness, anaemia and purulent ocular discharge, as well as producing fetal deformities if deficient in early gestation. In small ruminants it may also cause erosions at the corners of the mouth as well as alopecia, growth retardation, diarrhoea and death. In rodents and lagomorphs it has been reported as causing cataracts in addition to the above signs. In canids such as the fox, deficiencies have been reported to cause fetal deformities if they occur in early gestation, such as shortening of the limbs and reduced/fused numbers of digits. In wildcats, fetal deformities, weight loss, alopecia over the head and occasional cataracts are seen. In birds it can cause medial toe curling in developing chicks.

Recommended minimum dietary levels are shown in Table 26.4 (Wallach, 1970; Wallach and Hoff, 1982; National Research Council (NRC), 2006).

Vitamin B$_3$ (niacin)

This B vitamin is found widely in many foods, but the form which occurs in plants has low availability to the bird. It is used to manufacture

Table 26.4 Recommended minimum dietary levels of vitamin B$_2$.

Deer	20–30 mg/kg body weight per day
Foxes	0.03–0.1 mg/kg per day or 4 mg/kg of food fed on a dry matter basis
Wildcats	0.2 mg per day per cat or 0.7 mg per 1000 cal fed
Rodents/lagomorphs	8.8–13 mg/kg of diet fed

Table 26.5 Recommended minimum dietary levels of vitamin B_3.

Foxes	0.66 mg/kg body weight
Wildcats	60 mg/kg diet fed as dry matter
Rodents/lagomorphs	37–53 mg/kg diet fed as dry matter
Wild birds	50 ppm (50 mg/kg) of diet fed as dry matter

the coenzymes nicotinamide adenine dinucleotide (NAD) and nicotinamide adenine dinucleotide phosphate (NADP) which are required for many cellular metabolic processes. Birds or animals fed a high proportion of one type of seed, such as waterfowl overfed on sweetcorn, can become deficient with blackening of the tongue (pellagra) and oral mucosa, retarded growth, poor feather quality in birds, a lowered packed cell volume, diarrhoea and scaly dermatitis.

Recommended minimum dietary levels are shown in Table 26.5 (Wallach and Cooper, 1982; Wallach and Hoff, 1982; National Research Council (NRC), 2006).

Vitamin B_5 (pantothenic acid)

This B vitamin is needed to produce a compound known as acetyl coenzyme A which is vital for the entry of glucose and amino acids into the citric acid cycle (the chemical process whereby glucose is converted to the energy currency adenosine triphosphate or ATP which can be utilised by cells). It is found widely in plants and animals and so deficiency again rarely occurs. In birds deficiencies lead to crusting of the feet, eyelids and commissures of the beak, poor feather growth and general epidermal desquamation. In rodents and lagomorphs weight loss, hepatic lipidosis, diarrhoea, ataxia and alopecia occur. In canids diarrhoea, coat problems and terminal collapse, coma and death can occur especially in growing animals.

Recommended minimum dietary levels are shown in Table 26.6 (Wallach and Cooper, 1982; Wallach and Hoff, 1982; National Research Council (NRC), 2006).

Vitamin B_6 (pyridoxine)

This is a group of three compounds: pyridoxal is found in plants predominantly, with pyridoxamine and pyridoxal phosphate being found in animal tissues. The active form of B_6 is pyridoxal phosphate, which is vital for all areas of amino acid metabolism. Hence a deficiency, if it should occur, will result in retarded growth, hyperexcitability, convulsions, twisted neck and polyneuritis. Deficiencies have occurred in canids on a diet high in methionine as it is needed to metabolise this amino acid. In canids it has been shown to produce a microcytic hypochromic anaemia, with iron build-up in liver, spleen and bone marrow to the point where actual damage occurs (a condition known as haemosiderosis).

Table 26.6 Recommended minimum dietary levels of vitamin B_5.

Canids/felids	10 mg/kg of diet fed as dry matter
Rodents/ lagomorphs	15–22 mg/kg of diet fed as dry matter
Wild birds	20 ppm (20 mg/kg) for passerines of diet fed as dry matter

Table 26.7 Recommended minimum dietary levels of vitamin B_6.

Canids/felids	4 mg/kg of diet fed as dry matter or 0.1 mg/kg per day in wildcats
Rodents/ lagomorphs	6–14.15 ppm (6–14.15 mg/kg) of diet fed as dry matter
Wild birds	6 ppm (6 mg/kg) of diet fed as dry matter in passerines (watch toxicity issues in strict carnivores such as raptors)

A similar anaemia occurs in wildcats with a dietary deficiency, anaemia by this means being commoner than due to an iron deficiency. This is because raw meat diets are high in iron, but generally low in pyridoxine. Wildcats may also develop calcium oxalate urolithiasis. A deficiency is difficult to achieve.

Recommended minimum dietary levels are shown in Table 26.7 (Wallach and Cooper, 1982; Wallach and Hoff, 1982; National Research Council (NRC), 2006).

Vitamin B_7 (biotin)

This B vitamin is again widely distributed in animal and plant feeds, but at low levels. The digestive bacterial flora also produces biotin. True deficiencies are therefore rare. Biotin is responsible for preventing cellular degradation by helping form compounds which bind carbon dioxide in the body. Deficiencies can occur due to the antivitamin avidin, present in the albumen of raw unfertilised eggs of birds and amphibians.

Overconsumption of these foods produces exfoliative dermatitis, alopecia and ataxia, and toes may become gangrenous and slough off.

Recommended minimum dietary levels are shown in Table 26.8 (Wallach and Cooper, 1982; Wallach and Hoff, 1982; National Research Council (NRC), 2006).

Vitamin B_9 (folic acid)

Folates are widespread in foods and are necessary for the formation of three of the four nucleic acids which make DNA. A deficiency therefore leads to severely impaired cellular division. This can lead to a number of obvious problems such as non-maturation of the female reproductive tract, a macrocytic anaemia due to failure of red blood cell maturation and cellular dysfunction of the immune system. It can also lead to embryo toxicity and hydrocephalus if deficiencies occur in early gestation in rodents and lagomorphs and to cleft palates in canids. In addition, there are inhibitors of folic acid in some foods such as cabbage and other brassicas, oranges, beans and peas, and the use of trimethoprim sulfonamide drugs also reduces gut bacterial folic acid production.

Table 26.8 Recommended minimum dietary levels of vitamin B_7.

Canids/felids	0.07 ppm (0.07 mg/kg) of diet fed as dry matter
Rodents/ lagomorphs	0.12–0.34 ppm (0.12–0.34 mg/kg) of diet fed as dry matter
Wild birds	0.25 ppm (0.25 mg/kg) of diet fed as dry matter for passerines

Table 26.9 Recommended minimum dietary levels of vitamin B_9.

Canids/felids	0.8–1 ppm (0.8–1 mg/kg) of diet fed as dry matter
Rodents/ lagomorphs	1–4.4 ppm (1–4.4 mg/kg) of diet fed as dry matter
Wild birds	1.5 ppm (1.5 mg/kg) for passerines, of diet fed as dry matter

Recommended minimum dietary levels are shown in Table 26.9 (Wallach and Cooper, 1982; Wallach and Hoff, 1982; National Research Council (NRC), 2006).

Vitamin B_{12}

This is produced generally by intestinal bacteria and so deficiencies are uncommon but may occur iatrogenically after prolonged antibiotic medication. Vitamin B_{12} is required for many metabolic pathways and neurological function, and a deficiency may cause a deficiency in folic acid. Deficiencies produce slow growth, muscular dystrophy in the legs, renal atrophy, anaemia, anorexia, poor hatching rates, high mortality rates in young birds, and hatching deformities.

Recommended minimum dietary levels are shown in Table 26.10 (Wallach and Cooper, 1982; Wallach and Hoff, 1982; National Research Council (NRC), 2006).

Choline

Choline may be synthesised in the body, but not in sufficient quantities for the growing bird. Choline is essential for four functions: the formation of cell membranes, the maturing of the cartilage precursor of bone, for fat metabolism by the liver, and for the formation of the neurotransmitter acetylcholine. The need for choline is dependent on levels of folic acid and vitamin B_{12}. Excess protein or high-fat diets, as with folic acid, also increases choline requirements. Deficiencies cause retarded growth, disrupted fat metabolism, fatty liver damage in many species and perosis (slipping of the Achilles tendon off the intertarsal joint groove) in birds.

Recommended minimum dietary levels are shown in Table 26.11 (Wallach and Cooper, 1982; Wallach and Hoff, 1982; National Research Council (NRC), 2006).

Vitamin C

There is no direct need for this vitamin in birds other than one or two wild species (the red-vented bulbul and the willow ptarmigan) as vitamin C may be produced from glucose in the liver. A similar state exists for terrestrial mammals in the UK. However, during disease processes, particularly those which affect liver function, it may be beneficial to the recovery process to provide a dietary source of vitamin C. It is required

Table 26.10 Recommended minimum dietary levels of vitamin B_{12}.

Canids/felids	0.02–0.05 ppm (0.02–0.05 mg/kg) of diet fed as dry matter
Rodents/ lagomorphs	11–66 ppm (11–66 mg/kg) of diet fed as dry matter
Wild birds	0.01 ppm (0.01 mg/kg) in passerines of diet fed as dry matter

Table 26.11 Recommended minimum dietary levels of choline.

Canids/felids	1200 ppm (1200 mg/kg) of diet fed as dry matter
Rodents/ lagomorphs	880–1540 ppm (880–1540 mg/kg) of diet fed as dry matter
Wild birds	1500 ppm (1500 mg/kg) for passerines of diet fed as dry matter

for the formation of elastic fibres and connective tissues and is an excellent antioxidant similar to vitamin E. Deficiencies lead to scurvy where there is poor wound healing, increased bleeding due to capillary wall fragility and bone alterations.

Minerals

There are two main groups of minerals: macrominerals (i.e. those present in large amounts in the body such as calcium and phosphorus) and microminerals, also called trace elements, such as manganese, iron and cobalt, which are all necessary for normal bodily function.

Macrominerals

Calcium

Calcium has a wide range of bodily functions, the two most obvious being its role in the formation of the skeleton/mineralisation of bone matrix, and its requirement for muscular function. The active form of calcium in the body is the ionic double charged molecule Ca^{2+}. Low levels of this form, even though the overall body reserves of calcium are normal, leads to hyperexcitability, fitting and death.

Calcium levels in the body are controlled by vitamin D_3, parathyroid hormone and calcitonin. Low blood calcium causes release of parathyroid hormone from the parathyroid glands, which activates vitamin D_3 and stimulates increased calcium reabsorption from the kidneys at the expense of phosphorus, increases calcium absorption from the small intestine, and increases calcium mobilisation from bone reserves. Conversely, high blood calcium causes a release of calcitonin from the C cells of the thyroid which reduces kidney reabsorption of calcium and increases phosphorus retention and increases calcium deposition into the bone matrix.

The dietary ratio of calcium to phosphorus is therefore important: as one increases, the other decreases and vice versa. A dietary ratio of 2 : 1 calcium to phosphorus is therefore desirable in growing animals, and 1.5 : 1 for adults. However, in high egg-laying periods in birds and lactation in mammals, to keep pace with the output of calcium into shells and milk, respectively, a ratio of 10 : 1 may be needed. However, excessive calcium in the diet (>1%) reduces the use of proteins, fats, phosphorus, manganese, zinc, iron and iodine.

In seals (phocids) calcium deficiency is seen particularly in growing pups fed filleted fish or marine crustaceans without shells. Easily fractured and deformed limbs, difficulty moving and triple-phosphate uroliths are all seen with this condition in seals. In wildcats and mustelids, calcium deficiency is also a common problem for the same reason, that meat is a poor source of calcium on its own. In captive squirrels fed a high-sunflower-seed diet poor in calcium showed fibrous osteodystrophy, tooth loss and malocclusion problems. Persistent low levels of calcium will result in nutritional secondary hyperparathyroidism, with resultant elevated parathyroid hormone levels, parathyroid hypertrophy, bone demineralisation, renal disease and pathological fractures, paresis and paralysis.

Phosphorus

Phosphorus is, as with calcium, utilised in bones, but it is also used as the key component in the storage of energy as ATP, and as part of the structure of cell membranes. It is widespread in plants and animal tissues, but in the former may be bound up in unavailable forms as phytates. Levels of phosphorus are controlled in the body as for calcium, the two being in equal and opposite equilibrium with each other. Therefore, if dietary levels exceed calcium levels appreciably (a maximum of twice the calcium levels has been quoted), the parathyroid glands become stimulated to produce more parathyroid hormone and nutritional secondary hyperparathyroidism occurs which leads to progressive bone demineralisation and renal damage due to high circulating levels of parathyroid hormone. High dietary phosphorus also reduces the amount of calcium which can be absorbed from the gut as it complexes with the calcium present there. This can be a big problem in raptors, wildcats, mustelids and canids fed pure meat and no calcium/bone supplement, and in passerines/ruminants which are fed predominantly on seeds and cereals rather than herbage/grass as the former are high-phosphorus, low-calcium foods. Green vegetables or supplementation with calcium powders, or the practice of feeding whole mammalian/avian/fish prey to carnivores may therefore be necessary.

Lack of phosphorus in deer may result in reduced appetite and osteoporosis (weakening of the mineralised structure of the bones), with spontaneous fractures, damage to joint surfaces, abnormal feeding behaviour (pica) and paresis or ataxia.

Magnesium

Most of the magnesium in the body is bound up in the bone matrix. However, it is also essential for phosphorus transfer in the formation of ATP and cell membranes in soft tissues such as the liver. Most magnesium is absorbed in the small intestine and is affected by large amounts of calcium in the diet, which reduce magnesium absorption. Excessive levels in wildcats result in urolithiasis and urethral obstruction in males. A condition similar to 'staggers' in dairy cattle may be seen in the grazing species of deer (red, fallow) at certain times of the year when grass magnesium levels are low (autumn and early spring). This is typified by hyperexcitability, nervous muscle tremors and, in severe cases, collapse, fitting and death. Deficiencies in rodents and lagomorphs result in seizures and mineral precipitates in soft tissues, particularly the kidneys. Recommended levels are 8–10 mg/day for wildcats and a minimum of 0.6 g per 45.4 kg body weight in ruminants such as deer or 2 g/kg dry matter fed (Church, 1971; National Research Council (NRC), 2006).

Potassium

As with mammals this is the major intracellular positive ion, essential for maintaining membrane potentials; it is also the principal intracellular cation affecting acid–base reactions and osmotic pressure. Rarely is there a dietary deficiency, but severe stress can cause hypokalaemia due to increased kidney excretion of potassium due to elevated plasma proteins, which can lead to cardiac dysrhythmias, muscle spasticity, reduced appetite, shortened fur growth and neurological dysfunction. It is present in high amounts in certain fruits such as bananas and is controlled in the body in equilibrium with sodium under the influence of the adrenal hormone aldosterone, which promotes sodium retention and potassium excretion. Recommended minimum levels are 0.4% in passerines, 0.8–1.19% in rodents and lagomorphs and 80–200 mg/day in wildcats (Wallach and Cooper, 1982; Wallach and Hoff, 1982; National Research Council (NRC), 2006).

Sodium

This is the main extracellular positive ion and regulates the body's acid–base balance and osmotic potential. In conjunction with potassium, it is responsible for nerve signals/impulses. Rarely does a true dietary deficiency occur, but hyponatraemia may occur due to chronic diarrhoea or renal disease. This disrupts the osmotic potential gradient in the kidneys and water is lost leading to further dehydration. In canids, sodium deficiency leads to weight loss, dry skin, alopecia and death in 8 weeks. Recommended levels for canids are 0.33 g/kg body weight per day. In seals (phocids), however, relative sodium deficiencies are not uncommon, particularly if they are kept in fresh water. This results in leaching of sodium from the body. In addition, the practice of defrosting frozen fish in fresh water further reduces their salt content and contributes to sodium deficiencies. This leaching of sodium from the seal's body also takes with it body water and leads to dehydration. It is therefore necessary to add sufficient salt to the water to raise the sodium chloride levels to 3%, or to supplement the diet with sodium chloride at 3 g/kg food fed per day or even as high as 5.5% or 5.5 g/kg dry matter of food fed (Wallach and Hoff, 1982; Gili *et al.*, 2018). Other problems such as persistent conjunctivitis and corneal opacities will occur if the seal is kept in fresh water. Deficiencies may occur in deer where large amounts of cereals such as bran and oats are used without supplementing with a 0.5% salt ration.

Excessive levels of sodium in the diet (greater than 10 times the recommended 0.12% levels) lead to poor feathering, polyuria, hypertension, enteritis, oedema, neurological confusion and death in non-marine birds.

Chlorine

This is the major extracellular negative ion and is responsible for maintaining acid–base balance in conjunction with sodium and potassium. Deficiencies are rare outside the above-mentioned problems with seals, with 0.12% minimum requirements being advocated.

Trace elements

Cobalt

Cobalt deficiency may cause pernicious anaemia in canids (as does vitamin B_{12} deficiency) and may occur due to tapeworm damage to the small intestine where absorption occurs. In ruminant species such as deer, cobalt is needed for the synthesis of vitamin B_{12}, and deficiencies therefore lead to anorexia, anaemia and death. Levels of 0.055 mg/kg body weight per day in canids and 0.2–1 mg per 45 kg per day in deer have been quoted (Wallach and Hoff, 1982).

Copper

Copper is used for haemoglobin synthesis, collagen synthesis and the maintenance of the nervous system. Signs of deficiency include chronic anaemia/weakness, limb deformities/enlarged joints and hyperexcitability. In deer, coat abnormalities, as seen in cattle, with pale/light colouration of previously dark coats, particularly around the eyes (achromotrichia), and hindlimb ataxia similar to that seen in sheep ('swayback') have been reported and are more likely to occur in parts of the country where high molybdenum is present as this mineral can prevent copper absorption (Suttle, 2022). A milder form of the latter condition is thought to cause the excessive pacing seen in many captive exotic ruminants with copper deficiencies. Copper toxicity, on the other hand, will cause serious liver damage and jaundice. Recommended minimum requirements are 8 ppm in passerines, 13–20 ppm in rodents and lagomorphs, 17 ppm in deer and 10 mg/kg of dry matter fed in canids and felids (Wallach and Cooper, 1982; Wallach and Hoff, 1982; National Research Council (NRC), 2006).

Iodine

Iodine's sole function is in the synthesis of thyroid hormones, which affect metabolic rate. Deficiencies cause goitre which can have knock-on effects including reduced growth, stunting, abortions and neurological problems. Deficiencies can occur in herbivores fed large amounts of plants containing goitrogens, which interfere with iodine uptake, such as many brassica vegetables and pastures sprayed with nitrogen fertilisers. In canids, the incidence of thyroid adenocarcinomas is increased in cases of iodine deficiency. Levels of 0.6–2.2 ppm for rodents and lagomorphs and 1.5 mg/kg of diet for canids and felids have been quoted (National Research Council (NRC), 2006).

Iron

This is essential, as with mammals, for the formation of the oxygen-carrying part of the haemoglobin molecule. Absorption from the gut is normally relatively poor, as the body is very good at recycling its iron. In carnivores, deficiencies are rare, but can occur in the wild if the diet has been based on poor-quality white meat. A hypochromic anaemia is seen in these cases, with clinical lethargy. Levels of 200–350 ppm have been quoted for rodents and lagomorphs.

Manganese

This is primarily found in plant materials but is often present in unavailable forms. Efficient bile salt production is required for its absorption, so animals with hepatic/biliary dysfunction are at a disadvantage. Manganese is necessary for normal bone structure among other things and so dietary/functional deficiencies are shown by swelling and flattening of the lateral condyles of the intertarsal joint that allows the Achilles tendon to slip out of the groove created for it in passerines and raptors, and a shortening of long bones and poor growth in mammals. Recommended minimum requirements are 65 ppm in passerines, 40–120 ppm in rodents and lagomorphs and 7.5 mg/kg for canids and felids (Wallach and Hoff, 1982; National Research Council (NRC), 2006).

Selenium

Selenium's main role is as a constituent of the antioxidant enzyme glutathione peroxidase, vitamin E also being involved with the functions of this enzyme. The functions of selenium are therefore similar to those of vitamin E in that it helps neutralise peroxidases from attacking polyunsaturated fats in cell membranes. Therefore, there is some functional crossover and one compound will cover for a deficiency in the other. If, however, there is a general deficiency in both, a condition known as exudative diathesis will occur in birds. This is where oedema forms on the neck, wings and breast as the smaller blood vessels become more 'leaky' and fluid moves out into the subcutaneous spaces. This is often followed by stunted growth, limb weakness and death. In rodents and lagomorphs, liver necrosis has been reported, and in seals and deer the nutritional 'white muscle disease' is seen as described in the section on vitamin E. The selenium content of plants is dependent on where they are grown and the levels of selenium in the soil. Recommended minimum requirements are 0.1 ppm for passerines. Excessive levels of selenium (>100 mg/kg of dry matter fed) can cause ataxia, alopecia, fetal abnormalities and the loss of hooves in ruminants such as deer.

Zinc

This is a vital trace element for wound healing and tissue formation, being a constituent of a number of enzymes. Deficiencies can occur in young rapidly growing herbivores fed on plant material high in phytates, such as cabbage, wheat bran, beans and legume-based hay, particularly in deer. In addition, high dietary calcium decreases zinc uptake. Deficiencies produce retarded growth, poor feathering and enlarged intertarsal joints in birds, vomiting, conjunctivitis, dermatitis due to hyperkeratosis and teratogenesis. Minimum recommended requirements are 50 ppm in passerines, 20–122 ppm in rodents and lagomorphs, and 0.22 mg/kg/day in canids (Wallach and Hoff, 1982; Kollias and Kollias, 2010).

Requirements for young and lactating wildlife

Deer

A sheep milk replacer such as Lamlac® or Volostrum® (Volac Ltd) has been used with success in red deer to wean calves. It may be fed from proprietary lamb/calf or human infant bottles. Deficiencies of vitamin D_3 and magnesium have been seen in bottle-reared calves. The former will lead to bone growth retardation and possible deformities, the latter to the condition described above known as 'staggers'.

Lactating females experience a 1.5–2.5 times increase in maintenance energy requirements. Heavily pregnant females may suffer from pregnancy ketosis, particularly if they are fed on very coarse dry grasses only and are carrying more than one calf. This provides too little in the way of calories and the hind draws heavily on her fat reserves for energy. This fat mobilisation is then converted into glucose by the liver. However, for this to occur there must be glucose already in the body, and if there is not, as with this poor diet, the fats are converted into ketones. These create a state of metabolic acidosis, signs of which include anorexia, depression and unconsciousness. The hind affected may abort in an attempt to survive. Protein levels for the hind should also be around 18% to ensure the healthy growth of the calf during gestation and lactation.

Red foxes

Requirements for lactating vixens are approximately three times those needed for maintenance. Included in this is the need for greater supplies of calcium (the ratio of calcium to phosphorus should be 2 : 1 at this time) or eclampsia will occur. A feline growth diet for captive nutrition should therefore be considered, almost on an ad-libitum basis at this time, for its increased fat and calcium levels.

For unweaned fox cubs the requirements for a milk replacer most closely match those already available for the domestic cat. Feeding regimens mimic those devised for kittens, with 2-hourly feeding needed for the first few days, followed by a reduction to feeds every 4–5 hours by day 5, and every 6–8 hours by day 10. Weaning can be attempted at 5–6 weeks of age. Deficiencies in vitamin A can occur in young growing canids, with recommended levels being 198 IU/kg per day, otherwise there is an increased risk of gut and respiratory infections, along with stunted growth and development of hydrocephalus. Deficiencies are also seen in calcium, with a calcium/phosphorus ratio of 2 : 1 needing to be provided during early growth. The main problems with rearing the young of any wild species is the unnatural bond that forms between human and wild animal. This will severely reduce the chances of successful re-release of the fox cubs into the wild once fully weaned. A method that could be useful when rearing weaned fox cubs is to use proprietary domestic feline growth diets, fed in situ, but to allow the cubs to come and go as they please. Eventually as they become more adventurous, they will make fewer returns to the area for supplementary feeding and eventually will desert the den altogether.

Wildcats

Kittens of wildcats are weaned at 4–5 weeks of age. The milk replacer used logically would be the same as for domestic cats, with the same feeding pattern: every 2 hours for the first few days, dropping to every 4 hours for the first 10–14 days, and then four to five times daily until weaning. Kitten feeding bottles may be used for this purpose. Deficiencies in growing kittens include hypovitaminosis D_3, particularly at weaning when the young kitten cannot cope with whole prey and therefore only consumes the meat portion. Nutritional secondary hyperparathyroidism may ensue with concomitant poor calcium levels in as little as 30 days in a growing felid. Another deficiency is lack of iron and copper in kittens on unsupplemented all-milk diets. The minimum iron requirement is 5 mg/day and copper 0.2 mg/day.

European badgers

Esbilac® (Pet-Ag Inc.) has been used successfully to rear badger cubs with four to five feeds during the day being appropriate.

When attempting to wean badgers, the use of feline/canine proprietary growth/juvenile formulas has been advocated and this may be attempted at 8–10 weeks of age. This should be offered in the accommodation from which they may be released, preferably with other badger cubs. The cubs would, from the age of 3–4 months, be taken on expeditions away from the setts to forage for food, so attempts to mimic this should be tried in order that rehabilitation can be attempted.

Badgers should be reared with other badger cubs of the same or similar age as solitary hand-reared cubs frequently develop stereotypies such as limb sucking and fur chewing and can become overly tame which may lead to increased human conflict post release.

Wild mustelids

Esbilac (Pet-Ag Inc.) has again been used successfully to rear most small mustelids (Stocker, 2005). Weaning occurs in otters around 9–10 weeks, and around 5–6 weeks in most other mustelids. Higher levels of calcium, protein and fat are required for the mothers during lactation, and nutritional secondary hyperparathyroidism is common shortly after weaning if an all-meat diet is fed. Otters can be weaned onto a blenderised white-fish and milk replacer soup fed from a spoon. Addition of multivitamins (so-called 'fish eater' tablets) that contain vitamins A, E, D_3 and B_1 are typically added to the mix.

Seals (phocids)

Weaning may be performed from 4 weeks in the common seal and 15–17 days in the grey seal. A common clinical presentation in young seals is hypoglycaemia. This occurs most commonly in the very young pup which has been unable to suckle from its mother or receive the correct milk replacer. Initial signs are violent muscle rigidity and seizures, but death can rapidly ensue.

Treatment requires intraperitoneal injections of concentrated glucose solution. Prevention is to ensure that any pup at risk gets a rapid feed of a good-quality milk replacer. The latter can be difficult as seals have a poor tolerance of the lactose levels present in cows' milk. The common and grey seals are also better fed by gavage methods, which involves opening the seal's mouth and using a narrow-necked bottle and a mouth-gag pouring the formula into the back of the mouth. An alternative is to stomach tube the seal as described below. A good milk replacer powder is Multimilk® which is manufactured by the company Pet-Ag Inc. (Gage, 1993). Alternatively, a blended mixture of whipping cream (pretreated with a lactase enzyme to remove the lactose), whole fish, glucose solution, a mineral and vitamin supplement and safflower oil can be prepared, but it must be made fresh each day.

Microchiropterans

Again, a higher fat content than is found in cows' milk is advised; therefore the recommendation is to use a milk replacer such as Lamlac (Volac Ltd.) or one part full-fat cows' milk to three parts condensed milk, and then to add 6–7 g of skimmed milk powder to bring up the protein levels. When initially obtained, orphaned bats are frequently dehydrated and so initial feeds should concentrate on oral rehydration/electrolyte therapy. Once 24 hours has elapsed, the oral dog/cat electrolyte solution may be mixed in a four parts electrolyte to one part Lamlac formula, and dropper fed every 2 hours or so.

Stocker (2005) advises the use of Esbilac (Pet-Ag Inc.) one part powder to one part hot water and recommends that the bat remains at an environmental temperature of 25–30°C to aid digestion. The use of eyedropper pipettes or a paint brush is advised for feeding purposes as commercial cat/dog feeders are often too large. Milk feeding needs to occur for approximately 3 weeks from birth, which is the time the young bats start to fly but mealworms have been offered from 1 week of age blended with the milk formula (Constantine, 1993). It is important when changing to an all-mealworm/insect diet to supplement this with a calcium mineral and vitamin-containing powder on a daily basis.

Once bats have survived their first week on such a regimen, then solid insect foods such as small winged insects (e.g. the fruit fly *Drosophila* spp.) or mealworms may be blended into the formula a little more each day until it reaches a consistency which has to be fed on the end of a small spatula as it is too thick to go through a feeder.

Once this has been achieved at around 3 weeks, mealworms and winged insects including small moths may be hand fed to the young bat via a pair of forceps. It is often recommended that a drop of supplement such as BSP Vitamin Drops® or Avimix® (VetArk) is added every third day.

European hedgehogs

A useful milk substitute has been quoted as two parts goats' milk and one part goats' colostrum (Kirkwood, 1992) but understandably this may not be easy to source. Esbilac (Pet-Ag Inc.) supplemented for the first 3 weeks of life with a feline colostrum replacer in a ratio of 3 : 1 has also been suggested as sufficient (Stocker, 2005). Feeding frequency should be once every 2–3 hours in hedgehogs under a week of age dropping to once every 4–5 hours by week 2. Weaning can be tried from 21 days of age, roughly when teeth start to appear.

Hares

Leverets are very precocial, and are born with their eyes open, unlike rabbits. Their milk replacer needs are similar though, and a rough approximation may be achieved by using one-quarter full-fat cows' milk to three-quarters condensed milk, and to this adding 6 g skimmed milk powder per 100 mL made up to increase the protein content. This may be fed three to four times during the day, unlike rabbits which are frequently only fed once or twice. Alternatively, a mixture of one part Esbilac to two parts water can be fed. Feeding times are typically two to three times per day. The use of commercially available probiotics/prebiotics for domestic rabbits can help establish the gut flora.

Squirrels

Again, as with badgers, a milk replacer with a higher fat content such as Lamlac, or Volostrum (Volac Ltd.) should be considered. The use of puppy/kitten feeding nipples/syringes is easiest and the young may be kept in a darkened container with hay and a heat source such as a heat mat or hot water bottle/glove. The latter must be well protected from the young to prevent accidental burns. For very young squirrels, syringing every 3–4 hours is needed for the first 10–14 days. Weaning can be performed gradually onto a seed/pelleted rodent mix at 7–8 weeks of age. Stocker (2005) advises that milk-fed squirrels should be encouraged to lean forward or stand on all four feet to prevent too rapid consumption of milk resulting in bloat. At less than a week of age, feeding takes place every 2–3 hours, dropping to every 4 hours by 2 weeks of age and then four times daily by 3 weeks of age.

Wild birds

Young growing birds have a moderately high requirement for protein as an energy source, with Wallach and Cooper (1982) suggesting levels ranging from 17% in ducks and geese, 18% in raptors up to 30% in pheasants (see Figure 26.8).

Stocker (2005) recommends using a commercial food (Tropican Rearing Mix®, Hagen) for small garden birds such as buntings, tits, wrens, sparrows, etc., as well as Columbiformes and has created a homemade recipe for larger wild bird chicks (thrushes, corvids, starlings, woodpeckers, cuckoos, nuthatches) comprising:

- One tin Pedigree Chum Puppy Food®
- Water (volume equal to the above dog food tin)

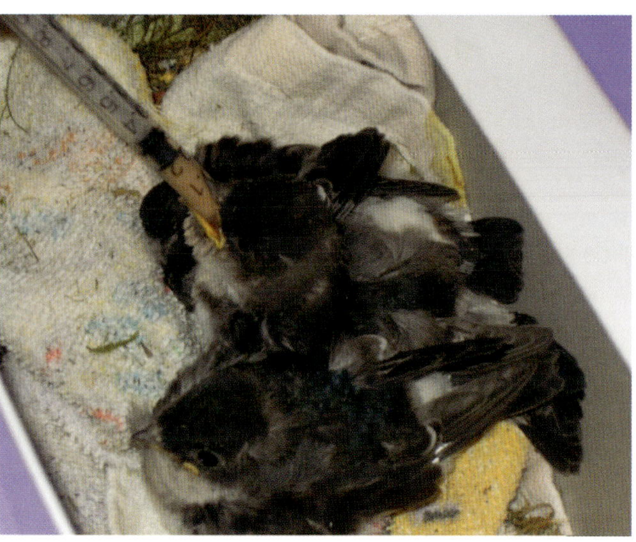

Figure 26.8 Syringe feeding juvenile swallows. Attention should be paid to hygiene with regular removal of faeces, and in altricial passerines removing the faecal sac post feeding.

- Dried insects (Prosecto®, Haith) (volume equal to the above dog food tin)
- Pinch of Pancrex-Vet® enzyme (Pharmacia Animal Health)
- Pinch of AviPro Paediatric® (VetArk Professional) probiotic/prebiotic.

This can be premixed and frozen. When fed it is often fed chilled to avoid spoilage; this appears not to cause any digestive issues for the hatchlings but avoids bacterial overgrowth and spoilage (Stocker, 2005).

Raptor chicks are more dependent on their parents and will require feeding with strips of raw meat supplemented with a calcium/vitamin/mineral supplement (e.g. Avimix®, VetArk) on a daily basis until they are 5–6 weeks old or older depending on the species.

Precocial omnivorous or carnivorous birds may be offered live insect feed to stimulate hunting activity. Altricial passerine birds will tend to produce a faecal sac from the vent (faeces wrapped in a clear sac) as soon as the crop is full; this should be removed. Once removed, the bird can immediately be fed again.

Requirements for debilitated wildlife

In all cases maintenance requirements may be doubled or tripled for severely debilitated animals. At the same time, care should be taken to ensure fluid requirements are considered (see Chapter 30).

Deer

Smaller or semi-tame debilitated deer may be gavage fed with a liquid slurry of cattle or preferably red deer pellets first crushed and suspended in water. Alternatively, products commercially available for critical care feeding of herbivores, such as the EmerAid® (Lafeber) range. This can be done by one handler restraining the rear end of the deer and the other grasping the head. One arm should be passed around the back of the head and the hand should grasp the end of the tongue and pull this to one side of the mouth. The other hand holds the liquid feed in a long-necked bottle (such as a wine bottle) which should be placed into the other side of the mouth, feeding small amounts frequently and allowing the deer to swallow each time.

Larger deer may be dangerous to approach in this manner; if assisted feeding is required and the animal is not too debilitated, a light sedative may need to be given first. After this a naso-reticular tube may be passed via the medial nasal passages. The head is held slightly flexed and the tubing (e.g. canine stomach tube) is passed slowly and should be felt to pass down the left side of the neck in the oesophagus. To check it is in the correct place, the operator may listen at the end of the tube for the absence of breathing noises and the possible presence of gas/gurgling noises of the forestomachs. The tubing may be inserted into the reticulum (the first of the forestomachs) at the level of the xiphoid sternal body, or merely advanced halfway down the oesophagus (although the latter option risks regurgitation of food given in some cases). The liquid formula may then be poured via a funnel into the end of the tubing after elevating the nose of the deer slightly. Small amounts should be placed at any one time, and watched to ensure the fluid is running away, as the risk of passive reflux is moderately high in these semi-sedated animals. In the main this technique is useful for the administration of probiotic ruminal products to replace or enhance the normal microflora of the fermenting forestomachs, which is essential to their normal function.

Red foxes

Debilitated and sedated/anaesthetised foxes may have a naso-oesophageal tube placed; measuring from extended nose tip to the level of the seventh rib gives an idea of the length of tubing required. A 3.5–4.5 French diameter tube is usually sufficient. The nose is first sprayed with lidocaine, and the tube is advanced via the medial aspect of the nasal passage. Care should be taken if the fox is under general anaesthesia as the tube may enter the trachea. Once advanced to the premeasured point, the end of the tube may be skin stapled, sutured or glued to the head of the fox and an Elizabethan collar applied, although these are not well tolerated in anything other than a debilitated animal. Liquid canine/feline rehabilitation formulas or critical care diets (see section Critical care preparations useful in wildlife rehabilitation) may then be syringed through the tubing. Care must be given to flush through the naso-oesophageal tube with sterile water prior to and after administering the liquid diet.

Wildcats

Naso-oesophageal/gastric tubes may be inserted under anaesthesia, premeasured from nose to the seventh rib in the manner described above. This species does not tolerate a lot of handling, or indeed collars, and it may be necessary to re-insert the tubing as and when it is required or just use it once to administer nutrition into the stomach. Volumes of 10–20 mL/kg body weight of a liquid cat/dog rehabilitation formula may be administered via this route. Warming food through gently and ensuring the nostrils are clear also helps to stimulate appetite.

European badgers

For debilitation purposes the same requirements as for foxes may be assumed. Examples of formulas used for liquid diets are given in the section Critical care preparations useful in wildlife rehabilitation. Naso-oesophageal tubes are less well tolerated than in foxes and are therefore uncommonly used.

Wild mustelids

Syringe feeding by mouth, as with ferrets, for the smaller species is advised. A standard cat rehabilitation liquid food may be used as nutrition. Scruffing the mustelid to ensure safe handling may well be necessary during this procedure, or wrapping the mustelid tightly in a towel by one handler while the other syringe feeds it. Feeds of 4–5 mL per stoat/marten and 1 mL per weasel may be given via this route, but frequent meals (every 3–4 hours) are often needed due to their high metabolic rates.

Seals (phocids)

These species may have a stomach tube passed orally. The tube should be measured from the nose tip to the xiphoid sternal body and a 1-cm diameter for seal pups is sufficient, although larger tubes can be used for adults. Two handlers are required, one to restrain the rear end of the seal by sitting astride the animal which is in sternal recumbency and then placing both hands onto the dorsal pelvic area. The other handler sits astride the seal in the shoulder area and, using a wooden block as a mouth gag (ideally one that bridges both jaws and has a hole drilled in the middle for tube insertion), inserts a well-lubricated stomach tube. Rehydration fluids may also be given by this route, such as canine electrolytes, or a slurry of fresh blended fish diluted with cooled, previously boiled water; 200 mL on average may be given at any one time to seal pups, anything up to a litre for adults.

In less severely anorectic seals, placing the fish into the mouth of the seal (being careful not to get bitten!) can be enough to stimulate swallowing, or throwing the fish just past the nose of the seal may trigger it to grab the prey and eat.

European hedgehogs

Naso-oesophageal tubes are very difficult to pass through the small passages of the hedgehog. Therefore, oral syringing with liquid dog/cat-based preparations should be attempted. Commercially available critical care formulas are also available and considered preferable in many cases (e.g. a 50 : 50 mix of the Intensive Care (IC) Carnivore and IC Omnivore EmerAid® (Lafeber)). The use of fruit purées can also be tried, although these contain no fats or calcium and so represent a supplement only.

Microchiropterans

Feeding mealworms via forceps is useful, as many bats will take them directly. Very debilitated specimens should be syringe fed from a 1-mL syringe, or eyedropper with either a solution of sugars/amino acids (see section Critical care preparations useful in wildlife rehabilitation) or a commercial carnivore/omnivore combined formula. The bat may be restrained for this by allowing it to grip onto a towel first. An avian crop tube attached to a syringe may be used to place food directly into the oesophagus in reticent individuals, although care should be taken to ensure gentle handling and insertion of the blunt-ended tube.

Hares

These may have a naso-oesophageal 3.5 French tube placed, premeasured to the level of the seventh rib. Again, it is advised that this be done with the animal conscious or lightly sedated if possible to ensure correct placement. A collar may not be tolerated, although glueing the tube to the back of the head and midline along the forehead is often tolerated. Through this a slurry of ground rabbit pellets or herbivore critical care formulas (see section Critical care preparations useful in wildlife rehabilitation) may be syringed, along with probiotics/prebiotics to recolonise or enhance the gastrointestinal tract with useful microflora. In severely debilitated cases simple sugar/amino acid preparations may also be utilised, as mentioned in the section Critical care preparations useful in wildlife rehabilitation.

Squirrels

It is almost impossible to place a naso-oesophageal tube in these species. Assisted feeding is therefore best performed using an oral syringing technique. Foods which may be utilised are non-lactose-containing vegetable baby foods, as these have more calories and less fibre than rabbit pellets, more closely mimicking the squirrel's natural diet which is largely seed based. Feeds of 4–5 mL at any one time two to three times a day is advised, but stress levels may dictate less frequent handling than this.

Wild birds

These may be crop tubed using standard cage bird metal tubes, volumes of 0.2–0.5 mL for small sparrow-sized passerines and up to 10–15 mL for some seagulls being administered. Formulas depend on the species, although the liquid sugar/protein digest formulas (see section Critical care preparations useful in wildlife rehabilitation) are useful in severely debilitated species. For raptors and seagulls, blended real prey (rodent/fish) or the use of commercially available carnivore rehabilitation formulas may be used. For herbivorous/granivorous species the use of ready-prepared commercial avian weaner/mash powders (such as Harrison's Bird Foods®), or the use of non-lactose-containing vegetable human baby foods can be tried. It is nearly always advisable to use a probiotic preparation as well, and feeding times can be reduced to two to three times daily due to the storage capacities of the crop. Some species, such as seagulls and raptors, do not have a crop but they can often use the whole length of the oesophagus as a storage receptacle.

Critical care preparations useful in wildlife rehabilitation

Some critical care preparations useful in wildlife rehabilitation. Please note the list is not intended to be exhaustive and comprises products used by the author.

Carnivores

Most would be suitable for strict carnivores such as wildcats, stoats, weasels, birds of prey, etc.

- Hills a/d®: a tinned rehabilitation diet for dogs and cats that may be mixed with cooled, previously boiled water to gain the correct consistency
- Lafeber Intensive Care Carnivore – EmerAid System® (NB: may be combined 50 : 50 with the omnivore version for insectivores such as hedgehogs)
- Oxbow Critical Care Carnivore®
- VetArk CCF Critical Care Formula®. This is a powder that can be reconstituted and contains dextrose for energy and protein which consequently is easily digested/absorbed. It is useful for initial emergency support, but is not designed for long-term use

Herbivores

Most would be suitable for lagomorphs, herbivorous rodents such as beavers, voles, etc., and potentially deer.

- Lafeber Intensive Care Herbivore – EmerAid System®
- Oxbow Critical Care Herbivore®
- Supreme Science Recovery Formula® for small herbivores
- VetArk CCF Critical Care Formula® (see above)

Pelleted foods for deer and domestic rabbits may also be blended and suspended in water and gavaged or tubed into less debilitated animals.

Prebotics/probiotics

These are helpful in herbivores in particular to speed up gut function recovery. A number of commercially available products exist, of which a few are mentioned below.

- Protexin Veterinary produce a range of probiotics for herbivores such as Bio-Lapis® which may be useful in wild lagomorphs for example
- Provita Eurotech produce a range of probiotics for ruminants (and others) such as Provita Protect® which may be useful at a dose of 3–5 mL per deer calf, orally, to encourage a positive bacterial flora in the gut for digestion to occur
- VetArk also produce a range of prebiotics and probiotics for small herbivores which can aid gut digestion

Omnivores

Most would be suitable for species such as the European badger and red fox and many of the passerines as well as some rodents such as rats and mice.

- Lafeber Intensive Care Omnivore – EmerAid System® (NB: combined 50 : 50 with the carnivore diet can be used for insectivores such as hedgehogs and bats)
- Oxbow Critical Care Omnivore®
- VetArk CCF Critical Care Formula® (see above)

References

Barboza, P.S., Parker, K.L. and Hume, I.D. (2009) *Integrative Wildlife Nutrition*. Springer, Berlin.

Buck, C.L. and Barnes, B.M. (2000) Effects of ambient temperature on metabolic rate, respiratory quotient, and torpor in an arctic hibernator. *American Journal of Physiology*, **279**, R255–R262.

Church, D.C. (1971) *Digestive Physiology and Nutrition of Ruminants*, vol. 1–3. Oregon State University Press, Corvallis.

Constantine, D.G. (1993) Chiroptera: bat medicine, management, and conservation. In: *Zoo and Wild Animal Medicine Current Therapy 3* (ed. M.E. Fowler), pp. 310–325. W B Saunders, Philadelphia.

Gage, L.J. (1993) Marine mammals: hand rearing pinnipeds. In: *Zoo and Wild Animal Medicine Current Therapy 3* (ed. M.E. Fowler), pp. 413–415. W B Saunders, Philadelphia.

Gili, C., Meijer, G. and Lacave, G. (2018) *EAZA and EAAM Best Practice Guidelines for Otariidae and Phocidae (Pinnipeds)*. Acquario di Genova, Genova, Italy.

Kirkwood, J.W. (1992) Wild mammals. In: *Manual of Exotic Pets* (eds P.H. Beynon & J.E. Cooper), pp. 122–149. BSAVA, Shurdington, Glos.

Kollias, G.V. and Kollias, H.W. (2010) Feeding passerine and psittacine birds. In: *Small Animal Clinical Nutrition Textbook* (eds M.S. Hand, C.D. Thatcher,

R.L. Remillard *et al.*), 5th edn, pp. 1255–1269. Mark Morris Institute, Topeka, Kansas.

Mateos, G.G., Garcia-Rebollar, P. and de Blas, C. (2020) Minerals vitamins and additives. In: *Nutrition of the Rabbit* (eds C. de Blas & J. Wiseman), 3rd edn, pp. 126–158. CABI, Wallingford, Oxford.

Mitchell, G.E. (1967) Vitamin A nutrition of ruminants. *Journal of the American Veterinary Medical Association*, **151**, 430–436.

National Research Council (NRC) (2006) *Nutrient Requirements of Dogs and Cats*, pp. 354–370. National Academies Press, Washington.

Sheldon, W.G. (1971) Alopecia of captive flying squirrels. *Journal of Wildlife Disease*, **7**, 111–114.

Stocker, L. (2005) *Practical Wildlife Care*, 2nd edn. Blackwell Publishing, Oxford.

Suttle, N.F. (2022) Copper. In: *Mineral Nutrition of Livestock* (ed. N.F. Suttle), 5th edn, pp. 259–300. CABI.

Wallach, J.D. (1970) Nutritional diseases of exotic animals. *Journal of the American Veterinary Medical Association*, **157**, 583–599.

Wallach, J.D. and Cooper, J.E. (1982) Nutritional diseases of wild birds. In: *Non-infectious Diseases of Wildlife* (eds G.L. Hoff & J.W. Davis), pp. 113–126. Iowa State University Press, Iowa.

Wallach, J.D. and Hoff, G.L. (1982) Nutritional diseases of mammals. In: *Non-infectious Diseases of Wildlife* (eds G.L. Hoff & J.W. Davis), pp. 127–154. Iowa State University Press, Iowa.

Chapter 27 Wildlife Handling and Chemical Restraint

HANDLING OF THE WILDLIFE PATIENT

Do we need to restrain the wildlife patient?

This question is particularly relevant to wildlife patients, as they are likely to be the most highly stressed of all the non-domestic species encountered in first opinion practice. Inappropriate handling/restraint of a wildlife case can lead to excessive stresses being placed on the patient, which at best will retard recovery and at worst may actually cause death as well as potentially exposing the handler to risk of injury.

There are a wide range of species to be considered but the following principles apply.

1. Always assess if restraint is absolutely necessary, for example does the animal need treatment at all? Most female deer will leave their fawns for long periods in an out-of-the-way spot, returning to feed them intermittently, and therefore an alert recumbent fawn is not necessarily an animal that needs restraint or interfering with. Alternatively, in a hospitalised wild animal, is it necessary to perform a vital physical exam/blood sample, or to provide medication, or can the procedure be performed without restraint, for example with in-feed medication as opposed to injection?
2. Consider the possibility that the wild animal may have underlying respiratory disease, and hence rigorous restraint may be contraindicated.
3. Consider how aggressive/hazardous that animal is to safely restrain.
4. Does the animal show evidence of physical trauma, such as a road traffic accident, in which case there may be multiple fractures, possibly of the ribcage with underlying lung pathology that will be considerably exacerbated by physical restraint.
5. Where is the restraint to be performed, and for how long? A short period of restraint in order to administer antibiotics in a purpose-built holding kennel is a different matter from attempting to capture an injured wild animal for transport to a treatment centre in a field situation.

Always assess if it is safe to restrain the patient. If the correct equipment and support staff are not available, then for the more hazardous species it is worthwhile postponing any handling.

Techniques and equipment involved in restraining wildlife patients

This section discusses the more commonly seen wildlife species. For rabbits, rodents, wild birds, amphibians and reptiles, please see Chapters 3, 11 and 19 which deal specifically with these groups. I shall therefore cover deer, foxes, badgers, wild mustelids (weasels, stoats, martens and otters), seals, bats, hedgehogs, hares and squirrels.

Deer

Among deer seen in the UK and Europe there is considerable size variation, from Chinese water deer weighing 9–12 kg as adults through to a red deer stag that may weigh up to 240 kg. This size variation, presence of antlers in many males and, in the case of Chinese water deer, the presence of tusks in males will alter the approach of the handler with regard to restraint. Another factor which will alter the ability to restrain deer is the time of year and the presence/absence of young at heel. The annual breeding season or rut in species such as red, fallow and sika deer can make the males particularly dangerous when they are in hard antler and aggressive. To reduce handler trauma, antlers may be wrapped in bandage material if they are small, as is the case with muntjac or roe deer, but they are extremely difficult to safely manage in adult male fallow and red deer without removal under anaesthesia, which has implications for the deer's short-term release as they may not be able to defend themselves against other stags. Prior to the rut itself the antlers are 'in velvet'. Trauma to or handling of the velvet leads to extensive bleeding and damage to the developing antler.

Methods for restraining wild-roaming deer often rely on remote darting techniques. In the UK, dart guns require a firearms licence to own and use and so may not be readily available. A series of gradually narrowing solid hurdle fences, creating a chute and placed in a curve so the deer cannot see the end, can be used to drive deer into a holding pen where more than one individual needs to be relocated. Nets or chemical immobilisation may then be performed. Once immobilised the deer may then be further restrained with ropes, forming either a head halter for those stags without extensive antlers, or neck halters with quick release knots that then extend around the deer's thorax and flank to create a casting system similar to that used in cattle. Hobbles can further prevent a deer from kicking out and injuring itself and the handler. This involves using padded ropes or bandages to tie the forelimbs and hindlimbs together separately and then tying forelimbs to hindlimbs.

For smaller species and orphaned young, restraint may be performed in a similar manner to domestic bovid calves. The easiest method is by placing one arm around the front of the neck and the other around the rear behind the thighs. Stocker (2009) refers to a sling system for muntjac and other small deer where the top of a surgical trolley is replaced with a cloth sling that the legs slot through and a strap is placed across the shoulders and rump so suspending

Veterinary Nursing of Exotic Pets and Wildlife, Third Edition. Simon J. Girling.

the deer allowing examination. Covering the eyes with a towel or cloth bag and, if possible, plugging the ear canals to minimise visual and auditory stimulation can reduce struggling.

To cast a small deer without antlers (i.e. to place it in lateral recumbency) from a standing position, the operator may reach over the deer's back/dorsum and grasp the carpus and tarsus of the two limbs nearest to their body in either hand. The hands are then brought upwards, allowing the dorsum of the deer to slide down the front of the operator's body until the deer is on its side. Pressure may then be applied with the operator's forearms across the deer's lower neck and flank while still grasping the underside carpus and tarsus. Deer can and will kick out and their hooves are razor sharp and can create deep cuts to the handlers and their skin.

More aggressive or lively individuals should be chemically immobilised before attempting restraint.

Any transport boxes or crates as well as housing should be well padded to avoid injury while catching debilitated deer, either with rubberised lower wall cladding, or by deep littering with straw. These boxes should be kept in dimmed/darkened conditions to further reduce stress during the holding periods. Domestic pet transport crates may be sufficient for transporting small deer but larger roe, fallow and sika deer will need a stretcher with strapping to prevent them getting off. Alternatively a cargo net may be used particularly for the larger red deer. Try to maintain deer in sternal or right lateral recumbency. Left lateral and dorsal recumbency will lead to ruminal regurgitation and potential aspiration with asphyxiation or pneumonia as a consequence.

It is important to remember that deer can also carry zoonotic diseases, the most concerning being bovine tuberculosis (*Mycobacterium bovis*).

Red foxes

A fully conscious fox is a significant biting hazard and so initial attempts at restraint should be directed towards neutralising this by effective control of the head. In aggressive individuals this is probably best achieved by using a dogcatcher pole snare, looping the snare over the head before pulling tight. The fox should then be swiftly moved to a pet carrier or other suitable container for transfer. It may be necessary to use long-handled nets as are used to restrain captive wild animals in zoos. Once in the net, an assistant can apply firm pressure via a broom to the neck area of the fox to then allow it to be carefully extracted and placed into a carry box. Gauntlets are advised to minimise the risk of being injured.

If the fox is severely debilitated, then the use of a large towel or blanket may be employed. The towel or blanket may be thrown over the fox and the neck grasped through the towel with both hands from either side to reduce lateral movement. Once trapped the fox may be transferred to a suitable container, or the towel carefully discarded and with one hand the handler takes a firm grasp of the fox's scruff high up behind the skull while the other hand grasps the skin over the rump. A tape muzzle or equivalent appropriately sized canine muzzle should be applied (see Figure 27.1) It is always worth remembering that the fox has a slender but athletic frame. They are therefore relatively strong for their size, but their bone density is more like a cat's rather than a dog's and so overzealous restraint may therefore cause fractures.

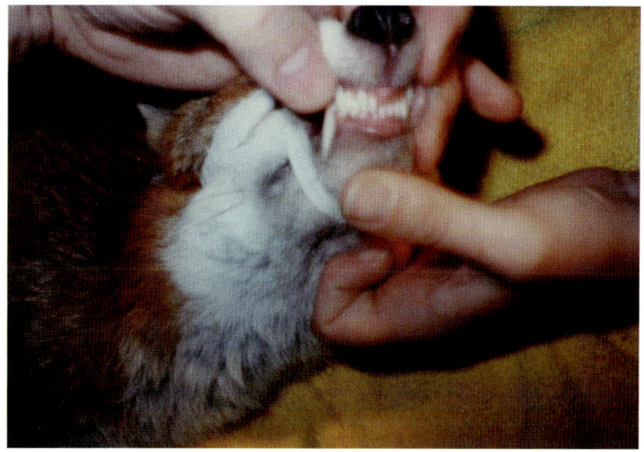

Figure 27.1 Juvenile red fox with tape muzzle applied.

European badgers

The European badger, although a similar size to the fox, is a much more densely built and powerful animal. Their main offensive weapons are the extremely powerful crushing jaws, but they can also produce severe scratches with their long forepaw claws. Trying to restrain a badger is much more difficult than the average fox, as they have a stout and thick neck, which is difficult to get a good scruff on.

Restraint in the average healthy adult badger therefore relies more on the use of equipment such as the dogcatcher pole snare. Indeed, two of these, or two noose leads may be needed to ensure full restraint, with the handlers pulling gently but firmly in opposite directions once looped over the badger's head.

Alternatively, in a severely debilitated badger that has been checked for a lack of responsiveness, a thick towel or blanket may be used to first cover the badger and then pin it to the ground with pressure applied either side of the neck region just in front of the shoulders. Thick, heavy-duty welder's gauntlets are advised. Transfer to a carry cage should occur quickly. Anything more than a cursory examination really necessitates some form of chemical restraint (anaesthesia). Even when anaesthetics are used always be wary when examining the oral cavity as even deeply sedated badgers can suddenly bite when something is placed close to or in the mouth. Application of a stout dog muzzle should be considered when examining a badger; however, care should be taken as a badger can remove a muzzle with their forepaws and, of course, a muzzle may be hazardous if the animal vomits or has respiratory difficulty.

Wild mustelids

All these species are carnivores by nature and so are invariably aggressive, their chief weapons being their teeth, although otters have powerful forelimbs and can inflict significant scratches.

The European otter is extremely difficult to restrain without sedation/anaesthesia and highly dangerous. Never restrain it by the tail as they can literally climb back up their own tail and then bite the handler! In severely debilitated otters where the risk has been assessed, physical restraint may be attempted using downward pressure either side of the neck just behind the head to immobilise the head end while another handler applies pressure to the pelvic region. This often allows enough time for the injection of an anaesthetic agent. Alternatively, the use of tubular sacking material which allows the head to protrude from one end may be employed to restrain the limbs while the handler's attention is directed to grasping the skin either side of the neck to prevent movement of the head. The use of dogcatcher pole snares may be necessary in order to capture a loose otter. It is worth noting that even the stoutest of leather gloves are no protection against an adult otter's bite.

Restraint of mustelids such as stoats and polecats should be the same as that for a more aggressive ferret. Their sinewy bodies make getting a firm hold extremely difficult, but grasping the scruff high up on the neck with one hand while grasping the musculature of the lumbar region with the other is one of the safer grips.

Weasels, because of their smaller size, may require more gentle handling, although they are equally ferocious when caught. A firm grip of the scruff between thumb and forefinger of one hand while supporting the rear with the other, or gripping loosely around the neck, using the thumb to push firmly up underneath the chin to prevent biting may also be useful. Alternatively, rapid transfer using a towel or box to an anaesthetic induction chamber for examination once anaesthetised can be performed.

If the mustelid is free in a larger space, then hooped pole nets using either fine netting for the smaller Mustelidae as one would use for birds and bats, or more coarse meshed netting for the stronger and larger otters may be used to control movement to allow chemical immobilisation (anaesthesia) and transferral to a container. The use of towels is preferable for other mustelids loose in boxes.

Seals (phocids)

Seals (phocids) are generally only brought to specific wildlife centres for treatment such as those run in the UK by the RSPCA/SSPCA, but disasters do occur such as outbreaks of phocine distemper virus, or marine oil spillages where additional support is required.

Restraint can be extremely hazardous as the two species are large, carnivorous and with few appendages to allow sufficient grip to ensure safe restraint. The grey seal is the larger species, with bulls weighing in around 270–320 kg, the common (harbour) seal bull weighing up to 150 kg. When in the open, large mesh cargo nets are best used to restrain seals for long enough to allow handlers to gain control using injectable anaesthetics. Chemical immobilisation (anaesthesia) should always be considered prior to any attempt to manually restrain them. For smaller debilitated seals, physical restraint may be achieved using at least two handlers: one controls the head with pressure either side of the neck immediately behind the head to prevent being bitten while this handler is astride the seal; the other handler puts downward pressure on the pelvic region. It is frequently useful to cover the seal's head with a towel during this process to calm the animal.

Seal pups may be restrained using canvas papooses with slits cut for the forelimbs to protrude through. The head is frequently left free for manual restraint as muzzles can be hazardous due to constriction of the nostrils which sit more dorsally in seals than in dogs or cats. A simple strap/tape muzzle to close the jaws may however be used. Alternatively, firm pressure to the back of the neck, associated with towels, may allow temporary restraint in a debilitated pup depending on its size (see Figure 27.2).

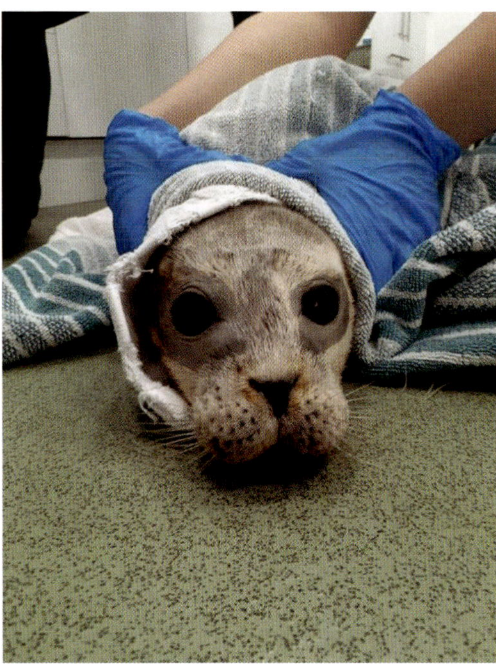

Figure 27.2 Restraint of seals is potentially hazardous. Smaller debilitated pups may be restrained using canvas papooses or towels with firm pressure behind the neck to prevent biting. *Source:* Courtesy of Diane Westwood RVN.

An implement known as a 'bull pole', resembling a dogcatcher with a rope noose on the end of a stout pole, may be used to part restrain smaller seals and guide them into containers. In addition, the use of boards, as with pigs, and heavy mesh netting can all be used as restraint aids to guide and direct seals.

An important consideration during restraint is the environmental temperature as they have excellent insulation in the form of blubber, and this can cause them to become overheated very quickly with physical exertion on a warm day. Buckets of cold water and minimising restraint as well as planning procedures for the cooler periods of the day (early morning or late evening in the warmer months) are advised.

The bite of seals is in itself extremely painful and may involve the loss of digits. In addition, many seals carry the bacterium *Erysipelothrix insidiosa* that induces an intense inflammatory reaction, a condition known as 'seal finger', as well as other unpleasant bacteria such as *Pasteurella* spp. Seals can also carry sealpox which can cause painful lesions in humans.

Microchiropterans

Microchiropterans are rarely brought to the attention of veterinary practices unless on an individual basis such as prey brought in by cats.

Handling should be performed with care, and a pair of lightweight leather gloves for the larger species, or latex gloves for the smaller ones is advised. Be warned, many bats will bite and they have sharp teeth. It is also possible for some bats to be carriers of rabies-related viruses (lyssaviruses) which can prove fatal to humans if not protected by rabies vaccination. For this reason it is advised that anyone handling microchiropterans has previously been fully immunised with the terrestrial rabies vaccine, which can provide crossover immunity to European bat lyssavirus and other lyssaviruses. Any bite from a bat, whether the handler is vaccinated or not, should have the wound immediately thoroughly irrigated with hot soapy/foaming antiseptic water and medical advice sought.

The use of a small hand-towel to allow the bat to clamber over while assessing them is helpful. When restraining, a thumb may be placed underneath the chin of the bat so pushing the lower jaw upwards and avoiding being bitten. The alternative is to encourage them to bite onto a wooden tongue depressor or other smooth object.

The wings may be extended for examination by grasping the point of the carpus (the second joint from the body attachment) and gently extending the wing. The wing membranes are extremely fragile and every attempt should be made to avoid tearing these.

If a bat escapes from restraint, it may be caught using a fine mesh aviary/butterfly net. The fine gauzes used do not seem to be detectable to bat radar and so they appear unable to avoid these nets. Care should be taken in unravelling them from these nets as they cling onto the gauze with the nails on their forelimbs and their bone structure is extremely fragile.

European hedgehogs

European hedgehogs are rarely aggressive, their defence being to roll into a protective ball. This can make examination extremely difficult and various techniques have been described to encourage a hedgehog to unravel.

The following are some methods which have been found useful (but note that leather gloves are advisable when handling hedgehogs to avoid being injured by the spines).

1. The hedgehog may be lightly 'bounced' in the hands, stimulating it to uncurl.
2. Firm backward stroking of the caudal dorsal area with a leather gauntleted hand has been described.
3. Holding the rolled-up hedgehog with both hands, with head downwards over a flat surface and applying pressure to the hip region either side and unrolling by pushing the thumbs downwards. Once the hindlimbs are exposed these may be grasped and so prevent the hedgehog from re-rolling up again.
4. Finally, some hedgehogs require chemical restraint (anaesthesia or sedation) to ensure minimal stress and a full clinical examination.

When examining a hedgehog, a pair of lightweight leather gardening gloves is useful, as is a thick towel to minimise trauma to the handler's hands. It is important to remember that ringworm is commonly carried on the skin/spines of even healthy hedgehogs. In addition, many hedgehogs are carriers for *Salmonella* spp. and *Escherichia coli* and many carry ticks so should be handled with care and due attention to hygiene.

Hares

The hare's main defence is their rapid turn of speed and occasionally their ability to fight, having powerful fore and hind limbs and sharp incisors.

Dimming room lights before approaching is extremely useful for these flighty creatures. The use of a heavy towel to papoose the hare, similar to the technique used for cats and aggressive domestic rabbits, just leaving the head free while the towel is tightly wound around the neck and rest of the body.

The hare may also be scruffed firmly with one hand, while the other restrains the hindlimbs around the hocks to prevent lashing out and damaging the hare's back. Alternatively, the hare may be scruffed with one hand, while the hare's head is placed into the crook of the elbow of the other arm, the forearm of this arm encircling the hare's rear. Long sleeves are advised as they may still kick and struggle. The advantage of this technique, though, is that the hare's eyes are placed into the dark again so reducing the stress somewhat.

Zoonotically speaking, hares may carry *E. coli* and the bacterium *Yersinia pseudotuberculosis*, which can cause a granulomatous intestinal disease with septicaemia in hare and human alike.

Squirrels

Restraint is performed in a similar manner to that employed for chipmunks and chinchillas. However, squirrels are more inclined to bite than the latter two species and so thick leather gauntlets should be worn, but be aware their sharp incisors can penetrate the thickest of leather gloves.

The squirrel may be scruffed at the nape of the neck with one hand, the other cupping the rear limbs or grasping the very base of the tail (do not grasp the end of the tail as you may inadvertently deglove the skin covering it). Alternatively, one hand may be placed around the neck with the thumb pushing up underneath the chin to close the mouth and pushing the head skywards while the other cups the rear limbs. Occasionally it may be necessary to get an assistant to distract the squirrel with a tongue depressor or other smooth object to prevent being bitten.

Finally, the use of thick towels to restrain an escaped squirrel is useful as are some of the larger aviary nets. Dimming the room lights also induces a calming effect, as it does with most diurnal species, combined with a reduction in environmental noise.

There is also, as with many small wild mammals, the zoonotic risks of catching leptospirosis from squirrels.

Wild birds

These may be handled and restrained in the same way as that described for cage and aviary birds. Dimmed lighting, reduction in environmental noise and the use of towels/cloths instead of heavy gauntlets is advised for most species. Large raptors are the exception, whereby heavy leather gauntlets are a must. A towel may be used to cover the head and enwrap the wings for physical examination to occur. Smaller birds of prey may be restrained without gauntlets but care should be taken to control the feet to stop the raptor from both 'footing' itself or the handler with its talons (see Figure 27.3).

With many birds of prey, frequently the beak and the talons are the offensive weapons, hence the need for gauntlets. However, with most other wild birds the beak is the only 'weapon', varying from the small beak of the house sparrow to the powerful bill of the grey heron. Control of the head is the first objective, with the covering of the eyes being useful, followed by firm but loose control of the wings to prevent self-inflicted damage. Again, the use of a cloth or light towel is best as this allows the weight of the material to restrict wing movement without fear of constricting the chest wall and so causing dyspnoea.

Aspects of chemical restraint

When dealing with species of wild animals, the need to provide chemical immobilisation is possibly greater than for any other group of animals encountered so far in this book.

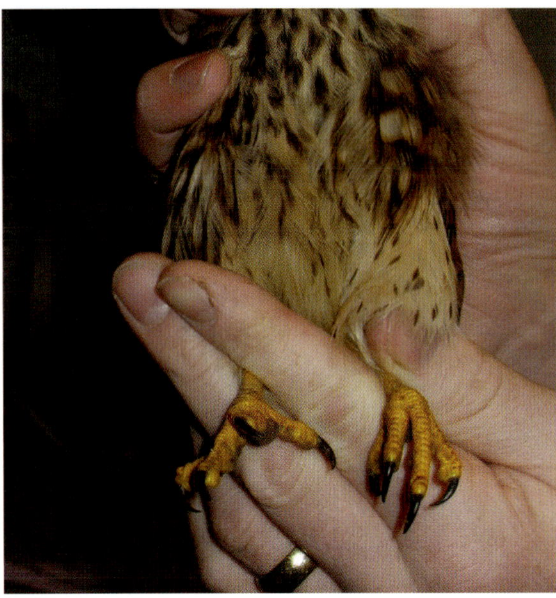

Figure 27.3 Smaller birds of prey such as this kestrel can be restrained manually but make sure the feet are constrained to prevent the bird grabbing itself or the handler and so causing trauma.

Assessments still need to be made with regard to an animal's health status.

- Is the animal gravid/pregnant?
- Is the animal suffering from obvious respiratory disease?
- Is the animal in shock after a road traffic collision?
- Does the animal have significant traumatic injuries/fractures?

However, we also have to take into consideration other aspects. These include an assessment of risk to the handler. An assessment should be made to determine if, for example, restraint of a roe deer stag or a grey seal bull is necessary or essential. In these cases chemical immobilisation would be the method of choice for any close inspection or invasive technique even if the animal is debilitated.

We also have to consider the physiological stress load we are placing the animal under. Many wild animals by definition are not used to close or prolonged human contact. The very act of restraint, whether the animal struggles or not, is likely to be physiologically stressful. This may have a deleterious effect which may be instantaneous. This can be exhibited by some small rodents or passerine birds which can literally die in the hand due to myocardial hypoxia associated with increased heart rates and underlying pathology. Alternatively, more long-term problems can be seen, such as the lowering of their immune system status so allowing secondary pathogens to cause disease. This condition is seen for example with the fungal infection aspergillosis in raptors and many other wild birds when they become stressed. It may therefore be desirable to use chemical immobilisation in order to render the patient insensible and so reduce stress levels during physical examination and of course during more invasive procedures.

Pre-anaesthetic preparation

Starvation

This is generally not possible in the majority of wildlife cases and so the risks of regurgitation and aspiration are increased. Where an elective procedure is carried out, withholding food for a period of time prior to the anaesthetic can minimise this and varies with the species from 2 to 4 hours in the case of most small birds and smaller mammal species through to 24–36 hours for ruminants such as deer. Clearly, species that have difficulty regurgitating or vomiting may not need a starve period such as lagomorphs and many rodents and indeed a starve period may have deleterious effects on gut motility as well as metabolism.

Weight measurement

This, as with any other species, is important to ensure accurate dosage. Absolutely accurate measurement is less vital for the larger species such as deer and seals, but it is extremely important in smaller mammals and wild birds, where a mistake of 10 g, a tiny amount, may lead to over- or under-dosage of anywhere from 10 to 50%.

The use of measuring scales accurate to a gram for the smaller species, or cotton sacks and a fine balance scale, is therefore advisable and obtaining an accurate weight measurement is important whenever an animal is anaesthetised.

Blood testing

This may not always be possible prior to anaesthesia for wildlife cases as immobilisation is frequently necessary in order to blood sample the patient. However, blood sampling can provide an important part of a wild animal's health status, whether performed before or after chemical restraint. Safe volumes that may be collected tend to be assumed to be around 0.5–1% of body weight in grams (i.e. a 450-g hedgehog may safely have 2.25–4.5 mL taken for sampling, more than enough for diagnostic testing). If very debilitated, clearly try to take the minimum needed for the test.

The following sections describe sites for venepuncture in the species mentioned above.

Deer

Blood samples may be taken easily from the jugular veins with 19–20 gauge needles under chemical or physical restraint in all species. The medial cephalic vein, medially located over the antebrachium, may also be useful although in the smaller species 21–23 gauge needles may be required. Alternatively, the ventral tail vein may be utilised in emergencies, although this is more of a plexus of vessels rather than a discrete vessel. Chemical immobilisation is almost always required unless the deer is very debilitated or immobilised.

Red foxes

The jugular veins are useful sites for blood samples of 1–2 mL using a 21–23 gauge needle. However, the cephalic veins may also be used with a 23–25 gauge needle for smaller samples. Samples are generally taken under anaesthesia to minimise stress but physical restraint may be possible in some smaller and younger individuals.

Wildcats

The jugular veins are useful sites for blood samples of 1–2 mL using a 21–23 gauge needle. However, the cephalic veins may also be used with a 23–25 gauge needle for smaller samples. Samples should always be taken under anaesthesia.

European badgers

Again, a jugular sample with a 21 gauge needle may be taken. Chemical restraint is required. In addition, samples may be taken from the cephalic and lateral saphenous veins.

Wild mustelids

Blood samples may be taken in a similar manner to that used for the ferret. In general the jugular veins are the most useful vessels to sample with a 21–27 gauge needle, depending on the species involved from otters to weasels. In larger species such as martens, the cephalic and lateral saphenous veins may be useful. As with ferrets, the cranial vena cava may also be used with the mustelid anaesthetised, placed on its back and the needle advanced through the thoracic inlet at the base of the neck from the left side. A longer needle is required, usually a 1 inch, and gauges from 23 to 27 depending on the species. Otters can be more difficult due to their layer of subcutaneous fat and thick fur coat but jugular or cephalic blood samples are preferred. Alternatively, the ventral tail vein can be used in otters. Chemical immobilisation is always required with wild mustelids.

Seals

A number of vessels may be used. The intravertebral vein can be accessed between the lumbar vertebrae from L4 to L7. At these positions the area of the intravertebral space is occupied by a sinus, and yet there is minimal nervous tissue to hit during venepuncture. Juveniles require a 2-inch 20-gauge needle, and adults an 18-gauge 3.5-inch needle, and this is inserted midline dorsally between the spinous processes. Alternatively, the hind flipper may be used. The target is the area where the phalanges of the flipper separate from each other, the approach being from the plantar aspect. A 20-gauge 2-inch needle is usually required. Chemical immobilisation is required in adult seals but it may be possible to blood sample smaller pups under light sedation or in some cases physical restraint.

Microchiropterans

In the larger species the median vein, which runs along the underside of the wing crossing the humerus, may be used. This vessel is fragile and blows easily, but is preferable to the smaller cephalic vein which runs along the leading edge of the propatagium. For small species, obtaining a decent volume of blood is fraught with difficulties. Apart from the difficulty of finding a large enough vessel, there is the problem of how much blood may be removed safely in even a healthy animal (generally no more than 1% of body weight). Chemical immobilisation, usually isoflurane or sevoflurane, is generally required as bats are fragile.

European hedgehogs

Sampling again requires chemical immobilisation to ensure the hedgehog remains uncurled during sampling. A jugular sample may be removed, as cephalic vessels are very small, and requires a 25–27 gauge needle and preferably a pre-heparinised syringe.

Lagomorphs

Blood sampling is similar to that for domestic rabbits. The lateral ear vein may be used with a 25-gauge needle. Alternatively, the cephalic or saphenous veins can be utilised. The jugular vessels should be avoided as they provide nearly the sole drainage for the eye and its orbit. Thrombosis of the jugular vessels is therefore inclined to cause ocular oedema or even loss of the eye.

Rodents

Most require chemical immobilisation to allow blood sampling due to their small size. However, the Eurasian beaver may be temporarily restrained in a hessian sack to allow blood sampling from the midline ventral tail vein. It may be difficult to take a blood sample from other rodents, although voles and many mice do have significant superficial jugular veins that 25–27 gauge needles can access. Mice and rats have lateral tail veins that may be easily seen. Squirrels may be blood sampled from the jugular vessels, or from the cephalic or saphenous veins under chemical immobilisation.

Wild birds

These are sampled from the same areas as cage and aviary birds. The easiest site and the largest volumes are from the right jugular vein, although in larger species the brachial vein under the wing parallel to the humerus can be used. In waterfowl, gulls and long-legged birds, the medial metatarsal vein can be used as it runs up the medial aspect of the lower limb across the intertarsal joint.

Pre-anaesthetic/anaesthetic medications

These are not often used in wild animals as they require the animal to be restrained on more than one occasion prior to anaesthesia being introduced. They are therefore often ‘combined’ with the sedative/anaesthetic drug or ignored.

It is probably easier to consider chemical restraint by species groups, as follows.

Deer

Tranquillisers

Tranquillisers such as diazepam, midazolam, acepromazine, azaperone, haloperidol and zuclopenthixol have all been used in cervids to reduce physiological stress when handling, immobilising and temporarily housing them. Some, such as diazepam, acepromazine and azaperone, are short-acting lasting a few hours; others, such as some formulations of haloperidol and zuclopenthixol, are longer acting. Most require an intramuscular (IM) injection of the medication for it to be fully effective as oral administration tends to have a dilution effect, considering these species have large rumens, and so uptake of the drug can be erratic. Diazepam has been used successfully by Stocker (2009) to calm fractious deer such as muntjac at 1 mg/kg IM but also noted that fallow deer do not respond well to this tranquilliser and so should be avoided. Azaperone has been used at 0.2 mg/kg intravenously (IV) on recovery from chemical immobilisation to facilitate short journeys (usually less than 6 hours) for release or treatment. Zuclopenthixol acetate at 1 mg/kg IM will last around 4 days and has been shown to increase water and food consumption as well as reducing flight distances in cervids (Reed *et al.*, 2000).

Injectable anaesthetics

Where general anaesthesia is required, reduction of external stimulation, such as blocking the ear canals and covering the eyes (see Figure 27.4), is important.

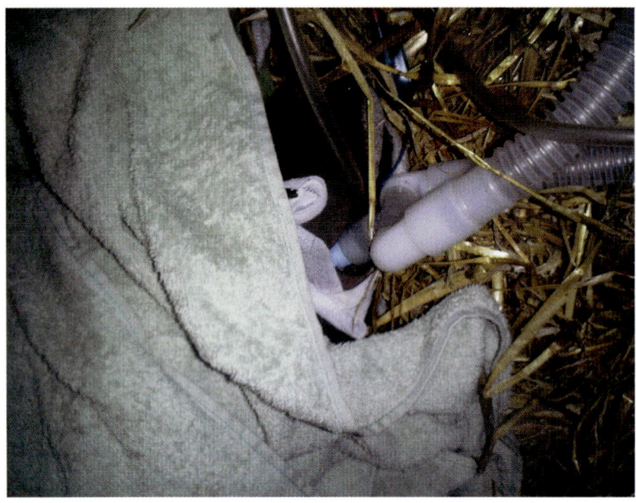

Figure 27.4 Blocking the ear canals and covering the eyes are important components of safe anaesthesia to reduce stimulation and arousal in ungulates.

Many have been described for deer and below are just some of those which may be utilised. Administration may be by straightforward injection intramuscularly if the deer is trapped or adequately physically restrained. Alternatively, the use of pole syringes (spring loaded or gas-powered injection devices) or in free-ranging deer remote delivery devices such as plastic darts fired from gas-powered guns and blowpipes may all need to be employed. Care should be taken not to chase or harry deer as they are prone to capture myopathy (see Chapter 30). Deer should not be chased as they are inclined to run straight into obstacles such as fences directly in their paths with fatal consequences (see Figure 27.5). In all cases, even if gaseous anaesthesia is not being used, it is helpful to supply intranasal or facemask oxygen to maintain blood oxygenation.

Deer should ideally be placed in sternal recumbency with the head extended and the nose pointing downwards in case of ruminal regurgitation and because they salivate profusely. Unfortunately, atropine does not inhibit this salivation in deer and so a suction device and the above-mentioned positioning until intubated may be required. If they are in left lateral recumbency the pressure on the rumen will increase and make ruminal regurgitation with subsequent aspiration much more likely. This should therefore be avoided and dorsal recumbency used wherever possible.

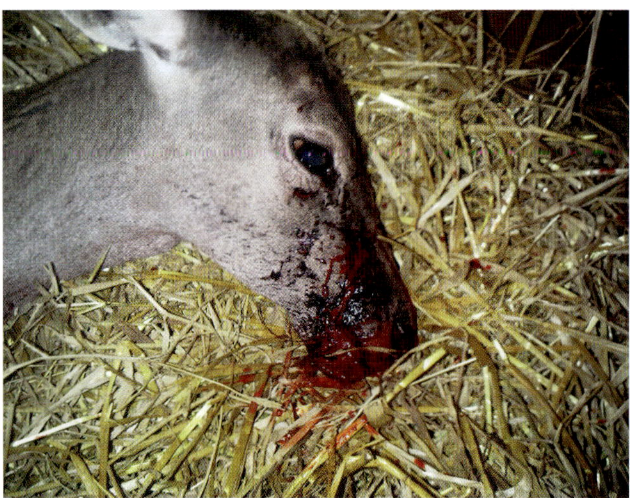

Figure 27.5 Deer should never be actively chased as they are highly likely to run straight into physical obstacles with often fatal results.

Ketamine and combinations: This can be combined at a dose of 7 mg/kg ketamine to 7 mg/kg xylazine and administered intramuscularly. Fallow deer may be sedated with 2–3 mL per 50 kg of a mixture of ketamine and xylazine known as the Hellabrun mixture. This is a combination of 4 mL of ketamine (of 100 mg/mL strength) and 500 mg of xylazine powder producing a mixture of 100 mg/mL ketamine and 125 mg/mL xylazine. Relaxation and surgical anaesthesia can be induced for 30 minutes or so. Reversal can be performed by the alpha-2 antagonist yohimbine 250 µg/kg IV.

Alternatively, ketamine 3 mg/kg may be combined with 0.1 mg/kg medetomidine. The medetomidine may then be reversed using atipamezole as with other species at 2.5–5 times the milligram per kilogram dosage of medetomidine used (in this instance, 0.25–0.5 mg/kg atipamezole).

M99® (etorphine 9.8 mg/mL): The opioid anaesthetic etorphine is used in a wide variety of wildlife species as well as farmed deer and larger zoo animals, particularly perissodactyls, although it should be used with caution in certain species of deer such as fallow deer. Etorphine is a potent morphine derivative and is used with xylazine or medetomidine to improve relaxation as etorphine on its own tends to produce a very rigid immobilisation. Like most morphine derivatives, etorphine causes respiratory depression and is highly dangerous to felines and primates including humans. Reversal of etorphine in deer is by using the partial morphine derivative diprenorphine (M5050®) which comes in the same pack as the M99 or by using naltrexone, a full opioid antagonist. Diprenorphine is administered intravenously or intramuscularly at the same volume dose as the M99 given (which equates to 1.3 mg diprenorphine per 1 mg etorphine administered), usually 50% reversal dose intramuscularly followed by 50% intravenously. However, in the case of accidental self-injection or contact with the handler's mucous membranes, the full morphine antagonist naloxone (Narcan®) at 2–3 mL given preferably intravenously and repeated every 2–3 minutes until the effects have been reversed is advised for humans. It is vitally important therefore when using etorphine that an assistant is available to administer any reversal agents should accidental self-injection arise.

In all instances the respiratory depression caused by etorphine makes it a more risky anaesthetic agent, and often intubation and intermittent positive pressure ventilation is necessary during prolonged anaesthetic procedures. It is also difficult and expensive to obtain due to its schedule 2 drug category and the fact that it is manufactured in South Africa currently; this, combined with its significant health and safety implications, makes it infrequently used in wildlife in the UK.

Propofol: This may be used to deepen anaesthesia after previous administration of ketamine and an alpha-2 drug. Intravenous access is necessary and often the medial cephalic vein is used. Boluses of 2–5 mg/kg are usually enough to allow intubation, although apnoea is common if administered rapidly.

Tiletamine/zolazepam: This combination is sold as Zoletil® (Virbac Ltd) in the UK and Europe and as Telazol® (Zoetis US) in North America and is a combination of a dissociative anaesthetic similar to ketamine (tiletamine) and a benzodiazepine (zolazepam). It comes as a powder that is reconstituted for one-time usage at a concentration of 100 mg/mL. It may be used on its own but is also often combined with an alpha-2 drug such as medetomidine. Dosages of 1 mg/kg tiletamine/zolazepam with 0.1 mg/kg medetomidine have been used in fallow deer and this combination was considered preferable to combining tiletamine/zolazepam with xylazine (Fernandez-Moran *et al.*, 2000). Tiletamine is not reversible but zolazepam may be reversed with flumazenil 0.11–0.77 mg/kg (Masters and Flach, 2015).

Gaseous anaesthetics

Isoflurane or sevoflurane: These may be used as an induction agent, particularly in more severely debilitated smaller and younger deer. Their advantages include rapid knock-down and minimal suppression of blood pressure and respiration. Their disadvantages include the ability to restrain the deer for long enough to get a face mask over its nose. However, these drugs may be used to deepen or prolong anaesthesia started with an injectable combination as above. It is preferable to intubate deer when doing this, but a face mask may be used in an emergency. Endotracheal intubation should be considered for anything other than a short procedure as ruminal regurgitation and aspiration and the profuse salivation that deer exhibit may occlude the airway, as mentioned above. Larger deer can be intubated with small equid endotracheal (ET) tubes of 14–16 mm internal diameter (ID) and muntjac and Chinese water deer with ET tubes of 4–8 mm ID depending on their sex and age. A long-bladed laryngoscope and a guide wire to stiffen the ET tube can be helpful. Intermittent positive pressure ventilation can then also be carried out if required at pressures around 15–20 mmHg and minute volume of 8–12 mL/kg.

Red foxes

Injectable anaesthetics

Acepromazine: This may be used as a sedative at doses of 0.075–0.1 mg/kg or in combination with ketamine at doses of 10 mg/kg ketamine to 0.05 mg/kg acepromazine. Its disadvantages include sometimes poor levels of sedation and the unavailability of a reversing agent leading to prolonged recovery times. It also lowers the seizure threshold and thus may be contraindicated in road traffic accidents where head trauma has occurred.

Ketamine and combinations: This may be combined with alpha-2 agonists such as medetomidine or xylazine to provide light planes of surgical anaesthesia as ketamine on its own provides poor muscle relaxation. Intramuscular doses of 10 mg/kg ketamine with 2 mg/kg xylazine have been reported as useful, although I prefer combining it with medetomidine.

Medetomidine 0.02 mg/kg plus butorphanol 0.4 mg/kg plus ketamine 4 mg/kg IM can provide light anaesthesia and may be reversed with atipamezole 0.1 mg/kg IM (Brash, 2003). This author also uses dosages of medetomidine 0.05 mg/kg with ketamine 5 mg/kg IM in this species, reversing with 0.25 mg/kg atipamezole when finished.

Medetomidine: This alpha-2 agonist drug may be used in combination with butorphanol to provide sedation during minor procedures at doses of 0.02 mg/kg medetomidine to 0.1 mg/kg butorphanol. This combination will not provide true surgical anaesthesia and intravenous propofol or gaseous anaesthetics would be required to top up the level of anaesthesia.

Propofol: This may be used as an intravenous induction agent, or for short-term anaesthesia by continuous slow infusion. Supplemental oxygen and intubation is recommended as apnoea frequently occurs. Doses of 4–6 mg/kg IV are required, with the lower doses required if the fox is debilitated or has received other medications.

Tiletamine/zolazepam: This dissociative anaesthetic/benzodiazepine combination has been used in foxes at similar dosages as used in domestic dogs, 10 mg/kg IM (Kreeger *et al.*, 1990). Recoveries can be prolonged and, in my experience, further deepening of the anaesthesia with gaseous anaesthetics or low-dose propofol is required to then allow intubation for surgical procedures.

Gaseous anaesthetics

Isoflurane or sevoflurane: Isoflurane is widely used in exotic species medicine and surgery. It is minimally metabolised in the body (0.3%) compared with halothane and respiratory arrest precedes cardiac arrest so it has high levels of safety in debilitated animals. Anaesthesia may be induced using face masks, or, preferably, after sedation with acepromazine, propofol or medetomidine. Induction as a sole agent takes 3.5–4%, maintenance usually being 1.5–2%. It is frequently used to prolong or deepen anaesthesia induced with injectable drugs such as ketamine and medetomidine.

Sevoflurane has excellent rapid knock-down effects and rapid recovery times. It is minimally metabolised and does not appear to induce cardiac arrhythmias. Induction is at 6–8% sevoflurane in 100% oxygen and maintenance at 2–3% sevoflurane in 100% oxygen when used as sole agent.

Intubation is relatively straightforward in foxes, being similar to the procedure in small domestic dogs (see Figure 27.6). Typically ET tubes of 3.5–7 mm ID are used.

Wildcats

Anaesthetic agents used in wildcats are very similar to those used in domestic felids.

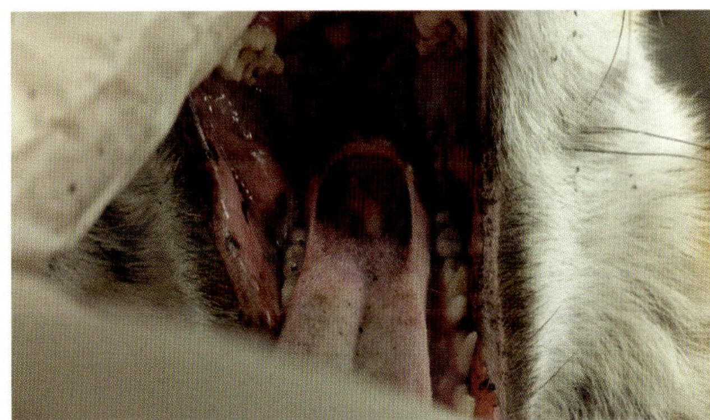

Figure 27.6 Endotracheal intubation in canids such as the red fox or felids such as the wildcat is similar to that in the domestic dog or cat, respectively.

Injectable anaesthetics

Alfaxalone: This may be used to increase the depth of anaesthesia when ketamine combinations previously used are insufficient to allow handling. See below for dosages.

Ketamine and combinations: This is commonly used intramuscularly in combination with medetomidine and butorphanol. Typical dosages would be 5 mg/kg ketamine plus 0.04 mg/kg medetomidine and 0.04 mg/kg butorphanol.

If the wildcat is very debilitated, medetomidine can be dropped and instead 5 mg/kg ketamine plus 0.25 mg/kg midazolam and 0.3 mg/kg butorphanol used but this may result in a cat being light. In this case alfaxalone 2.5–5 mg/kg IM can be introduced to allow a surgical plane of anaesthesia to be achieved.

For small sub-adults less than 1 kg and kittens, a quadruple intramuscular injectable combination, as with domestic cats where dosages are based on body surface area, can be used, typically a total dose of 5 mg ketamine plus 0.05 mg medetomidine plus 0.015 mg buprenorphine plus 0.5 mg midazolam.

Gaseous anaesthetics

Isoflurane or sevoflurane: Both gaseous anaesthetic agents have been used successfully to deepen and maintain anaesthesia in wildcats. Endotracheal intubation is recommended, with tube sizes of 1.5–5 mm ID typically being used. Intubation is the same as for domestic cats (see Figure 27.6).

European badgers

Injectable anaesthetics

Ketamine and combinations: Ketamine has been described as a sole agent in badgers at a dose of 20 mg/kg IM but I do not recommend it as it provides poor muscle relaxation (MacKintosh *et al.*, 1976). De Leeuw *et al.* (2003) compared ketamine as a sole anaesthetic agent in the European badger versus ketamine combined with medetomidine and butorphanol and found that ketamine alone resulted in more adverse effects (sneezing, muscle rigidity, excessive salivation and poor recovery).

Ketamine may also be combined with medetomidine as follows: 5–7.5 mg/kg ketamine and 0.04 mg/kg medetomidine IM; alternatively as a "triple" combination of 4 mg/kg ketamine plus 0.02 mg/kg medetomidine plus 0.4 mg/kg butorphanol IM. The medetomidine may be reversed with atipamezole at five times the milligram per kilogram dose of medetomidine.

Ketamine combined with midazolam in one study did not produce satisfactory anaesthesia and so should not be relied on as sole medication (Thornton *et al.*, 2005).

Medetomidine: This again may be used at 0.02 mg/kg combined with butorphanol 0.1 mg/kg IM to produce deep sedation. It also causes lowering of the blood pressure which may be problematic in shocked animals.

Propofol: This may be used to deepen anaesthesia induced with ketamine combinations where intravenous access is available. Dosages of 4–6 mg/kg IV can be used, but the need for vascular access makes this anaesthetic agent less favoured in this potentially aggressive species.

Gaseous anaesthetics

Isoflurane or sevoflurane: Isoflurane and sevoflurane can both be used as for foxes but rarely as induction agents due to the health and safety implications; rather they are used to deepen or prolong anaesthesia already started with an injectable combination.

Intubation may be performed but only once full anaesthesia has been induced due to the bite risk. The oral gape of badgers is narrower than that of foxes but still allows good visualisation of the glottis. ET tube sizes of 4–8 mm ID are typically effective in sub-adult to adult badgers.

Other wild mustelids

Injectable anaesthetics

Ketamine and combinations: Ketamine 10 mg/kg combined with medetomidine 0.2 mg/kg IM has been used in martens and 5 mg/kg ketamine and 0.1 mg/kg medetomidine in weasels and stoats (Kollias and Fernandez-Moran, 2015). Ketamine may also be used alone in many small mustelids at doses of 20–25 mg/kg but muscle relaxation and analgesia is poor and it is only advised for short-term restraint for non-invasive procedures.

In the Eurasian otter, ketamine on its own has been associated with problems of apnoea and hyperthermia due to muscle rigidity and the excellent insulative properties of otter's fur/subcutaneous fat. Ketamine has been combined with medetomidine in Asiatic otters at 4–5 mg/kg ketamine plus 0.1–0.12 mg/kg medetomidine to produce short-term anaesthesia (Lewis, 1991) and more recently in Eurasian otters with 5.1 mg/kg ketamine and 0.051 mg/kg medetomidine (Fernandez-Moran *et al.*, 2001). Transient apnoea occurs but respiratory efforts improve with stimulation. Ketamine 5 mg/kg plus medetomidine 0.08 mg/kg plus butorphanol 0.4 mg/kg produces good relaxation and excellent analgesia in otters (Simpson and King, 2003). This combination using medetomidine can be partially reversed with atipamezole 0.24–0.4 mg/kg. The use of atropine with alpha-2 agonists is not recommended unless heart block appears as it does not seem to reduce the bradycardia induced by xylazine and medetomidine, but hypertension often will occur; this is exacerbated by ketamine, which increases heart rate and cardiac output.

Gaseous anaesthesia

Isoflurane or sevoflurane: Isoflurane may be used as described above for red foxes. Sevoflurane provides an even faster knock-down and recovery. However, it is not generally advised that either anaesthetic is used to induce anaesthesia in otters unless dealing with small cubs due to the bite risk. Induction purely with isoflurane may be attempted in very debilitated otters and other mustelids; others, however, are better premedicated or sedated with acepromazine 0.2 mg/kg, or mixtures of ketamine, diazepam and medetomidine depending on the species. This reduces stress and breath-holding, and intubation and maintenance on gaseous anaesthesia may then be performed.

Once anaesthetised, otters in general may be intubated relatively easily, and this may well be necessary as they frequently become apnoeic during induction. Other mustelids are also easy to intubate, although weasels may require relatively small ET tubes (0.5–1 mm ID). Removal of the ET tube should be left for as long as possible on recovery in otters in particular due to their common apnoea problems. Therefore, it can be helpful to return them to a restraint cage while intubated, reverse the anaesthetic and tie a long piece of cord to the tube to allow its remote removal once the animal starts to swallow.

Seals (phocids)

Seal anaesthesia should always be performed during the cooler part of the day – early morning or late evening – as this will reduce the risks of hyperthermia induced by the stress of the procedure and some anaesthetics such as ketamine. In addition, the use of buckets of ice and cold wet towels over the extremities can be used to reduce the risk of hyperthermia for up to 4 hours after anaesthetic reversal. Finally, it is obviously important to ensure that any anaesthesia/sedation is only performed when the seal is on dry land and unable to gain access to water where a potentially life-threatening situation may arise.

Atropine is recommended in phocid seals at 0.02 mg/kg by deep intramuscular injection (the area laterally and just proximal to the flippers is useful with a 1–1.5 inch needle) 10 minutes prior to induction with a gas or injectable anaesthetic (Van-Bonn, 2015). This helps reduce the risks of bradycardia, which can be profound during induction, as well as reducing the oral/respiratory secretions.

Injectable anaesthetics

Ketamine and combinations: Combinations of ketamine 6 mg/kg and diazepam 0.3 mg/kg IM have been found to be useful in both grey and common seals. It is helpful to administer the diazepam first to induce muscle relaxation prior to injecting the ketamine, otherwise the ketamine can induce hyperthermia due to muscle contractions/rigidity combined with the insulative effects of the seal's blubber. This combination will give on average 20 minutes immobilisation time.

Other combinations with ketamine include the following.

- Medetomidine 0.06 mg/kg IM first followed by ketamine 2 mg/kg IM 15 minutes later in grey seal pups which usually gives around 1 hour of anaesthesia (Barnett, 1998).
- Medetomidine 0.025 mg/kg plus butorphanol 0.1 mg/kg followed by ketamine 2–2.5 mg/kg 15 minutes later in grey seal pups gives around 1 hour anaesthesia and better relaxation and analgesia (Barnett and Robinson, 2003).
- Midazolam 0.15 mg/kg first followed by ketamine 6 mg/kg plus midazolam 15 minutes later to avoid hyperthermia from muscle contractions associated with ketamine usage. Only provides short periods of anaesthesia (Barnett and Robinson, 2003).

Propofol: This has been used as an induction agent in phocids and for very short periods of anaesthesia. Its downside is its need to be given intravenously. Dosages of 5–6 mg/kg have been effective.

Tiletamine/zolazepam: This dissociative anaesthetic/benzodiazepine combination has been shown to be safe for common and grey seals, producing less risk of hyperthermia and less respiratory depression, with faster recovery times than ketamine/diazepam combinations when used at doses of 0.8–1.18 mg/kg IM (Langton *et al.*, 2011).

Gaseous anaesthetics

Isoflurane or sevoflurane: These are the anaesthetics of choice for maintenance of anaesthesia if a procedure is likely to last longer than 20 minutes. The seal may be intubated with a short-length, wide-bore ET tube as the trachea bifurcates into the two bronchi cranial to the thoracic inlet and so one-lung intubation is possible with long tubes. Alternatively, it may be possible to induce anaesthesia using isoflurane/sevoflurane via a face mask, and then attempt intubation. The downside to gaseous induction is that many grey and common seals can breath-hold, so making anaesthesia by this method alone difficult. It is advisable to intubate seals whenever anaesthesia is used as they have a lot of soft tissue at the back of the throat and a long soft palate. These can easily occlude the airway during injectable anaesthesia and so result in hypoxia.

Microchiropterans

Atropine 0.06 mg/kg or glycopyrrolate 0.01 mg/kg IM may be necessary prior to induction or shortly after induction to reduce oral secretions, which may become profuse.

Injectable anaesthetics

Very little has been published with regard to injectable anaesthetics in bats. The following have been briefly mentioned.

Ketamine and combinations: Used in combination with medetomidine intravenously, this has produced anaesthesia in flying foxes at 0.05 mg/kg medetomidine and 5 mg/kg ketamine (Epstein *et al.*, 2011). Medetomidine may be reversed with atipamezole at five times the dosage (in this instance, 0.25 mg/kg atipamezole). However, recovery may be prolonged.

Gaseous anaesthetics

Isoflurane or sevoflurane: These are the recommended anaesthetics for bats. Their disadvantage is the quick knock-down effect of the anaesthetic, which may cause the bat to become too deep too quickly. This may be a problem in the smaller species, but with experience they are both safe anaesthetics in microchiropteran bats. Pye (2001) views isoflurane as the anaesthetic of choice for microchiropterans.

European hedgehogs

Injectable anaesthetics

Alfaxalone: This has been used at 8–10 mg/kg IM on its own; alternatively, it can be combined with midazolam at doses of 3–5 mg/kg alfaxalone and 1 mg/kg midazolam IM, producing a light plane of anaesthesia at the lower alfaxalone dosage (Hawkins *et al.*, 2020).

Ketamine and combinations: This has been reported as useful for restraint but not full anaesthesia on its own at doses of 20 mg/kg IM but I do not recommend it. It has the disadvantage of poor muscle relaxation on its own, which makes unravelling the hedgehog difficult.

A combination of 2 mg/kg ketamine plus 0.2 mg/kg medetomidine plus 0.1 mg/kg fentanyl has been used in European hedgehogs and reversed with 1 mg/kg atipamezole and 0.16 mg/kg naloxone (Arnemo and Soli, 1995).

I have also used 0.08 mg/kg medetomidine with 5 mg/kg ketamine and found it to be effective. Reversal with atipamezole at five times the milligram per kilogram dose of medetomidine given is advised.

A combination of 30 mg/kg ketamine and 1 mg/kg midazolam has been used in African pygmy hedgehogs (Hawkins *et al.*, 2020).

PART IV: WILDLIFE

Gaseous anaesthetics

Isoflurane or sevoflurane: Isoflurane may be used for induction or maintenance or both. It is the more favoured anaesthetic as metabolism is minimal, knock-down is quick as is recovery, and so everything from quick procedures such as blood sampling through to more complicated procedures can be performed. In a curled-up state the hedgehog may be placed directly into an induction chamber. Once anaesthesia is induced the patient rapidly uncurls.

Sevoflurane may be used as for isoflurane via an induction chamber to induce anaesthesia at 5–6% and for maintenance at 3–4%.

Intubation may be complicated in some individuals as the size of the oral cavity is small and the epiglottis locked above the soft palate. An introducing/guide wire in the ET tube may help with intubation. Tube sizes required may vary from 1 to 4 mm ID in most individuals. In African pygmy hedgehogs a supraglottic airway device has been used successfully to maintain oxygen and gaseous anaesthetic supply and this may be an option for the European hedgehog when direct intubation is not possible (Huckins *et al.*, 2021).

Hares

Injectable anaesthetics

Ketamine and combinations: This may be used, as with domestic rabbits, in combination with medetomidine (20–35 mg/kg ketamine plus 0.3–0.5 mg/kg medetomidine) or with xylazine (20–35 mg/kg ketamine plus 5 mg/kg xylazine) intramuscularly to give 30–45 minutes of surgical anaesthesia. The lower doses are recommended for debilitated animals. As with many species the alpha-2 agonists cause blueing of the mucous membranes by peripheral vasoconstriction, which makes the assessment of hypoxia difficult. Apnoea can also easily occur.

Gaseous anaesthetics

Isoflurane or sevoflurane: This is best used after an injectable premedication as hares breath-hold like domestic rabbits. It is worthwhile pre-oxygenating the patient after premedication to ensure good haemoglobin saturation prior to induction, just in case apnoea occurs. Intubation is possible using a Wisconsin number 1 blade or similar paediatric laryngoscope, a rodent mouth gag and a 2–4 mm ID ET tube.

Sevoflurane may be used at slightly lower induction percentages than for foxes as lagomorphs still breath-hold at 8% sevoflurane. Therefore, induction is generally at 4–6% sevoflurane in 100% oxygen and maintenance at 2–3% sevoflurane in 100% oxygen.

Rodents

Injectable anaesthetics

Ketamine and combinations: Doses of 20–40 mg/kg may be used for immobilisation, although not for surgical anaesthesia due to the poor muscle relaxation and analgesic properties. It may be combined with xylazine at doses of 10–20 mg/kg ketamine to 2 mg/kg xylazine which considerably improves the muscle relaxation and analgesic properties and gives 30 minutes or so of anaesthesia. Alternatively, a combination of 5–7 mg/kg ketamine with 0.05–0.07 mg/kg medetomidine may be used. However, apnoea can be a problem with this combination and intubation is difficult in squirrels.

Gaseous anaesthesia

Isoflurane or sevoflurane: These are the anaesthetics of choice. Induction may be performed with 2–3% isoflurane or 5–6% sevoflurane via an induction chamber or face mask. In Eurasian beavers, placing the beaver into a hessian sack with its head in one corner allows a face mask to be placed over the muzzle safely without being bitten, with rapid induction times of 1–2 minutes.

Maintenance may then be performed by face mask at 1.5–2%. Intubation is possible but difficult in squirrels and small rodents due to their small oral cavity and long soft palate. It is relatively straightforward in Eurasian beavers but requires a long-bladed laryngoscope and 4–6 mm ID ET tube with preferably a guide wire to stiffen it for insertion. Recovery is rapid and though hypotension occurs it is minimal, with apnoea being transient during the initial induction phase. Pre-oxygenation without anaesthetic of the induction chamber first is a way to minimise hypoxia later on.

Wild birds

In general, it is advised that all wild birds, if they are to be chemically restrained, are so restrained using isoflurane or sevoflurane as the only source of anaesthesia. This is because knock-down times are very short, as are recovery times, and there is minimal hepatic metabolism of the anaesthetic. Both anaesthetics may be administered via a suitably sized induction chamber or via a face mask. Induction can be more difficult in long-beaked birds and requires adaptation of drinks bottles or other funnel-shaped devices (see Figure 27.7). Intubation is generally easy in birds and it is advisable to maintain a patent airway in all but the shortest of procedures. For more information please see Chapter 11.

Aspects of gaseous anaesthetic maintenance

Intermittent positive pressure ventilation

Where intubation is possible, then this may be required in any species, particularly reptiles and birds. However, some species are more susceptible to apnoea than others, including the otter, hares, and seals.

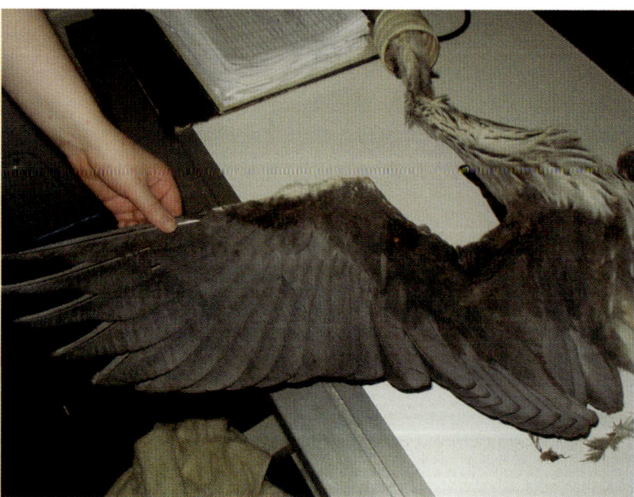

Figure 27.7 Induction of long-beaked birds, such as this grey heron with a wing injury, via inhalation anaesthesia can require adaptation of devices such as drinks bottles to provide a suitable shaped mask.

These species can all be intubated relatively straightforwardly after appropriate injectable/part gaseous induction, and the use of intermittent ventilation via manual expression of the rebreathing bag may well be required. Larger seals may benefit from mechanical respirators as they may require 20–30 mmHg pressure to inflate the lungs.

Anaesthetic circuits used

The smaller species such as hares, mustelids, foxes and hedgehogs may all be maintained on an Ayres T piece. Very small species, such as bats, some wild birds, and some mustelids such as the weasel, may require a Bethune, mini-Bain or Mapleson C circuit with minimal dead space. Larger species such as deer and seals may well require large animal circle circuits complete with soda-lime systems for prolonged anaesthesia.

Additional supportive therapy

Body temperature maintenance

This is very important for the smaller species such as wild rodents, hares, mustelids other than otters and smaller wild birds. Many methods can be used to provide heat for these animals:

- circulating water heat pads
- hot-water bottles/latex gloves filled with warm water
- bubble wrap or tin foil to conserve heat
- hot air circulating blankets.

It is also important to use as little water or surgical spirit as possible when preparing a patient in order to reduce heat loss. The administration of warmed fluids can also be very useful to maintain core body temperature.

However, the opposite difficulty may exist, with hyperthermia being a problem in seals and otters. Both have excellent insulation in the form of subcutaneous fat/blubber reserves and dense fur coats. Many of the injectable anaesthetic combinations involve the dissociative anaesthetic ketamine, which causes muscular rigidity that generates heat. The administration of other anaesthetics in combination with ketamine or before ketamine to allow muscle relaxation and the performance of these anaesthetic procedures at cooler times of the day (e.g. early morning) will all help. In addition, ice water and towels should be available for seals to be applied to the flippers if necessary.

Interestingly, elevated rectal temperatures in badgers during the early stages of anaesthesia (first 10 minutes) were associated in one study with sudden early recovery (McLaren *et al.*, 2005).

Fluid therapy

This, as with all species, is of vital importance for the full recovery of a patient, with particularly smaller species rapidly dehydrating during gaseous anaesthesia due to their large surface area to body weight ratio. In addition, many wild animals are severely debilitated on presentation and may have been anorectic and hence dehydrated for some time.

However, wildlife cases differ in one major respect from other animal patients in that they are less tolerant of persistently invasive procedures such as intravenous drip lines and repeated injections where restraint is required. Hence fluid therapy should always be considered at the time of any chemical restraint and the pros and cons of persistent re-administration of fluids weighed against the stress this may cause the individual animal.

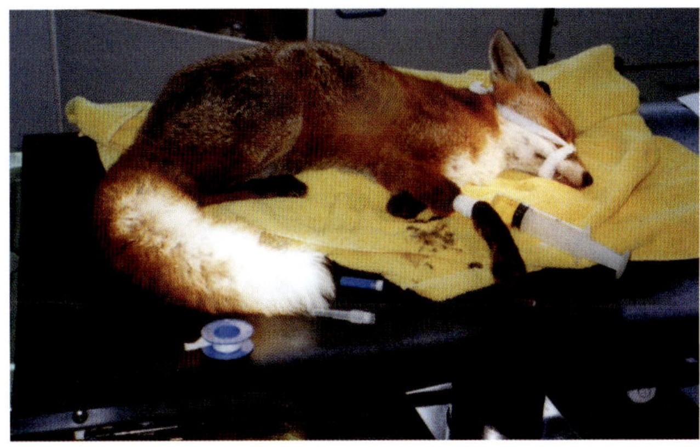

Figure 27.8 Intravenous fluid therapy can be administered via intravenous bolus or via syringe driver during general anaesthesia.

Routes of fluid administration vary from species to species. Most of the small mammals may have subcutaneous boluses of fluids administered when sedated/anaesthetised. However, this is not possible for seals as they have very little free subcutaneous space. Fluid therapy for seals must therefore be restricted to intravenous techniques via flipper veins during surgery, or more commonly by oral gavage/stomach tube along with nutritional support when awake.

Foxes, badgers and larger mustelids may have intravenous catheters placed in cephalic or saphenous veins, as for cats and dogs, during sedation/anaesthetic procedures, and relatively rapid rates of fluid administration may be given if severely dehydrated/shocked with hypotension (see Figure 27.8). Felids and rodents such as beavers are less tolerant of rapid fluid rates and so these should be administered with care while checking blood pressures. Duphalyte® (Zoetis UK Ltd.) or other intravenous amino-acid/B-vitamin complexes may be given at a rate of 1 mL/kg during this period.

For smaller mammals such as weasels and rodents, intraperitoneal fluids may be administered at a rate of 100 mL/kg per day (similar rates to domestic rodents).

Avian patients can receive boluses of fluids via the brachial vein or right jugular vein or, in long-legged birds, the medial metatarsal vein; alternatively, in severely shocked birds, the tibial crest or ulna bones may be utilised for intraosseous fluids (see Chapters 14 and 16). In bats, fluids may be administered via the brachial vein.

Deer may have jugular catheters placed, with flexible intravenous drip lines attached while they are kept in darkened holding pens during rehabilitation. However, these carry the risk of entanglement and so should be used for the shortest periods possible.

In all cases similar fluid compositions to those utilised in cat and dog medicine are best (i.e. lactated Ringer's or 0.9% saline). In hypoglycaemic animals, 50% dextrose solutions administered at 1–2 mL/kg body weight diluted 50 : 50 with 0.9% saline should be given intravenously. All fluids should be warmed to near core body temperature before administration. For a more in-depth discussion please see Chapter 29.

Monitoring of anaesthesia

Similar techniques to those used in other branches of veterinary medicine may be used. These include the traditional external and oesophageal stethoscopes, the use of respiratory monitors and capnographs attached to the anaesthetic circuit if intubation has occurred, and the use of Doppler techniques in smaller species to pick up faint heartbeats or peripheral pulses. In addition, ECG techniques may be used along with pulse oximetry. Most of the mammals will respond to anaesthesia in a similar way to cats and dogs or other small domestic mammals. Pulse oximeters will not give accurate SpO_2 measurements in neonatal mammals or in birds, amphibians and reptiles of any age due to the differing structure of haemoglobin. However, they may still be used to demonstrate changing trends in SpO_2 levels.

Blood pressure is relatively conserved across species and systolic pressures are generally around 120–140 mmHg in mammals, with the exception of Eurasian beavers whose systolic blood pressure is rarely above 75 mmHg. Avian species tend to have a systolic blood pressure between 120 and 200 mmHg and reptiles again are lower being typically 40–60 mmHg. Indirect measurement of blood pressure can be performed in mammals similar to the technique used in cats and dogs, with a Doppler placed over the ventral carpal area and a cuff 40% of the width of the forelimb placed above or below the elbow. Smaller species may be a challenge as cuff sizes are often too big. Direct blood pressure measurement may be performed if an artery can be cannulated.

The resting heart rate for mammals is calculated from the allometric equation (Schmidt-Nielsen, 1984):

$$\text{Heart rate} = 241 \times \left(\text{weight}\left[\text{kg}\right]\right)^{-0.25}$$

Hares and mustelids may be monitored by their response to pain stimuli such as toe withdrawal reflexes or tail/ear pinch reflexes. Eye position may be used for foxes, wildcats and badgers.

Deer and seals are difficult to monitor, the latter particularly so as pulse oximeters are best placed in the mouth on the underside of the tongue or per rectum in order to contact a blood vessel adequately and breath-holding frequently occurs. A response, or non-response, to pain stimuli is therefore useful as are heart rate and rhythm, as for cats and dogs; the colour of the mucous membranes also gives a good indication of blood oxygenation. ECGs and capnography (assuming they are intubated, which is recommended for seals) may also be used. It should be noted that while most mammals and birds would be expected to have capnography of 30–45 mmHg, seals may have very high levels of carbon dioxide, often reaching 70–80 mmHg in uncomplicated anaesthesia, and this is considered normal (Van-Bonn, 2015).

Body temperature should be monitored closely in those species prone to overheating, such as seals and deer. The core temperature of most eutherian mammals is between 36 and 38°C, with some exceptions such as the beaver and European hedgehog where it is often around 35°C and some of the rodents and smaller mustelids where it may be above 39°C (Schmidt-Nielsen, 1984; Reeve, 1994; Heard, 2014). Temperatures above 40°C should be treated as an emergency, with application of cold water enemas, cold intravenous fluids, wetting the fur with cold water and using fans to increase evaporative losses, all in the attempt to reduce core temperatures. Hyperthermia has also been reported in badgers, where elevated rectal temperatures (>38°C) that do not naturally fall within the first 10 minutes of induction may be associated with sudden early recovery (McLaren *et al.*, 2005). Avian species tend to have core temperatures between 37 and 42°C. Hypothermia is more commonly seen in smaller species, particularly birds and rodents, and associated with trauma and shock. If core temperatures drop below 34.4°C, the animal cannot then regulate its own body temperature through shivering, etc. and so will require emergency support with warmed fluids and other heating techniques until rectal temperatures for mammals achieve at least 36.9°C (Ko and Krimins, 2014).

Recovery and analgesia

In all cases where wildlife is concerned, the recovery period from anaesthesia is a critical time where if the animal starts to panic, severe trauma may be caused by the animal to itself. Therefore, the recovery period should be as stress-free as possible.

The recovery box/room should be darkened and all extraneous noises kept to a minimum. In particular it is vital to keep all sound and scent of predator animals, such as foxes and mink, away from prey species such as hares, etc., otherwise instant fright and flight responses will be triggered.

Anaesthetics are therefore chosen with a quick recovery in mind to ensure that as little time as possible is spent in a semi-conscious state, which is the most dangerous period. Therefore, gases such as isoflurane and sevoflurane and reversible injectable agents such as alpha-2 drugs, benzodiazepines and opioids may be preferred.

Analgesia plays an important role in the rehabilitation and recovery period. Inadequate or no analgesia may lead to death via unacceptably high stress levels and failure to eat, drink or indeed move on the part of the patient. Analgesics with long intervals between dosing are also favoured, hence the short-acting opioids such as pethidine and butorphanol are less favoured than the 12-hourly dosing intervals of opioid drugs such as buprenorphine or the 24-hourly intervals of non-steroidal anti-inflammatory drugs such as carprofen and meloxicam.

Doses of these drugs are frequently extrapolations from known doses in domestic species; for example, doses of 4–5 mg/kg carprofen are often used for small mammals and birds, doses of 0.01–0.03 mg/kg buprenorphine in small mammals, doses of 0.2–1.5 mg/kg meloxicam in small mammals, and doses of 0.3–0.6 mg/kg meloxicam in large mammals such as deer.

References

Arnemo, J.M. and Soli, N.E. (1995) Chemical immobilization of free-ranging European hedgehogs (*Erinaceus europaeus*). *Journal of Zoo and Wildlife Medicine*, **26**, 246–251.

Barnett, J. (1998) Treatment of sick and injured marine mammals. *In Practice*, **20**, 200–211.

Barnett, J. and Robinson, I. (2003) Marine mammals. In: *BSAVA Manual of Wildlife Casualties* (eds E. Mullineaux, D. Best & J. Cooper), pp. 182–201. BSAVA Quedgeley, Glos.

Brash, M. (2003) Foxes. In: *BSAVA Manual of Wildlife Casualties* (eds E. Mullineaux, D. Best & J. Cooper), pp. 154–165. BSAVA Quedgeley, Glos.

Epstein, J.H., Zambriski, J.A., Rostal, M.K. *et al.* (2011) Comparison of intravenous medetomidine and medetomidine/ketamine for immobilization of free-ranging variable flying foxes (*Pteropus hypomelanus*). *PLoS One*, **6**(10), e25361.

Fernandez-Moran, J., Palomeque, J. and Peinado, P.I. (2000) Medetomidine/tiletamine/zolazepam and xylazine/tiletamine/zolazepam combinations for immobilization of fallow deer (*Cervus dama*). *Journal of Zoo and Wildlife Medicine*, **31**(1), 62–64.

Fernandez-Moran, J., Perez, E., Sanmartin, M. *et al.* (2001) Reversible immobilization of Eurasian otters with a combination of ketamine and medetomidine. *Journal of Wildlife Disease*, **37**(3), 561–565.

de Leeuw, A.N.S., Forrester, G.J., Spyvee, P.D. *et al.* (2003) Experimental comparison of ketamine with a combination of ketamine, butorphanol and medetomidine for general anaesthesia of the Eurasian badger (*Meles meles L.*). *Veterinary Journal*, **167**, 186–193.

Hawkins, S.J., Doss, G.A. and Mans, C. (2020) Evaluation of subcutaneous administration of alfaxalone–midazolam and ketamine–midazolam as sedation protocols in African pygmy hedgehogs (*Atelerix albiventris*). *Journal of the American Veterinary Medical Association*, **257**(8), 820–825.

Heard, D. (2014) Rodents. In: *Zoo Animal and Wildlife Immobilization and Anesthesia* (eds G. West, D. Heard & N. Caulkett), 2nd edn, pp. 893–903. Wiley Blackwell, Ames, Iowa.

Huckins, G.L., Doss, G.A. and Ferreira, T.H. (2021) Evaluation of supraglottic airway device use during inhalation anesthesia in healthy African pygmy hedgehogs (*Atelerix albiventris*). *Veterinary Anaesthesia and Analgesia*, **48**(4), 517–523.

Kreeger, T.J., Seal, E.S. and Tester, J.R. (1990) Chemical immobilization of red foxes (*Vulpes vulpes*). *Journal of Wildlife Disease*, **26**(1), 95–98.

Ko, J.C. and Krimins, R.A. (2014) Thermoregulation. In: *Zoo Animal and Wildlife Immobilization and Anesthesia* (eds G. West, D. Heard & N. Caulkett), 2nd edn, pp. 65–68. Wiley Blackwell, Ames, Iowa.

Kollias, G.V. and Fernandez-Moran, J. (2015) Mustelidae. In: *Fowler's Zoo and Wild Animal Medicine* (ed. R.E. Miller), vol. 8, pp. 476–490. Elsevier, Philadelphia.

Langton, S.D., Moss, S.E., Pomeroy, P.P. and Borer, K.E. (2011) Effect of induction dose, lactation stage and body condition on tiletamine–zolazepam anaesthesia in adult female grey seals (*Halichoerus grypus*) under field conditions. *Veterinary Record*, **168**(17), 457.

Lewis, J. (1991) Reversible immobilisation of Asian small-clawed otters with medetomidine and ketamine. *Veterinary Record*, **128**, 86–87.

MacKintosh, C.G., MacArthur, J.A., Little, T.W.A. and Stuart, P. (1976) The immobilization of the badger (*Meles meles*). *British Veterinary Journal*, **132**, 609–614.

Masters, N. and Flach, E. (2015) Tragulidae, Moschidae and Cervidae. In: *Fowler's Zoo and Wild Animal Medicine* (ed. R.E. Miller), vol. 8, pp. 611–625. Elsevier, Philadelphia.

McLaren, G.W., Thornton, P.D., Newman, C. *et al.* (2005) High rectal temperature indicates an increased risk of unexpected recovery in anaesthetized badgers. *Veterinary Anaesthesia and Analgesia*, **32**(1), 48–52.

Pye, G.W. (2001) Marsupial, insectivore and chiropteran anesthesia. *Veterinary Clinics of North America: Exotic Animal Practice*, **4**(1), 211–237.

Reed, M., Caulkett, N.A. and McCallister, M. (2000) Evaluation of zuclopenthixol acetate to decrease handling stress in wapiti. *Journal of Wildlife Disease*, **36**, 450–459.

Reeve, N. (1994) *Hedgehogs. Poyser Natural History*. Academic Press, London.

Schmidt-Nielsen, K. (1984) *Scaling. Why Is Animal Size So Important?* Cambridge University Press, New York.

Simpson, V. and King, M.A. (2003) Otters. In: *BSAVA Manual of Wildlife Casualties* (eds E. Mullineaux, D. Best & J. Cooper), pp. 137–146. BSAVA Quedgeley, Glos.

Stocker, L. (2009) Deer. In: *Practical Wildlife Care*, 2nd edn, pp. 253–267. Wiley.

Thornton, P.D., Newman, C., Johnson, P.J. *et al.* (2005) Preliminary comparison of four anaesthetic techniques in badgers (*Meles meles*). *Veterinary Anaesthesia and Analgesia*, **32**(1), 40–47.

Van-Bonn, W.G. (2015) Pinnipedia. In: *Fowler's Zoo and Wild Animal Medicine* (ed. R.E. Miller), vol. 8, pp. 436–449. Elsevier, Philadelphia.

Chapter 28 Common Wildlife Disease

In an attempt to reduce repetition and due to the constraints on space, this chapter focuses primarily on mammalian diseases. The reader is referred to Chapter 13 (avian diseases) and Chapter 21 (reptile and amphibian disease) for more detailed information on other species.

ARTIODACTYLS: CERVIDS

Ectoparasites

Mites

Psoroptes spp. have been occasionally associated with pruritus, crusting, hyperkeratosis and fur loss in a range of wild ruminants. *Chorioptes* spp. mites, whilst considered less irritant than *Psoroptes* spp., may still infest wild ruminants such as deer, reindeer and bison causing patchy fur loss.

Lice

Deer are afflicted by both biting (mallophagan) and sucking (anopluran) lice. Biting lice are rarely pathogenic and include *Damalinia longicornis* in red deer, *Damalinia meyeri* in sika deer, *Damalinia tibialis* in fallow deer and *Damalinia indica* in muntjac.

Sucking lice are also rarely associated with primary disease but can induce anaemia in debilitated and young ruminants. Examples include *Solenopotes burmeisteri* in red, roe and fallow deer and *Solenopotes muntiacus* in muntjac.

Ticks

The sheep tick *Ixodes ricinus* is a common occasional ectoparasite of ruminants in Europe. It is often associated with the transmission of bacterial, viral and protozoal diseases in many species and may do so in deer. ‘Louping ill’ (a viral disease of deer and domestic ruminants), tick-borne fever (due to a blood-borne parasite *Anaplasma (Ehrlichia) phagocytophilum*) and babesiosis (a blood-borne protozoal parasite) as well as staphylococcal septicaemia/abscesses may all be transmitted.

Biting flies

Several species of fly may be found affecting wild ruminants. The commonest seen are the head fly (*Hydrotaea irritans*), which also afflicts domestic livestock, and the deer keds (*Lipoptena cervi*) which are a family of wingless (to be accurate reduced wing size) fly.

Nasal fly

Red deer bot fly (*Cephenemyia auribarbis*) is viviparous and active from July to September. The adult female bot fly squirts larvae up the nose of the red deer as she flies past and so cause disturbance, making the deer run about (‘gadding’). The larvae develop in the nasopharynx of the deer and eventually are sneezed out and develop into adult flies once again. Their main cause of debilitation in deer is loss of condition due to the increased exercise induced; rarely, sufficient numbers of bot fly larvae may be present in the nasopharynx of one deer to cause suffocation.

Warble fly

The deer warble fly is known as *Hypoderma diana*. The fly lays its eggs on the hair shafts of the deer. The eggs hatch and the larvae crawl to the hair follicle and migrate through the skin. They then continue their journey towards the spinal column of the deer, where the larvae remain throughout the winter months. They appear to cause no damage to the nervous tissues and generally no clinical signs are seen. In February and March, the larvae start migrating again, reaching a subcutaneous position over the dorsum of the deer where they sit in a raised swelling with a central breathing hole to the surface. Eventually the larvae mature and drop to the ground where they pupate into adult flies to complete the life cycle.

Endoparasites

Digestive tract nematodes

The Trichostrongyloidea are small, thin nematodes, and are the commonest intestinal and stomach worms affecting wild ruminants. Nematodes such as *Ostertagia* spp., *Haemonchus contortus* and *Trichostrongylus* spp. are all known to infest the abomasum or true stomach. They may be present in small numbers and cause no clinical disease or in greater numbers that result in damage to the lining of the abomasum and thus affect digestion. Clinically diarrhoea, dehydration and weight loss may be seen. *Haemonchus contortus* is particularly serious and can cause significant anaemia and hypoproteinaemia in affected individuals, with diarrhoea and sometimes oedema of the ventrum and limbs due to hypoproteinaemia.

Trichuris spp. (‘whipworms’) are seen in the large intestines of many ruminants, particularly roe deer, sika deer and Chinese water deer. They do not seem to be a cause of significant disease, but their characteristic oval bi-operculate eggs may be found in the faeces routinely.

Lungworms

The cattle lungworm *Dictyocaulus viviparous* has been recorded as a cause of lung disease in roe and Chinese water deer in the UK and wild ruminants in Europe. It may present as clinical dyspnoea and coughing and result in bronchitis with secondary pneumonia

Veterinary Nursing of Exotic Pets and Wildlife, Third Edition. Simon J. Girling.

and death of the infected roe deer. It is more commonly seen in the autumn in areas with high rainfall. Eggs are laid by adult worms in the bronchioles and then hatch immediately into the first-stage larva that are coughed up, swallowed and passed in the faeces. The larvae mature and are then taken up by grazing ruminants, where they migrate through the small intestinal wall and then migrate to the mesenteric lymph nodes. The larvae mature further and move in the blood and lymph fluids to the lungs to mature as adults.

Elaphostrongylus cervi has also been recovered from pneumonic lung lesions in red and roe deer. This parasite uses an intermediate host (the grey field slug) to complete its life cycle. Other lungworms (*Varestrongylus capreoli* and *V. sagittatus*) have been associated with lung infections in roe deer in south-west England (Simpson and Blake, 2018).

Trematodes (flukes)

Sheep and cattle liver flukes *Fasciola hepatica* and *Dicrocoelium dendriticum* have both been recorded in wild ruminants.

Fasciola hepatica has been seen in red, fallow, roe and occasionally muntjac deer. It is transmitted through an intermediate host, snails of *Lymnea* spp., commonly found in wet and boggy areas. Fluke eggs are shed in the faeces of the deer, taken up by the snail where they develop to form a motile cercaria that escapes from the snail and swims through surface water attaching to grass stems. There it forms an encysted stage (metacercaria) which is eaten by the next deer host. The metacercaria hatches in the deer's small intestine, penetrates the gut wall and heads for the liver. Flukes burrow through the liver to the bile ducts where they shed eggs into the biliary system and so into the gut and back out in the faeces. The whole life cycle takes approximately 17–18 weeks. Occasionally a deer may suffer from liver damage due to this fluke. Clinical signs include oedema of the ventrum and limbs due to a hypoproteinaemia (principally a hypoalbuminaemia from liver damage), and very occasionally jaundice.

Dicrocoelium dendriticum is another liver fluke, although the adult is very small, being only 1 cm long (unlike *Fasciola hepatica* which is 3–4 cm long). It again uses a land snail as the first intermediate host, then shed cercaria are consumed by ants, and develop further before the ant is consumed by grazing deer. The metacercaria in the ant hatches inside the deer's small intestine and again migrates to the liver via the bile duct and so rarely causes severe liver damage in wild ruminants.

Protozoa

Coccidiosis is a disease caused by coccidian protozoans such as *Eimeria*. Various *Eimeria* spp. have been recorded particularly in roe deer. In young, heavily infested deer, diarrhoea and poor weight gain may be seen. The coccidial parasites are small, oval in shape and can be shown easily on a faecal smear.

Toxoplasma gondii is an intestinal parasite of domestic and wild felids and may cause abortion in ruminants such as deer. It is also zoonotic and so care should be taken to use suitable personal protective equipment if dealing with any aborted materials.

Babesiosis

The blood-borne protozoal parasite *Babesia* spp. is transmitted by ticks and has caused disease in red and roe deer. The disease can cause intravascular haemolysis of erythrocytes, resulting in pyrexia and haemoglobinuria and giving the disease its more familiar name of 'redwater fever'. Most deer seem to recover and develop their own immunity, and the passage of passive immunity from hind to calf in the colostrum appears to occur, in much the same way as happens in cattle. The danger is when a calf fails to receive the natural colostrum from its mother, such as a hand-reared calf, and is then released into an infected area.

Bacterial diseases

Anthrax

This is due to the bacterium *Bacillus anthracis*. The disease is legally notifiable in many countries due to its zoonotic and highly dangerous potential for humans and, if suspected, government veterinary authorities should be contacted; in the UK this would currently be the Animal and Plant Health Agency (APHA). The spores of the bacterium will survive for many decades in the soil in areas that have been previously affected. Grazing animals may then be exposed to the spores, which may gain access to the bloodstream via cuts and grazes or inhaled into the lungs. The bacterial septicaemia which ensues is frequently rapidly fatal in ruminants. Diagnosis is made on finding blue-staining chains of bacilli on blood smears stained with methylene blue.

Bovine tuberculosis

Mycobacterium bovis is found in wild deer at low levels, with typically 1–5% of individuals being affected in south-west England for example (Delahay *et al.*, 2007). However, elsewhere in Europe in a more recent statistical review study it was estimated that up to 20% of fallow deer are likely to be affected, having the highest weighted mean disease incidence (Justus *et al.*, 2024). Transmission is via oral or respiratory routes, or occasionally cutaneous. In cattle, tuberculosis lesions produce a white caseous gritty nodule, although the abscesses produced in deer (and suids) can be more fluid and yellow-white, resembling abscesses due to other forms of less dangerous bacteria. This is important as any abscess seen in a wild deer could potentially be due to *M. bovis* and hence a zoonotic risk to the handler. Rarely will a wild deer show serious clinical signs of disease due to *M. bovis*, although a productive cough, cutaneous/subcutaneous abscesses and occasionally weight loss may be seen. If bovine tuberculosis is suspected in a wild deer, then the APHA in the UK should be contacted for further advice. APHA will make the diagnosis by culture of retropharyngeal, mediastinal and bronchial lymph nodes or any obvious granulomatous lesion, often in lung tissue.

Brucellosis

Brucella spp. infection has been reported in red, fallow, sika and roe deer as well as many wild bovids and ovids. It can cause abortion in domestic cattle, as well as orchitis in bulls and is a significant zoonotic disease. It is generally not life-threatening in ruminants, although fever, the above-mentioned abortion and anorexia may be observed, and in cervids often multiple joint swellings may be seen. There is currently no treatment for this condition but it is now rare, the last case in domestic cattle in the UK being reported in 2004.

Chlamydia spp.

Chlamydia spp. can, like *T. gondii*, result in abortion in ruminants. It may also affect breeding success. Clinical disease is poorly reported in the literature in wild ruminants, but seroprevalence in some populations may be high, 36.9% in European bison in Poland for example (Didkowska *et al.*, 2021). In roe deer in Italy one survey suggested levels of 4.6% (Ebani *et al.*, 2022). It is also a potential zoonosis and so care should be taken when handling any aborted material or where disease is suspected.

Clostridiosis

Clostridium spp. are known to cause a variety of diseases in grazing animals mainly through the release of potent exotoxins, which induce severe tissue damage, haemorrhagic enteritis and gangrene. *Clostridium* spp. are environmental organisms and more commonly affect young or immunologically naive animals. Treatment is rarely effective.

Coxiella burnetii (Q fever)

Seropositivity has been reported in a wide range of wild ruminants, from 0.58% in European bison, 1.2% in roe deer in Belgium, 2.4% in red deer and 6.8% in mouflon in Spain (Tavernier *et al.*, 2015; Fernández-Aguilar *et al.*, 2016; Didkowska *et al.*, 2021). It may also be detected by polymerase chain reaction (PCR) on tissue or blood samples. It produces an acute phase with fever and respiratory signs associated often with abortion in gravid females. It is a potential zoonosis and is highly infectious and can be transmitted via physical contact with infected tissues or by aerosol so extreme care should be taken around potentially positive cases.

Leptospirosis

This has been recorded in red deer, fallow deer and roe deer and may occasionally result in abortion or renal disease. As with any mammal, deer may become carriers of the bacterium and it is zoonotic being shed in urine and aborted placental or fetal material and gaining access through mucous membranes or wounds.

Paratuberculosis (Johne's disease)

Infection with *Mycobacterium avium* subsp. *paratuberculosis* can cause disease in a variety of large herbivores, including domestic cattle and sheep as well as wild ruminants. It produces an inflammatory, granulomatous intestinal disease resulting in weight loss and resultant poor coats and patchy alopecia (Fawcett *et al.*, 1995). Diagnosis is made on clinical signs and the demonstration of mycobacteria in the faeces using Ziehl–Neelsen acid-fast stains combined with PCR techniques. It is not treatable.

Pasteurellosis

Pasteurella haemolytica (now *Mannheimia haemolytica*) and *Pasteurella multocida* have both been isolated from the airways of deer affected with pneumonia (see Figure 28.1). The disease is thought to be spread via the oronasal route or as an aerosol. It is highly contagious, but generally only severely affects weaker debilitated individuals. Clinical signs include dyspnoea, coughing and nasal mucopurulent discharge. Abscesses, particularly in the cervical lymph nodes, may also be seen.

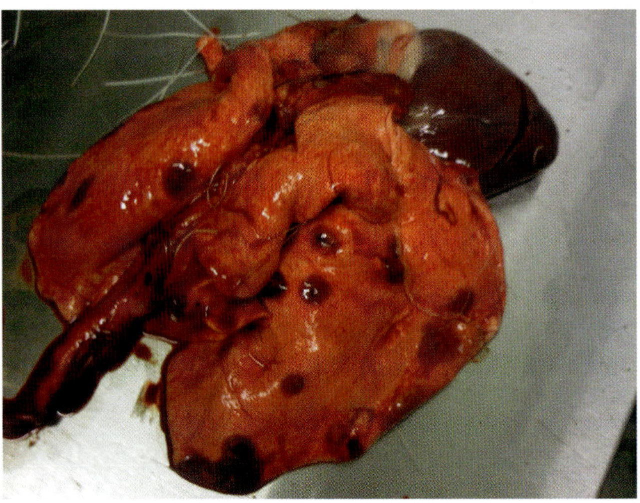

Figure 28.1 Pneumonia due to *Mannheimia haemolytica* is frequently reported in ungulates, particularly those affected by lungworm.

Yersiniosis

Yersinia pseudotuberculosis has been associated with intestinal disease in deer, particularly young muntjac where it causes gastroenteritis, although less commonly septicaemia may develop with lethargy, respiratory distress, and death. It is a potential zoonosis causing pharyngitis and enterocolitis. *Yersinia enterocolitica* was most frequently recovered in subclinically infected red deer (*Cervus elaphus*) in a study in Norway (4.7%), the prevalence of all *Yersinia* spp. being 5.9% (Aschfalk *et al.*, 2008).

Viral diseases

Bluetongue virus

This arbovirus has multiple serotypes and is found throughout Europe, Middle East and Africa. It is transmitted by midges and there are several strains. Clinical disease in many cervids appears mild and transient with a pyrexia, upper respiratory signs and very occasionally abortion. It is a notifiable disease in the UK and Europe similar to tuberculosis.

Bovine viral diarrhoea virus and border disease virus

These are pestiviruses related to classical swine fever virus. Bovine viral diarrhoea virus (BVDV) has been reported in a number of wild ruminants including cervids such as red, roe, fallow, sika and Chinese water deer, as well as reindeer and moose (Frolich, 2012). Clinical signs include diarrhoea, coronitis and laminitis in reindeer (Morton *et al.*, 1990). Infection of late term fetuses can result in persistently infected and infectious animals that perpetuate the disease, similar to domestic cattle. Haemorrhagic mucosal inflammation may be seen with acute infections with catarrhal enteritis and immunosuppression. Detection of the virus is by real-time reverse transcription (RT)-PCR or antibody enzyme-linked immunosorbent assay (ELISA).

Border disease virus (BDV) typically affects cervids, ovids and caprids. Antibodies have been demonstrated in roe deer (Marco, 2012). Alopecia and skin pigmentation has also been reported which can start on the head and neck and spread to the whole body. Neurological disease, anaemia and susceptibility to secondary infections (such as bacterial pneumonias) are also common. Detection of the virus is by RT-PCR or antibody ELISA.

Foot and mouth disease

This picornavirus is not currently present in the UK or Europe but deer like other ruminants are susceptible. It is highly infectious and a legally notifiable disease.

Herpesviruses

Cervid herpesviruses

This alpha-herpesvirus has two serotypes: cervid herpesvirus 1 (CvHV1) found throughout Europe in primarily red, but also roe and fallow deer; and cervid herpesvirus 2 (CvHV2) found predominantly in reindeer in Scandinavia. Both are spread by physical contact, aerosols and through mating and can demonstrate latency in their hosts, producing a mild keratoconjunctivitis and affecting the lips. They may be involved in abortions and cause a respiratory disease complex resulting in epithelial hyperplasia and destruction over time (Das Neves *et al.*, 2009).

Malignant catarrhal fever

This gamma-herpesvirus is spread from sheep by aerosol and can affect domestic cattle and deer. It causes a conjunctivitis, photophobia, a serous to purulent nasal discharge, fever, enlarged lymph nodes and sometimes diarrhoea. The signs in deer appear to be less severe than those seen in domestic cattle. There is no treatment for this virus.

Louping ill

This flavivirus is transmitted by ticks such as *Ixodes ricinus*. It has been found in young roe deer and red deer in particular. It may be subclinical but it can induce a non-suppurative meningitis and encephalitis that can lead to permanent damage to the central nervous system (CNS). There is no treatment available.

Paramyxovirus

The paramyxovirus parainfluenza virus 3 (PIV-3) affects roe deer in particular. Most infections produce no clinical signs, but it can produce a suppurative bronchopneumonia, particularly in a stressed individual. It is a respiratory spread virus is shed and highly infectious from animal to animal. There is no treatment.

Trauma

Road traffic collisions are extremely common for deer, particularly roe deer which are crepuscular to nocturnal in nature (see Figure 28.2). Injuries are often fatal or require the ruminant to be humanely destroyed as they frequently involve compound fractures to the limbs, and ruptured diaphragms. In addition, hindlimb lameness is often associated with pelvic fractures post road traffic collisions.

Trauma to the antlers when 'in velvet' in cervids can cause severe blood loss. There are no large vessels which can be ligated on the antler itself. Damage to the antler once the velvet has been shed tends to be less of a problem, as the antler will be shed after the rut and a new antler bud forms the following season.

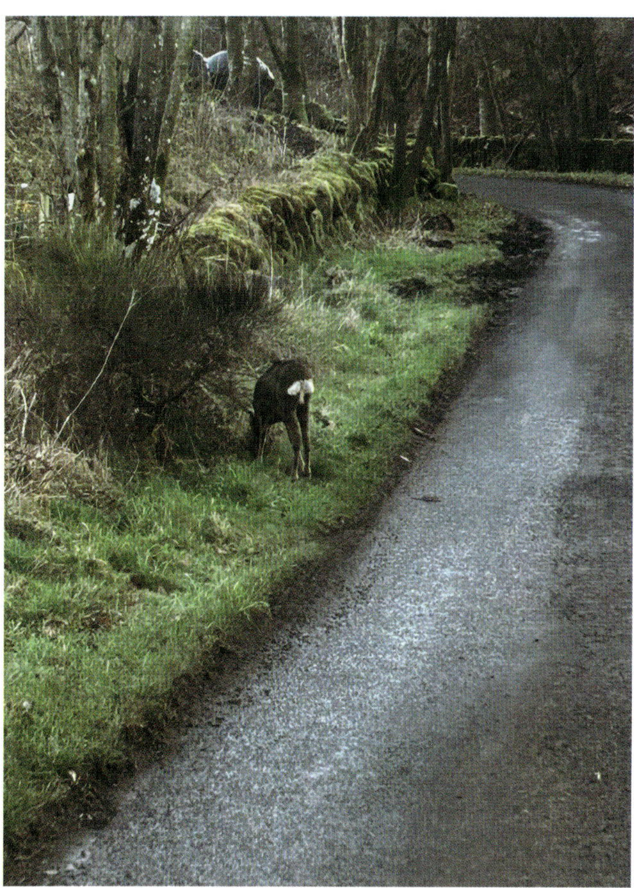

Figure 28.2 Road traffic collisions are common in deer, particularly in the late spring to summer and often in species such as roe deer, around dawn or dusk.

Poisoning

This is uncommon in wild ruminants. Cases of blue-green algae poisoning have been reported when deer have drunk from lakes/ponds containing this organism. Clinical signs include ataxia, diarrhoea, lethargy and convulsions in serious cases.

Other diseases

Neoplasia

Hepatocellular carcinomas are commonly seen in roe deer in the UK, but there is considerable regional variation. This is thought to reflect diet, with a suggestion that higher heather and spruce consumption may increase the risks (de Jong *et al.*, 2004).

Swayback

This is uncommon but has been reported on Scottish islands and areas with high molybdenum levels in the soil as this reduces copper absorption from the gut. Damage to the motor tracts of the spinal cord have been recorded, with clinical signs of hindlimb paresis, poor coat and loss of fur and high endoparasite burdens with anaemia. The condition once developed is irreversible. Liver copper levels are often below 20–30 ppm of dry matter and blood copper below 5 μmol/L.

CANIDAE: FOXES

Ectoparasites

Fleas

Cat and/or dog fleas *Ctenocephalides felis* and *C. canis*, as well as the rabbit flea *Spilopsyllus cuniculi*, are commonly found but rarely cause disease in their own right.

Mites

Sarcoptes scabiei is common in both rural and urban foxes. Urban foxes have been recently recorded as a main reservoir for infestation of domestic dogs. It is a widespread cause of mortality in the red fox. It is seen as both an acute form (intense pruritus, inflammation, papules and seborrhoea without alopecia) and a chronic form (tail base and dorsal body initially develop alopecia and lichenification).

Other mites commonly seen include the ear mite *Otodectes cynotis* which can cause severe ear infections and self-trauma, particularly again in *Vulpes* spp.

Diagnosis is made on skin scrapings and wax scrapings demonstrating the ectoparasite(s).

Ticks

Ixodes spp. ticks are common on debilitated foxes and may result in secondary skin infections and transmission of blood-borne parasites.

Endoparasites

Digestive system nematodes

Roundworms *Toxocara canis* and *Toxascaris leonina* are generally subclinical but in young cubs may lead to poor growth, or rarely a bowel blockage and death.

Hookworms such as *Ancylostoma tubaeforme* can result in clinical anaemia and poor growth and *Uncinaria stenocephala* (the northern hookworm) can cause diarrhoea and weight loss in young canids and pedal dermatitis, as the larval stages may migrate through the skin of the feet to gain access to the host's body (see Figure 28.3).

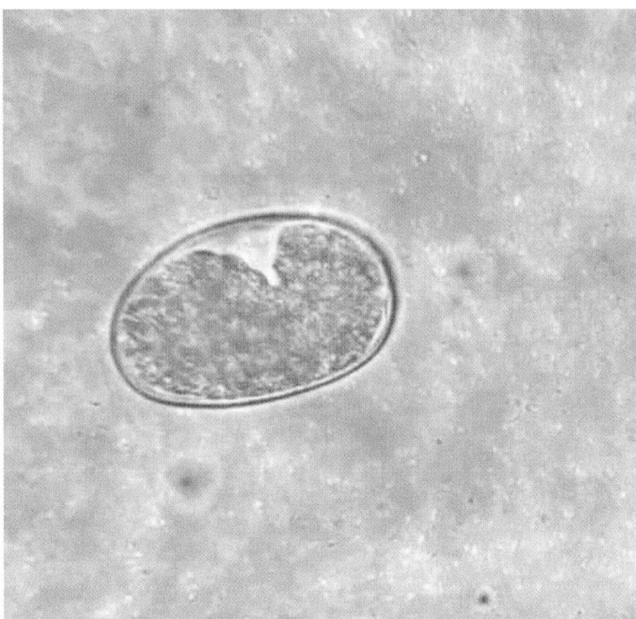

Figure 28.3 Oocyst of the northern hookworm *Uncinaria stenocephala* from a red fox.

Whipworms such as *Trichuris vulpis* has been known to cause diarrhoea in young cubs.

Spirocerca lupi has not been found in the UK but has recently been reported in a red fox in central Italy (Morandi *et al*., 2014). It has an indirect life cycle involving beetles and/or avian paratenic hosts before the infective L3 stage is consumed by the fox and develops in a granuloma in the wall of the oesophagus. This can lead on to oesophageal neoplasia or rupture of the aorta.

Digestive system cestodes (tapeworms)

These parasites rarely seem to cause pathogenicity in adult canids although, theoretically, large enough burdens could cause blockage of the small intestine, more likely in young animals. A few of the commonly seen ones are included in Table 28.1.

Table 28.1 Tapeworms of foxes.

Tapeworm	Intermediate stage (common host)	Notes
Echinococcus granulosus equinus	Hydatid cyst (equids)	Uncommon and only a few millimetres long in the definitive host
Echinococcus granulosus granulosus	Hydatid cyst (rodents usually voles)	Not currently in the UK and only a few millimetres long in the definitive host
Echinococcus multilocularis	Multilocular cysts (rodents usually voles)	Not currently present in the UK and a legally notifiable disease in the UK and only a few millimetres long in the definitive host
Taenia hydatigena	*Cysticercus tenuicollis* (sheep, cattle and pigs)	Up to 5 m long tapeworm in the definitive host
Taenia multiceps	*Coenurus cerebralis* (sheep)	Intermediate stage affects the brain of sheep. 1 m long tapeworm in the definitive host
Taenia ovis	*Cysticercus ovis* (sheep)	1.5–2 m long tapeworm in the definitive host
Taenia pisiformis	*Cysticercus pisiformis* (wild rodents, rabbits and hares)	1–2 m long tapeworm in the definitive host
Taenia serialis	*Coenurus serialis* (wild rabbits and hares)	50–70 cm long tapeworm in the definitive host

Lungworms

Capillaria (Eucoleus) aerophila may be found in the mucosa of the trachea, nasopharynx and bronchi of red foxes and causes a rhinotracheitis. It has a direct life cycle, the eggs being laid in the airways and then coughed up, swallowed and passed in the faeces. The eggs can survive for months in the environment where they are then ingested by the fox, or taken up by earthworms that are in turn eaten by foxes. The eggs hatch in the small intestine where they penetrate the mucosa and migrate to the lungs via the bloodstream. Diagnosis is based on clinical signs as well as finding the classical bi-operculate barrel-shaped eggs in respiratory secretions or the faeces.

Crenosoma vulpis can cause bronchopneumonia in red foxes, with coughing, sneezing and nasal discharge. Affected foxes may become emaciated if severely infested, and dyspnoeic. Snails are an intermediate host, which are then consumed by the fox. The larvae then migrate through the intestinal wall and into the bloodstream where they travel to the lungs. Once there they undergo two maturation changes to become the adult worm. Eggs are then shed into the airways, coughed up, swallowed and passed out in the faeces to restart the cycle, which altogether takes just 19 days. The adult has a spiny outer coat, which irritates the mucosa of the airways and so induces the bronchopneumonia and inflammatory response. The disease is commonest in the autumn when larger numbers of snails are present.

Aelurostrongylus abstrusus and *Filaroides osleri*, the cat and dog lungworms, can both infest wild foxes and may cause clinical signs including coughing, weight loss and increased susceptibility to other diseases such as sarcoptic mange.

Cardiovascular nematodes

Dirofilaria immitis (heartworm) may affect any canid in endemic areas of the northern hemisphere. Adult nematodes form in the right side of the heart and clinically animals show the same signs as domestic dogs, with right-sided heart failure, monocytosis and hyperchloraemia.

Angiostrongylus vasorum is a nematode that may be found in association with the pulmonary artery, right side of the heart and lungs of foxes. It has an indirect life cycle. The adult worm lays eggs in the airways which mature, are coughed up, swallowed and pass out in the faeces. They are taken up by a snail or slug and develop further. The snail/slug is then eaten by the fox, the activated larvae are freed and migrate through the intestinal wall into the bloodstream. Low levels of infection produce little or no clinical signs, but chronic large infestations may lead to right-sided heart failure and neurological disease. It is found throughout the UK and a survey in northern Europe recently suggested increasing levels in red foxes (Lemming *et al.*, 2020).

Urinary tract nematodes

A nematode of the urinary bladder of the red fox, *Capillaria plica*, has an indirect life cycle using the earthworm as its intermediate host. It is not known to cause any clinical disease and thus rarely needs treatment.

Other endoparasites

In one survey of foxes in Ireland, intestinal washes, faecal flotations and serological examinations for antibodies to *Toxoplasma gondii* and *Neospora caninum* were used to assess the prevalence of parasites in carcasses of foxes killed on roads or shot. Ascarids *Uncinaria stenocephala* and *Toxocara canis* were frequently recovered, as was the trematode *Alaria alata*, *Taenia* species, eggs of *Capillaria* species and sporocysts of *Sarcocystis* species. Only one fox out of 70 examined was seropositive for *N. caninum*, whereas 24 of 51 were seropositive for *T. gondii* (Wolfe *et al.*, 2001).

Bacterial diseases

Dental disease

Bacterial pulpitis and periodontal disease are common in red foxes and bacteria associated include *Pasteurella multocida*, anaerobes and *Streptococcus* spp. (see Figure 28.4).

Leptospirosis

The bacterium *Leptospira interrogans* has many different pathogenic varieties (serovars), and virtually any mammalian species may become a carrier or actively infected. The bacterium is shed in the urine, and gains access to the next host via breaks in the skin and mucous membranes. In unusual cases a red fox may develop clinical signs associated with an acute haemorrhagic form, with a severe fever and petechiae/ecchymoses being seen on the mucous membranes due to a vasculitis often with jaundice. Other signs include polydipsia, vomiting and diarrhoea. Death may ensue quickly, often due to acute renal failure. More chronic cases may show signs of chronic renal damage with weight loss, polydipsia and diarrhoea.

Salmonellosis

Salmonella spp. are commonly found in the digestive system of foxes. Disease states seen include haemorrhagic gastroenteritis, septicaemia and very rarely abortion. Generally, the fox is a subclinical carrier of these bacteria, and therefore all foxes should be treated as possible zoonotic sources of this disease.

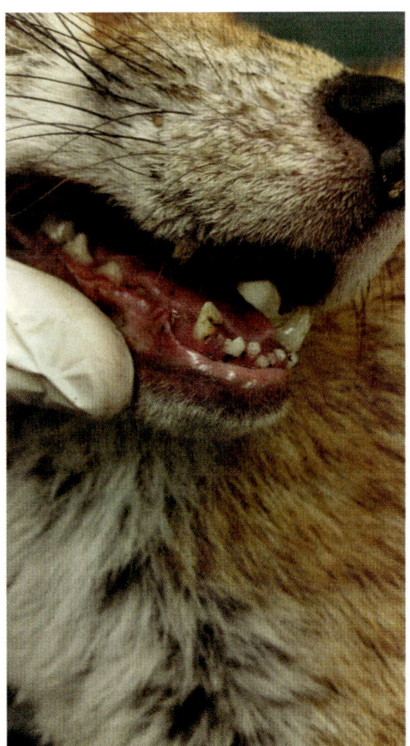

Figure 28.4 Dental disease with fractured teeth and dental loss are commonly seen in red foxes.

Other bacteria

Foxes may transfer potential zoonotic and domestic animal bacterial pathogens such as *Mycobacterium avium* subsp. *paratuberculosis* (the cause of Johne's disease in cattle) and *Yersinia pseudotuberculosis* as these are commonly also found in the gut of their principal prey, rodents and lagomorphs (Beard *et al.*, 2001). They are rarely clinically affected by these bacteria.

Fungal diseases

Dermatophytes such as *Trichophyton mentagrophytes* var. *erinacei* and *Microsporum canis* may be found on foxes. Disease is uncommon, but when it occurs it follows a similar pattern to that seen in domestic dogs and cats, with grey scaling areas over the muzzle and head, progressing into alopecic rings. The hedgehog has been blamed as a common cause of muzzle dermatitis in young inexperienced foxes that attempt to attack the curled-up creature, and receive many puncture wounds from the spines, all of which may impregnate the ringworm spores. It may also complicate scabies infections. Diagnosis is based on clinical signs, microscopy of affected hairs and culture on dermatophyte media.

Viral diseases

Adenovirus infections

Infectious canine hepatitis caused by canine adenovirus-1 can cause serious and even fatal infections in red foxes. It causes severe liver damage with clinical signs including anorexia and a nasal discharge in the first few days of infection. This progresses to a muco-haemorrhagic diarrhoea, jaundice, muscular tremors, seizures and death in extreme cases. The appearance of 'blue eye' due to corneal damage from the virus can occur in foxes surviving the disease. The virus is highly infectious and is spread in the urine, faeces and oral and nasal/respiratory secretions. It can remain viable in the environment for some months and recovered animals may continue to shed the virus for several weeks to months. There is no treatment for this disease available. A survey by Thomson *et al.* (2010) suggested a prevalence of 19% exposure on a study of cadavers in England and Scotland. Walker *et al.* (2016) reported two outbreaks of canine adenovirus-1 in red fox cubs in rehabilitation centres, highlighting the risk of increased transmission in such centres.

Aujesky's disease (suid herpesvirus-1)

Also known as pseudorabies this is not currently present in the UK but has been found in red foxes in Italy (Caruso *et al.*, 2014). It can produce motor incoordination, head scratching, biting and aggression with death occurring within 2–4 days. Aujesky's disease is legally notifiable in the UK, European Union and the USA.

Canine distemper virus

The red fox is not as susceptible to this paramyxovirus as the domestic dog. However, it can produce some clinical signs, with very young cubs being most severely affected. The incubation period is 1–2 weeks, with initial signs being anorexia, an oculonasal discharge that often becomes purulent, and a productive cough. Other signs may then appear as the fever sets in, with hyperpnoea, dyspnoea, diarrhoea and vomiting all being seen in severe cases. Red foxes can survive distemper, and those progressing through the acute phase of the disease may then go on to develop the typical skin lesions seen in domestic canids, with hyperkeratosis of the foot-pads. Neurological disease may also be seen, often 3–4 weeks after apparent recovery, with a variety of signs including seizures, muscular tremors, paresis and paralysis of limbs. The virus is shed in respiratory and digestive tract secretions and currently there is no treatment. Incidence varies from 4 to 17% of red foxes across Europe (Sobrino *et al.*, 2008; Santos *et al.*, 2009; Akerstedt *et al.*, 2010).

Diagnosis is based on clinical signs and the presence of intracytoplasmic acidophilic inclusion bodies. RT-PCR techniques and serology (virus neutralisation test) are also commonly used.

Parvovirus infections

This seems to be an unimportant virus family for the red fox. Serological tests have shown that the red fox can be infected by current members of the parvovirus family, although clinical signs do not become apparent. There is no need for treatment in the red fox.

Hantavirus

Hantaviruses are present in rats and voles in the UK and one serological survey in Belgium suggested an infection rate of 2.4% in red foxes (Escutenaire *et al.*, 2000).

Terrestrial rabies

Rabies viruses (family *Rhabdoviridae*) belong to the *Lyssavirus* genus and are RNA viruses. Terrestrial rabies excludes the bat *Lyssavirus* species and sometimes is referred to as classical rabies and belongs to genotype 1 with dog, fox and raccoon dog (*Nyctereutes procyonoides*) strains. Endemic European areas are now confined to Belarus, Ukraine, Russia, the Baltic states and Moldova (all due predominantly to the raccoon dog) with pockets in the Balkans and Turkey (predominantly due to the domestic dog genotype).

Carnivores develop a condition referred to as 'furious' rabies (as opposed to herbivores which frequently develop 'dumb' rabies) whereby the animal becomes hyperaggressive during the highly infectious stage. The virus is passed in blood and saliva and incubation periods can be prolonged. Most cases of terrestrial rabies globally occur in domestic dogs with other canids being the next most commonly affected animals. In the wild, different species of animal can maintain the sylvatic cycle.

There is no treatment for rabies once clinical signs have appeared. Post-exposure prophylaxis in humans involves vaccination and immunoglobulin therapy. Prevention is by vaccination and carnivores in collections where rabies is still endemic should be vaccinated using a killed rabies vaccine.

Any animal showing signs of hyperaggressiveness, neurological disease or profound stupor with no evidence of external trauma in a rabies endemic area should be treated as if infected and a hazard to human life.

Trauma

Road traffic collisions are a common source of trauma to red foxes, particularly with the urban fox population still on the increase. The majority of red foxes thus affected exhibit fractured limbs, pelvis and ribs to varying degrees. Evaluation and supportive therapy is along the same lines as that provided for cats and dogs, with the addition

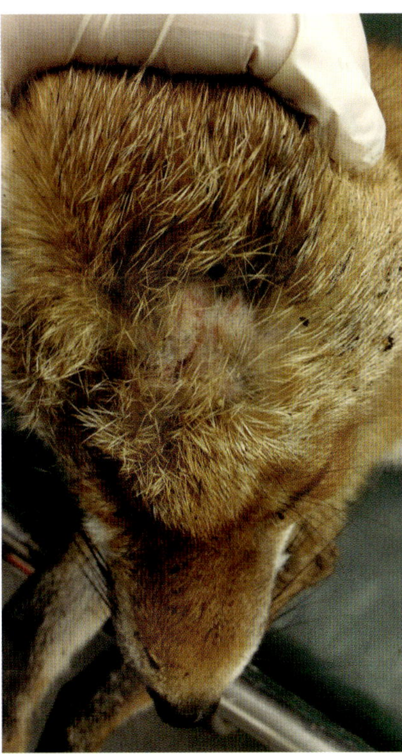

Figure 28.5 Intraspecific and extraspecific fight wounds may be seen in any wild animal and should be assessed along with other injuries.

that many red foxes which are still fully conscious will require sedation for radiographic evaluation.

Other causes of trauma include dog attacks, which may leave serious crushing and tearing injuries to the neck, muzzle and forelimbs, and intraspecific aggression which can leave scars to the head and rear (see Figure 28.5). Again sedation or anaesthesia is required to fully evaluate the extent of serious wounds.

Finally, gunshot wounds are also common, with both high-velocity rifle wounds (which may leave little external damage but cause massive internal shock damage as the bullet passes through) and low-velocity shotgun wounds (which produce obvious external damage) being seen.

Other conditions

Hydrocephalus

This is a common finding in young orphaned fox cubs and may be associated with vitamin A deficiency or genetic causes. It has been suggested that the development of this condition with its associated CNS signs may lead the vixen to abandon these cubs. Ljungan virus has also been implicated in Europe, a virus spread by rodents and causing hydrocephalus in humans. There is no treatment and euthanasia is advised.

FELIDAE: WILDCATS

Ectoparasites

Fleas

The cat flea *Ctenocephalides felis*, dog flea *C. canis* and rabbit flea *Spilopsyllus cuniculi* have all been recovered from wildcats. Rarely do they cause any problems, although young kittens may suffer from anaemia if heavily infested. They may also transmit *Mycoplasma haemofelis* (formerly known as *Haemobartonella felis*) and the tapeworm *Dipylidium caninum* amongst other diseases.

Lice

The cat louse *Felicola subrostratus* has been reported in small felids. This is a biting (mallophagan) louse, and rarely causes any problems although may result in fur loss.

Mites

Notoedres cati is a putative parasite but information on the disease is scarce. In addition it is possible for small felids to suffer from other domestic cat mites such as *Demodex cati* and *Sarcoptes scabiei* (Najera *et al.*, 2021).

Ticks

Commonly seen in Europe is the sheep tick *Ixodes ricinus*, although the hedgehog tick, *Ixodes hexagonus*, may also be recovered. In general, small numbers of ticks rarely cause a serious problem, although again they may be implicated in the transmission of blood parasites, viruses and bacteria such as the cause of Lyme's disease.

Endoparasites

Digestive system nematodes

Toxocara cati and *Toxascaris leonina* are common, particularly in young wild felids. Their life cycles are the same as for domestic cats, and generally do not produce any disease.

Lungworms

Aelurostrongylus abstrusus is commonly found in the small airways of wild small felids. It uses snails and slugs as an intermediate host, the cat then consuming the snail/slug, or a rodent which has consumed the snail/slug. Generally, such infections are rarely a problem, causing at most a mild cough; however, multiple infections may result in clinical disease (Stevanovic *et al.*, 2019; Diakou *et al.*, 2020). Other lungworms such as *Capillaria (Eucoleus) aerophila*, *Troglostrongylus brevior* and *Angiostrongylus chabaudi* may infect small felids and multiple species have been reported in single individuals resulting in severe cardiopulmonary disease (Diakou *et al.*, 2020).

Tapeworms

Taenia taeniaeformis is a tapeworm found in both wild and domestic cats, where the adult 50–60 cm long worm is formed. The intermediate hosts are rodents, where it forms pea-sized strobilocerci known as *Cysticercus fasciolarus* frequently in the liver.

Dipylidium caninum is also seen as in domestic cats. Its life cycle may involve the flea or louse as intermediate hosts.

Protozoa

Toxoplasma gondii is a common parasite of wildcats and is generally non-pathogenic to the Eurasian wildcat, but the sporocysts passed in the faeces, once activated after 2 weeks, can become infectious for other animals, and is zoonotic with a risk of abortion.

Coccidia such as *Cystoisospora felis* may be recovered from small wild felids and may result in clinical disease (diarrhoea and dehydration) particularly in young animals.

Bacterial diseases

Similar bacterial diseases seen in domestic cats may be seen in wildcats, from *Pasteurella* spp. and *Staphylococcus* spp. isolated from bite wounds and dental abscesses, to *Campylobacter* spp., *Salmonella* spp. and *Yersinia pseudotuberculosis* from the gastrointestinal tract. Treatments and diagnosis are the same as for domestic cats.

Chlamydia felis has been reported in Eurasian wildcats and should be considered whenever severe conjunctivitis and upper respiratory tract disease is present. It can of course be transmitted sexually and may affect multiple body organs in severely affected felids including the CNS and heart. Diagnosis by PCR is preferred due to the difficulty in culturing the organism.

Fungal diseases

The majority of wildcats are carriers of dermatophytes (ringworm) such as *Microsporum canis* and *Trichophyton mentagrophytes*. Rarely though do these organisms cause disease.

Viral diseases

Wildcats are afflicted by and susceptible to many of the viruses seen in domestic species including feline immunodeficiency virus, feline leukaemia virus (FeLV), feline panleukopenia virus (FPV), feline coronavirus, feline calicivirus, feline herpesvirus and cowpoxvirus. Their diagnosis, clinical signs and management is much the same as for domestic felines.

Feline herpesvirus and calicivirus appear to be a significant cause of morbidity and mortality in young small felids, with reported rates of 4–80% (Leutenegger *et al.*, 1999; Milan and Rodrigeuz, 2009).

Feline coronavirus appears to be commonly reported in Eurasian wildcats in captivity, but clinical disease and feline infectious peritonitis is uncommon. In Europe, prevalence of 4% is reported (Leutenegger *et al.*, 1999).

Feline immunodeficiency virus has been identified in mature male Eurasian wildcats in Scotland (my personal experience) but is uncommon elsewhere in Europe where it was not detected (Leutenegger *et al.*, 1999). However, the same survey found very high levels of antigen (49%) and antibody (75%) to FeLV but without clinical signs of disease.

FPV appears to be less commonly seen in Europe (10%) but may be more prevalent in small felids in Asia (80%) (Steutzer and Hartmann, 2014).

Canine distemper virus can affect small felids such as the Eurasian wildcat although its significance at this stage is not fully understood (Candela *et al.*, 2019).

Terrestrial rabies is less commonly seen in small felids in Europe and North America than it is in mustelids and canids and is not currently present in the UK.

Trauma

Road traffic collisions are common injuries for wildcats. The same protocols for treatment for shock and hypovolaemia as used for domestic cats are advocated. However, wildcats are much less tolerant of repeated medication and fluid therapy, which may need to be administered under sedation in bolus form.

Poisoning

Warfarin-style poisoning is not uncommon, due to the consumption of previously poisoned rodent prey. Clinical signs include petechiation of the mucous membranes, spontaneous internal bleeding, shock and death.

MUSTELIDAE: BADGERS

Ectoparasites

Fleas

Paraceras melis is commonly found and appears to not cause any serious disease, although heavy burdens in young debilitated individuals could cause anaemia. Other fleas such as the hedgehog flea *Archaeopsylla erinacei* and the mole flea *Histrichopsylla talpae* have both been recorded on badgers.

Lice

The main pathogenic louse is the biting (mallophagan) louse *Trichodectes melis*. It may be a cause of severe debility in a heavily parasitised badger, leading to scaling of the skin, pruritus and weight loss and general debilitation.

Mites

The sarcoptid mite *Sarcoptes scabiei* has been reported in badgers, and causes a severe pruritus, with hair loss, initially over the ears, limbs and face, but spreading over the whole body.

Ticks

Ixodes ricinus, *I. canisuga* and *I. hexagonus* have all been reported in the UK. They seem to cause little obvious disease, although all three ticks may be carriers of diseases such as Lyme disease, as well as being able to cause debilitation through anaemia.

Endoparasites

Lungworms

Crenosoma melesi has been identified in badgers in the UK and Europe. The life cycle of this parasite is direct, but there is evidence that paratenic hosts such as the earthworm and various dor beetles may provide a source of infection. Severe infestations can be fatal.

Other nematodes and cestodes

Intestinal *Strongyloides* spp. and *Angiostrongylus vasorum* can infect badgers. The hookworm *Uncinaria criniformis* has also been recorded although not with significant disease. Cestodes found in the badger's digestive system include *Taenia martis* which rarely causes disease in the badger but is potentially zoonotic.

Coccidiosis

Eimeria melis is a common finding in badgers of all ages but may reach particularly high levels in the spring in young cubs (Newman *et al.*, 2001). Like other *Eimeria* spp. the life cycle is short and direct. Damage, if caused, occurs in the small intestine chiefly, with the major clinical signs being stunted growth, unthriftiness, diarrhoea and in severe cases death. *Isospora melis* has also been identified as a cause of diarrhoea (Anwar *et al.*, 2000).

Giardiasis

This has been reported as a cause of mortality and diarrhoea in badger cubs in rehabilitation centres (Barlow *et al.*, 2010).

Bacterial diseases

Anthrax

Bacillus anthracis is a serious notifiable zoonotic disease and soil-associated bacterium. As a results, if badgers are present in an area that is contaminated, their fur may become coated in the spores. Most do not show clinical signs of the disease and treatment is therefore not indicated but care should be taken when handling them in an endemic area.

Brucellosis

The bacterium *Brucella abortus* is a notifiable disease in the European Union and USA affecting cattle. It is also a zoonotic disease, causing fever, septicaemia, orchitis and rarely abortion in humans. It has been recorded that the European badger may act as a carrier, spreading the bacteria from one herd of infected cattle to another. Corbel *et al.* (1983) showed that a carrier status could exist in the badger, recovering the bacteria 6 months after inoculation, although no conclusive proof exists of wild badgers carrying the disease.

Salmonellosis

Salmonella spp. have been isolated from the gastrointestinal tract of badgers, in some cases from as much as 7% of the population (Euden, 1990). Clinical signs vary, and badgers may act as subclinical carriers. Alternatively, haemorrhagic enteritis, septicaemia and abortion may be seen. Good personal protective equipment and biosecurity measures are therefore important.

Tuberculosis: *Mycobacterium bovis*

Badgers have been historically linked to outbreaks of bovine tuberculosis (TB) due to *Mycobacterium bovis*. Badgers may continue to harbour it within their family groups for many years and act as a recurrent source of infection for cattle (Neal and Cheeseman, 1996). Respiratory disease is predominantly seen but due to the presence of the mycobacteria in the respiratory secretions, these may be transferred to the oral cavity and so implanted into bite wounds on other badgers/animals. These can lead to open TB abscesses, which may allow further spread of the disease. The urinary tract can also be commonly affected, with bacteria being passed in the urine. However, many badgers infected may show few if any clinical signs of disease.

Numbers of badgers affected varies considerably with the location, with often localised specific 'hot spots', such as the south-west of England, where in parts of Gloucestershire, Cornwall and Avon levels may reach 7% of the badger population (Neal and Cheeseman, 1996). A statistical review article recently published suggested a badger weighted mean infection rate in Europe of around 11% (Justus *et al.*, 2024).

In the UK, a badger rehabilitation protocol to reduce the likelihood of disseminating TB via rehabilitated badgers has been drawn up with government support (Mullineaux, 2024). Testing involves serological (blood) sampling for antibodies using a test known as the Dual Path Platform VetTB® (DPP®) test (Ashford *et al.*, 2020). Sensitivity (the likelihood that the test will correctly identify a positive animal) has been shown to increase to over 91% by testing an individual a total of three times.

To prevent the spread of TB, adult badgers should be returned to the exact site found. Cubs can be triple tested (DPP) from 6 to 8 weeks of age (prior to this, maternal immunity may interfere with the test results) at 4-week intervals and only negative-testing cubs (on all three tests) should be released with positive cubs being euthanased. In the UK, APHA oversee testing and licensing of any euthanasia of cubs based on this test and their subsequent post-mortem. Because of the geographical variation in bovine TB incidence, if a cub cannot be released at their birth sett, it is essential to ensure that they are only moved to an area of equivalent bovine TB status or higher. Further information regarding testing and release measures in England can be found at the TB Hub website (Mullineaux, 2024).

Fungal diseases

The dermatophytes *Microsporum* and *Trichophyton* spp. have all been cultured from the fur of badgers. Actual ringworm lesions, though, are uncommon but where debilitated with other diseases such as bovine TB, grey scaling circular areas may be seen over the muzzle and other parts of the body, with hairs fracturing at the skin surface.

Viral diseases

Canine distemper

This viral disease, as with dogs, can result in a pneumonia with neurological signs, such as hyperaesthesia and disorientation, seizuring and death. There is no treatment or safe vaccine currently available. Some badgers do survive the condition and may develop foot-pad hyperkeratosis. Serological surveys have failed to identify it in UK badgers (Delahey and Frolich, 2000), but it has been reported elsewhere in Europe, Africa and the Middle East and so should be considered where neurological disease and pneumonia exist (Hammer *et al.*, 2004).

Herpesviruses

Mustelid gamma-herpesvirus 1 has been recovered from badgers in Europe by PCR and ELISA serology although no link to disease has yet been identified (Tsai *et al.*, 2022).

Parvovirus

This was recovered from five badger cubs that died in a rehabilitation hospital, likely contracted from domestic dogs (Barlow *et al.*, 2012).

Rabbit haemorrhagic disease virus

Infection with the calicivirus rabbit haemorrhagic disease virus 2 has been reported in badgers and linked to their death in Portugal (dos Santos *et al.*, 2022). This suggests the European badger may be an overspill host. The liver is the target organ with internal haemorrhages seen. There is no treatment.

Rabies

In Europe rabies is uncommon, but badgers may act as reservoir hosts for rabies virus in North America and Africa.

Trauma

Road traffic collision injuries can be extensive, and skull and pelvic fractures are common. As with domestic cats, the thick skin of a badger may hide serious signs of internal trauma, so chest and abdominal radiographs are routinely advised. Extreme care should still be taken with even an apparently comatose badger, as the potential for being severely bitten is still high.

Badger baiting is an offence in the UK and Europe. Injuries are often seen on the forelimbs and muzzle of the badgers, and the badger itself often inflicts severe crushing wounds to the forelegs and muzzle of dog(s) attacking it. Intraspecific (between badgers) fight wounds are often associated with large areas of skin trauma over the dorsal rump. These may require extensive treatment, skin flaps/grafts, analgesia and antibiosis to allow full recovery.

Snares and trapping injuries to the neck (snares) and feet (traps) are still reported and can be life-threatening. Treatment is often too late to affect the outcome as most affected individuals are found dead associated with the device. Loss of a limb will result in an animal unfit for release and so euthanasia is recommended.

Poisoning

Badgers have been reported as being poisoned by a wide range of chemical agents, including metaldehyde, paraquat, and warfarin and other rodenticides. Unfortunately the majority of these diagnoses were made post mortem, and it may be near impossible to ascertain the cause of poisoning quickly ante mortem. Metaldehyde poisoning has been reported as causing hyperaesthesia and avoidance of bright lights, and many rodenticides such as coumarin/warfarin derivatives may produce mucosal and internal haemorrhages.

Other conditions

Dental disease

This is common and occurs mainly due to fracture of canines leading to a pulp infection and root abscessation (Neal and Cheeseman, 1996). Serious disease may result in septicaemia, and mild disease may still restrict feeding so a dental check when anaesthetised is always advised as with other species.

MUSTELIDAE: MARTENS AND *MUSTELA* SPECIES

Ectoparasites

Mites

Otodectes cynotis has been recovered from wild mustelids, and causes intense irritation of the external ear and the skin around the ear base.

Sarcoptes scabiei can cause severe disease in the pine marten, producing alopecia and pruritus often initially over the head and feet but spreading over much of the body and limbs. Death can occur in adults, and particularly young kits. Mink seem to be relatively resistant to scabies in the wild.

Endoparasites

Nematodes

Skrjabingylus nasicola lives in the nasal sinuses of mustelids, particularly weasels, stoats, pine martens and polecats. In one study it was present in 37% of weasels, 39% of polecats and 41% of stoats (Simpson *et al.*, 2016). Some infections are subclinical but some cause deformity of the sinuses and severe nasal damage. The life cycle of the parasite is complex, with two intermediate hosts: molluscs (snails, slugs) and rodents. When the rodent is eaten, the parasite is released, migrates out of the gut and makes its way to the nasal sinuses via the spinal canal of the mustelid. However, no actual damage to the CNS seems to occur during this process.

There are several digestive system nematodes of mustelids, from both the strongylid and ascarid families, as well as some cestodes (tapeworms) but in general these are of little significance. *Angiostrongylus vasorum* has been reported in stoats and weasels, with adults in the right ventricle and juvenile stages in the lungs and may be pathogenic.

Flukes (trematodes)

Troglotrema acutum has been recorded in the European polecat. It has an indirect life cycle, using molluscs as the intermediate host. The adult fluke is small (1 cm) and migrates to the frontal sinuses of the head where it can cause damage by deforming the skull.

Cholecystitis has been reported in mink due to the fluke *Pseudamphistomum truncatum* which results in fibrosis and damage to the gall bladder (Simpson *et al.*, 2005b).

Other parasites

Bartonella spp. have been identified in small mustelids but disease is generally subclinical although hepatic pathology has been seen. It is thought to be contracted from rodent (principally vole) prey where *Bartonella* spp. infections are common.

Hepatozoon spp. infections in pine martens in Scotland have resulted in myocardial damage although this was not considered significant (Simpson *et al.*, 2005a).

Bacterial diseases

Zoonotic bacteria such as *Salmonella* spp. and *Campylobacter* spp. may be commonly recovered from the faeces of mustelids, although they rarely cause severe disease. Occasionally, though, diarrhoea may develop if the mustelid is stressed in captivity and then treatment may become necessary.

Yersinia pseudotuberculosis may result in a granulomatous enteritis, with abdominal pain, diarrhoea and weight loss. It is found in the gut of rodent and lagomorph prey. Occasionally it can cause septicaemia and death.

Mycobacterial disease with *Mycobacterium avium* subsp. *avium* has been recorded, and mustelids are suspected of acting as vectors for *M. avium* subsp. *paratuberculosis* due to their prey often being lagomorphs (Beard *et al.*, 2001). Lung granulomas due to *M. avium* complex and *M. kumamotonense* have also been reported in small mustelids (Simpson *et al.*, 2016).

Fungal diseases

Adiaspiromycosis – infections with the soil-associated organism *Emmonsia crescens (parva)* – has been reported in small mustelids. Most cases are subclinical, but pneumonia has been recorded, with small, grey, 2–4 mm abscesses in the lungs.

Viral diseases

Canine distemper

This disease is considered highly pathogenic, particularly in polecats and weasels. Clinically, signs resemble those seen in canids, with respiratory signs, nasal discharge, diarrhoea and often an ocular discharge. There may also be photophobia and hyperaemia over the head with thickening of the eyelids, lips and anus. These areas often become secondarily infected and pruritic. Neurological signs such as convulsions may also be observed. Death may occur within 7 days of infection. There is no treatment.

Influenza virus infection

Many mustelids are susceptible to influenza viruses, including the avian influenza type A virus and human influenza virus. This has been reported as an acute and sometimes fatal disease in domestic ferrets, but its true virulence in wild mustelids is unclear.

Parvovirus infection

In mink, mink enteritis virus (MEV) is a common cause of mortality. It is related to FPV, although mink can contract FPV as well. Clinical signs are worse in mink infected with MEV rather than FPV, and are often acute, with lethargy, fever, diarrhoea and death within 4–5 days. Young mink are more susceptible than adults. There is no treatment for this disease.

Other viruses

An aviadenovirus (marten adenovirus type 1, MAdV-1) has been identified in the tissues of dead pine martens, along with a mastadenovirus (marten adenovirus type 2, MAdV-2) (Walker *et al.*, 2017). The significance of these at the moment is not clear.

Trauma

Traumatic injuries to mustelids are not uncommon, although they rarely survive road traffic collisions. Domestic cat bites and trauma may be seen in the smaller species, with deep infected wounds that require flushing and antibiotic treatment, initially under sedation. Fractures associated with falls are reported in pine martens.

Poisoning

This is occasionally seen in mustelids and is usually secondary to consumption of a poisoned prey item, such as rodents or lagomorphs. Warfarin/coumarol-derived poisons are common causes of this sort of poisoning, with petechiation of the mucous membranes, melaenic faeces and haematuria being apparent.

Poisoning with strychnine may occasionally be seen, as this poison is still licensed for use as a mole poison, although its use for any other reason is prohibited. Affected animals show signs of seizuring, opisthotonus and rigidity, with death due to respiratory paralysis ensuing rapidly. There is no treatment.

MUSTELIDAE: OTTERS

Ectoparasites

Mites

Otodectes cynotis has been occasionally reported causing ear disease although scabies is uncommon.

Lice

Lutridia spp., a biting mallophagan louse, have been recorded in otters in Europe. They do not appear to be pathogenic although may reduce fur waterproofing with heavy burdens.

Ticks

Ixodes ricinus is commonly seen and may be important as a vector for diseases such as Lyme disease (*Borrelia burgdorferi*), other bacteria and protozoal parasites.

Endoparasites

Digestive system nematodes

Uncinaria stenocephala, the northern hookworm, has been reported in Eurasian otters. It may cause pedal dermatitis but seems to rarely cause serious disease in the wild state.

Trichuris spp. (whipworm) have also been recovered from otters. The life cycle is direct and clinically signs of infestation are uncommon.

Flukes (trematodes)

A severe enteritis due to *Cryptocotyle lingua*, which uses a marine fish *Tautogolabrus adspersus* as its intermediate host, has been observed (McCarthy and Hasset, 1993).

Cholecystitis has been reported due to the fluke *Pseudamphistomum truncatum* which results in fibrosis and damage to the gall bladder (Simpson *et al.*, 2005b). A study of the distribution of *P. truncatum* found it to be present in southern England and Wales but absent from the north of England, with an overall incidence of 11.7% (Sherrard-Smith *et al.*, 2009).

A second digenean, *Metorchis albidus*, was found in the biliary system of 6.6% of otters associated with cholecystitis (Sherrard-Smith *et al.*, 2009). This fluke appears well established in Suffolk, Norfolk and north Essex but was recorded elsewhere rarely.

Lungworms

Capillaria (Eucoleus) aerophila, the capillarian lungworm of many mammals, has been reported in otters, causing damage to the nasal, tracheal and bronchial mucosa. It has a direct life cycle, eggs being laid in the airways, coughed up and swallowed and passed in the faeces.

Urinary tract nematodes

Capillaria plica has also been recorded in the urinary bladder mucosa of otters. It seems to be non-pathogenic. *Dioctophyme renale*, a renal worm, has been found in the otter in the UK.

Protozoa

Various species of coccidia have been isolated from the gut of otters, mainly of the genus *Isospora*. Their significance is unclear, as no disease has been recorded from their presence, although these parasites may cause weight loss and diarrhoea in the young animals.

Bacterial diseases

Bacterial pneumonia

Bacteria include *Klebsiella pneumoniae*, *Bacteroides* spp., *Aeromonas hydrophila*, *Proteus* spp. and *Streptococcus* spp. and are common secondary to lungworm infection.

Dental disease

Fractured teeth and concurrent pulp infections are common in otters, particularly estuarine otters living off shellfish. These can lead to local abscesses and may need surgical intervention as well as antibiotic treatment. Bacteria involved include many anaerobes, as well as *Pasteurella* spp. and *Staphylococcus* spp.

Tuberculosis

Mycobacterium bovis and *Mycobacterium avium* have both been isolated from the digestive system of European otters. It is thought that the otter contracts the disease from eating infected prey. Infection may produce no clinical signs initially. Alternatively, diarrhoea, weight loss and death may occur in severe cases. There is no treatment.

Tyzzer's disease (*Clostridium piliforme*)

Clostridium (Bacillus) piliforme has been reported in the liver of a Eurasian otter leading to ascites and abscessation (Simpson *et al.*, 2008). It is carried by rodents.

Other bacterial infections

Otters may be subclinical carriers of the zoonotic bacteria *Salmonella* spp. but it may also cause diarrhoea, dysentery and septicaemia.

Other zoonotic bacteria which have been isolated from European otters include *Erysipelothrix rhusiopathiae*, which can cause skin nodules and fever in humans, *Plesiomonas shigelloides*, which caused abortion in an otter and has been known to cause diarrhoea in humans (Weber and Roberts, 1990), and *Leptospira interrogans* (leptospirosis), which has also been recovered in otters, occasionally associated with renal and liver damage and which is again zoonotic.

Fungal diseases

Adiaspiromycosis (infection with *Emmonsia crescens*) has been seen in otters as with other mustelids and can cause fatal pneumonias. It is difficult to diagnose ante-mortem, although a lack of response to antibiotic therapy, presence of miliary pneumonia on radiography and bronchioalveolar recovery of yeasts would all help a diagnosis.

Viral diseases

Clinical disease including a serous oculonasal discharge and fever with a mild skin erythema and papular rash has been reported with canine distemper virus (Giesel, 1979).

Feline panleukopenia virus has been seen in Eurasian otters and may produce a transient diarrhoea but may well be subclinical. Infection levels may be as high as 27.1% in North American otters which is believed to maintain the virus in the wild in Canada (Canuti *et al.*, 2020). Aleutian disease virus of mink has been linked to the death of one European otter (Wells *et al.*, 1989). A lutrine adenovirus type 1 was identified in one survey of European otter tissues but its significance is not known (Walker *et al.*, 2017).

Other diseases

Hydrocephalus

This is seen in some abandoned otter cubs and may be associated with hypovitaminosis A or a genetic component.

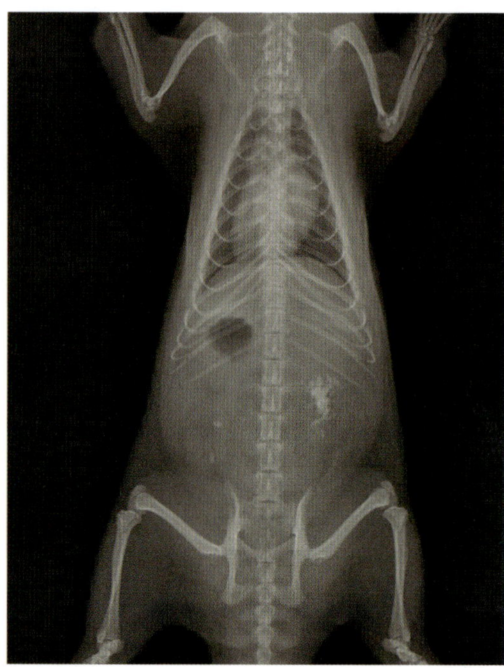

Figure 28.6 Renal, ureteral and bladder calculi in wild otters are relatively commonly seen.

Urolithiasis and renolithiasis

Calcium urate, calcium phosphate and ammonium urate crystals have all been recovered from the urinary system of European otters, including the kidneys. In the majority of cases the condition may be subclinical. One survey describes 10.2% of otters showing macroscopic renal calculi, with all of them composed of ammonium acid urate; the right kidney and males are more commonly affected (Simpson *et al.*, 2011). Uroliths and renoliths are radiodense and so show up well with radiography (see Figure 28.6).

Poisoning

Poisoning of watercourses by heavy metals affects the whole ecosystem and these will accumulate in the tissues of aquatic life and ultimately otters as they are top predators. Mercury poisoning has been reported in otters in Canada and Europe and levels of mercury seem to be highest in otters compared with other carnivores (Kalisinska *et al.*, 2016). Other poisons such as polychlorinated biphenyls are known to reduce fertility in a number of species. They are used as insulators and also as fireproofing materials. They tend to concentrate in fat depots inside the body, and so will reach higher levels of concentration in animals further up the food chain.

PHOCIDAE: SEALS

Ectoparasites

Mites

In the grey seal, the nasal mite *Orthohalarachne halichoeri* can cause signs of upper respiratory tract disease, with sneezing and a mucopurulent discharge in severe cases.

Lice
In both grey and common seals the louse *Echinophthirius horridus* is known to cause skin irritation.

Endoparasites
Lungworms
Two main lungworms are found, *Otostrongylus circumlitus* and *Parafilaroides gymnurus*, both having indirect life cycles through crustaceans and fish. They are common and often lead to secondary bacterial pneumonias, particularly in young seal pups. *Otostrongylus circumlitus* causes damage to the main airways and can cause blockage of bronchioles. It can also affect the pulmonary artery and right side of the heart. A productive cough with tachypnoea and a harsh-sounding chest on auscultation are common. *Parafilaroides gymnurus* causes more severe damage in the alveoli and lung parenchyma. Clinically the affected seal often shows signs of dyspnoea as demonstrated by flaring of the nostrils, a harsh-sounding chest with crackles and wheezes, and often coughing that occasionally produces blood-tinged sputum in which can be found the larvae.

Other nematodes
Contracaecum osculatum and *Terranova decipiens* can both lead to gastric and intestinal ulceration with resultant melaena, diarrhoea and secondary sepsis in young seal pups.

Protozoa: coccidia
Eimeria phocae can cause severe diarrhoea, dysentery and even death in young common seals, particularly if stressed by other diseases or prolonged captivity.

Bacterial diseases
Bacterial enteritis
Salmonella Bovismorbificans can cause haemorrhagic diarrhoea, especially in young pups and may circulate between seals and cattle. *Salmonella enterica* was found in the gut of 21% of live grey seal pups (although not in yearlings), being more common in pups exposed to seawater (Baily *et al.*, 2016).

Bacterial pneumonia
Bordetella bronchiseptica is often associated with lungworm infestations and causes a purulent bronchopneumonia. Other bacteria such as *Pasteurella haemolytica* can be seen which may cause septicaemia. Pups are most at risk, and develop tachypnoea, dyspnoea, sneezing and a mucopurulent oculonasal discharge.

Mycobacterium pinnepedii is the agent of seal tuberculosis and a member of the *M. tuberculosis* complex. Seals can become infected with *M. tuberculosis* and *M. bovis* as well. The respiratory tract appears to be the main organ affected but spread elsewhere is possible.

Mycoplasma phocacerebrale, *M. phocidae* and *M. phocarhinis* are associated in common seals with secondary infections, particularly pneumonias (Madoff *et al.*, 1982; Kirchhoff *et al.*, 1989). Diagnosis can be made on PCR or culture, but swabs require specialist media for transport. *Mycoplasma* spp. from seals can also be zoonotic and have resulted in so-called 'seal finger' cellulitis where bites or wounds of handlers become infected.

Dental disease
Severe periodontal disease or dental abscessation with fractured teeth from stone chewing has been reported.

Other bacterial disease
Infections of the umbilicus have been reported in young seals, causing local abscessation and associated liver disease, peritonitis and death.

Pseudomonas aeruginosa has been associated with melting corneal ulcers in grey seals (Fleming and Bexton, 2016).

Mycobacterium marinum infection usually results in skin abscesses.

Brucella spp. is a common potentially serious zoonotic pathogen and commensal of most marine mammals including seals. The nomenclature of species affecting seals is confusing and not yet fully understood but *B. pinnipedia* and *B. maris* have been suggested. It has been associated with skin and subcutaneous abscesses and pneumonias often in conjunction with lungworm. In dolphins it has been associated with abortion and meningoencephalitis so it potentially could result in abortions in seals.

Leptospira spp. have also been recovered from seals, particularly *L. interrogans* serovar *pomona*. It has produced interstitial nephritis in common seals with elevated liver enzymes, bilirubin, urea, creatinine and white cell levels.

Viral diseases
Influenza virus
Influenza A virus (family *Orthomyxoviridae*) has been recorded in the common seal, although the grey seal seems to be unaffected by the strains so far recovered. Transmission of the disease is via the respiratory and ocular secretion routes. Clinical signs include pneumonia, pyrexia, lethargy, incoordination, conjunctivitis and mucopurulent oculonasal discharge, which may progress to a blood-tinged frothy nasal discharge. Seals may also develop subcutaneous emphysema with swollen necks and chests, all similar to phocine distemper virus. It is seen particularly during periods of stress such as overcrowding.

Phocine distemper virus
This paramyxovirus is related to canine distemper virus. It first appeared in 1988 in northwestern Europe and was the cause of widespread mortalities in phocids. It is thought that the virus was brought across the Atlantic from Greenland by migrating harp seals (*Phoca groenlandica*) which seem to act as carriers without being affected by the disease. Transmission is by the respiratory, urinary, ocular and faecal routes. Clinical signs include mucopurulent oculonasal discharge, conjunctivitis, keratitis, coughing, dyspnoea, diarrhoea, pyrexia, lethargy, abortion, and neurological signs such as seizuring. The dyspnoea has in some animals been so severe that subcutaneous emphysema has occurred, leading to increased buoyancy in the affected seal, and an inability to dive.

Phocine herpesvirus

Phocid herpesvirus 1 infection has been associated with encephalitis, pneumonia, adrenocortical necrosis and hepatitis associated with high morbidity and sometimes mortality, especially in young seals. Clinical signs include vomiting, oral mucosal inflammation, diarrhoea, coughing and pyrexia. Disease is more severe in young seals and common seals.

Sealpox virus

This parapoxvirus causes raised pox lesions most frequently found on the flippers, although they can also be found on the thorax, lips and abdomen. These lesions may ulcerate and become secondarily infected with bacteria in young pups. In adults the condition will resolve on its own after 7–9 weeks but it is zoonotic so good biosecurity is important.

Trauma

Wounds can be due to other seal attacks, or from boats, or trauma in rough seas. Fractures of digits may be seen as well as skin injuries from fishing nets. Open wounds become quickly infected with environmental bacteria such as *Pseudomonas* and *Aeromonas* spp., and bite wounds often contain *Pasteurella* spp. and *Staphylococcus* spp. that can induce septicaemia.

Poisoning

Oil spills

Crude oil spills can cause intense irritation and inflammation of mucous membranes such as the eyes, mouth and nasal passages, as well as causing a general dermatitis. Any oil swallowed can also irritate the lining of the gastrointestinal system resulting in ulceration of the stomach lining, vomiting and diarrhoea. Absorption of the oil hydrocarbons may cause further toxic damage to the liver, nervous system and kidneys and cause haemolysis.

Polychlorinated biphenyl compounds

Polychlorinated biphenyls (PCBs) have been found in moderately high concentrations in seals similar to otters. They concentrate in fat, and will reach higher levels of concentration in animals further up the food chain. Clinical signs are vague, but it is known that PCBs can cause a reduced fertility rate and lead to CNS damage. Sufficiently high levels can kill.

CHIROPTERA: BATS

Ectoparasites

Bugs

Bugs are blood-sucking species of ectoparasite, of which several species of *Cimex* are reported in bats and may contribute to anaemia, disease transmission and debilitation (Frank *et al*., 2015).

Lice

Microchiropterans appear to have no natural sucking (anopluran) only chewing (mallophagan) lice but rarely has any serious disease been attributed to them.

Flies

Wingless flies of the family Nycteribiidae feed by sucking the blood of its host. The eggs are laid on the host, but may drop off into the area in which the bats roost. They are around 1 cm in length and their life cycle is around 2–3 weeks. When hatched the nymph has wings that allow it to find its host, but once attached to the bat the wings are shed, similar to the Hippoboscidae family comprising the sheep and horse 'keds'. They are known to bite humans and may transmit blood-borne parasites and viruses.

Fleas

Ischnopsyllid fleas have been reported in bats and may cause debilitation in large numbers.

Mites

Steatonyssus spp., *Dermanyssina* spp. and the nymphs of the harvest mite *Neotrombicula autumnalis* have been recovered from bats and may cause wing membrane irritation and damage in debilitated individuals that are not grooming properly.

Ticks

The bat tick *Argas vespertilionis* has been reported to be a vector for *Babesia vesperuginus*; *Ixodes ricinus* has also been reported.

Endoparasites

Cestodes

A variety of cestodes have been reported with high prevalence (e.g. *Vampirolepis* spp.). Cestodes typically use two hosts but high burdens in young bats have been recorded, suggesting auto-infection may occur in some species (Frank *et al*., 2015).

Nematodes

Members of the *Strongyloides* genus of nematodes are known to parasitise bats, and burdens can be large and some even found free in the abdominal cavity. Strongyles such as *Molinostrongylus* spp. have been reported in European bats and may debilitate young bats.

Haemoparasites

Babesia verperuginus has been reported in bats in Europe and may result in anaemia and splenomegaly. It is transmitted by the soft tick *Argas verpertilionis*.

Bacterial diseases

Salmonella spp. have been isolated from the faeces of bats including both *S. typhimurium* and *S. enteritidis*. These are thought to be transmitted from bat to bat when roosting or mutual grooming, or via the food source of insects. Many bats are subclinical carriers of the bacteria, but the possible zoonotic risk should be considered.

Other bacteria reported in bats include *Alcaligenes*, *Bacteroides*, *Borrelia*, *Campylobacter jejuni*, *Citrobacter*, *Clostridium*, *Enterobacter*, *Escherichia*, *Leptospira*, *Listeria monocytogenes*, *Mycobacterium*, *Proteus*, *Pseudomonas*, *Shigella flexneri*, *Staphylococcus* and *Yersinia* spp. (Muhldorfer, 2013). *Leptospira* spp. have also been recovered from bats with infectivity rates of up to 35%, the highest rates bring seen in the Vespertilionidae (Muhldorfer, 2013). Clinical disease is not commonly seen but clearly there is a zoonotic risk.

In one large study in Germany of over 500 vespertilionid bats, over 50% had bacteria-associated inflammatory lesions with pneumonia being the most commonly reported single body system disease (Muhldorfer *et al.*, 2011). Cat bite infections are common and Muhldorfer *et al.* (2011) demonstrated significant genetic diversity of *Pasteurella multocida* infections in bats suggesting a non-bat origin to many.

Fungal diseases

Histoplasmosis

Histoplasma capsulatum spores can be passed in the faeces of bats in warm damp climates. These spores easily become aerosolised when the faeces of the bats dry out and are inhaled by humans or other animals. This condition has not so far been recognised in the UK, although it has been seen elsewhere in Europe, the southern USA and Australia. However, the fungus does not seem to cause serious harm to the bats themselves, although those infected persistently shed the fungus from local infections of the gut.

White nose disease

Pseudogymnoascus (Geomyces) destructans causes white nose disease and mortalities, and has been reported in bat hibernacula in the UK (Barlow *et al.*, 2011, 2015). It likes cold (4–8°C) conditions and forms a white mat of infection, starting on the face, hence the name white nose disease. The conidia are sickle-shape on microscopy. There is some difference between its pathogenicity in North America, where mass die-offs of up to 80% mortality have been recorded, and Europe, where it is rarely associated with deaths.

Viral diseases

European bat lyssaviruses

Bats found in Europe are all possible carriers of the classical rabies virus (family *Lyssaviridae*). Other related lyssaviruses have been reported including European bat lyssavirus 1 (EBV-1) and European bat lyssavirus 2 (EBV-2); both are zoonotic and life-threatening infections to humans.

There is no treatment for rabies in the bat or human, or for rabies-related viruses in bats. Many bats will show no signs. It is for this very reason that all bats should be handled with care, and if any handler is bitten, medical advice should be sought immediately and the bat retained in captivity should the need for further testing be required. Bat handlers/rehabilitators should consider prophylactic vaccination against terrestrial rabies virus as this seems to provide cross-protection. In many countries bats are protected under laws that prohibit disturbance of any roosting bat, and which also prevent the killing of all species of bat found in the UK, unless it is seriously injured and is being humanely destroyed.

Other zoonotic viruses

Severe acute respiratory syndrome (SARS) coronaviruses 1 and 2 have been shown to infect bats. However. whether bats are the most important reservoir for human infection is not clear. Other zoonotic viruses worldwide affect bats including other lyssaviruses and Nipah, Hendra and Ebola viruses, so bats should always be considered a zoonotic hazard.

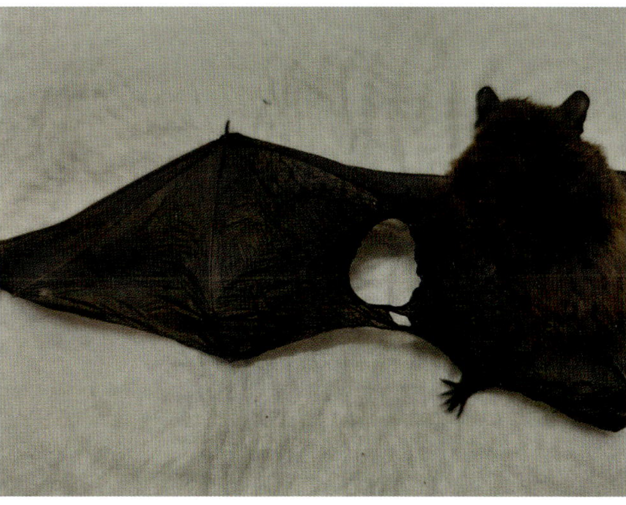

Figure 28.7 Wing defects in bats that do not extend to the wing edge tend to heal naturally and have a good prognosis. *Source:* Courtesy of Kelly Huitson RVN.

Trauma

Bats may be brought to rehabilitation centres and veterinary practices suffering from a variety of traumatic incidents, ranging from car collisions to injuries from domestic cats. Fractures of the smaller wing bones, such as the phalanges of the 'hands' which support the wing membrane, have been shown to heal of their own accord (Walsh and Stebbings, 1989). Fractures of the humerus or radius and ulna are more serious and may require splinting; in the larger species, Kirschner wires as the transcortical pins and polymethylmethacrylate as the crossbar are used to create an external fixator apparatus.

Tearing of the wing membrane has a considerable capacity to heal of its own accord if the tear is reasonably sized and is in the main body of the wing vane. If the tear is at the edge of a wing then healing potential is poor, but if contained within the wing itself then the prospect for recovery is good assuming no serious other debilitating condition (see Figure 28.7).

Suturing the membrane is extremely difficult, and due to the lack of a major vascular supply the wound frequently breaks down. The use of tissue glues may allow sufficient apposition of the edges of such a wound for long enough for re-epithelialisation to occur. If the wing membrane is irreparably damaged the bat is unlikely to be fit for release.

Poisoning

Bats are highly susceptible to the use of organophosphates and organochlorines. They also appear susceptible to the use of pyrethrins, which form the basis of many commercial ectoparasiticides. Their use should thus be avoided in bats.

Other conditions

Neoplasia

Cases of lymphoma have been reported in Microchiroptera (Andreasen and Dulmstra, 1996).

EULIPOTYPHLA: HEDGEHOGS

Ectoparasites

Fleas

Archaeopsylla erinacei is ubiquitous and may be differentiated from the cat or dog flea by the presence of only two spikes on the genal comb (cat and dog fleas, *Ctenocephalides* spp., possess eight or nine). Cat, dog and rabbit fleas (*Spilopsyllus cuniculi*), rat (*Nosopysllus fasciatus*) and avian fleas such as *Echidnophaga* spp., the latter two having no genal spines, have also been reported. *Archaeopsylla erinacei* is uniquely adapted to the hedgehog's lifestyle, coping with the long hibernation period. It also only reproduces in the nest of the breeding female hedgehog, where the pupae hatch, feed off skin debris and quickly develop into nymphs colonising young hedgehogs. The hedgehog flea can also only survive for limited periods away from the hedgehog, and cannot reproduce on any other animal species. Primary disease is uncommon but they can increase debilitation in sick hedgehogs.

Fly strike

The blowfly family of blue, green and black bottles can all cause blowfly strike in young, old or otherwise debilitated hedgehogs which can be life-threatening.

Mites

Four species of mite are commonly seen in the UK: *Sarcoptes* spp., *Notoedres cati*, *Demodex erinacei* and *Caparinia tripilis*. The psoroptid mite, *C. tripilis*, is the commonest cause of severe mange in UK hedgehogs. This mite may be seen with the naked eye as a white pinhead-sized surface mite. It is commonly found around the head and ears, but spreads to the whole body. Severe cases lead to a heavy white scurf, loss of spines, self-trauma (particularly to the pinnae which may become crusted and ripped due to repeated scratching), weight loss, secondary infections and death in severely affected individuals. Diagnosis is made on skin scrapings and/or tape strips. *Caparinia tripilis* has funnel-shaped suckers to the long legs, and pointed mouthparts, and is 0.5–1 mm in length.

Ticks

Ixodes hexagonus attaches to the hedgehog along the belly and around the anogenital area as well as around the ear base. The sheep tick *Ixodes ricinus* may also be commonly seen on hedgehogs in endemic areas. Both ticks may be a serious cause of blood loss in heavily infested individuals, as well as a potential transmitter of disease such as staphylococcal septicaemia, leptospirosis and Lyme disease; the saliva of the tick has also been known to contain neurotoxins which have produced paralysis in some individuals.

Endoparasites

Cestodes (tapeworms)

The tapeworm *Rodentolepis (Hymenolepis) erinacei*, a form of hymenolepid tapeworm, is found occasionally in hedgehogs. It may be a cause of weight loss and diarrhoea. Diagnosis is made on finding the egg sachets/segments in the faeces or on the fur around the anus.

Lungworms

Crenosoma striatum infestation may become so great as to cause blockage of the small airways and severe consolidation and damage to the lung structure allowing secondary infections to occur. The life cycle of the parasite involves an intermediate host, the slug or snail. Adult females in the bronchi of the hedgehog produce larvae, rather than eggs, which are coughed up, swallowed and passed out in the faeces where the motile larvae may be seen microscopically (300 μm long). The larvae then infect slugs and snails, in which they moult twice to become the infective organism, which when the slug/snail is eaten by the hedgehog, break out and migrate through the body into the lungs. The entire life cycle in the peak of summer takes 21 days. Signs of infestation include a dry cough, dyspnoea and weight loss. It can be a real health hazard, particularly when considering anaesthetising hedgehogs.

Another lungworm found in hedgehogs, called *Capillaria (Eucoleus) aerophila*, may infect the hedgehog at the same time as *Crenosoma striatum*. The life cycle is direct, but the eggs may be taken up by earthworms and beetles, which act as paratenic hosts, and are themselves eaten by the hedgehog. The eggs hatch in the gut of the hedgehog, releasing the worm which migrates to the lungs to form the adult.

Other worms

Capillaria erinacei and *C. ovoreticulata* are found in the stomach and intestines of the European hedgehog. Their life cycles are direct and generally few clinical signs are observed in hedgehogs infested. In very young hedgehogs, however, high burdens have been reported as causing severe diarrhoea, lethargy, weight loss and death.

Other nematodes that uncommonly cause clinical disease, but which are often seen in hedgehogs, include *Strongyloides* spp., ascarids, the oesophageal worm *Gongylonema neoplasticum* and the stomach worm *Physaloptera* spp.

Acanthocephalan (thorny-headed) worms such as *Oliganthorhynchus (Echinorhynchus) erinacei* amongst others have been reported affecting the stomach and intestines and may result in peritonitis (Gaglio *et al.*, 2010).

Protozoa

Cystoisospora (Isospora) rastegaivae is a common coccidial parasite in the European hedgehog. Most infections are subclinical, but occasionally with heavy infestations, or concurrent digestive system diseases, weight loss, diarrhoea and anorexia may be seen. Diagnosis is made on finding the oocysts which are round, approximately 20 μm in diameter, and when sporulated contain two circular bodies (sporocysts).

Trematodes (flukes)

Brachylaemus erinacei is found sporadically as an intestinal fluke, and like all digenean trematodes it requires an intermediate host, in this case snails. The parasite then develops and multiplies inside the snail, before reaching its infective stage known as the metacercaria. The snail is eaten by the hedgehog and the metacercariae develop into the adult flukes and live off the lining and blood supply of the small intestine causing haemorrhagic enteritis. Diagnosis is made on finding in the faeces the tiny trematode eggs, which are asymmetrically oval in shape, with a cap at one end.

Bacterial diseases

Bordetella bronchiseptica

This is commonly seen associated with respiratory tract infections, and often exacerbates lungworm infestations. It causes tracheitis that may progress to a bronchopneumonia and potential mortalities.

Leptospira interrogans

One serovar (strain) of *L. interrogans* in particular has been isolated from hedgehogs in the UK, serovar Bratislava. It appears not to cause a serious disease in hedgehogs, although histopathological damage to the structure of the kidney has been observed. It is shed in the urine, and is a zoonosis gaining access through mucous membranes and cuts.

Salmonellosis

This is commonly picked up from carrion or through beetles and maggots which have eaten carrion and then form part of the diet of the hedgehog. In general, most species of *Salmonella* may be said to form a 'normal' part of the flora of the hedgehog's gut, although the zoonotic aspects of this are important for handlers to consider. Biosecurity should be good, gloves worn when handling and hands thoroughly washed after handling hedgehogs. Enteritis and septicaemia have been recorded in hedgehogs and this should be considered as a differential diagnosis in any hedgehog presented collapsed, with or without diarrhoea.

Other bacteria seen in hedgehogs

Respiratory bacteria such as *Pasteurella multocida* and *Streptococcus* spp. may be associated with lungworm infections. Many abscesses from wounds in hedgehogs may be due to bacteria found in the environment or from their own digestive system and include *Corynebacterium pyogenes*, *Pseudomonas aeruginosa*, and *E. coli*. Occasionally some hedgehogs have been found to be contaminated with zoonotic tuberculosis, both bovine (*Mycobacterium bovis*) and avian (*M. avium*), although the hedgehog is not known to be a significant reservoir.

Yersinia pseudotuberculosis has also been seen in juvenile hedgehogs, with hindlimb weakness, chronic weight loss and occasionally diarrhoea. *Borrelia burgdorferi* has also been regularly recovered from ticks found on hedgehogs, and therefore Lymes disease may be present as a zoonotic reservoir and may also cause clinical disease in hedgehogs.

Dental disease is a very common problem in hedgehogs. In captivity the problem is often enhanced by the feeding of tinned commercial cat foods, which adhere to the teeth and cause a rapid build-up of tartar. The feeding of dry diets may therefore be useful in captivity, although fresh water should be made readily available at all times. Bacteria involved in dental abscesses include *Pasteurella* spp., *E. coli*, *Streptococcus* spp. and anaerobes.

Fungal diseases

Adiaspiromycosis

Emmonsia (parva) crescens can cause small grey multiple abscesses throughout the lung parenchyma leading to severe pneumonia, often complicating lungworm pneumonia or bacterial pneumonia (Seixas *et al.*, 2006).

Dermatophytosis (ringworm)

The dermatophyte *Trichophyton mentagrophytes* var. *erinacei* is a common commensal of hedgehog skin but can exacerbate *Caparinia tripilis* infection and produces grey crusting scale, particularly over the head, with fur and spine loss in severe cases. Diagnosis is by culturing the fungus on Sabouraud's media. *Trichophyton mentagrophytes* var. *erinacei* produces a fine white growth, with a yellow-green staining of the media.

Viral diseases

Foot and mouth disease

Hedgehogs are extremely susceptible to this disease and develop unpleasant mouth ulcerations, as well as ulcerations of the nose and perineum. In addition vesicles are often seen on the feet of hedgehogs. Some hedgehogs will survive the virus, but often the infection appears to be fatal. An interesting study by Hulse and Edwards (1937) showed that during hibernation of the hedgehog the virus failed to multiply and thus to cause severe disease. When the hedgehog reawakened the following spring, the virus was reactivated. The disease is of course notifiable and any hedgehog showing such signs should be isolated, and the APHA contacted for further advice.

Herpesviruses

These have been reported in Europe, the liver being the main target for damage, with intranuclear acidophilic inclusion bodies typically being seen in hepatocytes. Death has been recorded (Widen *et al.*, 1996). Erinaceid herpesvirus 1 is the main strain found in Europe.

Morbilliviruses

These have been isolated from the faeces of hedgehogs. Clinical signs involve thickening of the skin of the feet (similar to canine distemper, another morbillivirus), crusting of the eyes, sometimes blindness, incoordination, and other neurological signs. Some hedgehogs will die from this virus, and there is no known treatment or vaccination available.

Trauma

Hedgehogs are unfortunately frequently injured in gardens and in hedgerows and roadside verges, due to their habit of sleeping buried in deep leaf litter. Severe burns may be seen as they are often involved in fires, as they seek out hibernation sites in the autumn and burrow into ready-made bonfire night piles. Hedge strimmer and lawn mower injuries are also common. Injuries seen therefore will vary, but frequently involve tears or lacerations to the skin and subcutaneous layers over the dorsum (see Figure 28.8).

Subcutaneous emphysema is common after road traffic accidents and other traumas. Repeated deflation may be required to allow the condition to resolve. Another common feature of trauma is prolapse of the orbicularis muscle, where the muscle responsible for curling up the hedgehog everts as it slips off the edge of the pelvis caudally. This may be replaced after anaesthesia to its correct position.

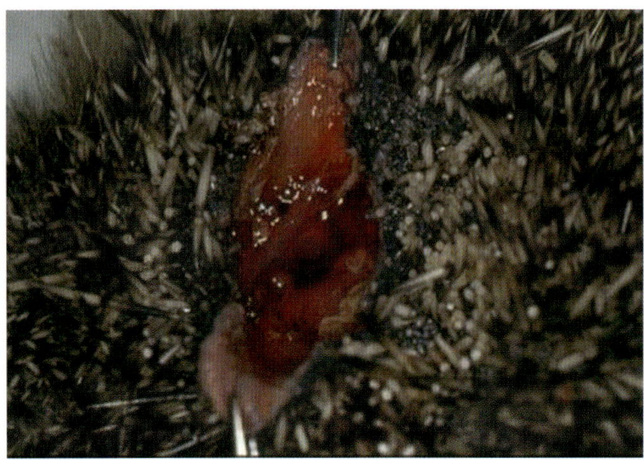

Figure 28.8 Strimmer injuries to the dorsum of wild hedgehogs are not uncommon.

Poisoning

The commonest cause of poisoning in hedgehogs is due to metaldehyde poisoning from slug-bait preparations. It appears that in many cases the hedgehog has actually consumed the pellets, rather than just the slug which has been killed by the pellets. Signs include increased activity/hyperaesthesia, occasionally vomiting and death.

Other diseases

Demyelinating paralysis

This syndrome involves spinal demyelination and posterior ascending paresis/paralysis and death (Palmer *et al.*, 1998). It is sometimes referred to as 'wobbly hedgehog' syndrome and may be seen in wild and captive hedgehogs. Clinical signs can include weakness, paresis or paralysis of hindlimbs, exophthalmos, wasting disease and seizures. A viral cause has been suspected but a toxin could not be ruled out.

Release weight

Do not release hedgehogs in the autumn if they are underweight as they may not have enough reserves to survive the hibernation period. There is some debate about weight, with some suggesting that if the adult hedgehog weighs less than 450 g or it is less than 560 g close to hibernation, then it has less chance of surviving (Morris, 1984, 1998; Stocker, 2005).

LAGOMORPHA: RABBITS AND HARES

Ectoparasites

Fleas

The rabbit flea *Spilopsyllus cuniculi* is commonly found on the ears of rabbits and is the main vector for myxomatosis.

Lice

The sucking louse *Haemodipsus ventricosis* is commonly found on the wild rabbit. In the brown hare it is the sucking louse *Haemodipsus lyrocephalus* which is frequently seen. Both lice may cause clinical anaemia if present in sufficient numbers and on a young host.

Endoparasites

Cestodes

The tapeworm *Mosgovoyia pectinata* has been reported in mountain hares (*Lepus timidus*) and in higher levels in woodland areas than on heather moorlands (Hulbert and Boag, 2001).

Nematodes

The stomach worm *Graphidium strigosum* is found in both hares and rabbits as is the small intestine worm *Trichostrongylus retortaeformis*, with the latter being more commonly seen in wooded environments than open moorland (Hulbert and Boag, 2001). However, Townsend *et al.* (2009) suggest that *T. retortaeformis* levels do not influence the population size of species such as the mountain hare, although Newey and Thirgood (2004) argue that while they do not reduce survival rates or body condition, heavy burdens do reduce fecundity in hares. *Graphidium strigosum* may cause gastric ulceration and secondary digestive upsets if present in large enough numbers.

In the large intestine the pinworm *Passalurus ambiguus* is a common finding. It rarely causes clinical problems.

Lungworms such as *Protostrongylus* spp. are well reported in mountain hares with high levels of infectivity (96%) and in brown hares at lower levels (60%), but in both cases with few clinical signs (Laakkonen *et al.*, 2006).

Protozoa

Coccidial organisms may cause significant problems, particularly *Eimeria* spp. such as *E. stiedae* which, as in domestic rabbits, may infest the liver as well as the small intestine. Weight loss, diarrhoea and failure to grow are all signs seen in young rabbits and hares.

Trematodes

Liver flukes have been reported in hares (both *Fasciola hepatica* and *Dicrocoelium dendriticum*) without clinical signs of disease but, theoretically, liver damage is a possibility.

Bacterial diseases

Borrelia burgdorferi

This is tick-transmitted and commonly seen in hares, which may act as a reservoir host. The European rabbit is one of the few animals that shows the cutaneous form of the disease (spreading erythema and pruritus around the tick bite) but will often mount an effective immune system response which clears infection. Clinical signs in hares are rarely seen and pathology poorly reported.

Clostridium spp.

Clostridium perfringens and *C. spiroforme* have both been implicated in peracute mortalities of lagomorphs.

Francisella tularensis

In central Europe, *F. tularensis* affects brown hares, which may act as a reservoir host. They are moderately affected with a more chronic form of the disease, small white 0.1–1 cm nodules being seen in the lungs, pericardium and kidneys. In mountain hares high mortality rates are seen, with typhlitis and splenomegaly at post-mortem. It is a significant zoonosis – the organism is the cause of tularaemia in humans. Transmission is via ticks or other blood-sucking arthropods but can be spread via the body fluids and excretions of infected animals. It is also transmitted via water. Diagnosis is by culture and PCR analysis, and in the UK it is a legally notifiable disease.

Pasteurella spp.

Pasteurella multocida can cause severe disease, with pneumonia, septicaemia and mortalities. In European brown hares it can cause a conjunctivitis that is often purulent. It can become systemic with pneumonia and splenomegaly. Related bacteria, such as *Mannheimia haemolytica*, can also cause disease in hares, usually causing a purulent bronchopneumonia. It can induce middle ear disease with torticollis and seizures and may result in reproductive tract infections and abortion. Diagnosis is based on clinical signs and culture.

Staphylococcus spp.

Staphylococcus spp. such as *S. aureus* and *S. xylosus* have been associated with skin infections and abscesses in mountain and brown hares. These can become systemic and result in septicaemia, multiple internal organ abscesses and mortalities. Diagnosis is by culture.

Yersinia spp.

Yersinia pseudotuberculosis is a common bacterium in the digestive system of wild lagomorphs, particularly hares, which seem to be very susceptible to the disease. Clinical signs include a gastroenteritis in mild cases, with incoordination, lethargy, collapse and death in cases which become septicaemic. *Yersinia enterocolitica* has also been recovered regularly from wild lagomorphs and may cause similar disease as *Y. pseudotuberculosis*. Both are zoonotic and their transmission is faeco-oral.

Fungal diseases

Pneumocystis spp.

Pneumocystis spp. have been recovered from the lungs of hares in Europe, with an incidence rate of 20% in brown hares and 16.9% in mountain hares (Laakkonen *et al*., 2006). Higher levels of infection were associated with lower body condition in young hares.

Trichophyton spp.

Ringworm (dermatophytosis) is occasionally reported in wild lagomorphs, although it can commonly be recovered from their fur where no clinical disease is present. It is usually self-limiting.

Viral diseases

European brown hare syndrome virus

This disease only affects the European hare (*Lepus europaeus*) and mountain hare (*Lepus timidus*). It is a member of the *Caliciviridae* family and so related to rabbit haemorrhagic disease virus (RHDV). It has a mortality rate that can vary considerably from 10 to 100%. Occasionally clinical signs are seen, ranging from depression, lethargy, anorexia and jaundice to neurological signs due to hepatic encephalopathy, where hares may run in circles and lose their fear of humans. The virus causes splenomegaly, kidney and liver damage including calcification and bile duct proliferation, and widespread cellular necrosis and haemorrhage. As with RHDV, young animals (<50 days old) appear to be innately resistant to infection. Chronic carriers are common. In Italy, 1% of the brown hare population had the virus (with 67–78% showing an immune response), while in Poland 7.6% had the virus (with 38% seroprevalence) (Frolich *et al*., 1996; Todone *et al*., 2008). PCR and haemagglutination serology tests have been used to diagnose the disease.

Myxomatosis

This parapoxvirus has been present in the UK since the 1950s and is now considered endemic in the wild rabbit population. It is transmitted by biting insects, principally the rabbit flea *Spilopsyllus cuniculi*. Clinical signs are similar to those seen in domestic rabbits, with oedema of the ear base, muzzle and periocular and anogenital areas (see Figures 28.9 and 28.10). Susceptible rabbits may die within 5 days of infection, while others may have a more protracted course and take 10–14 days to die depending on the virulence of the strain. An amyxomatous form of the disease has also been reported in Europe where rabbits infected die of respiratory disease with a few small skin nodules. Diagnosis may be made based on clinical signs, ELISA serology, agar gel immunodiffusion or PCR. Clinical disease is rare in European and mountain hares but has been reported.

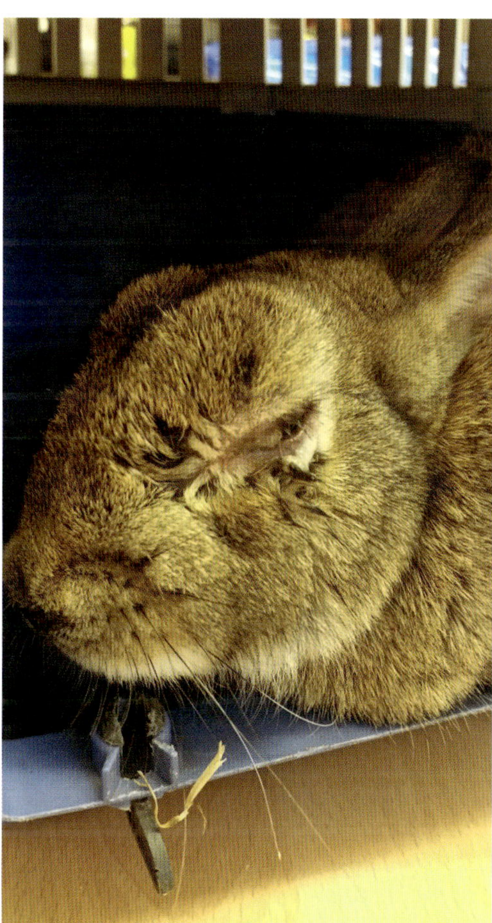

Figure 28.9 Myxomatosis in a European rabbit. Note the periorbital oedema and oculonasal discharge.

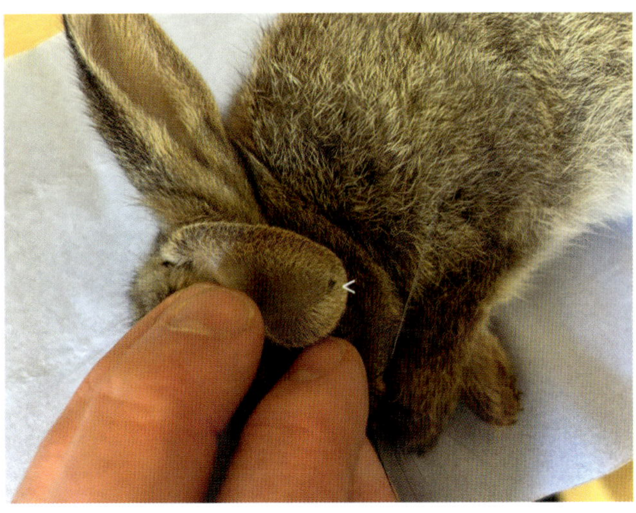

Figure 28.10 The rabbit flea *Spilopsyllus cuniculi* (white arrow) the principal vector for myxomatosis in its typical attachment site on the lateral ear vein.

Hare fibroma virus

Hare fibroma virus infection is seen rarely in European brown hares. Mortality rates are low, but morbidity can be 25–30% of the population during an outbreak. Clinically, tumours (fibromas) appear around the ears, head (particularly eyelid margins) and legs, but may spread to the body. They are 1–3 cm across and may be seen singly or in clusters. Spontaneous resolution occurs after 4–6 weeks, although as the tumours drop off, bleeding ulcers may be left. Virus isolation has been used to demonstrate the presence of a poxvirus. Histopathology of the fibromas shows fibroblasts with large nuclei and periodic acid Schiff-positive inclusions in the cytoplasm. There is no treatment.

Leporine dysautonomia

The cause of the condition is not really known. The clinical signs are similar to those seen in horses with grass sickness, where paralysis of the gut occurs leading to a wasting condition and eventually death. On examination of the nerve ganglia in the large intestine, pathologists have found, as with horses with grass sickness, a depletion in the number of nerves as compared with a healthy hare (Griffiths and Whitwell, 1993). There is no known treatment.

Rabbit haemorrhagic disease virus

There have been several epidemics in the wild in the UK. The virus is a member of the *Caliciviridae* family and is transmitted in faecal and respiratory secretions with an incubation period of 1–3 days. It is stable in the environment facilitating fomite spread. Rabbits are often found dead, sometimes with blood around the nares or anus. Internally significant haemorrhage is noted. The target organ is the liver, although the spleen is also often enlarged and death within 12–36 hours is common. Prior to death, fever in excess of 40°C may be seen as well as seizures, opisthotonus and vocalisation. Rabbits under 40 days of age appear innately protected. Two strains have been recorded in the UK, RHDV1 and RHDV2. There is some early evidence that brown hares, whilst not highly susceptible to it, can become infected with rabbit calicivirus, particularly RHDV2 (Velarde *et al.*, 2017). Currently in Europe RHDV2 strain k is causing problems in rabbits as it appears to be more virulent. PCR is available to help diagnosis and many rabbits will seroconvert even though it is usually ineffective.

Trauma

Road traffic collisions are common in hares and wild rabbits. The injuries are often terminal and frequently involve fractures of the spine. In addition, trauma from predator wounds are commonly seen. Small bite wounds around the neck and head are often the result of weasels and stoats, whereas larger flesh wounds may be associated with foxes, dogs and cats.

RODENTIA: BEAVERS, MICE, RATS, SQUIRRELS AND VOLES

Ectoparasites

Beetles

The Eurasian beaver can carry a host-specific beetle, *Platypsyllus castoris*. It appears to cause little or no clinical disease (see Figure 28.11).

Fleas

Orchopeas howardi is the common flea of the grey squirrel, and *Monopsyllus sciurorum* is the common flea of the red squirrel. Fleas in many rodents may act as vectors for haemoparasites and bacteria, including zoonoses such as *Yersinia pestis* the cause of plague although this is not seen in the UK.

Mites

Rodents may carry significant numbers of mites with high percentages of populations being affected, for example 43–47% of rodents sampled in Lithuania were positive, with up to eight species of parasitic mites from the Laelapidae family (Kaminskiene *et al.*, 2020).

Demodex spp. (e.g. *D. microti*) has been reported around the genital area of voles. It may result in mild alopecia but can be an incidental finding.

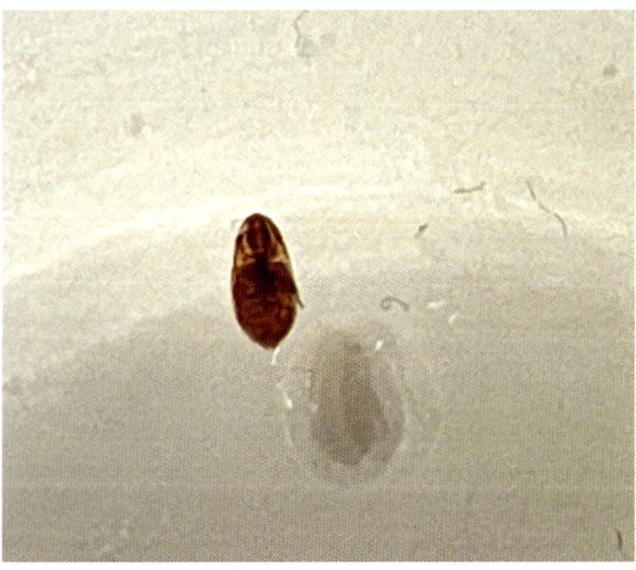

Figure 28.11 The beaver beetle *Platypsyllus castoris* less than 5 mm in length is a non-pathogenic parasite of the Eurasian beaver.

Chigger or harvest mites (Trombiculidae) may cause pruritus and fur loss particularly around the eyes and muzzle in a range of rodents.

Lice

Polyplax spp. are blood-sucking lice that may result in significant anaemia of rodents as well as acting as potential vectors of a range of blood-borne diseases, such as Q fever (*Coxiella burnetii*), *Borrelia*, *Bartonella*, *Acinetobacter*, *Anaplasma* and *Yersinia* spp. all of which are potential zoonoses. Both red and grey squirrels may be affected by the sucking louse *Neohaematopinus sciuri*, although in the healthy squirrel it appears to cause no disease.

Ticks

Ticks such as *Ixodes*, *Dermacentor* spp. and a range of fleas are commonly found on rodents and may act as significant vectors of blood-borne diseases such as those listed above under lice. In addition they can result in significant trauma to rodents and blood loss causing debilitation.

Endoparasites

Cestodes

Echinococcus multilocularis is a significant zoonotic disease, with the final/definitive host usually being a canid or sometimes a felid. It is currently not present in the UK and is legally notifiable. Rodents such as the common vole, water vole and bank vole are the most significant intermediate hosts of this parasite in Europe. The Eurasian beaver may also act as an aberrant intermediate host. As an intermediate host, rodents have to be consumed by a definitive host (felid, canid) for the adult cestode to form. Humans are therefore not at risk of contracting the disease from rodents (unless they consume them!). Diagnosis may be attempted by ultrasound, although it is often not possible to distinguish the disease from other cyst-forming agents. An ELISA blood test has been used in Eurasian beavers as has combined laparoscopy and ultrasound (Campbell-Palmer *et al.*, 2015). There is no treatment in the intermediate host.

The cestode *Rodentolepis nana* is small (5–6 cm) and only occasionally pathogenic, causing a blockage of the ileocaecal area. Egg packets may be found around the fur of the perineum of infected rodents. It is a potential zoonosis, although the closely related primate cestode *Hymenolepis nana* is of more concern.

Nematodes

Capillaria hepatica is common in many rodents. The eggs are consumed by the rodent and develop into larvae that migrate out of the intestine via the portal blood system to the liver where they mature, mate and produce more eggs. The cycle is completed by the consumption of the rodent by a predator when the eggs are released into the environment, or when the rodent dies and decomposes the eggs are again released. It is potentially zoonotic.

Trichostrongyles affecting the stomach such as *Travassosuis rufus* in Eurasian beavers have been associated with clinical disease. Diagnosis is by finding typical trichostrongyle eggs in the faeces.

Oxyurids such as *Syphacia* spp. and *Aspicularis* spp. are commonly seen in rodents. Faecal flotation techniques will demonstrate banana-shaped to ovoid eggs. Rarely does clinical disease develop as these are a large bowel nematodes.

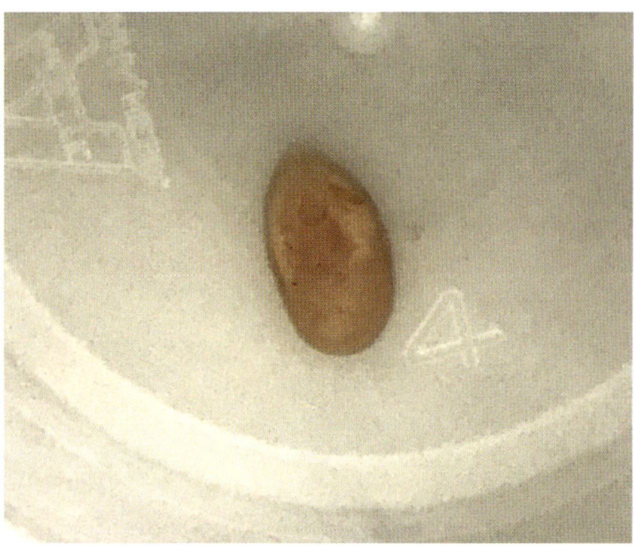

Figure 28.12 The adult trematode *Neostichorchis subtriquetrus* is non-pathogenic in the adult Eurasian beaver.

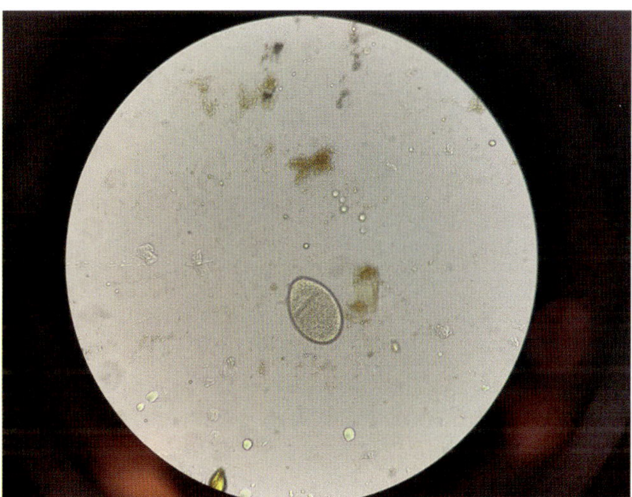

Figure 28.13 An oocyst of the non-pathogenic *Neostichorchis subtriquetrus* from a faecal sample of a Eurasian beaver.

Protozoa

Eimeria sciurorum is found in squirrels and is not often pathogenic on its own; rather it is an opportunist which will cause intestinal disease in the young or when the host is already debilitated.

Trematodes

Neostichorchis (Stichorchis) subtriquetrus is an intestinal fluke of beavers that is considered non-pathogenic and whose large oocysts may be found in faeces (Campbell-Palmer *et al.*, 2013) (see Figures 28.12 and 28.13). Liver fluke (*Fasciola hepatica*) has also been reported in rodents, although rarely with clinical disease.

Bacterial diseases

Bartonella spp.

Common in rodents, particularly mice (*Apodemus*, *Mus* spp.), voles (*Myodes*, *Clethrionomys*, *Microtus* spp.), rats (*Rattus norvegicus*) and shrews (Soricidae). They are spread by blood-sucking arthropods, fighting and faeces. Diagnosis can be made on blood smears, demonstrating bacilli in the cytoplasm of erythrocytes, and by PCR. Treatment is generally not necessary as infected rodents are rarely clinically affected but *Bartonella* spp. are zoonotic, causing conditions including cat scratch disease and vascular proliferative disease such as bacillary angiomatosis and peliosis hepatis.

Borrelia spp.

These are transmitted primarily by ticks. Two groups exist: Lyme borreliosis spirochaetes (LBS) and relapsing fever spirochaetes (RFS), comprising Old World relapsing fever spirochaetes (ORFS) and New World relapsing fever spirochaetes (NRFS). The LBS group are principally transmitted by hard body ticks such as *Ixodes* spp. and the RFS groups are transmitted by soft body ticks such as *Ornithodoros* spp. Rodents are significant reservoir hosts for many of these bacteria. Male rodents often have higher tick burdens than females and so may have higher burdens of spirochaetes. Experimental infection of mice (*Mus musculus*), American white-footed mice (*Peromyscus leucopus*) and hamsters (*Mesocricetus auratus*) showed evidence of persistent infection but without any pathological lesions. In some laboratory strains of rodents, pathological lesions reported are similar to those in humans, with multiple organ inflammatory disease (myocarditis, myositis, vasculitis, peripheral neuritis) and arthritis. Diagnosis is therefore difficult, the preferred methods being culture (which is challenging as they are microaerophilic and slow-growing) or PCR. Controlling ticks on rodents to avoid human or other animal spread is therefore important.

Brucella spp.

Brucella spp. are common in rodents and it is a potential zoonosis. *Brucella microti* has been isolated from voles in Europe and can survive for extended periods in the soil.

Chlamydiaceae and *Chlamydia*-like organisms

Chlamydia muridarum is the agent of mouse pneumonitis and has two strains, Nigg and SFPD. It affects all members of the Muridae producing a subclinical respiratory infection but can also be sexually transmitted and affect the reproductive tract.

Other organisms such as *Parachlamydia acanthamoebae* and *Waddlia chondrophila* are important emerging pathogens in animals with zoonotic potential and have resulted in abortions in cattle in Switzerland and Scotland (Ruhl *et al.*, 2009; Deuchande *et al.*, 2010). They have been isolated by PCR in several wild rodents including shrews (*Neomys anomalus* and *Crocidura leucodon*), voles (*Microtis arvalis* and *Arvicola scherman*) and house mice (*Mus musculus*) (Stephen *et al.*, 2014).

Clostridium piliforme

This causes Tyzzer's disease and most commonly affects the gastrointestinal system, particularly the terminal ileum and colon. Ulcerative typhilitis and colitis with haemorrhagic diarrhoea and small liver abscesses are common.

Leptospira spp.

Interstitial nephritis is commonly seen in rats and voles. Carriage with no obvious clinical signs is common in rats and so any wild rodent should be considered a potential zoonotic source for leptospirosis. Diagnosis of carriage is with a quantitative PCR, but seropositivity using microscopic agglutination tests to serovar pools 1–6 has been reported in rodents such as beavers and water voles (Girling *et al.*, 2019a).

Mycobacterium spp.

Mycobacterium microti is common in voles (*Microtus agrestis*). It can be a potential zoonosis. It most commonly affects the respiratory tract but may also be found in wounds and abscesses and skin lesions are common.

Mycobacterium bovis has also been reported in rodents such as voles (*Microtus agrestis*, *Clethrionomys glareolus*), mice (*Apodemus sylvaticus*, *A. flavicollis*) and shrews (*Sorex araneus*).

In the UK and elsewhere, *Mycobacterium avium* subsp. *paratuberculosis* (the cause of Johne's disease) has been isolated from red squirrels and *M. bovis* (bovine tuberculosis) has also been isolated from grey squirrels. *Mycobacterium lepromatosis* (the cause of human leprosy) has been isolated from red squirrel skin lesions (Meredith *et al.*, 2014). These are all zoonotic and so care should be taken if treating squirrels in particular.

Salmonella spp.

Salmonella typhimurium and *Salmonella enteritidis* are commonly carried subclinically in the gut of Muridae principally but in theory any rodent can transmit these bacteria and act as a zoonotic agent. Squirrels feeding from garden bird feeders are regularly exposed to *Salmonella* spp. from wild birds (see Figure 28.14).

Staphylococcus spp.

Staphylococcus stepanovicii has been recovered regularly from the skin, faeces and fur of rodents. *Staphylococcus aureus* has been associated with abscesses in rodents.

Yersinia spp. and *Francisella tularensis*

Yersinia pestis, the cause of bubonic plague, and *Francisella tularensis*, the cause of lemming fever, are commonly found in rodents in the Holarctic regions. Both are significant zoonoses and may be transmitted by tissue fluids and biting insects such as sucking lice, ticks and fleas that have previously been attached to the infected rodent. Neither disease is currently found in the UK and both are legally notifiable.

Yersinia enterocolitica and *Y. pseudotuberculosis* have also been recovered regularly from rodents (particularly rats, mice and voles) and are also zoonoses and are present in the UK. They may be carried with no clinical signs or, less commonly, may cause acute septicaemia or haemorrhagic diarrhoea. A chronic version of *Y. pseudotuberculosis* may produce granulomatous intestinal disease producing a wasting syndrome and is more commonly reported in voles. Transmission is via the faeco-oral route.

Fungal diseases

Candida albicans

This has been reported as a cause of oesophagitis and mortality in a red squirrel, although a suspected underlying undiagnosed stressor was suspected due to adrenal exhaustion (Simpson *et al.*, 2009).

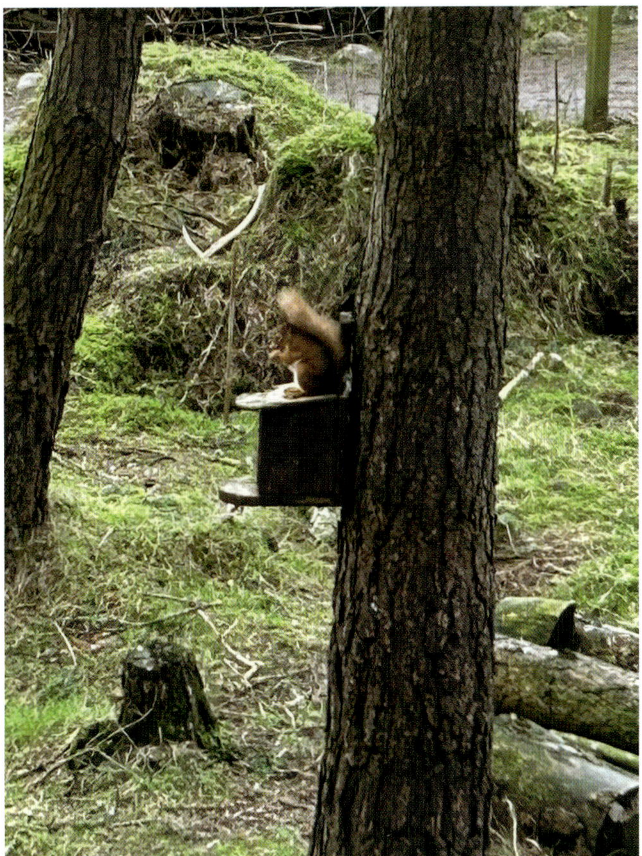

Figure 28.14 Bird nests and feeders can attract squirrels and wild birds and lead to an exchange of pathogenic bacteria such as *Salmonella* spp.

Emmonsia spp.

As with any semi-fossorial species, *Emmonsia* spp. yeast infection of the lungs resulting in pneumonia has been reported in rodents and may be advanced by the time of presentation.

Viral diseases

Cowpoxvirus

Cowpoxvirus is commonly recovered from rodents in the wild such as voles, lemmings, rats and mice. It rarely affects the host, but can of course cause disease in other mammals including humans. PCR testing of body tissues, particularly the spleen, has been used to diagnose the presence of the virus. There is no treatment.

Hantaviruses

These are members of the family *Bunyaviridae*. They rarely cause disease in rodents but they are significant zoonoses and can cause renal and cardiac damage in humans. In humans, hantavirus cardiopulmonary syndrome is reported in the Americas and haemorrhagic fever with renal syndrome in Asia and Europe.

Hantavirus has been diagnosed in rats and voles and wood mice (syn. long-tailed field mice) in the UK and elsewhere and is spread in the urine, saliva, blood and faeces of the rodent. It has not so far been reported in beavers and some voles such as water voles (*Arvicola amphibius*) (Girling *et al.*, 2019b).

Herpesviruses

Murine cytomegalovirus is seen commonly in the house mouse (*Mus domesticus*) in Europe.

Murine gamma-herpesvirus 4 (MuHV4) has been found in bank voles (*Clethrionomys glareolus*), wood mice (*Apodemus sylvaticus*) and shrews (*Crocidura russula*) in Europe, with wood mice being perhaps the main host with 13–24% seroprevalence (Blasdell *et al.*, 2003). It can cause bronchiolitis and B-cell lymphoma.

Ljungan virus

This picornavirus has a northern hemisphere Holarctic distribution and is found in a range of rodents particularly voles, lemmings and mice. It has been shown experimentally to cause type 2 diabetes and reproductive disease (resorptions, fetal malformations) in *Mus musculus* and is believed to be able to cause similar signs in humans, including type 1 diabetes mellitus, Guillain–Barré syndrome and myocarditis. It has also been suspected as a possible cause of hydrocephalus in the red fox (*Vulpes vulpes*), one of the main predators of these rodents (Barlow, 2012). Immunohistochemistry was used to diagnose the presence of the virus.

Squirrel adenovirus

The prevalence of virus shedding in faeces of red squirrels in one recent survey was 14.3% (Everest *et al.*, 2010). Diarrhoea, splenic necrosis and death have been associated with infections of red squirrels. There has been a suggestion that the grey squirrel may act as a reservoir, subclinical host to this virus (Everest *et al.*, 2009).

Squirrel parapoxvirus

Red squirrel parapoxvirus, now moved to an unassigned genus and known as squirrel poxvirus, causes squirrel poxvirus disease. It is subclinical in grey squirrels, which act as the reservoir host for the severe clinical disease in red squirrels. Up to 60% of the UK grey squirrel population is believed to be positive (Sainsbury *et al.*, 2000). In the red squirrel infection is usually fatal but recent work has shown there may be developing resistance (Everest *et al.*, 2016). Affected red squirrels develop pox-like lesions over the eyelids, mouth, anogenital area and the feet that become purulent with secondary bacterial infection. Nearly all develop a conjunctivitis with yellow ocular discharge and eyelid oedema. The disease also affects organs such as the liver and spleen. Transmission is by close physical contact via body fluids, although it is possible insect vectors may transmit the virus but this has yet to be proven. The virus can survive for weeks in the environment. Diagnosis is based on clinical signs and demonstration of the virus using PCR. There is no specific treatment available.

Squirrel rotavirus

This has been linked to diarrhoea and intussusception in young squirrels, with a reported infection level in one survey of 2.9% (Everest *et al.*, 2010).

Trauma

Trauma in rodents as with other wildlife is usually fatal. Larger rodents such as beavers may be shot and all may be subject to road traffic collisions.

Other diseases

Metabolic bone disease has been reported in the UK and suggestions have been made that it is associated with overfeeding at bird tables to the exclusion of a more natural wild-type diet.

WILD BIRDS

Many common avian diseases are covered in Chapter 13. The conditions below cover some aspects of disease not covered in that chapter.

Bacterial diseases

Avian tuberculosis

Mycobacterium avium or *M. avium-intracellulare* complex has been reported in most species of birds, particularly waterfowl such as ducks and geese but also finches and Galliformes. It is generally localised to the gastrointestinal system and liver and is therefore spread via faeces. Faecal PCR or acid-fast cytology may detect infection and an ELISA to detect antibodies has been used to screen waterfowl for avian tuberculosis. Treatment is not recommended and euthanasia should be performed.

Viral diseases

Pigeon paramyxovirus 1/Newcastle disease

Newcastle disease and pigeon paramyxovirus 1 disease are both legally notifiable diseases in Europe and the USA. Positive cases of Newcastle disease are compulsorily culled. Incubation periods are around 1 week with viral shedding at 1–6 weeks. Neurological signs including head tilt, torticollis, wing drooping and ataxia are typically seen. Polyuria is also a common feature. In falcons, anorexia, vomiting and paralytic ileus are seen. In pigeons, mortality rates are generally low with pigeon paramyxovirus 1 disease and all but the worst neurological cases can recover. Several vaccines exist for pigeons in the UK. Diagnosis is based on the signs and confirmation is made using viral hemagglutination inhibition tests.

Influenza virus disease

Avian influenza is an ever-present threat to bird and human health and wild-bird avian influenza infections have wiped out significant numbers of seabirds in particular over the last few years. It is also an emerging zoonosis and threat to mammalian species. Evidence of mutation of avian influenza viruses and infection with clinical disease in mammal species has occurred recently and includes sea lions, domestic cats and cattle as well as humans (Leguia *et al.*, 2023; Burrough *et al.*, 2024). This poses a significant zoonotic risk to wild bird handlers and risk assessments and personal protective equipment including face fitted masks during high-risk periods should be considered. No treatment for affected birds is currently available and preventative vaccination of wild birds is currently prohibited. More information on the virus can be found in Chapter 13.

Other conditions

Botulism

Clostridium botulinum is a soil-associated bacterium that can produce an exotoxin (types C and E) and be ingested by waterfowl in particular. Botulism is common after droughts that result in low levels of water in pools or ponds with consequent exposure of mud. It is also exacerbated by the presence of decomposing dead animals with resultant maggots that can concentrate the bacterium and its toxins and which provide a tempting food source for the bird. The exotoxins are neurotoxic and an affected waterfowl can be clinically graded in severity on a scale of 1 to 3:

1. Unable to fly but can walk and swim
2. Unable to fly or walk, but can swim and has a weak neck support (so-called 'limberneck')
3. Paralysed.

Lead poisoning

This is still a common problem in wild waterfowl, swans in particular. It is often due to the consumption of lead shot from shotgun discharges, or old lead weights from coarse fishing still present at the bottom of watercourses. In addition, commercial mining areas may also contribute occasionally to lead and other heavy metal discharges such as zinc and tin.

Diagnosis of lead poisoning can and should involve radiography of the affected bird to demonstrate radiodense particles, often in the gizzard/ventriculus of the patient. However, many affected birds no longer have lead particles in their digestive system, but are still suffering from lead poisoning. Therefore, a blood sample to demonstrate elevated levels of lead (normal levels are below 0.4 ppm, while anything over 0.5 ppm, particularly over 2 ppm is diagnostic for lead poisoning).

Clinically the bird presents in a number of ways but waterfowl will often be weak and may have wing droop and a curved S-shaped neck, particularly in swans as they have not got the strength to support the head.

Oil spills

Oil spills often affect large numbers of seabirds and shorebirds. Toxic effects can be associated with the failure of feather waterproofing resulting in hypothermia and drowning as well as a systemic toxicosis associated with the chemicals themselves, with effects that include gastrointestinal ulceration, neurological disease and haemolysis. Lighter petroleum-based fractions are often more acutely toxic than heavier crude oils but the latter are more likely to result in hypothermia and drowning through destruction of waterproofing.

Pesticide toxicity

Pesticide toxicity is the commonest form of poisoning and accounts for the majority of wildlife poisoning. Various chemicals have been associated including the following.

1. *Alphachloralose*: a small rodent poison causing hypothermia. Clinical signs in birds include lethargy, incoordination and stupor.
2. *Mevinphos*: an organophosphate and less commonly seen since most have been banned. Clinical signs include flaccid paralysis of the limbs although the head remains upright (unlike botulism), bradycardia, diarrhoea and dyspnoea.
3. *Strychnine*: still available as a mole poison. Clinical signs are rarely seen as death is usually peracute. After death, there is opisthotonus and rigor. The birds are often found adjacent to poisoned bait.

Trauma

Birds suffering from window or car strikes should receive a full physical examination and ideally a full-body radiographic assessment. They should also always receive a full ophthalmological examination, with care taken to check for evidence of detached retinas, hyphema, distortion of the globe or rupture of the pecten. The latter is the coiled blood supply to the retinal surface via the vitreous humour as there are no surface retinal vessels in birds. Therefore its rupture can cause retinal damage. In order to gain a better image of the retina, a mydriatic may need to be used but this is complicated by the presence of skeletal muscle in the iris which is under voluntary control in birds. Therefore rocuronium bromide can be used topically. One report in kestrels (*Falco tinnunculus*) and owls used 0.12 mg in each eye with consistent results and no side-effects (Barsotti *et al.*, 2012).

It is also worthwhile checking the external ear canal in birds, particularly in Strigiformes where it is large, for evidence of blood. If found, this often indicates a skull fracture and this almost always involves damage to the large globe of the eye. Any ocular deficits can be serious for wild bird rehabilitation, particularly in the case of binocular hunters such as many raptors.

References

Akerstedt, J., Lillehaug, A., Larsen, I.L. *et al.* (2010) Serosurvey for canine distemper virus, canine adenovirus, *Leptospira interrogans*, and *Toxoplasma gondii* in free-ranging canids in Scandinavia and Svalbard. *Journal of Wildlife Diseases*, **46**(2), 474–480.

Andreasen, C.B. and Dulmstra, J.R. (1996) Multicentric malignant lymphoma in a pallid bat. *Journal of Wildlife Diseases*, **32**(3), 545–547.

Anwar, M.A., Newman, C., MacDonald, D.W. *et al.* (2000) Coccidiosis in the European badger (Meles meles) from England, an epidemiological study. *Parasitology*, **120**(Pt 3), 255–260.

Aschfalk, A., Kemper, N., Arnemo, J.M. *et al.* (2008) Prevalence of *Yersinia* species in healthy free-ranging red deer (*Cervus elaphus*) in Norway. *Veterinary Record*, **163**, 27–28.

Ashford, R.T., Anderson, P., Waring, L. *et al.* (2020) Evaluation of the Dual Path Platform (DPP) VetTB assay for the detection of *Mycobacterium bovis* infection in badgers. *Preventative Veterinary Medicine*, **180**, 105005.

Baily, J.L., Foster, G., Brown, D. *et al.* (2016) *Salmonella* in grey seals. *Environmental Microbiology*, **18**, 1078–1087.

Barlow, A.M. (2012) Ljungan virus infection. In: *Infectious Diseases of Wild Mammals and Birds in Europe* (eds D. Gavier-Widen, J.P. Duff & A. Meredith), p. 179. Blackwell Publishing, Oxford.

Barlow, A.M., Mullineaux, E., Wood, R. *et al.* (2010) Giardiosis in Eurasian badgers (Meles meles). *Veterinary Record*, **167**(26), 1017. doi: 10.1136/vr.c7346.

Barlow, A.M., Jolliffe, T., Tomlin, M. *et al.* (2011) Mycotic dermatitis in a vagrant parti-coloured bat (*Vespertilio murinus*) in Great Britain. *Veterinary Record*, **169**, 614.

Barlow, A.M., Schock, A., Bradshaw, A. *et al.* (2012) Parvovirus enteritis in Eurasian badgers (*Meles meles*). *Veterinary Record*, **170**, 416.

Barlow, A.M., Worledge, L., Miller, H. *et al.* (2015) First confirmation of *Pseudogymnoascus destructans* in British bats in hibernacula. *Veterinary Record*, **177**(3), 73.

Barsotti, G., Asti, M., Giani, E. *et al.* (2012) Effect of topical ophthalmic instillation of rocuronium bromide on the intraocular pressure of kestrels (*Falco tinnunculus*) and little owls (*Athene noctuae*). *Journal of the American Veterinary Medical Association*, **255**(12), 1359–1364.

Beard, P.M., Daniels, M.J., Henderson, D. *et al.* (2001) Paratuberculosis infection in non-ruminant wildlife in Scotland. *Journal of Clinical Microbiology*, **39**(4), 1517–1521.

Blasdell, K., McCracken, C., Morris, A. *et al.* (2003) The wood mouse is a natural host for Murid herpesvirus 4. *Journal of General Virology*, **84**, 111–113.

Burrough, E.R., Magstadt, D.R., Petersen, B. *et al.* (2024) Highly pathogenic avian influenza A (H5N1) clade 2.3.4.4b virus infection in domestic dairy cattle and cats, United States, 2024. *Emerging Infectious Diseases*, **30**(7). doi: 10.3201/eid3007.240508.

Campbell-Palmer, R., Girling, S., Pizzi, R. *et al.* (2013) *Stichorchis subtriquetrus* in a free-living beaver in Scotland. *Veterinary Record*, **173**(3), 72.

Campbell-Palmer, R., Gottstein, B., Del-Pozo, J. *et al.* (2015) *Echinococcus multilocularis* detection in live Eurasian beavers (*Castor fiber*) using a combination of laparoscopy and abdominal ultrasound under field conditions. *PLoS One*, **10**(7), e0130842.

Candela, M.G., Pardavila, X., Ortega, N. *et al.* (2019) Canine distemper virus may affect European wildcat populations in Central Spain. *Mammalian Biology*, **97**(1), 9–12.

Canuti, M., Todd, M., Monteiro, P. *et al.* (2020) Ecology and infection dynamics of multi-host amdoparvoviral and protoparvoviral carnivore pathogens. *Pathogens*, **9**(2), 124.

Caruso, C., Dondo, A., Cerutti, F. *et al.* (2014) Aujesky's disease in red fox (*Vulpes vulpes*): phylogenetic analysis unravels an unexpected epidemiologic link. *Journal of Wildlife Diseases*, **50**(3), 707–710.

Corbel, M.J., Morris, J.A., Thorns, C.J. and Redwood, D.W. (1983) Response of the badger (*Meles meles*) to infection with *Brucella abortus*. *Research in Veterinary Science*, **34**, 296–300.

Das Neves, C.G., Mork, T., Godfried, J. *et al.* (2009) Experimental infection of reindeer with cervid herpesvirus 2. *Clinical and Vaccine Immunology*, **16**, 1758–1765.

De Jong, C.B., san Wieren, S.E., Gill, R.M.A. and Munro, R. (2004) Relationship between liver carcinomas and diet in Roe deer in Kielder forest and Galloway forest. *Veterinary Record*, **155**, 197–200.

Delahey, R.J. and Frolich, K. (2000) Absence of antibodies against canine distemper virus in free-ranging populations of Eurasian badger in Great Britain. *Journal of Wildlife Diseases*, **36**(3), 576–579.

Delahay, R.J., Smith, G.C., Barlow, A.M. *et al.* (2007) Bovine tuberculosis infection in wild mammals in the South-West region of England: a survey of prevalence and a semi-quantitative assessment of the relative risks to cattle. *Veterinary Journal*, **173**(2), 287–301.

Diakou, A., Dimzas, D., Astaras, C. *et al.* (2020) Clinical investigations and treatment outcome in a European wildcat (*Felis silvestris silvestris*) infected by cardio-pulmonary nematodes. *Veterinary Parasitology Regional Student Reports*, **19**, 100357.

Didkowska, A., Klich, D., Hapanowicz, A. *et al.* (2021) Pathogens with potential impact on reproduction in captive and free-ranging European bison (*Bison bonasus*) in Poland: a serological survey. *BMC Veterinary Research*, **17**, 345.

Dos Santos, F.A.A., Pinto, A., Burgoyne, T. *et al.* (2022) Spillover events of rabbit haemorrhagic disease virus 2 (recombinant GI.4P-GI.2) from Lagomorpha to Eurasian badger. *Transboundary and Emerging Diseases*, **69**(3), 1030–1045.

Deuchande, R., Gidlow, J., Caldow, G. *et al.* (2010) Parachlamydia involvement in bovine abortions in a beef herd in Scotland. *Veterinary Record*, **166**, 598–599.

Ebani, V.V., Trebino, C., Guardone, L. *et al.* (2022) Retrospective molecular survey on bacterial and protozoal abortive agents in roe deer (*Capreolus capreolus*) from central Italy. *Animals (Basel)*, **12**(22), 3202.

Escutenaire, S., Pastoret, P.-P., Brus Sojlander, K. *et al.* (2000) Evidence of Puumala Hantavirus infection in red foxes (*Vulpes vulpes*) in Belgium. *Veterinary Record*, **147**, 365–366.

Euden, P.R. (1990) *Salmonella* isolates from wild animals in Cornwall. *British Veterinary Journal*, **146**, 228–232.

Everest, D.J., Dastjerdi, A., Gurrala, R. *et al.* (2009) Rotavirus from red squirrels in Scotland. *Veterinary Record*, **165**, 450.

Everest, D.J., Stidworthy, M.F., Milne, E.M. *et al.* (2010) Retrospective detection by negative contrast electron microscopy of faecal viral particles in free-living wild red squirrels (*Sciurus vulgarus*) with suspected enteropathy in Great Britain. *Veterinary Record*, **167**, 1007–1010.

Everest, D.J., Dastjerdi, A., Cowan, D. *et al.* (2016) SQPV antibody detection in juvenile red squirrels. *Veterinary Record*, **179**, 101–102.

Fawcett, A.R.E., Goddard, P.J., McKelvey, A.C. *et al.* (1995) Johne's disease in a herd of farmed red deer. *Veterinary Record*, **136**, 165–169.

Fernández-Aguilar, X., Cabezón, Ó., Colom-Cadena, A. *et al.* (2016) Serological survey of *Coxiella burnetii* at the wildlife–livestock interface in the Eastern Pyrenees, Spain. *Acta Veterinaria Scandinavica*, **58**, 26.

Fleming, M. and Bexton, S. (2016) Conjunctival flora of healthy and diseased eyes of grey seals (*Halichoerus grypus*): implications for treatment. *Veterinary Record*, **179**, 99.

Frank, R., Kuhn, T., Werblow, A. *et al.* (2015) Parasite diversity of European *Myotis* species with special emphasis on *Myotis myotis* (Microchiroptera, Vespertilionidae) from a typical nursery roost. *Parasites and Vectors*, **8**, 101.

Frolich, K., Meyer, H.H.D., Pielowski, Z. *et al.* (1996) European brown hare syndrome in free-ranging hare in Poland. *Journal of Wildlife Diseases*, **32**, 280–285.

Frolich, K. (2012) Bovine viral diarrhoea. In: *Infectious Diseases of Wild Mammals and Birds in Europe* (eds D. Gavier-Widen, J.P. Duff & A. Meredith), pp. 152–157. Blackwell Publishing, Oxford.

Gaglio, G., Allen, S., Bowden, L. *et al.* (2010) Parasites of European hedgehogs (*Erinaceus europaeus*) in Britain: epidemiological study and coprological test evaluation. *European Journal of Wildlife Research*, **56**, 839–844.

Giesel, O. (1979) Distemper in otters. *Berliner und Münchener Tierärztliche Wochenschrift*, **92**, 304.

Girling, S.J., Goodman, G., Burr, P. *et al.* (2019a) Evidence of *Leptospira* spp. and their significance during re-introduction of Eurasian beavers (*Castor fiber*) to Great Britain. *Veterinary Record*, **185**(15), 482. doi: 10.1136/vr.105429.

Girling, S.J., McElhinney, L.M., Fraser, M.A. *et al.* (2019b) Absence of hantavirus in water-voles and Eurasian beavers in Britain. *Veterinary Record*, **184**, 253.

Griffiths, I.R. and Whitwell, K.E. (1993) Leporine dysautonomia: further evidence that hares suffer from grass sickness. *Veterinary Record*, **132**(15), 376–377.

Hammer, A.S., Dietz, H.H., Anderson, T.H. *et al.* (2004) Distemper virus as a cause of central nervous disease and death in badgers (*Meles meles*) in Denmark. *Veterinary Record*, **154**, 527–530.

Hulbert, I.A. and Boag, B. (2001) The potential role of habitat on intestinal helminths of mountain hares, *Lepus timidus*. *Journal of Helminthology*, **75**(4), 345–349.

Hulse, E.C. and Edwards, J.T. (1937) Foot-and-mouth disease in hibernating hedgehogs. *Journal of Comparative Pathology and Therapeutics*, **50**, 421–430.

Justus, W., Valle, S., Barten, O. *et al.* (2024) A review of bovine tuberculosis transmission risk in European wildlife communities. *Mammal Review*, **54**(3), 325–340.

Kalisinska, E., Lanocha-Arendarczyk, N., Kosik-Bogacka, D. *et al.* (2016) Brains of native and alien mesocarnivores in biomonitoring of toxic metals in Europe. *PLoS One*, **11**(8), e0159935.

Kaminskiene, E., Radzijevskaja, J., Stanko, M. *et al.* (2020) Associations between different Laelapidae (Mesostigmata: Dermanyssoidea) mites and small rodents from Lithuania. *Experimental and Applied Acarology*, **81**(1), 149–162.

Kirchhoff, H., Binder, A., Liess, B. *et al.* (1989) Isolation of mycoplasma from diseased seals. *Veterinary Record*, **124**, 513–514.

Laakkonen, J., Nyyssonen, T., Hiltunen, M. *et al.* (2006) Effects of *Protostrongylus* sp. and *Pneumocystis* sp. on the pulmonary tissue and the condition of mountain and brown hares from Finland. *Journal of Wildlife Diseases*, **42**(4), 780–787.

Leguia, M., Garcia-Glaessner, A., Munoz-Saavedra, B. *et al.* (2023) Highly pathogenic avian influenza A (H5N1) in marine mammals and seabirds in Peru. *Nature Communications*, **14**(1), 5489.

Lemming, L., Jorgensen, J.C., Nielsen, L.B. *et al.* (2020) Cardiopulmonary nematodes of wild carnivores from Denmark: do they serve as reservoir hosts for infections in domestic animals? *International Journal for Parasitology: Parasites and Wildlife*, **13**, 90–97.

Leutenegger, C.M., Hogmann-Lehmann, R., Riols, C. *et al.* (1999) Viral infections in free-living populations of the European wildcat. *Journal of Wildlife Diseases*, **35**(4), 678–686.

Madoff, S., Schooley, R.T., Ruhnke, H.L. *et al.* (1982) Mycoplasmal pneumonia in phocid (harbour) seals. *Reviews of Infectious Diseases*, **Suppl. 4**, 241.

Marco, I. (2012) Pestivirus of chamois and border disease. In: *Infectious Diseases of Wild Mammals and Birds in Europe* (eds D. Gavier-Widen, J.P. Duff & A. Meredith), pp. 147–152. Blackwell Publishing, Oxford.

McCarthy, T.K. and Hasset, D.K. (1993) *Cryptocotyle lingua* (Creplin) (Digenea: Heterophyidae) and other parasites of a coastal otter *Lutra lutra*. *Irish Naturalist's Journal*, **24**, 280–282.

Meredith, A., del Pozo, J., Smith, S. *et al.* (2014) Leprosy in red squirrels in Scotland. *Veterinary Record*, **175**, 285–286.

Milan, J. and Rodrigeuz, A. (2009) A serological survey of common feline pathogens in free-living European wildcats (*Felis silvestris*) in central Spain. *European Journal of Wildlife Research*, **55**(3), 285–291.

Morandi, F., Angelico, G., Verin, R. and Gavaudan, S. (2014) Fatal spirocercosis in a free-ranging red fox. *Veterinary Record*, **174**, 228.

Morris, P.A. (1984) An estimate of the minimum body weight necessary for hedgehogs (*Erinaceus europaeus*) to survive hibernation. *Notes from the Mammal Society*, **48**, 291–294.

Morris, P.A. (1998) Hedgehog rehabilitation in perspective. *Veterinary Record*, **143**, 633–636.

Morton, J.K., Evermann, J.F. and Dieterich, R.A. (1990) Experimental infection of reindeer with bovine viral diarrhoea virus. *Rangifer*, **10**, 75–77.

Muhldorfer, K., Speck, S. and Wibbelt, G. (2011) Diseases in free-ranging bats from Germany. *BMC Veterinary Research*, **7**, 61.

Muhldorfer, K. (2013) Bats and bacterial pathogens: a review. *Zoonoses and Public Health*, **60**, 93–103.

Mullineaux, E. (2024). Badger rehabilitation. Bovine TB Hub. https://tbhub.co.uk/ (accessed 13 June 2024).

Najera, F., Crespo, E., Garcia-Talens, A. *et al.* (2021) First description of sarcoptic mange in a free-ranging European wildcat (*Felis silvestris silvestris*) from Spain. *Animals (Basel)*, **11**(9), 2494.

Neal, E. and Cheeseman, C. (1996) *Badgers*. Poyser Natural History. T & D Poyser Ltd, London.

Newey, S. and Thirgood, S. (2004) Parasite-mediated reduction in fecundity of mountain hares. *Proceedings of the Royal Society B*, **271**(Suppl 6), S413–S415.

Newman, C., MacDonald, D.W. and Anwar, M.A. (2001) Coccidiosis in the European badger *Meles meles* in Wytham woods: infection and consequence for growth and survival. *Parasitology*, **123**(Pt 2), 133–142.

Palmer, A.C., Blakemore, W.F., Franklin, R.J.M. *et al.* (1998) Paralysis in hedgehogs (*Erinaceus europaeus*) associated with demyelination. *Veterinary Record*, **143**, 550–552.

Ruhl, S., Casson, N., Kaiser, C. *et al.* (2009) Evidence of *Parachlamydia* in bovine abortion. *Veterinary Microbiology*, **135**, 169–174.

Sainsbury, A., Nettleton, P., Gilray, J. and Gurnell, J. (2000) Grey squirrels have high seroprevalence to a parapoxvirus associated with the deaths in red squirrels. *Animal Conservation*, **3**, 229–233.

Santos, N., Almendra, C. and Tavares, L. (2009) Serological survey for canine distemper vírus and canine parvovirus in free-ranging wild carnivores from Portugal. *Journal of Wildlife Diseases*, **45**, 221–226.

Seixas, F., Travassos, P., Pinto, M.L. *et al.* (2006) Pulmonary adiaspiromycosis in a hedgehog (*Erinaceus europaeus*) in Portugal. *Veterinary Record*, **158**, 274–275.

Sherrard-Smith, E., Cable, J. and Chadwick, E.A. (2009) Distribution of Eurasian otter biliary parasites, *Pseudamphistomum truncatum* and *Metorchis albidus* (Family Opisthorchiidae) in England and Wales. *Parasitology*, **136**(9), 1015–1022.

Simpson, V.R. and Blake, D.P. (2018) Parasitic pneumonia in roe deer (*Capreolus capreolus*) in Cornwall, Great Britain, caused by *Varestrongylus capreoli* (Protostrongylidae). *BMC Veterinary Research*, **14**(1), 198.

Simpson, V.R., Panceira, R.J., Hargreaves, J. *et al.* (2005a) Myocarditis and myositis due to infection with *Hepatozoon* species in pine martens (*Martes martes*) in Scotland. *Veterinary Record*, **156**, 442–446.

Simpson, V.R., Gibbons, L.M., Khalil, L.F. and Williams, J.L.R. (2005b) Cholecystitis in otters (*Lutra lutra*) and mink (*Mustela vison*) caused by the fluke *Pseudamphistomum truncatum*. *Veterinary Record*, **157**, 49–52.

Simpson, V.R., Hargreaves, J., Birtles, R.J. *et al.* (2008) Tyzzer's disease in a Eurasian otter (*Lutra lutra*) in Scotland. *Veterinary Record*, **163**, 539–544.

Simpson, V.R., Davison, N.J., Borman, A.N. *et al.* (2009) Fatal candidiasis in a wild red squirrel (*Sciurus vulgaris*). *Veterinary Record*, **164**, 342–344.

Simpson, V.R., Tomlinson, A.J., Molenaar, F.M. *et al.* (2011) Renal calculi in wild Eurasian otters (Lutra lutra) in England. *Veterinary Record*, **169**(2), 49. doi: 10.1136/vr.d1929.

Simpson, V.R., Tomlinson, A.J., Stevenson, K. *et al.* (2016) Postmortem study of respiratory disease in small mustelids in south-west England. *BMC Veterinary Research*, **12**, 72.

Sobrino, R., Arnal, M.C., Luco, D.F. and Gortazar, C. (2008) Prevalence of antibodies against canine distemper virus and canine parvovirus among foxes and wolves from Spain. *Veterinary Microbiology*, **126**, 251–256.

Stephen, S., Guerra, D., Pospiscgil, A. *et al.* (2014) Chlamydiaceae and *Chlamydia*-like organisms in free-living small mammals in Europe and Afghanistan. *Journal of Wildlife Diseases*, **50**(2), 195–204.

Steutzer, B. and Hartmann, K. (2014) Feline parvovirus infection and associated diseases. *Veterinary Journal*, **201**(2), 150–155.

Stevanovic, O., Diakou, A., Morelli, S. *et al.* (2019) Severe verminous pneumonia caused by natural mixed infection with *Aelurostrongylus abstrusus* and *Angiostrongylus chabaudi* in a European wildcat from Western Balkan area. *Acta Parasitologica*, **64**(2), 411–417.

Stocker, L. (2005) Hedgehogs. In: *Practical Wildlife Care*, 2nd edn, pp. 200–215. Wiley Blackwell, Oxford.

Tavernier, P., Sys, S.U., De Clercq, K. *et al.* (2015) Serologic screening for 13 infectious agents in roe deer (*Capreolus capreolus*) in Flanders. *Infection Ecology and Epidemiology*, **24**(5), 29862.

Thomson, H., O'Keeffe, A.M., Lewis, J.C.M. *et al.* (2010) Infectious canine hepatitis in red foxes (*Vulpes vulpes*) in the United Kingdom. *Veterinary Record*, **166**(4), 111–114.

Todone, D., Bregoli, M., Favretti, M.A. et al (2008) A survey for European brown hare syndrome in Friuli Venezia Giulia region, North-Eastern Italy. *8th Conference of the European Wildlife Disease Association*, 2–5 October 2008, Rovinj, Croatia, p. 91.

Townsend, S.E., Newey, S., Thirgood, S.J. *et al.* (2009) Can parasites drive population cycles in mountain hares? *Proceedings of the Royal Society B*, **276**(1662), 1611–1617.

Tsai, M.-S., Francois, S., Newman, C. *et al.* (2022) Infection with a recently discovered gammaherpesvirus variant in European badgers, *Meles meles*, is associated with higher relative viral loads in blood. *Pathogens*, **11**(10), 1154.

Velarde, R., Cavadini, P., Neimanis, A. *et al.* (2017) Spillover events of infection of brown hares (*Lepus europaeus*) with rabbit haemorrhagic disease type 2 virus (RHDV2) caused sporadic cases of an European brown hare syndrome-like disease in Italy and Spain. *Transboundary and Emerging Diseases*, **64**(6), 1750–1761.

Walker, D., Abbondati, E., Cox, A.L. *et al.* (2016) Infectious canine hepatitis in red foxes (*Vulpes vulpes*) in wildlife rescue centres in the UK. *Veterinary Record*, **178**, 421.

Walker, D., Gregory, W.F., Turnbull, D. *et al.* (2017) Novel adenoviruses detected in British mustelids, including a unique Aviadenovirus in the tissues of pine martens (*Martes martes*). *Journal of Medical Microbiology*, **66**(8), 1177–1182.

Walsh, S.T. and Stebbings, R.E. (1989) Care and rehabilitation of wild bats. In: *Proceedings of the Inaugural Symposium of the British Wildlife Rehabilitation Council, London* (eds S. Harris & T. Thomas), pp. 64–72. BWRC, Horsham.

Weber, J.M. and Roberts, L. (1990) A bacterial infection as a cause of abortion in the European otter *Lutra lutra*. *Journal of Zoology*, **220**, 641–651.

Wells, G.A.H., Keymer, I.F. and Barnnett, K.C. (1989) Suspected Aleutian disease in a wild otter. *Veterinary Record*, **125**, 232–235.

Widen, F., Gavier-Widen, D., Nikiila, T. and Morner, T. (1996) Fatal herpesvirus infection in a hedgehog (*Erinaceus europaeus*). *Veterinary Record*, **139**, 237–238.

Wolfe, A., Hogan, S., Maguire, D. *et al.* (2001) Red foxes (*Vulpes vulpes*) in Ireland as hosts for parasites of potential zoonotic and veterinary significance. *Veterinary Record*, **149**, 759–763.

Chapter 29 An Overview of Wildlife Therapeutics

FLUID THERAPY

Maintenance requirements

Every mammal has a requirement for everyday fluid losses, such as urine output and insensible losses through sweating, panting, digestive system secretions and tears. In most small mammals, very little water is lost as sweat, as rodents and lagomorphs have little or no skin sweat glands, and most do not pant either. However, there are losses via this route in foxes, badgers, deer and other larger mammals.

In smaller mammals there are losses due to their increased metabolic rates over larger species, and the fact that their size is extremely small in most cases. This leads to a greater body surface area in relation to body volume, and this applies to the lung surface as well. Hence large amounts of fluids are lost due to normal respiration. Add to this the fact that a shrew at rest may have a respiration rate of 150–250 breaths a minute, which can likely double when stressed, then it is easy to appreciate where a lot of the water is going. Glomerular filtration rates are also higher due to the higher metabolic rates seen in small mammals. These factors account for maintenance fluid requirements being nearly double those seen in larger mammals such as cats and dogs (Table 29.1).

Disease influence on fluid requirements

Disease processes, as discussed in previous chapters, often increase urine output and may affect water absorption from the gut. Examples include the production of endotoxins in mammals such as foxes, hares or badgers with uterine infections such as *E. coli* pyometras and exotoxin release from clostridiosis in cervids.

Respiratory disease is common in debilitated wild mammals, especially hedgehogs, rabbits, hares and rodents. In these animals, chronic levels of lung infection occur, with increased respiratory secretions being the result. Fluid loss can therefore be appreciable via this route. In many mammals such as foxes, hedgehogs, mustelids and badgers, appreciable lung damage may be done by lungworms and other parasites which frequently migrate through the lung structure, causing damage, infection and fluid accumulation and loss in the process. Young seals are also prone to massive worm infestations which often migrate or live in the lung fields.

Gastrointestinal disease is also commonly seen and individuals suffering from diarrhoea will experience fluid loss and often metabolic acidosis due to the prolonged loss of bicarbonate. There may also be chronic losses of potassium, due to the reduced absorption of this electrolyte by the large intestine. These problems are particularly prevalent in wild deer which can suffer from a number of gut- and liver-associated parasites. Many wild mammals can vomit, the exceptions being the lagomorphs, cervids and many rodents, so the likelihood of fluid loss via this route and the development of metabolic alkalosis has to be considered.

Skin diseases may also create fluid and electrolytes losses, for example hares, hedgehogs, foxes, mustelids and squirrels suffering from skin or ear mites, or in squirrels with squirrel pox. Fox scabies may result in exudative skin lesions. Skin wounds, such as intraspecific fight wounds in badgers, may also create significant fluid and electrolyte loss.

Hypotension due to systemic inflammatory response syndrome (SIRS), where an organ or multiple organs are affected by sepsis or damage, can lead to rapid and life-threatening hypotension. Although this is not the same as dehydration, one of the effects (hypotension) is the same, resulting in tissue underperfusion and so ultimately starvation of nutrients and oxygen to vital organs. This syndrome can develop rapidly and go on to produce multiple organ failure and disseminated intravascular coagulation. All of these conditions are life-threatening. Correction clearly requires management of the underlying cause but in the acute patient focuses on maintenance of normotension (normal blood pressure), hence the importance of fluid therapy and associated blood pressure-modulating drugs.

Post-surgical needs

Surgery on an acute trauma victim may result in haemorrhaging during the procedure, necessitating vascular support with an aqueous electrolyte solution or, in more serious blood losses (>10%), colloidal fluids or even blood transfusions. Even if surgery is relatively bloodless there are inevitable losses via the respiratory route associated with the drying nature of the gases used to deliver the anaesthetics commonly used. Smaller-sized mammals and birds have a larger surface and lung area in relation to volume that exacerbates this. Patients are often not able to drink immediately after surgery, and so the period without water or food intake may stretch to a few hours, worsening dehydration. In trauma cases surgery, such as facial/jaw repair after road traffic accidents, will often lead to inappetence for a period.

Electrolyte replacements

These have already been mentioned but chronic cases of diarrhoea, such as coccidiosis in hares and deer or *E. coli*/*Salmonella* spp. in hedgehogs, foxes, badgers and mustelids, can result in gut pathology leading to maldigestion/malabsorption and fluid and electrolyte deficits. Electrolyte disturbances are often focused on bicarbonate and potassium, but sodium depletion can also be seen in seals and herbivores (see Figure 29.1).

Herbivores rarely vomit, particularly rabbits, hares, beavers and deer, and so metabolic alkalosis is less likely to occur in these species.

Veterinary Nursing of Exotic Pets and Wildlife, Third Edition. Simon J. Girling.

Table 29.1 Suggested maintenance fluid requirements for wild animals.

Species	Fluid maintenance values (mL/kg per day)
Badgers	50
Bats (Microchiroptera)	100
Deer	30–50
Lagomorphs	80–100
Foxes	50
Rodents/squirrels	90–100
Seals (phocids)	50
Wild small mustelids (weasels, stoats, polecats)	75–100
Wild birds	50

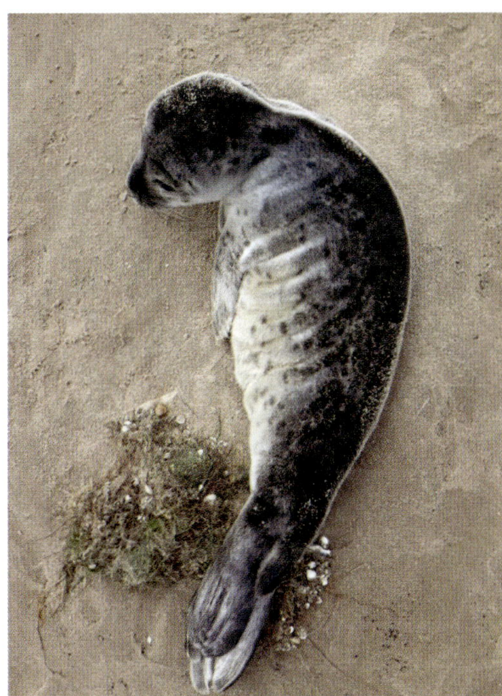

Figure 29.1 Dehydration is common in debilitated seal pups and can be accompanied by electrolyte imbalances. *Source:* Courtesy of Diane Westwood RVN.

The carnivorous species such as the mustelid, wildcat, fox and badger families will often regurgitate food or may have more serious problems with stomach ulceration due to stress or bacteria such as *Helicobacter* spp., and therefore may well develop metabolic alkalosis due to loss of hydrogen ions. However, if the vomiting persists, there is often bile reflux, and so loss of bicarbonate as well and thus a metabolic acidosis sets in.

Fluid types used in wildlife practice

Lactated Ringer's/Hartmann's

This is isotonic in birds and mammals (0.9%) and useful as a general-purpose rehydration as well as maintenance fluid. It is particularly useful for birds and mammals suffering from metabolic acidosis but can also be used for fluid therapy after routine surgical procedures. It may be less useful for chronic loss of potassium as a maintenance fluid as despite it containing some potassium it tends to result in depletion of potassium and excess of sodium.

Sodium chloride (0.9%)

Useful where metabolic alkalosis is present, as this fluid is acidifying in nature, and to replace fluid loss. It will however result in potassium depletion and so is not designed as a maintenance fluid, but additional electrolytes such as potassium may be easily added if required.

Glucose/dextrose and saline combinations

These are useful for small wild mammals and birds in particular as they may have been through periods of anorexia prior to treatment, and therefore may well be borderline hypoglycaemic. The principles of use for these fluids is the same as for cats and dogs. The concentration to start with when dehydration is present is 5% glucose, 0.9% saline. Once dehydration has been reversed, then for maintenance purposes the small mammal patient may be moved to the 4% glucose, 0.18% saline concentration but potassium will need to be added as depletion will occur. Glucose–saline combinations are also useful for cases of urethral obstruction such as mustelid urolithiasis where serum potassium may be elevated. Try not to use dextrose subcutaneously in birds as this tends to draw fluid to the injection site rather than allowing absorption so worsening dehydration (Martin and Kollias, 1989).

Protein amino acid/B-vitamin supplements

These are useful for nutritional support by using versions such as Duphalyte® (Zoetis) at the rate of 1 mL/kg body weight per day. They are particularly good in cases where the patient is malnourished or has been suffering from a protein-losing enteropathy/nephropathy to help replace some of the compounds needed for replenishment. It is also a useful supplement for patients with hepatic disease or severe exudative skin diseases such as scabies and burn wounds. Care should be taken in some species such as wild raptors and Columbiformes where such compounds that contain vitamin B_6 can be toxic when dosed above 5 mg/kg (Samour *et al.*, 2016).

Bicarbonate ions and capture myopathy

Bicarbonate may be added to isotonic fluid preparations if metabolic acidosis is suspected. Capture myopathy is a condition that results in acidosis and is worst, surprisingly, after relatively short bursts of intense activity such as occur in a flight or fright response when being pursued. It is most likely to be seen in deer and clinically raised heart and respiratory rates with hyperthermia may be seen. The anaerobic respiration of muscles due to the exertion results in rapid production of lactic acid and a resultant fall in blood pH, all of which causes further muscle damage. Skeletal muscle damage releases myoglobin and ions such as potassium (Chalmers and Barrett, 1982; Spraker, 1993). The result of all of this is a decrease in cardiac output, cardiac arrhythmias, fibrillations, a falling blood pressure and sometimes acute death. It may also result in muscle rupture and permanent lameness. If the animal survives this, then it may still die days to weeks later of renal failure as the myoglobin released causes progressive damage to the glomeruli, or of cardiac failure due to areas of myocardial

PART IV: WILDLIFE

infarction. The use of bicarbonate at doses of 400 mEq of sodium bicarbonate per 100 kg body weight (4 mEq/kg) has therefore been suggested where capture myopathy is diagnosed, and may be administered as a 1 mEq/mL solution of sodium bicarbonate, slowly over 5–10 minutes in deer until correction of the acidosis (Williams and Thorne, 1996).

Colloidal fluids

These have been used in wildlife practice only when direct venous access has been achievable, although there is some evidence that they can be used via the intraosseous route. This may limit their use as some small mammals and wild birds are just too small to gain full vascular access.

However, they may be used in lagomorphs, mustelids, foxes, badgers and even deer. They are used, as with cats and dogs, when a serious loss of blood occurs in order to support central blood pressure, with maximum dosage rates being equivalent at 20 mL/kg per hour; dosages of 40 mL/kg per day should not be exceeded. This may be a temporary measure whilst a blood donor is selected or, if none is available, the only means of attempting to support such a patient.

Hypertonic fluids

These are used in exotic animal practice and may be very useful for the larger wildlife species such as some of the deer and seals where profound hypovolaemia and hypotension exist. Their idea is to use the intravenous route to administer a concentrated electrolyte which then draws tissue fluids into the blood vessels by osmosis, so supporting the circulation. Doses of 4 mL/kg of a 7.2% solution are used, but these *must* be followed up by isotonic or hypotonic fluids. It is also vital that the animal be given access to fresh water after administration, as they will (hopefully) start drinking to reverse the dehydration once their circulation is supported by the osmotic effect of the hypertonic infusion. Without it, tissue fluids will remain depleted of water and permanent damage will be done. These fluids can also be used in smaller species (as already outlined in Chapters 6, 7, 13 and 14) where profound hypovolaemia/hypotension is present, as a bolus injection to rapidly increase blood pressure.

Oral fluids/electrolytes

These may also be used in wildlife cases for those patients experiencing mild dehydration, and for species such as seals which may be difficult to catheterise. Many products are available for farm animals, cats and dogs, and may be used for wildlife cases. Prebiotics and relevant probiotics can also aid digestion by encouraging growth of healthy gut bacteria, which are also often upset during periods of dehydration.

Blood transfusions

These are rarely performed, as the presence of a donor patient of the same species is necessary. However, if available, and the haematocrit drops below 0.20 L/L in small mammals such as foxes and badgers and below 0.15 L/L in birds and a donor is available, a transfusion may be considered although this does raise ethical issues regarding consent as a wild animal cannot give consent and has no 'owner'.

Little is known about cross-reactivity or the presence of defined blood groups in these species, and so there should be a close watch for signs of a recipient–donor reaction. These are similar to those seen in the cat or dog, and include:

- petechiation/ecchymoses in the mucous membranes
- increased heart rate/pulse
- signs of jaundice
- haemoglobinuria
- collapse
- hyperthermia, followed by hypothermia
- vomiting (in carnivorous species)
- urticaria
- frequent coughing (ruminants such as deer).

Wildcats are assumed to have similar blood groups to domestic species and the use of feline cross-matching kits may be of benefit in determining a safe donor. For other species a readily used test to assess compatibility is to mix two drops of donor blood in 2 mL of acid citrate dextrose (ACD) 3.85% solution and add two drops of this mixture to the recipient's serum on a glass slide. This is then gently agitated. If the two blood samples are incompatible, agglutination and microclots will be seen forming on the slide.

Blood is collected from an anaesthetised donor, usually from the jugular vein, into a bag containing the anticoagulant ACD at a ratio of one part ACD to nine parts blood. It is assumed that, providing the donor is healthy, 1% body weight (in grams) may be collected as the millilitre equivalent, so that a healthy 1000-g animal may safely donate 10 mL of blood. To transfuse into the recipient, a blood giving set with microfilter to remove clots is recommended. An initial slow rate of infusion of 1–4 mL/kg per hour can be employed to ensure no anaphylactic cross-reaction occurs, followed by a maximal rate of 15–20 mL/kg per hour once it is established that no reaction is occurring.

To calculate the volumes required for wild species, extrapolations may be made from companion and farm animal practice, so that for example in wildcats, badgers and mustelids, domestic cat rates can be used which may be approximated as:

$$\begin{array}{c}\text{Anticoagulated blood}\\ \text{volume required (mL)}\end{array} = \begin{array}{c}\text{body weight of}\\ \text{recipient (kg)} \times 70 \times\end{array} \frac{\begin{array}{c}\text{PCV desired in}\\ \text{recipient} - \text{PCV}\\ \text{currently in recipient}\end{array}}{\begin{array}{c}\text{PCV donor in}\\ \text{anticoagulant}\end{array}}$$

For foxes, and seals the use of the canine formula is perhaps more appropriate as:

$$\begin{array}{c}\text{Anticoagulated blood}\\ \text{volume required (mL)}\end{array} = \begin{array}{c}\text{body weight of}\\ \text{recipient (kg)} \times 90 \times\end{array} \frac{\begin{array}{c}\text{PCV desired in}\\ \text{recipient} - \text{PCV}\\ \text{currently in recipient}\end{array}}{\begin{array}{c}\text{PCV donor in}\\ \text{anticoagulant}\end{array}}$$

In deer, similar protocols as those used in cattle and horses may be employed, whereby if the patient/recipient's haematocrit is below 0.2 L/L (20%), then 10–15 mL/kg of blood is transfused, which will increase the haematocrit on average a further 0.15–0.2 L/L.

Although intravenous routes are preferred, the intraperitoneal route may be used instead (Blood and Radostits, 1989). This route has been shown to allow the uptake of whole red blood cells, at a rate of 48% over 24 hours and 65% over 48 hours. This route is much clearly slower than an intravenous one and should only be used in cases of non-hypovolaemic anaemia, but it may, by extrapolation, be useful in smaller mammals or in animals where venous access is not possible for the 2–3 hours needed for a full transfusion, either for the whole transfusion or to give the last 50–75% of the needed blood transfusion once a bolus of intravenous blood has been administered. Again, one should avoid the intraperitoneal route if there is evidence that abdominal haemorrhage has already occurred, or in the presence of peritonitis, ascites, abdominal distension, abdominal adhesions or recent abdominal surgery.

If an acute reaction is seen to be occurring, then dobutamine 1–5 μg/kg per minute and methylprednisolone (corticosteroids) 30 mg/kg should be administered intravenously if possible. Dobutamine acts on beta-1 receptors in the heart muscle, without affecting heart rate, thus increasing the force of contraction to support the blood pressure (a positive inotropic effect). In severe cases, 1 : 10 000 adrenaline at 20 μg/kg intravenously or subcutaneously can be used.

Equipment needed for administration of fluids to wildlife patients

Catheters of 27 gauge for the smaller mustelids, rodents, lagomorphs, bats, etc., through to catheters of 16 gauge or even larger for deer and seals may be required. In seals, needles and catheters may need to be 2–4 inches in length to reach some of the deeply located vessels.

Hypodermic/spinal needles

Useful for the administration of intraosseous or intraperitoneal/subcutaneous fluids or one-off intravenous boluses. Intraosseous fluids may be the only method of central venous support in very small patients. The proximal femur, tibia or humerus may be used in many mammalian species, the ulna and proximal tibiotarsus in avian species. Spinal needles have a central stylet to prevent clogging of the lumen with bone fragments after application and so may be more effective; 23–25 gauge needles are usually sufficient. Hypodermic needles may be used for the same purpose, although the risks of blockage are higher. Hypodermic needles may also be used of course for the administration of intraperitoneal and subcutaneous fluids. Generally, 23–25 gauge hypodermic needles are sufficient for the task.

Nasogastric and orogastric tubes

Nasogastric tubes are often used in small pet mammals in order to provide nutritional support. They are less useful in wildlife cases as there is no way that all the fluid deficits may be replaced via this route alone and many will not tolerate this method of administration unless they are anaesthetised. In seal pups, this method has been used in the conscious animal and an orogastric tube of 1 cm diameter may be used after wedging the mouth open with a metal/wooden gag, which ideally is placed across the mouth and has a central hole through which the tube may be threaded.

Syringe drivers

These can be useful for continuous intravenous or intraosseous fluid administration in smaller species.

Intravenous drip tubing

Particularly fine drip tubing is available for attachment to syringes and syringe driver units for the smaller species. It is useful if these are luer locking as this enhances safety and prevents disconnection when the patient moves. It may be necessary to purchase a sheath, such as is available for protecting household electrical cables, to cover drip tubing as most of the small herbivores are experts at removing/chewing through plastic drip tubing.

For foxes, badgers and larger mammals, standard cat and dog tubing may be used. When dealing with deer, the use of coiled extendable drip tubing is advised, as this allows some mobility of the patient with reduced risk of catheter displacement, allowing the drip bag to be suspended from a central point on the ceiling of the pen.

Routes of fluid administration available in the wildlife patient

As with cats and dogs the same medical principles broadly apply, with five main routes of administration available: oral, subcutaneous, intraperitoneal, intravenous and intraosseous. These routes all have their advantages and disadvantages and have been discussed in the previous chapters on small mammal, avian and reptile therapy, but broad principles apply.

The important points to consider in wildlife patients is that although certain routes are clinically the best for fluid therapy in certain conditions, constraints apply. Therefore, although intravenous fluid therapy may well be the best route for the patient, the nature of the patient prevents prolonged continuous fluid therapy from being carried out. **Advantage must be taken of any opportunity to administer intravenous/intraosseous fluids when the wildlife patient is being anaesthetised for diagnostic or surgical purposes.**

Fluid rates in dehydrated and hypotensive patients should therefore approach the maximum rates to achieve adequately administered volumes. Most anaesthetic rates for domestic mammals are around 2–10 mL/kg per hour. However, rates where systolic blood pressures are significantly less than 90 mmHg can be up to 90 mL/kg per hour for isotonic crystalloid therapy in canids and 45 mL/kg per hour for isotonic crystalloid therapy in felids and mustelids. Where low blood pressure species are encountered (reptiles and beavers), caution should be exercised and rates should not exceed 5 mL/kg per hour even with dehydration and hypovolaemia.

Subcutaneous or intraperitoneal depot injections are always to be recommended towards the end of the chemical restraint if considered safe and possible in order to continue fluid therapy during the recovery period with minimal further interference.

Access routes for deer

Oral

Nasogastric tube placement may be used to administer a bolus of fluids into the forestomachs and may be useful in animals where the gastrointestinal system is functioning and also require oral medication. It is not without risk and generally only considered under chemical restraint. Fluid volumes of 80–100 mL/kg may be administered via this route due to the large size of the forestomachs but passive reflux and the risk of aspiration pneumonia are possible. Permanent nasogastric tubes should not be used and are not tolerated.

Subcutaneous

This route is poorly tolerated in deer, as they have thick hides and relatively small subcutaneous areas.

Intraperitoneal

This route is avoided in adult deer, as the presence of the forestomachs on the left side of the abdomen makes the approach near impossible. The right side is also difficult to safely access due to the presence of the intestinal mass caudally and the abomasum cranially. It may however be utilised, caudally, in deer calves, where the forestomachs are poorly developed. Isotonic solutions may be given in the right caudal quadrant of the ventral abdomen, as with lambs. Volumes of up to half a litre may be administered in the larger species such as red and fallow deer calves. Glucose-containing solutions should be avoided via this route due to the increased risk of peritonitis.

Intravenous

An intravenous catheter can be placed in the jugular vein. It may also be used for hypertonic saline solutions, which are a rapid way of stabilising vascular pressure in larger species that are hypotensive. During this process the deer in question may need to be sedated or, if debilitated, the provision of a darkened sound-proofed room may be sufficient, along with the attachment of an extendable drip tubing to a fluid bag suspended from the ceiling in the centre of the room. A deer attached to an intravenous fluid giving set should be observed closely, as the likelihood of it becoming entangled in the drip tubing and/or displacing the catheter and haemorrhaging are high. The jugular vein runs in the jugular furrow or groove, a prominent depression running either side of the trachea between it and the muscles of the neck. Digital pressure may be applied at the base of the neck, and the jugular furrow will be seen to 'fill' as the blood dams towards the head. The catheter can be placed in a caudocranial fashion against the flow of blood and so is less likely to suck air into the vein should the connection detach. This means that if the connection detaches completely, blood from the jugular vein has a chance to flow out, so careful monitoring is essential. The catheter (gauges vary from 20 gauge in smaller breeds to 16 gauge in larger breeds, of 1–1.25 inch length) may then be taped and bandaged into place around the neck and attached to a coiled extendible drip set.

Intraosseous

This route is not used in conscious deer, as vascular access is rarely difficult and the stress of a permanent intraosseous catheter outweighs the limited benefits.

Access routes for foxes

Oral

Free access to oral rehydration therapies for dogs and cats may be employed if the fox is moderately (1–3%) dehydrated and has no severe gastrointestinal disease. The feeding of commercial cat or dog tinned foods will also aid fluid replacement as the majority of these (80% or so) is water. The placement of a nasogastric tube (3.5–5 French often fits) may be necessary if severe anorexia is present or trauma has occurred to the jaw preventing eating, but these are not always well tolerated. Volumes of up to 40 mL/kg body weight may be administered via this route at any one time, although this inevitably has to include any liquid feeding formula and may require sedation.

Subcutaneous

The skin overlying the thoracic wall is useful in young foxes where mild dehydration with no evidence of shock has occurred and where venous access may be difficult. Volumes of isotonic fluids of 10 mL at any one site may be administered, usually splitting the daily fluid requirement into two 12-hour doses.

Intraperitoneal

This may be useful where moderate dehydration occurs, and may be performed, using isotonic non-glucose-containing fluids, in the lower right quadrant of the ventral abdomen under anaesthesia or sedation. The fox will need to be placed on its back with the head down in order to allow the intestinal system to fall away from the injection site and so is generally only performed under anaesthesia. The needle is inserted at a shallow 45° angle in a caudocranial direction.

Intravenous

This is useful during initial stabilisation of the fox, particularly when sedated/anaesthetised for investigative or surgical procedures or when activity is reduced due to shock. Veins used are similar and found in the same places as the dog, including the cephalic, saphenous or jugular veins. Intravenous access allows blood transfusions to be given if necessary, as well as colloids in the case of hypovolaemic shock.

Intraosseous

This is useful in very young fox cubs with severe dehydration/shock as it allows direct access to the central venous system, when peripheral veins may be too collapsed or simply too small to catheterise. The proximal femur between the femoral head and the greater trochanter is the preferred site.

Access routes for wildcats

These are largely similar to those used for the red fox and domestic cat.

Access routes for badgers

Oral

As for foxes, this route may be used in mildly debilitated badgers with no evidence of serious gastrointestinal disease. Placement of nasogastric tubes is difficult due to the long snout of the badger, and tolerance is poor once in place.

Subcutaneous

This is possible in the badger, but the skin is extremely thick, particularly over the scruff area. Therefore, the subcutaneous route may not be an easy method for routine fluid administration. The area over the lateral ribcage is preferred as the skin is slightly thinner in this region.

Intraperitoneal
This is as described for the fox.

Intravenous
Similar vessels as described for the fox may be utilised. Again, the badger will need to be chemically restrained to apply the catheter, and often fluids are only administered during the period of anaesthesia/ sedation due to their poor tolerance of the drip lines and catheters when conscious.

Intraosseous
The proximal femur is the preferred site and is useful in severely debilitated cubs.

Access routes for hedgehogs

Oral
This route is useful in situations outlined for the fox. Placement of nasogastric tubes is not possible in the hedgehog due to the narrow nasal aperture and long muzzle.

Subcutaneous
The area around the 'skirt' of the spiny coat of the hedgehog may be used when conscious, particularly between the fore and hind limbs. This area has a degree of hypodermic space beneath the orbicularis muscle and small volumes (2–5 mL) may be given at each site. Elsewhere when the hedgehog is curled up, the skin is drawn tight and makes subcutaneous injections of moderate volumes difficult (see Figure 29.2).

Intraperitoneal
This is only really possible in the fully sedated/anaesthetised hedgehog, as the ventral abdomen may only be reached when the hedgehog is unconscious and unrolled. Isotonic fluids only may be given via this route, with maximum volumes of 15–20 mL given in the average adult.

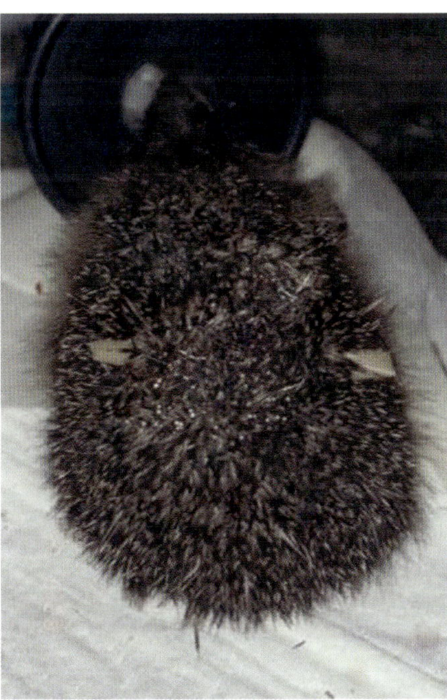

Figure 29.2 The subcutaneous route can be used around the edge of the 'skirt' of the spiny coat in hedgehogs that require fluid administration such as this individual recovering from a skin laceration.

Intravenous
Intravenous fluids in a hedgehog are difficult to administer due to their size and requirement for chemical restraint. The cephalic vein may be accessed using a 25–27 gauge catheter. In emergencies the jugular vein may be found running at an angle from the point of the shoulder to the base of the ear, but a cut-down technique may need to be employed.

Intraosseous
The proximal femur may be used, although access is through the mass of the panniculus carnosus covering the dorsum of the hedgehog, making visualisation more complex. The spines around the area may be clipped short prior to placement of the catheter due to the risk of displacement when the hedgehog rolls into a ball and the spines become fully erect.

Access routes for mustelids

Oral
This route may be used as described for the fox as some debilitated mustelids will tolerate nasogastric tubes for short periods, although they have to be placed in the anaesthetised animal. The smallest mustelids (e.g. weasel) are too small for these tubes, although the pine marten, polecat and even the stoat may be catheterised. Maximum volumes of 15–20 mL/kg may be fed at each sitting, preferably three to four times daily.

Subcutaneous
The skin over the thorax is the most readily available for use, with doses of 2–3 mL per site in weasels and up to 20 mL per site in pine martens being acceptable.

Intraperitoneal
See foxes.

Intravenous
The cephalic, saphenous and jugular veins may all be used in mustelids. Intravenous catheters must be placed under sedation/anaesthetic. The weasel and small stoats may be too small for easy venous access. Tolerance of the intravenous catheter and lines is moderately poor and species such as the pine marten are easily stressed and will only tolerate intravenous/invasive therapy when severely debilitated or anaesthetised.

Intraosseous
The proximal femur may be used but is only tolerated in anaesthetised or severely debilitated mustelids with adequate analgesia.

Access routes for otters

Oral
If drinking voluntarily and not severely dehydrated this may be possible but nasogastric tubes are poorly tolerated so this has to be voluntary.

Subcutaneous

The lateral thoracic areas may be used for isotonic fluid deposition sites but only when the otter is anaesthetised for another reason. Volumes of 30 mL may be placed at any one site.

Intraperitoneal

This route may be used in the anaesthetised otter if venous access is not possible and moderate dehydration exists. Volumes of 50–60 mL may be administered via this route in adult otters. As with all species this route should be avoided in cases of peritonitis, ascites, abdominal swelling and recent surgery.

Intravenous

The cephalic vein may be visualised across the dorsal aspect of the shaved antebrachium. The jugular vein runs from the point of the shoulder to the angle of the ramus of the mandible. Toleration of intravenous catheters in the conscious otter is extremely poor, and so this route should be reserved for periods when the otter is chemically restrained.

Intraosseous

This route should only be used in the young cub when central venous support is required but venous access is unavailable. The proximal femur may be used, but although the femur is very short and slightly curved, the same landmarks as in ferrets (i.e. the greater trochanter and the pelvis) may be used to guide the catheter into place.

Access routes for seals (phocids)

Oral

This route may be useful in seals as other access routes are limited. It is often combined with nutritional support to minimise handling and stress levels. A stomach tube may be used to administer an oral dog/cat electrolyte at a rate of 100–200 mL for common seal pups and 150–200 mL for grey seal pups (Barnett, 1998). This can be performed six times a day. Fluids are more important in the first instance, but gradually a slurry of blenderised fish and electrolytes may be fed after the first 24–48 hours.

Adult seals are generally too dangerous to administer via this route.

Subcutaneous

This is not a possible route in seals due to the large volumes of subcutaneous fat present.

Intraperitoneal

This is also a route rarely used in seals due to the thickness of the skin, subcutaneous fat and body wall, which makes accessing the peritoneal cavity difficult.

Intravenous

This route is possible via the extradural intravertebral vein. This is located through the lumbar intervertebral spaces L4 to L7. The spinal cord ends before this so the intravertebral space is filled with the venous sinus and therefore the risk of hitting nerves when catheterising the area is small. The needle/catheter is inserted midline, between the palpable spinous processes of the lumbar vertebrae concerned, and is therefore best performed under physical restraint in small seal pups or chemical restraint in larger specimens. The needle size varies from a 20-gauge 1.25-inch needle for animals under 10 kg to a 20-gauge 2-inch needle for 10–50 kg specimens and an 18-gauge 4-inch needle for animals over 50 kg (Sweeney, 1993). This route is useful for bolus treatment of severely dehydrated hypovolaemic cases, but is not useful for longer-term therapy.

Intraosseous

This route is not used due to the difficulty of accessing a bone marrow cavity.

Access routes for microchiropterans

Oral

This route may be utilised using oral electrolyte solutions. These may be administered via the bristles of a soft paintbrush in the smaller species, or via the end of a micro-pipette dropper in larger species. It is an effective method of rehydrating exhausted and mildly dehydrated bats.

Subcutaneous

This route has its limitations as bats are thin-skinned and the amounts which may be administered are small (0.2–0.75 mL) depending on the species. In addition, the skin is well attached to the underlying structures, particularly over the thorax, making subcutaneous injections difficult.

Intraperitoneal

This route is difficult due to the small size of species encountered. Small volumes (0.1–0.5 mL) may be given via this route, entering to the right of midline ventrally, just in front of the pelvis. A needle size of 25–27 gauge (0.25 inch) can be used with the bevel just pushed through the body wall to prevent puncture of vital organs.

Intravenous

The median (brachial) vein may be accessed as it passes over the ventral aspect of the mid-humerus. A 25–27 gauge catheter, preferably pre-heparinised to prevent clotting of blood, can be used under anaesthesia.

Intraosseous

This route is avoided due to their small size and fragility of the bones involved. The proximal femur is difficult to access in any case due to the normal anatomical 180° rotation of the hindlimbs.

Access routes for wild lagomorphs

Similar routes to domestic rabbits may be used but the tolerance of drip sets and catheters is markedly reduced in conscious animals.

Access routes for wild birds

See Chapter 14 for an overview of avian therapeutics. Typically, the distal ulna and proximal tibiotarsus bones may be used for intraosseous fluids (avoid the femur and humerus as these are pneumonised, i.e. connected to the airways and so can drown the bird). Intravenous access is via the medial metatarsal vein in long-legged birds or via the basilic vein on the underside of the wing caudal to the humerus or right jugular vein in short-legged species. Do not give intracoelomic fluids as the danger of puncturing an air sac and so drowning the patient is high.

TREATMENT OF WILDLIFE DISEASES

The following sections provide an overview of some common diseases and their treatments but are not intended to be exhaustive. It should be noted that there are no licensed products for use in wildlife cases.

Artiodactyls: bovids and cervids

The treatment of parasitic and bacterial diseases in cervids is shown in Tables 29.2 and 29.3.

Table 29.2 Treatment of selected cervid parasitic diseases.

Disease/parasite	Treatment
Babesiosis	Imidicarb 0.85 mg/kg IM once for treatment or 2.125 mg/kg once for prophylaxis Oxytetracycline (long-acting) 20–30 mg/kg IM
Coccidiosis	Sulfadimidine or sulfadimethoxine
Liver fluke	Triclabendazole 10 mg/kg IM
Mites	Ivermectin 0.2 mg/kg SC/PO Moxidectin 0.2 mg/kg SC
Parasitic gastroenteritis	Albendazole 10 mg/kg PO Ivermectin 0.2 mg/kg SC/PO Moxidectin 0.2 mg/kg SC
Ticks	Ivermectin 0.2 mg/kg SC/PO Deltamethrin spot-on
Warbles	Ivermectin 0.2 mg/kg SC/PO

PO, orally; SC, subcutaneously; IM, intramuscularly.

Table 29.3 Treatment of selected cervid bacterial diseases.

Disease/organism	Treatment
Anthrax	Long-acting amoxicillin 15 mg/kg IM Potentiated amoxicillin (amoxicillin clavulanate) 8.75 mg/kg IM SID for 5 days
Coxiella burnetii (Q fever)	Oxytetracycline 20–30 mg/kg IM
Leptospirosis	Oxytetracycline 20–30 mg/kg IM Dihydrostreptomycin-penicillin 25 mg/kg IM
Mannheimia haemolytica	Long-acting amoxicillin 15 mg/kg IM Potentiated amoxicillin (amoxicillin clavulanate) 8.75 mg/kg IM SID for 5 days Enrofloxacin 5 mg/kg SC SID
Mycoplasma spp.	Enrofloxacin 5 mg/kg SC SID
Salmonella spp.	Long-acting amoxicillin 15 mg/kg IM Potentiated amoxicillin (amoxicillin clavulanate) 8.75 mg/kg IM SID for 5 days Enrofloxacin 5 mg/kg SC SID
Yersinia spp.	Oxytetracycline 20–30 mg/kg IM

PO, orally; SC, subcutaneously; IM, intramuscularly; SID, once daily; BID, twice daily.

Trauma

Road traffic collisions are extremely common for deer, particularly roe deer, which are mainly nocturnal. Injuries are often fatal or require the deer to be humanely destroyed as they frequently involve compound fractures to the limbs, and ruptured diaphragms. In addition, hindlimb lameness is often associated with pelvic fractures.

Treatment of antler trauma when in velvet requires application of a pressure bandage around the area affected to stem blood loss. Surgical tie-off of any obvious arteries or even amputation may be needed under anaesthesia. Treatment with topical antibiotic sprays is also advised. Damage to the antler once the velvet has been shed tends to be less of a problem; the antler will be shed after the rut, and a new antler bud forms the following season.

Poisoning

There is no specific treatment for blue-green algae poisoning. Supportive therapy and the use of anticonvulsants such as diazepam may be helpful and the use of intravenous lipid emulsion therapy (see Chapter 30) could be considered. Relatively few other poisons are reported but theoretically deer can be poisoned by plants such as yew and rhododendron similar to domestic livestock. As both tend to be rapidly fatal should they be ingested, it is unlikely that an affected individual will be presented for treatment. Treatment would typically involve the use of oral adsorbents such as tannins for rhododendron poisoning (literally strong tea given orally) and removal where possible of plant material from the rumen through a left flank rumenotomy under general anaesthesia.

Canids and felids

Similar treatment regimens to domestic dogs and cats are often applied to foxes and wildcats, respectively (Tables 29.4 and 29.5).

Trauma

Causes of trauma in foxes include dog attacks and intraspecific fights, both of which may leave serious crushing and tearing injuries

Table 29.4 Treatment of selected red fox and wildcat parasitic diseases.

Disease/parasite	Treatment
Cestodes	Praziquantel 5 mg/kg PO/SC
Coccidiosis	Sulfadimidine or sulfadimethoxine
Fleas	Fipronil topically as per dog/cat Selamectin 6 mg/kg topically once
Mites	Ivermectin 0.2 mg/kg SC/PO repeated at 14 days Selamectin 6 mg/kg topically once
Nematodes	Fenbendazole 50 mg/kg PO for 7 days (lungworm and *Angiostrongylus vasorum*) Ivermectin 0.2 mg/kg SC/PO Moxidectin 2.5 mg/kg SC (*Crenosoma vulpis* and *Dirofilaria immitis*) Selamectin 6 mg/kg topically
Ticks	Manual removal and/or ivermectin 0.2 mg/kg SC/PO
Toxoplasmosis	Clindamycin 12.5–25 mg/kg PO BID

PO, orally; SC, subcutaneously; BID, twice daily.

Table 29.5 Treatment of selected red fox and wildcat bacterial and fungal diseases.

Disease/organism	Treatment
Chlamydia	Doxycycline 5 mg/kg PO BID
Leptospirosis	Doxycycline 5 mg/kg PO BID for 14 days
Ringworm	Topical enilconazole or miconazole Itraconazole 5 mg/kg PO as per domestic cats
Salmonella spp.	Long-acting amoxicillin 15 mg/kg IM Potentiated amoxicillin (amoxicillin clavulanate) 8.75 mg/kg IM SID for 5 days or 12.5 mg/kg PO BID for 5 days Enrofloxacin 5 mg/kg SC SID

PO, orally; SC, subcutaneously; IM, intramuscularly; SID, once daily; BID, twice daily.

to the neck, muzzle and forelimbs. Sedation or anaesthesia is required to fully evaluate the extent of serious wounds. Covering antibiotic therapy with broad-spectrum penicillins such as potentiated amoxicillin 8.75 mg/kg subcutaneously once daily (dosed as for cats and dogs) and analgesia with medications such as carprofen 4 mg/kg subcutaneously once daily (dosed as for cats and dogs) should be considered.

Finally, gunshot wounds are also common, both high-velocity rifle wounds (which may leave very little external damage but cause massive internal shock damage as the bullet passes through) and low-velocity shotgun wounds (which produce obvious massive external damage).

Road traffic accidents are common injuries for wildcats. The same protocols for treatment of shock and hypovolaemia as used for domestic cats are advocated. However, wildcats are much less tolerant of repeated medication and fluid therapy, and these may need to be administered under sedation via drip or in bolus form.

Poisoning

This is of a supportive nature for warfarin poisoning, with doses of phytomenadione (vitamin K_1) 3–5 mg/kg given intramuscularly daily for a minimum of 3–5 days. More potent anticoagulant pesticides such as hydroxycoumarin-containing compounds (e.g. brodifacoum) may require many weeks of vitamin K therapy and this should be taken into consideration when thinking about how long a species may be safely hospitalised. The use of charcoal adsorbents to prevent further absorption of poison from the gut may be helpful.

Other forms of poisoning, including strychnine poisoning, have been reported, although no treatment exists. The use of diazepam 1–2 mg/kg to effect intravenously or intramuscularly may help control seizuring.

Mustelids

Similar treatment regimens for domestic ferrets are commonly used in wild mustelids such as polecats, weasels and stoats (Tables 29.6 and 29.7). Otters may be more prone to conditions such as nephrolithiasis and stomach ulceration (particularly if associated with oil toxicity) and these should be considered when formulating a treatment plan to ensure appropriate fluid therapy and antacids for example are used.

Table 29.6 Treatment of selected mustelid parasitic diseases.

Disease/parasite	Treatment
Cestodes	Praziquantel 5 mg/kg PO/SC
Coccidiosis	Sulfadimidine or sulfadimethoxine
Fleas	Fipronil topically as per dog/cat Selamectin 6 mg/kg topically once
Mites	Ivermectin 0.2 mg/kg SC/PO repeated after 7–14 days Selamectin 6 mg/kg topically once
Nematodes	Fenbendazole 50 mg/kg PO for 7 days (lungworm and *A. vasorum*); 50 mg/kg PO for 10–14 days (sinus nematodes, [Roken, 1993]) Ivermectin 0.2 mg/kg SC/PO Moxidectin 2.5 mg/kg SC (*Crenosoma vulpis* and *D. immitis*) Selamectin 6 mg/kg topically
Ticks	Manual removal and/or ivermectin 0.2 mg/kg SC/PO
Toxoplasmosis	Clindamycin 12.5–25 mg/kg PO BID

PO, orally; SC, subcutaneously; BID, twice daily.

Table 29.7 Treatment of selected mustelid bacterial and fungal diseases.

Disease/organism	Treatment
Adiaspiromycosis	Itraconazole 5 mg/kg PO as per domestic cats
Dental disease	Dental extractions: antimicrobials effective against anaerobes such as clindamycin 5.5 mg/kg BID; potentiated amoxicillin (amoxicillin clavulanate) 8.75 mg/kg IM SID for 5 days or 12.5 mg/kg PO BID for 5 days
Campylobacter spp.	Potentiated amoxicillin (amoxicillin clavulanate) 8.75 mg/kg IM SID for 5 days or 12.5 mg/kg PO BID for 5 days
Leptospirosis	Doxycycline 5 mg/kg PO BID for 14 days
Ringworm	Topical enilconazole or miconazole Itraconazole 5 mg/kg PO as per domestic cats
Salmonella spp.	Long-acting amoxicillin 15 mg/kg IM Potentiated amoxicillin (amoxicillin clavulanate) 8.75 mg/kg IM SID for 5 days or 12.5 mg/kg PO BID for 5 days Enrofloxacin 5 mg/kg SC SID

PO, orally; SC, subcutaneously; IM, intramuscularly; SID, once daily; BID, twice daily.

Trauma

Intraspecific fight wounds are often associated with large areas of skin trauma over the dorsal rump. These may require extensive treatment, skin flaps/grafts and antibiosis to allow full recovery.

Snares and trapping injuries to the neck (snares) and feet (traps) are still also common and life-threatening. Treatment is often too late to affect the outcome as most affected individuals are found dead associated with the device.

Traumatic injuries to mustelids are not uncommon, although they rarely survive road traffic accidents. Domestic cat bites and trauma may be seen in the smaller species, with deep infected wounds that require flushing and antibiotic treatment, initially under sedation.

Poisoning

Oil spills may be an issue for otters and result in hypothermia, waterlogging of the fur, drowning, clinical anaemia and gastrointestinal tract ulceration as previously mentioned. Management should be similar to that described for management of oil spills in wild birds, with removal of the oil from the pelage and use of oral adsorbents and protectants and antacids. Other forms of poisoning are difficult to identify and so treatment is therefore often symptomatic, with activated charcoal, given orally to attempt to prevent further absorption of any poison, and fluid therapy, with seizure-modifying therapy such as diazepam 1–2 mg/kg intramuscularly being used when necessary. Doses of 3–5 mg/kg phytomenadione (vitamin K_1) given intramuscularly daily for 3–5 days may be necessary in cases of suspected warfarin/coumerol-related poisoning. However, see note above under wildcat poisoning regarding more potent hydroxycoumarin compounds such as brodifacoum which may require weeks of therapy due to their persistence in the body.

Phocids: common and grey seals

The treatment of parasitic and bacterial diseases in seals is shown in Tables 29.8 and 29.9.

Table 29.8 Treatment of selected phocid parasitic diseases.

Disease/parasite	Treatment
Coccidiosis	Sulfadimidine or sulfadimethoxine PO
Mites	Ivermectin 0.2 mg/kg IM/PO repeated after 7–14 days
Nematodes	Fenbendazole 50 mg/kg PO for 7 days Ivermectin 0.2 mg/kg IM/PO repeated after 10–14 days May require antacids for stomach worms where ulceration may be an issue (ranitidine, omeprazole) May require antimicrobials such as potentiated amoxicillin and mucolytics such as bromhexine with lungworm

PO, orally; IM, intramuscularly.

Table 29.9 Treatment of selected phocid bacterial diseases.

Disease/organism	Treatment
Brucellosis	Doxycycline 5 mg/kg PO BID
Dental disease	Dental extractions: antimicrobials effective against anaerobes such as clindamycin 5.5 mg/kg BID; potentiated amoxicillin (amoxicillin clavulanate) 8.75 mg/kg IM SID for 5 days or 12.5 mg/kg PO BID for 5 days
Campylobacter spp.	Erythromycin 10–20 mg/kg PO BID–TID for 3–5 days Enrofloxacin 5 mg/kg PO, IM SID for 3–5 days
Leptospirosis	Doxycycline 5 mg/kg PO BID for 14 days
Mycoplasma spp.	Enrofloxacin 5 mg/kg IM SID Doxycycline 5 mg/kg PO BID
Pseudomonas spp. ocular disease	Ofloxacin or gentamicin eyedrops Salt solution spray
Salmonella spp.	Long-acting amoxicillin 15 mg/kg IM Potentiated amoxicillin (amoxicillin clavulanate) 8.75 mg/kg IM SID for 5 days or 12.5 mg/kg PO BID for 5 days Enrofloxacin 5 mg/kg IM SID

PO, orally; IM, intramuscularly; SID, once daily; BID, twice daily; TID, three times daily.

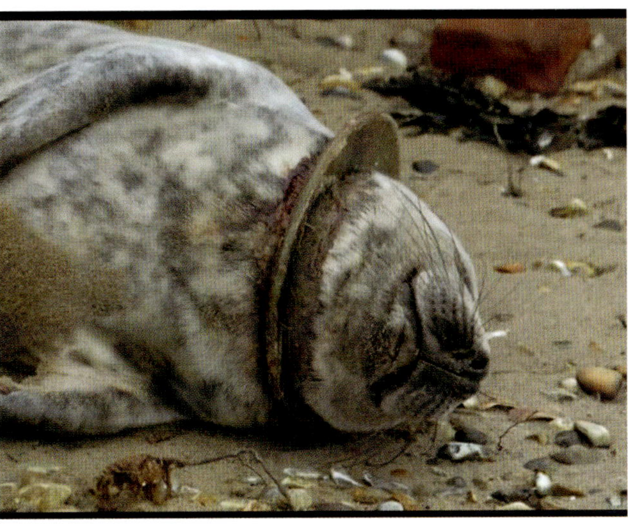

Figure 29.3 Old wounds are often infected and will need to be debrided under anaesthesia and appropriate antimicrobials used. *Source:* Courtesy of Diane Westwood RVN.

Trauma

Fresh wounds may need to be sutured under anaesthetic/sedation. Old infected wounds need to be debrided, and the seal placed on broad-spectrum antibiotics such as the potentiated amoxicillins 8.75 mg/kg intramuscularly once daily until culture and sensitivity results are known (see Figure 29.3). Topical treatment with thick oil-based antibiotic creams are also useful (e.g. Flamazine®), although the seal will need to be kept out of water until the wound has healed. See also Chapter 30 for a more general discussion on wound management.

Poisoning: oil spills

Fluid therapy and nutrition are necessary for young pups caught in oil. Treatment for conjunctivitis with topical eyedrops such as Maxitrol® (Alcon) is helpful but watch for melting corneal ulcers as topical corticosteroid-containing eyedrops should not be used in these cases. Oral adsorbents such as activated charcoal are necessary to prevent further absorption of oil. Oral gastrointestinal protectants such as sucralfate and antacids such as omeprazole may be helpful. Removal of the oil from the coat is best performed using a regimen similar to that used in wild birds (see also Chapter 14), with warm water and Fairy Liquid® (Proctor and Gamble) detergent being used until water beads on the fur.

Chiroptera: bats

The treatment of selected parasitic and bacterial diseases in bats is shown in Table 29.10.

Trauma

Fractures of the smaller wing bones, such as the phalanges of the 'hands' which support the wing membrane, have been shown to heal of their own accord (Walsh and Stebbings, 1989). Fractures of the humerus or radius and ulna are more serious and may require splinting or in the larger species the use of Kirschner wires as the transcortical pins and Technovit® as the crossbar to create an external fixator

Table 29.10 Treatment of selected bat diseases.

Disease/organism	Treatment
Cat bites	Enrofloxacin 10 mg/kg PO/SC BID: not effective against anaerobes and may cause injection site reaction so PO preferred if possible Potentiated amoxicillin 12.5 mg/kg PO BID: more useful for anaerobes as well as *Pasteurella* spp.
Mites	Ivermectin 0.2 mg/kg PO/SC Manual removal with paint brush dipped in milk
Nematodes	Ivermectin 0.2 mg/kg SC/PO
Ticks	Manual removal under anaesthesia
White nose disease	Itraconazole may be tried but little evidence of success Susceptible to ultraviolet light (Palmer *et al.*, 2018)

PO, orally; SC, subcutaneously; BID, twice daily.

apparatus. This is impossible in smaller species, and intramedullary pins tend to allow too much rotation of the bones when the bat moves its wing.

Other serious injuries to the wing are the tearing of the wing membrane itself. This has a considerable capacity to heal of its own accord if the tear is reasonably sized and is in the main body of the wing vane. If the tear is at the edge of a wing, then healing potential is poor. Suturing the membrane is extremely difficult, and due to the lack of a major vascular supply, frequently the wound breaks down. The use of tissue glues may allow sufficient apposition of the edges of such a wound for long enough for re-epithelialisation to occur. If the wing membrane is irreparably damaged, then flight will be affected and this must be considered before considering release of such a debilitated bat back into the wild.

Poisoning

Treatment of suspected organophosphate poisoning is supportive, with the use of atropine sulphate 0.2 mg/kg to counteract any bradycardia which might occur.

Other forms of poisonings are possible, such as the ingestion of insects carrying pesticides, as is the consumption of polluted water from ponds and rivers. These forms of poisoning are extremely difficult to diagnose and therefore to administer a specific treatment. Treatment is thus frequently of a supportive nature.

Eulipotyphla: hedgehogs

The treatment of selected parasitic and bacterial and fungal diseases in hedgehogs is shown in Tables 29.11 and 29.12.

Mites are commonly seen in hedgehogs and may be secondarily complicated with dermatophytosis (ringworm) (see Figure 29.4).

Blowfly strike can affect any animal and an underlying cause such as gastrointestinal disease leading to diarrhoea and debilitation should be identified (see Figure 29.5).

Trauma

Hedgehogs are unfortunately frequently injured in gardens and in hedgerows and roadside verges, due to their habit of sleeping buried in deep leaf litter. They are often involved in fires, as they seek out hibernation sites in the autumn and burrow into ready-made bonfire night piles. Severe burns are therefore not an uncommon injury in hedgehogs. Hedge strimmer and lawn mower injuries are also unfortunately not uncommon (see Figure 29.2), and are made worse by the hedgehog's survival tactic of not running from the danger but staying put and curling into a ball. Injuries seen therefore will vary, but frequently involve tears or lacerations to the skin and subcutaneous layers over the dorsum.

Subcutaneous emphysema is common after road traffic collisions and other traumas. Repeated deflation may be required to allow the condition to resolve. Another common feature of trauma is prolapse of the orbicularis muscle, where the muscle responsible for curling up the hedgehog everts as it slips off the edge of the pelvis caudally. This may be replaced after anaesthesia to its correct position but may prolapse again and may require surgery to attempt to secure though the prognosis is poor. A hedgehog that cannot roll up and defend itself is not safe to release back into the wild.

Table 29.11 Treatment of selected hedgehog parasitic diseases.

Disease/ parasite	Treatment
Blowfly strike	Fluid therapy and analgesia (NSAIDs, e.g. meloxicam) Manual removal of maggots and/or eggs under anaesthesia. Possible use of cyromazine topically if only eggs are present to prevent the larvae from pupating to the L2 stage that cause tissue trauma Ivermectin 0.2–0.4 mg/kg for larvae/maggots Broad-spectrum antimicrobial, e.g. potentiated amoxicillin, for secondary infection Identify underlying cause of likely debilitation that led to the animal being struck (e.g. gastrointestinal disease causing diarrhoea)
Cestodes	Praziquantel 7 mg/kg PO, may require repeat dose 14 days later
Coccidiosis	Sulfadimidine or sulfadimethoxine
Mites	Ivermectin 0.2 mg/kg SC/PO repeat 7–10 days later Selamectin 6 mg/kg topically once
Nematodes	Fenbendazole 10–30 mg/kg PO for 5 days Ivermectin 0.2 mg/kg SC/PO, repeated after 7–10 days for lungworm and after 10–14 days for intestinal nematodes. Dosage may need to be much greater for lungworms (typically 4–5 mg/kg have been used (see Van de Weyer *et al.*, 2023)) Levamisole 25–35 mg/kg orally once daily for 2 days for capillarid lungworm (Van de Weyer *et al.*, 2023) May require antimicrobials such as potentiated amoxicillin and mucolytics such as bromhexine with lungworm
Ticks	Manual removal under anaesthesia Ivermectin 0.4 mg/kg PO/SC
Trematodes	Praziquantel 7 mg/kg PO, may require repeat dose 14 days later

PO, orally; SC, subcutaneously; NSAID, non-steroidal anti-inflammatory drug.

Poisoning (e.g. metaldehyde)

This involves the oral administration of an activated charcoal slurry to absorb any further chemical remaining in the digestive system. Supportive treatment, such as fluid therapy, is advised and the use of diazepam 0.5–2 mg/kg intramuscularly if fitting occurs.

Table 29.12 Treatment of selected hedgehog bacterial and fungal diseases.

Disease/organism	Treatment
Adiaspiromycosis	Itraconazole 5–10 mg/kg PO BID Terbinafine 15 mg/kg PO SID
Dental disease	Dental extractions: antimicrobials effective against anaerobes such as clindamycin 5.5 mg/kg BID; potentiated amoxicillin (amoxicillin clavulanate) 8.75 mg/kg IM SID for 5 days or 12.5 mg/kg PO BID for 5 days
Bordetella bronchiseptica	Potentiated amoxicillin (amoxicillin clavulanate) 8.75 mg/kg IM SID for 5 days or 12.5 mg/kg PO BID for 5 days
Campylobacter spp.	Potentiated amoxicillin (amoxicillin clavulanate) 8.75 mg/kg IM SID for 5 days or 12.5 mg/kg PO BID for 5 days
Leptospirosis	Doxycycline 5 mg/kg PO BID for 14 days
Mycoplasma spp.	Enrofloxacin 5 mg/kg SC SID Doxycycline 5 mg/kg PO BID
Pseudomonas spp. ocular disease	Ofloxacin or gentamicin eyedrops Salt solution spray
Ringworm	Enilconazole/miconazole topically SID for 4–6 weeks Itraconazole 10 mg/kg PO BID, watch for toxicity as may require several weeks
Salmonella spp.	Long-acting amoxicillin 15 mg/kg IM Potentiated amoxicillin (amoxicillin clavulanate) 8.75 mg/kg IM SID for 5 days or 12.5 mg/kg PO BID for 5 days Enrofloxacin 5 mg/kg SC SID

PO, orally; SC, subcutaneously; IM, intramuscularly; SID, once daily; BID, twice daily.

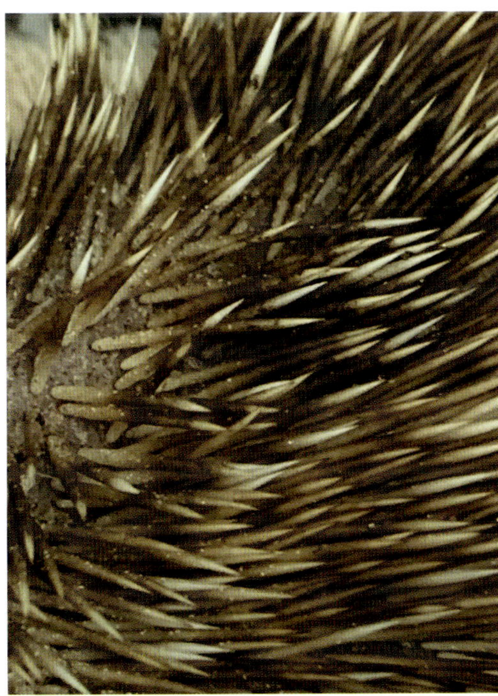

Figure 29.4 Mites such as *Caparinia tripilis* and dermatophytosis such as *Tricophyton mentagrophytes* are common in hedgehogs.

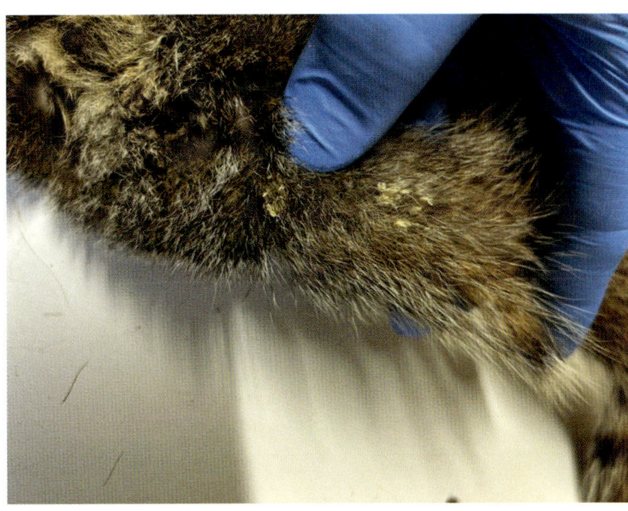

Figure 29.5 The eggs of blowflies (e.g. *Lucilia* and *Phormia* spp.) are often laid on debilitated animals, particularly those with gastrointestinal and urinary tract disease. Note that multiple respiratory infections (often lungworms and *Bordetella bronchiseptica*) and multiple gastrointestinal infections (trematodes, nematodes and often *Salmonella* spp.) may be seen in hedgehogs and so multiple therapies may be required at the same time (see Figure 29.6).

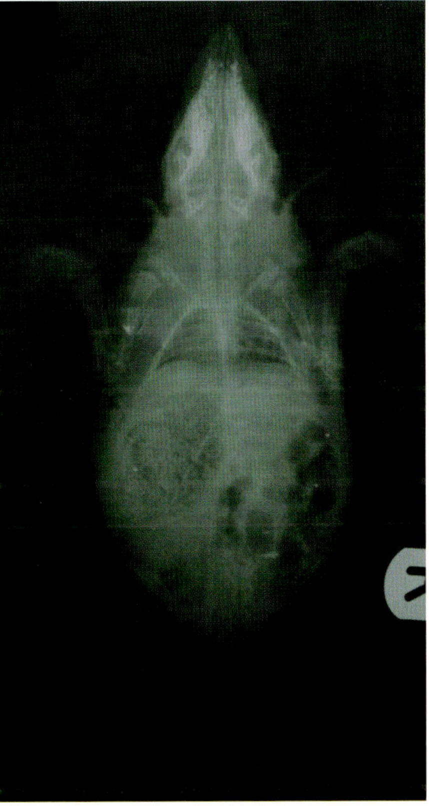

Figure 29.6 Bloat in hedgehogs can be seen with multiple infections of the gastrointestinal system and so may require multiple therapies at the same time.

Other poisoning cases are undoubtedly seen, but the problem is frequently being able to identify accurately the poison concerned.

Lagomorphs: rabbits and hares

Therapies are similar to those for the domestic rabbit. Many are presented in a state of decompensatory shock and will need to be warmed

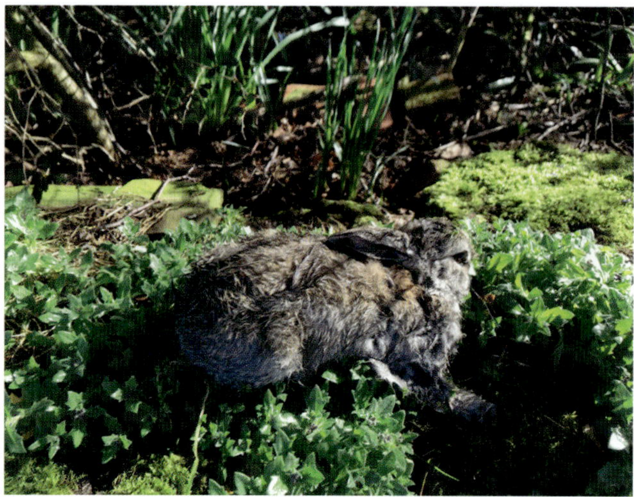

Figure 29.7 Lagomorphs often present in a state of decompensatory shock and are often hypothermic and hypoglycaemic.

thoroughly with fluid therapy often including intravenous glucose (see Figure 29.7). Please refer to Chapter 6 for further information on rabbits. Similar principles to domestic rabbits are used, with avoidance of oral penicillins, clindamycin, cephalosporins, etc., all of which can induce clostridial overgrowth within the large intestine and risk mortalities.

Rodents: mice, rats, voles, squirrels, beavers, etc.

Therapies are similar to those for the domestic rodents with some variations in drug toxicities. Herbivores such as beavers and voles should not be given oral penicillins, cephalosporins or clindamycin as these can lead to clostridial overgrowth and mortalities. Please refer to Chapter 6 for more information,

Wild birds

Therapeutic options for infectious diseases, fractures, oil contamination and lead poisoning among others are covered in more detail in Chapter 14. Fractures are common in wild birds and similar principles to captive birds can be used but the operative repair often needs to be perfect or the bird may not be able to manage after release (see Figures 29.8 and 29.9). Fractures close to the tip of the wing, where there is more movement, often require more accurate fixation. This is particularly so in birds that require complex or fine movements to hunt and manoeuvre, such as kestrels that hover above prey, an action that requires highly mobile carpal, metacarpal and digit movements. Birds that are gliders, such as buzzards, still require complete fracture fixation but may be less critically affected by some minor decrease in the range of wing movement after release. See also Chapter 30 for a discussion on acute management of avian (and mammalian) fractures.

Oiled seabirds are an emergency requiring intensive therapy and can rapidly swamp a rehabilitation centre with the sheer numbers of birds presented (see Figure 29.10). The specific issue regarding pesticide toxicity is mentioned in the following section.

Pesticide toxicity

- *Alphachloralose*: a small rodent poison causing hypothermia. Clinical signs in birds include lethargy, incoordination and stupor.

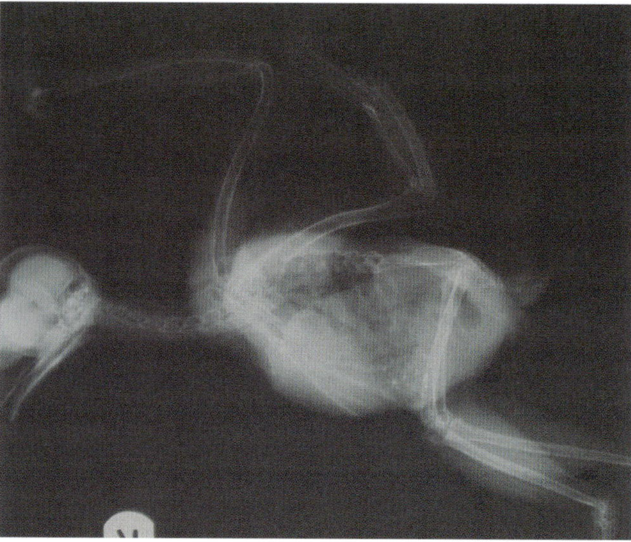

Figure 29.8 Fractures of the wing are common in wild birds such as this tawny owl. Care should be taken to ensure the bird has the best possible chance of being able to feed itself and evade predators after release.

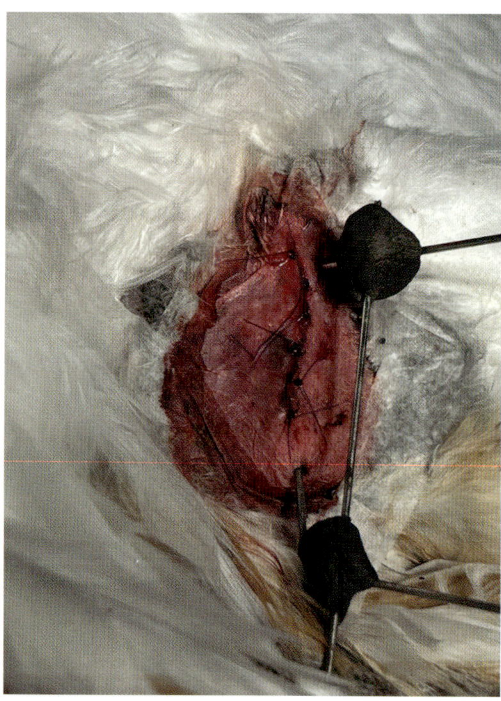

Figure 29.9 Primary fixation techniques such as external fixators, commonly used in captive birds, can be applied to some fractures in wild birds to ensure accurate fixation and a rapid return to full function.

  Treatment revolves around maintaining core body temperature, with recovery in 24–48 hours if this can be managed.
- *Mevinphos*: this and related organophosphates are less commonly seen although still used in sheep dips for treating sheep scab. Clinical signs of toxicity in birds include flaccid paralysis of the limbs although the head remains upright (unlike botulism), bradycardia, diarrhoea and dyspnoea. Treatment may be difficult and involves pralidoxine 10–20 mg/kg if seen less than 24 hours after

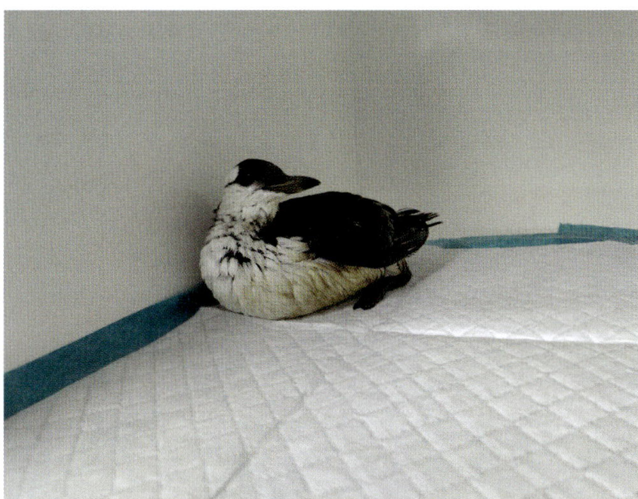

Figure 29.10 Oiled seabirds require intensive therapy before their return to the wild, including checking for anaemia and gastrointestinal ulceration as well as ensuring they are fully waterproofed. *Source:* Courtesy of Kelly Huitson RVN.

ingestion (unlikely) or atropine 0.2–0.5 mg/kg every 3–4 hours if seen more than 24 hours after ingestion.

- *Strychnine*: still available as a mole poison. Clinical signs are rarely seen as death is usually peracute. After death, grossly there is opisthotonus and rigor. The birds are often found adjacent to poisoned bait.

Reptiles and amphibians

Therapeutic options are covered in detail in Chapter 22.

References

Barnett, J. (1998) Treatment of sick and injured marine mammals. *In Practice*, **20**(4), 200–211.

Blood, D.C. and Radostits, O.M. (1989) Diseases of the blood and blood forming organs. In: *Veterinary Medicine* (eds D.C. Blood & O.M. Radostits), 7th edn, pp. 341–343. Bailliere and Tindall, London.

Chalmers, G.A. and Barrett, M.W. (1982) Capture myopathy. In: *Non-infectious Diseases of Wildlife* (eds G.L. Hoff & J.W. Davis), pp. 84–94. Iowa State University Press.

Martin, H. and Kollias, G.V. (1989) Evaluation of water deprivation and fluid therapy in pigeons. *Journal of Zoo and Wildlife Medicine*, **20**(2), 173–177.

Palmer, J.M., Drees, K.P., Foster, J.T. and Lindner, D.L. (2018) Extreme sensitivity to ultraviolet light in the fungal pathogen causing white-nose syndrome of bats. *Nature Communications*, **9**(35). doi: 10.1038/s41467-017-02441-z.

Roken, B.O. (1993) Parasitic diseases of carnivores. In: *Zoo and Wild Animal Medicine Current Therapy 3* (ed. M.E. Fowler), pp. 399–404. WB Saunders, Philadelphia.

Samour, J., Perlman, J., Kinne, J. *et al.* (2016) Vitamin B6 (pyridoxine hydrochloride) toxicosis in falcons. *Journal of Zoo and Wildlife Medicine*, **47**(2), 601–608.

Spraker, T.R. (1993) Stress and capture myopathy in artiodactylids. In: *Zoo and Wild Animal Medicine Current Therapy 3* (ed. M.E. Fowler), pp. 481–488. WB Saunders, Philadelphia.

Sweeney, J.C. (1993) Blood sampling and other collection techniques in marine mammals. In: *Zoo and Wild Animal Medicine Current Therapy 3* (ed. M.E. Fowler), pp. 425–428. WB Saunders, Philadelphia.

Van der Weyer, Y., Santos, M.C., Williams, N. *et al.* (2023) Efficacy of levamisole, ivermectin and moxidectin against *Capillaria* spp. in European hedgehogs (*Erinaceus europaeus*). *Journal of Helminthology*, **97**(e99), 1–9.

Walsh, S.T. and Stebbings, R.E. (1989) Care and rehabilitation of wild bats. In: *Proceedings of the Inaugural Symposium of the British Wildlife Rehabilitation Council, London* (eds S. Harris & T. Thomas). British Wildlife Rehabilitation Council, London.

Williams, E.S. and Thorne, E.T. (1996) Exertional myopathy (capture myopathy). In: *Non-infectious Diseases of Wildlife* (eds A. Fairbrother, L.N. Locke & G.L. Hoff), 2nd edn, pp. 181–193. Ames, Iowa.

Chapter 30 Wildlife Emergency and Critical Care Medicine

Assessment of the wildlife patient

Safety

Assessment of the patient should of course be done with caution as many are hazardous; even if they appear to be unconscious or stupefied, they may suddenly react aggressively to touch or interference. Male deer may be in antler or, in the case of muntjac and Chinese water deer, have significant canine teeth that can cause serious injuries. Carnivores can inflict serious bites and scratches. Wild birds of prey may cause injuries through talon strikes and in larger species from their bite; other wild birds may cause injuries to handlers through wing flapping or pecking.

Further caution should be taken in dealing with animals that may have significant zoonotic diseases. Deer, badgers and many other wild mammals may harbour bovine tuberculosis. Many carnivores and even hedgehogs can carry *Salmonella* and *Campylobacter* spp. Hedgehogs often carry significant burdens of ticks and ringworm. Rodents can carry bacteria such as *Salmonella* and *Leptospira* spp., viruses such as hantavirus and encephalomyocarditis virus, and parasites such as *Rodentolepis nana* (see Figure 30.1). Birds may harbour *Chlamydia* spp. and avian influenza virus and bats may carry rabies-like lyssaviruses. All mammals and some birds may be carriers of ticks such as *Ixodes ricinus*, which can act as a vector for a number of important zoonotic pathogens including Lyme disease (see Figure 30.2). In all cases appropriate personal protective equipment should be worn, risk assessments made and staff ideally should be vaccinated wherever possible, particularly against tetanus, tuberculosis and rabies virus.

Initial steps

An initial assessment of avian patients should focus on similar points to those in captive birds (see Chapter 16), such as evidence of dyspnoea (tail bobbing, open beak breathing, audible respiratory noise) and abnormal carriage of wings or legs that may indicate an underlying skeletal injury or fracture.

An initial assessment of mammalian patients should focus on:

1. Degree of alertness
2. Evidence of dyspnoea (increased chest movement, audible respiratory noise)
3. Limb carriage and ability to use all limbs
4. Obvious wounds and skin deficits
5. Evidence of blowfly strike/maggots (see Figure 30.3)
6. Evidence of external haemorrhage
7. Unusual behaviours (lack of fear for example, which might indicate central nervous system dysfunction).

Detailed examination of the collapsed wildlife patient

If examining the patient 'in the field' then a decision has to be made as to whether the patient needs to be brought into a clinic for further treatment, whether it is fit to release immediately or whether it is not safe to move, carries a poor prognosis and may need to be euthanased. This will often require sedation or anaesthesia for safety, although wild birds, many rodents, reptiles, amphibians and sometimes lagomorphs may often be examined without anaesthesia, but stress levels may be significantly reduced if this is kept to a minimum. Examination should be thorough but quick and can focus on the following.

1. Oral examination to check mucous membrane colour, presence of dental disease, oral ulceration, excess fluid from the glottis and entrapment of linear objects (e.g. fishing lines in birds).
2. Examination of the nares for evidence of discharge that may indicate respiratory disease or parasites (leeches, flukes, nematodes, etc.).
3. Examination of the external ear canal for evidence of infection and parasites.
4. Examination of the genitalia and anus for evidence of diarrhoea, blowfly strike and haemorrhage.
5. Palpation of the limbs for evidence of crepitus that may indicate a fracture or infection.
6. Auscultation of the chest for evidence of respiratory noise that may indicate infection and the heart for evidence of cardiac murmurs. (NB: some murmurs may not be associated with disease, e.g. wildcats and beavers requiring further examination such as echocardiographic assessment.)
7. Assessment of the femoral or peripheral pulse to see whether it matches the heart rate and the intensity of its output.
8. Assessment of the rectal or cloacal temperature (see Table 30.1) for hypothermia or hyperthermia.
9. General overall physical examination of the body surface for evidence of wounds, infection, neoplasia or parasitism.
10. Assessment, if possible, of weight and body condition score.
11. Always consider radiographing the patient, as many have underlying issues that may not be always apparent on initial examination (see Figure 30.4).

Triage

With wild animals, triaging is particularly important and a critical and realistic appraisal of the patient, early on in the course of the assessment, should be made. The correct decision in many cases is sadly to humanely euthanase the patient. This is particularly the case where a course of treatment is likely to result in medium- to

Veterinary Nursing of Exotic Pets and Wildlife, Third Edition. Simon J. Girling.

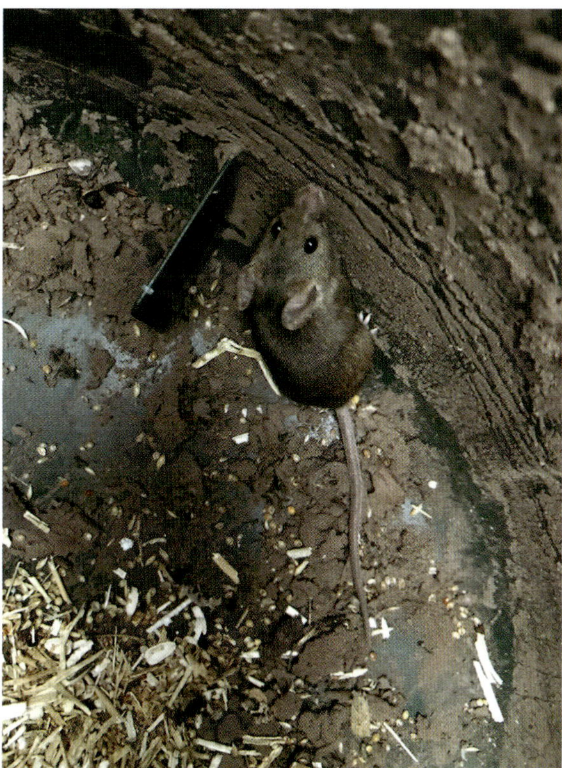

Figure 30.1 Many wild animals can carry zoonoses, particularly rodents.

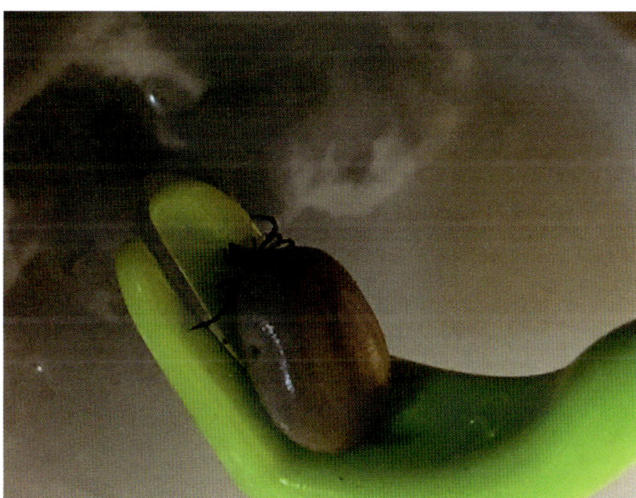

Figure 30.2 Ticks, such as *Ixodes ricinus*, are commonly found on wildlife and can act as significant vectors of zoonotic disease including Lyme disease (*Borrelia burgdorferi*).

long-term confinement and where animals have been injured in a way that is likely to reduce their survivability in the wild post release. For example, the release of owls with only one functional eye, or deer with only three functional limbs is likely to lead to unnecessary suffering of the animal after release and probably its early demise. It should also be noted that in the UK the current legislation prohibits the release of an animal that is not fit to cope with its newly found wild state. Best and Mullineaux (2003) have suggested that there are six stages in dealing with a wildlife patient:

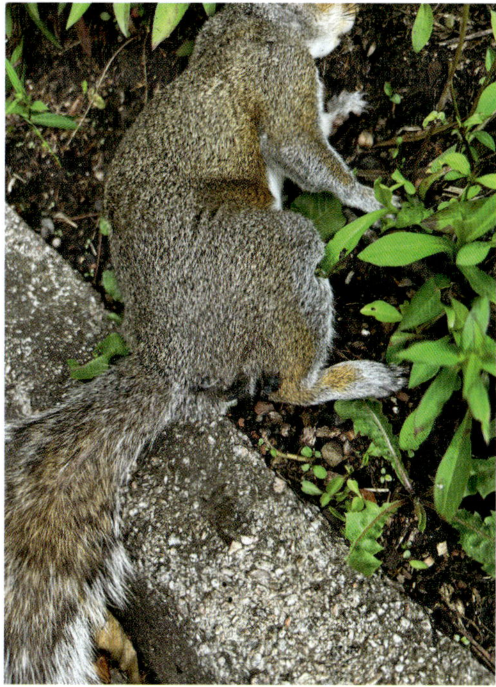

Figure 30.3 Evidence of blowfly strike is never a good sign as it suggests not only a life-threatening parasitic condition but also points to an often serious underlying cause of debilitation.

Table 30.1 Some typical rectal/cloacal temperatures of wildlife.

Species	Rectal/cloacal temperature (°C)
Badger	37.8–38.5
Birds	40–42
Deer	38–39
Eurasian otter	37.5–38.9
Fox	37.8–39
Hedgehog	35.4–37
Lagomorphs	38.5–40
Seal	36–38
Squirrel	37.4–38.5
Wildcats	37.5–39.2

1. Initial location, capture and translocation
2. Examination and assessment for rehabilitation
3. First aid and stabilisation
4. Treatment
5. Recuperation and rehabilitation
6. Release.

Making an educated assessment of the age of the patient is also important. Many juvenile birds are believed to be abandoned or unwell, but may simply have recently fledged and actually need to be returned quickly to the place where they were found to be reunited with their parents. Fawns, seal pups and leverets are usually left alone by the mother for long periods, only reuniting for feeding and when the mother decides to move to another area; fox cubs will often leave

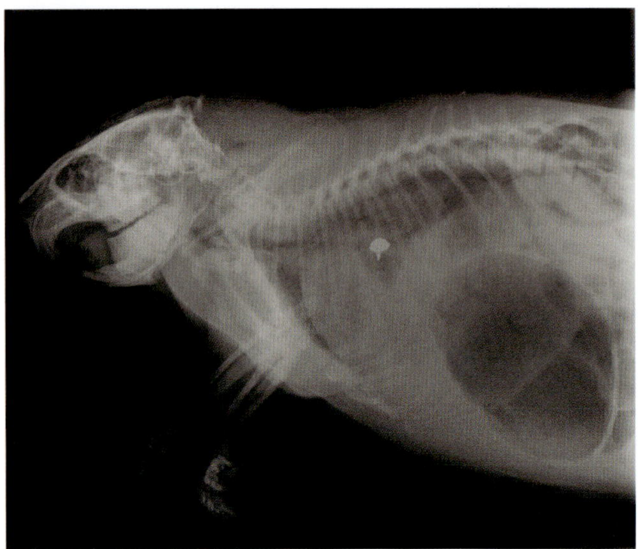

Figure 30.4 Radiography of the wildlife patient is always advisable as many have underlying issues, such as this beaver with a piece of bullet casing lodged in its chest.

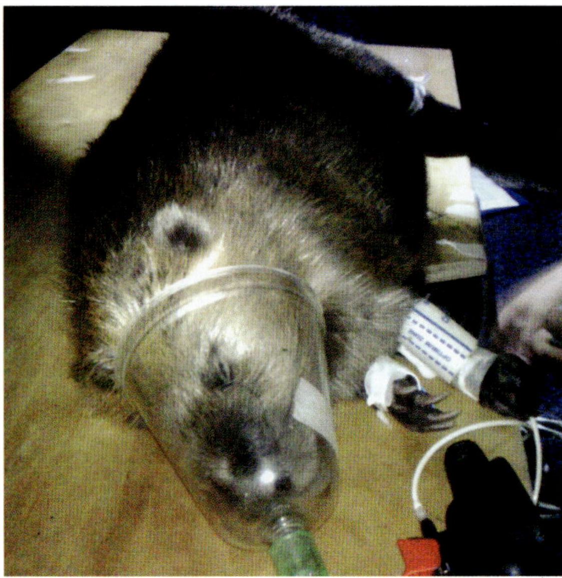

Figure 30.5 Indirect blood pressure assessment may be possible where the patient is large enough. Most mammal's systolic blood pressure should be over 90 mmHg but there are some exceptions such as the Eurasian beaver, whose systolic blood pressure is often around 60 mmHg normally.

the den when the vixen is away and so such individuals, although alone, are not abandoned.

Very young animals requiring hand rearing can bring their own problems, not least of which is the time and effort required to prepare them for release back into the wild, particularly for predators. Deer can become hazardous to humans if hand reared in a way that results in them losing fear of humans, particularly male deer when they go through the breeding season. Many young animals do better if socialised with their own kind early on, badgers being a typical example; therefore, if no other cubs of a similar age are being cared for when a new cub is handed in for treatment, other rehabilitators should be contacted to see if they have cubs being reared that could pair up and, if not, euthanasia may again be the preferred decision.

Emergency ABC protocol

A for airway and B for breathing

Provision of a quiet environment and an increased oxygen level through the use of oxygen tents may be all that is required in some cases. Incubators designed for commercial poultry or small vivaria can be set up to provide heat as well as an oxygen-enriched environment. Areas dedicated to this should be quiet, have dimmed lighting and where possible have an increased humidity for smaller patients to reduce further dehydration. Maintaining animals in sternal recumbency is important; in the case of birds, taking the weight off the sternum by using a doughnut-shaped piece of towelling and placing the bird in the centre can help ease breathing.

Intubation should be attempted in an animal that stops breathing but extreme care should be taken not to get bitten in the case of some more hazardous species (e.g. badgers and foxes). I have also used **v-gel**® Advanced Rabbit (Docsinnovent Ltd, www.docsinnovent.com) laryngeal cuffed tubes in wild lagomorphs. Some species are relatively straightforward to intubate (e.g. birds, foxes, wildcats) while others are more difficult due to the narrow oral aperture and caudally located larynx and sometimes longer skull shape (e.g. deer, beavers, rabbits) and some are difficult due to their small size (e.g. most rodents and sometimes hedgehogs). Paediatric Wisconsin 0 blades for the smaller species and large-animal long-bladed laryngoscopes for deer and beavers can help.

If intubation is not possible, then either a tight-fitting face mask connected to an anaesthetic circuit may be applied with a high flow rate of oxygen (4–5 L/minute), or an Ambu bag used to force ventilate, although this may result in air being pushed into the stomach, which can impede inspiration particularly in lagomorphs and many rodents (see Figure 30.5).

In deer, breathing rates of 10 breaths per minute with a tidal volume of 10 mL/kg have been suggested (Newhard *et al.*, 2021).

In birds, an air sac tube may be placed should the trachea become blocked (see Chapter 16 for further information).

Puncture of the thorax is often associated with secondary infection due to a bite wound (common in smaller species) or a goring or other traumatic incident (common in deer). In all cases the prognosis is poor as clostridial or anaerobic infection is often present by the time the animal becomes clinically affected by it and presented for examination. Pyothorax and severe systemic sepsis may be present and euthanasia should be considered. In the acute cases, repair of the chest wall injury under anaesthesia and drainage via simple three-way tap and syringe or, for more severe injuries in a compliant species such as hedgehogs, a water trap drain for pneumothorax or active suction for pleural effusion may be adopted similar to domestic species.

C for cardiovascular

In mammals weighing less than 10 kg, direct cardiac massage by compressing the chest directly over the heart is most effective at increasing thoracic pressure and forcing blood through the arterial vasculature (Henrik, 1992). Heart compression rates of 100 beats per minute need to be achieved in most rodents, hedgehogs and lagomorphs; the technique recommended to maximise cardiovascular output is circumferential chest compression, as is used in human infants, where the chest is compressed over the heart from both sides at once (Costello, 2004). Even in deer, the recommendation is chest compressions from both sides of the heart, at a rate of 100 compressions per minute for a cycle of continuous compressions for 2 minutes with a pause of around 5 seconds before again commencing 100 compressions per minute for a further 2 minutes (Newhard *et al.*, 2021).

D for drugs

Relatively few data are available on emergency drug usage in wild animals but broad principles apply. Table 30.2 lists some typical emergency drugs used in wild mammals (see also Chapter 16 for birds).

Table 30.2 Some commonly used emergency drugs in wildlife mammal patients.

Drug	Dosage	Notes
Adrenaline (1 : 1000 = 1 mg/mL formulation)	0.01 mg/kg IC 0.01–0.1 mg/kg IV, IT, IO	Dilute to 1 : 10 000 before IV or IC use
Atropine	0.05–0.2 mg/kg IV, SC	Used where bradycardia detected. May not be effective in some species, e.g. lagomorphs due to atropinesterases in their serum; consider using glycopyrrolate instead 0.15–0.5 mg/kg IV has been used for organophosphate toxicity
Calcium gluconate	10–11 mg/kg IV	Suspected or confirmed hypocalcaemia or as a cardioprotectant where hyperkalaemia is diagnosed
Diazepam	0.3–1 mg/kg IV, IM 0.5–1 mg/kg rectally (mammals)	Higher dosages where seizuring occurring. Lower dosages may be used to facilitate handling in herbivorous species in particular
Furosemide	0.5–1 mg/kg IV	Congestive heart failure (left-sided)
Glycopyrrolate	0.01 mg/kg IV 0.02–0.1 mg/kg SC, IM	Used in herbivores in particular where atropinesterases are present or suspected
Intravenous lipid emulsion therapy	1.5 mL/kg of a 20% solution over 1 minute IV; followed by a continuous rate infusion 0.25 mL/kg per minute for next 30–60 minutes	Used where toxicity suspected, such as consumption or administration of ivermectin, permethrins, organophosphates, pentobarbitone, etc.
Lidocaine	1–2 mg/kg IV 2–4 mg/kg IT	Used for supraventricular tachycardia. Do not use where heart block and bradycardia is present
Midazolam	0.5–2 mg/kg IV, IM	Higher dosages where seizuring occurring.

IC, intracardiac; IM, intramuscularly; IO, intraosseously; IT, intratracheally; IV, intravenously.

Poisoning

A number of cases of oral poisoning can be seen in wildlife. Some basic principles apply to managing these such as the following.

1. Reduce the amount of poison that can be further absorbed either by inducing vomition with apomorphine (not in the case of suspected alkali or acid poisons where stomach wash may be preferable) or by preventing further absorption (by the use of gastrointestinal adsorbents such as activated charcoal; or in clostridial cases colestyramine; or in diquat and paraquat poisoning Fuller's earth [bentonite clay]; or the use of intravenous lipid emulsion therapy, see below), or by simply physically removing the toxin (as in oil-contaminated animals).
2. Manage the clinical effects of the poison.
3. Administer antidotes to poisons where they are available.

Further information about avian lead and oil poisons can be found in Chapters 14 and 16. Specific antidotes to other poisons include the following.

1. *Coumerol- and warfarin-related rodenticides*: vitamin K_1 can be used at 2.5–5 mg/kg subcutaneously every 6–12 hours for the first week, then orally at 1–2.5 mg/kg for a further 1–3 weeks depending on the pesticide formulation.
2. *Organophosphates and carbamates*: pralidoxime 10–20 mg/kg intramuscularly can be used but only if it is given within 24 hours of consumption/exposure which is unlikely and only where organophosphate (not carbamate) toxicity occurs. Atropine sulphate 0.2–0.5 mg/kg IM/SC every 3–6 hours can be given in both cases.

Intravenous lipid emulsion therapy is used in domestic dogs and cats where suspected lipophilic drug toxicity has been diagnosed, such as ivermectin or permethrin poisoning. In wild mammals it may be used in similar situations and has even been used in marine turtles affected by algal toxins such as brevetoxicosis and birds where oral consumption of rodenticides and pentobarbitone has occurred (Perrault *et al.*, 2021; Schmidt *et al.*, 2023).

E for ECG

Principles for wild mammals are similar to those for domestic species. ECG traces can help confirm heart rates and potentially identify the causes of arrhythmias. Heart block is commonly seen in birds and small species of mammal, particularly herbivores. Myocardial hypoxia is often reflected with a change in polarity of the T wave on lead II during anaesthesia. Lead placement for mammals is similar to that in cats and dogs. Lead placement in wild birds is similar to captive ones, the forelimb leads typically being applied to the propatagium and the hindlimb leads applied to either the fold of skin from thigh to body wall or to the foot. Sticky pads are preferred for attachment as alligator clips can cause skin trauma.

Monitoring of cardiopulmonary resuscitation responses

Capnography

End tidal CO_2 ($ETCO_2$) levels measured by capnography may be used to monitor cardiac output during cardiopulmonary resuscitation (CPR). A steady increase in $ETCO_2$ is more likely to be associated with a successful outcome; conversely, if the $ETCO_2$ does not increase above 10 mmHg after a resuscitation time of

15–20 minutes, then resuscitation is unlikely to be successful (Marino, 1997). In dogs and cats, the RECOVER guidelines suggest that an $ETCO_2$ of 15 mmHg or more is indicative of good CPR responses (Fletcher *et al.*, 2012). Use of the capnograph requires that the patient be intubated.

Blood pressure

Blood pressure can be measured in a non-invasive manner using techniques similar to those used in domestic cats. A cuff (width 40% circumference of the limb applied to) is placed proximal to the elbow. The plantar carpal area is clipped and a Doppler probe attached. The cuff is inflated until the pulse is cut off and then deflated. The pressure is noted when the pulse returns (this is the systolic pressure). Usually five readings are taken and the average recorded. Normal mammalian blood pressures ranges from 90 to 120 mmHg (although there are outliers such as the Eurasian beaver whose systolic blood pressure may be as low as 60 mmHg; see Figure 30.5). Systolic pressures less than 80 mmHg are considered significantly hypovolaemic in felids, canids, lagomorphs, mustelids, deer, etc. and anything less than 90 mmHg will likely require intravenous or intraosseous fluid therapy. Invasive blood pressure methods may be applied using an artery such as the central ear artery in lagomorphs and deer, dorsal pedal or branch of the radial artery in canids, felids and larger mustelids or the carotid artery in smaller species. The central ear artery can result in kinking of the vessel and erroneous results as well as potential damage to the artery and ear tip sloughing.

Mucous membrane colour should be assessed where possible; the lining of the mouth or the anus are the two best sites in small mammals. Rectal temperature may also give an indication of peripheral perfusion.

Critical care blood analysis

Blood gas analysis and electrolyte assessment is also an important aspect of monitoring the emergency case and wildlife patients are no different. Arterial sampling is preferred and the central ear artery is the vessel of choice. Point-of-care analysers such as the i-STAT® 1 Analyser (Abbott) and epoc® Blood Analysis System (Siemens) are commonly used. Whilst little has been published about normal blood gases, acid–base balance and metabolite levels in wildlife species, some broad principles apply. For example some very general assumptions can be made.

1. For the majority of species considered here, the blood pH of a healthy individual should be somewhere between 7.4 and 7.5.
2. Arterial PO_2 should be between 75 and 110 mmHg and PCO_2 between 30 and 40 mmHg.
3. Bicarbonate levels are usually between 18 and 27 mmol/L.
4. Plasma sodium levels are usually between 135 and 145 mmol/L and potassium between 3 and 5.5 mmol/L.
5. Glucose levels are between 2.5 and 6 mmol/L.
6. Haematocrit (packed cell volume) is usually between 27 and 45%.

Most trauma cases will present with acidosis (i.e. arterial pH <7.4) and many will be hypoxic or hypercapnic and some may be hypoglycaemic. Low levels of sodium (<129/130 mmol/L) are known to be associated with poor survivability in species such as rabbits, dogs and humans assuming no other pseudohyponatraemic conditions are present (such as hyperproteinaemia) or hyperglycaemia that will draw water into the bloodstream and so falsely reduce sodium levels (Bonvehi *et al.*, 2014; Burton and Hopper, 2019). In wildlife, in my experience, most hyponatraemic animals are also hypovolaemic, having lost fluid and sodium through gastrointestinal tract disease or haemorrhage.

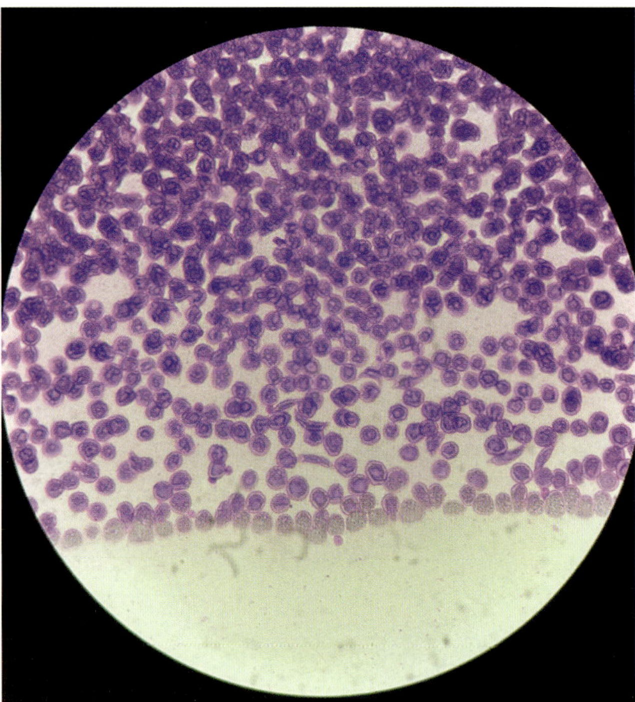

Figure 30.6 Blood smear from a deer showing sickling of some erythrocytes which is normal in cervids.

A blood smear can also be useful as a rapid test to assess for polychromasia, anisocytosis, blood parasites and an inflammatory response (left shift neutrophilia or monocytosis). However, some species variations are seen which are actually normal (see Figure 30.6).

Pulse assessment

Pulse assessment is a basic test but in experienced hands can provide a rapid interpretation of blood pressure, heart–pulse mismatches (so-called dropped beats) and peripheral circulation. Femoral pulses are commonly used in smaller mammalian species. The pulses of larger species may be detected on vessels at the angle of the jaw (maxillary artery in deer for example).

Cardiac and respiratory auscultation

The position of the heart in the thorax in wild mammals has similarities to many domestic ones. For example, wildcat anatomy is broadly similar to that of the domestic cat, and cardiac position in polecat, weasel and stoat is similar to that in the domestic ferret. Heart size varies considerably with larger species of deer, although having a large heart can ironically sometimes make locating it with a stethoscope more tricky than in a smaller species such as a rabbit, where the diaphragm of the stethoscope covers most of the chest and so by default the heart. In most cases heart location is caudodorsal to the elbow area between ribs 4 and 6. Cardiac murmurs may be normal for certain species, for example wildcats and beavers, so critical evaluation with additional modalities such as echocardiography may be required to elucidate whether the murmur is pathological or not.

However, it is important to listen thoroughly across the whole of both sides of the chest for evidence of respiratory sounds (absence, as with domestic animals, may indicate pneumothorax) and abnormal respiratory sounds (crackles, wheezes, whistles, etc.).

Neurological assessment

An assessment of the animal as to whether it is in control of all limbs and responding appropriately to its environment is critical before treatment begins and certainly before release back to the wild is considered. Prey species may conceal illness and disease and so not clearly demonstrate their neurological or other disease states. Some animals may present with severe neurological conditions, although they may be difficult to separate from musculoskeletal problems (fractures, muscle rupture) and so further imaging tests may be necessary. Some species (e.g. bats) may be susceptible to neurological diseases (e.g. lyssaviruses) which may cause them to behave differently and this needs to be taken into account when assessing the individual. Other species are more likely to be affected by chemicals that can affect the central nervous system such as deer, lagomorphs, rodents, insectivores and birds (e.g. organophosphates in sheep dips; lead consumption in waterfowl and raptors; diquat and paraquat poisoning in hedgehogs and carbamate insecticides in a wide range of species).

Pulse oximetry

Pulse oximeters can be useful to assess blood oxygen saturation but it should be noted that they are not calibrated to the species considered here, therefore absolute values may be misleading. Trends however can be helpful when assessing response to resuscitation.

Monitoring and treatment of acute hypovolaemia

For routine fluid maintenance and dehydration corrections please see Chapter 29. Shock is something commonly seen in birds and mammals following severe trauma or infection. Many species are presented in decompensatory shock, either because they do not experience a significant phase of compensatory shock (e.g. mustelids, wildcats, lagomorphs, many birds) or because they are often presented later in the course of the condition. This means such patients are hypovolaemic, bradycardic, hypothermic and sometimes hypoglycaemic as well.

Keeping the patient warm and ideally within its normal expected body temperature range is important as adrenergic receptors will not respond well to fluid therapy if the patient is hypothermic (Lichtenberger, 2007). One study suggested that hypothermic rabbits on admission were three times more likely to die, with the odds of death doubled for each decrease of 1°C below the references range (37.9–39.9°C) (Di Girolamo *et al.*, 2016).

Fluids should therefore be warmed to close to or at expected body temperature before administration and heat mats, hot hands, hot air circulating blankets, etc., used. If hypovolaemic, a slow intravenous bolus of fluids such as hypertonic saline (7.2–7.5%) at 3 mL/kg to draw fluid rapidly into the circulation can be used (Lichtenberger and Lennox, 2010). This can be maintained by follow-up administration of a colloid (3 mL/kg) over 10 minutes but care should be taken not to use a colloid where there is ongoing bleeding or renal failure. The patient should be warmed plus isotonic crystalloids at 3–4 mL/kg per hour administered. It is important to measure systolic blood pressure during this procedure (see section Monitoring of cardiopulmonary resuscitation responses). Once the patient has been warmed, the aim is to get the systolic blood pressure above 90 mmHg. This may require further boluses of isotonic crystalloids (10 mL/kg) with a colloid (5 mL/kg). Once normovolaemia has been achieved, replacement of fluid deficits may be started (see Chapter 29).

Alternatively, if hypotensive with a systolic blood pressure below 90 mmHg, a dopamine drip may be used at 10 µg/kg per minute to rapidly increase. Do not use this in species that naturally have low blood pressures (e.g. beavers, reptiles, amphibians) or those whose systolic blood pressure is above 90 mmHg.

Calculation of fluid requirements for wildlife patients

See Chapter 29 for fluid therapy and blood transfusions in wildlife patients.

Supportive therapy

Environmental temperature needs are one area of supportive therapy that should be considered in the wildlife patient. Thermoneutral zones (i.e. where a normothermic animal can maintain its body temperature without shivering or other activities to raise its temperature) for wildlife have been quoted as 15–25°C for birds over 0.5 kg; 22–35°C for birds less than 0.5 kg; 15–24°C for mammals; 22–30°C for UK reptiles; and 15–30°C for UK amphibians (Mullineaux and Keeble, 2017). As noted above, if the patient is hypothermic, then fluid therapy is unlikely to have significant positive effects on blood pressure and organ perfusion.

Ongoing medication

As with all animals, adequate analgesia is essential where trauma or significant disease is seen. Non-steroidal anti-inflammatory drugs (NSAIDs) are commonly used and are appropriate in many cases but care should of course be used where renal disease or gastric ulceration is suspected. Opiates may commonly be used but may in some cases have depressive effects on respiration and cause gut hypomotility and so similar principles used in domestic animals should be applied. Corticosteroids have been historically used in shock cases and their effects have sometimes been positive but many feel that their use in wildlife cases is now less appropriate due to the risks of immunosuppression and the fact that NSAIDs cannot also be used in conjunction (Mullineaux and Keeble, 2017).

Use of antimicrobials is likely in many wildlife cases with wounds or severe debilitation. Birds are prone to aspergillosis and cat bites in birds and mammals are commonly infected with anaerobes and *Pasteurella* spp. Hedgehogs may have underlying lungworm with secondary *Bordetella bronchiseptica* infections necessitating the use of potentiated amoxicillin. Careful selection of antimicrobial drugs is increasingly important with the growing resistance seen and campaigns for good antimicrobial stewardship. Ideally, culture and sensitivity testing, where possible, should be carried out prior to antimicrobial usage; however, some cases are more acute and may need medication before test results are available.

Critical care nutrition including calculation of energy requirements

Little has been published on specific nutritional energy requirements for UK native species wildlife. However, some broad principles can be assumed and extrapolation from domestic animals may help. The basal maintenance requirement (BMR, sometimes referred to as the resting energy requirement, RER) can be calculated using the following formula:

$$\mathrm{BMR} = k \times \left[\mathrm{weight}\left(\mathrm{kg}\right)\right]^{0.75}$$

where k is a factor that varies according to species. Where data for a specific species do not exist, then there are some broad principles that can be applied and k has been assumed to be 70 for placental mammals, 78 for a non-passerine bird and 129 for a passerine bird. When an animal is sick, the BMR/RER can be multiplied by a factor of approximately 1.5 to achieve the maintenance energy requirements, or even higher if the patient has significant wounds, is growing/juvenile or has significant sepsis.

A number of commercially available critical care foods have been developed relevant to domestic animals and wildlife which may be used. See Chapters 4, 8, 12, 16, 20 and 24 for further relevant details.

Nursing of wounds, assisted feeding techniques and foods

Nursing of wounds

Types of wound

A number of differing types of wounds are commonly seen in wildlife cases. The majority are associated with interspecific or intraspecific fighting and road traffic collisions. Domestic dog attacks are not uncommon (see Figure 30.7). Many are therefore grossly contaminated wounds and by the time they are presented for treatment some are seriously infected. Added complications can be open fractures and secondary blowfly strike.

Occasionally burns, either chemical or heat associated, may be seen. Finally some wounds can be associated with avascular necrosis and these can include frostbite and of course ligatures associated with plastic netting, fences and in some instances snares.

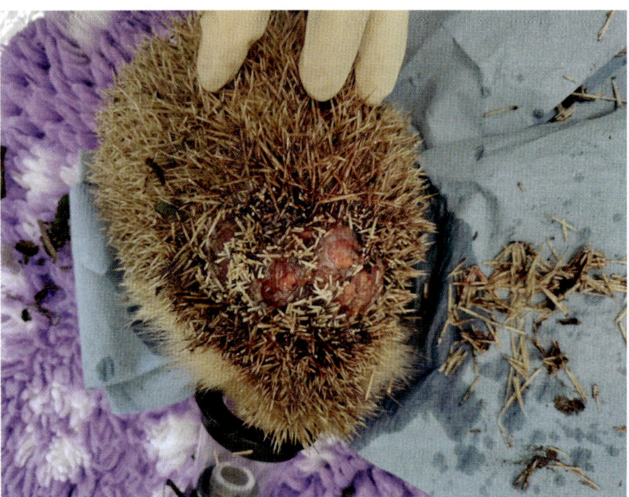

Figure 30.7 Dog attacks on hedgehogs are not uncommon and result in significant wounds often contaminated with bacteria. *Source:* Courtesy of Kelly Huitson RVN.

Initial management

Initial management should be to stabilise the patient in shock with fluid therapy, prevent bleeding and provide adequate analgesia and, if required, antimicrobial medication. Wounds may be protected in the short term using aqueous wound gels to prevent desiccation.

Once stabilised, wound management should be started, likely requiring anaesthesia of the patient. Fur and feathers around the wound can be carefully removed prior to removing the aqueous gel. Feathers are best plucked rather than cut as plucking results in their rapid replacement. The process of plucking is painful to the bird and so should always be performed under anaesthesia and care should be taken not to tear the skin in the process.

This can be followed by thorough flushing of the wound to remove gross contamination and dead tissue using techniques familiar to domestic animal medicine. Typically, flushing with isotonic fluids such as lactated Ringer's in a 60-mL syringe attached to a 19 gauge needle provides the correct force to remove debris without significantly damaging fibroblasts. Be aware that skin disinfectants are generally not helpful with open wounds, causing cellular damage and in some cases may be toxic (e.g. many birds and reptiles can have an adverse reaction to chlorhexidine). Any necrotic tissue should be thoroughly debrided under anaesthesia and a realistic assessment made of the extent of functional damage which is likely to impact the animal's release. It may be better to euthanase an animal at this stage if the damage to tissues is so severe that release is unlikely to be successful or retention of the animal in captivity is likely to be prolonged. Clearly this also depends on the species as some cope with confinement better than others. Cases of blowfly strike can be particularly challenging to manage as all larvae/maggots and eggs need to be removed and the wound's depth thoroughly assessed; if it penetrates a body cavity, euthanasia should be performed.

Fracture stabilisation

Any long bone fractures in birds and mammals will require some form of emergency stabilisation to prevent excessive soft tissue trauma and pain.

Birds

Wing fractures in birds can be managed for the first couple of days using figure-of-eight bandages and temporary splints as described in Chapter 14. A simple circular body bandage to tie the wing to the chest wall is most appropriate for a humeral fracture. Figure-of-eight bandages are more appropriate for suspected radius and ulna fractures. Simple tape applied to the primary feathers can be used to stabilise carpal and metacarpal fractures. All of these fractures will need to have a more rigorous fixation process applied once the bird is stabilised (an overview can be found in Chapter 14).

Leg fractures in birds may also require stabilisation. Tibiotarsal and tarsometatarsal fractures may be stabilised using finger splints or gutter splints with bandaging in the larger species and simple zinc oxide tape (so-called 'Altman splint') in small passerines. Femoral fractures are often splinted by the muscle mass and so, providing the bird does not move the limb too much, no further temporary support is given, although surgical fixation will be required.

Mammals

Limb fractures in mammals may require support using aluminium finger splints, gutter splints and Robert Jones bandages; in the smaller species simple bandage material with smaller splints such as paper-clips or cotton buds can be used. In deer, Velpeau slings for forelimb fractures and Ehmer slings for hindlimb fractures have been described as temporary stabilisation techniques (Stocker, 2009). A peculiar phenomenon can be seen in male deer with a severely damaged forelimb, particularly where amputation or part amputation occurs, whereby the next season's antler growth on the contralateral side of the body is often abnormal and may result in an ingrowing antler that causes eye or skull damage (Antony-Davis, 1983).

Pelvic fractures may be particularly problematic as they take considerable time (4–6 weeks) to heal and in female animals may significantly reduce the diameter of the pelvic canal and so may lead to dystocia in the future.

Jaw fractures are common particularly in mammals involved in road traffic collisions. Surgical options used in domestic dogs and cats can be applied to wild mammals, whether wiring or plating or using epoxy splints glued to teeth. All should be removed once the jaw has healed and prior to release, and again consideration should be given to how quickly the patient can resume mastication of food postoperatively before the process is attempted.

Where any metal implants are used, such as plates, screws and intramedullary pins, these should be removed from the patient prior to release.

Euthanasia

Euthanasia, as mentioned throughout this chapter, is an important consideration to prevent suffering and should be actively considered in any wildlife case where the prospects of a quick and full recovery and release are not possible. In a veterinary clinic it is always preferable to euthanase an animal through anaesthetic overdose, not just because this will be more familiar to veterinary staff and is available, but also because it is likely to result in a more rapid and less stressful process to remove suffering than a physical method. In small rodents, small mustelids and birds, inhalation anaesthesia in an induction chamber or, if safe to restrain, via face mask using isoflurane or sevoflurane will render the animal unconscious. To then euthanase, pentobarbitone is injected intravenously, intraosseously or, if these routes are not available, intraperitoneally in mammals. For larger mammals, injectable anaesthesia using drugs such as those described in Chapter 27 followed by pentobarbitone injection intravenously is recommended.

Physical methods are legally permitted for wildlife seriously injured and suffering and where chemical means are not readily available such as in a field situation. For most small avian patients, cervical dislocation is straightforward. For lagomorphs, rodents and larger bird species, cervical dislocation may be performed but is more difficult and should only be carried out by someone experienced in the technique. Captive bolts, firearms and shotguns can of course be used for larger species where the marksman is correctly licensed and has permission to use the weapon safely on that land, but care should be taken to ensure the correct gauge of shot/bullet is used appropriate to the size of the wild animal.

References

Antony-Davis (1983) Antler asy'mmetry caused by limb amputation and geo-physical forces. In: *Antler Development in Cervidae* (ed. R.D. Brown), pp. 223–230. Caeser Kleberg Wildlife Research Institute.

Best, D. and Mullineaux, E. (2003) Basic principles of treating wildlife casualties. In: *BSAVA Manual of Wildlife Casualties* (eds E. Mullineaux, D. Best & J.E. Cooper), pp. 6–28. BSAVA, Quedgeley, Glos.

Bonvehi, C., Ardiaca, M., Barrera, S. *et al.* (2014) Prevalence and types of hyponatraemia, its relationship with hyperglycaemia and mortality in ill rabbits. *Veterinary Record*, **174**(22), 554.

Burton, A.G. and Hopper, K. (2019) Hyponatremia in dogs and cats. *Journal of Veterinary Emergency and Critical Care*, **29**, 461–471.

Costello, M.F. (2004) Principles of cardiopulmonary cerebral resuscitation in special species. *Seminars in Avian and Exotic Pet Medicine*, **13**(3), 132–141.

Di Girolamo, N., Toth, G. and Selleri, P. (2016) Prognostic value of rectal temperature at hospital admission in client-owned rabbits. *Journal of the American Veterinary Medical Association*, **248**(3), 288–297.

Fletcher, D.J., Boller, M., Brainard, B.M. *et al.* (2012) RECOVER evidence and knowledge gap analysis on veterinary CPR part 7. Clinical guidelines. *Journal of Veterinary Emergency and Critical Care*, **22**(Suppl. 1), S102–S131. doi: 10.1111/j.1476-4431.2012.00757.x.

Henrik, R.A. (1992) Basic life support and external cardiac compression in dogs and cats. *Journal of the American Veterinary Medical Association*, **200**, 1925–1931.

Lichtenberger, M. (2007) Shock and CPCR in small mammals and birds. *Veterinary Clinics of North America: Exotic Animal Practice*, **10**(2), 275–291.

Lichtenberger, M. and Lennox, A. (2010) Updates and advanced therapies for gastrointestinal stasis in rabbits. *Veterinary Clinics of North America: Exotic Animal Practice*, **13**(3), 525–542.

Marino, P.R. (1997) Cardiac arrest. In: *The ICU Book* (ed. P.L. Marino), pp. 260–298. Lippincott Williams and Williams, Philadelphia.

Mullineaux, E. and Keeble, E. (2017). In: *BSAVA Manual of Wildlife Casualties* (eds E. Mullineaux & E. Keeble), 2nd edn, pp. 37–55. BSAVA Quedgeley, Glos.

Newhard, D.K., Bayne, J.E. and Passler, T. (2021) Diseases of the cardiovascular system. In: *Sheep, Goat and Cervid Medicine* (eds D.G. Pugh, A.N. Baird, M.A. Edmondson & T. Passler), 3rd edn, pp. 439–460. Elsevier, Edinburgh.

Perrault, J.R., Barron, H.W., Malinowski, C.R. *et al.* (2021) Use of intravenous lipid emulsion therapy as a novel treatment for brevetoxicosis in sea turtles. *Scientific Reports*, **11**, 24162.

Schmidt, L.K., Keller, K.A., Tonozzi, C. *et al.* (2023) Intralipid emulsion therapy for the treatment of suspected toxicity in 2 avian species. *Journal of Avian Medicine and Surgery*, **36**(4), 394–399.

Stocker, L. (2009) Deer. In: *Practical Wildlife Care*, 2nd edn, pp. 253–267. Wiley.

Chapter 31 Wildlife Rehabilitation and Release Considerations

Welfare and ethics of animal releases

In my opinion and currently the way the UK animal welfare legislation is formulated the decision on whether to attempt treatment or to euthanase an animal on humane grounds should always focus on the individual animal's welfare. Other considerations may also play a part in this, such as the welfare of the animal's offspring, the rarity of the species and the impact its demise has on the ecosystem it derives from, but the individual animal's experience of welfare should *always* be taken first.

Any wild animal that is taken into captivity should immediately receive a hypercritical assessment of its chances of full recovery. The ultimate goal of any rehabilitation procedure is to return that animal to the wild. The animal should therefore be in as fit a state as possible to ensure its survival in the wild, in terms of its ability to feed itself, avoid predators and to compete with conspecifics.

Care should also be taken not to introduce novel infections into the ecosystem via the introduction of an otherwise healthy animal and to avoid overloading an environment with animals that do not have a sufficient local food source to maintain them.

There is also a wider philosophical aspect to rehabilitating every injured or sick individual wild animal as we are perhaps interfering with natural selection and so falsely selecting potentially weaker and less 'fit' animals. This could over time result in a weakening of the genetic make-up of the species. Clearly, however, day-to-day human impact on wild animal disease and debilitation may counteract this philosophical view and drive a more ethical imperative to preserve wild animals wherever we can.

Release considerations

Legality of release

This can be fraught with complications. It is important to understand the legislation that applies to the species and location where a proposed release is to occur. Perhaps the most important legislation in the UK regarding wild animals releases are the Wildlife and Countryside Act (WCA) 1981 and the various pieces of legislation applying to invasive non-native species. These outline what species can be released and what cannot (see Figures 31.1–31.3). Other pieces of legislation, such as the Animal Health Act and those applying to the control of bovine tuberculosis, may prohibit the release of certain species such as the badger in certain areas. Release of birds may be prevented during periods of increased avian influenza outbreaks. Finally, no animal that is not fit for release should be released into the wild as this is an offence under the Animal Welfare Act 2006 and Animal Health and Welfare (Scotland) Act 2006. Further advice can be found through the British Wildlife Rehabilitation Council, Natural England, NatureScot, DEFRA and the Welsh Government websites and an overview can be found in Appendix 2.

Release site

Rehabilitated adult animals should be released within the animal's normal home range, or within 10 miles (16 km) from the point of capture, when possible and reasonable. This practice minimises the spread of diseases, and genetic material, among wild populations and maximises the animal's chance of survival. Exact release location and time should be chosen at the discretion of the rehabilitator, based on the appropriateness of the habitat and the condition of the animal. Adult mammals are generally best released as close to the spot where they were found as possible in order to minimise territorial conflicts and maximise their chances of finding a suitable food source. When circumstances allow, rehabilitated adult birds should be released in a suitable habitat as close as possible to the point of their capture except during migration. If migration has occurred while the bird has been in captivity, the bird should be released in the area of the migratory destination (see Figures 31.4 and 31.5). Studies have shown that rehabilitated reptiles and amphibians should be released within half a mile (0.8 km) of the point of capture to maximise their chance of survival.

Juvenile animals, especially those that were brought into rehabilitation as infants, do not have to be released at the site of capture to ensure survival; however, efforts should still be made to release these animals within 10 miles (16 km) of the capture site, if possible. If not possible to release at the same site, then an assessment of the habitat should be made to assure adequate food source, hides and water source and absence of significant predators (see Figure 31.6).

The area where an animal is released clearly needs to be safe and permission to release may need to be sought from the landowner and, depending on the species, potentially governmental bodies. Some species are considered non-native and their release is prohibited and this should be taken into consideration before attempts to treat the animal are made (see Appendix 2).

Pre-release conditioning

Prior to release for animals that have been in captivity for a period longer than a few days, it may be helpful, if available, to provide larger appropriate outdoor housing that allows an assessment of the animal's

Veterinary Nursing of Exotic Pets and Wildlife, Third Edition. Simon J. Girling.

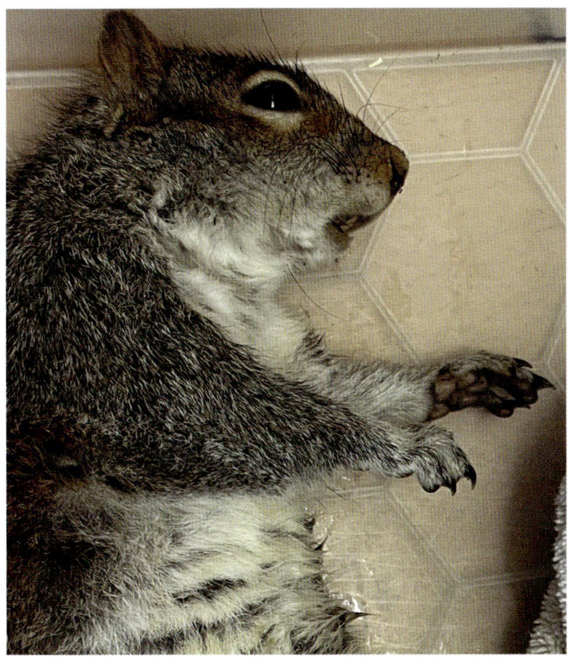

Figure 31.1 Grey squirrels (*Sciurus carolinensis*), while common in the UK since the 1930s and previously able to be released under licence in certain areas, are currently not able to be released in the UK (or European Union) due to recent changes in invasive non-native species legislation.

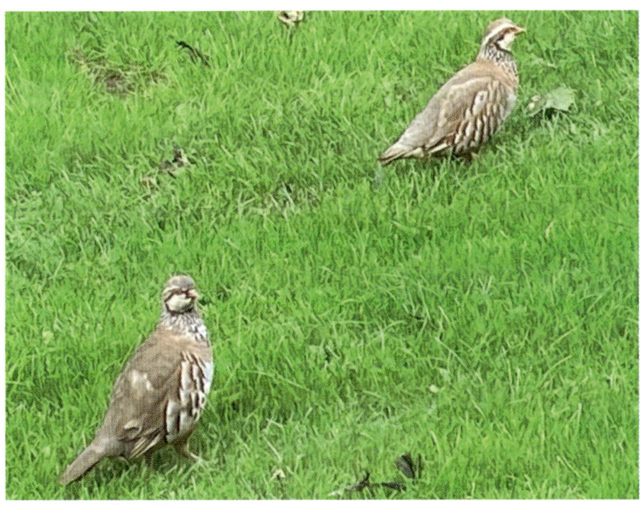

Figure 31.2 Although non-native, red-legged partridge (*Alectoris rufa*) are allowed to be released in the UK providing certain general licensing conditions are met, as they are a game bird.

mobility and behaviours. For birds this may include moving them to a flighted aviary to allow them to build up flight muscle strength as well as allowing an assessment of their flight capabilities. For waterfowl, provision of a pond to allow an assessment of waterproofing is important.

The health of the animal should be monitored, including weight and general condition. Provision of appropriate nutrition should continue while introducing a more natural diet in the lead up to release. Any medical issues should be evaluated and treated and, if severe, the prospect of release abandoned.

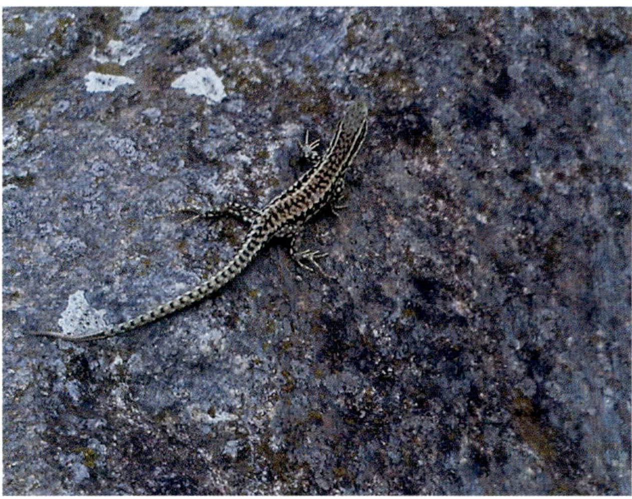

Figure 31.3 Non-native species such as this wall lizard (*Podarcis muralis*) are found in several sites, mainly in southern England. While not specifically listed in the invasive non-native species legislation, they are covered by a blanket ban on the release of non-native species under the WCA.

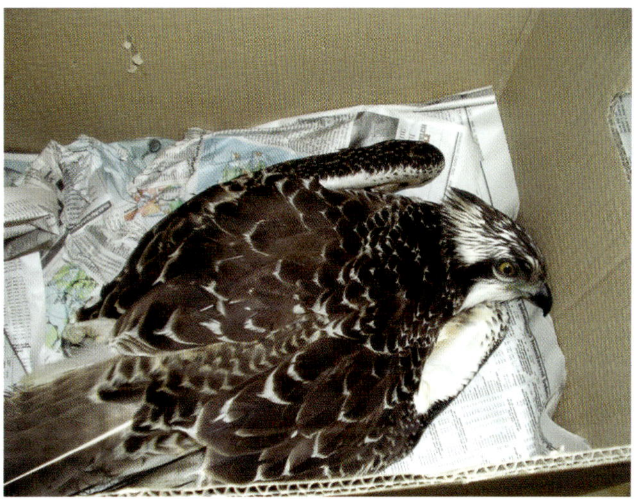

Figure 31.4 Ospreys are a migratory species and so when considering release the bird should be released at the migratory destination appropriate for the time of year.

Pre-release evaluation

It is important that the animal's ability to self-feed is assessed. Normal mobility and function, reasonable level of physical fitness and stamina necessary for foraging, breeding, or territory defensive behaviour should all be reviewed.

Clearly there should be no evidence of disease, and the weight of the animal optimal for the species, age, sex and time of year (see Figures 31.7 and 31.8). In many cases additional testing such as radiography, haematology and biochemistry may need to be performed to ensure the animal is as healthy as possible.

The minimum standards for wildlife rehabilitation (Miller, 2012) suggest that the following criteria are met before the release of an animal.

1. Have a full recovery from the original injury or from injuries incurred while in care.
2. Be no longer in need of medical care.

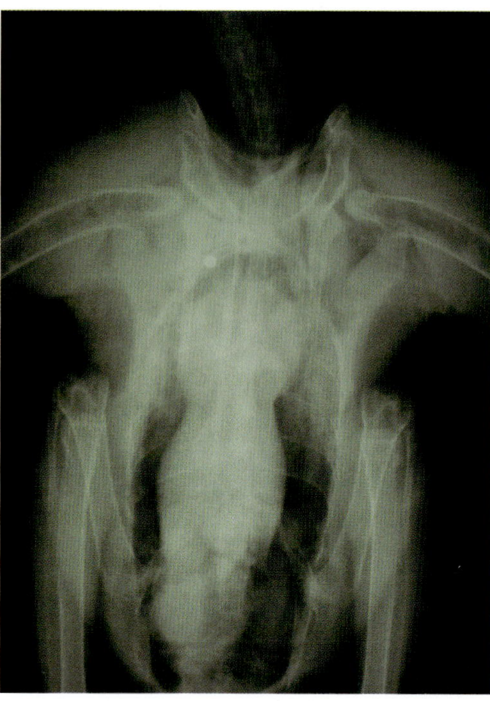

Figure 31.5 Radiograph of the osprey in Figure 31.4 with evidence of lead shot pellet associated with its collapse and presentation, highlighting the importance of a thorough examination before attempting to release a wild animal.

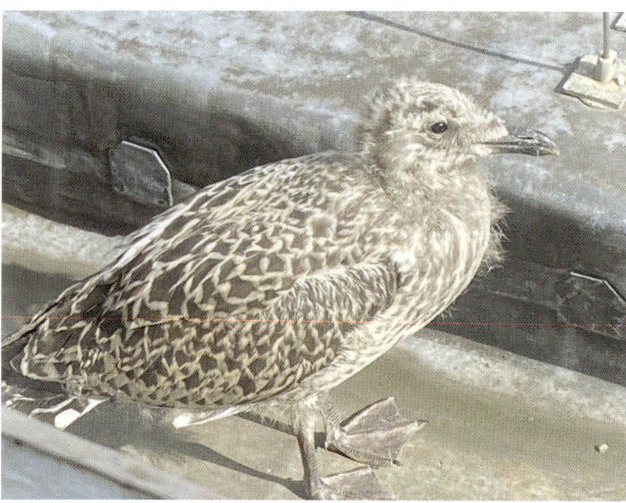

Figure 31.6 Juvenile birds and mammals should be released ideally at the site of capture but can be released elsewhere if a habitat assessment has been made and permissions gained.

3. Exhibit no signs of active disease.
4. Have normal biochemical and haematological values for the species.
5. Possess pelage or plumage that is adequate for that species to survive, including exhibiting waterproofing sufficient for that species.
6. Possess adequate vision to find/catch food and manoeuvre in a normal manner.
7. Exhibit locomotive skills necessary for that species to survive.
8. Demonstrate the fight or flight behavioural response.

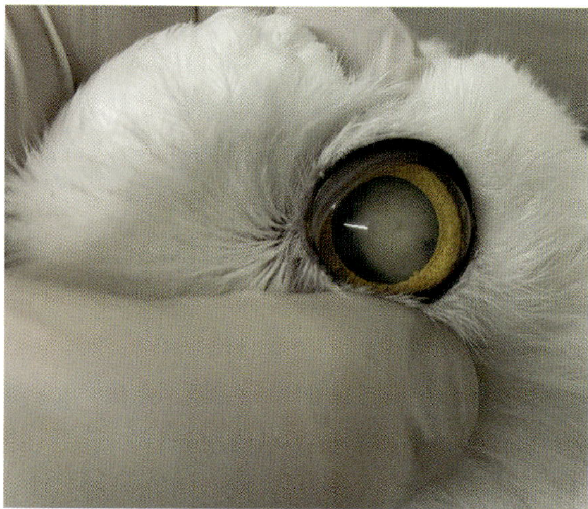

Figure 31.7 Pre-release assessment should always be critical of their abilities to hunt and fend for themselves. A mature cataract in this owl makes it unlikely that it will be able to catch prey successfully post release.

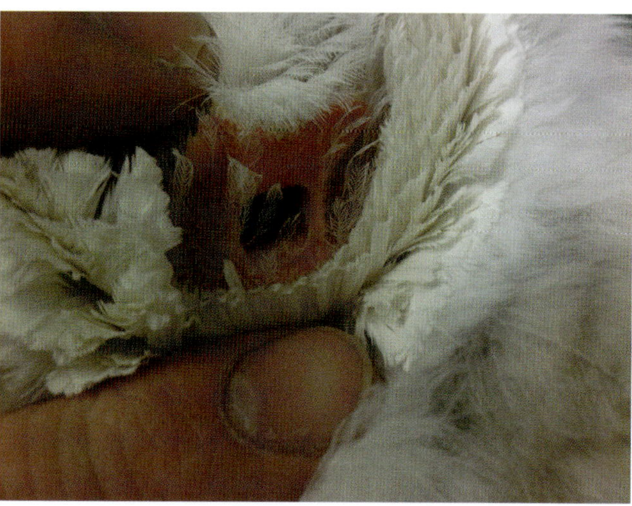

Figure 31.8 Pre-release assessment should be thorough and include a full body examination. The ear canal of owls is large and on its cranial edge runs around the eye socket so it is useful to examine not only for ear disease, but in case of head trauma, bleeding in the ear canal suggests a skull fracture and likely ocular damage.

9. Demonstrate proper foraging behaviour (self-feeding if raised in captivity).
10. Demonstrate proper species behaviour (e.g. not improperly imprinted).
11. Be of correct age for independent survival.
12. Be of correct weight for that sex, species, age and season.

Other pre-release testing may include screening for specific diseases. For example, in badgers in the UK, three separate serological tests for the presence of antibodies to bovine tuberculosis with negative results has been advocated prior to their release (Ashford *et al.*, 2020; Mullineaux, 2024). Pre-release faecal parasitology may also be advisable to ensure that the patient does not have a high parasite burden that may affect its survival and also to check for novel parasites that may be inadvertently released into the environment (see IUCN best practice guidelines below).

Finally, an assessment of the animal's behaviour should be made. This may be particularly difficult as not only does it depend on the rehabilitator knowing what is 'normal' for that species but in the artificial environment of captivity the animal may naturally fail to exhibit normal behaviours without there being a pathological reason. However, malprinting is one behaviour that may be seen, most commonly in young animals that have been hand reared. Attempts should always be made to limit human contact to a minimum when treating wildlife to prevent this. A lack of fear of humans is one of the more significant negative behaviours that this process can produce and which may then result in either animals becoming harmed or, less commonly, animals harming humans. In order to avoid malprinting, minimising human contact and time spent in rehabilitation are two important steps. If a young animal, its return to its parents or mixing with conspecifics of a similar age when safe to do so can also help reduce malprinting and the development of stereotypies such as tail and paw sucking in badger cubs. Rapid weaning of young animals to again minimise the time spent in captivity may also help prevent malprinting. In some cases exposing the young developing animal to familiar sounds can help, for example in passerines playing appropriate birdsong has been shown to be beneficial during the rehabilitation process (Spencer *et al.*, 2007).

Hard release

This is the most common form of release in wildlife rehabilitation practice. The release is immediate once the animal is deemed fit to do so. There is no support of the animal post release. Hard release is therefore best suited to adult animals, released back into the exact environment that they have previously come from, after a short period of captivity/treatment (see Figure 31.9).

Even though hard release requires minimal theoretical preparation to carry out, attention should still be paid to some key factors. The time of day the release occurs is important. For example, nocturnal species such as badgers should be released after dark. Diurnal species should be released early in the day to allow sufficient time to feed before nightfall. The weather will also influence the success of the release of an animal, as will the presence or absence of potential predators.

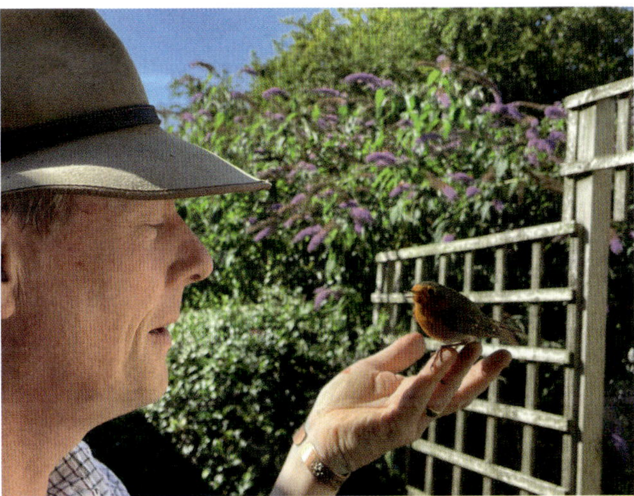

Figure 31.9 Hard release is best suited to adult animals released to the exact spot they were found after a short period of rehabilitation.

Soft release

This is less commonly performed as it is more labour intensive and inevitably complicated and costly. Release is not immediate but gradual. The animal is supported by additional feeding at the release site, which is carefully chosen to provide the resources necessary for the animal with minimal dangers and/or absence of predators. The release site may involve the use of shelters and a period of captivity at the release site to orientate the animal. An example would be release of a raptor into a new environment or as a young bird. It is also suited for release of groups of young similar-aged animals such as badger cubs. This technique is used in wildlife reintroduction projects and has been used successfully to introduce white-tailed sea eagles to eastern Scotland in 2007 by the Royal Society for the Protection of Birds (RSPB). Chicks were transferred under licence from the wild in Norway and then housed in aviaries at the release sites in Scotland. They were fed with minimal exposure to humans, within the aviaries which had a commanding view of the surrounding landscape to orientate the birds. Once fledged and sufficiently strong/healthy, the aviaries were opened but the birds fed at the site until the eagles dispersed. Radio transmitters were attached to the birds to track their movements post release.

Another reintroduction project (undertaken by the *Royal Zoological Society of Scotland)* utilised soft release of European wildcats which were bred in captivity with minimal human contact. Wildcats were released into the Cairngorms of Scotland successfully from pens built at the release site. Adult wildcats were held in the pens for a few days and fed. Once released, food was provided at the release site until the cat dispersed. Radio-transmitter collars were used to monitor the cats post release.

For rehabilitating some raptors, the use of lures and a creance (a fine line attached to a jess on the bird's leg) to prevent escape until the bird can demonstrate satisfactory hunting skills may be used. This tends to be uncommon, though, as it requires specialist training for the handlers/rehabilitators.

Post-release monitoring

As mentioned in the two examples above, this is more commonly carried out for soft release and reintroduction projects where money and resources are allocated as part of the process. However, some form of post-release monitoring as a kind of clinical audit is good practice even for hard-released animals. It does not necessarily require tracking equipment or other technology, but can be as simple as returning to the release site regularly after the release of the animal(s) or the use of camera traps to determine if there are, for example, field signs, mortalities and changes to the environment that can give a clue as to whether the release has been successful or not. The use of rings on the legs of birds is commonplace and depending on the ring type can sometimes allow identification of the bird from a distance. Care should be taken to ensure the correct size of ring is picked relative to the bird to prevent limb damage or debilitation. The British Trust for Ornithology are experts on bird ringing and will record the ringing of rehabilitated birds. If collars are used in mammals, the weight and size of the collar should be assessed in relation to the animal. Kenward (2000) suggested that collars should be less than 3% of body weight, harnesses less than 5% of body weight and tags glued to fur or feathers less than 1–2% of body weight

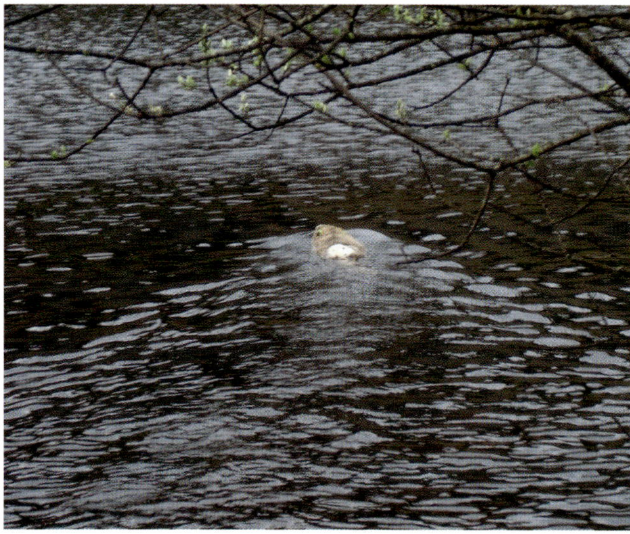

Figure 31.10 Tracking devices may be applied via collars or, as in this beaver, glued to the pelage, but they should not be so heavy as to result in potential harm to the animal through increasing energy requirements or inhibiting movement.

(see Figure 31.10). Care should be taken to check whether a licence is required to place a collar on an animal; badgers for example are protected by the Protection of Badgers Act (1992) making it necessary to obtain a licence before marking or collaring them.

If evidence emerges of mortalities at a release site, post-mortem examination to determine the cause should be carried out to ascertain if this is the fault of the release site, underlying pathology that was not identified prior to release or other significant issues. This information should then be fed back into the rehabilitation process to critically evaluate procedures and make changes where necessary.

Organisations providing guidance and best practice for wildlife reintroductions

International Union for the Conservation of Nature

Reintroduction of a species is not the same as rehabilitation. The International Union for Conservation of Nature (IUCN, 1987) has provided a definition of reintroduction of a species as:

The release of an organism into an area that was once part of its range but from which it has been extirpated.

Reintroduction of a species therefore increases the potential risks of introducing novel pathogens to an environment as the animals released clearly originate from a separate place, whether wild translocated or captive bred. Reintroduction is much more likely to require a soft release methodology and significant post-release monitoring. Guidance on release or reintroduction of wildlife and its best practice are outlined in the *IUCN Guidelines for Reintroductions and Other Conservation Translocations* (IUCN/SSC, 2013).

The IUCN is involved in worldwide conservation, assessing species vulnerability and also providing guidelines on processes around reintroductions. An IUCN commission, the Species Survival Commission (SSC), provides information on biodiversity conservation, the inherent value of an individual species including their role in ecosystem health and functioning. In addition it gives information on a species requirements for provision of ecosystem services, and their support to human livelihoods.

A separate IUCN group is the Conservation Planning Specialist Group (CPSG) that assists in the development of conservation plans involving over 250 species through more than 600 workshops held in 71 countries. Their motto is 'Changing the Future for Wildlife'. The CPSG's website can be found at http://www.cpsg.org.

World Organisation for Animal Health

The World Organisation for Animal Health (WOAH) was founded in 1924 and was originally known as OIE (Office Internationale des Epizooties) but changed its name to WOAH in 2003. For reintroduction of species, one important consideration should be the potential for disease spread. WOAH has a working group on wildlife disease and considers the risks associated with inadvertent reintroduction of disease with wildlife translocations. WOAH produces guidance on how to carry out risk analyses as well as factual information regarding specific diseases of concern to wildlife, humans and domestic animals. In conjunction with the IUCN/SSC, OIE published disease risk assessment guidelines for reintroduction of a once-native species (World Organisation for Animal Health (OIE) and International Union for Conservation of Nature (IUCN), 2014). These were used in producing disease risk assessments for Eurasian beaver and Eurasian wildcat reintroductions to Scotland and mainland Britain (Girling *et al.*, 2019). More information can be found on their website at www.woah.org.

References

Ashford, R.T., Anderson, P., Waring, L. *et al.* (2020) Evaluation of the dual path platform (DPP) VetTB assay for the detection of *Mycobacterium bovis* infection in badgers. *Preventative Veterinary Medicine*, **180**, 105005.

Girling, S.J., Naylor, A.N., Fraser, M.A. and Campbell-Palmer, R. (2019) Reintroducing beavers to Britain: a disease risk analysis. *Mammal Review*, **49**(4), 300–323.

IUCN (1987) *IUCN Position Statement on the Translocation of Living Organisms: Introductions, Re-Introductions, and Re-Stocking*. IUCN, Gland, Switzerland Available at https://portals.iucn.org/library/efiles/documents/PP-002.pdf (accessed 29 September 2024).

IUCN/SSC (2013). *Guidelines for Reintroductions and Other Conservation Translocations*. Version 1.0. Gland, Switzerland: IUCN Species Survival Commission. Available at https://www.iucn.org/resources/publication/guidelines-reintroductions-and-other-conservation-translocations (accessed 26 June 2024).

Kenward, R. (2000) *A Manual of Wildlife Radio Tagging*, 2nd edn. Academic Press, London.

Miller, E.A. (2012) *Minimum Standards for Wildlife Rehabilitation*, 4th edn. National Wildlife Rehabilitators Association, St. Cloud, Minnesota.

Mullineaux, E. (2024) Badger rehabilitation. Bovine TB Hub. https://tbhub.co.uk/ (accessed 13 June 2024).

World Organisation for Animal Health (OIE) and International Union for Conservation of Nature (IUCN) (2014). *Guidelines for Wildlife Disease Risk Analysis*. OIE, Paris. Published in association with the IUCN and the Species Survival Commission. Available at https://portals.iucn.org/library/sites/library/files/documents/2014-006.pdf (accessed 26 June 2024).

Spencer, K.A., Harris, S., Baker, P.J. and Cuthill, I.C. (2007) Song development in birds: the role of early experience and the potential effect on rehabilitation success. *Animal Welfare*, **16**, 1–13.

Appendix 1 Utilising Nursing Care Plans in the Care of Exotic Pets and Wildlife

When nursing a case, you will need to bring together many different aspects of veterinary nursing: husbandry, nutrition and anaesthesia alongside specific care for individual animals and the conditions they present with. To complicate things further, cases may present with comorbidities, meaning that life can get complicated.

You are probably familiar with the basic concepts of nursing care plans for cats and dogs, such as the Orpet and Jeffery model (Orpet, 2008). These frameworks can be applied to birds, small mammals, reptiles and wildlife with a few adaptations.

The basic nursing care plan can link the care of the patient to the normal activities of that animal, focusing on:

- Eating
- Drinking
- Elimination/toileting
- Exercise
- Sleep
- Breathing
- Grooming
- Normal behaviour.

When faced with a patient for the first time, there are four main steps to consider:

1. Assessment
2. Plan
3. Implement
4. Observe and evaluate.

Following on from this, as care progresses:

5. Change the care plan accordingly
6. Implement those changes
7. Observe and evaluate
8. Change as necessary, and repeat.

What is normal for an individual animal will depend on the age, breed, species and home environment. What is normal for a working bird of prey will be different to that of a parrot kept as a pet. Normality for a wild rabbit will be different to that of a pet rabbit.

So, the first thing to address is to find out more about the individual animal, and their history. Building up a picture of normality for that animal, gives us something to aim for.

Assessment

Before handling a patient, it is helpful to read through the clinical notes/history to get a better understanding of any current and previous health conditions.

Then, observation of the patient from across the room can provide lots of information before we change the behaviour by handling the animal. Information that can be collected includes the following (but see also Chapters 8, 16, 24 and 30 for more species-specific assessments).

1. How are they behaving?
2. How are they holding themselves?
3. Do they look in pain? Carry out a pain scoring assessment if possible.
4. Are there any obvious sores or discharges?
5. How is the animal breathing?
6. What is the body condition of the animal? Might not be obvious if lots of fur or feathers are covering the animal.

Then handling the patient:

1. What does the animal weigh?
2. What is the body condition/body score?
3. Temperature, pulse, respiration (TPR): is this normal or abnormal?
4. Urination/defecation: is this normal or abnormal?
5. Any other obvious problems?

Pulling all of this information together gives us the information that we need to decide on the care that the patient needs.

Plan

When considering the nursing care that is required it can be helpful to have a checklist to ensure that all parameters are covered. This could include the following:

1. Analgesia
2. Medication
3. Nutrition
4. Hydration
5. Elimination
6. Environment/housing
7. Exercise
8. Other, for example wound or fracture care.

Within each of these points you need to think about how these will be addressed.

1. Analgesia
   a. Which medication should be given, dose, route, side-effects.
   b. How quickly improvements should be seen.
   c. How often ongoing pain scoring needs to be carried out.
2. Medication
   a. Which medication should be given, dose, route, side-effects.

Veterinary Nursing of Exotic Pets and Wildlife, Third Edition. Simon J. Girling.

3. Nutrition
   a. Energy calculations, type of food to be given, route, frequency, and volume.
   b. Whether food is given to be eaten ad lib, or assisted feeding is required.
   c. If ad lib then the amount eaten or left needs to be accurately measured/assessed.
   d. If assisted feeding then which route, and what care does this require?
4. Hydration
   a. Does the patient require ad lib fluids, or parenteral?
   b. If ad lib, when do they drink from a bowl, bottle or other method?
   c. If giving fluid therapy, what route is going to be used?
   d. If intravenous, then which vein will be used and what care will be required?
   e. It is also important to think about what problems could be encountered, what to watch out for, and to manage any problems.
5. Elimination
   a. Is the patient passing urine/faeces?
   b. What is the amount/volume/frequency of elimination?
   c. Do these appear normal?
   d. If not normal, then what is the problem?
6. Environment
   a. What sort of housing/bedding does the patient require?
   b. Where is this situated in relation to other animals/noise/lighting.
7. Exercise
   a. For inpatients would exercise be beneficial for the patient?
   b. How could this be provided in a safe, secure manner?
8. Other
   a. There are many other conditions that could require nursing care, e.g. wounds or fractures. You also need to plan the care that will be given here, the frequency, how it will be monitored, and think about possible problems and how they could be prevented or dealt with.

Implementation

Putting in place the care, and recording what is happening.

Assessment

For some aspects of care, assessment will take place continuously, or every time the patient is handled. Other aspects, such as weight, may be monitored every 24 hours. The frequency will depend on the individual case. The important thing is to record everything, and discuss ongoing care with the team.

Re-evaluation

Depending on the response to therapy, it is likely that care will change over time. Fluids may only be required for 24 hours, or analgesia requirement may decrease in the days following surgery. But equally the patient may deteriorate and require new therapy. This is where monitoring and recording build up a picture of how the patient is progressing, and allow us to determine what is required next.

For some cases care will be very simple, while others can get very complicated. In order to give some structure to this, and a starting point, the following checklists have been developed. They are only a starting point, and every case will have extra factors that should be added to the list.

The above process can be summarised in the infographic shown in Figure A1.1.

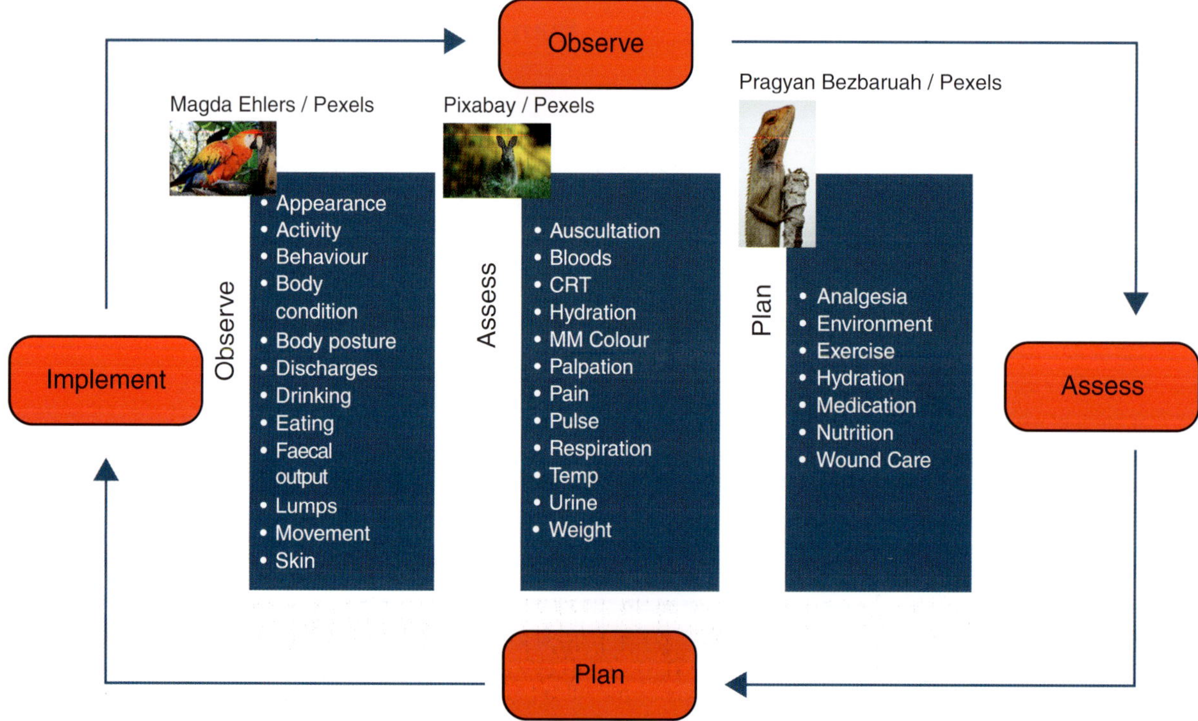

Figure A1.1 Example exotics nursing care checklist. *Source:* adapted from Girling and Fraser nursing care plan (Adapted from Fraser, 2020).

Patient details

Time	a.m./p.m.	a.m./p.m.	a.m./p.m.
OBSERVE			
Activity			
Appearance			
Behaviour			
Body condition			
Body posture			
Discharges			
Drinking			
Eating			
Faecal/urine output			
Integument			
Lumps or bumps			
Movement			
ASSESS			
Auscultation			
Bloods			
CRT			
Hydration			
Mucous membranes			
Palpation			
Pain			
Pulse			
Respiration			
Temperature			
Urine			
Weight			

Source: adapted from Girling and Fraser nursing care plan (Fraser, 2020).

Main areas of concern

	General	Ongoing	Re-evaluation
Date/time			
Environment			
Exercise			
Nutrition			
Hydration			
Medication			
Analgesia			
Wound care			
Other			

Example case: rabbit presenting with fly strike

History and clinical presentation

A 3-year-old female, neutered, lop-eared rabbit is brought into the practice one morning, as the owner has noticed that she is not eating, and is very quiet. The veterinary surgeon examines it and informs you that they are going to admit the patient for work-up and treatment. On examination it is clear that the rabbit has faecal soiling and maggots are evident around the tail. The rabbit stays with another rabbit in the house and is fully vaccinated.

Assessment

Time	8 a.m.	a.m./p.m.
OBSERVE		
Appearance	Very quiet and still, good body condition but obvious maggots around the tail	
Activity	Very quiet and still, not moving much	
Behaviour	Very quiet and still, not acting normally	
Body condition	Good 3/5	
Body posture	Hunched and looks uncomfortable	
Discharges	Oozing from the skin around the tail where maggots are seen. No other discharges	
Drinking	Not seen drinking over the past 24 hours	
Eating	Not seen eating over the past 24 hours	
Faecal/urine output	None evident, although there is faecal soiling around the tail	
Integument	Skin damaged around the tail	
Lumps or bumps	None	
Movement	Not moving so cannot assess	
ASSESS		
Auscultation	Lungs clear	
Bloods	Vet has taken these to check, waiting for results	
Blood pressure	Lower than normal (85 mmHg)	
CRT	Pale and slower than normal	
Hydration	Skin tenting evident, estimate 7% dehydration	
Mucous membranes	Tacky, and pale pink	
Palpation	No bloating of the stomach, and no obvious pain on palpation	
Pain	Grimace scale parameters indicate that the rabbit is in pain	
Pulse	180 bpm, weaker than normal	
Respiration	40 bpm	
Temperature	38.5°C	
Urine	No urination	
Weight	4 kg (was 4.5 kg when seen 6 months ago for vaccinations)	

Main areas of concern

1. Maggots in skin: wound, skin damage and infection.
2. Quiet, pale mucous membranes, dehydrated: possibly going into shock.
3. Not eating so likely to develop gastric stasis.
4. Obviously in pain.

Plan

		Ongoing				
Date/time	**General**	**8 a.m.**	**2 p.m.**	**8 p.m.**	**2 a.m.**	**Re-evaluation**
Environment	Quiet cage away from cats, ferrets and dogs					Keep in current location
Exercise	Not yet but could be useful in coming days					Cage rest for now
Nutrition	Calculate energy requirement (see Chapters 4 and 8)					
	Assisted feeding, decide on method	Feed ¼ of daily allowance	Feed ¼ of daily allowance	Feed ¼ of daily allowance	Feed ¼ of daily allowance	Continue until eating voluntarily
Hydration	Place intravenous catheter into cephalic or lateral ear vein	Check catheter	Check catheter	Catheter has blocked, place new catheter in other leg or ear	Check catheter	
	Calculate fluid rate (see Chapter 6)					
	Decide on best fluids (see Chapter 6)	Start on shock dose for 30 min then review	Maintenance fluids continued	Maintenance fluids continued	Maintenance fluids continued	Repeat bloods to check biochemistry
	Monitor hydration	Improving	Within normal limits	Within normal limits	Within normal limits	Responding well. Continue until starts drinking
	Monitor auscultation	No evidence of fluid overload	No evidence of fluid overload	No evidence of fluid overload	No evidence of fluid overload	
	Monitor blood pressure	Lower than normal	Normal	Normal	Normal	Improving, but continue to monitor
Medication	Antibiotics (avoid oral penicillins, cephalosporins, clindamycin, etc.)	Administered				Continue course
	Gut motility (e.g. cisapride, metoclopramide and/or ranitidine)	Administered				Continue course
Analgesia	Decide on best medication and frequency of administration (e.g. NSAID ± buprenorphine or tramadol)	Administered	Pain scoring (see Chapter 3 for further information)	Pain scoring More medication administered	Pain scoring	Responding well to analgesia
Wound care	Assess wound: decide if can be debrided consciously or require anaesthetic. Stabilise first			Topical therapy applied, wearing gloves	Topical therapy applied, wearing gloves	
Other	General demeanour	Quiet and hunched	A little brighter	Slowly improving	Brighter and moving	Improving
	Elimination	None	None	None	Passed faecal pellets and urinated	Improving

Treatment begins and the patient starts to look a little brighter. A more detailed examination of the skin around the tail shows that the wounds are quite superficial, and so surgery is not required. Now that analgesia is in place, the rabbit allows cleaning and removal of maggots, and then topical therapy. The rabbit receives assisted feeding for the first couple of days, and then by day 3 is seen eating hay which was left in the cage with them. The rabbit is then given 30 minutes of exercise in the kennel room, under observation, and is seen to be much brighter, and moving normally. The rabbit is then sent home on medication, and the owner is provided with information about how to prevent fly strike in the future.

You can see that one case can bring together many different aspects of nursing. This case combines:

- Husbandry
- Nutrition/assisted feeding
- Fluid therapy
- Pain scoring/analgesia
- Wound care
- Monitoring and intensive care nursing.

References

Fraser, M.A. (2020). Implementing a nursing care plan for exotic pets. *VN Times* 20 (10): 4–5.

Orpet, H (2008). Advances in the delivery of practical nursing care: practical examples. *World Small Animal Veterinary Association World Congress Proceedings*, 20–24 August 2008, Dublin. Available at https://www.vin.com/apputil/project/defaultadv1.aspx?pid=11268&catid=&id=3866664&meta=generic&authorid=

Appendix 2 Legislation Affecting Exotic Pets and Wildlife in the UK

This appendix is intended to provide an overview of the legislation affecting the keeping and treatment of exotic pets and wildlife in the UK. Since the creation of regional governments for Scotland, Northern Ireland and Wales, some legislation has become devolved, and animal welfare and wildlife are just two of these.

UK animal welfare acts

In England and Wales, the Animal Welfare Act 2006 and in Scotland the Animal Health and Welfare (Scotland) Act 2006 cover the welfare of captive vertebrate animals. This definition extends to vertebrate wild animals when they are brought into temporary or permanent captivity. It is not only an offence to cause harm to a vertebrate animal under these pieces of legislation, it is also an offence to omit to do something that could then lead to harm (e.g. omitting to feed or provide suitable water sources). It is also an offence to release back into the wild a wild animal that is not fit to survive. Further information on the Acts can be found at https://www.legislation.gov.uk/.

UK wildlife specific legislation

The UK wildlife legislation is complicated. Several overarching pieces of legislation exist in the different areas of the UK covering wildlife, its protection and management. Some cover the period in which wild animals can be held. The Wildlife and Countryside Act 1981 restricts the holding of many birds of prey (see Schedule 4) to less than 15 days for rehabilitators and 6 weeks for veterinary surgeons before a licence has to be applied for (and the licence should be applied for in the first 4 days of captivity where it is predicted the bird will be held longer than these times). Some of the more general wildlife legislation in the UK can be summarised as follows.

1. Wildlife and Countryside Act 1981 covers Scotland, England and Wales.
2. The Conservation of Habitats and Species Regulations 2010 covers Scotland, England and Wales.
3. The Conservation (Natural Habitats, etc.) Regulations 1994 covers Scotland.
4. The Wildlife and Natural Environment (Scotland) Act 2011 covers Scotland.
5. The Wildlife (Northern Ireland) Order 1985 covers Northern Ireland.
6. The Wildlife and Natural Environment Act (Northern Ireland) 2011 covers Northern Ireland.
7. The Conservation (Natural Habitats, etc.) Regulations (Northern Ireland) 1995 covers Northern Ireland.

In addition there are species-specific pieces of legislation that protect individual species of wild animal.

1. Protection of Badgers Act 1992 covers Scotland, England and Wales and deals with badgers.
2. The Wildlife (Northern Ireland) Order 1985 covers Northern Ireland and deals with badgers, deer and seals.
3. The Wildlife and Natural Environment (Northern Ireland) Act 2011 covers Northern Ireland and deals with badgers, deer and wild birds.
4. Deer Act 1991 covers England and Wales and deals with deer.
5. Regulatory Reform (Deer) England and Wales Order 2007 covers England and Wales and deals with deer.
6. The Wildlife and Natural Environment (Scotland) Act 2011 covers Scotland and deals with deer.
7. Conservation of Seals Act 1970 covers England and Wales and deals with seals.
8. Marine Scotland Act 2010 covers Scotland and deals with seals and other marine animals.
9. The Wild Mammals (Protection) Act 1996 covers Scotland, England and Wales and deals with the protection of wild mammals. This Act does permit the killing of a protected species of wild mammal if it can be shown that this is an act of mercy due to the animal being so seriously disabled that there is no chance of recovery.
10. Wildlife and Countryside Act 1981 covers Scotland, England and Wales and deals with protection of wild bird species in particular but also covers some mammals, reptiles and amphibians in Schedule 5.

Further information regarding wildlife legislation in the UK can be found through the websites of the Joint Nature Conservation Committee at https://jncc.gov.uk/ and the British Wildlife Rehabilitation Council at https://www.bwrc.org.uk/.

Non-native species

Some species of animal, including wildlife, are considered non-native and an invasive species, for example the grey squirrel, muntjac deer, red-eared terrapin, coatimundi and raccoon. Their keeping, movement and release is therefore strictly controlled under the Invasive Species (Enforcement and Permitting) Order 2019 for England and Wales, which enforces European Union Invasive Alien Species (IAS) Regulation 1143/2014. Currently this means that the release of muntjac and grey squirrels is not permitted, revoking previous licences that allowed this. In Scotland, the EU legislation is enforced through the Invasive Non-native species (EU Exit) (Scotland) (Amendment, etc.)

Veterinary Nursing of Exotic Pets and Wildlife, Third Edition. Simon J. Girling.

Regulations 2020. More information can be found through the websites of the British Wildlife Rehabilitation Council (see above) and NatureScot (see https://www.nature.scot/professional-advice/protected-areas-and-species/protected-species/invasive-non-native-species).

UK veterinary health relevant legislation

The Veterinary Surgeons Act 1966 dictates that in the UK only a veterinary surgeon (and therefore a current Member or Fellow of the Royal College of Veterinary Surgeons) can diagnose, carry out surgery and treat mammals, birds and reptiles. Registered and student veterinary nurses may carry out the care of any animal, including medical treatments and minor surgery, providing they act under the conditions and supervision of Schedule 3 of the Act.

The Veterinary Medicines Regulations govern the use of veterinary medicines in the UK. Most of the animals considered here have few if any specifically licenced medications for their treatment in the UK and therefore the use of medicines in these species commonly follows the 'cascade'. More information can be found at the Veterinary Medicines Directorate website (https://www.gov.uk/government/organisations/veterinary-medicines-directorate).

The Animal Health Act 1981 (Scotland, England and Wales) and the Diseases of Animals (Northern Ireland) Order 1981 (Northern Ireland) and linked legislation control so-called notifiable diseases (e.g. avian influenza, bovine tuberculosis, foot and mouth disease, bluetongue virus) amongst other things. This means that if such a disease is diagnosed or suspected in an animal, including wildlife, the relevant government authority should be notified, which in England and Wales currently is the Animal and Plant Health Agency (APHA) and in Scotland the relevant APHA field office and in Northern Ireland the Department of Agriculture, Environment and Rural Affairs (DAERA) Direct regional office.

Health and safety

The Health and Safety at Work Act 1974 as amended covers all aspects of health and safety in the workplace in the UK. Many of the animals discussed in this textbook may carry zoonotic disease and some pose a physical risk to handlers and veterinary staff. Some drugs mentioned in this textbook can also be harmful and in some cases be potentially lethal should accidental self-administration occur. All veterinary staff have an obligation to avoid hazards and prevent accidents and accidental cross-infection in the workplace. In addition, an employer has an obligation to ensure that facilities and training of staff are sufficient to minimise the risks of handling and treating these animals. The British and Irish Association of Zoos and Aquaria (BIAZA) in conjunction with the Health and Safety Executive have produced their own set of guidelines for zoos and aquaria that cover many aspects of zoonotic disease and working with hazardous species (see https://biaza.org.uk/policies-guidelines/ for further information).

Convention on international trade in endangered species (CITES)

This is internationally recognised and in the UK is enforced through the Control of Trade in Endangered Species (Enforcement) Regulations 2018 (COTES). They require the licencing of the sale or display of species listed in Annex A of Commission Regulation 750/2013 and include, for example, species of Mediterranean tortoise such as *Testudo graeca*, *T. hermanni* and *T. marginata* as well as the sale of captive-bred European birds of prey including owls. It should be noted that several wild UK animals such as the European otter (*Lutra lutra*) are also CITES 1 and COTES Annex A listed protected species.

Dangerous Wild Animals Act 1976

This piece of legislation covers Scotland, England and Wales and as its name suggests requires the keeping of animals listed within the amended legislation to be licenced, currently by the local authority government. Many venomous species of snake, crocodilians, many exotic wild carnivores, most of the larger primates and exotic ungulates are included. It does not apply to a licenced zoo premises or to pet shops. More information, including the current list of species covered, can be found at https://www.legislation.gov.uk/ukpga/1976/38/contents.

Appendix 3 Useful Resources

Association of Avian Veterinarians
This association welcomes veterinary nurses/technicians and produces a quarterly peer-reviewed journal as well as holding an annual conference.
Website: www.aav.org

Association of Reptile and Amphibian Veterinarians
This association welcomes veterinary nurses/technicians and produces a quarterly peer-reviewed journal as well as holding an annual conference.
Website: www.arav.org

Association of Zoo and Exotic Veterinary Nurses
Website: www.azevn.org

British Veterinary Zoological Society
This society welcomes veterinary surgeons, students and veterinary nurses alike and holds conferences and workshops.
Website: www.bvzs.co.uk

British Wildlife Rehabilitation Council
This organisation has online resources around ethics and legislation for the UK regarding wildlife rehabilitation.
Website: www.bwrc.org.uk

European Association of Zoo and Wildlife Veterinarians
This organisation hosts the free-access Transmissible Diseases Handbook and the EU Animal Health Law Handbooks.
Website: www.eazwv.org

Girling and Fraser Ltd Training and Consultancy
Resources and training for veterinary nurses/technicians including the Advanced Programme in Veterinary Nursing of Zoo, Wildlife and Exotics, accredited by City & Guilds, and comprising five programmes: Avian, Reptile and Amphibian, Small Mammal, Wildlife and Zoo Nursing.
Website: www.girlingandfraser.com

IUCN SSC Conservation Translocation Specialist Group
This organisation has a number of free-access resources including their Guidelines for Reintroductions and Other Conservation Translocations.
Website: www.iucn-ctsg.org

National Centre for the Replacement, Refinement and Reduction of Animals in Research (NC3Rs)
This website has details of grimace pain-scoring systems for rodents and lagomorphs.
Website: www.nc3rs.org.uk/3rs-resources/grimace-scales

Rabbit Welfare Association and Fund
Website: www.rabbitwelfare.co.uk

TBhub The Home of UK TB Information
This website has useful sections on bovine tuberculosis in wildlife.
Website: https://tbhub.co.uk/tb-in-wildlife/

Tortoise Trust
Website: www.tortoisetrust.com

Wildlife Disease Association
Website: www.wildlifedisease.org

Veterinary Nursing of Exotic Pets and Wildlife, Third Edition. Simon J. Girling.

Index

Veterinary Nursing of Exotic Pets and Wildlife, Third Edition. Simon J. Girling.

B

C

F

M

N

O